20.00

N D Johnson
1983

A COMPANION TO DENTAL STUDIES
Volume 1 Book 1

Editorial Board

A COMPANION TO DENTAL STUDIES
Editors in Chief/A.H.R. Rowe & R.B. Johns
Volume 1 Book 1

Anatomy, Biochemistry and Physiology

Edited by

J.W. OSBORN

WITH

W.G. ARMSTRONG

AND

R.L. SPEIRS

Blackwell Scientific Publications
OXFORD LONDON EDINBURGH
BOSTON MELBOURNE

© 1982 by
Blackwell Scientific Publications
Editorial offices:
Osney Mead, Oxford OX2 0EL
8 John Street, London WC1N 2ES
9 Forrest Road, Edinburgh EH1 2QH
52 Beacon Street, Boston
    Massachusetts 02108, USA
99 Barry Street, Carlton Victoria 3053,
    Australia

First published 1982

Set by Southline Press,
Ferring, W. Sussex
Printed in Great Britain by
Butler & Tanner Ltd,
Frome and London

DISTRIBUTORS

USA
    Blackwell Mosby Book Distributors
    11830 Westline Industrial Drive
    St Louis, Missouri 63141

Canada
    Blackwell Mosby Book Distributors
    120 Melford Drive, Scarborough
    Ontario M1B 2X4

Australia
    Blackwell Scientific Book Distributors
    214 Berkeley Street, Carlton
    Victoria 3053

British Library
Cataloguing in Publication Data

A Companion to dental studies.
    Vol. 1
    Bk. 1: Anatomy, biochemistry and
    physiology
    1. Dentistry
    I. Osborn, J.W.   II. Armstrong, W.G.
    III. Speirs, R.L.
    617.6 RK51

ISBN 0–632–00797–4

Contents

(continued overleaf)

Contributors to Volume 1 Book 1

W.G. Armstrong   MSc MSc PhD
Professor of Biochemistry in Relation to Dentistry, Department of Biochemistry,
Royal Dental Hospital of London School of Dental Surgery, Cranmer Terrace,
London SW17 0RE

M. Armstrong-James   BSc PhD
Department of Physiology, The London Hospital Medical College, Turner Street,
London E1 2AD

L. Bannister   BSc PhD
Department of Biology, Guy's Hospital Medical School, London SE1 9RT

K. Clarke   BSc PhD BDS MIBiol
206 Sutton Road, Mansfield, Nottinghamshire NG18 5HL

D. Cotterrell   BSc PhD
Department of Physiology, The University, Leeds LS2 9JT

D.J. Cove   MA PhD
Professor of Genetics, The University, Leeds LS2 9JT

K.W. Cross   MB BS DSc FRCP
Professor of Physiology, The London Hospital Medical College, Turner Street,
London E1 2AD

B.N. Davies   BSc PhD
Department of Physiology, St. Bartholomew's Hospital Medical College,
Charterhouse Square, London EC1M 6BQ

A. D'Mello   MSc PhD
Department of Pharmacology, The London Hospital Medical College, Turner Street,
London E1 2AD

Barbara Dodd   MSc PhD DSc
Professor of Blood Group Serology, The London Hospital Medical College, Turner Street,
London E1 2AD

Mary Dyson   BSc PhD
Department of Anatomy, Guy's Hospital Medical School, St Thomas' Street,
London SE1 9RT

G. Embery BSc PhD
Department of Dental Sciences, University of Liverpool, Pembroke Place,
PO Box 147, Liverpool L69 3BX

Wendy Ewart BSc PhD
Department of Physiology, The London Hospital Medical College, Turner Street,
London E1 2AD

D.B. Gower DSc PhD CChem FRSC FIBiol
Department of Biochemistry, Guy's Hospital Medical School, St Thomas' Street,
London SE1 9RT

J.M. Graham MA BM BCh MFCM
Department of Health and Social Security, Hannibal House, Elephant and Castle,
London SE1 6TE

M.K.S. Hathorn BSc MB BCh PhD
Department of Physiology, The London Hospital Medical College, Turner Street,
London E1 2AD

A.F. Hayward BSc MB BS PhD
Reader and Head of Department of Anatomy, Royal Dental Hospital of London School of
Dental Surgery, Cranmer Terrace, London SW17 0RE

Karen M. Hiiemae BDS PhD
Interim Dean, Graduate College, University of Illinois at the Medical Center,
808 S. Wood Street, Chicago, Illinois 60612, USA

F.J. Imms BSc PhD MB BS
Department of Physiology, Guy's Hospital Medical School, St Thomas' Street,
London SE1 9RT

J. Joseph MD DSc FRCOG
Professor and Head of Department of Anatomy, Guy's Hospital Medical School,
St Thomas' Street, London SE1 9RT

W.R. Keatinge MA MB BChir PhD
Professor of Physiology, The London Hospital Medical College, Turner Street,
London E1 2AD

R.A. Lee MB BS LRCP MRCS DO(Eng)
Department of Physiology, The London Hospital Medical College, Turner Street,
London E1 2AD

Moya Meredith Smith BSc PhD
Department of Anatomy in Relation to Dentistry, Royal Dental Hospital of London School
of Dental Surgery, Cranmer Terrace, London SW17 0RE

B. Moreland BSc PhD
Department of Biochemistry, Guy's Hospital Medical School, St Thomas' Street,
London SE1 9RT

R.L.B. Neame MA PhD MB BCh
Department of Human Physiology, Faculty of Medicine, The University of Newcastle,
New South Wales 2308, Australia

R.E.S. Prout BSc PhD
Department of Biochemistry, The University, Sheffield S10 2TN

F.B. Reed BSc PhD
Department of Biochemistry, Royal Dental Hospital of London School of Dental Surgery,
Cranmer Terrace, London SW17 0RE

E.L. Rees MB BS
Department of Anatomy, Guy's Hospital Medical School, St Thomas' Street,
London SE1 9RT

N. Robinson PhD
Department of Anatomy, The London Hospital Medical College, Turner Street,
London E1 2AD

L.H. Smaje BSc MB BS PhD
Professor of Physiology, Charing Cross Hospital Medical School, Fulham Palace Road,
London W6 8RF

J.A. Sofaer BDS PhD
Department of Oral Medicine and Oral Pathology, Old Surgeon's Hall, High School Yards,
Edinburgh EH1 1NR
and University Department of Human Genetics, Western General Hospital,
Edinburgh EH4 2XU

R.L. Speirs BSc PhD
Professor of Physiology in Relation to Dentistry, The London Hospital Medical College,
Turner Street, London E1 2AD

S.M. Standring BSc PhD
Department of Anatomy, Guy's Hospital Medical School, St Thomas' Street,
London SE1 9RT

A.J. Thexton BDS FDSRCS BSc PhD
Department of Physiology, Royal Dental Hospital of London School of Dental Surgery,
Cranmer Terrace, London SW17 0RE

A.J. Wade BSc BVSc PhD
Department of Physiology, The London Hospital Medical College, Turner Street,
London E1 2AD

P.J. Warren   BSc PhD
Department of Biochemistry, The London Hospital Medical College, Turner Street,
London E1 2AD

P.J. Wells   BSc PhD
Department of Biochemistry, Royal Dental Hospital School of Dental Surgery,
Cranmer Terrace, London SW17 0RE

R.Wong   BSc
Department of Physiology, The London Hospital Medical College, Turner Street,
London E1 2AD

J.A. Veinman   BA PhD ABPsS
Unit of Psychology as Applied to Medicine, Guy's Hospital Medical School,
St Thomas' Street, London SE1 9RT

Foreword

A Companion to Dental Studies has been written to provide both the undergraduate and the recent graduate with a comprehensive and integrated text of dentistry. We hope that the series will provide the background for an appreciation of the scientific foundation of dentistry, as well as the techniques and philosophies necessary for its practice.

The Companion will be published in three volumes and integrated in a manner which it is hoped will give balance to the increasing complexity of the undergraduate dental course. The Editors and authors are all experienced teachers and well qualified to understand the needs of the students and can help them explore the plethora of information now available.

While there are many excellent texts on the different elements of the dental course, these have inevitably led to much duplication of subject matter. Furthermore, it is difficult for the student to assess the relative importance of each discipline, each teacher tending to feel that his particular subject is at the heart of dentistry. The Companion seeks to avoid unnecessary repetition and yet to provide the reader with an opportunity to appreciate the many facets within the subject and their relevant importance and perspective.

The authors and contributors have shown the utmost forebearance in having their texts modified and revised in order to conform to the overall style and limitations that a project of this complexity requires. The Editors, however, take responsibility for any errors or imbalance which have persisted into the final text.

At the end of each chapter there is a short reading list which is to be regarded as a stimulus to further study of a particular subject.

There have been important changes in nomenclature in some fields, such as anatomy, and the modern terminology has been adopted throughout. SI units have been used, except in a few instances, for example for blood pressure, where the old unit still appears to be appropriate.

The idea that a sister publication to the successful *Companion to Medical Studies* should be written was that of Per Saugman, and he should be given full credit for this inspiration.

The Editors-in-Chief wish to acknowledge the invaluable support of the publishers, particularly Miss Helen Varley, who has been responsible for the sub-editing, under the guidance of Mr Peter Saugman. The artists have diligently drawn and redrawn many of the illustrations and Mr Frank Wallis has been responsible for preparing the indices.

Finally we wish to express our appreciation to the many secretaries who have been responsible for producing innumerable drafts of the texts.

A.H.R. Rowe　　　　　　　　　　　　　　　　　　　　　　　　　　　　　　*July 1981*
R.B. Johns

Preface

This book is designed to present in an integrated text the corner stones of the basic medical sciences. It is hoped that the understanding and relevance of these subjects to the study of dentistry will be readily apparent, as will the relationships of the individual subjects to each other.

For the last decade integration has been a major source of discussion. From a student's point of view, is it easier and more helpful to be taught fundamentals in somewhat isolated compartments and then learn to apply them in different situations, or to be given an integrated approach from which to abstract fundamentals? We are persuaded that to a university student most fundamentals are more important than their applications and should therefore generally, but not always, be given pride of place. For this reason we have attempted in this text to develop a 'first order' of integration. Descriptions of the anatomy, physiology and biochemistry of each topic have been separately contributed and then integrated to the level we judged appropriate. The degree of integration can be assessed by studying the page of contents. Whilst there are a number of texts on each of these subjects, we hope that by combining them in one volume we have reduced repetition to a minimum.

All the authors are experienced teachers of students of dentistry and their original texts reflected what they considered should be included in the dental course. However, in an integrated text, the position, weight, and the content of each topic are matters of fine judgement. The authors have shown great forebearance with the editors, who in their efforts to produce a book which will both stimulate and educate the undergraduate, have modified or pruned the original manuscripts.

New disciplines appear at intervals and a glance at the contents page shows that we have been influenced by these trends: less than some would like and more than others would condone. Furthermore contributors must decide whether recent and hence more controversial findings should be included. Need the concepts which are described be supported by experimental evidence? While acknowledging the educational merit of including both, space considerations have weighted our decision in favour of a rather didactic presentation of well-established facts.

In summary this book contains discrete anatomy, physiology and biochemistry courses and several interdisciplinary sections. In our view, the subjects should still be taught separately. By 'interleaving' the subject matter of each discipline in a single text, we hope to encourage students to break down those apparent barriers between disciplines which evolve during teaching. Real barriers will always exist because the philosophies inherent in the major disciplines are so different.

Finally it is important to stress the role of the basic sciences in relation to the rest of the dental course. Most agree that the practice of dentistry cannot achieve its highest level without a sound foundation in basic science. The word 'foundation' is carefully chosen. Foundations are there to be built upon and clinical teachers should be constantly referring to and using the implications of basic science.

J.W. Osborn   *December 1981*
R.L. Speirs
W.G. Armstrong

A Companion to Dental Studies

Volume 3   Clinical Dentistry

CHAPTER 1

The Basis of Scientific Investigation

WHAT USE ARE THE PRECLINICAL SUBJECTS TO ME AS A DENTIST?

The distinguished British dental surgeon, the late Sir Wilfred Fish, suggested that should a dental student fail to find interest or excitement in the scientific background of his professional activities, he or she would be well advised to seek out another career before becoming too committed along the path leading to a dental qualification.

It is likely that a majority of dental students would agree that they should be interested in the scientific background of their subject. However, one might also predict that in practice they are unlikely to heed Sir Wilfred's advice! Why indeed should they? Is the scientific background really so important for the clinician? Perhaps it is no more than a fashionable irrelevance or spicing injected into a preclinical course, forced on the student by General Dental Council edicts and university regulations, to be endured until one gets on to the real business of the prevention and treatment of oral disease? Need we really bother with the basic sciences as chairside dental surgeons? This chapter attempts to answer these questions from a general consideration of the nature of scientific enquiry and activity. Some answers from a biochemical viewpoint are provided on pp. 25–7, and the text throughout illustrates the need for a knowledge of the basic sciences.

The history of science is by and large a history of progress; there are few other fields of human endeavour of which this can be unequivocally said. Science works for us and continues to reveal a wealth of insights concerning ourselves and our environment which can be used for good or ill. For the student there are useful lessons to be learnt from the scientist's approach to problem-solving which are equally applicable to academic dentistry and chairside diagnosis and treatment; more than this there is the opportunity to share in this remarkable aspect of mankind's development.

WHAT IS SCIENCE?

In its very broadest sense, science is man's systematic attempt to seek order and meaning in a seemingly chaotic universe. The pursuit of science implies a refusal to be content with the bare welter of facts; for man the facts have to be incorporated within some coherent consistent picture of 'how things are'.

But what are the facts? How do we perceive them? As human beings we are flooded with information by our environment. We are bombarded with electromagnetic radiation (light), air density oscillations (sound), chemical substances (smells) and pressures (tactile sensations). In order to extract a coherent arrangement of thoughts we have to abstract or filter this mass of information. To abstract is to summarize, remove, select, and the resulting abstractions provide the basis for conscious thought.

Perception is a highly complex, automatic construction. It is a decision-making system which sifts through information according to programmed criteria as to what is important. Recently, a man, blind from birth, had an operation which allowed him to see for the first time in his life. This man had to be taught how to recognise simple shapes such as a square, triangle or circle. At first he was unable to distinguish between them because he was not programmed with criteria as to what differentiated these simple shapes. But it is not only the newly-sighted who have such a problem. For instance it is no use telling someone to 'observe'. They will have to ask 'what is it that you want me to observe?' Observation is selection and we select according to criteria that reflect what we believe to be important. As the American philosopher of science Thomas Kühn puts it, 'I'll see it when I believe it!' Facts may often seem to be a matter of commonsense but as the biologist C. H. Wad-

1

dington reminds us ' . . . commonsense is the philosophy which your parents or peers have soaked you in when you weren't realizing what you were absorbing.' Here of course Waddington is referring to the 'common agreement about what is sensible' that is held by people in society at large. He is not criticizing it but drawing attention to its ad hoc character and therefore its limitations.

Thomas Kühn has suggested that scientific communities share implicit assumptions, (or 'agreements about what is sensible') which he calls paradigms (pronounced 'para-dimes'). A paradigm is an agreed concept of what is possible; a prevailing orthodoxy. It sets the boundaries of acceptable inquiry and determines those facts which are selected as illustrations of the paradigm. He points out that a paradigm allows a certain stability of knowledge at the cost of some insensitivity to new knowledge because a boundary implies exclusion.

The commonsense of science (which Kühn might call its collection of paradigms) is derived from a heritage that has its roots in Hellenic culture. The Greek philosophers were not scientists in the sense in which we now use the word. They were however lucid, logical thinkers with a passionate interest in understanding nature. To later generations they bequeathed a number of clear-cut philosophical ideas which provided mental scaffolding for the subsequent development of science. After a period of gestation, modern science was launched into being during the seventeenth century by a number of men of genius including Galileo, Newton and Descartes. Their achievements marked the flowering of the mentality that is at the heart of science and is the motivating force behind all scientific investigations — *that scientists perform their experiments with the conviction that there is in existence an order of things.* This widespread acceptance that nature has a pattern that can be revealed is really an article of faith, but the assumption has worked with great success.

Another characteristic of this scientific tradition is that it is one of the very few human activities where participants readily agree on shared areas of experience regardless of social or political barriers. The physicist von Weizsäcker in his book 'The Relevance of Science' tells how Western and Soviet physicists met for the first time, in 1955, at the first Geneva conference on the peaceful use of atomic energy.

'It was a great experience to see that the numerical values of the same atomic constants, measured in deep secrecy in different countries under opposed political systems and creeds, when compared, turned out to be identical down to the last decimal. The Soviet physicist and his colleague from the West are united by a bond which no political dissension can touch; they are united by a common truth.' Nothing of the sort happened with respect to theories on society.

The establishment of reliable observations about phenomena (the *facts*) is an important task in science, but facts are valueless without a subsequent evaluation of their significance within the context of a *theory*. Science is *not* a static welding of fact to theory. Nor is it a collection of dusted and polished certainties, like so many archaelogical exhibits in a museum. The many exhibits in a museum. The essence of science is problem-solving via the never-ending critical dialogue between immediate observations of things which seem important and the theories incorporating them, which at the same time can suggest new methods of observation.

Science describes the world but it also interprets this description in terms of an intelligible theory. Facts and theory must come to grips with each other: both are essential in the development of scientific ideas. Science is a complex self-correcting enterprise concerned not with individual events, but with classes of events as illustrations of general principles.

Classes of events are groups of repeatable observations. In recent years some interest has been regenerated in the idea, first suggested by the French naturalist Lamarck, that living organisms can transmit acquired characteristics to their progeny. A lively debate has developed, initiated by results apparently in support of Lamarck's view, though attempts to repeat these have failed. The validity or otherwise of this hypothesis is not our concern, but a 1981 contribution to this debate in the American journal, *Science*, nicely expressed the attitude of the scientific community to such observations which do not fit the current paradigms when it concluded: 'If these results cannot be repeated independently . . . they must be said to be not generalizable and therefore not very interesting.' It is *classes* of events that count, not independent ones.

The subject of parapsychology — extrasensory perception (ESP) and psychokinesis (PK) — illustrates another facet of the scientific dialogue. Some university departments study ESP, but parapsychology has not yet found general acceptance within the scientific community because its implications cannot be reconciled with our present knowledge of the physical world. This is not necessarily a rejection of parapsychology; perhaps people can influence dice, read minds or bend spoons — perhaps not. Future work in extending our mental machinery for coping with these results (if they are valid) may one day bring the subject fully into the scientific arena. At present there is no theoretical framework wherein such data can be incorporated, and unless one can be found, parapsychology cannot be justifiably accepted into the domain of 'science.'

We have seen that fact and theory are inseparable partners in science. Nevertheless the existence of this marriage in some areas of investigation does not automatically qualify that discipline as a science. The philosopher Karl Popper distinguishes between science and non-science by requiring that scientific theories make potentially testable (and thereby refutable) statements. Initially Popper was concerned with the problem of the scientific status of certain political theories and the theories of human behaviour due to Freud and Adler. These theories are open to the criticism that they may use any fact to illustrate the general principles enshrined in their particular theory. This implies that no fact can fail to illustrate their theoretical basis, which therefore becomes irrefutable. A theory which does not make risky predictions is thereby immune to criticism and cannot participate in the critical dialogue that is the main source of new ideas in genuine science. While denying such theories scientific status and emphasizing their relative sterility, Popper stresses that they may not necessarily be valueless but can stimulate the development of better theories that *are* testable.

HOW ARE SCIENTIFIC PROBLEMS SOLVED?

Scientific progress results from critical analysis of imaginative ideas. How does this occur in practice? The classic scientific method was held to operate in the following chronological sequence:

1 *Observation.* An objective detached examination, collection and determination of relevant facts relating to a particular area of knowledge.
2 *Hypothesis.* The formulation of a supposition, a conceptional framework, put forward to explain the facts observed.
3 *Testing of hypothesis (experiment).* The setting up of experiments designed to test the truth of the hypothesis or hypotheses proposed. Much

of modern science involves accurate measurements and comparisons, and the experiments are designed to ask specific questions, the answers to which will support, confirm or invalidate an hypothesis proposed.
4 *Theory.* The establishment of an hypothesis as an accepted explanation of the facts observed, on the basis of experimental data obtained.

This explanation of the scientists' approach to solving a problem is a misleading representation of the ways in which research is actually approached and conducted. The classic scientific method is not a recipe for solving problems, but an objective record, written with hindsight, of the ways and means by which facts are observed and ideas formulated.

Such a presentation is logically appealing and is probably the best framework for presenting the problem investigated, the results obtained, and the consequences of examining these in relation to each other. It has certainly for instance dictated the form in which the great majority of scientific publications are cast:
1 *Introduction.* Defining the theoretical background and area under investigation.
2 *Materials and Methods.* The techniques and experimental approaches used.
3 *Results.* The facts deriving from observation and/or the answers to the questions asked in a particular experiment.
4 *Discussion.* An examination of the facts obtained in the context of the hypothesis examined, and, where appropriate, the formulation of alternative explanations (hypotheses) to explain new facts not accommodated within the older explanation.
5 *Conclusions.* A summary of the result of the investigation — a confirmation or querying of the proposals and hypotheses tested.

This implied chronology does not in fact represent the way in which scientists conduct their research investigations. Individual scientists vary in the degrees of caution in approach, and conceptual visualizing, that their particular personalities bring to a problem. An amalgam of intelligence, intuition, imagination, serendipity and chance will contribute to the experimental design and results. Hunches and intelligent guesses may well form the major basis for an investigation or interpretation, rather than the detached objective appraisal of facts and related testing of hypotheses that the scientific method implies.

The following account, which allows a role for such imagination, intuition and chance, more accurately represents the scientists' way of tackling problems.

1 The problem is identified as clearly as possible, a task unfortunately not always given the critical attention it demands.

2 A number of likely explanations or hypotheses, even guesses, are formulated.

3 A crucial experiment is designed. This is an experiment with a number of possible outcomes which will as nearly as possible exclude one or several of these explanations.

4 The experiment is carried out in such a way that it attempts to guarantee an unambiguous result. Any unexpected finding should be considered in the context of the axiom that chance favours the prepared mind.

5 Finally the problem is reassessed in the light of a critical examination of the results obtained.

This outline of the general approach that scientists use in their investigations can be seen as a way of setting up and maintaining the critical dialogue which is the essential ingredient of scientific progress. The approach implies firstly that results and theories are not regarded as sacrosanct (the possibility of error or oversight is always present) and secondly a readiness to examine any new data which may modify or invalidate current thinking about a subject. Both these attitudes are encouraged by the ready interchange of ideas between scientists. Science is very much a communal activity and much of the impetus behind the recent spectacular advances in the natural sciences has come from the mutual constructive and destructive criticism which has taken place through the abundance of publications and personal encounters within the international scientific community in the postwar years.

evaluate chairside problems and the novel or contentious issues that will be presented to the practising dentist in his professional life. In dental science there is currently agreement favouring for example the acidogenic theory of caries and the role of fluoride in caries prevention. But the history of science is littered with the wreckage of discarded or obsolete theories abandoned in the wake of new discoveries. In the event that evidence is presented to challenge or shift emphasis within a particular theory or treatment, the dental surgeon should be both prepared and able to assess the validity and significance of new facts and concepts. The stamp of certainty enshrined in the phrase 'scientifically proven' belongs to the world of advertising rather than of science.

Awareness and experience of the scientific approach to problems provides a strong basis for reaching the right decisions and conclusions about any issues that may be argued on the grounds of newly presented evidence. The scientist's approach to problem-solving is not peculiar to science. It can be applied to many other problems. There is no magic formula that has been vouchsafed only to scientists. Their method of 'conjecture and refutation,' as Popper has called it, may seem rather obvious. It may seem just commonsense but it is also true that most people have a natural reluctance to accept criticism. Few of us enjoy having our cherished personal, political, religious or other beliefs called in question. Science's major contribution to human thought has been to emphasize how progress can be achieved when we are prepared to give up entrenched opinions and welcome new ideas that are better adapted to the facts.

THE ROLE OF SCIENTIFIC THOUGHT IN DENTISTRY

To return to the original question which prompted this examination of the nature and method of science — what does the study of the basic sciences offer to the dental undergraduate and practitioner? Firstly, it is essential to an understanding of many clinical aspects of dentistry. Fish makes the point that the clinician might well accept that it is worth making the effort to discover better clinical procedure based on a constantly growing awareness of the disease processes he daily observes. Secondly, a study of the basic sciences encourages the ability to

FURTHER READING

FISH, SIR WILFRED (1976) The framing and testing of hypotheses. In *Scientific Foundations of Dentistry*, pp. 669–76. Editors R.H. Kramer & B. Cohen. London, Heinemann.

MAGEE, BRYAN (1973) *Popper*. London, Fontana.

MEDAWAR P.B. (1981) *Advice to a Young Scientist*. London, Pan.

MONOD, JACQUES (1979) *Chance and Necessity*. Glasgow, Collins.

WADDINGTON C.H. (1977) *Tools for Thought*. St Albans, Paladin.

VON WEIZSACKER C.F. (1964) *The Relevance of Science*. Glasgow, Collins.

CHAPTER 2

Biological Variation and its Measurement

Variation is a fundamental characteristic of all biological processes, and it is only through a study of variation and its underlying causes that insight can be gained into the ways in which biological systems operate. This chapter is concerned with types and sources of variation, where variation occurs, and some elementary statistical ideas that can be used in the interpretation of observed differences.

VARIATION AND WHERE IT COMES FROM

Variation can be categorized according to the nature of the differences that are observed, and also according to the underlying basis for these differences.

Types of variation

The majority of biological variation falls into one of the following four categories: discrete, continuous, quasicontinuous or discontinuous variation.

Characters that show discrete variation exist in two or more qualitatively different forms. Those existing in two forms only, such as sex, are known as dimorphisms, and those for which there are more than two forms, such as ABO blood type, are known as polymorphisms. Using blood type as an example, individuals are either of one type or another, there is no continuum of intermediates, no variation within each type and no continuous scale of measurement against which different types can be compared. Discrete variation between individuals usually has a simple genetic basis, different forms of the same character being produced by different alleles at the same locus (see Book 2, Chapter 2).

Continuous variables, such as height, weight, tooth size, rate of tooth eruption or the activity of an enzyme, are characters that can be measured against an appropriate continuous scale.

Continuous variation is quantitative rather than qualitative, and levels of expression of the same continuously variable character in different situations can be compared by means of the common scale of measurement. Continuous variation usually has a multifactorial basis, several genes and environmental influences, each with a relatively small effect, contributing to the level of expression.

Characters that are either present or absent, but when present vary continuously, are called quasicontinuous variables (or threshold characters). An example is the accessory feature on the mesiolingual surface of the crown of upper molars, known as the cusp of Carabelli (or Carabelli's trait). It is present on some teeth but not on others, and when present it may appear as anything from a small pit or groove to a pronounced extra cusp. The accepted explanation of quasicontinuous variation rests on the assumption that there is an underlying scale of continuous variation of some attribute (the result of a combination of all the genetic and environmental factors involved) that is immediately related to the development of the character. The character is absent in situations where the level on the scale fails to reach a critical threshold value, and present when the level exceeds this threshold value. The greater the distance above the threshold the more intense is the expression of the character. A quasicontinuous character can therefore be regarded as a continuous variable whose expression has a 'visible' and a 'nonvisible' range. Quasicontinuous variation, like continuous variation, usually has a multifactorial basis.

Variation in number of similar items is discontinuous in that the number of items must always be an integer (whole number); for example, the number of teeth an individual possesses or the number of children in a family. Variation occurs about a modal number, the number that is found more frequently than any other, but only in decreasing or increasing integer steps. For example, the modal number of teeth in a fully developed human permanent dentition is thirty-two. In other words, individuals with thirty-two teeth make up the largest category. Other individuals have thirty-one, thirty or even fewer teeth, and still others have thirty-three, thirty-four and sometimes even more. Development never produces, for instance, thirty-one and a half teeth. Each structure formed is a whole tooth even though teeth vary continuously in size. It is sometimes useful to think of discontinuous variation as an extension of quasicontinuous variation, with the underlying scale divided by several thresholds, each threshold separating one integer value from the next. Discontinuous variation, like continuous and quasicontinuous variation, usually has a multifactorial basis.

Sources of variation

Differences may occur for either genetic or environmental reasons, or some combination of both. Observed variation is also contributed to by errors of observation or measurement and by differences due to chance. However, even if all the observed variation can reasonably be attributed to measurement error and chance, undisclosed biological differences may still exist.

HEREDITY AND ENVIRONMENT

The variation observed among living things is composed of hereditary and environmental components. Heredity supplies the potential and the environment determines how this potential is expressed. Variation may also be broken down into other causal components, either subdivisions of heredity or environment, or components that contain both hereditary and environmental fractions.

Every individual, with the exception of identical twins, has a unique genetic constitution. There is therefore enormous genetic diversity, and this is partly responsible for the observed differences between individuals. Differences between 'normal' individuals may be discrete differences under simple genetic control (as in the case of blood type); or multifactorially controlled differences leading to continuous variation (as for body height), quasicontinuous variation (as for a dental morphological variant), or discontinuous variation (as for tooth number). Gross differences from the population norm

may be caused by single genes with major effects or by chromosomal abnormalities. For example, in achondroplasia, an abnormality of cartilage controlled by a single gene, there is reduced epiphyseal growth resulting in dwarf stature. Achondroplastics fall well outside the normal range of body height. In Down's syndrome (mongolism) several abnormalities, from the characteristic facial appearance to mental retardation and congenital heart defects, stem from the presence of one small additional chromosome, or sometimes only part of it.

One of the major subcomponents of normal genetic variation is the difference between the sexes, a difference that ultimately rests on the different sex chromosome complements (XY and XX) of males and females. In addition to the more obvious differences between the sexes there are less common but nevertheless interesting ones, particularly in the expression of certain developmental and metabolic abnormalities. For example, cleft lip with or without a cleft of the palate affects males more frequently than females (about 60% of cases are males), and also tends to be more severe in males than in females. A more extreme difference between the sexes is found in congenital dislocation of the hip, where there are about six times as many female cases as male cases. A good example of a metabolic disorder affecting the sexes differently is gout, where the afflicted are predominantly males.

All individuals are, of necessity, exposed to at least slightly different environments, simply because more than one individual cannot be in exactly the same place at the same time. Extreme environmental differences of, for example, climate, altitude or availability of food, are understandably likely to have definite biological effects, but even minor environmental variation within a population occupying a restricted area often contributes considerably to observed differences between individuals. Environmental effects are superimposed on genetic differences. Thus individuals with the same hereditary potential may grow to different heights, depending on the environments to which they have been exposed during the growth period. Similarly, individuals with different hereditary potentials may grow to the same height if an environmental difference exactly compensates for the hereditary one. Some ways of estimating the relative contributions of genetic and environmental differences to the observed variation between individuals are described elsewhere (Book 2, Chapter 2).

For most characters studied, members of the same family tend to be more alike than unrelated individuals. This resemblance between relatives can usually be attributed largely to the fact that relatives have a proportion of their genes in common. However, particularly for characters showing continuous, quasicontinuous or discontinuous variation, the common environment experienced by members of the same family may also contribute to the resemblance between relatives. Members of a family group may therefore be alike not only because they have inherited the same genes but also because they are exposed to similar environmental influences.

For some characters a given change in the environment produces different observed effects in individuals with different genetic constitutions. Many examples of this kind of interaction between heredity and environment are found in the field of disease susceptibility. There may be inherited variation of susceptibility to a disease produced by a specific extrinsic factor, for example a particular microorganism, making individuals with different inherited susceptibilities react differently to the same level of the same pathogenic agent.

MEASUREMENT ERROR AND CHANCE VARIATION

Most measuring procedures are not absolutely accurate; that is, measurements made of an identical situation on more than one occasion may give slightly different answers. Some proportion of the variation that is recorded by measurement can therefore arise from measurement error. The importance of the error in a given situation can be assessed by measuring the same set of items on two occasions and by comparing the differences between first and second sets of measurements with the variation within each set of measurements. If the differences between first and second measurements are very small compared with the variation between one item and the next, measurement error can be ignored.

In addition to the differences ascribable to major or minor inherited or environmental differences or to measurement error there is always a small residual component of variation due to chance. This is the variation that would be recorded, if it were possible to do so, between genetically identical individuals in identical environments with a perfect measurement technique. It is the result of random variation of cell function and interaction.

HETEROGENEITY

Absence of observed variation, other than that attributable to measurement error and to chance, does not imply absence of variation at a more fundamental level. Different combinations of hereditary and environmental factors may produce the same end result, so a group of individuals with, for example, a particular developmental malformation may be heterogeneous; that is, what appears to be the same condition may have been produced in a number of different ways. Any attempt to analyze such a group as a whole can only lead to misleading or nonsensical conclusions. Every effort should be made to subdivide it into more homogeneous classes using whatever information is available. For instance, clefts of the palate may occur either in association with cleft lip (cleft lip with or without a cleft of the palate, CL(P)), or alone (isolated cleft palate, CP). When studied further, these two classes of cleft palate cases are found to differ in other respects also. First, different developmental processes are involved. Cleft palate in CP cases results directly from an abnormality at the stage of secondary palate (hard palate) formation, whereas in CL(P) cases it is a consequence of failure of fusion of the primary palate (lip and alveolus) at an earlier stage of development. Second, many CL(P) cases have affected relatives but fewer CP cases do; and affected relatives of CL(P) cases have CL(P) not CP. There are therefore grounds for believing that CL(P) is a separate entity from CP and has a larger genetic component in its aetiology.

WHERE VARIATION OCCURS

Differences exist not only between individuals but also within individuals, between tissues or regions of the body, and with time. Differences are also found between populations or groups of individuals.

Variation within individuals

All the somatic cells of an individual contain, at some stage, the same complement of genes, yet differences within an individual begin to appear early in development when cells or groups of cells start to differentiate along a variety of developmental pathways. The basis for this differentiation seems to be that only particular genes are 'switched on' in particular cells, the remaining majority of genes in each cell type being inactive for most of the time. Discrete differences between tissues can be detected by immunological techniques, each tissue type having a unique set of chemical specificities that is presumably a direct consequence of the activity of a particular set of genes. These discrete differences may be expressed at a different level through variation in such characters as cell size, shape and staining intensity, characters that can be measured on continuous scales.

A second kind of variation that occurs within individuals is that between right and left sides of the body. In bilaterally symmetrical organisms many structures are represented on both sides and develop as mirror images of each other. However, perfect symmetry is rarely attained, minor differences between sides being the general rule. It is reasonable to assume, barring exceptional circumstances, that at any given stage of development the same genes are active in the same tissues on both sides of the body. Failure of bilaterally represented structures to form as exact mirror images of each other is therefore an expression of imprecise genetic control over development.

Variation within individuals may also occur with time. There may be changing levels of expression of a character, either over the growth period or from day to day due to cyclic changes of physiology. For instance, there is the continuous change in body height through infancy, childhood and adolescence into adulthood, and diurnal variation throughout life caused by postural fatigue, individuals tending to be taller in the morning and shorter in the evening. Parallel instances can be found within developing systems. During tooth formation, for example, cells of the internal enamel epithelium become progressively more columnar as they differentiate into ameloblasts, reaching a maximum height when enamel formation is in progress. A continued rhythmic variation of ameloblast function then occurs as enamel matrix is being laid down, variation that results in the incremental lines (brown striae) of Retzius, visible in sections of fully formed enamel.

Variation between individuals and between groups of individuals

DISCRETE VARIATION

Discrete variation between individuals means that some individuals show one form of a charac-

ter whereas others show other forms. Differences between groups are measured in terms of relative frequencies of the different forms. For example, there is variation both within and between racial groups for ABO blood type. About 45% of caucasians are of blood type A, whereas only 28–29% of individuals from mongoloid or negro groups are of blood type A (Table 2.1).

Table 2.1. Percentage frequencies of ABO blood types in large samples from different racial groups.

	A	B	AB	O
Caucasian (North Europe)	45	8	3	44
Negro (Africa)	29	17	4	50
Mongoloid (China)	28	24	7	41

CONTINUOUS VARIATION

Continuous variation results in individuals occupying different positions on the scale of measurement. In any range on any scale there is theoretically an infinite number of possible values, but for practical purposes measurements are made in terms of a chosen size of subdivision. A population is described by the number of individuals falling within each subdivision; that is, by the distribution of individuals over these subdivisions of the scale. Examples of two such distributions are shown in Fig 2.1 a and b. They are distributions of third molar size in two genetically different groups of mice, measured to the nearest hundredth of a millimetre. The horizontal scale is marked off in the chosen subdivisions and the vertical scale shows how many teeth fell into each one. The pictures shown in Fig. 2.1 a and b are called histograms.

Each of these histograms approaches the most commonly encountered type of distribution for continuous variables, the normal distribution, whose 'ideal' shape is described by the bell-shaped normal curve. Normal curves corresponding to the two histograms are shown in Fig. 2.1 c and d. The horizontal scale for these curves, though still a scale of tooth size, is not subdivided, and the vertical scale measures the relative frequency with which teeth of particular sizes are found in each 'idealized' group. These 'ideal' curves can be regarded as histograms that would be produced if the groups were infinitely large, and if tooth size were measured in infinitesimally small subdivisions. Other aspects of these distributions will be referred to later.

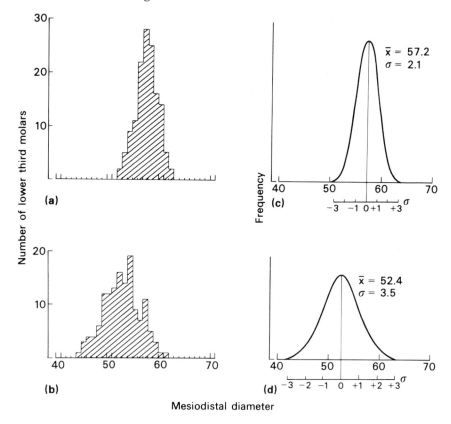

Fig. 2.1. Histograms showing the distribution of mesiodistal diameters of lower third molars in two groups of mice (a (n = 139) and b (n = 141)), and corresponding normal curves (c and d). 1 unit = 10 μm.

The normal curve has quite specific mathematical properties, and many statistical procedures are based on them. Before going into some of these properties a few symbols commonly used in the analysis of continuous variation must be introduced.

The average, or mean, of several measurements is equal to the sum of all the measurements divided by the number of measurements. If each measurement is given the symbol X, the sum of all the measurements can be represented by ΣX, where Σ (the Greek capital sigma) means 'sum of'. If there are n measurements altogether, and if $\bar{X}$ ('X-bar') stands for the mean of all these measurements, then $\bar{X} = \Sigma X/n$. The mean is an indication of the most fundamental property of a distribution, its position on the scale.

The second important property of a distribution is its spread on the scale. This can be expressed by the deviation of a 'typical' or 'standard' measurement from the mean of the distribution. The deviation of one measurement from the mean can be given the symbol x, so that $x = X - \bar{X}$. For measurements that fall above the mean x is positive, whereas for measurements that fall below the mean x is negative. It is a characteristic of the mean that Σx, the sum of all the deviations from it, is equal to zero. Therefore the average of all the deviations, which in other situations might be considered the 'typical' value, is also equal to zero and provides no information about the spread of the distribution on the scale. The way in which this difficulty is overcome is to take, instead of the deviations themselves, the squared deviations, which are all of necessity positive. The average of these squared deviations, known as the variance, is an indication of spread. However, since the quantity required here is an expression of deviation (rather than squared deviation) the square root of the variance is used. This is known as the standard deviation and is given the symbol σ (the Greek lower case sigma). Thus, $\sigma = \sqrt{\Sigma x^2/n}$. Table 2.2 illustrates how a value for σ is calculated. The variance will be referred to again later, but for the present it should be noted that the variance is given by $\sigma^2 = \Sigma x^2/n$.

Table 2.2. Calculation of σ for ten lower third molar diameters (under X) from distribution b of Fig. 2.1. All values are in units of one hundredth of a millimetre.

X	$x = X-\bar{X}$	x^2
48	−4.7	22.09
54	+1.3	1.69
51	−1.7	2.89
58	+5.3	28.09
53	+0.3	0.09
50	−2.7	7.29
57	+4.3	18.49
54	+1.3	1.69
50	−2.7	7.29
52	−0.7	0.49
$\Sigma X = 527$	$\Sigma x = 0.0$	$\Sigma x^2 = 90.10$

$n = 10$
$\bar{X} = \Sigma X/n = 527/10 = 52.7$
$\sigma = \sqrt{\Sigma x^2/n} = \sqrt{90.1/10} = 3.0$

Consider the proportion of a normal distribution that falls within the range bounded by a given number of standard deviations, say w, on each side of the mean. If the mean is given the value zero on the scale this range extends from $-w\sigma$ to $+w\sigma$. As w increases, and therefore as the range on the scale increases, so does the proportion of the distribution falling within the range. It is a characteristic of the normal distribution that the area under the curve bounded by a given number of standard deviations on each side of the mean always contains the same proportion of the distribution, no matter what the degree of spread in terms of units on the scale of measurement (Table 2.3). One, two and three standard deviations on each side of the mean are shown for the two normal curves in Fig. 2.1. For each of these curves the area under the curve falling within the range -3σ to $+3\sigma$ amounts to 99.8% of the total (Table 2.3).

QUASICONTINUOUS VARIATION

With this in mind the third type of variation' between individuals, quasicontinuous variation, can be considered in greater detail. In a population of individuals, some of whom show a quasicontinuous character and others of whom do not, the distribution on the underlying continuous scale is divided by the threshold. The shape of the whole distribution is therefore not fully disclosed, but unless there is reason to think otherwise it is often useful to assume it is normal. Fig. 2.2 (a and b) shows two histograms, the distributions of two groups of mice affected or nonaffected by the presence of a supernumerary cusp on the lower first molar. The zero category contains mice without the cusp and is separated from category 1 by the threshold. The arbitrarily defined categories 1 to 4 contain mice with progressively more extreme levels of expression of the cusp. In one of the groups most of the mice are affected. The histogram of this group (a) bears some resemblance to a normal distribution because most of the animals are allotted an appropriate value on the scale above the threshold. The histogram for the other group (b)

Table 2.3. The proportion of a normal distribution falling below, within and above the range bounded by different numbers of standard deviations from the mean. The ranges are expressed relative to a mean at position zero (see, for example, standard deviation scales in Fig. 2.1 c and d).

	Percentage of distribution			
Range	Below range	Within range	Above range	Total outside range
$-0.5\sigma - +0.5\sigma$	31.0	38.0	31.0	62.0
$-1.0\sigma - +1.0\sigma$	15.9	68.2	15.9	31.8
$-1.5\sigma - +1.5\sigma$	6.6	86.8	6.6	13.2
$-2.0\sigma - +2.0\sigma$	2.3	95.4	2.3	4.6
$-2.5\sigma - +2.5\sigma$	0.6	98.8	0.6	1.2
$-3.0\sigma - +3.0\sigma$	0.1	99.8	0.1	0.2

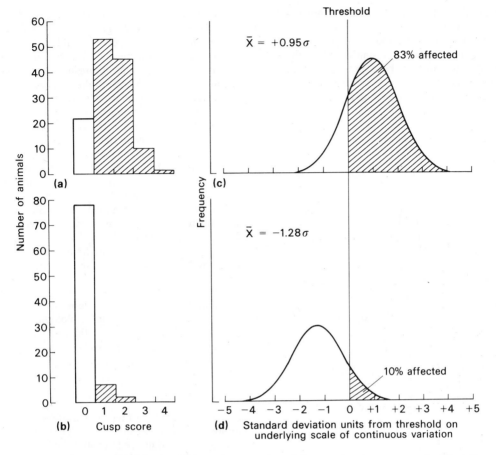

Fig. 2.2. Histograms showing the distribution of scores for a supernumerary cusp on the lower first molar in two groups of mice (a (n = 131) and b (n = 87)), and corresponding normal curves (c and d), assuming the same standard deviation for both groups. The shaded areas indicate affected and the non-shaded areas non-affected animals.

does not resemble a normal distribution because all unaffected mice, the majority in the group, are lumped together into the single zero category, even though they may occupy different positions below the threshold on the presumed underlying continuous scale. However, if it is assumed that both these groups are normally distributed on an underlying continuous scale, it is possible to establish the distance between the threshold and the mean for each group in terms of a number of standard deviations. This is done simply by applying the proportion of affected individuals in each group to tables of the normal distribution, like that shown in Table 2.3. Fig. 2.2 c and d show the normal curves corresponding to the two groups of mice, assuming that they both have the same standard deviation, with the means of both distributions expressed relative to

the threshold on the standard deviation scale (for example, $\bar{X} = -1.28\sigma$, Fig. 2.2d). The difference between groups can now be given by the distance between means on the underlying continuous scale rather than simply by a difference in the proportion affected.

A simple comparison between groups can be made in terms of means arrived at in this way, but such a comparison suffers from the possible unjustified assumption that the standard deviations of the groups being compared are the same. In order to compare the spread of different groups, and also to make a better comparison of means, the quasicontinuous variable must be capable of being scored in three categories rather than two: nonaffected, minimally affected, and moderately to maximally affected. In such a situation there are therefore two thresholds. Threshold 1 separates nonaffected from minimally affected, and threshold 2 separates minimally affected from moderately to maximally affected. The standard deviations of the groups can then be expressed in terms of what is assumed to be a constant interval between the two thresholds. Fig. 2.3 illustrates how

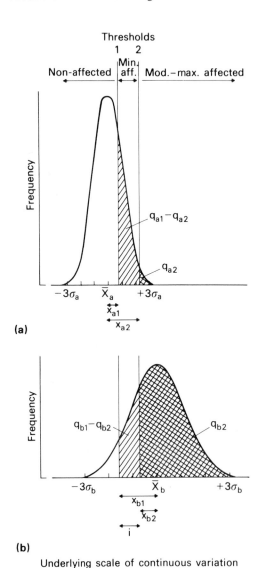

Fig. 2.3. Quasicontinuous variation with two thresholds. A value for x can be derived from tables given the appropriate proportion, q; and standard deviations and means can be compared in terms of the threshold interval, i.

comparisons of this sort can be made. Applying proportions (q) of each group to tables of the normal distribution, q_{a1} gives x_{a1}, the distance of threshold 1 from the mean of distribution a; and q_{a2} gives x_{a2}, the distance of threshold 2 from the mean of distribution a. Both these distances are in terms of σ_a, the standard deviation of distribution a. A similar procedure is adopted for distribution b. Thus the interval between the two thresholds, i, is given by $i = (x_{a2}-x_{a1})\sigma_a = (x_{b2}-x_{b1})\sigma_b$. If, for the sake of simplicity, i is defined as unity, or one threshold unit, the standard deviations of the two groups are: $\sigma_a = 1/(x_{a2}-x_{a1})$ threshold units, and $\sigma_b = 1/(x_{b2}-x_{b1})$ threshold units. It follows that the mean of distribution a, $\bar{X}_a$, is given by $\bar{X}_a = -x_{a1}\sigma_a$ threshold units from threshold 1, and the mean of distribution b, $\bar{X}_b$, is given by $\bar{X}_b = -x_{b1}\sigma_b$ threshold units from threshold 1.

Defining the position and spread of groups on the underlying continuous scale is perhaps one step closer to understanding the biological basis of quasicontinuous variation than simple consideration of the proportions of groups falling into two or three different classes.

DISCONTINUOUS VARIATION

An example of the last type of variation, discontinuous variation, is found in the dentition of the rice rat, a rodent native to central America. In a particular strain of these animals the molars, instead of remaining separate, frequently become fused together during development. Fusion may affect the molars of one, two, three or all four quadrants (each quadrant being the right or left side of the upper or lower jaw in each animal), or no quadrants at all. The number of quadrants affected is therefore always an integer. Table 2.4 shows the distribution of a large group of rice rats from the 'fused molar' strain over these five categories. Assuming that the number of quadrants affected is dependent on an individual's position on an underlying scale of continuous variation divided by four thresholds, and that the group of animals is normally distributed over this scale, reference to tables of the normal distribution can locate each threshold relative to the mean of the rice rat distribution in terms of this distribution's standard deviation. This is illustrated in Fig. 2.4. A point of interest to emerge is that the one-quadrant and three-quadrant categories, those categories that necessarily contain asymmetrical individuals, each occupies a range on the scale

Table 2.4. The distribution of a group of rice rats from the 'fused molar' strain according to the number of quadrants affected by molar fusion.

	Quadrants affected					
	0	1	2	3	4	Total
Number of animals	113	101	453	304	1209	2180
Percentage	5	5	21	14	55	100

about half the size of the two-quadrant interval. The two-quadrant category contains predominantly individuals with either two upper or two lower quadrants affected, in other words symmetrically affected animals. The level on the underlying scale therefore has to change twice as much to move from one end of this symmetrical category to the other as it does to move across either the one-quadrant or the three-quadrant interval, implying greater developmental stability of the symmetrical condition.

DIFFERENCES OF POSITION AND SPREAD

The general features of biological variation described in previous pages have been discovered by observation and experiment in a very large number of situations. It is appropriate now to consider how to interpret a particular observed difference, the basis of which is not yet understood. The approaches to this problem given here are largely concerned with differences between individuals or groups of individuals for continuous variables, but similar principles can be applied to quasicontinuous and discontinuous variables and to differences operating within individuals. A later section deals with the analysis of differences between groups for discrete variables.

Sampling

It is usually quite impractical to study an entire population or every example of a particular biological situation. Investigators must therefore be content to take samples; but how representative of an entire population, or every situation of a particular type, is a sample likely to be?

Suppose that the group of teeth in Fig. 2.1 b represents a complete population from which samples are drawn at random. The distributions of five random samples of ten teeth and five random samples of fifty teeth from this 'popula-

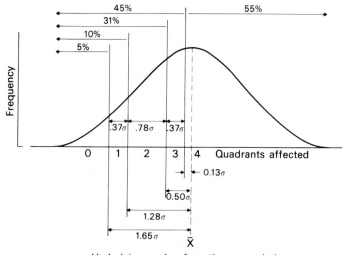

Fig. 2.4. The assumed normal distribution of the group of rice rats from Table 2.4 on an underlying scale of continuous variation divided by four thresholds. The distance of each threshold from the mean, $\bar{X}$, is shown in terms of σ, the standard deviation, as are the sizes of the intervals between adjacent thresholds.

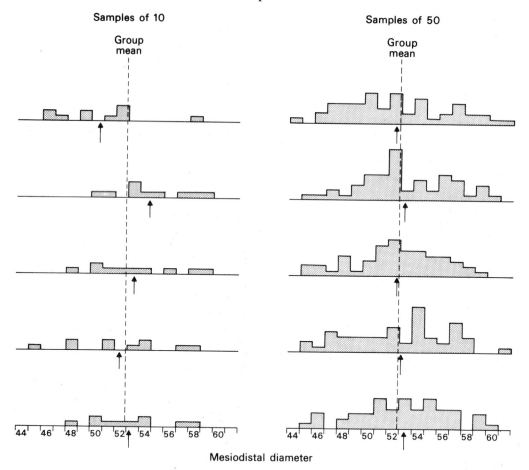

Fig. 2.5. Samples of ten and fifty taken at random from the group of teeth shown in Fig. 2.1b. The mean of the group from which the samples were drawn is shown by the broken vertical lines, and the samples means are shown by arrows. The average spread of samples of ten is 12.0 units, and the average spread of samples of fifty is 16.4 units of the scale. 1 unit = 10 μm.

tion' are shown in Fig. 2.5. The most obvious finding is that the means of the large samples agree much more closely with the mean of the whole group than the means of the small samples. In other words, the standard deviation of sample means from the true mean of the group is smaller for larger samples. The standard deviation of sample means from the true mean of a population is known as the standard error of the mean, and is symbolized by $\sigma_{\bar{x}}$. If the population is normally distributed (or nearly so), the means of samples of a given size are also normally distributed. The standard error is therefore exactly the same kind of statistic as the standard deviation. For instance, if in the present example each sample were composed of only one tooth, the standard error would be equal to the standard deviation, σ, of teeth in the group as a whole. It can be shown that the standard error decreases from this maximum value with increasing values of $\sqrt{n}$, the square root of sample size. The standard error is therefore given by $\sigma_{\bar{x}} = \sigma/\sqrt{n}$.

The standard error is used in attaching a level of reliability to the mean of a sample as an indicator of the true mean of the population from which the sample was drawn. The larger the standard error, the more unreliable the sample mean. Reliability is expressed by giving a range of values together with an associated level of confidence that the true mean of the population lies within the range. This can be accomplished using Table 2.3, where the values for standard deviations also apply to standard errors (because the standard error is itself a standard deviation, that of sample means). The implication of Table 2.3 in this context is that when a large number of samples is taken from a given population their means fall, for example, within the range $-\sigma_{\bar{x}}$ to $+\sigma_{\bar{x}}$ (that is, one standard error on each side of the true mean) 68.2% of the time. The converse must also apply, namely that the true mean lies somewhere within one standard error on each side of the sample mean, also in about sixty-eight samples out of every 100. A greater level of confidence can be given if the range is widened. The true mean lies within two standard errors on each side of the sample mean in about ninety-five samples out of every 100, or within three standard errors in very nearly all samples (Table 2.3). Thus, once a value for $\sigma_{\bar{x}}$ has been calculated from a sample, the reliability of the sample mean can be expressed in terms of ranges on the scale of measurement.

A further point to notice in Fig. 2.5 is that the average spread of each sample on the scale, the distance on the scale between the smallest and largest items in the sample, is smaller for small samples than for large samples. Thus, whereas the mean of a sample is an unbiased estimate of the true mean of the population from which it comes, the standard deviation calculated from a sample is biased, always tending to underestimate the true spread of the population. This underestimation becomes more marked as sample size is reduced.

It has already been shown that the standard deviation of a complete group is given by $\sigma = \sqrt{\Sigma x^2/n}$, but it is apparent now that if this formula is applied to a sample it will underestimate the true standard deviation of the population from which the sample was drawn. What is needed is some sort of correction for this bias that will have a larger effect in smaller samples. It can be shown that a good correction for bias is achieved by substituting $n-1$ for n, so that the corrected, unbiased estimate of the standard deviation of a population, made from a sample of size n, is given by $\sigma = \sqrt{\Sigma x^2/(n-1)}$. The larger the sample the less effect the correction will have.

The quantity $n-1$ is known as the number of degrees of freedom. The reason for this may be illustrated as follows. Suppose that the mean of ten measurements is 100. Values for nine of these can be freely assigned; that is, each of nine measurements could theoretically take on any value from a very large negative number to a very large positive number, but the tenth can only have the value that makes the mean of all the measurements equal to 100. In a sample of n items there are therefore $n-1$ degrees of freedom.

Variance

As already mentioned, the square of the standard deviation, σ^2, is known as the variance. It is also sometimes symbolized by V. (The symbols σ^2 and V are normally used in slightly different contexts, but this distinction is not made here). The unbiased estimate of the variance of a population, made from a sample of size n, is therefore given by $V = \sigma^2 = \Sigma x^2/(n-1)$. The variance, like the standard deviation, is an indication of spread on the scale, but the variance has particular properties that make it useful for certain kinds of statistical analysis. The most important of these properties is the additive nature of the variance. This is best explained using an example. The diameter of the crown of a tooth is dependent both on the width of the dentine core and on the combined thickness of enamel on opposite faces of the crown. The width of the dentine core and enamel thickness vary from one individual to another, so there is a variance for dentine width, say V_d, and a variance for enamel thickness, say V_e. Assuming V_d and V_e to be independent of each other, the variance of crown diameter, say V_c, which is equivalent to the variance of the sum of the two measurements, symbolized by V_{d+e}, is simply the sum of the two variances. Thus $V_c = V_{d+e} = V_d + V_e$. What may appear surprising is that the variance of the difference between dentine width and enamel thickness, symbolized by V_{d-e}, is the same, that is, $V_{d-e} = V_d + V_e$. The reason for this is that two sources of variation contribute to the difference between dentine width and enamel thickness, as well as to their sum. These properties of variance are referred to later.

Differences between samples

There are two common kinds of statistical tests. First, there are tests for deciding whether a particular sample is likely to have been produced by the same general set of circumstances as that prevailing in a known situation; in other words, whether the sample is likely to have come from a known 'population'. Second, there are tests for deciding whether two samples are likely to be results of common influences, even though the nature of these influences may not be understood; or, put another way, whether the two samples are likely to have come from a single 'population'. In the sense used here and in the rest of this chapter, 'population' refers to groups not only of living individuals but also, for example, of fossil jaw bones or red blood cells.

THE NULL HYPOTHESIS

The samples in Fig. 2.5 obviously differ from each other. However, since they have all been made by random choice of individual teeth from the same group of third molars, the differences between them are due to nothing more than random sampling variation. Another way of saying this is that the differences are due to chance alone. The procedure for interpreting a difference of unknown origin, for example a difference between two samples, is to start with the hypothesis that the two samples are in fact derived from the same population. This is known as the null hypothesis, the hypothesis that there is no 'real' difference between the samples. A statistical test is then made, and if the result shows that the difference can reasonably be accounted for by chance alone the null hypothesis is accepted; that is, it is concluded that the samples come from the same source. Alternatively, if the test indicates that the observed difference is unlikely to have arisen by chance alone the null hypothesis is rejected and the difference between samples is said to be statistically significant. When this occurs, it is reasonable to accept that the difference is due, at least in part, to a real difference of circumstances that produced the different samples. Some simple statistical tests will now be described.

DIFFERENCES INVOLVING MEANS

Between the mean of a single sample and a known value
Suppose that an investigator wants to know whether the mean, $\bar{X}$, of a sample is significantly different from a value A, the known mean of a population. In other words, in terms of its position on the scale, is the sample likely to have come from this population? To answer this question the observed 'error', the difference between the sample mean and the mean of the known population, is compared with the standard error associated with the sample mean. (It will be recalled that the standard error is the difference from the true mean of the source population that is exceeded by sample means 31.8% of the time—Table 2.3). Under the null hypothesis, the population from which the sample was drawn is taken to be the known population itself. The

investigator can therefore decide whether the observed error, in terms of the standard error assumed to apply to the known population, is small enough to be accounted for by chance alone. If so, he must conclude that there are no grounds for suspecting that the given sample has come from any other than the known population.

The ratio of the observed error to the standard error is distributed in the same way as a statistic known as Student's t; 'Student' being the pseudonym of W. S. Gosset, who introduced the statistic in 1908. Thus, $t = \lceil \bar{X} - A \rceil / \sigma_{\bar{X}}$, where $\lceil \bar{X} - A \rceil$ stands for the absolute value of the difference between the sample mean and the mean of the known population, a positive value no matter whether $\bar{X}$ is larger or smaller than A. The larger the difference between the sample mean and the mean of the known population the larger the value of t. Tables have been drawn up to show values of t for different degrees of freedom and different levels of confidence. The t values for, say, the '5% level' (the 5% level of significance, or the 95% confidence limits) are those which would be exceeded by chance alone in only 5% of samples. In other words, the mean of one in every twenty samples taken from the same population, when tested against the population mean, is expected to give a t value greater than that shown for the 5% level and the appropriate number of degrees of freedom. Yet another way of saying this is that the probability of this difference occurring by chance alone is less than 5%, symbolized by $P < 0.05$. Samples giving probabilities of less than 5% are generally regarded as being significantly different from the population against which they are being tested, and are therefore accepted as coming from a different source. Table 2.5 lists values of t for the 5% and 1% levels of significance (the 95% and 99% confidence limits) and for a few selected degrees of freedom.

Between the means of two samples
Suppose now that an investigator is comparing two samples, one with the other, and wants to know whether the difference between their means can be attributed to chance alone. In other words, is it likely that the two samples have been drawn from the same source? It is relevant here to have in mind the kind of distribution that results from plotting the difference between two sample means for a large number of pairs of samples drawn at random from the same population, a distribution that expresses the relative frequency with which differences of various size

Table 2.5. Values of t for two levels of significance and a few selected degrees of freedom.

Degrees of freedom	Probability of a larger t value occurring by chance alone	
	5% (0.05)	1% (0.01)
1	t = 12.71	t = 63.66
2	4.30	9.93
3	3.18	5.84
4	2.78	4.60
5	2.57	4.03
6	2.45	3.71
7	2.37	3.50
8	2.31	3.36
9	2.26	3.25
10	2.23	3.17
20	2.09	2.85
50	2.01	2.68
100	1.98	2.63

occur. If the population is normally distributed (or nearly so), so that the distribution of means of samples of a given size is also normal, the difference between sample means is normally distributed too. Consequently, a standard deviation of the difference between sample means, known as the standard error of the difference, can be calculated. The investigator can therefore assess the difference between his two samples in a way similar to that used for testing a single sample against a known population; by comparing the observed difference between sample means with the standard error of the difference. One standard error (of the difference) is the difference that would be exceeded in about thirty-two pairs of samples out of every 100 drawn from the same population (Table 2.3).

The standard error of the difference between sample means is calculated as follows. The variance of sample means is the square of the standard deviation of sample means (the square of the standard error), that is, $\sigma_{\bar{X}}^2$. Because of a property of variances already referred to, the variance of the difference between two sample means, symbolized by σ_d^2, is given by the sum of the variances of sample means. Thus, $\sigma_d^2 = \sigma_{\bar{X}1}^2 + \sigma_{\bar{X}2}^2$, where the variances $\sigma_{\bar{X}1}^2$ and $\sigma_{\bar{X}2}^2$ are the squares of the two standard errors, $\sigma_{\bar{X}1}$ and $\sigma_{\bar{X}2}$, calculated for the two samples being compared. The square root of the variance of the difference, σ_d, is the standard deviation of the difference between sample means, and this is the standard error of the difference. The ratio of the observed error (the difference between sample

means) to the standard error (of the difference) is again distributed as Student's t. Thus, $t = |\bar{X}1 - \bar{X}2| / \sigma_d$. The appropriate number of degrees of freedom is $n_1 + n_2 - 2$, where n_1 and n_2 are the sizes of the two samples being compared.

DIFFERENCES BETWEEN VARIANCES

A comparable test can be applied to variances. What is required is simply the ratio of the two variances being compared. The larger variance is always divided by the smaller so that the variance ratio, symbolized by F, is always greater than unity. Tables of F values are available for different levels of significance and various degrees of freedom. Two different degrees of freedom are required for each comparison, $n_1 - 1$ and $n_2 - 1$, where n_1 and n_2 are the sizes of the groups being compared. Table 2.6 shows values of F for the 5% and 1% levels and for a few selected degrees of freedom. The F values for, say, the 5% level are those which would be exceeded by chance alone in only one out of every twenty pairs of samples drawn from the same population.

As an example, consider again the two groups of mouse lower third molars illustrated in Fig. 2.1. For the two groups n = 139 and 141, and σ^2 = 4.5 and 12.3. The variance ratio is given by $F_{139}^{141} = 12.3/4.5 = 2.73$. Reference to Table 2.6 shows that this ratio exceeds the value given for F_{100}^{100} at the 1% level (that is, the value given for degrees of freedom closest to but less than 139 and 141), so the probability of this difference occurring by chance alone must be less than 1%. There is therefore good reason to believe that the variances of the two groups have been produced by sets of biological circumstances that are fundamentally different.

Problems of scale

Table 2.7 shows the mean and standard deviation of upper first molar width in one human and one mouse sample. Measured in millimetres, the standard deviation for the mouse molars is less than one tenth that for the human molars. Does this mean that upper first molars vary much less from one mouse to another than they do from one person to the next? In purely numerical terms this is certainly so. However, a given difference between two teeth, say a difference of 0.2 mm, has a much greater biological implication in mice than it does in man. This is a difference of four standard deviations in the quoted mouse sample, one that would be exceeded only

Table 2.6. Values of F for two levels of significance and a few selected degrees of freedom. Values in the upper row for each number of degrees of freedom correspond to a probability of 5%, and those in the lower rows to a probability of 1%; that is, values of F larger than those shown occur by chance alone only 5% and 1% of the time.

Degrees of freedom for smaller variance	Degrees of freedom for larger variance									
	5	6	7	8	9	10	20	50	100	200
5	5.05	4.95	4.88	4.82	4.78	4.74	4.56	4.44	4.40	4.38
	10.97	10.67	10.45	10.27	10.15	10.05	9.55	9.24	9.13	9.07
6	4.39	4.28	4.21	4.15	4.10	4.06	3.87	3.75	3.71	3.69
	8.75	8.47	8.26	8.10	7.98	7.87	7.39	7.09	6.99	6.94
7	3.97	3.87	3.79	3.73	3.68	3.63	3.44	3.32	3.28	3.25
	7.46	7.19	7.00	6.84	6.71	6.62	6.15	5.85	5.75	5.70
8	3.69	3.58	3.50	3.44	3.39	3.34	3.15	3.03	2.98	2.96
	6.63	6.37	6.19	6.03	5.91	5.82	5.36	5.06	4.96	4.91
9	3.48	3.37	3.29	3.23	3.18	3.13	2.93	2.80	2.76	2.73
	6.06	5.80	5.62	5.47	5.35	5.26	4.80	4.51	4.41	4.36
10	3.33	3.22	3.14	3.07	3.02	2.97	2.77	2.64	2.59	2.56
	5.64	5.39	5.21	5.06	4.95	4.85	4.41	4.12	4.01	3.96
20	2.71	2.60	2.52	2.45	2.40	2.35	2.12	1.96	1.90	1.87
	4.10	3.87	3.71	3.56	3.45	3.37	2.94	2.63	2.53	2.47
50	2.40	2.29	2.20	2.13	2.07	2.02	1.78	1.60	1.52	1.48
	3.41	3.18	3.02	2.88	2.78	2.70	2.26	1.94	1.82	1.76
100	2.30	2.19	2.10	2.03	1.97	1.92	1.68	1.48	1.39	1.34
	3.20	2.99	2.82	2.69	2.59	2.51	2.06	1.73	1.59	1.51
200	2.26	2.14	2.05	1.98	1.92	1.87	1.62	1.42	1.32	1.26
	3.11	2.90	2.73	2.60	2.50	2.41	1.97	1.62	1.48	1.39

rarely if pairs of teeth were drawn at random many times from this group of mice; whereas it represents less than one third of a standard deviation in the human sample, a difference that would be exceeded frequently if pairs of teeth were drawn at random many times from this human group. Any biological deductions made from the spread of a distribution on the original scale of measurement must therefore take into account the position of the distribution on the scale. The usual way in which this is done is to indicate the level of variability by the coefficient of variation, the standard deviation in terms of (divided by) the mean. When expressed as a percentage the coefficient of variation is therefore given by CV% = $100\sigma/\bar{X}$. Table 2.7 shows

Table 2.7. The mean ($\bar{X}$), standard deviation (σ) and coefficient of variation (CV%) for the width (buccolingual diameter) of upper first molars in one large human sample and one large mouse sample. Measurements for both samples were made in millimetres.

Sample	$\bar{X}$	σ	CV%
Human	12.05	0.71	5.9
Mouse	1.06	0.05	4.7

that the coefficients of variation of the human and mouse groups, although not the same, are very much more alike than the standard deviations. For their size, mouse molars therefore vary among themselves about as much as human molars.

Sometimes comparable scale effects operate within a single group spread over a wide range of the scale, resulting in an asymmetrical or skewed distribution with, for positive measurements, the highest point of the distribution curve shifted to the left of centre. Logarithmic transformation of the measurements may be effective in eliminating skewness to produce a more or less normal distribution, allowing statistical procedures based on the normal curve to be applied. Other kinds of transformation may be appropriate under other circumstances.

VARIATION FROM MORE THAN ONE SOURCE OR WITH MORE THAN ONE EFFECT

A single variable may be subject to more than one influence. As already mentioned, tooth crown size is dependent both on the size of the dentine core and on enamel thickness. However, restricting considerations to the outside of the crown alone provides no information about the dentine and enamel of which it is composed. Demonstration of a significant difference, for example between two groups for tooth size, therefore provides no information about the sources of variation that are responsible for the difference, or the relative sizes of their contributions. Conversely, two or more variables may be affected by a single common source of variation. The size of the dentine core and the thickness of enamel are probably dependent to some extent on common nutritional and metabolic factors, but studying the dentine and enamel separately will not disclose such an association between them. Statistical methods are therefore available for assessing the relative importance of different sources of variation, and for analyzing the way in which two or more characters vary together.

Before going into this in a little more detail, it should be mentioned that if dentine width and enamel thickness are found to have a common source of variation, the equation $V_c = V_d + V_e$, referred to earlier, does not apply (unless the common source can be shown to have a relatively small effect). This is because the commom source variance contributes to both V_d and V_e, causing it to be represented twice instead of only once in the right hand side of the equation. The size of V_c therefore becomes progressively smaller than $V_d + V_e$ as the common source variance increases.

Components of variance

In many other situations too, the total observed variation can be partitioned into components associated with different sources of variability. For example, two examiners may be scoring dental caries in children of the same age group at a number of different schools. To check on the accuracy of the scoring procedure they may choose to score each child on two separate occasions. If all caries scores collected in this way were considered together there would be an overall variance of caries score, but differences between scores may have arisen for three different reasons. First, there may be a real difference between schools, perhaps due to a preponderance of different dietary habits. Second, there may be a difference between examiners, one examiner consistently recording higher scores than the other because of slightly different scoring criteria. Third, the caries score for each individual may not be exactly the same for the two

occasions on which it was recorded, a difference due to imperfect repeatability.

The relative importance of different sources of variation in a situation of this kind can be assessed by what is known as analysis of variance. As already shown, the unbiased estimate of the variance of a population, made from a sample of size n, is given by $V = \sigma^2 = \Sigma x^2/(n-1)$. The quantity Σx^2, the sum of squared deviations from the mean, is often referred to as the sum of squares. The variance is therefore equal to the sum of squares divided by the number of degrees of freedom. Suppose that there are s samples each composed of n items, so for the sake of simplicity only two possible sources of variation are being considered, 'within sample' and 'between sample' variation. Under the null hypothesis there is no real difference between samples; in other words the assumption is that they have been drawn from the same population. Sums of squares and degrees of freedom are first computed for each sample separately. For each of the s samples, this gives a value for Σx^2 (the sum of squared deviations from their own sample mean) with $n-1$ degrees of freedom. The variance within samples, V_W, is the sum of all these within sample sums of squares, symbolized by $\Sigma\Sigma x^2$, divided by the sum of all their degrees of freedom, $s(n-1)$. Thus, $V_W = \Sigma\Sigma x^2/s(n-1)$. Assuming the null hypothesis to be correct, this observed within sample variance provides an estimate of σ^2, the true variance of the population from which the samples were drawn. It has already been shown that the variance of the means of samples drawn from the same population is given by $\sigma_{\bar{x}}^2 = \sigma^2/n$. Thus, if the null hypothesis is correct, the observed variance of sample means, $V_{\bar{x}}$, should not differ significantly from V_W/n, the expected variance of sample means if all samples come from the same population. This difference can be tested using the variance ratio $F = V_{\bar{x}} : V_W/n = nV_{\bar{x}}/V_W$, with $s-1$ degrees of freedom associated with the variance of sample means and $s(n-1)$ degrees of freedom associated with the within sample variance. If the F test shows that there is a significant difference between these variances it can be concluded likely that the samples have been drawn from more than one population with means that differ from each other.

The difference between the observed variance of sample means, $V_{\bar{x}}$, and that predicted by the null hypothesis, V_W/n, is the between sample component of variance, V_B. Thus, $V_B = V_{\bar{x}} - (V_W/n)$. Once the null hypothesis has been rejected it is concluded that individuals are different partly because of within sample variation and partly because of variation between samples. The relative size of these two components indicates the relative importance of within and between sample sources of variation. Other forms of analysis of variance can be applied to more complex situations where several sources of variation are considered at the same time.

Regression and correlation

So far only a single variable, symbolized by X, has been considered. Suppose now that there is some reason for studying two variables, X and Y, at the same time. For example, does an individual with a large upper jaw also have a large lower jaw; and likewise, does a small upper jaw go with a small lower jaw? In more general terms, do the sizes of upper and lower jaws tend to vary together from one individual to another?

Consider how the two variables X and Y might be related. The simplest (and luckily the most frequent) kind of relationship can be represented graphically by a straight line. It could be that Y is simply proportional to X, so that Y is equal to X multiplied by some unknown constant, say b. In such a case $Y = bX$. For example, if $b = 1$ the value of Y is always equal to the value of X, if $b = 2$ the value of Y is always twice that of X, and if $b = \frac{1}{2}$ the value of Y is always half that of X. The value of b is known as the slope of the line (Fig. 2.6a). If the relationship between X and Y is always exact, only one pair of corresponding X and Y values is required to find b (from the equation $b = Y/X$). However, this is extremely unlikely. The general trend of the association between X and Y may be described by a straight line, but the association is almost never perfect

so that different X,Y pairs usually give different values of b. A series of X and Y values is therefore required to arrive at a slope for the line that is representative of the situation as a whole.

Furthermore, straight lines expressing the relationship between two variables do not always pass through the origin, the point corresponding to zero on both axes of the graph. The full equation for a straight line is given by $Y = bX + a$, where a is the point where the line intersects the Y axis (Fig. 2.6b). Values for both a and b are required to describe a straight line relationship fully. The question is how to arrive at values of a and b for a sample of X and Y measurement pairs. The values required are those specifying the 'best straight line' for the particular set of data. One thing that can be seen intuitively is that this line must pass through the point $(\bar{X},\bar{Y})$, corresponding to the means of X and Y values, but a second point through which the line passes must be known before the line can be drawn.

Returning for a moment to the case of a single variable, X, it can be shown that the sum of squared deviations of individual measurements from any point selected on the scale is a minimum when the selected point is at the mean, $\bar{X}$. If deviations are taken from any other point on the scale their sum is larger than Σx^2. This principle of least squares is used to arrive at the best fitting straight line. The value of b, the regression coefficient, for the best straight line is known as the regression of Y on X and is given by $b = \Sigma xy/\Sigma x^2$, where $x = X - \bar{X}$ as before, and where $y = Y - \bar{Y}$. The quantity Σxy is the sum of products of the deviations x and y for each pair of X and Y measurements. Since the value of b can be calculated in this way, and

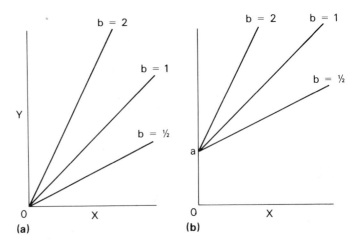

Fig. 2.6. Different straight line relationships between two variables, X and Y. The slope of the line is given by b.

since $\bar{X}$ and $\bar{Y}$ are known, the value of a can be found from the equation $a = \bar{Y} - b\bar{X}$. There are now two points through which the best straight line is known to pass, $(\bar{X},\bar{Y})$ and $(X=O, Y=a)$, so the line can be drawn. The line produced in this way is that from which the sum of squared deviations of Y values is at its lowest.

The null hypothesis here is that Y is unrelated to X. In other words, variation in Y has nothing to do with variation in X, and the true value of the regression coefficient, b, is zero; but how is an investigator to know whether the value of b he has calculated reflects a real relationship between X and Y or whether it occurred by chance alone in a situation where no real relationship existed? The level of confidence in the estimated value being significantly different from zero is taken from tables of F values, the same tables that are used to test variance ratios. The value of F is given by

$$F = \frac{b\Sigma xy(n-2)}{\Sigma y^2 - b\Sigma xy}$$

where n is the number of pairs of X and Y measurements. One degree of freedom is associated with the numerator and $n-2$ degrees of freedom with the denominator. The standard error of the regression coefficient, given by $b/\sqrt{F}$, can be used to test for a difference between regression coefficients calculated for two samples.

The regression coefficient indicates the direction (in graphical terms) of the association between X and Y rather than its strength. The most usual way of expressing the strength of an association is by means of the correlation coefficient. This is a quantity that always falls between -1 and $+1$. A value of zero means that there is no association; a value of $+1$ means that there is perfect association, with Y increasing as X increases; and a value of -1 means that there is perfect association but that Y decreases as X increases. Different correlation situations are illustrated in Fig. 2.7. The correlation coefficient, symbolized by r, is given by

$$r = \frac{\Sigma xy}{\sqrt{\Sigma x^2 \Sigma y^2}} .$$

The level of confidence that a calculated value of r is significantly different from zero is taken from special tables drawn up for this purpose (Table 2.8). There are also ways of testing for a difference between correlation coefficients calculated from two samples of unknown origin, but these are too involved to be mentioned here.

There are three kinds of reason for a significant correlation coefficient, and the investigator must use whatever other facts are available to decide which one applies in any given situation. The first is that the association stems from a direct cause and effect relationship as, for instance, between physical exertion and heart rate. Second, the two variables may not be directly related but affected by a common influence. For example, human development can be divided into stages according to either the state of ossification of the skeleton or the degree of calcification of the forming teeth. The developmental stages defined by ossification are highly correlated with those based on dental calcification, but not because the skeleton influences the dentition directly, or vice versa. Both are affected by the general body changes associated with growth and development. Third, the association may be entirely spurious, with no causal relationship between the two variables, either direct, or indirect through the operation of a common influence. This spurious association is what the significance test is designed to reduce to an acceptable level of probability.

DIFFERENCES OF FREQUENCY

Populations or groups of individuals may be characterized by the frequencies of the different forms of discrete variables (see, for example, Table 2.1). There are two kinds of question that can be asked here, analogous to those for which the two kinds of t test are used. The first is, are the frequencies in a sample compatible with the null hypothesis that the sample has come from a

Table 2.8. Values of the correlation coefficient at the 5% and 1% levels of significance. For an observed correlation to be regarded as significantly different from zero it must be equal to or larger than the value shown for the chosen level of significance and the appropriate number of degrees of freedom. The table applies to negative as well as positive values.

Degrees of freedom	5% (0.05)	1% (0.01)
5	0.75	0.87
6	0.71	0.83
7	0.67	0.80
8	0.63	0.77
9	0.60	0.74
10	0.58	0.71
20	0.42	0.54
50	0.27	0.35
100	0.20	0.25
200	0.14	0.18

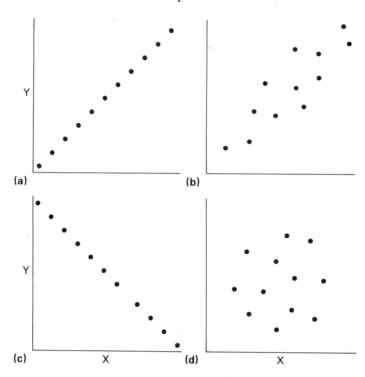

(a)

(b)

(c)   X   (d)   X

Fig. 2.7. 'Scatter diagrams' showing different kinds of association between two variables, X and Y. (a) shows perfect positive association, with r = 1 (and b = 1); (b) shows strong positive association, with r between 0.8 and 0.9 (and b = 1); (c) shows perfect negative association, with r = −1 (and b = −1); and (d) shows no association, with r = 0.

known population where the overall frequencies of the different forms have been established? For example, prior knowledge leads to the expectation of a 1:1 female to male ratio in human populations. The ratio of females to males in samples of human populations should therefore not differ significantly from a 1:1 ratio unless there are factors involved in making up the samples that tend to alter the ratio in one direction or the other. Suppose that in a class of dental students nineteen are females and thirty-one are males. Some of us may be all too ready to ascribe this difference to superior academic achievement of males, and others to poorer opportunity for females. (There are, of course, other possible reasons for a difference also.) However, before jumping to any rash conclusion, the data should be properly analyzed to see if there is any justification for accepting that the difference from a perfect 1:1 ratio is likely to be due to anything other than chance.

Table 2.9 shows how such an analysis is carried out. The observed numbers, O, are nineteen females and thirty-one males, with a total of

fifty. The expected numbers, E, are based on the expected proportions (1:1) and the total (fifty), and so are twenty-five females and twenty-five males. The appropriate number of degrees of freedom is equivalent to the number of categories whose frequencies can be assigned arbitrarily. For example, in this case the frequency of females could take on any value, but

Table 2.9. The calculation of chi-square expressing the difference between observed and expected numbers. The symbol χ_1^2 means chi-square with one degree of freedom. The probability of this particular difference occurring by chance alone is greater than 5%, and the difference is therefore not regarded as statistically significant.

	Females	Males	Total
Observed (O)	19	31	50
Expected (E)	25	25	50
O–E	−6	6	
(O–E)²	36	36	
(O–E)²/E	1.44	1.44	2.88

$\chi_1^2 = \Sigma((O-E)^2/E) = 2.88 \quad P>5\%$

once the female frequency is decided the frequency of males is fixed by the total. In these two categories there is therefore only one degree of freedom. (More than two categories are allowed in such a test, and the number of degrees of freedom is always one less than the number of categories.) The sum of the squared differences between observed and expected numbers, each squared difference expressed relative to the expected number for its own category, is given the symbol χ^2 (chi-square). Thus, chi-square is given by $\chi^2 = \Sigma((O-E)^2/E)$. Tables of chi-square values are available for different degrees of freedom and different levels of significance. The values of χ^2 for, say, the 5% level (the 95% confidence limits) are those which would be exceeded by chance alone in one out of every twenty samples drawn from the known population. Samples giving larger values are therefore regarded as significantly different from the expected proportions against which they are being tested, and are accepted as coming from a different source. Values of χ^2 for the 5% and 1% levels, and for a few selected degrees of freedom, are shown in Table 2.10. It can be seen that the value calculated from the example given in Table 2.9 would be exceeded by chance alone more often than 5% of the time. The difference between the sex ratio in the class of students and the expected 1:1 ratio is therefore not statistically significant, and there is no reason to suppose, on statistical grounds, that anything other than chance is responsible for the difference.

The second question is, given the frequencies of the different forms of a discrete variable in two samples, is it likely that the two samples have come from the same source? For example, suppose that a new treatment for a particular disease has been developed, and everyone is anxious to know whether it is better than the old treatment. Patients are assigned at random to the two treatment groups and the results of the treatment, in terms of the numbers of patients cured and uncured, are set up in the form of a contingency table, as shown in Table 2.11. The contingency table in Table 2.11 is a 'two-by-two' table, that is, it has two rows and two columns, but more than two rows and two columns are allowed. For instance, if three treatments were being tested there would be three rows, and if some of those individuals left uncured suffered a toxic reaction to treatment a third column could be added. The number of degrees of freedom in a contingency table is given by $(R-1)(C-1)$, where R is the number of rows and C is the number of columns. The numbers of patients in Table 2.11 have been represented by symbols. Using these sympols, chi-square is given by

$$\chi_1^2 = \frac{n(ad-bc)^2}{(a+b)\ (c+d)\ (a+c)\ (b+d)}$$

Values that exceed those given for the 5% level are generally taken to indicate that the two samples have been drawn from different sources; in other words, in this case, the treatments had different effects.

Table 2.11. A 'two-by-two' contingency table for calculating chi-square that expresses the difference between two samples. The symbols a, b, c and d stand for different numbers of patients.

	Patients cured	Patients not cured	Total
Old treatemt	a	b	a+b
New treatment	c	d	c+d
Total	a+c	b+d	a+b+c+d=n

$$\chi_1^2 = \frac{n(ad-bc)^2}{(a+b)\ (c+d)\ (a+c)\ (b+d)}.$$

Table 2.10. Values of χ^2 for two levels of significance and a few selected degrees of freedom.

Degrees of freedom	Probability of a larger χ^2 value occurring by chance alone	
	5% (0.05)	1% (0.01)
1	$\chi^2 = 3.84$	$\chi^2 = 6.63$
2	5.99	9.21
3	7.81	11.34
4	9.49	13.28
5	11.07	15.09

CONCLUDING REMARKS

Whenever anything is measured numerically, some procedure is required for giving meaning to the numbers obtained. Statistical tests have been devised for this purpose. Statistics is concerned with probabilities that are invariably greater than zero (complete impossibility) and less than unity or 100% (absolute certainty). Statistical tests can therefore neither prove nor disprove anything absolutely. They can only indicate the relative likelihoods of alternative explanations. It is up to the investigator to decide what level of probability he will regard as providing acceptable evidence for or against a particular hypothesis.

There are two problems for the user of statistical procedures. The first is the choice of an appropriate test for the situation in hand, and the second is the interpretation of the results of the test. The tests dealt with in previous pages are among the simplest and most commonly used in biology, and it is hoped that the explanations given are sufficient to provide the reader with some insight into a few relevant fundamentals of statistics. There are, however, many more tests in use, the application and interpretation of which may be difficult for anyone other than a professional statistician. This should not deter the biologist from using more sophisticated tests, since professional statisticians can easily be consulted when all but the simplest of procedures are being contemplated.

Finally, it may encourage the critical faculties of the reader to ponder on the following. Every year in the research literature thousands of results significant at the 5% level are quoted and taken as evidence of real differences. Five out of every hundred of these are suggesting a difference where no real biological difference exists. Which results are the misleading ones?

Biochemistry and its relevance to dental science

Biochemistry is the science which studies the chemistry of the components that constitute living matter. It is about their nature, composition and structure and the myriad changes that are wrought upon them by the process of life — how they are assimilated, broken down, changed and transmuted to the vast complex of intermediates and derivatives essential for the correct functioning and biological activities of the organism concerned. It investigates, dissects and describes the intricate intermeshed complexities of metabolic pathways and cycles whereby energy is drawn from the environment to be stored and used to drive the activities of life. It examines the mechanisms and pathways whereby organisms, tissues, cells, synthesize the complex fabric of innumerable molecular components, both large and small, essential for the maintenance and perpetuation of the life form involved, and it determines how unwanted or dangerous products are disposed of. It describes how inheritable information is chemically coded and locked up in the cell nucleus and copied and passed on when cells divide, and the means whereby such genetic information is transmitted and expressed in the phenotype.

Life on this planet manifests itself in a bewildering complexity of ways. Hundreds of thousands of species abound in the bacterial, plant and animal kingdoms with an incredible range and diversity of form and function. Yet within this wide diverse complexity the underlying biochemistry shows a surprising similarity. Essentially the same 20 amino acids are found in the proteins of all life forms, and the same 2 purines and 3 pyrimidines are used to form their nucleic acids. The same select few energy-capture and transfer components (e.g. adenosine triphosphate, ATP) and hydrogen carrier molecules (e.g. nicotinamide adenine dinucleotide, NAD) occur in virtually all organisms: yeast cells will break down carbohydrates by steps essentially similar to those used in vertebrate muscle and liver tissue: the mechanism of inheritance is fundamentally similar in principle in bacteria, bees and bohemians. This fundamental unity in biochemistry is more than a coincidence, and points to and supports the concept of a single origin to earthly life from which all other forms have derived.

For the dental undergraduate or practitioner a study of these aspects of living matter and tissues may seem remote from the chairside activities of a practising dental surgeon. Nevertheless dentistry is a medico-biological subject and the practitioner throughout his professional life will be concerned with various aspects of the hard and soft tissues in health and disease. Heredity and environment will determine the growth and development of the form of an individual mouth and jaw. Possibly inheritable factors may predispose the gingival tissues of certain individuals to a greater degree of susceptibility to the various environmental and nutritional factors involved in the diseases of the gingiva. Dental caries is a bacterial disease which ravages two of the toughest tissues nature has produced, first bringing about the removal and dissolution of the tooth's mineral component which has added hardness and strength to the already intrinsically tough structural proteins of enamel and dentine: these proteins in turn are ultimately destroyed. In effect the disease dismantles the carefully engineered product of a series of complex biochemical pathways, evolved and designed to function as the first stage in food ingestion. Both periodontal diseases and dental caries result from the activities of oral microorganisms, and are a consequence of their utilization of dietary components in their own metabolism to form products injurious to the tooth and gingival tissues. The nature of the tissues attacked—their composition and metabolism—and the specific activities of the disease-producing microorganisms involved is the business of the dental surgeon. So also is a knowledge of saliva functions and components and the role they may play in the protection of the dental tissues and their maintenance in a healthy condition: the saliva also plays prominent roles in taste, digestion, swallowing and the cleansing of tooth surfaces. Biochemical modifications to salivary proteins are involved in more than one theory of dental plaque formation, not to mention the role the physico-chemical properties of saliva may play in denture retention. Also important is a knowledge of nutrition and how dietary factors and deficiencies may contribute to, or manifest themselves in, the oral environment.

We do not know enough yet of the details of the biological factors involved in the maintenance of the dental tissues and their supporting structure in the healthy state, nor have we a very complete picture of the biochemical mechanisms involved in their diseases or of the various means that can or may be employed to minimize the ravages of dental caries and periodontal disease. Several questions remain unanswered, or partially so, on both fundamentals and details. What is the actual mechanism of action of fluoride ion in limiting dental caries? Is the role of the saliva in forming proteinaceous films on the enamel a protective one or alternatively the first stage of the development of plaque? Are the main causative agents in caries exclusively a group of streptococcal species with specific biochemical, metabolic and synthetic properties and can we then immunize human beings against the disease? If so what might be the consequences in ecological terms to the oral environment of such an immunization procedure? From a knowledge of the physics and chemistry of the surface of the enamel or enamel mineral crystals can we design a biological adhesive which will adhere to and provide a protective covering for the tooth surface against adverse oral agencies? Would such a chemical barrier, sealing off the tooth from the oral environment, create problems in relation to the physiology of the tooth itself?

Today's—and tomorrow's—dental surgeon will need to assess and evaluate new knowledge, new interpretations and new theories in such subject areas vital to his professional interests. He cannot achieve this without an adequate grounding in the fundamental principles and facts relevant to these topics. Thus he will require to know the nature of protein structure and metabolism with particular reference to the calcified and soft connective tissues and the salivary secretions. He will need to understand the nature of mineralization mechanisms and the physico-chemical properties of the mineral component of

bones and teeth and the physiology and biochemistry of the calcified tissues in general. A knowledge of the structure of carbohydrate polymers and intermediary sugar metabolism is essential to an appreciation of plaque biochemistry and methods of caries control. In this context he will also need to know how enzymes work and the essentials of immunochemistry. When teeth are extracted the wounded tissues bleed. The student should know how clots form and the nature of the inheritable biochemical deficiencies which may affect some individuals in this and other contexts. Dental diseases, extractions and tooth conservation procedures all involve pain and some knowledge of the physiology or neurochemistry involved is needed in an understanding of tooth sensation and the action of local anaesthetics.

These and other topics are directly related to dental matters and problems and it is the intention in this text to stress and indicate their dental relevance. These considerations apart the study of the subject involves, with the other medical sciences, an insight into the complexities of the fascinating means whereby life functions, maintains and reproduces itself whatever the form it may take. Man's understanding of these activities grows apace each year and with due diligence and application the sympathetic student, undergraduate and postgraduate, should find himself caught up with the fascination and excitement of discovery as the frontiers of biological science advance.

FURTHER READING

At the end of appropriate sections, short lists of Further Reading recommendations are provided. Some of these are short booklets amplifying a particular topic, others are more comprehensive texts for consultation by those further interested or requiring more specialized information and background.

Listed immediately below is a selection of general biochemistry text books, both introductory and advanced. Each has been chosen and recommended as providing lucid and interesting reading to complement or amplify the text. Several, for example Stryer's book and the *Scientific American* publications, benefit from some really excellent illustrations in addition to a stimulating prose style. The two Penguin books are recommended for pre-2nd BDS course reading and as a basis for previewing chosen areas of study.

General textbooks

INTRODUCTION TO BIOCHEMISTRY

CLOWES R. (1967) *The structure of life.* Penguin Books, Harmondsworth.

EDWARDS N. A. & HASSALL K. A. (1980) *Biochemistry and physiology of the cell.* (2nd Edition). McGraw Hill, New York.

LOEWY A.G. & SIEKEVITZ P. (1970) *Cell structure and function* (2nd Edition). Holt, Rinehart & Winston (Open University text), Eastbourne, Sussex.

ROSE S. (1979) *The chemistry of life* (2nd Edition). Penguin Books, Harmondsworth.

Readings from *Scientific American.* 1. *The living cell,* J. Brachet (1961) (only available as an offprint) 2. *Organic chemistry of life*, Calvin Prior (1973) 3. *The chemical basis of life*, H. Hanawait (1973) W. H. Freeman & Co., San Francisco.

MORE ADVANCED TEXTS

BOHINSKI R. C. (1976) *Modern concepts in biochemistry* (2nd Edition). Allyn & Bacon, Boston, Mass.

LEHNINGER A. L. (1975) *Biochemistry: the molecular basis of cell structure and function* (2nd Edition). Worth, New York.

MCGILVERY R. W. (1979) *Biochemistry: a functional approach* (2nd Edition). W. B. Saunders, Eastbourne, Sussex.

METZLER D. E. (1977) *Biochemistry: the chemical reactions of living cells.* Academic Press, New York.

ORTEN J. H. & NEUHAUS O. W. (1975) *Human biochemistry* (9th Edition). C. V. Mosby, St Louis.

STRYER L. (1981) *Biochemistry* (2nd Edition). W. H. Freeman & Co., San Francisco.

WHITE A., HANDLER P., SMITH E. L., HILL R. L. & LEHMAN I. R. (1978) *Principles of biochemistry* (6th Edition). McGraw Hill, New York.

CHAPTER 3

The Biopolymers

The range of biochemistry embraces the function and biological roles of chemical entities as small as the hydrogen ion (H^+) the molecules of oxygen (O_2), nitrogen (N_2) and carbon dioxide (CO_2), and anions and cations such as chloride (Cl^-) and carbonate (CO_3^{2-}) and sodium (Na^+), potassium (K^+), magnesium (Mg^{2+}) and calcium (Ca^{2+}). At the other extreme are giant protein and carbohydrate molecules with molecular weights which can run into millions. These large molecules are termed macromolecules by virtue of their size and this description is generally applied to molecules with molecular weights of from a few thousand (10^3) upwards to a thousand million (10^9). The term is generally applicable to all such giant molecules and includes such man-made products as nylon and polythene.

The biological macromolecules are the proteins, the carbohydrate polysaccharides, and the nucleic acids. The molecular weights of individual lipids, in the range 750–2500, are by comparison low but as they can spontaneously associate into high molecular weight aggregates they may be included, somewhat arbitrarily, in the category of macromolecules.

These large biological molecules are made up of units linked in chains, formed by joining the units together through elimination of a molecule of water between each pair–a condensation reaction. As such they are polymers made up from what have been termed *building block* molecular units whose molecular weights are in the region of 100–350. Proteins are made from amino acid building blocks, the nucleic acids from mononucleotides, and the polysaccharides are formed by polymerization of monosaccharides. Many of the lipids consist of long-chain fatty acid units condensed with glycerol, or glycerol derivatives.

The biological macromolecules are therefore biopolymers, a term virtually synonymous with biomacromolecules, the latter term describing the physical nature of the giant molecules or molecular aggregations involved (Table 3.1).

The macromolecular biopolymers and their building block monomer molecule constituents are two levels in the ordered hierarchy of the *biomolecules*—the chemical compounds which have been selected by evolution as the best designed and fitted for their respective functions in life processes (Fig. 3.1).

The plant kingdom, utilizing the sun's energy, takes the primordial precursors and, along with a handful of trace elements, builds them up via intermediates to the building blocks from which the complex array and organization of the cell macromolecules and organelles are formed. The other life forms (animal, bacterial, fungal, viral) are ultimately dependent on these photosynthetically produced stores of chemical energy, both to draw upon for their own energy requirements and to provide the carbon skeletons and frameworks from which they can synthesize their own specific molecules.

The primordial CO_2, N_2 and H_2O are converted through various metabolic intermediary forms to the building block molecules, from which the next hierarchy of complexity, the biomacromolecules, are formed. These are then further organized into supramolecular assemblies such as the cell ribosomes and enzyme complexes. At an even higher complexity of organization are the cell organelles, the mitochondria, nuclei, lysosomes, and the chloroplasts of plant cells. All these cell components are futher ordered and arrayed within the cell at specific locations.

Before exploring the intricate networks of the metabolic processes that constitute life's various activities, and the structures and functions of the innumerable biomolecules involved, it is important to be aware of their relationships within the living cell structures. The microcosm of life is to be found in the cell (Fig. 3.2). In this figure are indicated key structural features of the cell components with a summary of the metabolic activities and biomacromolecules associated with them.

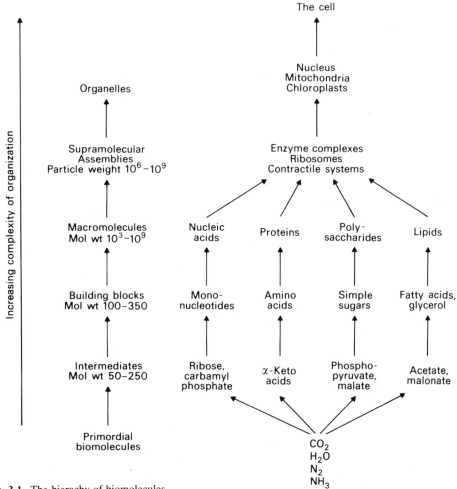

Fig. 3.1. The hierachy of biomolecules.

Table 3.1. The biopolymers and their building block units.

Building blocks (R)	Biopolymer (biomacromolecule)
Amino acids	Proteins
Simple sugars (monosaccharides)	Polysaccharides
Mononucleotides	Nucleic acids (polynucleotides)
Fatty acids, glycerol	Lipids

The monomer building block units (R) link together in chains by condensation reactions.

The specific functions of the different categories of biomacromolecules are the same whatever the form of life involved, whether microbial, animal or plant. The nucleic acids store and transmit genetic information to successive generations. The polysaccharides store energy in chemical form upon which virtually all life ultimately depends: in addition they can fulfil a structural role such as that of cellulose in plant cell walls. The lipids function primarily as important reserve fuel stores locked up as chemical energy and in addition are key components in the organization of biological membrane structures. The proteins play many roles in the biochemical arena: some act as chemical messen-

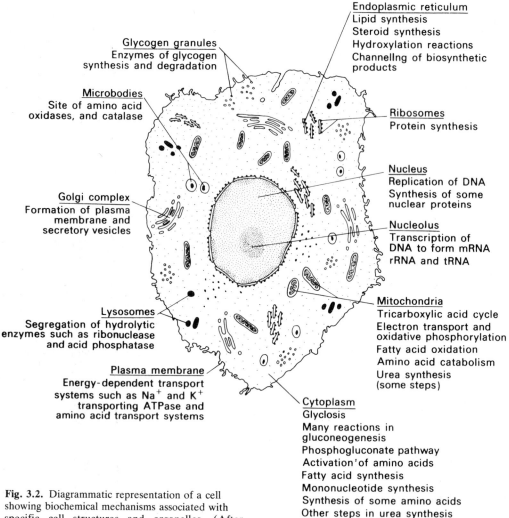

Fig. 3.2. Diagrammatic representation of a cell showing biochemical mechanisms associated with specific cell structures and organelles. (After Lehninger A.L. (1975) *Biochemistry*, 2nd edn. New York, Worth.)

gers (the hormones), others as oxygen carriers, and others are found in association with the nucleic acids of the genes, in chromosomes. Proteins function also in immunological defence mechanisms and in muscle contraction, but possibly their most prominent activities lie in their roles as biological catalysts (the enzymes), and as prime structural elements in the scaffolding and architecture of the cell and the body tissues.

The proteins, then, occupy a central position in the architecture and function of living matter, qualifying perhaps as the most versatile category of the biomolecules, and so form an appropriate point of entry to a study of biochemical principles in greater depth and detail.

THE PROTEINS

AMINO ACIDS: THE BUILDING BLOCKS OF PROTEINS

Before the wide range of protein activities can be examined it is necessary to know something of the composition, structure and properties of their constituent amino acids, the building blocks of proteins. The ordered sequence in which the amino acids are joined together in chains ultimately determines the actual three-dimensional shape and properties of a particular protein molecule.

Chemical structure of the amino acids

The amino acid molecules all contain the elements carbon, hydrogen, oxygen and nitrogen, and two of them contain sulphur. Some 20 are involved in protein structure and their molecular weights range from glycine, the simplest (mw 75) to tryptophan (mw 204). There are several other amino acids found in nature not involved in protein structure, but which play important roles in metabolism. Examples are the hormone thyroxine; ornithine, which is an intermediate in urea synthesis; and β-alanine, a component of pantothenic acid an important member of the vitamin B complex.

All amino acids are built upon the same structural plan:

$$
\begin{array}{c}
H \\
| \\
R - C - COOH \\
| \\
NH_2
\end{array}
$$

The business end of the molecule is the α-carbon atom (more correctly called the carbon-2 atom), to which is covalently bonded the basic amino (NH_2) group and the acidic carboxyl (COOH) group. Hence the term α-amino acid which, strictly speaking, should exclude *proline* and *hydroxyproline* as they are actually α-imino acids.

The amino NH_2 (and imino NH) groups and the acidic COOH group on the α-carbon atom of amino acids become linked to adjacent amino acids by the elimination of a molecule of H_2O to form a peptide link or bond. These peptide bonds constitute the backbone of the polypeptide chains which form the fundamental primary structural units of protein molecules.

Amino acid types

Variations in the chemical nature of the R group on the carbon atom account for the differences between the amino acids found in nature (Table 3.2). When R is a single H atom then the amino acid is *glycine*, the simplest amino acid possible.

$$
\begin{array}{c}
H \\
| \\
H - C - COOH \\
| \\
NH_2
\end{array}
$$

THE ALIPHATIC AMINO ACIDS

When the R groups consist of straight or branched saturated aliphatic hydrocarbon chains, the group of amino acids is classified as aliphatic (Table 3.2). Inspection of the formulae shows that *alanine* is derived from *glycine* by substituting a methyl (CH_3-) group for one of the H atoms on the α-carbon: similarly *valine* is characterized by the substitution of an iso-propyl ($\begin{array}{c}CH_3\\CH_3\end{array}>CH-$) group and *leucine* by the presence of an iso-butyryl group. Although chemically relatively inert, these non-polar aliphatic side arms play important roles in determining the three-dimensional structure of proteins due to their shape and size and their hydrophobic (water-hating) character (pp. 50, 985).

THE AROMATIC AMINO ACIDS

The aromatic amino acids *tryptophan*, *phenylalanine* and *tyrosine*, also have side-chains which are predominantly non-polar and hydrophobic. *Tyrosine* however does bear a reactive ionizable phenolic OH group. *Tryptophan* is classified as an aromatic amino acid because of the benzenoid ring in its indole structure.

THE HYDROXY AMINO ACIDS

The hydroxy amino acids *threonine* and *serine* carry an alcoholic (OH) group on their side-chains. These endow their molecules with physical and chemical properties important in their metabolism as free amino acids and also when incorporated into a protein structure.

THE ACIDIC AMINO ACIDS

In the acidic amino acids the side-chains bear terminal acidic carboxyl groups. These can give the molecules negatively charged polar sites, in addition to those on the carboxyl groups on the α-carbon atom, and are important in many aspects of protein structure and function. The two acidic amino acids, *aspartic* and *glutamic acid*, also occur in their amide forms, either in a free state or incorporated in proteins, when their $-CONH_2$ terminal side-arm groups are effectively non-ionized. These amide forms are termed respectively *asparagine* and *glutamine*.

THE BASIC AMINO ACIDS

In the basic amino acids the R side-chains have either amino groups attached, as in *lysine* and

Table 3.2. Structures and characteristics of the amino acids.

Side chain (R. Group) Characteristic	Chemical structure	Amino acid
Aliphatic, non Polar		Glycine
		Alanine
		Valine
		Leucine
		Isoleucine
Alcoholic, aliphatic and aromatic		Serine
		Threonine
Aromatic		Tyrosine
		Phenylalanine
		Tryptophan
Carboxylic (acidic)		Aspartic acid

Side chain (R. Group) Characteristic	Chemical structure	Amino acid
	$\overset{O}{\underset{HO}{\diagup}}C-CH_2-CH_2-\overset{H}{\underset{NH_2}{C}}-\overset{O}{\underset{OH}{C}}$	Glutamic acid
Amine bases (basic)	$NH_2-CH_2-CH_2-CH_2-CH_2-\overset{H}{\underset{NH_2}{C}}-\overset{O}{\underset{OH}{C}}$	Lysine
	$NH_2-CH_2-\underset{OH}{CH}-CH_2-CH_2-\overset{H}{\underset{NH_2}{C}}-\overset{O}{\underset{OH}{C}}$	Hydroxylysine
	$NH_2-\underset{NH}{C}-NH-CH_2-CH_2-CH_2-\overset{H}{\underset{NH_2}{C}}-\overset{O}{\underset{OH}{C}}$	Arginine
	$HC=C-CH_2-\overset{H}{\underset{NH_2}{C}}-\overset{O}{\underset{OH}{C}}$ $N\underset{C}{\diagdown}NH$ $\underset{H}{}$	Histidine
Sulphur containing	$HS-CH_2-\overset{H}{\underset{NH_2}{C}}-\overset{O}{\underset{OH}{C}}$	Cysteine
	$CH_3-S-CH_2-CH_2-\overset{H}{\underset{NH_2}{C}}-\overset{O}{\underset{OH}{C}}$	Methionine
Amides	$\overset{O}{\underset{NH_2}{\diagup}}C-CH_2-\overset{H}{\underset{NH_2}{C}}-\overset{O}{\underset{OH}{C}}$	Asparagine (AspNH$_2$)
	$\overset{O}{\underset{NH_2}{\diagup}}C-CH_2-CH_2-\overset{H}{\underset{NH_2}{C}}-\overset{O}{\underset{OH}{C}}$	Glutamine (GluNH$_2$)
Imino	$\underset{H_2C}{\overset{H_2C}{\diagdown}}\overset{H_2}{\underset{N}{C}}\underset{H}{\diagup}\overset{H}{\underset{}{C}}-\overset{O}{\underset{OH}{C}}$	Proline
	$\underset{H-C}{\overset{H_2C}{\diagdown}}\overset{H_2}{\underset{N}{C}}\underset{OH}{\diagup}\overset{H}{\underset{H}{C}}-\overset{O}{\underset{OH}{C}}$	Hydroxyproline

hydroxylysine, or a basic guanidyl group ($-NH-C\lessgtr^{NH_2}_{NH_{3+}}$), as in *arginine*. These give rise to additional positively charged sites in the molecule which when incorporated in proteins contribute to determining the spatial form of their molecules. *Histidine* is classified as a basic amino acid because of the proton acceptor nature of the $-NH-$ group, a part of the five-membered imidazole ring.

THE SULPHUR AMINO ACIDS

The sulphur containing amino acid *methionine* has a side-chain S atom in an ether-type linkage with a terminal methyl group (CH_3-), and is involved in important metabolic reactions involving the transfer of methyl groups. Rather different is the S-containing amino acid *cysteine* bearing on its side-arm a terminal $-SH$ group. Cysteine, either as a free amino acid or incorporated within a protein structure, is important because of this highly reactive $-SH$ group. A major role of cysteine in proteins is to link with other cysteine molecules by oxidation reaction to form important protein cross-linking structures, the disulphide bonds (p. 48). This dimeric form of cysteine is called *cystine*.

The presence of free SH groups in the cysteine molecules of certain enzymes is essential for their catalytic activity.

THE IMINO ACIDS

Proline and *hydroxyproline* are exceptional in amino acid structure because their nitrogen atom, covalently linked to their α-carbon atom, is locked up in a heterocyclic pyrrolidine ring as an imino group. These two imino 'amino' acids are of considerable importance in the connective tissue protein collagen, together constituting about 25% of its amino acid content. The regular repeat involvement of their pyrrolidine ring structures along the polypeptide backbone of collagen imposes on it a rigid and unique coiling structure (p. 66).

Only some 20 amino acids commonly occur in proteins, reflecting the highly specific nucleic acid coding arrangements which direct the incorporation of these amino acids during protein synthesis (p. 238). However, many more than these 20 amino acids exist in nature, most derived from one or other of these parent amino acids, and they usually occur free, often in special cells or tissues. Exceptions are hydroxy-

proline and hydroxylysine, found almost exclusively in the collagen group of proteins: these are not synthesized as separate entities but are initially built into protein polypeptide chains as proline and lysine and then subsequently converted to their hydroxy derivatives. Similarly, the dimeric cystine molecules develop post-ribosomally by oxidation reactions which form covalent disulphide bridges between two appropriately situated cysteine molecule residues in polypeptide chains.

THE AMINO ACID POOL

Amino acids are found free in the cell cytoplasm, in tissues, in tissue fluids, and in blood, where they constitute an 'amino acid pool' as the source for all reactions requiring their participation.

Physico-chemical properties of amino acids

OPTICAL ISOMERISM AND CONFIGURATION
(see Appendix)

With the exception of glycine, each amino acid α-carbon atom has its 4 valencies satisfied by 4 different groups or atoms. The glycine α-carbon atom bears two hydrogen atoms; one NH_2 and one COOH group in contrast to, for example, alanine with one CH_3 group, one NH_2, one COOH group and one hydrogen atom attached to the same α-carbon. This tetrahedral arrangement of the 4 carbon valencies dictates that there are two possible non-superimposable (mirror-image) arrangements in space of the 4 different substitutional groups or atoms for all amino acids with the exception of glycine.

Fig. 3.3 shows a diagrammatic representation of the two optical isomers of alanine referred to as enantiomers (p. 986). The differences in optical properties observed reflect the two different configurational arrangements of the constituent atoms. These different configurations are often represented by planar formulae termed Fischer projections (p. 112) (in which an asterisk is used to designate the asymmetric carbon atom).

$$N_2H - \overset{\overset{\textstyle COOH}{|}}{\underset{\underset{\textstyle CH_3}{|}}{C^*}} - H \qquad H - \overset{\overset{\textstyle HOOC}{|}}{\underset{\underset{\textstyle H_3C}{|}}{C}} - NH_2$$

One of these forms turns the plane of polarized light to the right (dextro-rotatory) whereas the mirror image (laevo-rotatory) form turns it an exactly equivalent amount to the left (p. 987). The dextro-rotatory amino acids are designated by the symbol (+), and the laevo-rotatory by (−). Of the naturally occurring amino acids in proteins some are (+), others (−): for example alanine, isoleucine, glutamic acid and lysine are dextro-rotatory (+), whereas leucine, phenylalanine, serine and proline are laevo-rotatory (−).

It is important to remember the difference between the property of optical isomerism and D and L *configuration*. The latter refers specifically to the particular spatial arrangement of the 4 groups around the asymmetric carbon atom (the stereochemistry) and not the direction of rotation of any associated optical properties. It is possible, and does happen, that the biomolecules of the L-configuration may be dextro-rotatory (+) in terms of optical properties (such a compound is alanine) and vice versa.

These optically active compounds are related stereochemically to a single compound, the 3-carbon sugar, glyceraldehyde.

Stereochemistry refers to the actual arrangement in space of the groups and atoms in their molecules. Alanine, with its central asymmetric (C*) atom, like glyceraldehyde has two possible non-superimposable, spatial arrangements of the 4 groups or atoms attached to it (Fig. 3.3).

The left-hand arrangement of glyceraldehyde is the stereoisomer with laevo-rotatory (−) optical properties and was by convention adopted as the L-configuration. Conversely the right-hand representation is dextro-rotatory (+) and is called the D-configuration. The naturally occurring glyceraldehyde has been shown to be of the D-configuration and is therefore designated D(+)-glyceraldehyde.

At the time the decision was first made to allocate this D-configuration (the formula below which places the OH group on the right of the asymmetric carbon) to the dextro-rotatory form, it was not known whether this was the correct absolute configuration, and the choice made was in fact an arbitrary one. Subsequent X-ray diffraction studies on the glyceraldehyde enantiomers showed the choice to have been the correct one–a lucky guess even if the odds were as low as 1:1! (Unlike the early days of electricity when it was uncertain whether it flowed from positive to negative or in the opposite direction

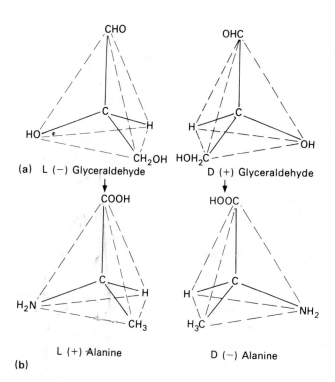

(a) L (−) Glyceraldehyde
D (+) Glyceraldehyde

(b) L (+) Alanine
D (−) Alanine

Fig. 3.3. The configurational relationship between glyceraldehyde and alanine: (a) glyceraldehyde enantiomers, (b) alanine enantiomers.

and the arbitrary choice then was for the former—which turned out to be wrong. You can't win them all!)

When the two diagrammatic representations of alanine are compared with glyceraldehyde (Fig. 3.3), it can be seen that theoretically the former could be derived from the latter by

1　Oxidizing the −CHO aldehyde group to an acidic −COOH.

2　Substituting the −OH group for an −NH₂ group.

3　Reducing the CH₂OH group to a CH₃ group.

Such theoretical conversions can and have been confirmed in practice, and are applicable to all stereoisomers. Stereoisomers structurally related in this way to L-glyceraldehyde are said to be of the L-configuration and those related to D-glyceraldehyde are of the D-configuration—this is irrespective of any dextro- or laevo-rotatory optical properties they may possess.

All the naturally occurring amino acids in proteins belong to the L-configuration. The alanine in proteins is L(+)-alanine indicating that it is of the L-configuration series with respect to L-glyceraldehyde but with dextro-rotatory optical properties. Conversely, naturally occurring L(−)-proline, also belonging to the L-configuration series, is laevo-rotatory. D-configuration amino acids do occur rarely in nature, as in the cell walls of certain micro-organisms and in some antibiotics, such as gramicidin. In contrast to the naturally-occurring L-configuration amino acids, nearly all naturally-occurring carbohydrate molecules belong to the D-configuration (p. 113). Some-where in the early stages of biomolecule evolution some selective advantage may have favoured the D-configurational series for the carbohydrates and the L-form for the amino acid proteins. However it may have been just a chance selection in either instance.

Diastereoisomers (also p. 986)

Some amino acids, such as threonine, isoleucine, hydroxyproline and hydroxylysine possess two asymmetric carbon atoms and as a result can exist as four stereoisomers:

D-Threonine　　　　L-Threonine

D-Allothreonine　　　L-Allothreonine

The allothreonine forms are diastereoisomers. By convention the groups attached to the α–C atoms are used to classify them as belonging to either D or L-configurations. Only the ordinary L-threonine isomer occurs in nature.

AMINO ACIDS AS ACIDS AND BASES

So far, the amino acids have been represented by strictly organic molecular formulae, with the amino groups as NH₂ and the carboxyl as COOH. In living cells and tissues however the free amino acids are dissolved in an aqueous environment and the functional groups exist as ionizable forms. The acidic carboxyl group dissociates into a hydrogen ion (H^+) and a negatively charged carboxylate ion (COO^-), and the basic amino group acquires an H^+ ion to become a positively charged $-NH_3^+$ group.

Before examining these ionic forms of amino acids in detail, and the important consequences of the properties they impart to the amino acid molecules, it is necessary first to recall in general terms the concepts of ionic dissociation, acids, bases and pH. It is essential that Appendix 1 (pp. 996–999) be studied or revised before proceeding further.

The Bronsted concept of acids and bases as proton donors and acceptors respectively, the logarithmic functions pH and pK as measures of hydrogen ion concentration and ionic dissociation, and the related Henderson–Hasselbalch equation are all important to an understanding of the behaviour of the amino acids as electrolytes and buffers. These properties are essential for our consideration not only of the behaviour of the amino acids themselves but also of the proteins. Various separation and analytical techniques involved in determining the amino acid composition and their arrangement in protein molecules are dependent on the behaviour of the amino acids as electrolytes.

As indicated above the state of amino acids in aqueous solutions is more accurately represented by the following form:

$$R—\overset{\overset{\displaystyle H}{|}}{\underset{\underset{\displaystyle NH_3^+}{|}}{C}}—COO^-$$

or more conveniently as $NH_3^+ - CH(R)COO^-$. Thus they are capable of functioning both as acids and bases since each contains at least one carboxyl group (a proton donor) and one amino group (a proton acceptor). Such substances, whose molecules possess both proton donor (acid) and proton acceptor (base) sites are called ampholytes (or sometimes amphoteric compounds).

In some ways it is useful to think of amino acids as fully ionized, internally neutralized salts, with protons from the carboxyl groups (COOH) having directly transferred to the amino groups (NH₂) until the negative charges ($-COO^-$) exactly balance the number of positive charges ($-NH_3^+$). Their properties of easy solubility in water, high melting points, and high dielectric constants, all conform to such a salt-like character. When ampholytes such as amino acids are dissolved in water, they exist in their ionic, electrically neutral, dipolar forms, and are called zwitterions (from the German zwitter meaning hybrid or bastard, although their formation would seem to be more incestuous than illegitimate).

Let us now examine in more detail the amphoteric properties of a simple mono-amino, mono-carboxylic acid with a non-polar aliphatic side-chain, such as alanine (where $R = CH_3$)

$$^+H_3N–CH(CH_3)–COO^-$$

When dissolved in pure water the zwitterionic alanine molecule is electrically neutral, the positive charge on the $-NH_3^+$ group exactly counter-balancing the negative charge on the $-COO^-$ group. In this condition the molecule is said to be in its iso-electric state for, bearing neither excess positive or negative charge, it will not migrate in solution to either cathode or anode when subjected to the influence of an electric field. The pH of the solution at which a dipolar ion, such as alanine, does not migrate in either direction because there is no net charge, is called its *iso-electric point* (or *iso-electric pH*), designated by the symbol pI (for alanine the pI is 6.02 and most of the non-polar amino acids have iso-electric points around pH 6, as the pI column in Table 3.3 shows.

Next consider the effect of the addition of some H^+ ions from an acid solution, such as HCl, upon the alanine molecules in their iso-electric state. The higher H^+ concentration suppresses the ionization of the carboxyl groups by a mass action effect:

$$^+H_3N–CH(CH_3)–COO^- + H^+ \rightleftharpoons$$
$$^+H_3N–CH(CH_3)–COOH$$

Table 3.3. Dissociation constant (pKa) and isoelectric point (pI) values for amino acids.

Amino acid	Residue code	pKa¹ (COOH)	pKa²	pKa³	pI
Alanine	Ala	2.34	9.69	—	6.02
Arginine	Arg	2.12	9.04 (NH₃⁺)	12.48 (guanidinium)	10.76
Asparagine	Asn	2.02	8.80	—	5.41
Aspartic acid	Asp	1.88	3.65 (COOH)	9.60 (NH₃⁺)	2.77
Cysteine (30°)	Cys	1.96	8.18 (SH)	10.28 (NH₃⁺)	5.07
Cystine (30°)	CyS	<1.0	1.7 (COOH)	7.48 and 9.02 (NH₃⁺)	4.60
Glutamic acid	Glu	2.19	4.25 (COOH)	9.67 (NH₃⁺)	3.22
Glutamine	Gln	2.17	9.13	—	5.65
Glycine	Gly	2.34	9.60	—	5.97
Histidine	His	1.82	6.00 (imidazole)	9.17 (NH₃⁺)	7.59
Hydroxyproline	Hyp	1.92	9.73	—	5.83
Isoleucine	Ile	2.36	9.68	—	6.02
Leucine	Leu	2.36	9.60	—	5.98
Lysine	Lys	2.18	8.95 (α-NH₃⁺)	10.53 (ε-NH₃⁺)	9.74
Methionine	Met	2.28	9.21	—	5.74
Phenylalanine	Phe	1.83	9.13	—	5.48
Proline	Pro	1.99	10.60	—	6.30
Serine	Ser	2.21	9.15	—	5.68
Tryptophan	Trp	2.38	9.39	—	5.89
Tyrosine	Tyr	2.20	9.11 (NH₃⁺)	10.07 (OH)	5.66
Valine	Val	2.32	9.62	—	5.96

The negatively charged carboxylate ions (–COO⁻) of the alanine combine with the H⁺ ions, losing their charge to form the unionized carboxyl groups (–COOH). The amino acid molecule is here acting as a base by virtue of its carboxylate ion accepting the proton H⁺. An important consequence of this neutralization of the –COO⁻ is that the molecules acquire an increasing net positive charge and become cations because the positively charged –NH₃⁺ groups remain unchanged. As a result the molecules will now move in the direction of the cathode if an electric current is passed through the solution.

Conversely as alkali is added to the iso-electric zwitterion solution the amino acid molecules will have their positively charged –NH₃⁺ groups discharged.

$$OH^- + H_3^+N-CH(CH_3)-COO^- \rightleftharpoons$$
$$H_2N-CH(CH_3)-COO^- + H-OH$$

The NH₃⁺ group acts as an acid, donating an H⁺ to the OH⁻ to form water. The overall effect is to give the amino acid molecules a net negative charge, causing them to become anions which will move towards the anode when a current is passed. The effects of these changes in pH on the charge on the molecules is the basis of various techniques for their separation to be discussed later.

Thus an amino acid will act as either base or acid, according to the environmental conditions. Note that the positively charged amino group (as NH₃⁺) is potentially active as an acid, in Bronsted–Lowry sense, because it is a potential proton (H⁺) donor. Conversely the negatively charged carboxylate ion (–COO⁻) is a base, by virtue of its ability to accept a proton. In illustration of these properties consideration is given to the effect of adding alkali stepwise to alanine over the pH range 1–13.

A molar alanine solution is adjusted to pH 1 by making it approximately 0.1 M with a strong acid such as HCl. At this pH all the alanine molecules are in a positively charged cationic form, because the carboxylate ions (–COO⁻) have accepted H⁺ ions to form undissociated carboxyl groups, (–COOH), i.e.

$$H_3^+N-CH(CH_3)-COOH$$

Measured amounts of alkali are added stepwise and each corresponding pH value determined and plotted against the equivalents of alkali added. From the data a pH-titration curve of alanine is constructed (Fig. 3.4). The particular ionic species present at key points are indicated on this graph. It is important that the significance of the double sigmoid nature of this titration curve be understood. From pH 1–6 the carboxyl group ($pKa^1 = 2.34$) of alanine is being titrated. The pH rises steeply at first for small additions of alkali but above pH 1.5 the curve flattens out as the –COOH are increasingly

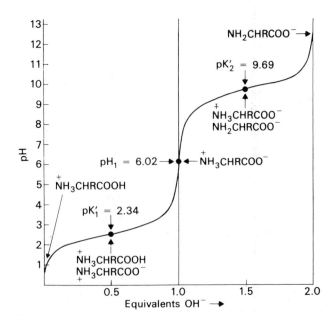

Fig. 3.4. Titration curve of alanine. The predominant ionic species at key points on the titration is indicated by arrows. (After Lehninger A.L. (1975) *Biochemistry*, 2nd edn. New York, Worth.)

titrated to –COO⁻ by addition of the alkali.

The midpoint of this dissociation range of the alanine carboxyl group is at the pH numerically equal to its pKa^1 value, when equimolar quantities of the ionized and unionized forms present.

This follows from the Henderson–Hasselbalch equation (p. 999) of which the pH-titration curves are a graphical form. This equation states that:

$$pH = pKa^1 + \log_{10} \frac{[proton\ acceptor]}{[proton\ donor]}$$

or

$$pH = pKa^1 + \log_{10} \frac{[ionized\ acid]}{[unionized\ acid]}$$

For the carboxyl group in alanine this becomes

$$pH = 2.34 + \log_{10} \frac{[H^+_3N\ CH(CH_3)\ COO^-]}{[H^+_3N\ CH(CH_3)\ COOH]}$$

When the carboxyl groups and carboxylate ions are present in equal amounts the logarithimic ratio on the right hand side of the equation becomes $\log_{10} \frac{[1]}{[1]}$ and since $\log_{10} 1 = 0$ then the $pH = pKa^1 = 2.34$

In other words the pKa for any acid can be defined as the pH at which the dissociated and undissociated molecules are present in equal amounts. Put another way this means that if a solution of a weakly dissociable acid contains equimolar parts of its dissociated and undissociated molecules then the pH of the solution will have the same numerical value as the pKa of the acid.

AMINO ACIDS AS BUFFERS

The above considerations apply not only to amino acid titration curves but are characteristic of all weak acid dissociations and as such provide the theoretical basis for all buffer action (p. 748). It follows that the amino acids can function as buffers and so tend to resist changes in pH when acid or alkali is added in the appropriate ranges governed by the dissociation of their ionizable groups. For example a solution of 0.01 M HCl has a pH of 2 and the addition to this of 0.01 moles of strong base will bring the pH to 7, a shift of 5 pH units. Therefore, in a 0.1 M solution of alanine with equimolar concentrations of ionized and unionized carboxyl groups:

$$pH = 2.34 + \log_{10} \frac{[0.1]}{[0.1]}$$

$$= 2.34 + 0$$

On addition of 0.01 mole of strong base an additional 0.01 moles of carboxylate ion will be formed by ionization of 0.01 moles of unionized carboxyl group. The pH of the solution will therefore be:

$$pH = 2.34 + \log_{10} \frac{[0.11]}{[0.09]}$$

$$= 2.34 + \log_{10} 1.02$$
$$= 2.34 + 0.09$$

This upward shift of only 0.09 pH units contrasts strongly with the shift of 5 pH units which would have occurred if the alanine had not been present. Similar calculations show that the addition of 0.01 M of strong acid will only reduce the pH of the buffer system by 0.09 units to 2.25. For all buffer systems the maximum buffering effect is at the mid point of its titration curve when the pH is equal to its pKa value. The buffering range is most effective up to 1 pH unit on either side of this pKa value.

Returning to the pH-titration curve for alanine (Fig. 3.4) its carboxylate group is an effective buffer over the range pH 2.34 ± 1.0 but at pH 6.02, when 1 equivalent of alkali has been used up, all the carboxyl groups will have been ionized (to –COO⁻) and all the amino acid molecules will then be in their zwitterionic isoelectric state, i.e.

$$^+H_3N–CH(CH_3)–COO^-$$

At this point further small additions of alkali produce sharp increases in pH until the buffering range of the α-amino group in the molecule is reached. With the addition of alkali continued from pH 6 upwards the second proton donor/acceptor group in the alanine molecule, the NH_3^+, is titrated until the molecule exists entirely in its anionic form:

$$H_2N—CH(CH_3)—COO^-$$

As with the carboxyl group/carboxylate ion leg of this biphasic titration curve of alanine, so the $-NH_3^+/-NH_2$ side also has a mid point (at pH 9.69), corresponding to the pKa value for the dissociation of the basic amino group. At this point there are equimolar amounts of the ionized ($-NH_3^+$) and undissociated ($-NH_2$) forms and, therefore, alanine solutions can effectively buffer in the range pH 9.69 ± 1.0 as well as pH 2.34 ± 1.0.

Thus the complete pH-titration curve of

alanine over the pH range 1–13 contains titration curves of two proton donor/acceptor sites—the carboxyl group and the amino group. At the point of inflection between these two separate titration curves the alanine molecules will be at their iso-electric point (pI 6.02). This is calculable as the mean of the pKa values of the carboxyl and amino groups respectively.

i.e. $pI = \frac{1}{2}(pKa^1 + pKa^2)$
$= \frac{1}{2}(2.34 + 9.69)$
$= \frac{1}{2}(12.03)$
$= 6.02$

The above considerations are equally applicable in principle to all amino acids.

All the mono-amino, mono-carboxylic amino acids with uncharged R groups have similar pKa^1 values and pKa^2 values (Table 3.3). With pKa^1 values around 2.3 and pKa^2 values of 9.6, and buffering ranges up to ± 1.0 pH units on each side, these amino acids can clearly have no significant buffering role to offer at physiological pH ranges.

The pH-titration curves for amino acids with polar groups on their R side-chains are more complex as the curves for the different titration groups overlap. pK of R group is designated pK_R

The complete titration curves for glutamic acid (with an additional −COOH at the end of its R group), lysine (with an additional −NH₂) and histidine (with a basic imidazole side-chain) are shown in Fig. 3.5. The imidazole −NH group has a pKa^2 of 6 which means that histidine alone of the amino acids can buffer within the physiological pH range.

For amino acids with more than two ionizable centres, the pI is calculated as the mean of the two pKa values on one side of the iso-electric zwitterion state. Thus the pI for glutamic acid is (2.19 + 4.25)/2 = 3.22 and for lysine it is (8.95 + 10.53)/2 = 9.74 (Table 3.3).

The principles of dissociation and buffer action discussed above are the same whether concerned with the buffering properties of serum, or urine, the regulation and disturbances of acid-base balances in the body, or the buffering capacity of saliva (which is statistically related to caries experience).

Some chemical reactions of amino acids

Organic chemistry text books list numerous reactions involving the chemistry of the amino, carboxyl and side-chain groupings of amino acids. It suffices here to describe briefly only

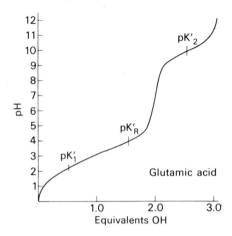

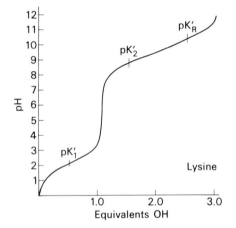

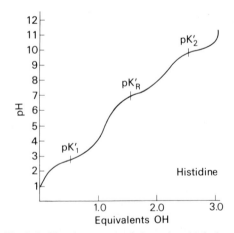

Fig. 3.5. Titration curves of glutamic acid, lysine, histidine. (After Lehninger A.L. (1975) *Biochemistry*, 2nd edn. New York, Worth.)

those relevant to the identification of amino acids in the laboratory and to studies of protein structure.

THE NINHYDRIN REACTION

Ninhydrin (indanetrione hydrate) reacts with the amino groups of all amino acids to give a characteristic blue–violet colour, and with the imino acids proline and hydroxyproline with which it yields yellow products. Ninhydrin reacts similarly with ammonia, amines, peptides and proteins and is widely used as an agent for both locating and quantitatively estimating amino acids in colorimetric, chromatographic and electrophoretic separation procedures.

THE FLUORODINITROBENZENE (FDNB) REACTION

This yellow reagent (1, fluoro-2, 4-dinitrobenzene) reacts with the amino and imino groups of amino acids and has been of particular value in studies of protein structure, where it is used to label and so identify, the amino acid at the end of the polypeptide chain which bears the free amino group. The reaction covalently links a yellow 2, 4-dinitrophenyl grouping (DNP) to the terminal $\alpha -NH_2$ group. Subsequent acid hydrolysis of the polypeptide breaks it down to its constituent amino acids but with the terminal amino acid still labelled as a DNP derivative. Its yellow colour usually assists in its chromatographic identification (p. 43).

This technique was first used with remarkable success by Sanger in elucidating the complete structure of insulin (p. 52), the first protein to be so characterized.

A more recent development is the use of the reagent *dansyl chloride*, which reacts similarly with amino groups, but the fluorescent property of the dansyl group increases the sensitivity of the chromatographic detection and quantitation by 100-fold.

THE EDMAN REACTION (Fig. 3.6)

This too has been a major tool in studies of protein structure. Phenylisothiocyanate (Edman's reagent) couples with the free amino group present at one end of a polypeptide chain to give the phenylthiocarbamoyl (PTC) derivative. Under acid conditions this is cleaved from the terminal amino acid, forming a ring structure derivative, a phenylhydantoin (PTH) amino acid.

Each amino acid forms a unique PTH derivative (because of its characteristic R group) which can be identified usually by chromatographic methods. The Edman reaction has the additional and distinct advantage that the process can be repeated many times over on the same protein chain, nipping off each amino acid one by one as its specific PTH derivative, each of which is then

The FNDB reaction.

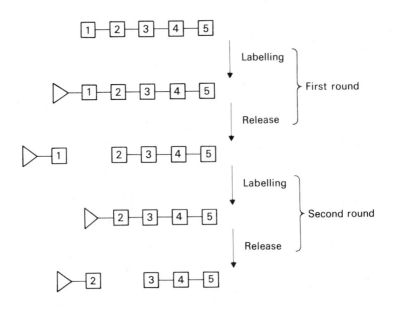

Fig. 3.6. The Edman degradation. The labelled amino-acid residue (PTH-alanine in the first round) is removed without hydrolyzing the rest of the peptide. The N-terminal residue of the shortened peptide (Gly-Asp-Phe-Arg-Gly) is determined in the second round. Three more rounds of the Edman degradation reveal the complete sequence of the original peptide. (After Stryer L. (1981) *Biochemistry*, 2nd edn. San Francisco, W. H. Freeman.)

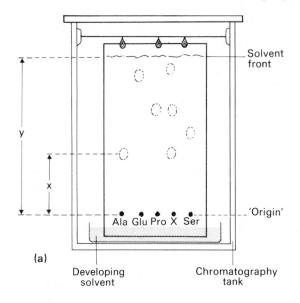

(a)

Developing solvent

Chromatography tank

Solvent front

'Origin'

Ala Glu Pro X Ser

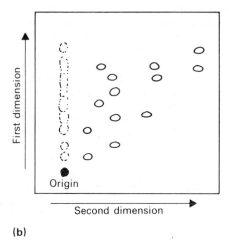

First dimension

Second dimension

Origin

(b)

Fig. 3.7. (a) Single dimensional chromatogram (ascending method): The 'unknown' mixture of amino acids (X) is placed on the origin line as indicated, with known 'marker' amino acids Ala, Glu, Pro and Ser as adjacent spots on the same line. The paper is dipped into the developing solvent tray and hung vertically from a suitable support in the chromatography tank, which is closed with an airtight lid. After the solvent has soaked up to a point near the top (the solvent front) the different amino acids will have travelled different distances (their positions indicated by the dotted circles). Removal of the sheet, evaporation of the solvent, and reaction with ninhydrin reveals their exact position. This particular example shows that the mixture X contains the 3 amino acids Ala, Glu, Pro (but not Ser). The Rf. value of Ala is x/y. (b) two dimensional chromatogram. The complex mixture (e.g. protein hydrolysate, urine sample) is applied near one corner of a square or rectangular sheet of chromatography paper, and developed in one direction by one solvent system as for single dimension chromatography (the partial separation of the components is indicated by the dotted perimeters). The paper is taken out of the tank, the solvent removed and the process repeated with a different solvent in a direction at 90° to that of the first separation. This results in development of a 2D 'map' of the amino acids, revealed by ninhydrin treatment following removal of the second solvent. Most, if not all, of the 18–20 amino acids in a protein hydrolysate may be separated by this means.

identified. In this manner it is possible to determine the sequence of amino acids along a protein polypeptide chain in a stepwise manner. Automated apparatus can now carry out 40 or more stepwise Edman degradations in 24 hours.

Separation techniques for amino acids

Determination of the types and amounts of the component amino acids present is essential to an understanding of the properties of proteins and polypeptides and is a necessary prerequisite to further considerations of their structure.

Proteins are routinely hydrolysed to their constituent amino acids with 6N HCl under nitrogen, in sealed tubes for 18–24 hours at 110°C.

Estimations of the free amino acid levels in body fluids such as blood, urine and cerebrospinal fluid are important in various aspects of clinical biochemistry. The main techniques used for the separation and estimation of amino acids are as follows.

CHROMATOGRAPHIC METHODS

Paper chromatography (Fig. 3.7)

More correctly termed filter paper partition chromatography (FPPC), this technique has proved invaluable in the separation and identification of amino acids. The method is based on the partition coefficient a particular substance possesses in relation to a given immiscible or partially miscible two-phase liquid solvent system. One of these liquids is almost invariably water, and termed the *stationary phase* because it is held tightly in the microinterstices of the paper sheet support medium. The organic solvent which flows through the support medium via capillary action is called the *mobile phase*, carrying with it, at different rates, the various biomolecules being separated. The technique can be either ascending or descending and is carried out in an air-tight glass tank.

Complete separation of all 20 amino acids in a protein hydrolysate is not usually obtainable with a solvent run in only one direction, but can be achieved where the amino acid mixture is initially applied near one corner of a square sheet of chromatography paper, first developed in one direction with a one solvent system. The solvent is then removed by drying off, the paper turned through 90° and developed again with a second different solvent system.

After removal of solvents the chromatograms are sprayed with a ninhydrin solution and briefly heated in an oven to 'develop' the colour reaction amino acids give with ninhydrin (p. 41). Each separated amino acid then shows up on the paper as a discrete coloured spot (Fig. 3.7). The ratio of the distance travelled from the origin by a particular substance in FPPC to the distance travelled by the solvent is called its Rf value

$$Rf = \frac{\text{distance of substance from origin}}{\text{distance of solvent front from origin}}$$

The paper chromatogram technique is applied in the separation of many other biochemical compounds (carbohydrates, lipids, nucleotides, etc.), employing a wide range of different solvent systems. Although essentially a qualitative method, an approximate quantitative estimation of components is often possible.

Thin layer chromatography (TLC)

Like FPPC the TLC technique involves separation in one plane, using a single or two dimensional method. In TLC the support medium can be a variety of inert components–celluose, aluminium oxide, silica gel, etc., which are spread as an even slurry on a glass plate and baked hard on to this backing. (Plastic-backed TLC plates are also made.) Essentially the same principles of sample application, separation and location of component positions apply. The separations are considerably faster, and the spots much smaller, so aiding resolution. The scope of the separations obtainable is wider due to the much greater choice of support media and the related developing solvent systems available.

Ion-exchange chromatography

A most useful technique for both separation and exact quantitation of amino acids is column ion-exchange chromatography, where the support medium is not inert (as in FPPC and TLC) but a synthetic resin, bearing exchangeable anions or cations. For amino acid separation the ion-exchange resins most used are cationic sulphonated ($-SO_3H$) polystyrene resins, and running these columns through with a succession of buffers of increasing pH and strength can separate all the amino acids on a single column, one by one. The separated amino acids are collected as they elute individually from the column and assayed quantitatively by the colorimetric ninhydrin reaction. Various automated instruments are available and complete analyses of a few micrograms of protein hydrolysate can be achieved within an hour (Fig. 3.8). (This includes automatic calculation and print out!)

ELECTROPHORETIC METHODS

High voltage electrophoresis (HVE) (Fig. 3.9)

Electrophoretic separation techniques utilize the net charge distribution on amino acids molecules in relation to the pH of the system. At pH 6 acidic amino acids such as glutamic and aspartic acid will bear net negative charges, because their pI values are around pH 3 (see p. 40), and will move to the anode: conversely the basic lysine (pI 9) and arginine (pI c. 12) molecules, with a net positive charge, will move towards the cathode. 'Neutral' amino acids such as alanine, with pI about 6, will remain effectively stationary. By using different pH systems it is possible to achieve separation of most of the amino acids, as their net charges will vary

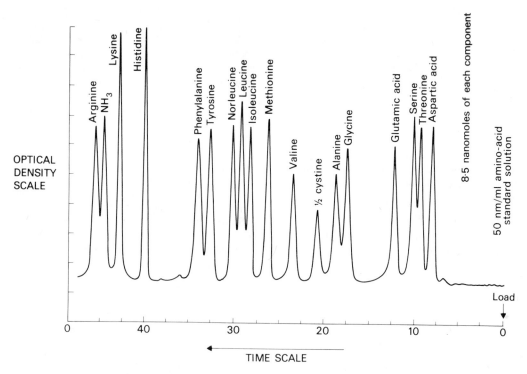

Fig. 3.8. Chromatogram of amino acids separated and assayed on automated ion exchange amino acid analyser column.

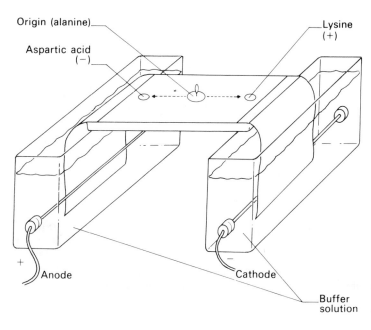

Fig. 3.9. High voltage electrophoresis technique. At pH 6.02 the alanine molecules will not move from the origin on passage of current: the aspartic acid molecules have a net negative charge and will move towards the anode, whilst the positively charged lysine molecules move towards the cathode.

slightly according to their particular pI and ionizable group pKa values. The support medium is sheets or strips of paper, and to achieve effective separation of each amino acid into a discrete area, voltages in the region of 1000–2000V are employed: hence the name high voltage electrophoresis (HVE) for the technique.

PROTEINS

The bonds and forces of interaction which determine the structure and shapes of protein molecules

COVALENT FORCES

These are the strongest forces involved, with bond strengths in the region 30–100 kcal/mol (130–420 kJ/mol) (p. 983).

The peptide bond
In proteins the most important covalent linkage is the peptide bond, formed by a condensation (dehydration) reaction which eliminates a molecule of water from between the amino group of one amino acid and the carboxyl group of its neighbour. This is the means whereby amino acids join together to form the long unbranched polypeptide chains that constitute protein molecules. When incorporated in polypeptide chains in this way the amino acids are referred to as *residues*. The hypothetical linking together of the amino acids leucine, aspartic acid, proline and histidine to form a tetrapeptide is represented in Fig. 3.10.

Some important features which arise from a consideration of this tetrapeptide can be applied to protein polypeptide chains involving hundreds of amino acids linked together. These are

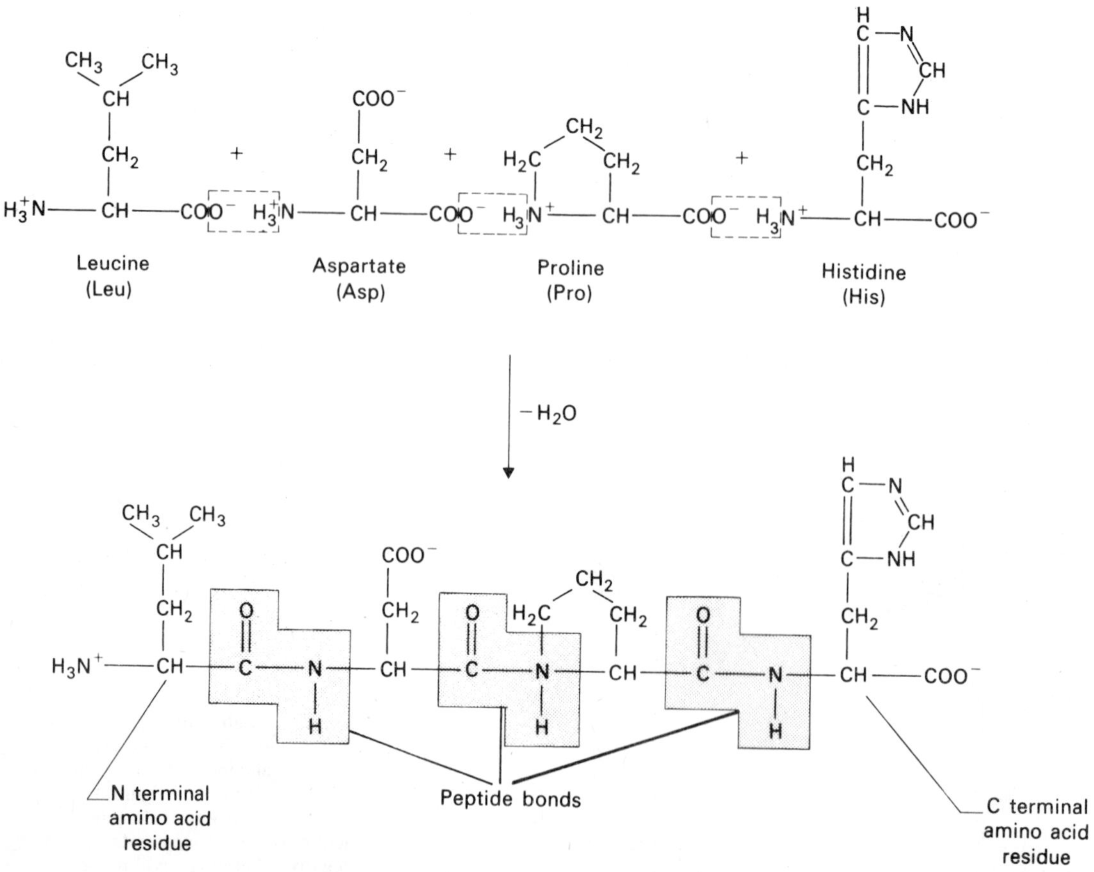

Leucine (Leu)　　Aspartate (Asp)　　Proline (Pro)　　Histidine (His)

$-H_2O$

N terminal amino acid residue　　Peptide bonds　　C terminal amino acid residue

Fig. 3.10. Hypothetical tetrapeptide formed by formation of peptide bonds between the amino acids leucine, aspartic acid, proline and histidine. The Leu residue forms the N-terminal amino acid and His the C-terminal one. Note how the *whole* Pro ring structure becomes part of the peptide backbone.

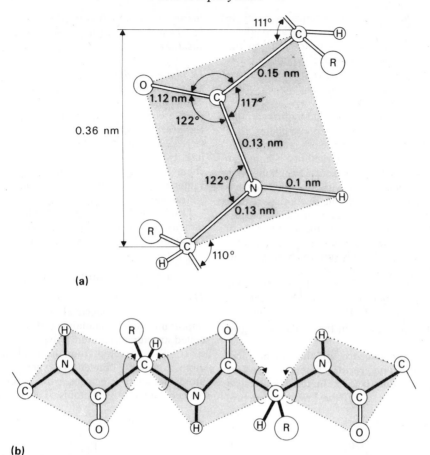

(a)

(b)

Fig. 3.11. Limited rotation in peptide chain backbone. (a) The peptide bonds joining amino acids in protein chains have a rigid planar structure.

(b) This imposes a corresponding rigidity and limited rotation on the backbones of polypeptide chains.

as follows:

1 Each polypeptide chain has a free α-amino group at the N terminal end, which by convention is always written starting on the left, and a free α-carboxyl group at the C-terminal end, written at the right end of the polypeptide.

2 The peptide bond itself has none of the ionization properties associated with the original amino (NH_3^+) and carboxylate ($-COO^-$) groups of the free amino acids from which the link was forged. The nitrogen atom of the

$$\begin{matrix} & O \\ & \| \\ -C&-N- \\ & | \\ & H \end{matrix}$$

(amide type) peptide bond has no tendency to give up its attached hydrogen as a proton ($H+$) nor to accept one. However, these hydrogen atoms do play a most important role in forming the *hydrogen bonds* (p. 984), which

are key interaction forces controlling protein structure.

3 Each peptide bond has a rigid planar structure because it cannot rotate around its central $-C-N-$ bond (Fig. 3.11a). This property, therefore, gives the polypeptide chains a backbone structure consisting of a series of relatively rigid planes alternating with substituted methylene (CHR) groups around which rotation may occur (Fig. 3.11b).

The rigidity of the peptide bond structure is due to its existence in a resonance hybrid form. This imparts some double bond characteristics to the link which has the effect of 'freezing' the entire amide group in a single plane. As a result the only possibility for free rotation in the molecule is around the two bonds on each side of the α-C atoms which join each peptide link to the next, but even here the presence of bulky R side-chains may impose steric hindrance effects on rotation. These various restrictions on the flexibility and rotation within polypeptide backbones helps to determine the particular three dimensional forms ultimately assumed by different protein molecules.

4   The imino acids proline and hydroxyproline are incorporated in polypeptide chains in a rather different way from the other amino acids. Their heterocyclic ring structures become an integral part of the polypeptide backbone (Fig. 3.10). This feature as will be seen later has important consequences in disrupting regular α-helix type structures in protein chains, and as a major determining factor in the architecture of collagen molecules (p. 66).

5   The nature of each R side-chain brings to its site on the polypeptide its own particular properties. Examples of this are: the hydrophobic aliphatic side-chain of leucine; the negatively charged terminal $-COO^-$ ion of aspartate; the charged $-\overset{+}{N}H-$ group in the imidazole ring of histidine.

The actual sequence of the amino acid residues in a polypeptide chain is termed its *primary structure* (p. 52). In the hypothetical tetrapeptide (Fig. 3.10) the primary structure

therefore is Leu-Asp-Pro-His, with Leu its N-terminal and His its C-terminal amino acid residues.

Disulphide bridges
Closely approximated $-SH$ groups from the R side-chains of different cysteine residues may join together by oxidation reactions which remove the hydrogen atoms to form disulphide ($-S-S-$) links (Fig. 3.12). These may cross-link two different polypeptide chains (inter-chain crosslinks) or join different parts of the same polypeptide chain folded back on itself (intra-chain crosslink).

Disulphide bonds help to stabilize the three dimensional shapes of proteins and to impart mechanical strength, as in the keratins.

NON-COVALENT FORCES

The hydrogen bond
Hydrogen bonds collectively provide the most important forces maintaining the folded and coiled structures of protein polypeptide chains in space. They develop from the tendency of H atoms covalently bonded to oxygen or nitrogen atoms to share electrons with other nearby oxygen and nitrogen atoms. The H-bonds so

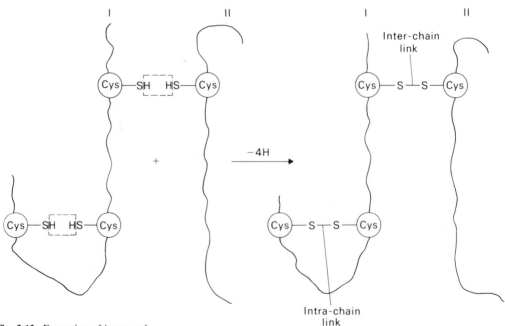

Fig. 3.12. Formation of inter- and intra-chain disulphide bridges (S-S).

Example   Type

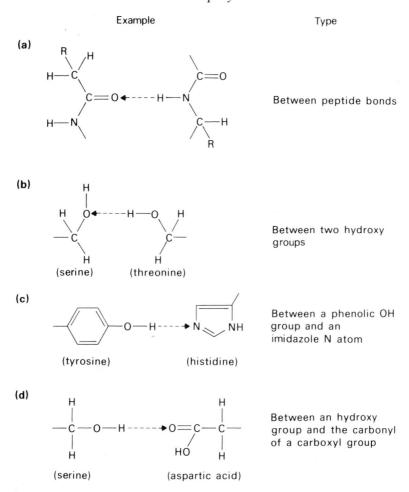

(a) Between peptide bonds

(b) Between two hydroxy groups

(serine)   (threonine)

(c) Between a phenolic OH group and an imidazole N atom

(tyrosine)   (histidine)

(d) Between an hydroxy group and the carbonyl of a carboxyl group

(serine)   (aspartic acid)

Fig. 3 13. Examples of hydrogen bonds formed in biomolecules.

formed are relatively weak, with bond energies of the order 3–7 kcal/mol and bond lengths in the range 0.26–0.31 nm. Examples are shown in Fig. 3.13.

Aliphatic and aromatic hydroxy (−OH) and amino (−NH) groups made good H-bond donors. Carbonyl ($>$C=O) groups, alcoholic (OH) groups, and nitrogen atoms in the imidazole rings of histidine act as receptors.

The −NH− group in one peptide bond provides a good H-bond donor site for the carbonyl group of another peptide bond (p. 56). The regular spacing of the peptide bonds causes their associated H-bond interactions to pull polypeptide chains into corresponding regular shapes. One such form is the *α-helix* where the hydrogen bonds form between each peptide bond and the

fourth residue further along in sequence. This causes the chain to coil like a spring (Fig. 3.14).

The α-helix is one example of the *secondary structure* spatial arrangement that a polypeptide chain can take up. It is the configuration they tend to assume spontaneously because energetically it is the most stable form possible. Particular R groups may interfere and disrupt α-helix formation.

An alternative pattern of H-bonds contributes to the shape and stability of the *β-pleated sheet*, a secondary structure form found in several proteins (Fig. 3.23).

Although individually weak, the presence of a large number of H-bonds in a structure is a source of great overall strength and stability.

In summary the −CO−NH− peptide bond in

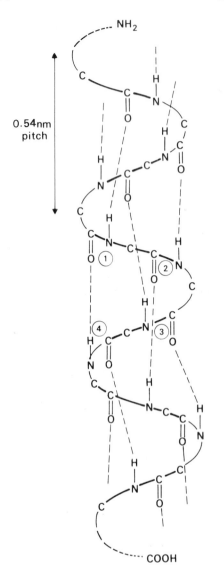

0.54nm
pitch

NH₂

COOH

Fig. 3.14. Hydrogen bonds stabilizing α-helix form of a polypeptide chain.

The ionic bond

In the physiological pH range the ionizable R groups of lysine and arginine residues and the N-terminal amino acid α-amino groups bear positive charges. Conversely the side-arms of aspartyl and glutamyl residues, and the C-terminal carboxylate ions, bear negative charges. When appropriately juxtaposed in space coulombic attractions between these oppositely charged centres form inter- and intra-chain stabilizing forces (Fig. 3.15).

Since such charged $-NH_3^+$ and $-COO^-$ groups are normally hydrated, they can only function effectively as ionic bonds in regions in the molecule protected from water; these will occur in the hydrophobic regions involving the non-polar amino acid residue side-chains which tend to be located within the central cores of protein molecules. The attractions and repulsions between unlike and like charges respectively will eventually influence the shape taken up by polypeptide chains.

Hydrophobic 'bonds'

Another major determinant in protein structure derives from the tendency of the non-polar R side-chain residues of the aromatic and aliphatic amino acids to cluster together towards the centre of protein molecules. This is due not to any mutual attractive forces between them (they are non-polar and unreactive), but rather to their ability to exclude water because of their hydrophobic (water-hating) nature (p. 985). This can lead to large regions of the peptide chains where these non-polar side-chains are grouped as tightly organized internal structures, with the hydrophilic (water-loving) R chains, ionic groups such as on aspartyl, lysyl and argininyl residues orientated at the surface (Fig. 3.16).

With some proteins the whole molecules form globular or ovoid shapes with the non-polar side-chains located predominantly to the interior, and the ionic groups on the surface. Such structures have been likened to 'an oil drop with a polar coat', an arrangement which is similar to the lipid micelle aggregations (p. 156).

Van der Waals forces

These include London forces (a man's name not the UK capital), are the weakest forces operating to regulate protein shapes but are important because potentially so many abound. They involve induced charge effects between molecules and tend to make the molecules nestle together (p. 984).

proteins joins the amino acids together; stabilizes protein molecules by virtue of its rigid planar form; and provides a battery of stabilizing hydrogen bonds throughout the length of a polypeptide chain.

Other H-bonds which contribute to protein structures involve donor OH groups (Ser, Thr, Tyr, Hyp), and $-NH_2$ and $-NH_3^+$ groups (Asn, Gln, Arg, Lys and N-terminal amino acids). Groups acting as acceptor sites for H-bonds include the $-COO^-$ groups on aspartic and glutamic residue side-arms, and $-S-S-$ links.

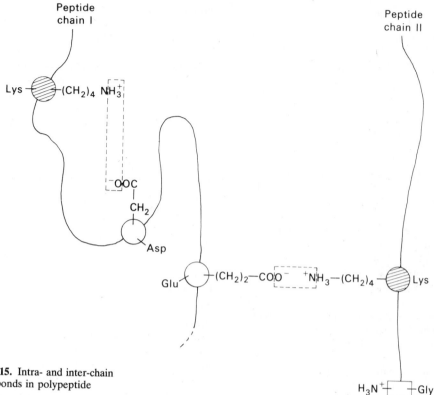

Fig. 3.15. Intra- and inter-chain ionic bonds in polypeptide chains.

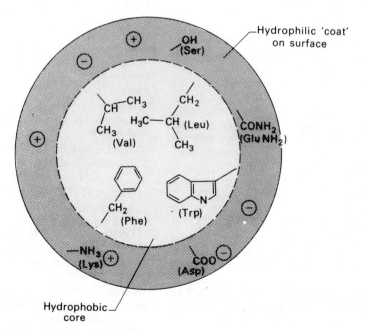

Fig. 3.16. Hypothetical picture of the cross-section of a protein showing a hydrophilic 'coat'. (After Yudkin M. & Offord R. (1973) *Comprehensible Biochemistry*. London, Longman.)

Shapes of proteins in space

With knowledge of the various bonds and forces of interaction operating it is now possible to examine in greater detail the shapes assumed by protein molecules. There is hierarchy in the complexity of their organization to which most, if not all, conform. The levels in the hierarchy are know as the *primary, secondary, tertiary* and *quaternary* structures.

The primary structure of a protein is the specific ordered sequence in which the amino acids are actually arranged along the entire length of its polypeptide chain(s). Primary structure refers not only to the order but also to the number and type of amino acid. The important bonding force in the primary structure is the covalent peptide link joining the amino acids together (p. 46). Primary stucture determines the particular form of secondary, tertiary and quaternary structure a protein takes up in space.

The secondary structure is the form into which the primary polypeptide chains themselves fold or coil. The most common secondary structures are the *β-pleated sheet* (p. 58), the *α-helix* (p. 57), and the *random coils*, which shows no regular form or pattern. The rigidity of the peptide bond is important in the form and stabilization of secondary structures, braced by the intra-chain H-bonds (p. 50) and disulphide bonds (p. 48).

The *tertiary structure* is the further folding the already folded and/or coiled secondary structures may develop to form the molecule into its final characteristic and unique shape. In summary the final shape is maintained in space by ionic bonds, hydrogen bonds, intra- and inter-chain disulphide bridges, intra-chain peptide bonds, Van der Waals forces and the hydrophobic 'bond' effects of the non-polar amino acid side-chains (Fig. 3.17a).

The term 'conformation' is often used to refer to the secondary and tertiary states together. It describes the overall form and shape of the molecule in space.

The quaternary structure denotes the form only taken by some proteins, when tertiary sub-units aggregate or associate with similar or identical protein subunits (Fig. 3.17b). Quaternary structures are usually loosely held together by non-covalent forces (ionic bonds, hydrogen bonds and Van der Waal forces) and because of this they readily dissociate into their constituent subunits.

The subunits are termed protomers, and the whole structure an oligomeric protein. Haemo-globin is an oligomeric protein whose structure has been determined in great detail. Its quaternary form consists of four protomers of two identical α-chains and two identical β-chains, each consisting of about 140 amino acid residues. The four protomers aggregate in an approximately globular shape with a complex non-protein haem molecule lodged in each like a lozenge in the centre. Considerable lengths of the primary structure take up an α-helix form.

The very simplified diagrammatic representation of haemoglobin structure (Fig. 3.18) illustrates and summarizes the general features of these different levels of protein structure organization. Haemoglobin structure and function are discussed in greater detail later (pp. 73, 505).

THE PRIMARY STRUCTURE OF A PROTEIN: INSULIN

The elucidation of the primary structure of the pancreatic hormone insulin (Fig. 3.20) published in 1955 by Sanger, marked a milestone in biochemistry. Frederick Sanger and co-workers in Cambridge spent ten years establishing this first complete amino acid sequence of a protein, introducing new techniques and approaches which heralded a whole new era of protein structure studies. The work received a justly deserved Nobel Prize. Insulin is one of the smaller proteins with only 51 amino acid residues in its molecule and a molecular weight of 5733. Impairment of its production causes diabetes mellitus (p. 799).

In working out the primary structure of a protein chain (Fig. 3.19) the following need to be determined:

1 The identity of the N-terminal amino acid(C_t)
2 The identity of the C-terminal amino acid(N_t)
3 The number, identity and sequential arrangement of the amino acids residues.

In his studies on insulin Sanger introduced the use of the reagent 2, 4-fluoro-dinitrobenzene (FDNB) to identify the N-terminal amino acid. The FDNB labels or 'tags' this amino acid residue with a yellow dinitrophenyl radical (DNP). The DNP-amino acid derivative survives acid hydrolysis of the peptide chains and is identified chromatographically (p. 41).

Using this method Sanger found that insulin had two N-terminal amino acids, *glycine* and *phenylalanine*, and therefore concluded that insulin must contain two polypeptide chains which he called A and B respectively.

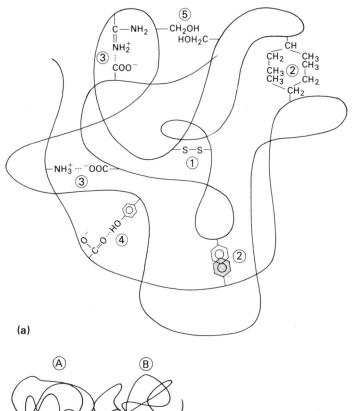

(a)

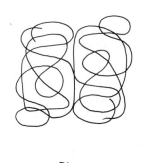

(b)

Tetramer
(composed of two different
subunits A and B)

Dimer
(composed of identical
subunits)

Fig. 3.17. (a) Stabilization of the tertiary structure of a protein by (1) covalent disulphide bonds formed by the oxidation of two cysteine residues; (2) hydrophobic interactions; (3) ionic interactions (salt linkages); (4) hydrogen bonds; and (5) dipole-dipole interactions. (b) The association of tertiary-structured subunits to form a dimer and a tetramer quaternary structure. The subunits of an oligomer are not always identical. (After Segal I.H. (1976) *Biochemical Calculations*, 2nd edn. New York, John Wiley.)

Various chemical and enzymic methods were used to identify the C-terminal amino acids. The enzyme *carboxypeptidase* (p. 610) specifically cleaves off C-terminal residues which can then be identified by paper chromatography. With insulin they turned out to be *asparagine* and *alanine* for the A and B chains respectively. Following removal of the C-terminal amino acid the

enzyme continues to clip off further amino acid residues one by one, and their identification gave the amino acid sequence reading inwards from the C-terminal end of the A polypeptide chain.

Sanger first separated the two A and B chains of insulin (which are joined by disulphide bridges) by a performic acid reaction which

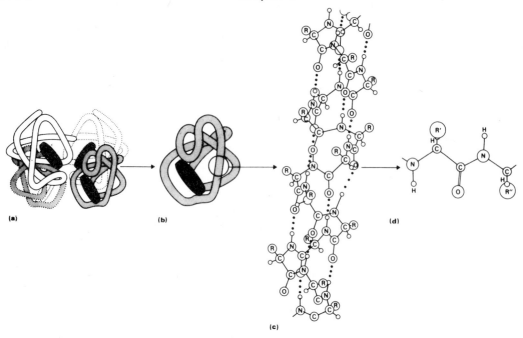

Fig. 3.18. Levels of structural organization in haemoglobin. (a) quaternary, showing aggregation of α- and β-chain subunits; (b) tertiary, showing folding of β-chain helix; (c) secondary, composition of helical structure; (d) primary, peptide bond structure. (After Bennett T.P. & Frieden E. (1970) *Modern Topics in Biology.* London, Macmillan.)

broke the bridges, oxidizing each half to a cysteic acid residue (CySO₃H).

The next—and monumental—task was to work out the order of the actual amino acids in each chain. The complete primary structure of insulin as worked out by Sanger is shown in Fig. 3.20.

The means he employed in deducing this structure were as follows. The isolated A and B chain were individually broken down to di-, tri-, tetra-, and penta-peptide fragments using partial acid hydrolysis and a proteolytic enzyme such as trypsin. The resultant peptides were chromatographically separated and the C- and N- terminal amino acids for each identified and their amino acid compostion determined. Then the A and B chains were each broken into a different series of peptide fragments using a different proteolytic enzyme (e.g. pepsin) or a chemical method. (This method relies on the use of proteolytic enzymes which break the peptide chains at different specific places. In more recent years the reagent cyanogen bromide (CNBr) which specifically breaks polypeptide chains at methionyl peptide links, has proved particularly valuable.)

The end result of these various procedures was the production of a series of peptide jig-saw pieces. The amino acid sequences in the di- and tri-peptides were obvious from a knowledge of their composition and end group analyses. However, the larger peptide fragments usually required further degradation into smaller units and similar analysis, to enable the amino acid sequences of the large peptides to be unequivocally established.

An examination of the sequences in all the fragments showed a sufficent amount of over-

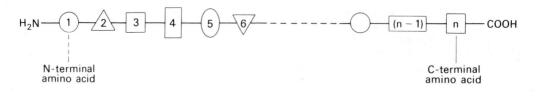

Fig. 3.19. Primary structure of hypothetical polypeptide.

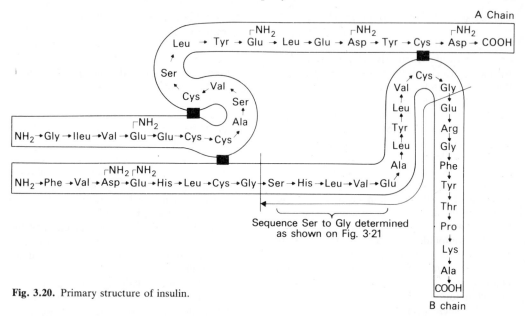

Fig. 3.20. Primary structure of insulin.

lapping of individual structures to allow logical deductions to be made of the sequences in large sections of the A and B chains (Fig. 3.21). For obvious reasons, this approach was known as the overlapping method. Using it, Sanger was able to reconstruct the whole sequence and structure of the two-chain insulin molecule shown in Fig. 3.20.

An alternative, and complementary, approach is step-wise fragmentation with carboxy-peptidase enzyme, clipping off amino acid residues inwards from the C terminal end (p. 41). However, this carboxypeptidase method is limited to detection of only a few sequence steps before interpretation becomes difficult. Much more rewarding has been a combination of the CNBr reagent to produce relatively large peptide fragments coupled with use of the

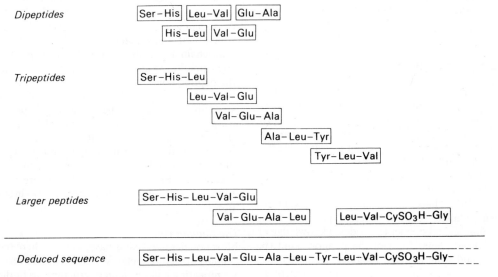

Fig. 3.21. Deduction of amino acid sequence (primary structure) of a polypeptide from smaller peptide fragments using the overlapping method.

Edman degradation method (p. 41) to subtract amino acids one by one inwards from the
N-terminal ends of these peptides. This technique has proved particularly valuable in studying
the larger protein and peptide fragments where
the overlap technique becomes increasingly difficult to apply and interpret.

Studies on the amino acid sequences such as
those of insulin, are not merely of academic
interest. With its primary structure determined it
is possible to design experiments in which known
parts of the insulin molecule are removed and
the residues tested for biological activity.
Although it is not yet certain which amino acids
constitute the active centre of the molecule it is
known that:

1   The disulphide ($-S-S-$) bridges must be
intact for biological activity to be retained.

2   The sequence of amino acids in the disulphide ring of the A chain (Fig. 3.20) is not
important for biological activity and its sequence
varies between species.

3   Removal of the 8 amino acid residues from
the C-terminal end of the B chain of bovine
insulin reduces the biological activity to 15%.

4   The carboxyl group of the C-terminal
asparagine residue on the A chain is necessary
for full biological activity.

THE SECONDARY STRUCTURE OF A PROTEIN: KERATIN

The keratins constitute an important group of
structure proteins and are found in hair, nails,
wool and epidermis. They were among the first
proteins to be investigated by X-ray diffraction
by Astbury in the 1930s, and they all showed
similar distinctive patterns, indicating an
ordered arrangement of their constituent atoms,
with evidence of a regular repeat pattern in their
structure at intervals of 0.5–0.55 nm. After
steaming, stretched hair produced a different
X-ray diffraction pattern and a repeat pattern
interval of 0.7 nm. Astbury concluded that the
keratin molecules are differently arranged in the
normal and stretched states. The former was
designated the α-keratin, and the latter the
β-keratin state.

In 1939 Linus Pauling and R. B. Corey, utilizing detailed X-ray diffraction patterns from
amino acid crystals and peptides, a knowledge of
the rigid planar form of the peptide bond (p.
47) and scale molecular models examined the
possible ways in which α-keratin polypeptide
chains could twist or fold. They found that the
simplest form which could accommodate their

data and account for the 0.5–0.55 nm repeat in
α-keratins was a structure they called the α-helix.

The α-helix

As indicated previously, the rigid planar form of
peptide bonds and their ability to form H-bonds
induces many proteins to adopt α-helix form
secondary structures. Various features and
aspects of the structure are shown in Fig. 3.22.

Theoretically an α-helix can form from either
L or D-amino acids, but never from a mixture.
The naturally occurring L-amino acids can form
right-handed or left-handed helices but so far
naturally occurring proteins have been found to
form right-handed α-helices.

The α-helix is ideally suited for creating the
long fibrous molecules found in α-keratins, but it
is also found routinely as part of the structure of
many globular proteins.

In keratins such as hair or wool, right-handed
α-helices may wind round each other to give a 3
or 7 stranded 'rope' structure, the molecular
basis for much of the strength and stability exhibited by these tough fibrous proteins. Many
interchain covalent disulphide bridges stabilize
the structures. Human hair for example contains
14% cystine residues.

The β-pleated sheet

As described α-keratin fibres when subjected to
moist heat can be stretched to twice their length
and in this form possess an X-ray diffraction
pattern different from the α-type. This change
is due to the breakage of the intra-chain H-bonds
which stabilize the α-helix conformation, and a
consequent stretching of the polypeptide coils
which then link together in a different way by
inter-chain H-bonds to give the pleated sheet
conformation (Fig. 3.23). As in the α-helix all
the peptide bonds participate in H-bond formation, and so form sheet structures of great
strength. In β-pleated sheets the R groups can
project above or below the plane of the sheet.
β-pleated sheets exist in nature in two forms:
one where the constituent polypeptide chains
line up parallel to each other (as in hair
α-keratins) (Fig. 3.23a); the other where they
run in opposite anti-parallel directions (as in silk
fibroin) (Fig. 3.23b).

The random coil

Most polypeptide chains have regions where the
primary structure dictates that there is no regular repeating coil or pleated structures as in the
α-helix and β-pleated sheet conformations. In
these regions the polypeptide chains are more

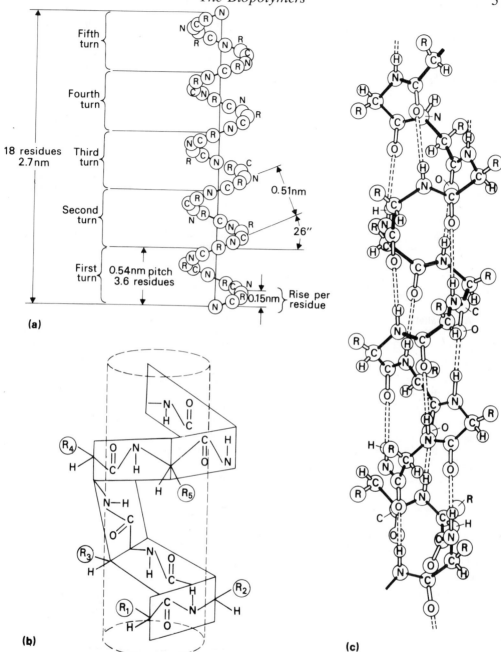

Fig. 3.22. The α-helix configuration: (a) illustrates the number of amino acids residues per turn of the coil, major pitch between each turn, distance between each amino acid residue, (b) indicates how the planar form of the peptide bond imposes rigidity on the α-helix coils, (c) ball and stick model (broken lines indicate hydrogen bonds).

flexible and able to randomly fold and bend: hence the term random coil structures.

Amino acid residues which contribute to random coil region formation are called α-helix (or

β-pleated sheet) breakers. For example, proline and hydroxyproline, whose pyrrolidine ring structures are actually part of the polypeptide backbone (see Fig. 3.10), form distinct kinks at

(a) Parallel

(b) Antiparallel

(c)

0.695nm

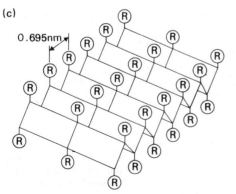

their sites in a molecule. Their regular arrangement in a protein molecule such as collagen not only prevents any α-helix formation but also imposes a quite different helical structure on the molecule (see Fig. 3.26).

Glycine, with its absence of an R side-arm, also favours the formation of bends in peptide chains which can disrupt α-helix formations.

LYSOZYME STRUCTURE

Lysozyme, an enzyme present in tears and saliva, is an example of a protein molecule which contains all three types of secondary structure and shows how the α-helical and β-pleated sheet regions give strength and form to the shape the molecule takes up in its tertiary state (Fig. 3.24).

The molecule also illustrates how the hydrophobic side-arms of non-polar amino acid residues tend to cluster towards the central parts of the molecule, with the polar hydrophilic side-arms orientated more to the molecule surface, so rendering it soluble in an aqueous environment–'an oil drop with a polar coat' (p. 50).

Classification of proteins

A widely used and generally acceptable system of classification divides proteins into two broad categories–*fibrous* and *globular* proteins. To a large extent this distinguishes them on the basis of (a) their molecular shape and/or microscopic appearance and (b) their solubility, composition and functional properties.

THE FIBROUS PROTEINS

These are long thin molecules, relatively insoluble and chemically inert, often forming long fibres visible under the microscope. As they are mainly concerned with the structural features of tissues they are also often referred to as the structure proteins. Examples are the connective tissue proteins collagen and elastin.

THE GLOBULAR PROTEINS

These spheroid, ovoid or ellipsoid shaped molecules are generally soluble in water, dilute salts, acids, and bases. Some are concerned with catalysing metabolic processes (the enzymes), others

Fig. 3.23. β-pleated sheet structures: (a) parallel, and (b) antiparallel. (c) A schematic representation showing adjacent polypeptide chains with the R-groups projecting above and below the plane of the sheet. (After Segal I.H. (1976) *Biochemical calculations*, 2nd edn. New York, John Wiley.)

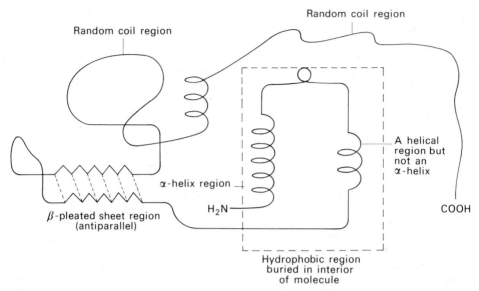

Random coil region

Random coil region

A helical region but not an α-helix

α-helix region

β-pleated sheet region (antiparallel)

H₂N

COOH

Hydrophobic region buried in interior of molecule

Fig. 3.24. Simplified diagram of tertiary structure of lysozyme; a protein containing α-helix, β-pleated sheet and random coil secondary structures in its molecule. These each contribute to the conformation of the molecule in which the hydrophobic regions are mostly buried inside. The charged hydrophilic groups lie on the surface of the molecule, exposed to its aqueous environment. (After Bhagavan (1978) *Biochemistry*, 2nd edn. Philadelphia, Lippincott.)

with biological roles involving transport (e.g. oxygen carrying), hormone activities and immunological defence mechanisms. They are sub-classified on the basis of differential solubility and chemical composition, i.e.

1 *Albumins* are water soluble and are coagulated by heat. Examples are serum and egg albumin.

2 *Globulins* are soluble in water with difficulty, but are soluble in dilute salt solution–a property used in their extraction from tissues. They are also heat coagulable. The immunoglobulins are an example of this class.

3 *Histones* are water soluble basic proteins with a high content of lysine and arginine residues.

4 *Protamines* are low molecular weight basic proteins characterized by high levels of arginine and by the absence of tyrosine, tryptophan and sulphur amino acids.

THE CONJUGATED PROTEINS

These proteins are characterized by their chemical combination with non-protein moieties, a property which forms the basis of their sub-classification. Some are fibrous and others are globular proteins and, therefore, classifiable under two headings: collagen is both a fibrous protein and a glycoprotein.

1 *Nucleoproteins.* Proteins in combination with nucleic acids.

2 *Glycoproteins (Mucoproteins).* Combinations of proteins with carbohydrates. Mucoproteins used to be distinguished from glycoproteins on the basis that they contained less than 4% carbohydrate: however, recent development in the knowledge of these structures has made this distinction arbitrary and unacceptable. Examples are serum albumin, the immunoglobins, salivary glycoproteins and collagen.

3 *Lipoproteins.* Proteins in combination with a lipid. They are water soluble, e.g. serum lipoproteins.

Physicochemical properties of proteins

Protein molecules are of colloidal dimensions and possess in their structures a battery of negatively and positively charged ionizable sites. It is these two properties, size and charge, which largely determine the various physicochemical characteristics of protein behaviour. These form the basis for many protein separation techniques.

AMPHOTERIC NATURE OF PROTEINS

Like their constituent amino acids proteins are amphoteric, bearing both proton-donor and proton-acceptor sites, although in protein molecules these are counted in hundreds rather than the two or three ionizable groups found in amino acid molecules. For example human serum albumin (mw 69 000) has 144 basic group (proton-acceptor) sites and 135 acidic (proton-donor) sites.

These ionizable sites in protein molecules, derive mainly from the following side-chains:
1 The β- and γ-COOH groups at the ends of Asp and Glu residues.
2 ϵ-NH$_2$ groups terminating the Lys residues.
3 The imidazole ring structure of His residues.
4 The guanidinium groups terminating Arg residues.

Table 3.4 shows that the pK values of the acidic and basic groups as observed in proteins. Comparison with Table 3.3 shows that these values differ slightly from those in their free amino acid forms. Theoretically the free SH groups in proteins (pK 8.49) contribute, but in practice they are usually present in such small amounts as to prove negligible. In tyrosine-rich proteins the phenolic OH groups (pK 9.5–10.4) contribute significantly to the overall charge distribution in the molecule.

ISO-IONIC POINT, ISO-ELECTRIC POINT AND TITRATIONS CURVES

As with the amino acids, the degree of ionization of the acidic and basic groups is related to the surrounding pH (p. 36). At one specific pH the protein molecules will exist in a state where the total number of negatively charged sites exactly balances those of the positive charged sites. This pH is termed the *iso-ionic point* (or iso-ionic pH) and in amino acids it is identical to the experimentally determined iso-electric (pI) value. In proteins however, the measured iso-electric point, pI, differs slightly from the iso-ionic pH because of the effect of

ions absorbed from the buffers necessarily involved in electrophoretic techniques (see Fig. 3.9).

Proteins give characteristic titration curves, though the large number of ionizable groups contributing causes the curves to be obtained composite in form, deriving from overlapping titrations of the numerous participating component groups.

Like the amino acids (p. 39), proteins act as effective buffers; it is one of their major functional roles in numerous biological systems (cells, blood, saliva etc.). From Table 3.4 it can be seen that the only titratable group ionizing significantly in the physiological pH range is the −NH− group in the imidazole ring of histidine residues (pK 5.6–7.0). Thus *histidine residues in proteins play a major buffering role in cells and tissues.* The α-NH$_2$ group of the single N-terminal amino acid on each polypeptide chain will obviously only contribute a negligible buffering effect, similarly with the C_t carboxylate group.

ION BINDING BY PROTEINS

The various charged sites in a protein molecule give it the property of being able to bind both cations and anions. The binding of ions from the buffers used in electrophoresis experiments will neutralize some of the charged sites in a protein molecule and this is the reason that its measured pI value (i.e. pH at which it will not move in an electric field because its net charge is zero) does not exactly coincide with its iso-ionic point.

At pH values strongly on the alkaline side of their pI, proteins will be predominantly in their anionic (negatively charged) state and will readily bind heavy metal ions such as mercury, silver, zinc, barium, etc., to form insoluble salts. Similarly when proteins are strongly on the acid side of their pI they will more readily bind anions

Table 3.4. pK values of acidic and basic groups in proteins.

Amino acid residue	Group	pK
Acidic		
C-terminal amino acid (C_t)	α –COOH	3.0–3.2
Asp	β –COOH	3.0–4.7
Glu	γ –COOH	4.4
Basic		
N-terminal amino acid	α –NH$_2$	7.6–8.4
His	Imidazole ring	
	(–NH–)	5.6–7.0
Lys	ϵ –NH$_2$	9.11–10.6
Arg	Guanidinium	11.6–12.6

such as phosphotungstate, trichloracetate and picrate, also to form insoluble salt complexes. Both methods are routinely used as laboratory techniques for deproteinizing solutions.

The binding of Ca^{2+} ions to anionic sites in collagen has been suggested as a possible means for accumulating calcium in the calcifying tissue prior to mineralization proper (p. 389). Calcium ion binding may possibly play a role in salivary glycoprotein aggregation and enamel formation, also in *in vivo* enamel remineralization processes.

SOLUBILITY OF PROTEINS: 'SALTING-OUT'

A classification of proteins, based in part on their differential solubilities in salt solutions, has already been outlined (p. 58). Individual proteins have characteristic solubilities in strong inorganic salt solutions of defined concentration and pH and use is made of this in the primary purification stages of many proteins. The solubility of a protein is at a minimum at its pI value because it is at this pH that the electrostatic repellant forces between molecules are at a minimum. The presence of strong salt concentrations (e.g. $(NH_4)_2SO_4$) at this pH favours the formation of insoluble, sometimes crstalline, precipitates in this so-called 'salting out' technique. The added salt removes water from the protein molecules, further favouring their precipitation. With mixtures of proteins of differing pI values, a sequential salting out, giving partial purification of each component, can be achieved by a succession of shifts in pH value and/or salt concentration.

DENATURATION

Similarly partial protein purification may sometimes be achieved by careful addition of organic solvents such as alcohol or acetone. With these the danger is that the proteins may suffer permanent disruption of their secondary, tertiary or quaternary structures. The possibility of irreversible denaturation is minimized by carrying out the procedures around or below 0°C.

This denaturation involves the unfolding and uncoiling of the uniquely characteristic 3-dimensional architecture of protein molecules. A most sensitive index of it occurring is the loss of any biological activity of the protein concerned (e.g., enzymes). Though usually an irreversible change it may occasionally be reversed if the disruption of the molecule has not been too savage.

Addition of strong alkali or acid will also denature protein structures because of the effect of discharging the positively charged sites or the negative sites respectively. This disturbs the finely balanced array of electrostatic forces, which help hold the molecule together in space, to such an extent that the molecule distorts and collapses to an insoluble or inactive form.

OSMOTIC PRESSURE

The phenomenon of osmosis has been summarized in general terms in another section (p. 994) and this should be referred to in the context of the ensuing discussion.

Because of their large size protein molecules will by definition not pass through semipermeable membranes, which freely pass water and low molecular weight substances. A protein solution contained within a semi-permeable sac (as in a cell) will therefore induce a flow of water inwards from the external aqueous surroundings, with the osmotic pressure (Π) as a measure of the force needed to exactly balance this flow.

The following relationship exists between Π and the molecular weight of a protein:

$$\Pi . V = \frac{g/ RT}{M}$$

When Π = Osmotic pressure
V = Volume of solvent
g = Weight of solute (protein) in grams
M = mw of solute (protein)
R = Gas content
T = Absolute temperature

It is possible, therefore, to determine the molecular weight of a purified protein by an osmotic pressure method. Since the pressure changes involved are very small, and equilibrium must be rapidly attained, specialized apparatus is required. The results obtained give the average molecular weight of all the protein molecules present, and do not indicate the degree of heterogeneity of the protein molecules involved.

Proteins can also exhibit Gibbs–Donnan equilibria effects (p. 995) and to minimize this effect the Π values must be determined at the pH of the protein's iso-electric point.

Separation and purification of proteins

Reference has already been made to the use of the 'salting out' technique as a means of obtaining an initial partial purification of proteins. A whole battery of further techniques can be brought to bear in the preparation of purified

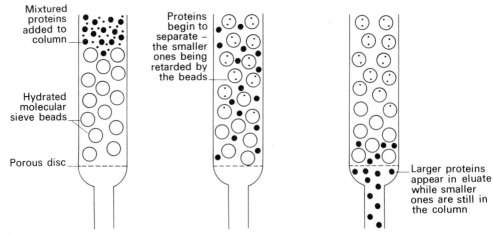

Mixtured proteins added to column

Hydrated molecular sieve beads

Porous disc

Proteins begin to separate – the smaller ones being retarded by the beads

Larger proteins appear in eluate while smaller ones are still in the column

Fig. 3.25. The principles of molecular sieving in gel filtration chromatography.

homogeneous protein samples. These fall broadly into three major categories:

1 Electrophoretic (based on charges on molecules)
2 Chromatographic (based on size and charge on molecules)
3 Ultracentrifugation (based on size and shape of molecules)

Several of these are used routinely for analysis of protein mixtures and as tests for homogeneity. Scaled up they may be used for preparative purposes.

ELECTROPHORETIC METHODS

Paper and cellulose acetate strips
The simpler analytical techniques include paper and cellulose acetate strip electrophoresis in apparatus similar in design principles to that used for amino acid separation (HVE, p. 44). The voltage and current used are much less than those needed for amino acid HVE and the separated proteins may be stained and quantitated on the strips.

Polyacrylamide gel electrophoresis (PAGE or 'disc' electrophoresis)
Similar in principle to strip electrophoresis the support medium is a small semi-rigid cylindrical gel in a closed tube or a flat slab in which, under the influence of a suitable current, the protein components in a preparation separate into discrete bands, which in the tubes are also, in effect, thin cylindrical discs. After separation on the gels the protein bands are stained with a suitable reagent (Amido black, Coomassie blue).

The technique provides a most valuable method for assessing the homogeneity, or otherwise, of protein preparations. It has also been scaled up for use as a preparative technique.

Iso-electro focussing
This method depends on the addition to the electrophoretic system of substances (trade name Ampholines) which, under the influence of a current, set up a permanent pH gradient. Proteins present in the system will move to the appropriate pH zones corresponding to their individual iso-electric (pI) values and stay there—hence the name iso-electro focussing.

The method is capable of providing a high degree of resolution and can also be used in cylindrical gel or flat slab forms, with polyacrylamide as the support medium. The method is invaluable for establishing the purity and homogeniety of protein preparations. Iso-electric focussing can also be used on the preparative scale.

CHROMATOGRAPHIC METHODS

Gel filtration
This is a column chromatographic method, where the support medium is either a highly cross-linked fine particle form of special polysaccharides, dextrans (trade name Sephadex), or a similar polyacrylamide gel (Biogel) fine bead preparation. Both act as 'molecular sieves' with the smaller protein molecules penetrating the particles deeper and being held back (retarded) on the column, whilst the larger protein molecules elute faster. Fig. 3.25 illustrates the principles involved. Gel filt-

ration is a widely used preparative method and uses water or salt solutions as the eluants. Because the method is based on a molecular sizing principle it may be also used to give reasonably accurate estimates of molecular weights by reference to a previously constructed 'map' of elution times for a range of substances of known molecular weight in the particular column system used.

Ion-exchange chromatography

This is essentially the same in principle as that used in amino acid ion exchange chromatography (p. 44) except that for proteins the ion-exchange materials used are modified dextrans or cellulose preparations bearing appropriate anion or cation exchange sites. Buffer solutions of varying pH and molarity are used to elute the proteins and the method is often used in conjunction with the other preparative techniques finally to attain homogeneous protein samples.

Affinity chromatography

This technique makes use of the 'affinity' a particular protein has for some specific related biomolecule. A chromatographic column is set up based on this property for the selective isolation of the protein. For example the solid phase column support medium can have bound to it the substrate for a specific enzyme it is required to purify or isolate. When a crude preparation of the enzyme is placed on the column it binds to the solid phase substrate, and the other components and contaminants are then removed by an appropriate column elution. The specific enzyme itself is then freed and eluted separately using an eluant of higher ionic strength and/or suitable pH.

Ultracentrifugation methods

Modern ultracentrifuges operate at speeds of up to 75 000 rpm, which exert forces up to 400 000 times that of gravity on protein molecules, normally held in equilibrium suspension as colloidal sols. Under the influence of these high 'g' values the protein molecules will move at different rates dependent on their size, weight and shape. Use is made of this in the separation of proteins (preparative ultracentrifugation) and in the determination of their homogeneity and molecular weight values (analytical ultracentrifugation).

In preparative ultracentrifugation the heavier protein molecules will sediment out faster than the smaller, and selection of the appropriate centrifugal force and sedimentation time permits collection of individual protein components.

Molecular weight determination by analytical ultracentrifugation involves measurement, by optical means, of the sedimentation rate at which a specific protein moves under a high 'g' force. This rate (expressed as S values), used in conjunction with the determination of other parameters (viscosity or diffusion rates), permits calculation of the molecular weight.

Somewhat similar is the sedimentation equilibrium method using rather lower 'g' forces. With these a point is reached where the tendency for specific protein molecules to sediment towards the bottom of the centrifuge tube is exactly balanced by their rate of diffusion back to the lower concentration regions in the upper part of the tube. This equilibrium point is dependent on the mass and density of the protein, and with accurate knowledge of the latter the molecular weight of the protein concerned can be calculated with a high degree of accuracy.

Thus the molecular weight determination of proteins can be made by the sedimentation rate method and the sedimentation equilibrium method in the analytical ultracentrifuge. In addition, as explained above, osmotic pressure measurement and gel filtration chromatography are also techniques for estimation of molecular weight values.

PROTEINS IN ACTION

In living matter the proteins carry out numerous functions (Table 3.5). They may be information proteins concerned with the control, transmission and expression of genetic information (chromosomal and ribosomal proteins). Some are involved in the structural integrity of connective and skeletal tissues (the fibrous proteins); others act as transport agencies carrying essential material from one site to another (respiratory and cell transport proteins); they can act as chemical messengers (hormones) controlling metabolism and some are concerned with bodily defences against foreign invasion (immunoglobulin molecules). A large and important group (the enzymes) have conformations specifically designed for catalysis of the thousands of chemical reactions involved in metabolism.

The ensuing text gives examples of proteins in action in different ways at different levels: how they work, and how a specific protein molecule is constructed to carry out its particular job, i.e. its *structure-function* relationships.

A protein of prime importance in connective tissues—*collagen*—is dealt with as a specific example of a structural or fibrous protein. Another fibrous protein *keratin*, in epidermal structures, has already been discussed, mainly to illustrate the α-helix and β-pleated sheet conformations in proteins (p. 56).

Table 3.5. Classification of proteins on basis of function.

General protein groups and types	Functions and/or occurrence
Structural proteins	
Keratin	Epidermis
Collagen	Connective tissues: dermis, bones, teeth, tendon
Elastin	Connective tissues, ligaments.
Glycoproteins (mucoproteins)	Cell walls and mucous secretions: saliva
Myosin, actin	Muscle contraction
Enzymes	
Oxido/reductases	Oxidation reduction reactions
Hydrolases	Hydrolysis reactions
Transferases	Transporting of groups
Phosphorylases	Addition of phosphoryl radicals
Isomerases	Isomerization changes
Respiratory proteins	
Haemoglobin	O₂ transport in vertebrate blood
Myoglobin	O₂ transport in vertebrate muscle
Cytochromes	O₂ transport in tissues
Protective proteins	
Immunoglobulins	Antibody activity
Thrombin	Blood clotting chains
Hormones	
Insulin	Carbohydrate metabolism
Growth	Bone growth
Storage proteins	
Ovalbumen	Egg white
Casein	Milk protein
Nucleoproteins	
Cell nucleoproteins	Control of heredity and transmission
Ribosomal proteins	Protein synthesis

✕ PROTEINS IN ACTION I ✕

A structural protein: collagen

IMPORTANCE AND DISTRIBUTION

Collagen is of paramount importance throughout the animal body. It is the most abundant protein in the body constituting some 25–30% of the total protein and therefore 6% of the total body weight. It is a mesodermal extracellular protein produced by fibroblasts (skin, tendon), osteoblasts (bone), chondrocytes (cartilage), cementocytes (cementum) and odontoblasts (dentine) and as such becomes the primary structural element of connective tissues. It is present to some extent in most organs, where its function is to act as scaffolding.

Collagen is the protein that dental surgeons are most concerned with both directly and indirectly, in their role as practitioners. It is the major structural (fibrous) protein of the tooth dentine, whose ravaging by dental caries is the disease most commonly requiring treatment in the dental surgery. Collagen is also a key structural protein in the periodontal and gingival tissues and its breakdown is a major factor in the development of periodontal disease.

The structural feature which fits collagen molecules for these various roles (its structure-function relationship) is its particular molecular conformation which is ultimately expressed in the form of long insoluble fibres whose tensile strength (100 kg/cm²) matches that of a steel cable of the same weight. In addition it possesses a small degree of extensibility. It has been likened to a ship's anchor cable—flexible enough to be coiled when not in use, yet strong enough to take the strain and hold a ship at anchor as required.

This high tensile strength of collagen gives functional integrity to bones, teeth, skin and tendons and combined with its low solubility, relative inertness to chemical change within the normal range of physiological conditions. Its low rate of metabolic turnover produces tissue of great strength and stability. In skeletal structures such as bone, and tooth dentine, the tensile strength is fortified by the presence of a mineral component, *calcium hydroxyapatite* (p. 346), the two in combination resembling in structure reinforced concrete. Such a material is superbly designed to cope with the strains and stresses imposed upon the teeth and skeleton. Collagen is also involved in tissue repair and regeneration, as in the formation of scar tissue and bone resorption and remodelling.

Various pathological conditions can be related to defective or inadequate collagen structures. The formation of scar tissue can lead to adhesions and a variety of diseases, such as osteo- and rheumatoid arthritis and heart valve lesions, are essentially collagen diseases. Certain genetic defects result in the formation of imperfect collagens and are the underlying cause of various genetic diseases as in Marfan's syndrome, scleroderma, homocystinuria, dermatosporaxis (in cattle) and the Ehlers–Danlos syndromes (p. 251).

Not least of the changes in collagen affecting the efficient functioning of tissues and organs is the process of ageing. There are various theories concerning the mechanisms involved in this (Vol 1, Bk 2). Whatever the causes one of the inevitable tolls of the ageing process is that tissue collagen molecules become increasingly rigid. The tensile strength increases and there is an associated resistance to solubility (*in vitro*) and to dissolution by collagenolytic enzymes. These altered properties have been ascribed to an increased degree of crosslinking between collagen molecules, although the exact identity of these have not yet been fully worked out. The net effect is a more inflexible collagen structure which contributes to skin changes in ageing: the skin of the old no longer springs back as in youth and the rigidity also sets in patterns of wrinkles and folds. Collagen changes are also involved in the arterial walls' loss of elasticity and contractability, which contributes to the cardiovascular diseases that increasingly take their toll of life as age progresses.

PROPERTIES

Solubility

The insolubility of collagen for many years impeded its chemical investigation. However it was eventually found that soluble collagen fractions could be readily extracted from the tissues of young animals using neutral salt conditions (1M NaCl), weak acids (acetic acid, pH 3–4), and H-bond breaking reagents (such as strong urea solutions). This opened the way to the detailed study of the structure and chemistry of collagen using young skin and tendon extracts. Calcified tissue collagens in bone and dentine cannot be extracted in this way, even in demineralized form. This indicates that some structural difference exists between the collagen fibres of calcified tissues and the soft tissue collagens of skin and tendon.

The collagen subunit macromolecule: tropocollagen

Soluble collagen tissue extracts contain a basic structural unit, common to all collagen fibril structures—a thin rod, some 300 nm (3000 Å) long by 1.5 nm (15Å) wide with a molecular weight of 285 000. This collagen macromolecule structural unit is called *tropocollagen*, and consists of three polypeptide chains wound round one another, each about 1000 amino acid residues long. It is the longest protein molecule known.

Amino acid composition

Data from some typical collagen analyses are summarized in Table 3.6. The predominant amino acid is the simplest known, *glycine*, which contributes about a third of the total amino acid residues. Because of its relatively low molecular weight (80), glycine only contributes one quarter of the weight of the total protein. *Proline* (c.120/1000 residues) and *4-hydroxyproline* (c.100/1000 residues) together contribute another fifth of the amino acids, so that these three amino acids (Gly, Pro, Hyp) therefore constitute more than half the collagen molecule. One in every three amino acid residues is glycine, one in every $8\frac{1}{2}$ is proline and 1 in 10 is hydroxyproline.

Collagen has a relatively high content of acidic amino acids residues, *aspartate* and *glutamate* together totalling some 120/1000 residues. It is low in aromatic and sulphur amino acid residues: it probably contains no cysteine, and methionine contributes only a few residues/1000 to the total.

The amino acid *5-hydroxylysine* is present in small amounts: 0.5–1.5% according to tissue and species. However it is important in that it is virtually specific to collagen molecules and, with its parent lysine, forms sites for inter- and intramolecular crosslinkages in collagen (p. 69). Specific hydroxylysine residues also provide the sites where hexose units (glucose and galactose) are covalently linked to collagen molecules (p. 71).

Hydroxyproline is almost as specific to collagen as hydroxylysine although it does occur in smaller amounts in a few other proteins. Nevertheless, the detection of hydroxyproline in tissue preparations, either chemically or histochemically, is virtually a fingerprint indicating the presence of collagen.

Collagen is also found in invertebrates, e.g. sea-urchins (Table 3.6). In these animals, and the more primitive vertebrates, the proline and hydroxyproline content is significantly lower.

Thus evolution to higher forms has been associated with an increase in imino acid levels in their collagens.

STRUCTURE

The collagen helix

Extraction and heating of tropocollagen preparations, and examination of the products by electrophoresis and gel chromatography, show that three types of denatured collagen (the gelatins) are formed; α-gelatin (mw 95 000); β-gelatin (mw 190 000); and γ-gelatin (mw 285 000). This implies a trimeric structure for the tropocollagen. The tropocollagen macromolecules in bone, dentine, skin and tendon consist of three polypeptide chains termed the α-chains. Two of these are identical (the α_1 chains) and one (the α_2 chain) differs slightly in length and amino acid sequence. There are different α_1 chain primary structures in cartilage, aorta and basement membrane tissue within the same species. There are also differences between species.

The tropocollagen structure of skin, bone and tendon is designated $[\alpha_1(I)]_2.\alpha_2$ to indicate that it consists of two Type I α_1 chains with one α_2 chain. The collagen in cartilage, $[\alpha_1(II)]_3$, consists of three α_1 chains of a Type II form which contains more hydroxylysine and less lysine than Type I. Dermis and aorta contain a collagen species with three Type III α_1 chains designated $[\alpha_1(III)]_3$, and basement membrane contains three Type IV α_1 chains, $[\alpha_1(IV)]_3$ or possibly two $[\alpha(IV)]$ chain types.

Sequence studies have revealed two important features in the primary structure of collagen. The first is that throughout most of each α-chain every third amino acid is glycine. Second, amino acid sequence triplets, Gly-X-Y, are regularly repeated, of which Gly-Pro-Pro and Gly-Pro-Hyp forms predominate. The ring structures of imino acids such as proline and hydroxyproline actually become incorporated into the polypeptide backbone when they are joined by peptide bonds (Fig. 3.10). These impose on the chains a rigidity and a characteristic secondary structure in the form of a left-handed kinked helical coil (Fig. 3.26a), *which is quite distinct from an α-helix*, (Fig. 3.22). Its pitch, the distance between each turn of the collagen helix, is greater, 0.93 nm (compared to 0.54 nm) and the distance from one amino acid residue to the one above is 0.31 nm (compared to 0.15 nm). The coil of the α-chain helix in collagen is maintained by its rigid imino acid backbone structure in contrast to the intra-chain hydrogen bonds which are the main forces stabilizing the α-helix of keratins (Fig. 3.14 and 3.22). However, the peptide bonds deriving from glycine residues do contribute to *inter*-chain hydrogen bonding, and the hydrogen from the OH group of the hydroxyproline residues may also be involved in collagen helix stabilization.

Table 3.6. Collagen amino acid analyses (expressed as residues per 1000 total residues).

| Amino acid | Dentine | | Cementum | Tendon | Bone | | Echinoderm |
	Human	Bovine	Bovine	Bovine	Human	Bovine	Sea urchin
3-Hydroxyproline	—	—	1	2	—	—	—
4-Hydroxyproline	99	99	105	90	99	101	54
Aspartic acid	46	50	50	47	46	50	76
Threonine	17	17	19	17	18	20	51
Serine	33	38	39	34	36	38	55
Proline	116	118	124	120	123	119	81
Glutamic acid	74	71	80	74	74	76	101
Glycine	329	326	307	331	319	314	308
Alanine	112	125	115	112	113	110	114
Valine	25	21	21	23	24	21	21
Half-cystine	0	0	<0.5	0	0	0	0
Methionine	5	4	3	5	5	5	7
Isoleucine	9	11	12	12	13	12	13
Leucine	24	25	27	27	25	28	28
Tyrosine	6	4	3	5	4	3	11
Phenylalanine	16	12	14	14	14	16	11
Hydroxylysine	10	9	11	9	5	6	5
Lysine	22	19	25	22	28	26	12
Histidine	5	5	—	5	6	6	5
Arginine	52	47	51	51	47	49	46

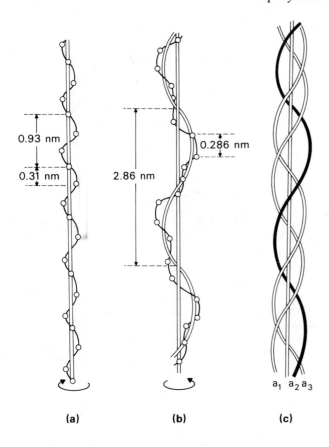

0.93 nm

0.31 nm

0.286 nm

2.86 nm

(a)

(b)

a_1 a_2 a_3

(c)

Fig. 3.26. The triple helix of collagen. (a) Single polypeptide chain wound in a left-handed helix of pitch 0.93 nm with three amino acids per turn. (b) Here the axis of the simple helix in (a) is wound in a right handed helix of pitch 2.86 nm, so that the polypeptide chain itself forms a compound helix. (c) Three units of the type shown in (b) arranged to form a triple helix called the collagen super helix. For simplicity only the three axes are shown.

As with other proteins the primary structure (amino acid sequence) determines the secondary, tertiary and quaternary forms of collagen.

In tropocollagen the three individual α-chains are further wound around each other in a right hand helix and the whole structure is called a *super helix* whose pitch is 10.4 nm (Fig. 3.26c).

The small glycine residues at every third place along each chain make this close intertwining possible, and the hydrogen bonding between the glycine peptide bonds and adjacent chains provides the inter-chain stabilization of the super helix.

This super helix occurs over 96% of the length of the macromolecules and is characterized by the triplet Gly-X-Y residue patterns. However, at the C-terminal head end of the α-chains there are regions some 25 residues in length which lack the characteristic triplet sequences and helical coiling: these are called the *telopeptide regions*. A similar telopeptide region of some 16 residues is found at the N-terminal tail ends of α-chains and it is here that considerably different sequences can be found and where collagen antigenicity is determined. This antigenic effect is more marked in the α_2 chains. The C-terminal telopeptide regions appear to determine antigenic differences between collagens of different species.

Tertiary and quaternary structures

Electron microscope pictures of collagen fibres from all higher vertebrates are characterized by regularly repeated bands (Fig. 3.27). The distance between the major bands is variously reported between 64 and 70 nm depending on the technique used in the tissue or collagen preparation. More accurate recent assessments lie in the range 67-68 nm (670–680 Å). It is possible to reconstitute· collagen fibrils from soluble tropocollagen extracts but different reagents precipitate fibrils with different bandings and spacings (Fig. 3.28; FLS & SLS collagens).

In-vitro studies on the mineralizing potential of these various artificially reconstituted collagens were important in the development of the

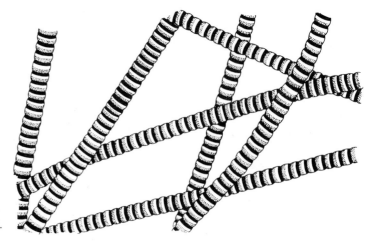

Fig. 3.27. Drawing from electron microscope picture of collagen fibrils, showing regular repeated bonds 67–68 nm apart.

seeding (nucleation) hypothesis of calcification (p. 392).

Coupled with X-ray diffraction data these observations led to the hypothesis that in native collagen protofibrils the tropocollagen macromolecules are laid longitudinally head to tail, but laterally the head of each molecule is placed back approximately one quarter the length of the neighbour at its side. This is termed the quarter-staggering array for collagen. Thus the tropocollagen heads (and tails, and other regions) are laterally aligned at repeat positions

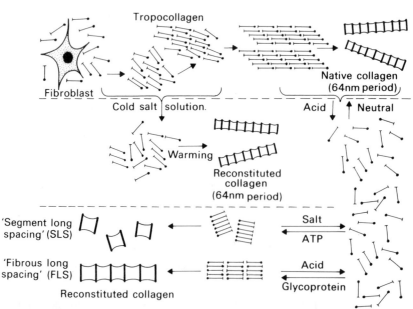

Fig. 3.28. Aggregation of tropocollagen to form collagen fibres. Tropocollagen arranges itself in parallel linear arrays in which each N-terminus is displaced by about one-quarter the length of the molecule from that on either side ("quarter-staggered"). The resulting fibres show the characteristic 64 nm spacing. If soluble, young collagen is dissolved it will realign normally if warmed.

In the presence of ATP, reaggregation occurs with the tropocollagen units in perfect register (SLS form). In the presence of glycoprotein molecules, the parallel strands may be in register but oriented randomly (FLS form). The quarter-staggered array is the normal arrangement in all native collagens. (After J. Gross (1961) *Scientific American* **204**, (May) 120).

about ¼ the length of each molecule, i.e. about 70 nm, which is the approximate major banding distance found in native collagen.

More recent studies have contributed refinements to this arrangement (Fig. 3.29). It is now envisaged that a space or 'hole' of about 61 nm in diameter separates the head from the tail of each tropocollagen molecule ahead. The length of each tropocollagen molecule is assigned 4.4 D units, where D=67 nm, and laterally each head region overlaps an adjacent tail region by 0.4 D units. These are the *hole* and *overlap* regions respectively.

This modified quarter-staggering hypothesis more exactly fits the 67 nm banding characteristic of native collagen fibrils, and it has been suggested that the hole regions may be the sites where mineralization of calcified tissues such as bone and dentine begins.

In nature tropocollagen molecules do not exist as flat sheets extending laterally indefinitely and/or lying piled upon each other. To account for the fibrillar structure of collagen it has been suggested that primary filaments are formed from 5 or 7 chains of tropocollagen molecules (each quarter-staggered in relation to its neighbours on either side). These primary filaments roll up to form hollow cylindrical filaments (p. 251).

CROSS-LINKS IN COLLAGEN

It will be recalled that in keratin fibres the polypeptide chains are joined to adjacent chains by disulphide bridges formed from cysteine residues (p. 56). The almost complete absence of cystine in native collagen means that no such $-S-S-$ bridges exist. Instead, the collagen polypeptide chains are braced and stabilized by covalent crosslinkages involving lysine and hydroxylysine residues. There are two categories of these cross-links:

1 *Intra*-molecular, which form between the three helices which constitute the tropocollagen super helix.

2 *Inter*-molecular, which link adjacent tropocollagen superhelices, and stabilize the quarter-stagger arrays.

The intra-molecular cross-links

These involve specifically located lysine or hydroxylysine side-chains whose terminal amino (NH₂) groups are first oxidised by the enzyme *lysyl oxidase* to aldehydic form, which then form covalent links between chains by an aldol type condensation reaction illustrated overleaf (Fig. 3.30).

The above example shows the intra-molecular *aldol* cross-link formed between two lysine residues from different α-chains within a single tropocollagen super-helix molecule. Since they can form between lysine or hydroxylysine side-arms there are theoretically four possible aldol type linkages between two adjacent but separate chains:

	on chain A		on chain B
1	LysCHO	to	LysCHO
2	LysCHO	to	HylCHO
3	HylCHO	to	LysCHO
4	HylCHO	to	HylCHO

Intra-molecular aldol type links occur in the non-helical 16 residue N-terminal telopeptide

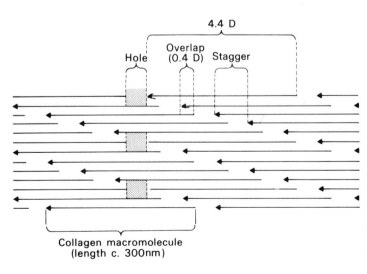

4.4 D

Hole | Overlap (0.4 D) | Stagger

Collagen macromolecule (length c. 300nm)

Fig. 3.29. Current concept of quarter-stagger alignment between tropocollagen molecules. Each molecule, 4.4D in length, has a space or *hole* 0.61 nm long, separating it from the one in front and behind it. Each molecule is also approximately ¼ staggered in relation to its neighbour by 1D (67 nm) but its head 'overlaps' the adjacent tail region by 0.4D.

α-chain A   α-chain B

AA₁   AA₁

Lys   Lys
residue   AA₂   AA₂   residue
(AA₃)   NH   H₃N⁺   N

H—C—(CH₂)₂—CH₂—CH₂—NH₃⁺   CH₂—CH₂—(CH₂)₂—CH

O=C   C=O

AA₄   AA₄

Lysyl oxidase

AA₁   AA₁

AA₂   AA₂

NH   NH

H—C—(CH₂)₂—CH₂—C   HCH—(CH₂)₂—CH

O=C   C=O

AA₄   AA₄

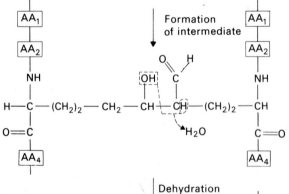

AA₁   Formation   AA₁
             of intermediate

AA₂   AA₂

NH   NH

H—C—(CH₂)₂—CH₂—CH—CH—(CH₂)₂—CH

O=C   C=O

AA₄   AA₄

Dehydration
(−H₂O)

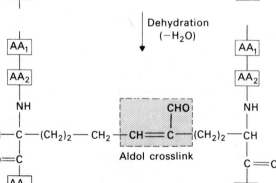

Fig. 3.30. Formation of aldol
crosslink between two collagen
α-chains.

AA₁   AA₁

AA₂   AA₂

NH   NH

H—C—(CH₂)₂—CH₂—CH=C—(CH₂)₂—CH

O=C   Aldol crosslink   C=O

AA₄   AA₄

region of α-chains. The lysine residues in position 9 near the N-terminal ends of α_1-chains, and residue position 6 in the α_2-chains are specifically involved in intra-molecular cross-links.

The inter-molecular cross-links
These types of linkage form between lysine and hydroxylysine residues in adjacent quarter-staggered tropocollagen units by means of a reaction involving the formation of a Schiff base type compound (Fig. 3.31). Here the derived aldehyde form on the side-arm of one residue reacts with the unaltered amino group on the side-arm of a nearby Lys or Hyl residue on a neighbouring α-chain.

There are therefore, theoretically, four Schiff base *aldimine* cross-link formations possible:

	on chain A		on chain B
1	LysCHO	to	NH₂Lys
2	LysCHO	to	NH₂Hyl
3	HylCHO	to	NH₂Lys
4	HylCHO	to	NH₂Hyl

Linkages of types 1, 2 and 4 have all been identified in skin collagen and it appears that type 4, known as *syndesine*, is involved as a major intermolecular cross-link in the collagens

of tendon, cartilage and bone (and presumably dentine also).

Another important cross-linkage is formed by histidine residues which first join two α-chains by an aldol cross-linkage and then form a Schiff base type link with a hydroxylysine residue from a third chain. Thus three collagen α-chains are covalently linked to one another via one histidine residue.

The inter-molecular cross-links discussed above appear to be mainly associated with maturation stages as fetal collagen changes to a young adult form. After this they reduce in number and are presumably replaced by other cross-links which account for the known ageing changes in collagen. As yet little is known of the nature of these hypothetical cross-links. It has been suggested that they may involve collagen molecules linking with the glycoproteins and proteoglycans in the ground substance.

Collagen as glycoprotein
Certain hydroxylysine residues at specific sites in tropocollagen covalently bind small amounts of hexose with the result that collagen can justifiably be classified as a glycoprotein as well as a fibrous protein. Either a galactose molecule or

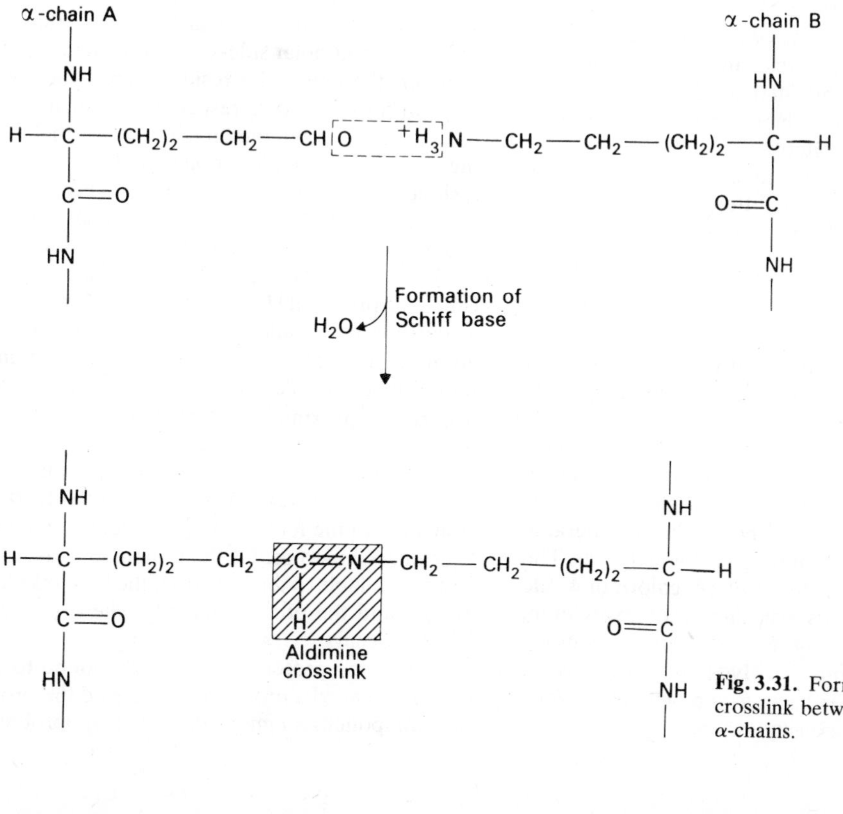

Fig. 3.31. Formation of aldimine crosslink between two collagen α-chains.

a glucose–galactose disaccharide unit joins to these residues (p. 249). The amounts vary in different tissues. Skin and tendon, for example, contain about 6 hexose residues per collagen molecule. Cartilage has 16–30/1000 amino acid residues and it is thought that this is probably related to the much higher levels of hydroxy-lysine found in this tissue. The function of these carbohydrate moieties has not been established. One suggestion is that they may link collagen to ground substance components.

PROTEINS IN ACTION II

Transport molecules, myoglobin and haemoglobin

Lower organisms such as Amoeba and Paramecium acquire their molecular O_2 by a process of simple diffusion from the environment, but this method is necessarily limited to organisms whose volume is less than 1 mm³. Evolution to higher life forms overcame this limitation with the development of circulatory systems for carrying dissolved O_2 to the various parts of the organism. This involved the associated evolution of carrier molecules to transport O_2 in much larger quantities than fully saturated water could carry.

In vertebrates these O_2 transport (or carrier) molecules are *haemoglobin* in red blood cells and *myoglobin* in muscle, and they can increase the payload up to 50–70 times. Both proteins are globular proteins as their names imply (p. 58), and since haemoglobin closely resembles an aggregation of four myoglobin-like subunits (with certain important differences) it is appropriate to begin with an account of the myoglobin molecule.

MYOGLOBIN

Myoglobin is a comparatively small protein molecule, 153 amino acid residues long (mw 17 600), and is located in muscle where its function is to store and facilitate the transport of oxygen. It is of paramount importance to diving mammals such as the whale, porpoise, seal and walrus who need a considerable reservoir of oxygen during prolonged dives. The very dark brown, almost black, colour of whale meat is due to its rich supply of myoglobin, likewise accounting for the dark colour of human heart muscle. Myoglobin contains an iron-porphyrin or haem group, where a reversible binding of oxygen occurs.

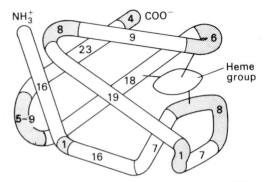

Fig. 3.32. Conformation of the myoglobin chain. The haem group is the shaded flat section at upper right. The eight straight portions are α-helical regions interrupted by seven nonhelical corners of different degrees of tightness. The numbers represent the number of amino acids in a given region. (After Loewy A.G. & Siekevitz P. (1970) *Cell structure and function*, 2nd edn. New York, Holt, Rinehart & Winston.)

The myoglobin molecule is very compact, $45 \times 35 \times 24$ Å in size, with barely sufficient space within to accommodate four water molecules. Its polypeptide chain consists of eight straight portions, each of which is a right handed α-helix, connected by seven bends at the nonhelical, random coil corner regions (Fig. 3.32). The inside of the molecule consists almost entirely of non-polar side-arms from amino acid residues, the only polar residues being the *histidine* at sites 63 and 93 respectively, which play a key role in oxygen binding. The outer shell of the molecule contains polar and non-polar residues. A Fe-haem group 'lozenge' (Fig. 3.33) sits in a cleft and is attached to the much folded protein molecule at three points, via residues 39 (Ile) and 138 (Phe) and 93 (His). The latter is called the proximal His, and the histidine residue at position 63 is called the distal His. The iron atom is centrally placed within the haem molecule and displaced slightly out of its plane towards the proximal His (93): when O_2 binds to the site on the opposite side.

The haem molecule is a planar structure made up of four substituted pyrrole rings with a central iron atom in the ferrous (Fe^{2+}) state, bonded to four nitrogen atoms. Of the remaining two valencies available to the iron atom the first links to His 93 and the other is the site where the O_2 binding occurs.

Such a non-protein group tightly bound to a protein is called a *prosthetic group* and the protein component an *apoprotein*. The apoprotein

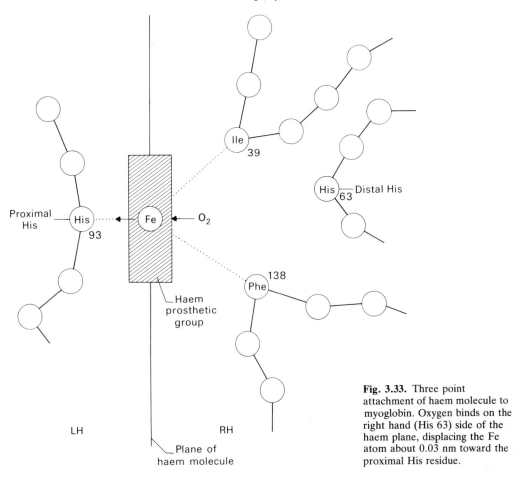

Proximal His

His 93

Fe

O_2

Ile 39

His 63 — Distal His

138 Phe

Haem prosthetic group

LH

RH

Plane of haem molecule

Fig. 3.33. Three point attachment of haem molecule to myoglobin. Oxygen binds on the right hand (His 63) side of the haem plane, displacing the Fe atom about 0.03 nm toward the proximal His residue.

part of the myoglobin molecule stabilizes the iron of the haem prosthetic group in the ferrous state, which is required for the reversible O_2 binding, whilst the haem molecule aids in determining the shape assumed by the apoprotein.

HAEMOGLOBIN

Haemoglobin is the blood-borne protein which is the carrier vehicle that transports O_2 from the lungs to the tissues. It is contained exclusively within the red blood cells, the erythrocytes, and constitutes 90% of their total protein.

Haemoglobin is an *oligomeric* globular protein (p. 52) because its quaternary structure is composed of two or more aggregated *protomer* sub-units. In fact it is made up of four such sub-units, each of which closely resembles the myoglobin conformation. Of these, two are identical α-chains (141 residues long), and two

are identical β-chains (146 residues long). Each of the four subunits contains a haem molecule identical to that in myoglobin and bound in virtually the same way. Thus there are four O_2 binding sites per haemoglobin molecule. The $\alpha_2\beta_2$ structure which constitutes *Haemoglobin A* is the primary haemoglobin in adults. Fetuses manufacture a succession of different haemoglobins. One known as *Haemoglobin F ($\alpha_2\gamma_2$)* has a much higher affinity for O_2 than Haemoglobin A and promotes the movement of O_2 across the placental barrier to the fetus.

Haemoglobin is a compact, near spherical, aggregate molecule, $6.4 \times 5.5 \times 5.0$ nm, mw 65 000. Its four protomer sub-units are packed in such a way that each of the four haem prosthetic groups lie in clefts opening to the outer surface of the oligomer (Fig. 3.34). Thus the architecture of the molecule facilitates its O_2 exchange functional property.

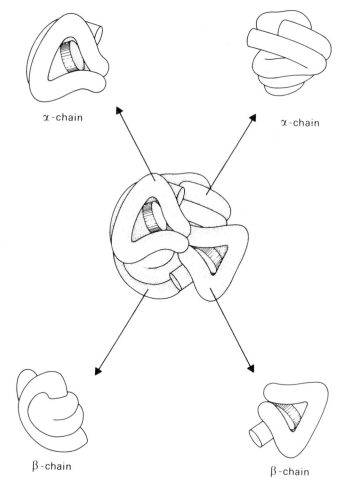

α-chain

α-chain

Fig. 3.34. A schematic drawing of adult haemoglobin. The molecule contains parts of each of two kinds of peptide chains, termed α and β, which are also shown in exploded view at the approximate orientation they have in the complete molecule. Two of the four haem units are visible in pockets formed by folds of the peptide chains. (After McGilvery R.W. (1979) *Biochemistry*, 2nd edn. New York, W. B. Saunders.)

β-chain

β-chain

Although the shapes of each of the four sub-units in haemoglobin are nearly identical to myoglobin, there are many differences between the primary amino acid sequences in each molecule. There are also differences between the primary structures of the α and β-chains in haemoglobin.

Comparison between myoglobin and the haemoglobin α and β-chain primary structures shows that only 24 of the total amino acid residue positions in the three polypeptide chains coincide. Thus very different primary sequences can form similar tertiary structures, each with the same functional properties.

The amino acid sequences of haemoglobin molecules from over 20 species have now been mapped and although considerable differences in primary structure were found, they all had the same nine amino acid residues in sequence that were important in the molecule's O_2 binding property. Thus biochemical evolution, whilst producing different primary structures for various species O_2 carrier molecules, has retained unchanged the region where the gas exchange occurs.

The differences between the structure of haemoglobin and myoglobin lead to marked differences in their O_2 dissociation curves, whose significance is described later (the Bohr effect, p. 506).

A BIOCHEMICAL DETECTIVE STORY—
THE SICKLE CELL ANAEMIA MYSTERY

The account which follows illustrates how studies on protein structure were successfully applied to the solution of a medical problem in biochemical terms. Knowledge of genetics;

primary and secondary structure of proteins; amino acid sequencing; ionization properties of amino acids; the role of polar amino acid side-arms in conformation; and use of electrophoresis and chromatographic techniques, all contributed to the final answer.

The malady

The condition of sickle cell anaemia was first reported as a distinct disease by a Chicago doctor, James Herrick, in 1910. The symptoms presented are weakness, dizziness, palpitations and dyspnoea (shortness of breath), enlarged lymph nodes, heart enlargement and murmurs and the general symptoms of anaemia (with haemoglobin counts 50% of normal). Indeed the whole blood picture is abnormal—the red blood cell (erythrocyte) count is half to one-third of normal and the number of white cells is doubled. Many of the blood cells are peculiar in shape: Herrick described them as 'irregular in shape' and noted in particular the 'large number of thin elongated sickle-shaped and crescent-shaped forms'. Hence the name *sickle cell anaemia*. It was usually a fatal disease, sufferers dying of thrombosis or cardiac or renal failure usually before they reached their thirties.

The clues

One distinctive feature was that the disease was more or less exclusively confined to the black races of the world. In Africa 60 000–80 000 children die annually and many more are incapacitated by it. A few cases occur in India (primarily in primitive tribes) and in some Mediterranean areas.

The causes of death—usually cardiac or renal failure—were found to be due to the clumping of the sickle shaped erythrocytes, especially when deoxygenation occurred, so blocking capillaries carrying blood to vital tissues. Such events, if not fatal, produce clinical crises characteristic of sickle cell patients.

Early investigations failed to trace the condition to any obvious cause as there were no related blood borne or intestinal parasites involved: no bacterial disease such as TB could be found as a causal agent. However, the red cells of sufferers were always of this curious sickle shape. It had to be, as Herrick said, due to 'some unrecognised changes in the composition of the corpuscles'.

A curious feature was that on the African continent sufferers seemed to have a greater resistance to malaria than their fellows.

The investigations

The first important piece of evidence was the establishment, 40 years after Herrick's first report, that the condition was an inheritable genetic disease. Some 8–9% of black Americans were found to be carriers of an abnormal gene although only 1 in every 70–300 manifested the disease. Some were homozygous for the condition (i.e. they had received one mutant abnormal gene from each parent, to give them a heterozygous gene state). However, individuals carrying one abnormal and one normal gene (heterozygotes) can manifest symptoms if under rather more than normal O_2 stress situations (as when flying in aircraft pressurized for an altitude of 5000 ft.). These individuals are said to show the *sickle cell trait* as only 1% of their erythrocytes are sickled compared with 50% in homozygous patients. This sickle cell trait has an important consequence in medicine and dentistry in relation to use of general anaesthesia. If given anaesthetics with attendant O_2 stress then sickle cell trait symptoms may manifest themselves. For this reason it is routine practice to carry out sickle cell blood tests on all black patients recommended for general anaesthesia.

Microscopic examination of the red cells of sickle cell patients confirms the role of low O_2 tension, because they sickle at low O_2 partial pressures. Furthermore the deoxygenated sickle cell haemoglobin (HbS) has an abnormally low solubility, 25 times less than normal deoxygenated haemoglobin A. The haemoglobin of sickle cell patients was therefore suspected as being different from normal.

Attention was next given to examination of the electrophoretic mobility patterns obtained for the haemoglobin of sickle cell anaemia patients (HbS) compared with normal (HbA). Linus Pauling and his co-workers showed in 1949 that the isoelectric points of the sickle cell oxygenated and deoxygenated HbS forms each differed by being 0.22 pH higher than their normal HbA counterparts. These results indicated that there was a difference in the number of ionizable groups in the normal and sickle cell haemoglobins. Next the acid-base titration curves were constructed for the HbA and HbS and comparisons showed that the HbS had between 2 and 4 extra positively charged groups per molecule.

The next step was to find where these charge differences were. X-ray data exonerated the haem groups as suspects as they were the same in normal and sickle erythrocytes. So this narrowed the search down to the apoprotein part of the molecule.

Preparations of HbS and HbA were then broken down to peptide fragments by digesting with the proteolytic enzyme *trypsin*. These peptides were then separated by a 2-dimensional paper chromatography/electrophoresis procedure (Fig. 3.35). The peptide mixtures from each trypsin digest (HbS and HbA) were applied to one corner of a large sheet of chromatography paper for the separation in the first dimension to be carried out by FPPC chromatography. This separated the peptides on the basis of their different relative solubilities in a mobile solvent phase (e.g. butanol or phenol) and the aqueous phase held in the paper.

Passage of the solvent resulted in a partial separation of the components in the first dimension but there were too many peptides (28) to allow complete resolution. Therefore, the paper was removed and dried and the peptides further separated in the second dimension at 90° to the first. This was achieved by passage of an electric current which separated the components, this time on the basis of their varying mobilities as determined by their net charges. A suitable pH (4 or 9) was chosen so that all or most of the peptides had a net positive charge (at pH 4) or negative charge (at pH 9) (see p. 60). On completion of development in this second dimension the paper was removed and the peptide spots visualized by the ninhydrin reaction. The result was a 2D 'fingerprint' map, of the peptide components in the digests. Fig. 3.35 shows the respective fingerprint maps obtained for tryptic digests of HbA and HbS.

Each map contained 28 peptide spots but with one difference—the peptide in position X in the HbA digest was absent in the HbS digest but a new peptide in position Y was present in its stead. The two peptides, X from HbA and Y from HbS digests, were isolated and analysed. They each contained 8 amino acids but differed in their valine and glutamic acid content levels.

Futher investigations showed the the difference in HbS resided in the β-chains and sequencing of the two peptides X and Y showed the following:

```
        1     2     3     4     5     6     7     8
```

X peptide (from HbA)
    Val−His−Leu−Thr−Pro−Glu−Glu−Lys
Y peptide (from HbS)
    Val−His−Leu−Thr−Pro−Val−Glu−Lys

Thus the only difference between HbA and HbS was in the switch from glutamic acid in HbA

to valine in the abnormal HbS at position 6 of the peptide. Subsequently it was shown that this was also the position of residue 6 in thé Hb β-chain itself: thus the X and Y peptides constituted the first 6 residues from the N-terminal valine end of the polypeptide chain.

The genetic mutation responsible for this switch changed the normal polar positively-charged glutamyl residue side-arm to a non-polar aliphatic valine side-arm. It is thought that

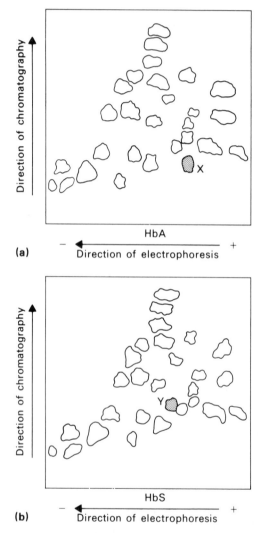

Fig. 3.35. Peptide 'fingerprint' maps of tryptic digests of (a) normal haemoglobin (HbA) and (b) sickle cell haemoglobin (HbS). The only difference is the appearance of the peptide Y in the HbS digest and the corresponding absence of peptide X found in digests of the normal haemoglobin, HbA. This is due to the substitution in X of one valine residue for a glutamic acid residue.

this Val in HbS joins with the N-terminal Val to form a hydrophobic association, causing the HbS conformation to distort. This produces an area known as a 'sticky patch' on the HbS molecules which considerably reduces the solubility of their deoxidized forms and also causes them to form long aggregations that disrupt the cell to produced the characteristic sickle shape. In turn this sickling leads to red cell clumping and when this leads to capillary blockage a local area of O_2 lack is set up, encouraging the further formation of deoxy HbS with more sickling and clumping. Thus a kind of chain reaction effect is set up with the blockage becoming progressively larger and more severe.

The solution

Thus the mystery was solved. Sickle cell anaemia with all its manifest unpleasant symptoms and consequences was due to just one amino acid being changed in the synthesis of the 146 residue long β-chains of the Hb oligomer. But like most true mystery stories there still remain ends to draw together and problems left to explain. How, for instance, does the possession of the genetic defect actually protect against malaria? This is as yet unanswered but the curious consequence is a preserving of the mutant gene in African populations. Although homozygous sickle cell anaemia patients will have mostly died young, the heterozygotes (showing the 'sickle cell trait') have a protective selective advantage over their normal fellows against the highly lethal indigenous forms of malaria. Thus their survival rate against malaria is better and the recessive HbS gene is maintained and passed on from generation to generation.

The cure?

There are reports that some African tribes drink cow's urine to ameliorate the disease! There may just be a method in this apparent madness. The urine contains urea, a well-known protein denaturant and H-bond breaker. There is just the possibility that this may be helping to reduce the hydrophobic Val–Val interactions which presumably cause the insolubility of HbS, for quite independently some medical workers have proposed a high urea ingestion therapy for the condition.

More recently low concentrations of potassium cyanate (KCNO 5×10^{-3} M) have been shown to inhibit the sickling of sickle cells and it is suggested that this acts by blocking the N-terminal Val 1 of HbS β-chains so breaking

its hydrophobic association with the aberrant Val 6. Whether this therapy can assist sickle cell anaemia patients without causing toxic side effects is the subject of contemporary studies.

Other abnormal haemoglobin mutants

The sickle cell anaemia case is but one of over 150 similar mutants where abnormal haemoglobins of genetic origin are known—mostly shown to be due to single amino acid changes in protein synthesis. These have been detected using the fingerprinting and sequencing studies described above. It has been estimated that about 0.5% of the population carries a mutant haemoglobin form.

PROTEINS IN ACTION III

Defence agents

THE IMMUNOGLOBULINS

Strip electrophoresis of the proteins present in plasma separates them into six major fractions (Fig. 3.36, Table 3.7).

Of these the γ-globulin fraction includes most of the heterogeneous group of proteins, the immunoglobulins (Ig), involved in body defence mechanisms against pathologic effects due to foreign proteins and other macromolecules associated with invading pathogens (the antigens). In response to a specific antigen stimulus appropriately constructed immunoglobulins are synthesized (the antibodies), tailor-made to combine with and so activate the destruction of the specific antigens involved.

Ultracentrifugation, chromatographic and electrophoretic techniques, have now shown that millions of different immunoglobulins are contained within the human γ-globulin fraction. These fall into five major groups—IgG, IgA, IgM, IgD and IgE.

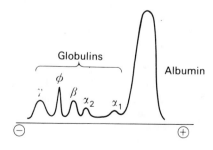

Fig. 3.36. Densitometric tracing of normal plasma protein electrophoretogram.

Table 3.7. The protein components of blood plasma.

Plasma protein	As % of total protein	Some functions
Albumins	50–60	Osmoregulation: transport of organic ions
α_1–globulins	4–7	Binding and transport of thyroxine and corticosterone: fat transport (high density lipo-proteins)
α_2–globulins	7–12	Haemoglobin transport: Cu^{3+} transport
β –globulins	9–15	Binding and transport of Fe^{3+}: fat transport (low density lipo-proteins)
Fibrinogen (ϕ)	7	Blood clotting
γ –globulins	13–20	Antibody reactions

Each immunoglobulin molecule is constructed of four polypeptide chains held together by numerous intra- and inter-chain disulphide bonds and noncovalent forces (Fig. 3.37). Each molecule consists of two identical 'light' chains (mw 23 000 c. 200 residues). The molecules are glycoproteins, glycosylated at various points on the heavy chains and contains 3–13% total carbohydrate (Table 3.8). Antigens bind to the N-terminal regions.

The heavy chains are divided into five types on the basis of their amino acid sequences, each one corresponding to an Ig class as follows:

Heavy chain type	*Ig Class*
α (alpha)	A (IgA)
μ (mu)	M (IgM)
γ (gamma)	G (IgG)
δ (delta)	D (IgD)
ϵ (epsilon)	E (IgE)

Light chains are of two types only, κ (kappa) and λ (lambda) also on the basis of amino acid sequence. Either type can associate with each of the heavy chain types. The κ:λ ratio is species-specific, the figures for human and mouse sera, for example, being 2:1 and 20:1 respectively.

The different Ig classes are made up of subunit aggregates in much the same manner as haemoglobin is oligomeric (p. 52).: thus IgG exists in a monomer form whereas IgM is a pentameric molecule (Fig. 3.39). The five Ig classes have different biological functions.

Immunoglobulin G (IgG)
This, the major class of antibody in serum, is a monomeric molecule and is important in the secondary response to antigen. It is the only Ig capable of crossing the placenta to help protect the fetus against infection in the early weeks of life.

The structure of IgG was elucidated by Porter and Edelman (1972), and this classic and elegant work forms the basis of our understanding of immunoglobulin structure and function.

Incubation of IgG with the proteolytic enzyme papain split the molecule into three fragments. Two were identical (mw 52 000), still contained the antigen binding sites and were therefore termed the Fab fragments (fragment-antigen-binding). The third fragment, Fc (fragment-crystallizable), mw 48 000, constituted the remaining core of the molecule (Fig. 3.38). Further investigations using other proteolytic enzymes and disulphide bond reduction led to the formulation of the Ig structure represented in Fig. 3.37.

Immunoglobulin M (IgM)
This large molecule, composed of five Ig sub-units (Fig. 3.39c), is important as an early line of defence in the body's response to infection (the primary response). It is present in serum and in monomer form on the surface of certain lymphocytes it plays a role in the initial recognition of an antigen as alien.

Immunoglobulin A (IgA)
IgA occurs in serum as a monomer and a dimeric form, secretory IgA, is found in saliva and other secretions of the gastro-intestinal tract, in tears, in nasal fluids and in mother's milk (Fig. 3.39). It helps defend the exposed external surfaces of the body from colonization by microorganisms, and in this context it has been suggested that salivary IgA may prevent bacteria from adhering to the enamel surface: alternatively it may act by preventing formation of dextran in dental plaque through inhibition of microbial glucosyl transferase activity. The formation of the highly branched dextran polymers of glucose by these microbial enzymes is considered to be a major determinant in dental caries, giving adhesive and cohesive properties to dental plaque.

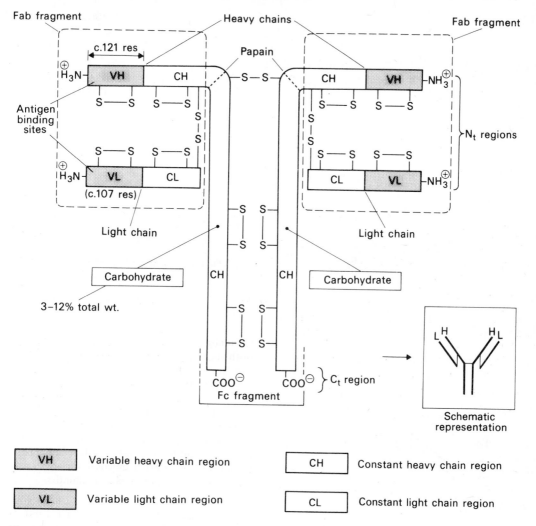

Fig. 3.37. Structure of an immunoglobulin molecule.

Table 3.8. Properties of the five major immunoglobulin classes.

WHO designation	IgG	IgA	IgM	IgD	IgE
Molecular weight	150 000	160 000 + dimer (390 000)	900 000 (pentamer)	185 000	200 000
Carbohydrate content (%)	3	8	12	13	12
Concentration in normal serum (mg/cm³)	8–16	1.4–4	0.5–2	0–0.4	$17–450 \times 10^{-6}$
Concentration in unstimulated whole saliva (mg/100cm³)	1.4	19.4	0.2	trace	trace

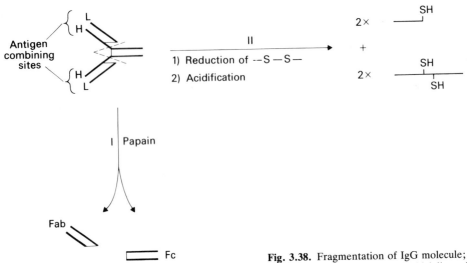

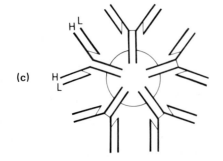

Fig. 3.38. Fragmentation of IgG molecule; polypeptide chains indicated by thick lines, disulphide bonds by thin lines.

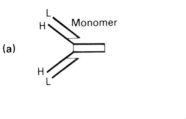

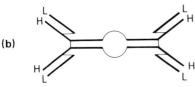

Immunoglobulins D and E (IgD, IgE)

Both are only minor components of serum. IgD, together with IgM, may be involved in lymphocyte activation and suppression. IgE molecules bind to mast cells which degranulate on contact with antigen, and in this manner grass pollen as antigen (or allergen) causes hay fever in susceptible individuals. However, the normal role of IgE is thought to be in assisting IgA in the protection of the external mucosal surfaces from infection by such parasites as helminths.

THE GENERATION OF ANTIBODY DIVERSITY

The N-terminal regions of both heavy and light chains exhibit considerable variation of amino acid sequences, whereas the C-terminal portions have a relatively constant primary structure. The capacity to bind specifically to a particular antigen arises from the variation in amino acid sequence in *variable* regions of both heavy and light chains (V_H and V_L). Other 'effector' properties

Fig. 3.39. Schematic representation of polymeric human immunoglobulins. Polypeptide chains indicated by thick lines, disulphide bonds by thin lines. (a) Serum IgA (dimer), (b) Secretory IgA (dimer), (c) IgM (pentamer). (After Fudenberg H.H. *et al* (1980) *Basic and Clinical Immunology*, 3rd edn. Los Altos, Calif., Lange.)

of antibody, for example activation of complement or macrophage binding, are determined by the regions of *contant* amino acid sequence.

It has been estimated that the immune system has a potential repertoire of between 10^7 and 10^8 different antibody molecules, and this figure provides a potential range of defence against the total universe of all possible antigen structures, as required.

In protein synthesis (p. 238) the formation of a specific protein structure is determined by a corresponding specific gene polynucleotide structure in the form of a code in the chromosomal DNA (p. 244). In the human, heavy and light Ig chains are coded for on different chromosomes: furthermore the individual H or L polypeptide chains are each coded for by more than one gene. A V gene codes for the variable portion of a particular polypeptide chain (V_H or V_L) and a C gene codes for its portion of constant amino acid sequence (C_H or C_L).

Part of the diverse potential range of the antibody repertoire arises from the fact that there can be as many as 400 different V genes for each C gene. In embryonic cells the V and C gene loci are separated from each other by considerable lengths of DNA molecule. As the embryo develops and lymphocytes differentiate, much of the DNA molecule between the V and C gene loci is spliced out. This occurs at various positions along the DNA molecule, resulting in the production of a corresponding number of different B lymphocyte cell lines each differing from the other in that a different one of the 400 V genes is juxtaposed to the same C gene. Ultimately this results in 10^7–10^8 different B lymphocyte cell-lines (or clones) being present in the adult, each one with a unique immunoglobulin molecular structure as determined by its specific V_H and V_L primary structures.

With each of these Ig molecules uniquely associated with a single cell line capable of synthesizing a particular antibody shape there is, therefore, a range of 10^7–10^8 different Ig forms potentially available. This is more than enough to match any variant of antigenic structure which may present. When this occurs that specific B lymphocyte clone capable of producing the Ig structure matching the antigen concerned is 'triggered' in some way so that it selectively grows up and synthesizes increasing amounts of the appropriate antibody.

PROTEINS IN ACTION IV

As catalysts: the enzymes

Probably the most important general category of proteins in living matter is that group involved with the catalysis of the innumerable metabolic chemical reactions which underly the activities of living matter. These biological catalysts, the enzymes, are all proteins constructed from the same 20 or so amino acids that constitute other proteins. Each enzyme has its characteristic primary, secondary and tertiary, and sometimes quaternary, structure whose design and conformation biochemical evolution has shaped so that each can catalyse a particular chemical reaction. Enzymes differ from simple catalysts, as involved in laboratory and industrial chemical reactions, in their much higher degree of specificity, with enzyme catalysts limited in most instances to reaction with one or two specific substances, or at most a few closely-related compounds. With these restrictions a very fine control of metabolic processes is attained. Enzymes such as *urease*, act only on certain substances (i.e. urea) whereas the proteolytic digestive enzymes such as *pepsin* and *trypsin* have a broader specificity, hydrolysing peptide bonds in various proteins: even so the peptide bonds attacked have specificity in that they involve only specific types of amino acids.

The substance(s) involved in the specific reaction catalysed by a particular enzyme is called the enzyme's *substrate*. Thus urea is the substrate for the enzyme *urease*.

It is probable that man's first intensive interest in enzyme activity dates from the discovery that a ferment of yeast converted grape juice into wine. For many centuries, indeed millenia, he was apparently more interested in the product and its effect on human metabolism and behaviour, than the exact nature of the agencies producing this remarkable brew. Ultimately however it was man turning his attention to the fermentation process which gave birth to modern enzymology.

In 1835 a Swedish chemist Jan Jacob Berzelius first coined the term catalysis to describe the phenomenon whereby reactions were made to go more quickly. He cited a number of instances of chemical catalysis but also included some biological examples, notably that an extract from potatoes broke down starch more quickly than strong acids. With remarkable insight he predicted that virtually all reactions occurring in living matter were probably catalysed.

These observations led to the 'vital force'

controversy culminating in a long drawn out argument between the German chemist Justus von. Liebig (of the condenser), and the French chemist Louis Pasteur (of 'pasteurization') whose later work formed the basis for fermentation chemistry and the germ theory of disease. Pasteur claimed catalysis was the property of intact living cells only (a vital force) whereas Leibig found that plant tissue extracts were capable of biological catalysis (a mechanistic action).

It was around this time (1878) that the German, Kühne, coined the word enzym (from the Greek for 'in yeast') to indicate the source of these fermentation catalysts, and the anglicized form enzyme entered the English vocabulary three years later.

In 1897 Edward Buchner (of the funnel) and his brother Hans broke up yeast cells by grinding them with sand and obtained a cell free extract capable of fermenting sugar, thus settling the vital force controversy in favour of Liebig's mechanistic interpretation. From this simple experiment developed the 50–60 year explosion of biochemical exploration during which hundreds of enzymes were isolated, purified, even crystallized, and their mode of action and structure elucidated. The ensuing text is concerned with the main features of these discoveries.

Nomenclature and units of activity

Most enzymes have a common name indicating the nature of the substrate catalysed. Duclaux in 1898 proposed the elegantly simple suggestion that each enzyme be named by adding the suffix '-ase' to the name of its substrate. Thus *urease* catalyses the hydrolysis of urea to NH_3 and CO_2 and *collagenase* hydrolyses peptide bonds in collagen substrates.

The reactions catalysed by enzymes may also be designated more generally. For example, the group of *oxido-reductases* which includes a large number of enzymes concerned with various types of oxidation and reduction reactions, of which a specific example is *lactic dehydrogenase (LDH)* catalysing the reversible removal of two H atoms from lactic acid to form pyruvic acid.

$$CH_3CH(OH)COOH \xrightarrow[LDH]{2H} CH_3-\overset{O}{\overset{\|}{C}}-COOH$$

Lactic acid   Pyruvic acid

However, many enzymes still have trivial names which are chemically uninformative—such as the proteolytic digestive enzymes *pepsin, trypsin* and *chymotrypsin*. With the ever

growing number of enzymes discovered, it became necessary to formulate a rational and unambiguous system for naming them. This was achieved by an International Enzyme Commission (EC) set up in 1956 whose proposals were adopted in final form by the International Union of Biochemistry (IUB) in 1964.

Each enzyme is first referred to one of the six major categories listed in the left-hand column of Table 3.9. These six groups are each divided into subclasses relating to the reaction catalysed: subclasses then further define the reaction details. In this way each enzyme is assigned an unambiguous classification number. The EC also recommended that each enzyme be given (or retain) a short everyday use recommended name and in addition a more specific systematic name to indicate the nature of the reaction catalysed by the enzyme.

The first row of Table 3.9 will suffice to illustrate the above principles. In the last column *lactic dehydrogenase* is shown as the common usage name of an oxidoreductase enzyme (main class 1) which acts on the $-CH(OH)-$ groups in specific molecules (subclass 1) and requires a coenzyme NAD (placing it in sub-subclass 1). Lactic acid is the 27th substrate listed under this sub-subclass in the IUB tables. Hence its classification number 1.1.1.27. Its systematic name is L-Lactate:NAD oxidoreductase.

Enzyme activities are expressed in terms of international units (I.U.); one I.U. is the amount of enzyme which will catalyse (under standard conditions) one μmol of substrate per minute. A new unit now recommended by the IUB is the *katal* (kat.) which is the quantity of enzyme that converts one mole per second of substrate to product (1 kat. = 6×10^7 I.U. : 1 I.U. = 16.67 nanokat).

How enzymes work

As indicated above, enzymes are proteins specially constructed so that they are able to catalyse changes in other compounds. How is this achieved and what environmental factors and specific properties of the enzyme determine the specificity of the reactions involved? Various features of the structure and properties of enzyme molecules which account for their specific catalytic functions are discussed below.

LOWERING THE ACTIVATION ENERGY OF A REACTION

The significant property of enzymes is their ability to make reactions in living matter proceed

Table 3.9. Enzyme classification and nomenclature.

Main class	Reactions catalysed	Subclass examples	Sub-subclass examples	Examples of specific enzymes with common name (and classification number)
1. Oxidoreductase	Oxidation–reduction	1.1. Acting on CH(OH) group of donors	1.1.1. With NAD or NADP as acceptor	Lactic dehydrogenase (1.1.1.27)
		1.4. Acting on CH–NH$_2$ group of donors	1.4.3. With O$_2$ as acceptor	Amino acid oxidase (1.4.3.2)
2. Transferases	Transfer of groups from one molecule to another	2.1. Transfer of C$_1$ containing groups	2.1.1. Transfer of methyl (CH$_3$) group	Guanidoacetate methyl transferase (2.1.1.2)
		2.6. Transfer of N-containing groups	2.6.1. Transfer of amino groups	Aspartate amino transferase (transaminase) (2.6.1.1)
3. Hydrolyases	Hydrolysis of bonds	3.4. Cleaving peptide bonds	3.4.4. Peptidases	Pepsin (3.4.4.1)
4. Lyases	Non-hydrolytic cleavage of bonds	4.1. –C–C– lyases	4.1.1. Carboxyl group removal	Pyruvic decarboxylase (4.1.1.1)
5. Isomerases	Intramolecular rearrangements	5.1. Racemases and epimerases	5.1.1. Amino acids and derivatives	5.1.1.1. Alanine racemase
6. Ligases or synthetases	Formation of bonds with utilization of energy	6.3. Forming C–N bonds	6.3.2. Amino acid ligases	Glutathione synthetase (6.3.2.3)

briskly, under relatively mild conditions, around neutral pH and temperatures of 0–40°C, which, uncatalysed, would be so slow as to be virtually nonexistent. Some of the increases in reaction rates achieved by enzymes are numerically astronomical in size. Thus *carbonic anhydrase*—an important enzyme in red blood cells involved with respiration (p. 507) catalyses the reaction:

$$CO_2 + H_2O \underset{\text{Carbonic anhydrase}}{\rightleftharpoons} H_2CO_3$$

Without the rapid transfer of CO$_2$ from tissues to the blood by the forward reaction, and its subsequent expiration from the lungs by the reverse reaction, respiration would be sluggish and incomplete. Carbonic anhydrase is one of the fastest acting enzymes known; one enzyme molecule joins six million molecules of CO$_2$ and H$_2$O in one second! The catalysed rate is 10 million times faster than the uncatalysed. Similarly the enzyme *catalase* is required to rapidly destroy hydrogen peroxide, H$_2$O$_2$, produced in some metabolic reactions (p. 219) and a potential hazard to life processes if not immediately converted to some harmless form.

$$2H_2O_2 \underset{\text{Catalase}}{\rightleftharpoons} 2H_2O + O_2$$

Each catalase molecule deals with some 5 million molecules of H$_2$O$_2$ a minute, an acceleration of 10^{14} over the uncatalysed rate.

The catalytic power of enzymes is therefore prodigious. How is this achieved?

For chemical reactions to proceed two things must happen: firstly the reactants involved must come together in correct orientation and secondly they must possess sufficient energy to bring about the breaking (or forming) of the bonds involved. The reaction has to go through a transition state which has higher energy than either the substrate A or the product B. Thus for the reaction A⟶B to proceed as in Fig. 3.40a an intermediate energy hump or barrier (*the activation energy*) has to be surmounted in order to bring about bond breakage to form the product(s) B. The energy of the system after this reaction is less than at the start, the difference being the *energy of reaction*. The reaction can only proceed if sufficient energy is introduced into the system to ride over the activation energy barrier and one way of achieving this is to add

heat energy so raising the temperature of the system. By increasing their thermal energy and motion more molecules are able to enter the transition state. A 10°C rise in temperature will approximately double the reaction rate. However life processes operate within fairly narrow temperature ranges and sharp increases beyond these are usually destructive and therefore not desirable.

With living matter the activation energy barrier is made easier to surmount by lowering its value for a particular reaction, and this is achieved by the intermediate combination of enzyme(E) with its substrate(S). Fig. 3.40b shows how in the enzyme catalysed reaction the E_{Act} energy hump barrier is reduced to E'_{Act}. It is important to note that the energy of reaction, i.e. the energy difference between the beginning and

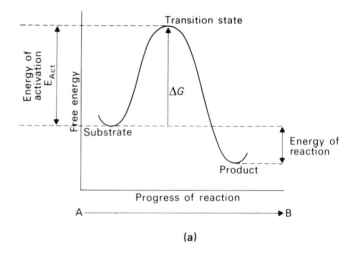

(a)

Fig. 3.40. Energy states and changes associated with catalysed and non-catalysed reaction A→B. The energy of activation, E_{Act}, barrier is much less in the catalysed reaction, although the energy of reaction (difference of energy states before and after reaction) is the same.

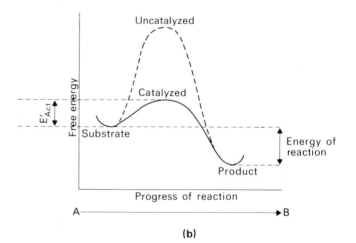

(b)

end of the reaction A——→B, is the same whether the reaction is catalysed or not.

In other words the enzyme-substrate union allows the same reaction to proceed via a new transition state which has a much lower activation energy value.

THE ENZYME-SUBSTRATE COMPLEX

As indicated the catalytic effect of enzymes is achieved through an intermediary union of enzyme and substrate molecules, represented as follows:

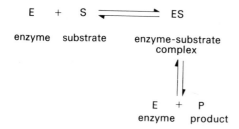

The concept of a specific union of substrate and enzyme was originally put forward by Emil Fischer in 1894 who postulated his *lock and key* model to explain enzyme specificity long before the actual nature of enzymes was understood. The model conceived an enzyme molecule fitting its substrate as a key fits a lock. Similarly shaped locks may take the enzyme key but not be able to turn. Only the enzyme key whose notches exactly fit the substrate lock can turn the tumblers and in the analogy catalyse the specific reaction.

The first experimental evidence for an enzyme–substrate union occurring came in 1936 when it was shown that mixing of an enzyme with its substrate was accompanied by a change in light absorption properties of the solution, a change which was reversed by addition of agents known to reverse the enzyme reaction involved. This was strong presumptive evidence for occurrence of an E–S combination but only in recent years has it been convincingly demonstrated by electron microscopy and X-ray crystallography that E–S complexes are actually formed. Furthermore kinetic analysis of enzyme action, which will be discussed shortly, necessarily involves the assumption that an E–S complex is formed and the theoretical results derived from this assumption are fully in accord with the experimental data from studies on enzyme activity.

The lock and key analogy provides a basis for an understanding of the very high degree of specificity of most individual enzymes, which can distinguish not only between similarly shaped molecules but even between the D and L configurations of the same molecule.

More recent studies suggest that the docking of substrate with enzyme is not initially the direct fit of one rigidly shaped molecule (the substrate) into an equally rigidly shaped mould of it on some part of the enzyme surface. Instead it is now considered that the shape of the key (more like a pocket) on the enzyme surface is a rather more flexible structure which does not match the substrate in an exactly complementary fashion until after the substrate has been bound. In effect the substrate induces the enzymic pocket shape to fit it perfectly as it combines with it. This process of dynamic recognition is termed the *induced-fit* model of E–S union, to distinguish it from the earlier more rigid lock and key model. Fig. 3.41 illustrates the essential differences between the older and more recent concepts. This more flexible structure, the induced fit model, also suggests how changes in enzyme shape induced by the substrate may bring active groups on the enzyme surface to their optimum positions for the most effective catalysis of a reaction (Fig. 3.42). This 'induced fit' hypothesis can explain, therefore, why larger or smaller analogue compounds, though very similar to the true substrate, either may not be acted on by the enzyme at all, or may be catalysed at lower reaction rates.

THE ACTIVE SITES OF ENZYMES

The specific recessed pocket region of an enzyme molecule which is involved in the E–S combination is called the *active site* of the enzyme. It is at this site that the catalysed reaction occurs. It has been suggested that the active site binds the substrate and enzyme in mutually strained forms which lowers the energy of the transition state for reaction (Fig. 3.40), so easing the pathway over the activation energy barrier.

The active site is small in relation to the total size of the whole enzyme. In those enzymes whose structures have been studied in detail the active sites have been found to consist of recessed grooves, or pockets on the molecule surface shaped from many different parts of the intricately folded polypeptide primary structure of the enzyme involved. In lysozyme for example, the active site is a long thin recessed groove on the surface which contains groupings from residues 35, 52, 62, 63, and 101 of the primary structure sequence exactly folded into this

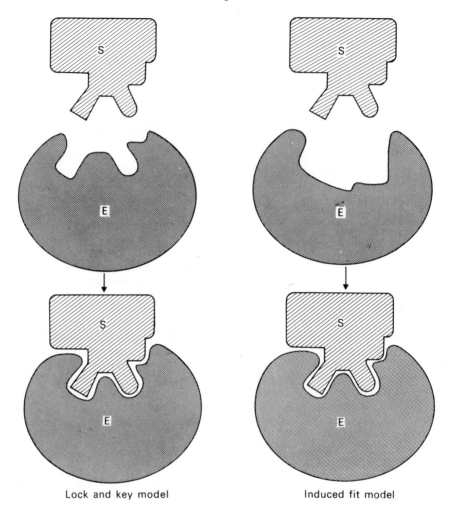

Lock and key model   Induced fit model

Fig. 3.41. 'Lock and key' and 'induced fit' models of enzyme-substrate union.

groove on the tertiary structure surface of the long polypeptide chain (129 amino acids) of the enzyme (Fig. 3.43).

In all known enzyme examples the cleft or crevice of the active site is dominated by hydrophobic amino acid residue side-arms, which ensures the exclusion of water, an important factor in the binding of substrate to enzyme. However these active sites do include residues with polar side-arms, essential for binding the substrate, and for the catalysis mechanism.

Some authorities distinguish the binding or specificity sites concerned with the substrate recognition from the active site region where the actual catalysis occurs. However these binding sites generally overlap with a part of the active site. Thus the actual catalysis site on lysozyme is only a small central region of the long grooved recess (Fig. 3.43). The rest of the groove contains the binding or specificity sites. It is probably simpler to consider the active site as embracing both functions.

The exclusive ability to recognize and catalyse only one of a pair of enantiomers is readily understood in terms of the specific form of one of the optically active isomers as being the only one capable of fitting the corresponding mould at the active site on the enzyme surface. Less easy to explain is how a substrate without an asymmetric carbon atom, such as glycerol, is

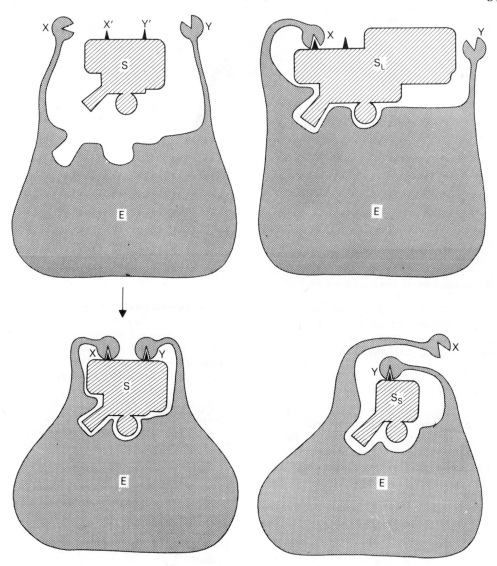

Fig. 3.42. The induced fit model of enzyme-substrate union. The induced fit model envisages E–S union as also bringing important active groups X and Y on the enzyme molecule into 'correct' orientation with the right substrate (S) but not with the closely related small (S_S) and larger substrate (S_L) analogues.

phosphorylated on only one of its $-CH_2OH$ groups by *glycerolkinase* in the formation of glycerol–3–phosphate. In other words, how can symmetric molecules apparently behave asymmetrically? The answer is provided by the hypothesis that such substrates have a *3-point attachment* to the enzyme surface (Fig. 3.44). With such an orientation it can be seen that only one of the substrate's primary alcoholic groups will be involved at the active site.

THE FORCES BINDING ENZYME–SUBSTRATE COMPLEXES

The forces that can bind enzyme to substrate in the E–S complex are the same as those which maintain the conformations of proteins (p. 46). These are: *electrostatic forces* between oppositely charged sites on both participants; *hydrogen bonding*—of which enzymes are a rich potential source; and the weaker *Van der Waals*

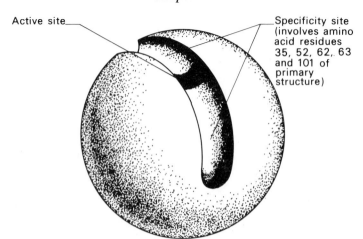

Active site

Specificity site
(involves amino
acid residues
35, 52, 62, 63
and 101 of
primary
structure)

Fig. 3.43. Representation of the active site 'groove' of lysozyme, this 'recognises' the molecules that can react. The *active* (or catalytic) *site* is a small part of the groove where the reaction is catalysed. The term *active*

site is often used to describe the binding and catalysis sites together. (After Yudkin M. & Offord R. (1973) *Comprehensible Biochemistry*. London, Longman.)

forces. The latter are particularly important as the close steric fit between substrate and enzyme provides the opportunity for numbers of these short distance attractions and repulsions to occur.

COFACTORS AND COENZYMES IN ENZYME ACTION

Some enzymes require a non-proteinaceous partner, a cofactor, for their catalytic function. Inorganic examples include metal ions such as manganese (Mn^{2+}), magnesium (Mg^{2+}), zinc (Zn^{2+}), iron (Fe^{2+} : Fe^{3+}) etc. which are essential for the activity of the enzyme. These may form coordination complexes, important in maintain-

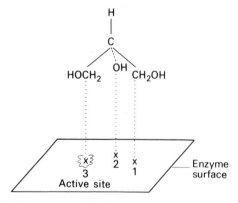

Fig. 3.44. The three-point attachment of glycerol to the glycerokinase enzyme surface. Each alcohol group binds to a separate site, only one of which (3) is active as far as phosphorylation is concerned (the active site). There is only one way in which the glycerol can bind in this manner.

ing specific structural features of an enzyme at its active site, or they may help link substrate directly to enzyme. Such enzymes are sometimes referred to as *metalloenzymes*. In many *in vitro* studies it is necessary to add small amounts of a specific metal ion cofactor before the enzyme will act. An example is the enzyme *enolase* in glycolysis which catalyses the formation of phosphoenol pyruvate from 2-phosphoglycerate (p. 185) and requires Mg^{2+} for its activation. One hypothesis put forward to explain the action of fluoride in limiting dental decay suggests that the fluoride forms an insoluble complex with Mg^{2+} ion so inactivating the enzyme and limiting glycolysis by oral bacteria on the tooth surface. This reduces the quantity of lactic and other fermentation acids formed, the products thought mainly responsible for dental decay (Volume 3).

Coenzymes are relatively small, non-proteinaceous organic cofactor molecules which play a key role in the reaction mechanisms of certain enzymes. For example *lactic dehydrogenase* (LDH) requires a coenzyme NAD^+ (nicotinamide adenine dinucleotide) for its catalytic removal of two hydrogen atoms from lactic acid to form pyruvate. In the process NAD^+ is reduced to NADH which is then regenerated by another oxido/reductase system and recycled for a repeat performance. By this means coenzymes can couple separate enzyme reactions. In the glycolysis–fermentation pathway, the LDH system is linked by NAD/NADH to the triosephosphate dehydrogenase enzyme (see Fig. 4.16).

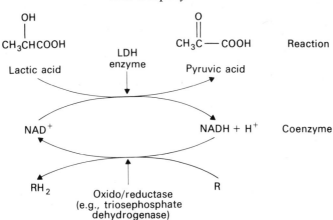

Note that one of the two hydrogen atoms from lactic acid goes to form NADH and one is released as H^+. Electroneutrality is maintained because the loss of the positive charge on NAD^+ is balanced by appearance of an H^+ ion. Thus the NAD/NADH coenzyme system is a hydrogen carrier-system essential for the functioning of the LDH dehydrogenation mechanism.

When a coenzyme is involved, the enzyme must bind the coenzyme close to or at its active site, because the coenzyme, in essence, functions as a cosubstrate.

Coenzymes by definition are readily separable from their enzyme by dialysis, but some enzymes have their cofactors firmly (covalently) attached and are not removable by dialysis. In the latter situation the coenzyme is referred to as the *prosthetic group* of the enzyme (as the haem group in haemoglobin (p. 72) is a prosthetic

group for that molecule). The functional differentiation between a coenzyme and a prosthetic group is made solely on the basis of its separation by dialysis.

An enzyme molecule with an attached prosthetic group is termed the *holoenzyme*, but when denuded of its prosthetic group, and hence inactive, it is called the *apoenzyme*.

Some enzymes may require both organic coenzymes and inorganic metal ions as their cofactors in order to function.

An important example of a coenzyme as a prosthetic group is the pyridoxal phosphate attached to *transaminase* (*aminotransferase*) enzymes: these catalyse transfer of an amino group from an amino acid to a keto(oxo-) acid to form another amino acid (p. 217). In this system the coenzyme acts as an amino group carrier, and is transiently changed to its amino form pyridoxamine phosphate in the process:

CH$_3$—C(H)(NH$_2$)—COOH

Alanine

CH$_3$—C(=O)—COOH

Pyruvic acid

Pyridoxal-(P)
(—CHO group)

Pyridoxamine-(P)
(—NH$_2$ group)

Transaminase
(amino transferase)

COOH
|
CH$_2$
|
H$_2$N—C—H
|
COOH

Aspartic acid

COOH
|
CH$_2$
|
O=C
|
COOH

Oxalacetic acid

The alanine substrate combines with the transaminase–pyridoxal–Ⓟ complex and first transfers its α-amino group to the prosthetic group to form pyridoxamine–Ⓟ.

In this process the amino acid is converted to the keto acid, pyruvic acid. A second keto acid, e.g. oxaloacetic acid, then picks up the –NH₂ group from the pyridoxamine–Ⓟ to form aspartic acid. This latter reaction regenerates the pyridoxal–Ⓟ ready for the next alanine molecule transamination.

The relationship between coenzymes and vitamins

It is an important fact that most coenzymes are closely related structurally to a specific vitamin. For example, the NAD^+ coenzyme for LDH is derived from the B group vitamin *niacin* (or nicotinic acid) (p. 813), and the pyridoxal of transaminases is formed from *pyridoxine* (vitamin B6) (p. 814). Neither coenzyme can be synthesized directly by the body and their structural cores have to be supplied by the corresponding essential components in the diet. The symptoms of vitamin deficiency are related to impaired or lost function of the enzymes requiring the missing coenzyme.

Table 3.10 lists some important vitamin–coenzyme relationships with their related functions and the disease states associated with the vitamin deficiency.

THE EFFECT OF pH ON ENZYMES: OPTIMUM pH

The majority of animal enzymes are active in the range pH 6–8 where pH shifts will not affect the positively charged side-arm ε-amino groups (pK$_a$ values 9–10) or negatively charged γ-carboxyl groups (pK$_a$ values 3–4) (Table 3.5, p. 64). An earlier section has discussed the ionization of these charged proton donor and acceptor sites on protein residue side-chains (p. 61). The presence of these charged sites at strategic positions on the enzyme surface plays a vital role in anchoring the substrate (binding site) and in the actual catalysis at the active site. Their charges will only be changed at extreme acid or alkaline pH values when the enzyme structure could be denatured anyway.

However the charged α-amino groups terminating polypeptide chains in enzymes (pK$_a$ values 7.6–8.4) and charged histidine residues in the molecule (pK$_a$ 5–7) are affected by pH shifts within the physiological range. Since the exact state of such charged groups plays an important role in enzyme specificity and action, it is to be expected that pH shifts in the physiological range will affect the level of enzyme activity. For each enzyme there is a pH at which maximal activity is observed and this value is called the optimum pH for the enzyme.

Table 3.10. Vitamin coenzyme relationships and functions.

Vitamin	Coenzyme form	Function	Deficiency disease symptoms
Thiamin (B₁)	Thiamine pyrophosphate	Decarboxylation α-keto acids	Beri-beri
Riboflavin (B₂)	Flavins (FAD, FMN)	H atom (electron) transfer	Dermatitis, stomatitis
Niacin (nicotinic acid)	NAD^+, $NADP^+$	H atom (electron) transfer	Pellagra
Pyridoxine (B₈)	Pyridoxal phosphate	Amino acid transaminase decarboxylation: Tyr synthesis	Dermatitis, stomatitis, convulsions
Pantothenic acid	Coenzyme A	Acylation reaction (TCA cycle)	Anaemia
Folic acid	Tetrahydrofolic acid	Transfer 1C (formyl) fragments: purine biosynthesis	Macrocytic and megaloblastic anaemia, sprue
Cobalamin (B₁₂)	Cobamin coenzyme	Transfer 1C (methyl) fragments: purine biosynthesis	Pernicious anaemia, sprue
Ascorbic acid (C)	not known	Collagen (hydroxylation) biosynthesis	Scurvy: delayed wound healing

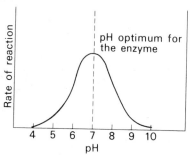

Fig. 3.45. The effect of pH on enzyme activity: the optimum pH of chymotrypsin.

Animal enzymes usually possess optimum pH values within a relatively narrow band around pH 7.4. For example the proteolytic digestive enzyme *chymotrypsin* has an optimum pH of 7 (Fig. 3.45). The enzyme is virtually inactive at pH 4 and 10 and only approximately half as efficient at 6 and 8 as at 7. Most enzyme activity/pH curves of enzymes are bell-shaped though they can vary considerably in form. The shape of the curve is in one sense a measure of the effect of pH on those ionizable groups, titratable within the physiological pH range, in both enzyme and substrate. The curve maximum (the optimum pH) is the pH value at which both sets of ionizable groups are best suited for formation of the E–S complex and the catalysis. When a substrate has ionizable groups it will usually have a particular charged state, determined by pH, best suited for its union with the enzyme. Similarly with the enzyme where the physiologically ionizable sites are the single α-NH$_2$ group terminating each polypeptide chain and the –NH$^+$– groups in the imidazole side-chains of the histidine residues. These latter therefore play a most important role in enzyme specificity and activity.

Returning to the activity/pH curve for chymotrypsin (Fig. 3.45) we can attempt to interpret it in the light of this knowledge.

The structure of chymotrypsin has been worked out in some detail and Fig. 3.46 is a planar diagrammatic representation of features of the tertiary structure which make up the active site region (shown contained within the circle).

Two histidine residues and an N-terminal isoleucine NH$_3^+$ group are involved and it has been found that the latter is an important substrate binding site. The histidine residue at 57 plays a vital role in the actual catalysis. At pH 7, 90% of the terminal α-amino groups are in –NH$_3^+$ form and 90% of the imidazole groups are uncharged: these are the optimal conditions for enzyme activity. A shift to either side of pH 7 alters the correct balance of charged and uncharged groups and so lowers the binding and catalytic efficiency of the enzyme molecules. The optimum pH/activity curve reflects these factors, and may also depend on other effects, such as the state of SH groups in substrate and enzyme.

This is a simplified model and explanation of what may be happening 'on site', as it is uncertain whether the environmental pH is exactly the same as that which occurs at the active site. In addition the shape of the pH/activity curve often varies with substrate concentration.

EFFECT OF TEMPERATURE ON ENZYME ACTIVITY

Enzymes are susceptible to temperature changes, their optimum working temperatures usually being in the region of 37–40°C (Fig. 3.47).

With any chemical reaction the rate initially increases with temperature, approximately

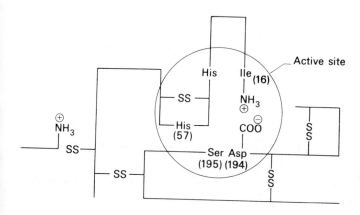

Fig. 3.46. Representation of amino acid residues constituting active site of chymotrypsin.

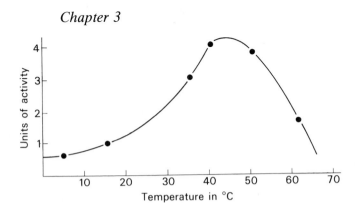

Fig. 3.47. The effect of temperature on enzyme activity.

doubling per 10°C rise, but with enzyme-catalysed reactions this falls away at higher temperatures because of the denaturation of the catalyst. Globular protein molecules such as enzymes are very susceptible to denaturation above about 40°C, their structures becoming increasingly modified by the alterations in the stability of the various weak bond forces holding them in their correct conformation. Thus boiling an enzyme destroys its catalytic activity by disrupting its unique architecture.

THE ACTIVATION OF ZYMOGENS

The proteolytic digestive enzymes pepsin, trypsin and chymotrypsin are initially secreted in inactive forms called zymogens—*pepsinogen*, *trypsinogen*, and *chymotrypsinogen* respectively (p. 610). This is nature's way of ensuring that the secreting cells do not digest themselves. Such an enzyme's proteolytic potential is made available by modification of its zymogen: the conversion of chymotrypsinogen to chymotrypsin is an example.

Chymotrypsinogen, synthesized in the pancreas, is a single polypeptide chain 245 residues long, and cross-linked by five cystine disulphide intrachain bridges. After secretion the peptide bond between residues 15–16 is cleaved by trypsin to form π-chymotrypsin which in turn acts on other π-chymotrypsin molecules removing two dipeptides—Ser–Arg (residues 14–15) and

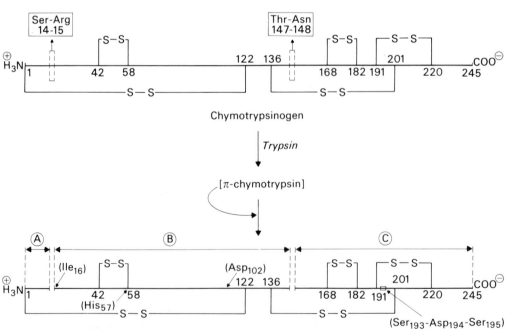

Fig. 3.48. The activation of chymotrypsin.

Thr–Asn (residues 147–148). The end product of this process is the active chymotrypsin enzyme molecule which now, therefore, consists of three polypeptide chains A, B and C joined together, still with the same five disulphide bridges but now with three as intrachain and the remaining two as interchain joining A to B and B to C. These chymotrypsin molecules are folded into a new tertiary form which brings together the amino acid residues that constitute the enzyme's active site (e.g. Ile_{16}, His_{57}, Asp_{102}, Ser_{193}, Asp_{194}, Ser_{195}) (Fig. 3.46).

ENZYME KINETICS

Some energy aspects of enzyme action
All biological reactions and changes must conform to the first and second laws of thermodynamics and with the free energy and entropy concepts (p. 988). As will be seen later (p. 238) light energy from the sun is captured in chemical bond energy form by the process of photosynthesis to form the plant products which both directly and indirectly provide most animal food and energy requirements. It is important to appreciate that the energy locked up in this chemical form in substrates for many biochemical reactions is released with the help of enzymes with very great efficiency.

The free energy of small molecules, in the form of these 'locked up' energy stores is tapped in such cellular organelles as the mitochondria where, through oxidation of fat (p. 205) and carbohydrate (p. 195) molecules, the energy is transferred to a new currency in the form of 'high energy' Ⓟ bonds such as are found in ATP. These 'high energy' compounds then provide a bank of readily available energy for various biosynthetic, and mechanical energy-requiring activities in animal tissues.

All these energy transformations are catalysed by enzyme molecules which therefore play a key role in the utilization of chemical energy sources.

Since an enzyme is by definition a catalyst, it can only speed up the rate of a reaction—it cannot alter its equilibrium.

For example in the reaction:

$$S \underset{k_2}{\overset{k_1}{\rightleftharpoons}} P$$

where S is the substrate and P the product

Then $k_1 [S] = k_2 [P]$

and $\dfrac{k_1}{k_2} = K_{eq} = \dfrac{[P]}{[S]}$

Consider an equilibrium point at which the concentration of P is 10 times that of S, i.e.

$$K_{eq} = \frac{[P]}{[S]} = \frac{10}{1}$$

(K_{eq} is the equilibrium constant)

The addition of an enzyme makes this equilibrium state attainable in a fraction of the time taken by the uncatalysed system. But the equilibrium state is still the same with 10 times as many P molecules present as S at the equilibrium point.

The concept of an activation energy barrier to be surmounted in reactions has already been considered (Fig. 3.40), and here it is only necessary to examine this in terms of the free energy (ΔG) of the system. The change from S to P requires passage through a transition state and the rate of this forward reaction (k_1) will depend on both the temperature and the difference in free energy (ΔG) between the reactant S and its transition state, i.e.

$$\begin{array}{cccc} \Delta G_{Act} & = & (G_T & - & G_S) \\ \text{Free energy} & & \text{transition} & & \text{reactant} \\ \text{of activation} & & \text{state} & & \end{array}$$

As explained above the effect of enzymes on catalysis is to reduce the energy barrier between the transition state and the reactant(s) (Fig. 3.40) and so make the reaction go faster. This is because more of the reactant molecules will then have an energy content sufficient to permit them to ride over the lower activation energy barrier of the new transition state.

Effect of enzyme and substrate concentrations on enzyme activity
Studies on the relationship between the rate of reaction and enzyme concentration and substrate concentration were made in 1913 by Leonor Michaelis and Maud Menten in investigations which have become a classic milestone in the history of biochemistry.

Michaelis and Menten investigated the hydrolysis of sucrose by invertase and found that the reaction rate increased in direct linear relationship to the enzyme concentration (Fig. 3.49). Because enzyme concentration [E] is the sole determinant of the rate, the reaction is said to be of the *first order* type in relation to [E] (see p. 994).

However when the enzyme concentration was kept constant it was found that a maximal rate (V_{max}) was approached as the substrate concentration [S] was increased (Fig. 3.50).

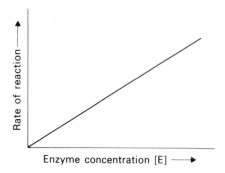

Fig. 3.49. Relationship between rate of catalysed reaction and enzyme concentration [E].

The rate constants for the forward and reverse reactions for the E–S complex formation are k_1 and k_2 respectively. The rate constant for E and P formation from ES is k_3 and for the reverse reaction it is k_4.

The amount of enzyme–substrate complex formed will be proportional to the concentrations of the participants, i.e. [E] and [S].

Thus $[ES] \propto [E][S]$

or $[ES] = k_1[E][S]$

(where k_1 = rate constant for E–S formation)

$$(1)$$

When the substrate S is present in large (and therefore effectively constant) amounts, any increase in [E] increases [ES] linearly and the rate of formation of product P will also be linear, as shown in Fig. 3.49. This is because the rate of formation of the product P is effectively determined by the enzyme–substrate complex concentration [ES].

or $P = k_3[ES]$ (2)

Thus at low substrate concentrations the rate is initially linear—*a first order reaction* with respect to [S]. However as substrate concentration increases this changes progressively until ultimately at V_{max} it is independent of substrate concentration. The reaction is now said to be a *zero order reaction* with respect to substrate.

To explain these results Michaelis and Menten postulated the now well known concept that an enzyme–substrate complex (E–S) is first formed which subsequently breaks down to the reaction products (P) with regeneration of the enzyme (E), i.e.

Alternatively when [E] is kept constant and [S] increased a level is reached when all the enzyme molecules available will be in union with the substrate. Since the [ES] present determines the rate of product P formation, there will be at this [S] level a maximum reaction rate. This is the maximum velocity, V_{max}, when all the enzyme molecules present are saturated with substrate molecules and no further increase in rate of formation of P is possible.

$$E + S \underset{k_2}{\overset{k_1}{\rightleftharpoons}} ES \underset{k_4}{\overset{k_3}{\rightleftharpoons}} E + P$$

enzyme   substrate   enzyme-substrate   enzyme   product
                           complex

Fig. 3.50. Relationship between rate of enzyme reaction and the substrate concentration [S].

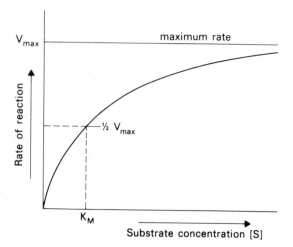

This concept of formation of an ES complex therefore provides a reasonable explanation of the observed effects of enzyme and substrate concentrations on the kinetic patterns of enzyme–catalysed reactions. Michaelis and Menten were led to postulate such an ES complex on purely theoretical grounds long before direct experimental evidence in support of the hypothesis became available.

Kinetics of enzyme action: the Michaelis constant
These considerations are less formidable than they might seem at first sight. They are important in that they develop a rational basis for understanding enzyme function, and at the same time provide mathematical support for the reality of the E–S complex concept. In addition they explain enzyme inhibition and show how different types of inhibition may be distinguished. Such knowledge has provided the basis for understanding drug action and even helped direct research in the design of new drugs. It has also contributed to furthering our knowledge of how metabolism is controlled.

The model for formation of E–S complex (Stage 1) and its breakdown to products P (Stage 2) is abbreviated as follows:

$$[E] + [S] \underset{k_2}{\overset{k_1}{\rightleftharpoons}} [ES] \qquad \text{Stage 1}$$

$$k_4 \updownarrow k_3$$

$$[P] + [E] \qquad \text{Stage 2}$$

The amount of ES in Stage 1 is envisaged as that present after a steady state condition has been attained—that is when the rates of formation and breakdown of the ES complex are equal. It can be assumed that none of the product P reverts to initial substrate S via E–S (i.e. initially the rate constant k_4 is negligible). Then V, the rate of formation of P, becomes

$$V = k_3[ES] \qquad (2a)$$

The rate of E–S breakdown is made up of two components:
1 Its dissociation back to E + S (whose rate = $k_2[ES]$).
2 Its breakdown to P + E (where the rate = $k_3[ES]$).
∴ total rate of breakdown of ES
$= k_2[ES] + k_3[ES]$
$= (k_2 + k_3) [ES] \qquad (3)$

The rate of formation of ES is given by equation (1), i.e.

$$[ES] = k_1[E][S] \qquad (1)$$

In the steady state therefore when rates of formation and breakdown of ES are equal:

$$k_1 [E] [S] = (k_2 + k_3) [ES]$$

This can be rearranged as:

$$[ES] = \frac{[E] [S]}{(k_2 + k_3)/k_1}$$

The denominator, made up of the three constants k_1, k_2 and k_3, is designated by the symbol K_m, and called the *Michaelis constant*. This is a most important constant, specific to each enzyme under defined conditions. Its significance will be discussed below.

$$K_m = \frac{k_2 + k_3}{k_1} \qquad (4)$$

$$\therefore [ES] = \frac{[E] [S]}{K_m} \qquad (5)$$

As it is usually the case that [S] is very large compared to [E], the amount of substrate bound to enzyme in the complex is numerically negligible compared to total [S].

Furthermore the amount of free enzyme $[E]_{free}$ present at equilibrium will equal the total enzyme, $[E]_t$, less the amount bound to the ES complex, the latter being numerically equal to [ES].

$$\therefore [E]_{free} = [E]_t - [ES]$$

Substitution of this value for [E] in equation 5 gives:

$$[ES] = \frac{([E]_t - [ES]) [S]}{K_m}$$

which can be rearranged as follows:
$$K_m [ES] = [E]_t [S] - [ES] [S]$$
or $$K_m [ES] + [S] [ES] = [E]_t [S]$$
or $$K_m + [S] = \frac{[E]_t [S]}{[ES]}$$

which becomes
$$[ES] = \frac{[E]_t [S]}{K_m + [S]} \qquad (6)$$

The velocity of formation of P (from equation 2a) is
$$V = k_3[ES] \ .$$

Rewriting this as [ES] = V/k_3 and substituting for [ES] in equation (6) gives:

$$V = \frac{k_3[E]_t [S]}{K_m + [S]} \qquad (6a)$$

The observed maximal reaction rate V_{max} will be attained when all the enzyme is saturated with substrate and $[E]_t$ becomes virtually the same as $[ES]$.

Since $[ES] = V/k_3$ (2a)

Therefore equation (6a) becomes

$$V = \frac{V_{max}[S]}{K_m + [S]} \qquad (7)$$

This is the *Michaelis-Menten equation* whose graphical form coincides with the rectangular hyperbole curve found experimentally for the relationship between substrate concentration and reaction rate (Fig. 3.50). The mathematical treatment of the formation of an E–S complex therefore provides an explanation of the laboratory data.

If in equation (7) we make $V = \frac{1}{2} V_{max}$

then $\dfrac{V_{max}}{2} = \dfrac{V_{max}\ [S]}{K_m + [S]}$

$\therefore \quad K_m + [S] = 2[S]$

or $\quad K_m = [S]$ (8)

Thus the K_m is equal to the substrate concentration at half the maximum reaction rate.

This therefore provides a ready means of measuring the Michaelis constant K_m for an enzyme in a specific reaction. From Fig. 3.50 it can be seen that dropping a perpendicular from the intersect on the curve with the $\frac{1}{2} V_{max}$ value gives the K_m value on the $[S]$ axis.

The *Michaelis–Menten equation* evolved above (equation 7), and the *Michaelis constant* K_m are of fundamental importance in the study of enzymes. It may not be necessary to reproduce, under examination conditions, the steps involved in their derivation but it is essential to have followed these and understood them in order to appreciate their significance and application.

The importance of K_m and V_{max} values
Table 3.11 lists selected K_m values for some important enzymes, expressed in substrate molarity concentration values.

K_m values mostly lie between 10^{-1} and 10^{-6} M. It should be realised that K_m for a particular enzyme is not really a 'constant' in the usually accepted sense because its value can change with the pH, ionic strength and temperature of the system. It also varies in relation to different substrates (compare the K_m values for the different chymotrypsin and aspartate transaminase substrates in Table 3.11).

K_m values provide extremely valuable information. As discussed above the K_m value for a given reaction is the substrate concentration corresponding to half the V_{max}, which occurs when half the active sites are occupied. Thus with a knowledge of the K_m the proportion of sites filled at any substrate concentration can be simply estimated.

K_m is also defined in terms of rate constants, i.e.

$$K_m = \frac{k_2 + k_3}{k_1} \qquad (4)$$

In a situation where the dissociation of ES $\underset{}{\overset{k_2}{\rightleftharpoons}}$ E + S is much greater (say 50–100 times) than the product formation ES $\overset{k_3}{\rightleftharpoons}$ P + E, then the K_m value will approximate to k_2/k_1.

Table 3.11. K_m values for some enzymes, expressed in substrate molarity concentration values.

Enzyme	Substrate	K_m value
Chymotrypsin	N-acetyl tyrosinamide	3.2×10^{-2} M
	N-formyl tyrosinamide	1.2×10^{-2} M
	Glycyl tyrosinamide	1.2×10^{-1} M
	N-acetyl tryptophanamide	5×10^{-3} M
Aspartate amino transferase (transaminase)	Aspartate	9×10^{-4} M
	α Ketoglutarate	1×10^{-4} M
	Oxaloacetate	4×10^{-5} M
	Glutamate	4×10^{-3} M
Catalase	H_2O_2	2.5×10^{-2} M
Lysozyme	Hexa-N-acetyl glucosamide	6×10^{-6} M

For the dissociation of the ES complex

$$ES \underset{k_1}{\overset{k_2}{\rightleftharpoons}} E + S$$

the dissociation constant,

$$K_{ES} = \frac{[E]\,[S]}{[ES]} = \frac{k_2}{k_1}$$

Under these conditions then $K_m \simeq K_{ES}$ and the Michaelis constant K_m provides therefore a measure of the tendency of the enzyme and substrate to form an E–S complex. Low values mean strong binding and vice versa. It must be emphasized that this is only under those specific conditions when k_2 is much greater than k_3.

The V_{max} rate, which is the rate when all the active sites are saturated, is a measure of the turnover rate of an enzyme. When all the active sites are saturated with substrate

$$V_{max} = k_3[E]_t \qquad (9)$$

Knowing $[E]_t$, the total enzyme concentration, k_3, the *turnover number* of the enzyme, can be calculated. Also called the molar or molecular activity, this is defined as the number of substrate molecules converted to the product by a single enzyme molecule in unit time (seconds, or minutes according to authority) when the active sites are fully saturated with substrate. Reference has already been made to such rates for *catalase* and *carbonic anhydrase* (p. 83) whose turnover numbers label them as two of the fastest acting enzymes known. The turnover number of carbonic anhydrase tops the league at 36 000 000 per second compared with catalase, 5 600 000. *β-amylase*, an enzyme attacking glycosidic bonds, does well at 1 100 000 per minute but an enzyme such as *succinic dehydrogenase* is down to 1150 per minute, with *lysozyme* by comparison a positive sluggard at 30!

Lineweaver–Burk plots
Fig. 3.50 shows that there are problems in obtaining accurate measurements of enzyme K_m values for a particular system because of the difficulties in accurately assessing the V_{max} value from such graphs. The rectangular hyperbole form of the curve approaches a maximum value but there are practical difficulties in determining its exact value accurately. For this reason it is more convenient to express the Michaelis–Menten equation in a form which will give a straight line graph. This is easily achieved by taking reciprocals on both sides of the equation 7.

Thus
$$V = \frac{V_{max}\,[S]}{K_m + [S]} \qquad (7)$$

becomes
$$\frac{1}{V} = \frac{K_m + [S]}{V_{max}\,[S]}$$

This is rearranged to the form

$$\frac{1}{V} = \frac{K_m}{V_{max}\,[S]} + \frac{[S]}{V_{max}\,[S]}$$

$$\therefore \qquad \frac{1}{V} = \frac{K_m}{V_{max}\,[S]} + \frac{1}{V_{max}} \qquad (10)$$

Equation 10 is known as the *Lineweaver-Burk Equation* and the graphical form of this double reciprocal plot is shown in Fig. 3.51.

Its gradient is K_m/V_{max}. It cuts the ordinate at $1/V_{max}$ and the abscissa at $-1/V_{max}$. Thus both V_{max} and K_m values can be readily and accurately determined by measuring a series of reaction rates for different substrate concentrations and plotting them against each other in their reciprocal form.

These Lineweaver–Burk plots have proved particularly useful in the interpretation and identification of various types of enzyme inhibitor action.

Reversible inhibition of enzymes
Using Lineweaver–Burk plots three major types of reversible enzyme inhibition have been distinguished from the way in which different inhibitors may affect the kinetics of enzyme action in terms of the Michaelis–Menten equation. These are *competitive, non-competitive* and *uncompetitive* inhibition.

Competitive inhibition. In this type of inhibition the inhibitor combines with the enzyme at the active site and forms an enzyme–inhibitor complex (EI) in the same way as the ES complex forms with the natural substrate. These competitive inhibitor molecules usually have a similar chemical form to the substrate and as such are partially 'recognized' by the enzyme in such a way that the inhibitor molecules, (I), compete with the substrate molecules (S) for places at the active sites of the enzyme molecules. As a result the rate of catalysis is lowered because only a proportion of the total active sites are available for the correct substrate molecules.

A classic example of competitive inhibition is that of malonic acid on *succinic dehydrogenase*, which normally catalyses dehydrogenation of succinic acid, but in the presence of malonate has its catalytic power (i.e. turnover number) reduced proportionately.

COO⁻ CH₂ CH₂ COO⁻ — Succinate ion

COO⁻ CH₂ COO⁻ — Malonate ion

COO⁻ COO⁻ — Oxalate ion

From the formulae it can be seen that malonate differs from succinate in lacking one $-CH_2-$ group. Similarly oxalic acid lacks yet one more $-CH_2-$ group but is still recognizably out of the same molecular stable of small dicarboxylic organic acids. Oxalic acid is also a competitive inhibitor of succinic dehydrogenase but to a much less extent than malonate.

When a competitive inhibitor (I) such as malonate is present the following situation arises:

$$E \underset{}{\overset{+S}{\rightleftharpoons}} \{ES\} \longrightarrow E + P$$

enzyme-substrate complex

inhibition overcome by an increase in [S]

+I k_4 k_5

EI

enzyme-inhibitor complex

S and I compete for the active sites on enzyme E with the formation of the ES and EI complexes respectively.

The dissociation constant K_I for the (EI) complex is given by:

$$K_I = \frac{k_5}{k_4} \qquad (11)$$

Applying similar considerations to those used in deriving the Michaelis–Menten equation an expression for the velocity of the inhibited reaction V_I can be obtained.

$$V_I = \frac{V_{max}}{1 + \frac{K_m}{[S]} \left(1 + \frac{[I]}{K_I}\right)} \qquad (12)$$

Expressed in Lineweaver–Burk reciprocal form this becomes:

$$\frac{1}{V_I} = \frac{K_m}{V_{max}} \left(1 + \frac{[I]}{K_I}\right) \cdot \left(\frac{1}{[S]}\right) + \frac{1}{V_{max}} \qquad (13)$$

Comparison of equation (13) with equation (10) shows that the difference is an increase in the K_m/V_{max} value by a factor $(1+([I]/K_i))$, which in in effect increases the slope of the line by this amount. But the intersect on the y axis will still be at the $1/V_{max}$ value (Fig. 3.52).

Therefore two important features of competitive inhibition are that V_{max} *does not change* and the K_m *value increases*.

As the substrate concentration [S] increases (theoretically to infinity when 1/[S] becomes 0) so the substrate molecules increasingly outnumber the inhibitor molecules competing with them for the active sites. Thus a third major characteristic feature of competitive inhibition is that a sufficient *increase in the substrate concentration can overcome the inhibition*.

The experimental data for the 'inhibitor-present' curve in Fig. 3.52 is obtained by using a fixed inhibitor concentration [I] and varying the [S]. In practice this procedure is repeated for a series of different inhibitor concentrations to provide a family of inhibitor curves, each with increasing gradient as [I] increases, but all cutting the ordinate at the $1/V_{max}$ intercept. However the intercept on the abscissa, $-1/K_m$, decreases in value as [I] increases. Thus the effect of increasing inhibitor concentration is to increase the apparent K_m value of the enzyme for the substrate, because, of course, the enzyme will require higher substrate concentrations to achieve its maximum velocity effect.

Non-competitive inhibition. Non-competitive inhibitors combine reversibly either with the

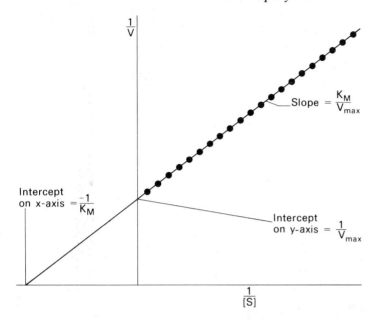

Fig. 3.51. Lineweaver–Burk double reciprocal plot of 1/V against 1/S. The K_m value is determined from the negative intercept on the x-axis.

free enzyme E or the ES complex, interfering with the action of both. They bind to sites other than the active site or binding sites in such a way that rate of ES formation (k_1) is reduced and once formed the ES complex does not break down to its reaction products at the normal rate (k_3). Because the inhibitory effect is not on the active sites, increasing the substrate concentration has no effect on non-competitive inhibition.

Examples of non-competitive inhibitors are heavy metal ions such as Ag^+, Hg^{2+}, Pb^{2+} which can affect SH groups in the enzyme.

The Lineweaver–Burk plot for non-competitive inhibition is shown in Fig. 3.53.

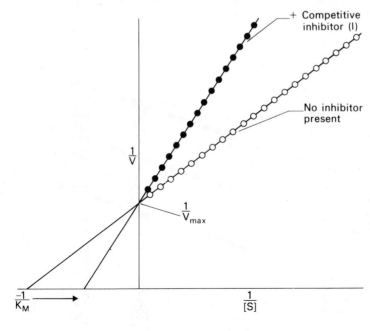

Fig. 3.52. Lineweaver-Burk double reciprocal plot of enzyme kinetics in presence (–•–•–•–) and absence (–o–o–o–o–) of competitive inhibitor (I). With inhibitor the negative intercept on the x-axis ($-1/K_m$) is lower in value, therefore K_m is increased.

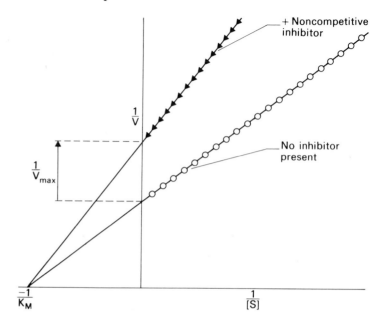

Fig. 3.53. Lineweaver–Burk double reciprocal plot for non-competitive inhibitor. The $1/V$ intercept on the y axis is greater, therefore V_{max} is lower. The $-1/K_m$ value is unchanged, i.e. K_m is unaltered.

The intercept on the ordinate (I/V) axis is higher because the V_{max} of the inhibited reaction is always reduced. The slope of the inhibited reaction is:

$$\frac{K_m}{V_{max}} \cdot \left(1 + \frac{[I]}{K_I} \right)$$

At all [I] concentrations the abscissa is cut at the same $-1/K_m$ value. The K_m is unaffected because the active site of the enzyme is not involved. Thus the effect in non-competitive inhibition is to reduce V_{max} with no effect on K_m.

This is the opposite of a competitive inhibitor effect.

Uncompetitive inhibition. In this ineptly named type of reversible inhibition the inhibitor combines with the ES complex to give an inactive complex:

$$ES + I \rightleftharpoons ESI.$$

It is not reversed by increasing substrate concentration and is easily recognized from the form of its Lineweaver–Burk plot (Fig. 3.54).

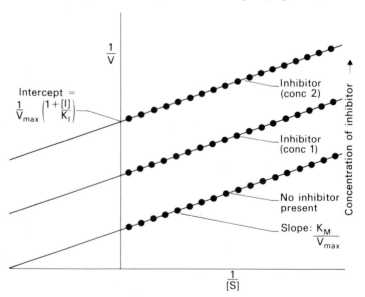

Fig. 3.54. Lineweaver–Burk double reciprocal plot for uncompetitive inhibitor. V_{max} decreases with increasing I but slopes are identical.

Typically V_{max} decreases with increasing [I] but the slope of each line remains unchanged. This type of inhibition is rare in one-substrate reactions but common in two-substrate reactions.

Irreversible enzyme inhibition

The previously discussed forms of inhibition are reversible in the sense that the inhibitors can be removed by prolonged dialysis, as the EI or ESI complexes formed are reversibly dissociated. With irreversible inhibition the inhibitor is permanently bonded to the enzyme.

An example is the effect of di-isopropyl fluorophosphate (DFP) on chymotrypsin, and here reference should be made to the representation of the enzyme's active site (Fig. 3.46). The importance of the role of the histidine residue in the active site at position 57 was referred to earlier, but here attention must be directed to the nearby serine residue at position 195. There are 27 serine residues in the chymotrypsin molecule but this one is involved in the active site. Serine residues have an alcoholic OH group on their side-arms which appear to play an important role in the active sites of several other enzyme structures, the so-called *serine enzymes* which include chymotrypsin, trypsin, elastase and thrombin. The DFP reaction with such serine residues is shown in Fig. 3.55.

Each molecule of DFP completely and irreversibly inactivates the proteolytic activity of one molecule of chymotrypsin and the bonding is so strong that it is possible to break down the enzyme molecule stepwise and isolate the phosphorylated serine residue. Indeed this was how the actual involvement of residue 195 in the active site was first discovered.

A rather more sinister use of DFP and similar compounds is in chemical warfare as a nerve gas. Serine residues form an essential part of another enzyme *acetyl cholinesterase* which breaks down the substance acetylcholine, released as nerve impulses pass across nerve synapses (p. 288). If these enzymes are inactivated the animal's nervous system is effectively knocked out. Minute quantities of the substance absorbed into the body cause the muscles to contract as if receiving a continual series of nerve impulses.

Allosteric enzymes

These are enzymes whose activity is affected by the binding of a low molecular weight compound, the *effector*, which is usually a metabolite or coenzyme not directly involved in the reaction catalysed by the allosteric enzyme. Effectors modify the binding of substrate to the enzyme by altering the latter's conformation. They do not bind to the active site and can be positive (activatory) or negative (inhibitory). Allosteric enzymes therefore play a key role in metabolic control mechanisms (p. 269), and for this reason are also referred to as *regulatory* enzymes.

Many examples of their action in this context are given in the text and index. They usually have

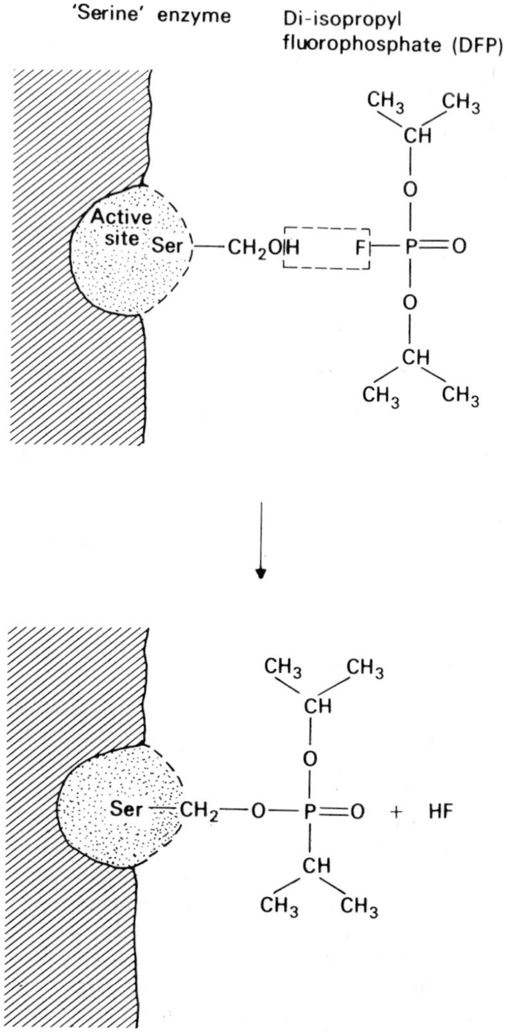

Fig. 3.55. Irreversible inhibition. Reaction of 'serine' enzyme with DFP (di-isopropyl fluorophosphate).

a quaternary structure, comprising two or more subunits; their kinetics are often characterized by S-shaped Michaelis-Menten curves (Fig. 3.56).

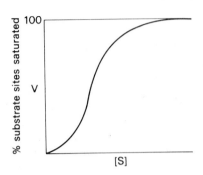

Fig. 3.56. The signed curve relationship between V and [S] produced by an allosteric enzyme.

THE NUCLEIC ACIDS

The nucleic acids constitute one of the most important areas of study in contemporary biochemistry. As their name suggests they are located in the nuclei of cells but in addition are present in the cell cytoplasm: they usually occur naturally in association with proteins as nucleoproteins. The nucleic acid macromolecules are among the largest known with molecular weights in the millions and ranging up to the thousand million mark in bacteria. As major components of all cells they constitute 5–15% of the total dry weight.

They have been isolated from living matter by a series of extraction and precipitation preparative procedures and subjected to an elaborate array of physical, chemical and biological investigations. The resultant detailed knowledge of their structure has provided the basis for a growing insight into the manner in which cells transmit heritable factors, synthesize many essential biomolecules, and also direct and control the innumerable metabolic steps which constitute the functional activities of living organisms. They act as storers and transmitters of genetic information and the study of their highly complex chemical structure is a classic example of structure–function relationships at the molecular level.

THE MONOMERIC UNITS OF NUCLEIC ACIDS (MONONUCLEOTIDES)

The nucleotides (or more correctly the mononucleotides) are the monomeric building block units from which the polymeric nucleic acids (polynucleotides) are constructed. Apart from their role as constituents of the nucleic acids in addition they have important independent roles in intermediary metabolism.

Nucleotides are compounds made up of a nitrogenous base, a sugar, and a phosphoric acid molecule.

Complete acid hydrolysis of nucleic acids yields a mixture of these three chemical components:

1 The *purines* and *pyrimidines*.
2 The *pentose sugars* (ribose or deoxyribose).
3 Phosphoric acid.

Milder treatment, such as enzymic degradation, breaks the nucleic acid molecules (or polynucleotides) into a mixture of smaller nucleotide and nucleoside units and phosphoric acid.

PYRIMIDINES

The pyrimidine bases are so named because of their derivation from the parent structure *pyrimidine* which is a nitrogenous single ring compound, originally identified by Emil Fischer in 1880. The conventional numbering of positions in the basic ring structure are as shown. The principal pyrimidines found in nucleic acids are *thymine, cytosine* and *uracil*. (*5-methylcytosine* and *5-hydroxymethylcytosine* are also found in certain nucleic acids).

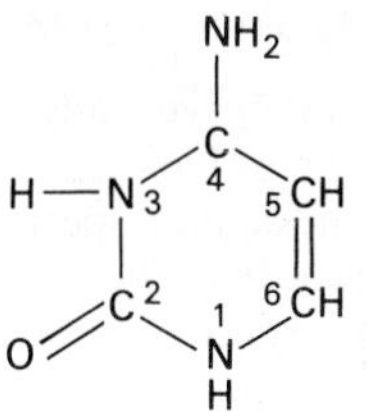

Cytosine (C)

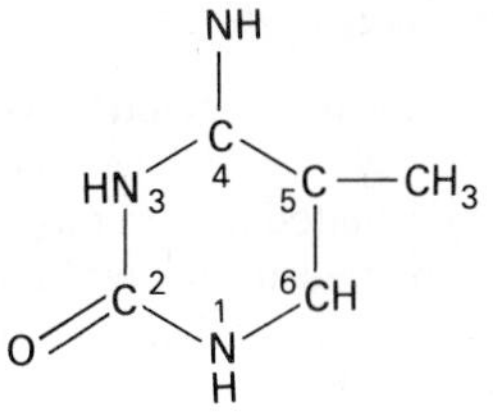

5-Methylcytosine (MC)

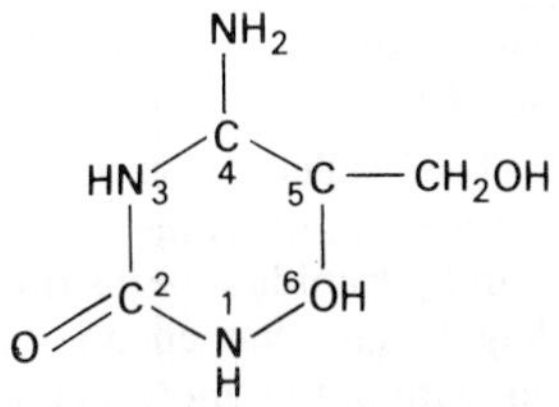

5-Hydroxymethylcytosine

The pyrimidines all demonstrate a lactam-lactim tautomerism, as they are weakly basic compounds, although at physiological pH values and below the lactam forms predominate.

PURINES

These bases are derived chemically from the parent *purine* which is a pyrimidine ring fused to a five-membered imidazole ring. The major purine constituents of nucleic acids are *adenine* (A) and *guanine* (G).

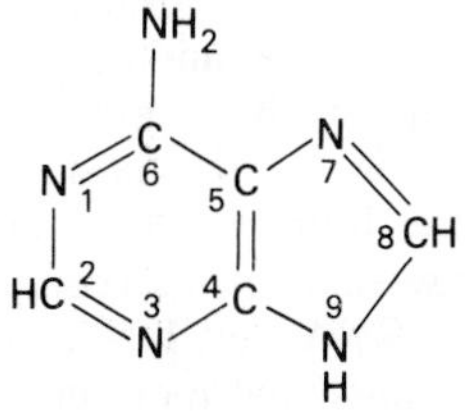

Adenine (A')

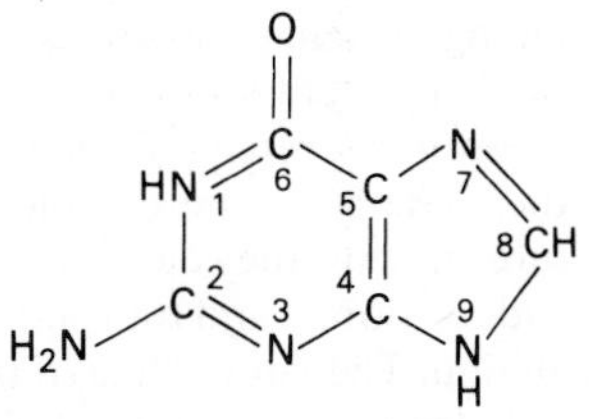

Guanine (G)

Hypoxanthine and certain methylated derivatives of adenine and guanine have a limited distribution, the latter forms being present in minor quantities in the DNA of bacteria and bacterial viruses (bacteriophages).

THE NUCLEOSIDES

The nucleoside structures formed by partial hydrolysis of nucleic acids are compounds in which pentose sugar molecules are covalently linked to one or other of the purine or pyrimidine bases. The important sugars in nucleic acid biochemistry are the two pentoses, *D-ribose* and *D-2-deoxyribose* and the two main classes of nucleic acids, *ribonucleic acid* (RNA) and *deoxyribonucleic acid* (DNA), take their names from their respective sugar constituents.

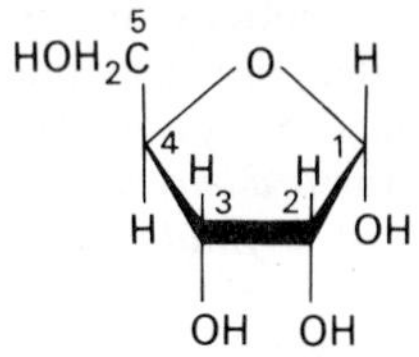

D-Ribose
(α-D-ribofuranose)

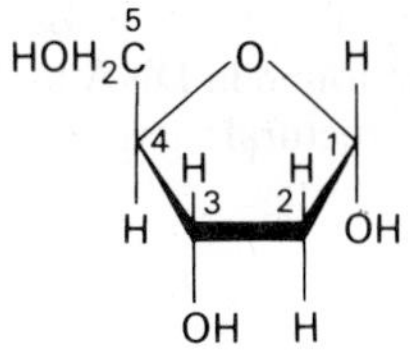

D-2-Deoxyribose
(α-D-deoxyribofuranose)

Chemically a nucleoside is an N-glycoside of a heterocyclic base. The glycosidic linkage is of the β-form linking the N1 of pyrimidines and N9 of purines to the carbon-1 of the sugar, which is in the furanose (5-membered ring) form. Thus the nucleoside *adenosine* is 9-β-D-ribofuranosyladenine and there is a corresponding deoxyadenosine. Similarly there are guanine nucleosides termed *guanosine* and *deoxyguanosine* respectively. The deoxyribonucleoside of thymine is termed *thymidine* and not deoxythymidine since this pyrimidine is located predominantly in DNA. The corresponding pyrimidine nucleosides are *cytidine, deoxycytidine, uridine* and *deoxyuridine*.

Deoxyadenosine

THE NUCLEOTIDES

The nucleotides are sugar-O-phosphate ester derivatives of the nucleosides, also obtained by mild chemical or enzymic hydrolysis of the nucleic acids. The mononucleotides are the structural units from which the polynucleotides (or nucleic acids) are assembled. They are strong acids and are therefore termed *adenylic acid, guanidylic acid, cytidylic acid, thymidylic acid* and *uridylic acid*.

The *deoxyribose* nucleotides can only bond phosphate groupings at carbon 3′ and 5′, since carbons 1′ and 4′ are involved in their furanose structures and carbon 2′ of deoxyribose does not, of course, carry any hydroxyl group. Both types of phosphate ester are found in DNA hydrolysates and are of major structural significance in deoxypolynucleotide chemistry.

Deoxy-5-adenylic acid

Conversely, the ribonucleotides can be phosphate ester-linked at carbons 3′, 5′ and 2′ since only carbon 1′ and 4′ are not available for esterification.

The polymeric structure and function of DNA

DNA was subjected to its first intensive study in 1869 by Friedrich Miescher, a Swiss biochemist, who isolated it from pus cells and salmon sperm. He named it 'nuclein' and more than 70 years were to elapse before attempts at the full elucidation of its composition and structure and function became successful. Up to 1944 it had been assumed that the genetic material was chromosomal protein, with DNA of secondary importance, but work on bacterial and viral nucleic acids established unequivocally the genetic role of DNA.

DNA has been called the 'molecule of heredity'. It is the actual sequential arrangements of the purine and pyrimidine bases throughout its long winding length that encodes the genetic information within the molecule in chemical form. The actual sequence of bases constitutes the variable part of DNA molecules, whereas the backbone of deoxyribose molecules, linked by phosphate ester bridges, is of constant form in all DNA molecules. Thus the sugar and phosphate groups in DNA play an essentially passive structural role.

Chemically the deoxyribonucleic acids are polynucleotides in which the phosphate residues of each nucleotide unit form internucleotide phosphate diester linkages between the deoxyribose residues. As described above, in DNA the diester bridges are formed between carbon 3′ and carbon 5′.

The four deoxyribonucleotides found in DNAs differ only in terms of their nitrogenous base components, the purines adenine and guanine, and the pyrimidines cytosine and thymine. Similarly there are four different ribonucleotides in the RNAs deriving respectively from the four bases adenine, guanine, cytosine and uracil. In terms of component structure therefore RNA and DNA differ only in their pentose units (ribose or deoxyribose) and the presence of uracil in RNA and thymine (5-methyl uracil) in DNA.

Just as a knowledge of amino acids and peptide bond formation is a necessary basis for understanding protein structure, so a consideration of the component structures of the nucleic acids is an essential prerequisite to any appreciation of their characteristic complex molecular architecture and how they determine the roles of nucleic acids as storers and transmitters of genetic information. The unravelling of this fascinating story of structure-function relationships is a fundamental cornerstone of modern biology.

Numerous investigations have established DNA as the universal genetic information material for all life forms (with the exception of certain viruses which appear to possess RNA as their only functional genetic substance). In nearly all living organisms, plants and animals, it is found in the chromosomes in the form of nucleoprotein. Up to about 1947 it was not known how DNA molecules existed spatially, nor was it understood how they actually carried stores of information specific to each cell type and organism. The pieces began to fall into place in 1947 when, as a result of chemical analyses carried out on DNA obtained from a number of sources, certain regularities of base compostition were observed by Erwin Chargaff and his co-workers.

Four fundamental features of base composition in DNA were observed:

1 In DNA the sum of the number of the purine nucleotides was equal to the sum of the pyrimidine nucleotides

adenine + guanine = thymine + cytosine
(+ methyl cytosine
if present)

or A + G = T + C + (MC?)   (1)

In other words the ratio of purines to pyrimidines was unity, i.e.

$$\frac{(A + G)}{(T + C)} = 1 \qquad (1a)$$

2 Of perhaps greater significance was the finding that the ratio of adenine to thymine was also equal to 1 — as was the ratio of guanine to cytosine, i.e.

$$\frac{A}{T} = 1 \qquad \frac{G}{C} = 1 \qquad (2)$$

This equality between numbers of bases in the molecule proved to be of fundamental importance in the ultimate deciphering of nucleic acid structure and has been called *Chargaff's Rule*.

3 It was also observed that the sum of the 6-amino (purine) and 4-amino (pyrimidine) group-containing bases (A and C) was numerically equal to the sum of the 6-keto (purine) and 4-keto (pyrimidine) group-containing bases (G and T respectively).

4 The base ratio $(A + T)/(G + C)$, called the *dissymmetry ratio*, was found to be unique and characteristic for a particular species, and varied in value between species.

A great impetus to structural studies on DNA

derived from the X-ray diffraction analysis of native DNA fibres made by Maurice Wilkins and Rosalind Franklin in the early 1950s. A consideration of their experimental results in relation to various possible model constructions led them to the conclusion that the purine and pyrimidine bases were spaced regularly along the molecule at 0.34 nm distances apart, in the form of a coil, each turn containing 10 nucleotide units. Density measurements showed that the DNA molecule probably consisted of more than one nucleotide chain.

A number of workers suggested that hydrogen bonding between inward-facing bases probably helped to stabilize the molecules. However it was James Watson and Francis Crick who in 1953 incorporated the data and various ideas in the construction of their now famous 'double helix' model of the DNA molecule for which they, together with Wilkins, were awarded the 1962 Nobel Prize for medicine and physiology.

The validity of this proposed DNA structure is now firmly established and provides a rational explanation of how genetic information is stored, transferred and expressed. The 'double helix' structure for DNA proposed by Watson and Crick is illustrated in Fig. 3.57a.

The structure consists of two polynucleotide chains coiled round each other in a double helical arrangement. The main backbone of each chain consists of deoxyribose residues linked by 3'–5' phosphodiester bonds as shown in Fig. 3.58a. The two chains are wound round each other so that the ribose-phosphate backbones lie on the outside, and the bases are on the inside pointing towards the central axis of the structure (Fig. 3.57).

The two chains are held together in part by hydrogen bonding between the inward-facing bases, bonding occurring between the amino group of one base on one chain and the keto group of another base on the other chain. This *base-pairing* is very specific and occurs only between adenine and thymine (A-T) and guanine and cytosine (G – C) (Fig. 3.58b).

These associations are not only in accord with Chargaff's findings, but are also a structural necessity since 3-dimensional models show that no other pairings will either allow the correct spatial arrangement for a regular helix to occur, or permit hydrogen bonding between the bases in the two coils to become possible.

The two chains of the helix are coiled to allow the necessary hydrogen bonding. The chains are not identical but are said to be *complementary* in terms of the specific base-pairing

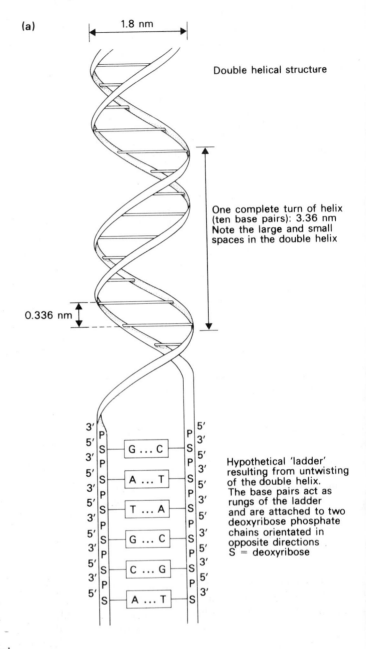

(a)

1.8 nm

Double helical structure

One complete turn of helix
(ten base pairs): 3.36 nm
Note the large and small
spaces in the double helix

0.336 nm

3′ P   P 5′
5′ S   S 3′
3′ P — G ... C — P 5′
5′ S   S 3′
3′ P — A ... T — P 5′
5′ S   S 3′
3′ P — T ... A — P 5′
5′ S   S 3′
3′ P — G ... C — P 5′
5′ S   S 3′
3′ P — C ... G — P 5′
5′ S   S 3′
   P — A ... T — P 3′
   S   S

Hypothetical 'ladder'
resulting from untwisting
of the double helix.
The base pairs act as
rungs of the ladder
and are attached to two
deoxyribose phosphate
chains orientated in
opposite directions
S = deoxyribose

Fig. 3.57. (a) The 'Watson and
Crick' double helix structure for
DNA. (After Edwards N.A. &
Hassall K.A. (1980) *Biochemistry
and Physiology of the Cell*, 2nd
edn. New York, McGraw Hill.)
(b) One of the strands of the DNA
double helix, viewed down the
helix axis. The bases are inside and
the sugar-phosphate backbone is
outside. (After Stryer L. (1981)
Biochemistry, 2nd edn. San
Francisco, W.H. Freeman.)

(b)

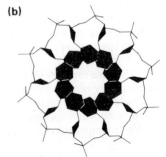

rules defined above. For example if one chain sequence is adenine–guanine–cytosine–thymine (A–G–C–T) then the corresponding chain complement will be thymine–cytosine–guanine–adenine (T–C–G–A).

The chains of the helix are *antiparallel* in the sense that if the adenine–cytosine region runs 3′–5′ then the complementary sequence of the thymine–guanine in the other chain will run 5′–3′. In addition to hydrogen bonding, hydrophobic interactions between the stacked purines and pyrimidines also help maintain the rigid, double-stranded structure.

Difficulties were encountered in assigning the correct molecular sizes to DNA molecules because of the presence, during their isolation, of nucleases, which break down the molecules and also the disruptive shearing forces involved in certain necessary preparation procedures. Despite such problems the evidence is that in prokaryotic cells with a single chromosome, such as the bacteria, all the DNA is present as a single molecule exceeding 2×10^9 in molecular weight. In the microorganism *E. coli*, the DNA is known to be circular in form. In the polychromosomal eukaryote cells of higher plants and animals DNA molecular weights of the order of 10^6 are found.

In the diploid eukaryotic cells of higher organisms, such as man, the DNA is nearly all associated with the cell nucleus where it is combined with strongly basic proteins called *histones*. In addition there are small amounts of cytoplasmic DNA which differs in molecular size and base composition from nuclear DNA. The histones contain large amounts of the basic amino acids lysine and arginine, which are involved in some way in their association with DNA to form nucleoproteins. One role for histones suggested is as repressors of cellular genetic activity: an alternative hypothesis implicates them in binding together the genetic units of DNA within the chromosome to form nucleosomes.

The functional roles of the nucleic acids

As indicated, the nucleic acids are concerned with the storing, transmission and cellular expression of heritable information. First, consideration must be given to how this stored information is reproduced (*replication*), then how this information is carried in message form to the cytoplasm (*transcription*) and finally how it is expressed phenotypically in terms of cellular activity (*translation*).

REPLICATION OF DNA

The term *replication* describes the processes whereby DNA molecules are exactly copied to form identical 'daughter' molecules. Such DNA synthesis occurs during the latter part of the interphase stage of cell nucleus division. The observation by Watson and Crick in 1953 that their double helical model of DNA could readily account for DNA molecule replication with consequent conveyance of identical genetic information to the daughter cells during mitotic and meiotic cell division has been confirmed experimentally. The unwinding of the two polynucleotide chains coupled with the formation of complementary DNA strands on the separating chains is termed *semi-conservative replication*: this process leads to the formation of two identical DNA double helix daughter molecules, each containing one polynucleotide chain derived from the parent DNA molecule.

Evidence confirming the semi-conservative replication mechanism was produced by the classic experiment of Meselson and Stahl in 1972. *E. coli.* bacterial cell cultures were grown first in a medium containing the heavy isotope of nitrogen, ^{15}N. DNA containing the ^{15}N isotope can be readily separated by density gradient centrifugation on account of its greater density than DNA containing the normal ^{14}N isotope. After allowing several generations of *E. coli* to divide in the ^{15}N medium the ^{15}N-labelled bacteria were harvested, transferred, and allowed to divide in a medium containing ^{14}N, the normal isotope. The DNA synthesized in the latter medium contained an intermediate form consisting of one ^{15}N and one ^{14}N-labelled strand of polynucleotide combined in one double helical DNA molecule (Fig. 3.59). On centrifugation this hybrid form sedimented at a point intermediate between the heavy and the normal types of DNA.

The replication process is also under careful metabolic control as was shown by Kornberg in 1958 when he established that a specific enzyme, *DNA polymerase*, was required to link the new nucleotide units on to each of the unwound template strands to form the new complementary continuous strand. A certain amount of DNA was required to prime the system as no synthesis of DNA occurred in its absence, a feature giving strong support to the semi-conservative replication theory.

The DNA polymerase copies in only one direction from the 3′ terminal to the 5′ terminal, with the synthesis necessarily functioning in short bursts. The short lengths are linked up by a

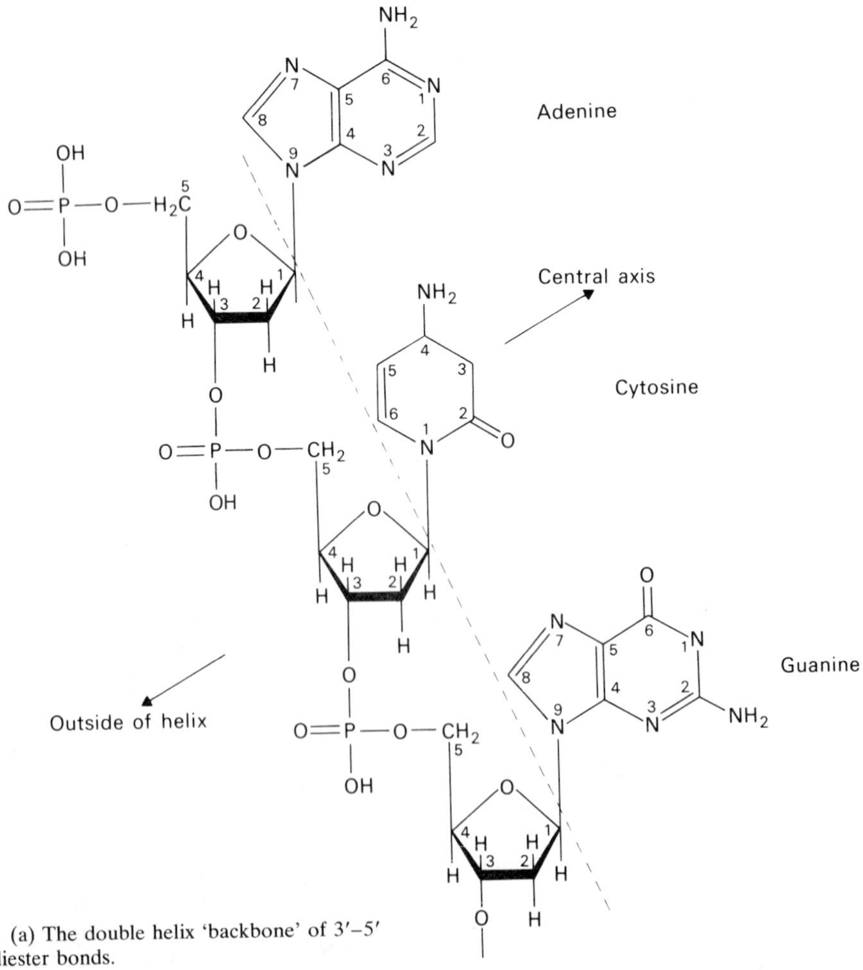

Fig. 3.58. (a) The double helix 'backbone' of 3′–5′ phosphodiester bonds.

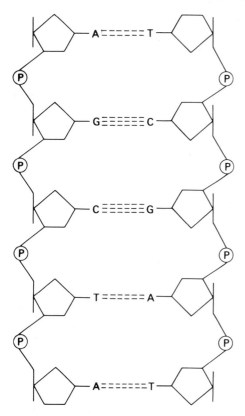

Fig. 3.58. (b) A sequence of base pairs between two strands of DNA.

DNA-joining enzyme called DNA-ligase, whose primary function, however, is to join the two ends of a single DNA-chain to form a circular model of DNA providing the ends of the chains are duplexed to a complementary strand. The DNA-ligase enzyme may also be considered to be of importance in repairing DNA molecules damaged by external factors, such as ultraviolet and ionizing radiations. It is thought that this activity may be its true function *in vivo* with alternative DNA polymerases being involved in the normal replication process.

The mechanics of the DNA replication process concern the actual unwinding of the double helix. It is now understood that the two processes of unwinding and synthesis occur simultaneously. As the molecule unwinds, torsion must be built-up in the structure until a point is reached at which further unwinding becomes increasingly difficult. Cairns has suggested that a swivel point exists near the growing point allowing that part of the molecule to rotate with respect to the remainder, thus keeping torsion to a minimum.

STRUCTURE AND SYNTHESIS OF RNA

Whereas the biological role of a DNA molecule is as a master file-index of genetic information, carefully reproduced and transmitted at each cell division, it is the task of the RNA molecules to translate these banks of coded data into tangible forms. They function both as working copies of the DNA information bank and as the tools which manufacture the specific protein molecules a particular DNA molecule encodes.

In contrast to the DNA molecules which usually exist as a single type in a given cell, three different kinds of RNA are present. These are *messenger RNA*, (mRNA), *transfer RNA* (tRNA) and *ribosomal RNA* (rRNA). This classification is both structural and functional, as will be evident later. In the liver cell approximately 11% of the total cell RNA is in the nucleus, mostly as precursors of mRNA; 15% is in the mitochondria; 50% is in the ribosomes, mainly as rRNA, and about 24% is in the cytosol as tRNA. In bacterial cells nearly all RNA is free in the cytosol (bacterial cells have no nucleus). RNA is present in plant viruses and in some animal and bacterial viruses.

Like DNA, the RNA molecules are long-chain polynucleotides made up of four different purine and pyrimidine bases and linked by 3′–5′ phosphate diester linkages. In contrast to DNA, the sugar component of RNA is *D-ribose*. RNA contains only three of the bases found in DNA, namely *adenine, guanine* and *cytosine*, the place of thymine being taken by *uracil*. Each of the three RNA types has a characteristic range of molecular weight values and each type exhibits further sub-division. In a given species three or more rRNA forms exist, there can be up to 60 different tRNA molecules, and there are many thousands of different mRNA types in a given cell. In addition the rRNA and tRNA molecules found in mitochondria differ from the extra-mitochondrial molecules.

The early observations of Casperson, Brachet and other workers indicated that the initiation of protein synthesis was accompanied in nearly all instances in intact cells by a parallel increase in

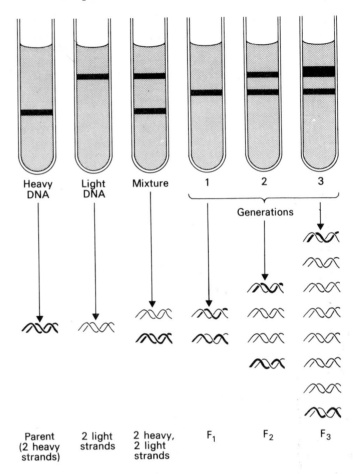

Fig. 3.59. The Meselson and Stahl experiment showing semi-conservative replication. (After Lehninger A.L. (1975) *Biochemistry*, 2nd edn. New York, Worth.)

Heavy DNA	Light DNA	Mixture	1	2	3

Generations

Parent (2 heavy strands)	2 light strands	2 heavy, 2 light strands	F_1	F_2	F_3

the amount and turnover of cytoplasmic RNA. Moreover cells which produce much protein, such as the salivary glands, contain large amounts of RNA, whereas cells producing little protein are low in RNA content. Thus there is a relationship between cell RNA content and protein synthesis. Bautz and Hall in 1962 found that cytosine and guanine, which are base-pairs in DNA (see p. 105), existed in differing proportions in an RNA produced in bacteriophage-infected *E. coli* cells. This implied that RNA chains did not pair in a complementary manner as in DNA. The results also suggested that RNA existed as a single-stranded molecule copied from a single-strand of the DNA molecule.

RNA is copied and synthesized from DNA in a manner analagous to that in which the enzyme DNA polymerase mediates DNA formation. The RNA synthetic process requires the involvement of *DNA-directed RNA polymerases* and in mammalians cells there are three of these enzyme types. Type I is in the nucleolus and responsible for synthesis of large precursor molecules of rRNA. Type II in the nucleoplasm is involved in synthesis of mRNA precursors, and the similarly located Type III enzyme is thought to be involved in the manufacture of the tRNA precursors. The production of messenger RNA by this DNA directed process is the basis of the important mechanism of transcription, whereby the genetic formation coded in the DNA base sequences is transcribed to a more mobile RNA carrier form.

The RNA-polymerase enzymes are very similar in action to DNA-polymerase. All four nucleotide 5'-triphosphates are required to be present simultaneously. Reaction proceeds with the release of pyrophosphate and adds nucleotide units at the 3'-OH terminal so that RNA is constructed in a 3' to 5' direction. The presence of such an enzyme in mitochondria is associated with the transcription of mitochondrial DNA.

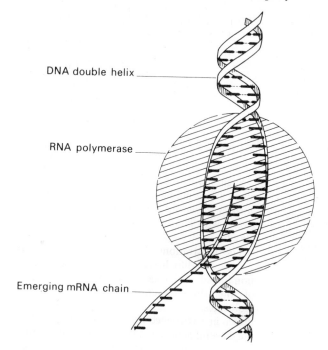

DNA double helix

RNA polymerase

Emerging mRNA chain

Fig. 3.60. The synthesis of RNA on a DNA template. The DNA unwinds some 4–8 nucleotides under the influence of RNA polymerase and the single RNA strand is produced from $5' \rightarrow 3'$ DNA polynucleotide. The diagram exaggerates the amount of DNA double helix unwinding.

For the formation of RNA the DNA double helix must partially unwind to expose the base sequence to be transcribed. After synthesis the RNA strand formed readily detaches itself from the DNA single-strand template probably because the DNA-RNA hybrid is less energetically stable than the DNA-DNA association (Fig. 3.60) which has a preferential affinity between its polynucleotide strands. The reason why only one strand of the DNA is selected for copying is as yet an unsolved problem but presumably must depend in some way on the physical states of the DNA template and the RNA polymerase.

THE CARBOHYDRATES

Carbohydrates are a major class of cell components. The simpler ones are involved in energy production in the cell and in the synthesis of noncarbohydrate constituents. They also occur as components of nucleic acids and of many cofactors essential in biochemical conversions. Polymeric carbohydrates are important sources of energy for organisms, both within the cell and, for many animals, as part of the diet. Carbohydrates form some 50% of the average human diet. They are constituents of supporting tissues in animals and especially in plants, which contain 60–90% carbohydrate. The structural properties of the plant carbohydrates are utilized by Man in the manufacture of materials such as rayon, linen, cotton, wood and paper.

Chemically, carbohydrates are a group of organic molecules which characteristically contain carbon, hydrogen and oxygen, usually exclusively so, in the ratio approximately represented by the empirical formula $C_x(H_2O)_y$ (where x may be equal to y). They have molecular weights which range from about 100 to several million. The larger carbohydrates are polymers which can be broken down to smaller units or monomers. Carbohydrates are classified according to their size. Two categories are recognized:

1 *Monosaccharides* are often called simple sugars. This term sugar is also used as a synonym for carbohydrate, though it is more generally reserved for the smaller molecules that have a characteristic sweet taste. Monosaccharides cannot be broken down into smaller units by hydrolysis with weak acid such as 1M HCl.

2 *Polysaccharides.* These are polymeric carbohydrates which on hydrolysis release their constituent monosaccharides. The smaller polysaccharides, containing between two and ten monosaccharides, are collectively termed the *oligosaccharides*.

A precise definition of the carbohydrates in chemical terms follows in the section devoted to monosaccharide structure.

Three important general points to note are:

1   Carbohydrates are not 'hydrates of carbon' in the way that $CuSO_4 . 5H_2O$ is a hydrated compound.

2   A substance with the empirical formula $C_x(H_2O)_y$ is not necessarily a carbohydrate. Thus acetic acid (CH_3COOH) has an empirical formula of $C_2(H_2O)_2$ while lactic acid, $CH_3CH(OH)COOH$, has an empirical formula of $C_3(H_2O)_3$, yet neither of these substances is a carbohydrate.

3   A number of widely distributed carbohydrates contain nitrogen, sulphur and phosphorus in addition to carbon, hydrogen and oxygen.

THE MONOSACCHARIDES

Definition

Of the 80 or 90 naturally occurring amino acids, only some 20 are used as the monomeric building blocks of proteins. Similarly, of the 100 naturally occurring monosaccharides only about 10 of these are found in natural polysaccharides, or occur to any great extent as free sugars.

Compared with the amino acids, the monosaccharides are a much more closely related group of substances. They all contain from three to nine carbon atoms though the majority are five- or six-carbon compounds. The smaller sugars with three or four carbons occur typically as phosphate esters in the metabolic sequences involved in the synthesis and breaking down of larger carbohydrates. Chemically, *monosaccharides, are polyhydroxy alcohols containing potentially active aldehyde or ketone groups.* 'Potentially active' is used because most monosaccharides containing five carbon atoms or more exist predominantly in ring forms in which the aldehyde $-C {\overset{H}{\underset{O}{\diagdown}}}$ or ketone $> C = O$ group is not normally free to participate in the reactions typically associated with these functional groups. However the two simplest monosaccharides, the three-carbon sugars, glyceraldehyde and dihydroxyacetone are straight-chain compounds. These sugars are termed *trioses* (the suffix *-ose* denotes a sugar). Glyceraldehyde is an *aldotriose* (or less specifically, an aldose) because it is a three-carbon polyalcohol containing an aldehyde group.

Dihydroxyacetone is a *keto-triose* because it contains a keto group:

Glyceraldehyde   Dihydroxyacetone

Sugars with four, five, six, seven, eight and nine carbon atoms are called *tetroses, pentoses, hexoses, heptoses, octoses* and *nonoses* respectively, with aldo- or keto- prefixes as the case may be.

The illustrations shown above for glyceraldehyde and dihydroxyacetone are called projection formulae. These are planar representations of the three-dimensional structure of the molecules. Projection formulae are always drawn in accordance with certain rules and they are a useful means of enabling the configuration and some of the salient features of the conformation of a molecule to be accurately and easily represented. It will be recalled that *conformation* is the three-dimensional arrangement of a molecule in space. *Configuration* refers to different molecular arrangements whose interconversion requires the breaking and reformation of covalent bonds.

Fischer projection formulae for carbohydrates

The convention used above for representing the two trioses was introduced by Emil Fischer (1852–1919). The rules for interpreting these projection formulae are as follows:

1   The carbon chain is written vertically with the most highly oxidized group uppermost.

2   The chain is numbered starting with the carbon of the aldehyde group as carbon-1, or in the case of the ketoses, labelling the carbon of the carbonyl group carbon-2.

3   Each carbon atom in the chain should be *viewed in turn* as if the horizontal bonds project towards the reader out of the paper while the vertical bonds linking neighbouring carbon atoms project away from the reader into the paper.

4   The formulae may be rotated 360° in the plane of the paper but never rotated out of this plane. (Occasionally difficulties arise in understanding a structural feature because this limitation is not appreciated).

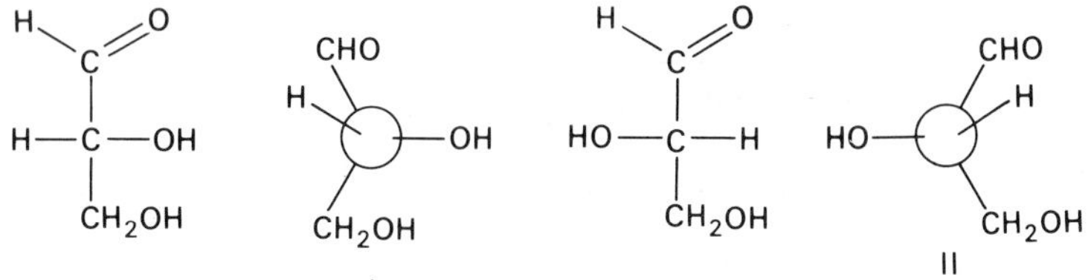

Fig. 3.61. Fischer and ball and stick representations of D- and L-glyceraldehyde.

Using these rules the molecular configuration is unambiguously defined, but it must be borne in mind that the Fischer formula does not represent the conformation that a sugar molecule adopts in solution.

Stereoisomerism and configuration in the monosaccharides

In glyceraldehyde carbon-2 is attached to four different substituents and is therefore an *asymmetric* carbon atom (see p. 34).

Accordingly, glyceraldehyde has two stereoisomers, distinguished by the use of the prefix D or L. It has been accepted by convention that in the Fischer formula, D-glyceraldehyde be represented with the hydroxyl group at carbon-2 projecting on the right-hand side. Similarly, in L-glyceraldehyde the hydroxyl group extends to the left-hand side. The two molecules are shown using both the normal Fischer formula and a ball-and-stick version (following the same rules) (Fig. 3.61).

There are no stereoisomers of dihydroxyacetone or of glycerol (the reduced form of glyceraldehyde) because they have no asymmetric carbon atom, as the following projection formulae show:

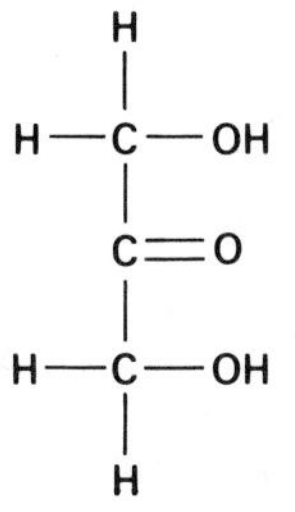

Dihydroxyacetone 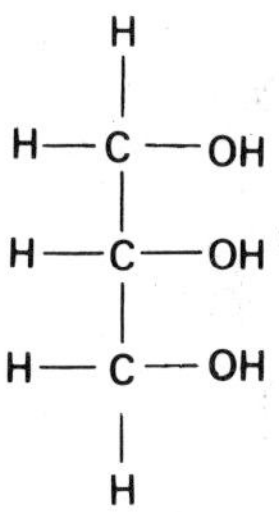   Glycerol

The D and L convention is applied to the nomenclature of all other monosaccharides no matter how many carbon atoms they contain. This follows from envisaging all the aldose sugars as structurally derived from either D-glyceraldehyde or L-glyceraldehyde. The decision as to which configurational family a given sugar belongs is made from an inspection of its projection formula, by observing the substituents on the highest-numbered asymmetric carbon atom. When the attached hydroxyl group on this atom is on the right then that sugar is called a D-series sugar (i.e. it is said to be of the D-configuration because it is structurally related to D-glyceraldehyde). Conversely, if the hydroxyl group is on the left in the Fischer formula it is an L-series sugar. Exactly the same rule applies to the ketoses (e.g. fructose). Dihydroxyacetone itself does not contain an asymmetric carbon atom but the ketotetrose formed by adding another carbon atom to dihydroxyacetone is asymmetric at its carbon-3 atom (its highest numbered asymmetric carbon atom) and therefore will exist in D and L forms, i.e.

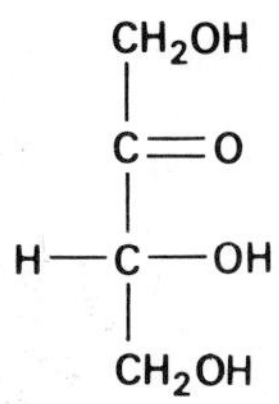

D-erythrulose 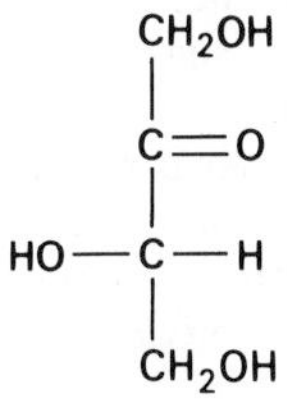   **L-erythrulose**

Larger D series sugar molecules such as the tetroses, pentoses. etc. are constructed by addition of further carbon atoms to the carbon-1 atom of the 3-carbon chain of D-glyceraldehyde. An L-sugar is defined similarly by reference to an analogous relationship with L-glyceraldehyde. No matter how much the carbon chain-length is increased, the structural orientation of the groups about that part of the molecule which was originally the carbon-2 of D-glyceraldehyde remains the same. Replacement of the OH group of this penultimate atom by any other group does not alter the fundamental configurational arrangement.

On the basis of this D and L series convention, all monosaccharides belong to one or other of four families based on the four sugars, D-glyceraldehyde, L-glyceraldehyde, D-erythrulose and L-erythrulose. The complete D-aldose and D-ketose series of sugars containing three, four, five and six carbon atoms are shown in Fig. 3.62 and Fig. 3.63.

As the carbon chain length is increased so the number of asymmetric carbon atoms also increases. For each asymmetric atom added a new enantiomeric pair is formed and the number of possible isomers for any given sugar is 2^n, where n is the number of asymmetric carbon atoms in the molecule. Thus, in the case of an aldohexose, n is 4, and there will be $2^4 = 16$ isomers in all, 8 in the D-series and 8 in the L-series. An L-series sugar is written using the Fischer convention by writing the D-series sugar in its mirror-image form. This is illustrated for D-glucose and L-glucose in Fig. 3.64.

Most of the naturally occurring carbohydrates belong to the D-series, although this rule is not absolute. Natural vitamin C (ascorbic acid) is a carbohydrate derivative related to L-glucose and in its D-isomer form will not prevent or cure scurvy (p. 248). A number of other L-series sugars occur naturally, and many glycoproteins contain L-series sugars.

It is evident then that biological systems must distinguish between these different configurations. Generally this is achieved by the involvement of sugars in metabolic processes where enzymes (p. 86) will only 'recognize' one isomer. As a result, living organisms generally contain only one configurational type of carbohydrate isomer and cells do not synthesize isomeric mixtures of molecules.

Optical isomerism in monosaccharides

Molecules with asymmetric centres exhibit the property of *optical activity*. Naturally occurring glucose, as in mammalian blood sugar, is designated D-(+) glucose, and the sweet tasting component in honey and many fruits is D-(−) fructose. Both are D-series sugars in terms of

their configurational stereochemistry but glucose is dextrorotatory (+), whereas fructose is laevorotatory (−).

The ring structure of the monosaccharides

The aldose and ketose families are shown in Figs. 3.62 and 3.63 and stress the structural similarities of the monosaccharides. All sugars are variations on a theme. The theme is a carbon chain containing carbonyl (aldehyde or keto) and alcohol groups. The variations arise from a lengthening of the carbon chain with the consequent addition of new asymmetric centres. The total number of isomers up to and including those containing six carbon atoms amounts to 30 aldoses and 15 ketoses. However, in 'performance', to use a musical analogy, only a few of these variations are usually encountered. The biologically important sugar molecules have been underlined.

The following discussion considers the theme in more detail and describes the ring structure—a feature which arises from the polyfunctional nature of carbohydrates. To understand monosaccharide ring structure it is helpful to consider first the ways which the functional groups of sugar molecules may interact when they are not part of the same molecule. Aldehydes and ketones both react reversibly with alcohols to form addition compounds called *hemiacetals* and *hemiketals*. Acetaldehyde and methanol, for instance, form the hemiacetal, methoxyethanol. The general reaction is:

$$R-C{\overset{O}{\underset{H}{\big\backslash\!\!/}}} \ + \ R'OH \ \rightleftharpoons \ R-\underset{OR'}{\overset{OH}{\underset{|}{\overset{|}{C}}}}-H$$

Aldehyde   Alcohol   Hemiacetal

Hemiacetals combine irreversibly with a further alcohol molecule to form an acetal:

$$R-\underset{OR'}{\overset{OH}{\underset{|}{\overset{|}{C}}}}-H \ + \ R''-OH \ \longrightarrow \ R-\underset{OR'}{\overset{OR''}{\underset{|}{\overset{|}{C}}}}-H$$

Hemiacetal   Alcohol   Acetal

Acetal formation is catalysed only by acids, whereas the formation of a hemiacetal or hemiketal is catalysed by either acid or base.

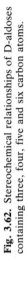

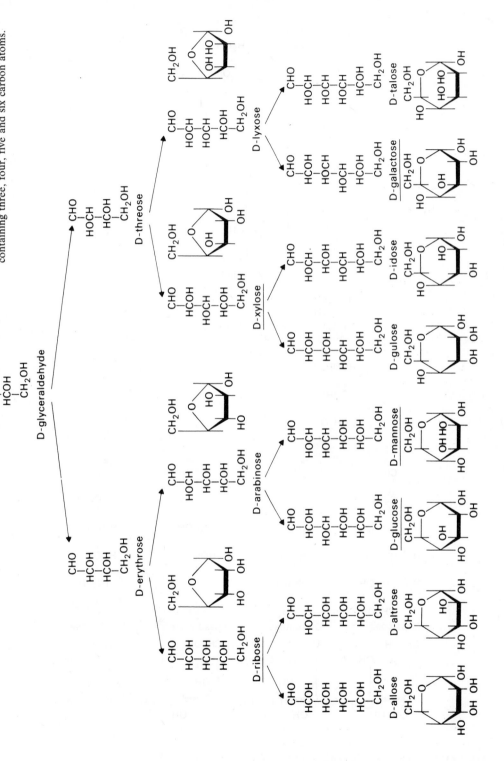

Fig. 3.62. Stereochemical relationships of D-aldoses containing three, four, five and six carbon atoms.

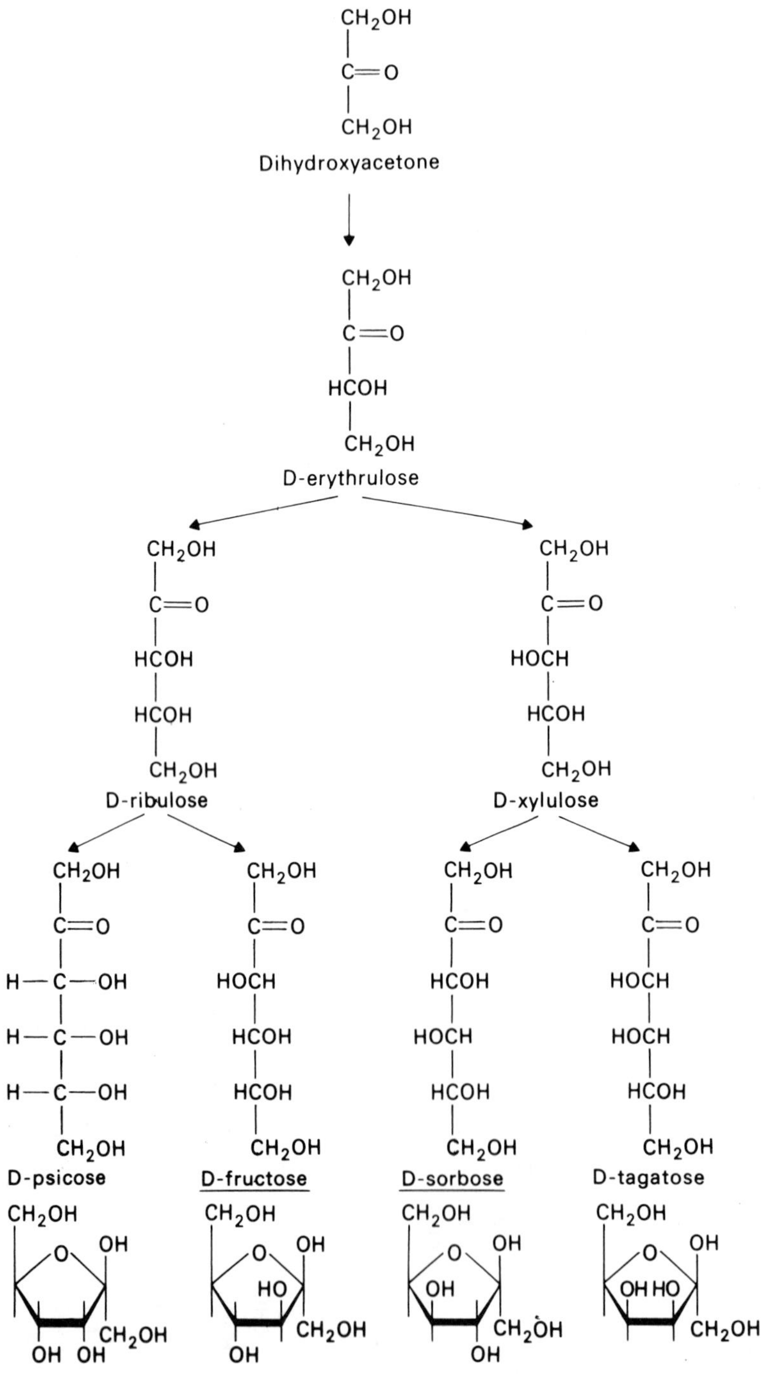

Fig. 3.63. Stereochemical relationships of D-ketoses containing three, four, five and six carbon atoms.

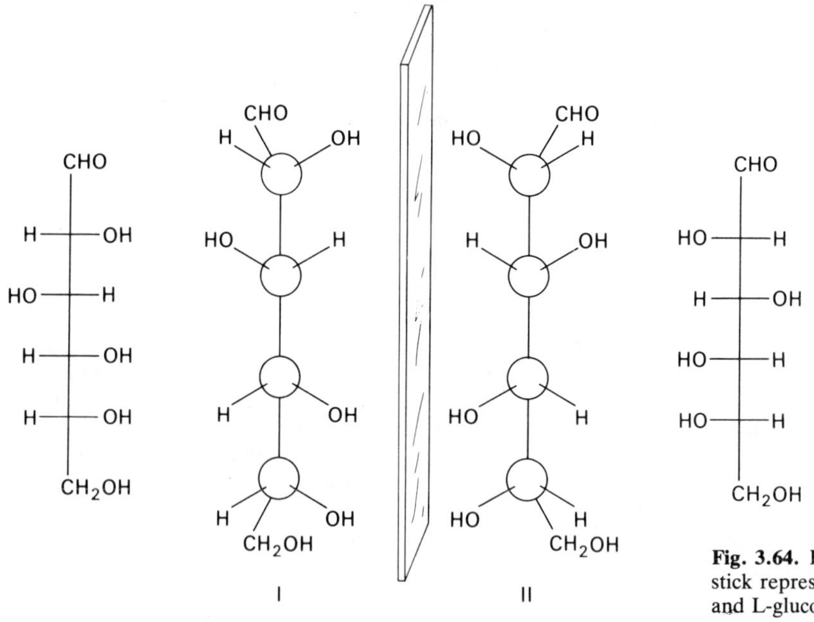

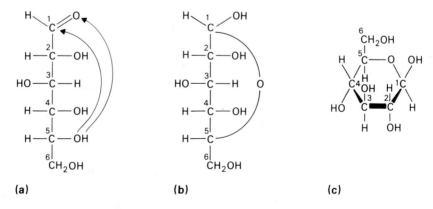

Fig. 3.64. Fischer and ball and stick representations of D- (I) and L-glucose (II).

Since monosaccharides contain both carbonyl and hydroxyl groups within the same molecule sugars where the carbon chain is sufficiently long to permit two such groups to come into close proximity can form *internal* hemiacetals and hemiketals. Both intramolecular and intermolecular reversible reactions of this type occur, but the latter involve unfavourable entropy changes. These thermodynamic considerations dictate that monosaccharides containing a chain of five or more carbon atoms exist more stably in ring forms. Thus, in the six-carbon

chain of D-glucose, the carbonyl group at carbon-1 reacts with the alcohol group at carbon-5 and so forms a 6-membered ring consisting of five carbon atoms and a single oxygen atom. This hemiacetal form of D-glucose is shown in Fig. 3.65b using the Fischer projection formula, which presents an exaggerated length for the oxygen bridge. A more realistic projection formula (Fig. 3.65c) was suggested by Walter Haworth (1883–1950) and formulae of this type are now widely used.

It is important to know that the oxygen joining

Fig. 3.65. Projection formulae for D-glucose. (a) Open-chain Fischer formulae. (b) The cyclic Fischer formulae. (c) The Haworth formulae.

carbon atoms 1 and 5 is derived from the hydroxyl group of carbon-5 and not from the oxygen attached to carbon-1 (Fig. 3.65a).

On inspection, the relationship between the Fischer and Haworth formulae may not be apparent. The cyclic Fischer projection formula is slightly misleading in that it seems to imply that the oxygen bridge extends from the back of carbon-1 to the front of carbon-5. However, if carbon-5 is rotated about the carbon-4–carbon-5 bond (a →b in Fig. 3.66), an operation which readily takes place in the open chain form, then structure (c) results, in which the oxygen bridge is clearly seen to extend from the back of carbon-1 to the back of carbon-5. The Haworth structure (d) can then be seen to be identical with (c).

This re-interpretation of the Fischer formula does not involve the breaking of any chemical bonds and so does not imply any change in the configuration of the molecule.

INTERPRETATION OF THE HAWORTH FORMULA

In D-glucose, the ring of five carbon atoms and one oxygen atom lies approximately in a single plane. Using the Haworth formula, the orientation of this plane is at right angles to the plane of the paper and so projects directly towards the reader. This is suggested by the thickened lines representing the bonds joining carbon atoms 1, 2, 3, and 4. The hydrogen, hydroxyl and the primary alcohol groups project either above or below this plane, as their bond lines indicate.

The D and L configuration is indicated in a 6-membered ring aldohexose such as D-glucose by the position of the carbon-6 primary alcohol group ($-CH_2OH$) relative to carbon-5. This group is drawn above the plane for D-sugars and below for L-sugars, as illustrated for the stereoisomers of galactose (Fig. 3.67). Imagine the D-galactose molecule as suspended above a horizontal mirror.

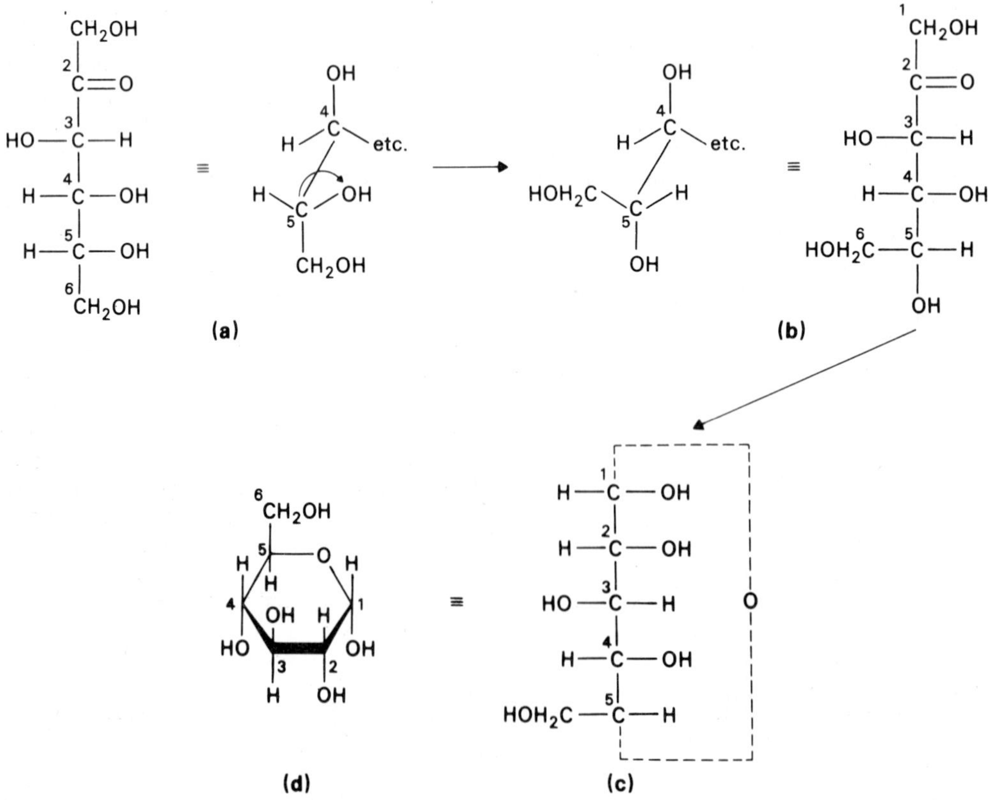

Fig. 3.66. Relationships between the Fischer open-chain and Haworth formulae.

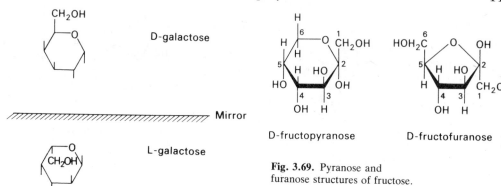

CH₂OH

D-galactose

/////// Mirror

CH₂OH

L-galactose

Fig. 3.67. Stereoisomers of galactose.

D-fructopyranose   D-fructofuranose

Fig. 3.69. Pyranose and furanose structures of fructose.

Most of the aldohexoses form ring structures by the interaction between the functional groups on carbon-1 and carbon-5. However, the aldehyde group at carbon-1 can also react with the –OH group at carbon-4 to form a 5-membered ring. The monosaccharide ring structures are classified on the basis of their similarity to the heterocyclic organic compounds tetrahydropyran and tetrahydrofuran, and the 5- and 6-atom rings found in the sugars are referred to as *furanose* and *pyranose* rings, respectively (Fig. 3.68).

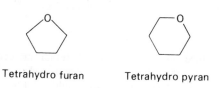

Tetrahydro furan   Tetrahydro pyran

Fig. 3.68. Furanose and pyranose ring structures.

As D-glucose usually forms a six-membered ring it may also be designated as *D-glucopyranose* to take account of this fact. D-fructose in its free state generally adopts the pyranose form (hence *D-fructopyranose*), but when combined with other monosaccharides it exists as a furanose ring and is called *D-fructofuranose*. The two forms are shown below (Fig. 3.69). Since fructose is a ketose, the –OH at carbon-5 reacts with the keto function which is at carbon-2 (not carbon-1).

THE CONFORMATION OF MONOSACCHARIDES

Projection formulae are merely symbols which record only some of the important characteristics of the molecules they represent, and are inadequate in various respects. The Haworth formulae for instance show the carbon chain and oxygen bridge as a planar ring but this is true only for the furanose ring system, not for the pyranose form. The pyranose rings adopt conformations which are generally variations on what is known as the *chair form*, as shown for β-D-glucopyranose below (Fig. 3.70).

ANOMERISM—STEREOISOMERISM ARISING FROM RING FORMATION

The Haworth or Fischer ring formulae for D-glucose show that the carbon-1 (in contrast to its open-chain form) carries four different substituents and is therefore asymmetric. As a result, D-glucose in its ring form (and indeed all other cyclic sugars) can exist as two optically active isomers which differ in their configuration about carbon-1 (Fig. 3.71). This special type of isomerism arising from ring closure is called anomerism. The two resultant isomers are termed the α- and β-anomers. These anomers are differentiated by reference to the configuration of their hydroxyl groups. In the Haworth formulae the hydroxyl group carbon-1 of the α-anomer has a *cis*-relationship (see p. 988) to the hydrogen at carbon-5, which acts as a reference carbon, whilst the hydroxyl group of the β-anomer has a *trans*-relationship with the carbon-5 hydrogen.

For the D-sugars this rule means that α-anomers are represented by formulae in which the –OH group at carbon-1 is below the plane of the ring and vice versa for the β-anomers.

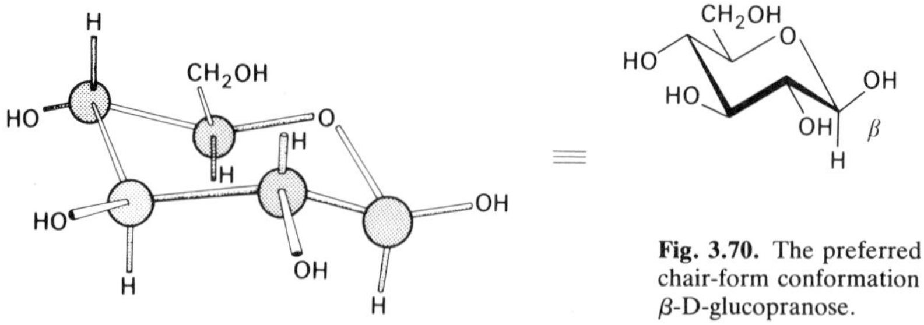

Fig. 3.70. The preferred chair-form conformation for β-D-glucopranose.

MUTAROTATION—THE INTERCONVERSION OF ANOMERS

The reversible nature of hemiacetal and hemiketal formation has already been stressed and this is so also for such intramolecular reactions occurring within sugar molecules. As a result a sugar solution usually contains three molecular species; an α-anomer; a β-anomer; and an open-chain form, which constantly interconvert, i.e. the conversion of β-D-glucose to α-D-glucose:

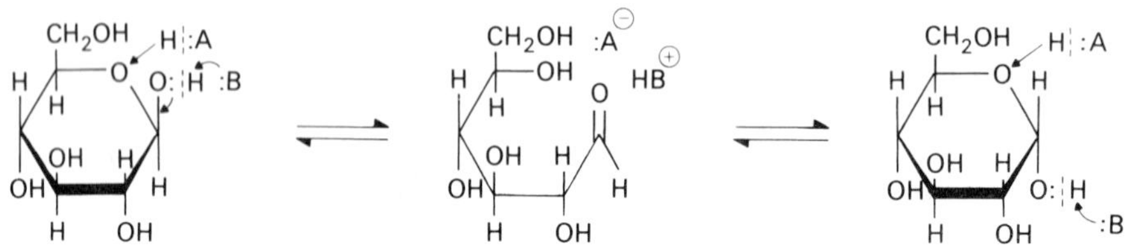

D-fructose does not form an α-anomer. Presumably it is too unstable.

Reactions of the monosaccharides

Aldose and ketose sugars can undergo various chemical changes. The more important of these reactions, together with a number of the commonly encountered sugar derivatives, may be categorized under the following headings; *reduction, oxidation, dehydration, rearrangement, glycoside formation,* and *hydroxyl group substitution.*

β-D-Glucose   Aldehyde form   α-D-Glucose

In solution D-glucose exists as an equilibrium mixture containing less than 0.05% of the open-chain form, up to 70% of the β-anomer and 30% of the α-anomer.

This interconversion phenomenon is called *mutarotation* for the following reason. Both α and β anomers are optically active but have different rotational (α_D^{20}) values. On dissolving one or other of the anomers in water the interconversion to an equilibrium mixture of the α, β and open-chain species is observed by recording changes in optical rotation against time. In the case of D-glucose this can readily be followed (Fig. 3.72) as a decrease in the optical rotation of the α-anomer (+112°) or an increase for the β-anomer (+18.7°) until the equilibrium value of +52.7° is reached. Several hours must elapse before equilibrium is attained.

Since sugars are polyfunctional molecules containing both carbonyl and hydroxyl groups it could be thought that they should react in ways characteristic of both. However, this is true for the open-chain forms only. Hemiacetal ring formation involves interaction of the carbonyl group with a hydroxyl group in the same molecule, and so prevents their full expression. Hence sugars do not give all the reactions typical of aldehydes or ketones. For example, glucose does not form a disulphite addition compound and does not give a positive result with Schiff's test, both characteristic aldehyde reactions. Nor does glucose have the pungent odour associated with aldehydes and ketones, such as formaldehyde and acetone.

In monosaccharide chemistry it is important to recall the reversible nature of hemiacetal for-

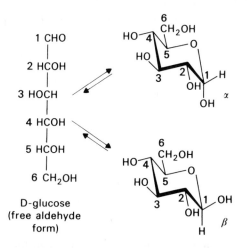

	6
1 CHO	
2 HCOH	
3 HOCH	
4 HCOH	
5 HCOH	
6 CH₂OH	

D-glucose
(free aldehyde
form)

Fig. 3.71. The anomeric forms of D-glucose.

mation. Thus, the small fraction of glucose molecules present in any equilibrium solution as the open-chain aldehydic form can undergo reactions characteristic of aldehydes. Continual removal of this open-chain form by such a reaction disturbs the equilibrium so that eventually all the hemiacetal form will be utilized via its conversion to the open-chain molecule, i.e.

Hemiacetal   Open-chain   Modified
sugar 99.95% at ⇌ sugar 0.05% at ⟶ sugar
equilibrium   equilibrium

In the above equation it is assumed that the reaction to form the modified sugar is not itself reversible.

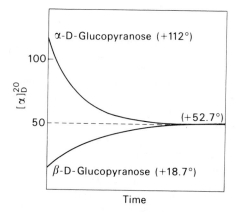

Fig. 3.72. The change in $[\alpha]_D^{20}$ with time on adding pure α-D-glucose and β-D-glucose to water.

The preponderance of hydroxyl groups in carbohydrates makes sugars strongly polar substances. Consequently they are readily soluble in polar solvents such as water, and insoluble in non-polar solvents such as ether or benzene. Moreover, these hydroxyl groups also provide for the possibility of extensive hydrogen bond formation. The crunchy texture of ordinary domestic sugar (sucrose) results from this hydrogen bonding which contributes to the dense packing of the sugar molecules within the crystal.

THE REDUCTION OF MONOSACCHARIDES

Sugar alcohols

Monosaccharides possess several hydroxyl groups but only one carbonyl group. The reduction of this carbonyl group to a hydroxyl group converts the sugar to a polyhydric alcohol.

Polyhydric alcohols exist as either open-chain or cyclic compounds. The former are called *sugar alcohols* and may be formed by simple reduction of sugars using, for instance, hydrogen and a platinum catalyst. The ring compounds are called *cyclitols* and are quite distinct from the open-chain sugars because they do not result from hemiacetal formation. Hence they are unable to exist in equilibrium with open-chain forms and they cannot be synthesized by reduction of sugars. The best known example of a cyclitol is myo-inositol whose hexaphosphoric acid ester is called phytic acid and occurs in many cereals. There is evidence that this substance interferes with calcium absorption from the gut. Myo-inositol itself is incorporated into the phospholipid, phosphatidyl inositol, which occurs in plants and nervous tissue.

Myo-inositol

The open-chain sugar alcohols formed from aldoses and ketoses are known as *alditols* and *ketitols*. The simplest example, glycerol, can form from glyceraldehyde or dihydroxyacetone. Glycerol is important as the alcohol moiety of neutral fats (p. 150).

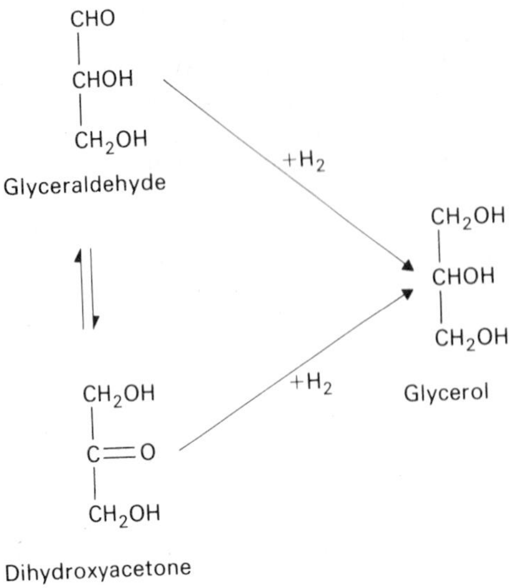

CHO
|
CHOH
|
CH₂OH

Glyceraldehyde

+H₂

CH₂OH
|
CHOH
|
CH₂OH

Glycerol

+H₂

CH₂OH
|
C=O
|
CH₂OH

Dihydroxyacetone

obtained by the acid hydrolysis of xylan, an important structural polysaccharide in wood:

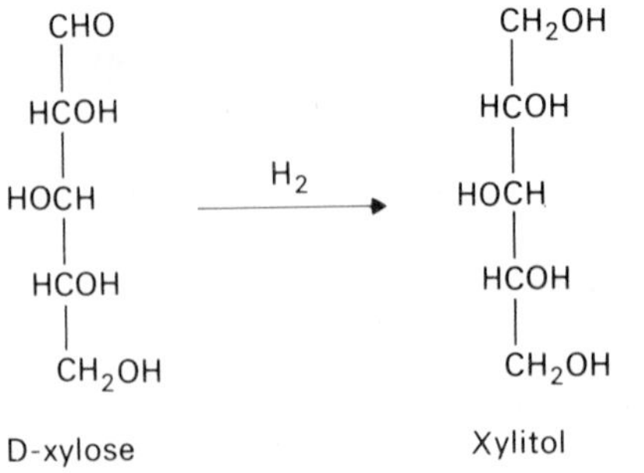

CHO
|
HCOH
|
HOCH
|
HCOH
|
CH₂OH

D-xylose

H₂ →

CH₂OH
|
HCOH
|
HOCH
|
HCOH
|
CH₂OH

Xylitol

Reduction of either glucose or fructose results in the same product—the open-chain sugar alcohol with the trivial name of sorbitol.

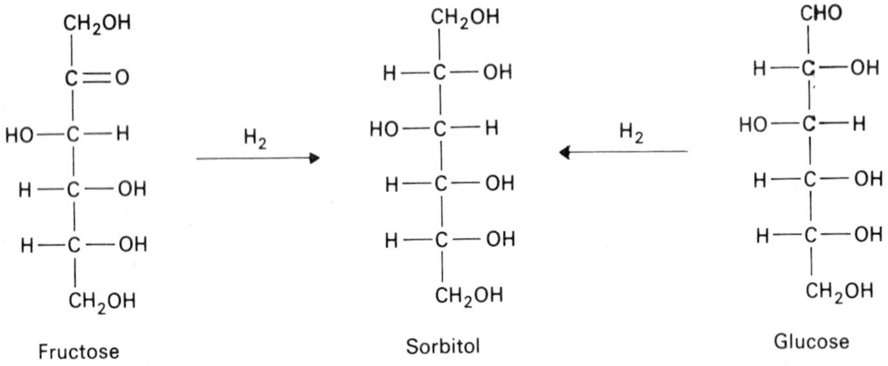

Both xylitol and sorbitol are used in foods for patients suffering from diabetes mellitus. Neither sugar is actively absorbed from the gut and so their ingestion in food has only a very minor influence on the blood sugar level. However, excessive intake disturbs the osmotic balance in the gut and results in diarrhoea.

CH₂OH
|
C=O
|
HO—C—H
|
H—C—OH
|
H—C—OH
|
CH₂OH

Fructose

H₂ →

CH₂OH
|
H—C—OH
|
HO—C—H
|
H—C—OH
|
H—C—OH
|
CH₂OH

Sorbitol

← H₂

CHO
|
H—C—OH
|
HO—C—H
|
H—C—OH
|
H—C—OH
|
CH₂OH

Glucose

The five-carbon alcohol xylitol has aroused considerable interest recently due to its recommended use as a dietary substitute for sucrose in the control of dental caries. This sugar is not attacked by those oral bacteria thought responsible for tooth decay, and is not, therefore, fermented in the mouth to form organic acids which dissolve hydroxyapatite in enamel and so initiate and develop carious lesions. Since xylitol is at least as sweet as ordinary sugar, and appears to be well tolerated in the human diet, it has been recommended by some authorities as a non-cariogenic substitute for ordinary sugar. A main objection to its widespread use at present is its very high cost compared with sucrose. Xylitol is manufactured by the reduction of xylose, a sugar

Deoxy-sugars

Deoxy-sugars result from reduction at positions in the carbon chain other than at the carbonyl function. As the name implies, they have fewer oxygen atoms than carbon atoms. One example is the pentose deoxy-D-ribose (p. 103) which is a component of the deoxyribose nucleic acid (DNA) (p. 103). This sugar and the parent aldopentose ribose (in RNA) are two carbohydrates involved in the inheritance and expression of genetic information (p. 239).

Two other important deoxy-sugars are L-fucose (6-deoxy L-galactose) and L-rhamnose (6-deoxy L-mannose). L-fucose occurs as a component sugar in many glycoproteins (p. 60) including the immunoglobulins, the blood group antigens, some of the pituitary hormones (LH and FSH) and many salivary and plasma glycoproteins. L-rhamnose is confined to plants and bacteria, and its appearance in dental plaque is therefore directly related to the bacterial content. L-fucose, although originally present in salivary glycoprotein components, is largely absent from plaque, which implies their degradation during plaque formation.

Amino sugars (glycosamines)

Like the deoxy-sugars, amino sugars occur naturally in many plant and animal polysaccharides. With one exception they contain a single amino group substituted in the carbon-2 position. The amino group is more usually present in an acetylated form, i.e.

Chitin, the tough, inert, protective, outer casing of insects, spiders and crabs is a polysaccharide constructed from N-acetyl glucosamine (p. 139).

THE OXIDATION OF MONOSACCHARIDES

Sugar acids

All monosaccharides are reducing sugars. For example, they can reduce cupric ions (Cu^{2+}) to cuprous ions (Cu^+) and during this process themselves become oxidized. This characteristic reaction is utilized in the Fehlings', Benedicts' and Folin–Wu laboratory tests for reducing sugars. These involve linked reactions that allow visualization of the reductive formation of Cu^+. Thus in the Folin–Wu reaction, cuprous oxide

$$Sugar - NH_2 \longrightarrow Sugar - \underset{\underset{H}{|}}{N} - \overset{\overset{O}{\parallel}}{C} \diagdown CH_3$$

Amino sugar   N-acetylated amino sugar

In animals they occur mostly as constituent monomers of connective tissue polysaccharides. Three important amino sugars are N-acetyl glucosamine found in hyaluronic acid and keratan sulphate (p. 141); N-acetyl galactosamine, a constituent of the chondroitin sulphates (p. 141), and N-acetyl neuraminic acid which is one of a small group of important carbohydrates known as the *sialic acids* (p. 345). These substances are N− or O− substituted derivatives of neuraminic acid (Fig. 3.73). N-acetyl neuraminic acid is a derivative of a nine-carbon sugar although it contains a six-membered ring only. In effect it is a condensation product formed between N-acetyl mannosamine and pyruvic acid. It is an important constituent of glycoproteins and its bacterial enzymic removal from salivary glycoproteins is the basis of one hypothesis of dental plaque formation (Vol 3). Sialic acids are also components of the ground-substance of bone, dentine, cementum, etc.

Both non-acetylated and N-acetylated amino sugars occur in the oligosaccharide antibiotics streptomycin, kanamycin and neomycin.

(Cu^+ state) is reoxidized by phosphomolybdous acid with the formation of blue phosphomolybdous acid which can be measured spectrophotometrically. This type of oxidation can occur only with sugar containing a hemiacetal linkage since it is the open-chain form that is responsible for this reducing action. Thus oxidation of reducing sugars takes place via the continual shifting of equilibrium mentioned earlier.

The reducing sugar tests described above, all involve the conversion of the sugars to various derivatives. With more gentle oxidation the basic sugar structure can be retained and conversion to a carboxyl function can occur at different positions as shown in Table 3.12.

Periodic acid oxidation

Periodic acid (HIO_4) is a powerful oxidant which breaks carbon–carbon bonds in various structures where there are adjacent carbons carrying hydroxyl groups (i.e. a 1, 2-glycol group). The cis 1, 2 glycols are oxidized more rapidly than the trans glycols, i.e.:

$$\begin{array}{c} CH_2OH \\ | \\ (CHOH)_n \\ | \\ CH_2OH \end{array} + (n+1)\, H^+IO_4^- \longrightarrow \begin{array}{l} 2HCHO \\ + n(HCOOH) \\ + H_2O \\ + n+1\ (HIO_3) \end{array}$$

Table 3.12. Oxidation of aldoses to different sugar acids.

Position of oxidation	General name for product	Specific example		
Carbon–1	Aldonic acid	D-gluconic acid	1	COOH
			2	HCOH
			3	HOCCH
			4	HCOH
			5	HCOH
			6	CH₂OH
Carbon–6	Alduronic acid	D-glucuronic acid	1	CHO
			2	HCOH
			3	HOCH
			4	HCOH
			5	HCOH
			6	COOH
Carbon–1 and Carbon–6	Aldaric acid	D-glucaric acid	1	COOH
			2	HCOH
			3	HOCH
			4	HCOH
			5	HCOH
			6	COOH

From this equation it can be seen that primary alcohol groups are converted to aldehyde groups while secondary alcohol groups are converted to formic acid. Since carbohydrates contain many such pairs of hydroxyl groups this reaction has been of great importance in carbohydrate chemistry. Where the sugars are bound in polysaccharides the resulting aldehydes are not further oxidized. Such polysaccharides can then be localized histochemically in tissue sections by condensation with Schiff's reagent (a dye containing an amino group) to give a substituted product which is red in colour. This is the basis of the periodic acid–Schiff (PAS) reaction (p. 71).

Glycogen, starch, cellulose, most glycoproteins, and many complex lipids all give positive reactions.

The lactones

In some instances oxidation involves the formation of an internal ester known as a *lactone*. These are usually either 5 (γ) or 6 (δ) membered ring compounds. Here the Greek lettering designates the carbon atom to which the car-

boxyl group is esterified. 6-phospho glucono-δ-lactone occurs as an intermediate in the oxidation of glucose-6-phosphate to gluconic acid 6-phosphate (see p. 210 on the pentose shunt oxidation of glucose).

A biologically very important lactone is 2,3-didehydro-L-gulonolactone (a γ-lactone) better known as *vitamin C* or *L-ascorbic acid*. As it is sometimes difficult to see how vitamin C is related to the aldose sugars, Fig. 3.74 shows the relationship of vitamin C to D-gulose, one of the sixteen isomeric aldoses shown in Fig. 3.62.

Vitamin C biosynthesis in animals, such as rat, proceeds via the conversion of D-glucuronic acid to L-gulonic acid, however man cannot synthesize it—hence its importance as a vitamin for humans and its associated deficiency disease of scurvy (p. 248). Ascorbic acid is also widely used as an antioxidant to prevent oxidative discolouration in frozen food. These reducing properties are due to its enediol ($-CHOH=CHOH-$) grouping. Since ascorbic acid is a strong reducing agent it is readily oxidized to dehydroascorbic acid. This reversible reaction is undoubtedly responsible for several of its physiological properties.

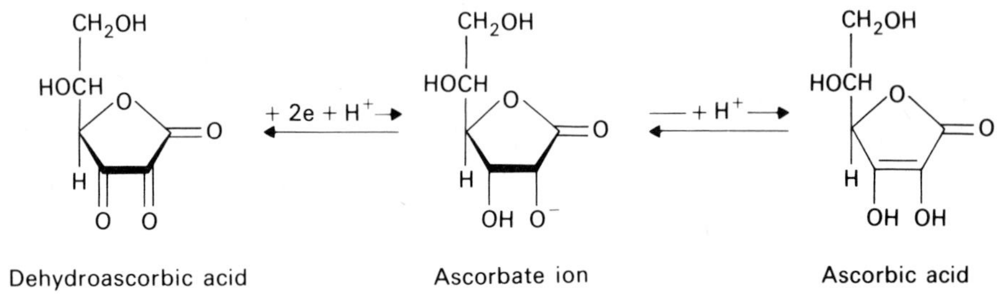

The oxidation of ascorbic acid to dehydroascorbic acid.

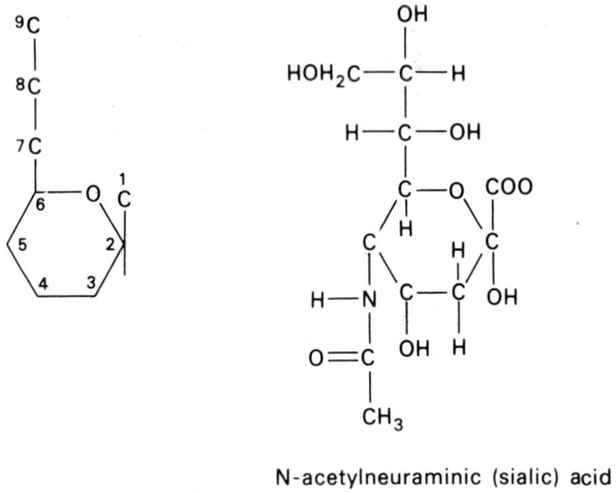

N-acetylneuraminic (sialic) acid

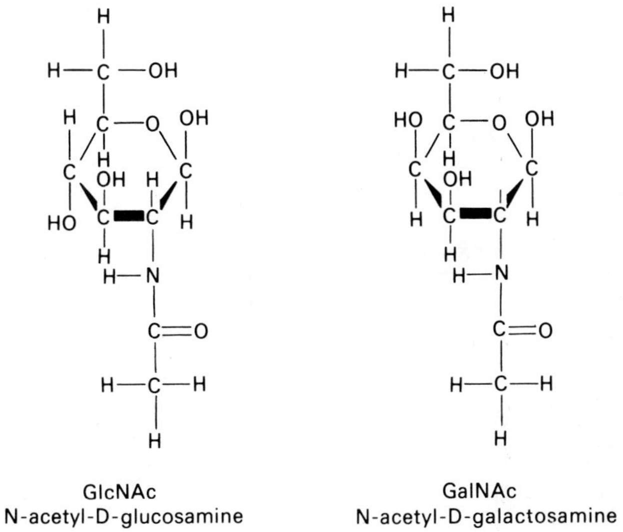

GlcNAc
N-acetyl-D-glucosamine

GalNAc
N-acetyl-D-galactosamine

Fig. 3.73. Three important N-acetylated glycosamines.

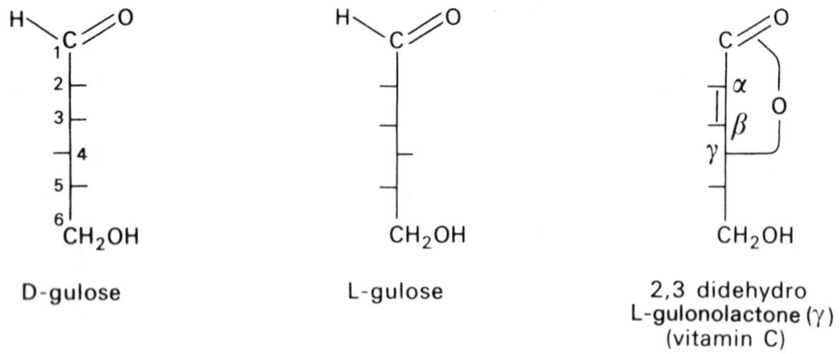

D-gulose   L-gulose   2,3 didehydro
                                                        L-gulonolactone (γ)
                                                        (vitamin C)

Fig. 3.74. The relationship of D-gulose to ascorbic acid.

DEHYDRATION REACTIONS

The Maillard reaction and the melanoidins
The elimination of water from glucose molecules
by the prolonged action of concentrated sulphuric acid provides a dramatic illustration of
the fact that this carbohydrate has been called a
'hydrate of carbon' for the product formed is
pure carbon. Less severe acid conditions (e.g. 6

N HCL) form dehydration products which by
their condensation with specific phenols provide
the basis for a number of colour tests for carbohydrates (e.g. the anthrone reaction and
the Molisch test). In these tests the primary
condensation products of carbohydrate dehydration formed are *5-hydroxy-methyl-*
2-furaldehyde (HMF) from aldo- or keto-

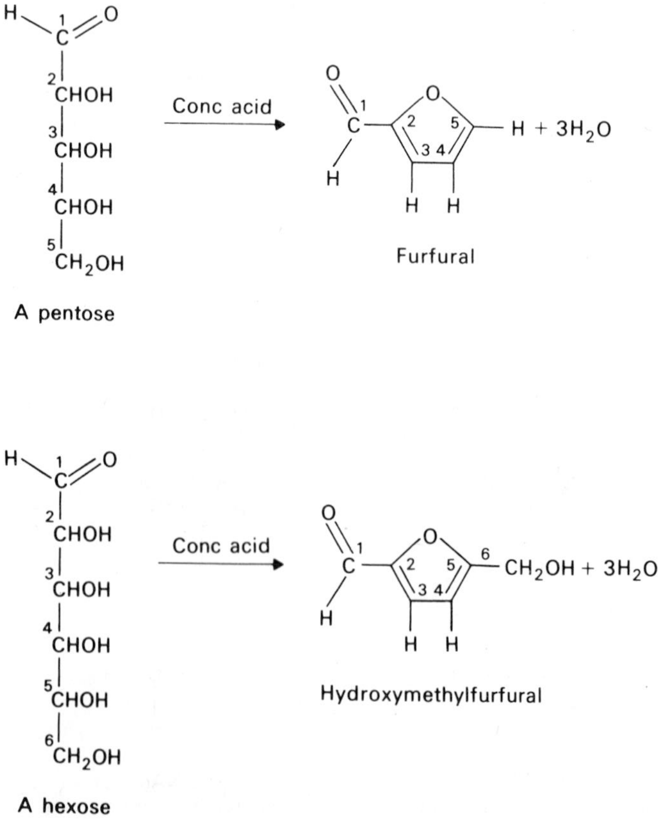

A pentose   Furfural

Fig. 3.75. Dehydration of
pentose and hexose to form
furfural and hydroxy-
methylfurfural.

A hexose   Hydroxymethylfurfural

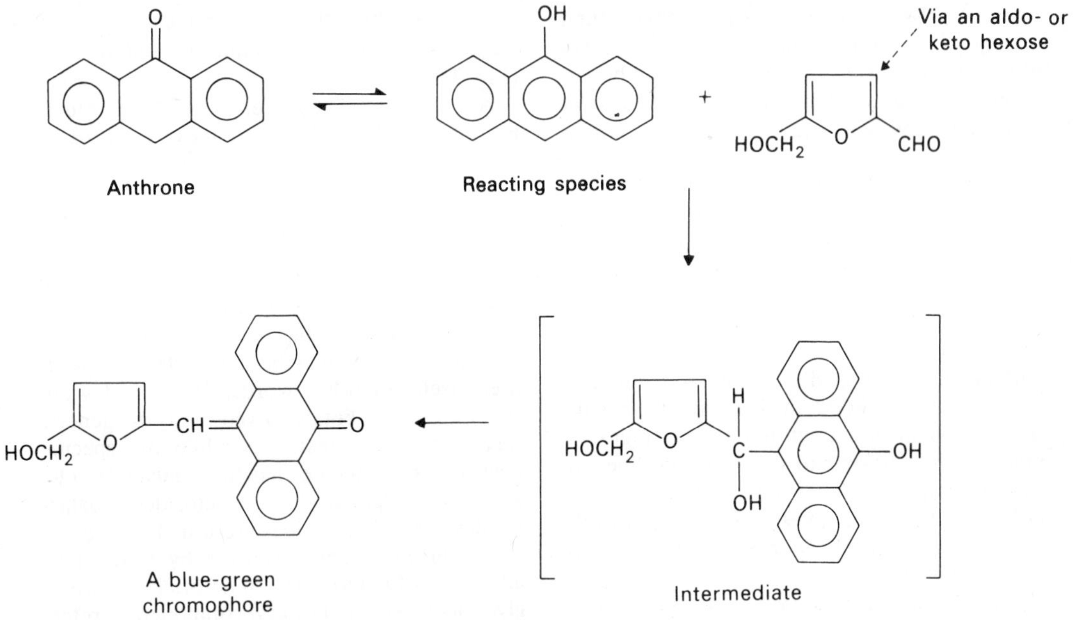

Fig. 3.76. The anthrone reaction.

hexoses and *furaldehyde* (also termed furfural for furfuraldehyde) from aldo- or keto-pentoses (Fig. 3.75).

A widely used colour test for carbohydrates is the *anthrone reaction* shown in Fig. 3.76.

A positive result (a blue-green colour) is given by any carbohydrate which forms furfural (e.g. from pentoses) or hydroxymethylfurfural (e.g. from hexoses, disaccharides, glycosides, carbohydrate ethers and esters). In Molisch's test, α-naphthol instead of anthrone is used in an analogous reaction, which results in a purple complex.

With prolonged heating under strong acid conditions both hydroxymethyl furfuraldehyde and furfuraldehyde undergo further condensation reactions leading to the formation of dark coloured complex polymers of unknown structure (humins).

The Maillard reaction is responsible for the undesirable browning that occurs when natural products such as milk, eggs, fruit juices and others are dried for conservation and storage. Initially interaction between the amino group of an amino acid, peptide or protein and the carbonyl group of a reducing sugar forms an N-substituted glycosylamine (Fig. 3.77).

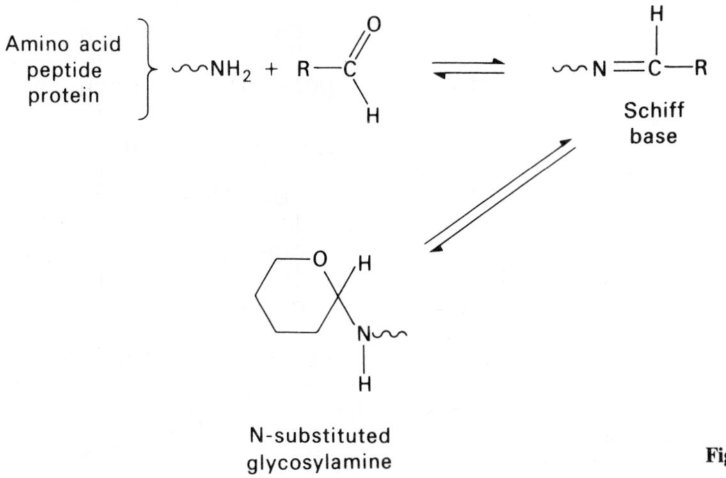

Fig. 3.77. The Maillard reaction.

These N-substituted glycosylamines then undergo a series of complex reactions, as yet little understood, leading to formation of brown polymer products called *melanoidins* (as distinct from melanins, see p. 275) which are humin-like substances.

As an example of its deleterious effects, dried egg, containing 83%protein and 3% glucose, will deteriorate both in nutritional value and in flavour during prolonged storage. Removal of this glucose prevents deterioration.

On the other hand, the Maillard reaction is responsible for many of the attractive colours and flavours developed in baking, roasting, frying and toasting. Foods such as biscuits, breakfast cereals, meat extract and malt extract owe much of their flavour to this reaction. Specific flavours can sometimes be created. Glucose heated with glycine gives a flavour of freshly baked bread, and with hydroxyproline a flavour of potato is produced.

The brown discolouration in carious dentine has been attributed to the formation of such compounds involving reaction with the ε-amino groups of the lysine side-chains of the exposed collagenous matrix of dentine.

MONOSACCHARIDE REARRANGEMENTS

Glucose, when dissolved in dilute alkali, undergoes rearrangement, forming an equilibrium solution containing 60% D-glucose, 30% D-fructose and 3% D-mannose. D-glucose and D-mannose differ only in their configuration at carbon-2 (Fig. 3.78). Molecules related in this manner are called *epimers*.

The transformation shows the close relationship between glucose, mannose and fructose (Fig. 3.78).

Another important rearrangement, mutarotation, has been discussed above (p. 120).

O- AND N- GLYCOSIDES

O-glycosides are derivatives of sugars where the hydrogen atom of the hydroxyl group of the hemiacetal function has been substituted by an alkyl group which may be substituted and modified itself. In other words, O-glycosides are sugar acetals or ketals. Glycoside is the generic term for these substances while the specific derivatives of glucose, fructose, galactose, etc. are termed 'glucosides', 'fructosides', 'galactosides', etc. N-glycosides are usually named as such, whilst the term 'glycoside' by itself generally means 'O-glycoside'. In naturally occurring glycosides, the alkyl or aryl component is referred to as the aglycone.

The common structural feature of all glycosides is the glycosidic link (Fig. 3.79).

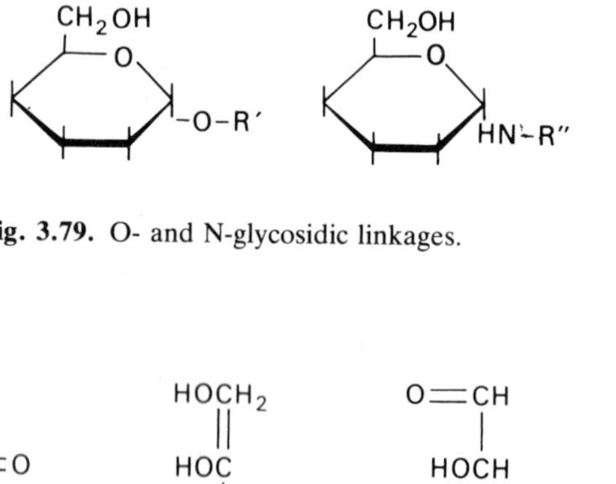

Fig. 3.79. O- and N-glycosidic linkages.

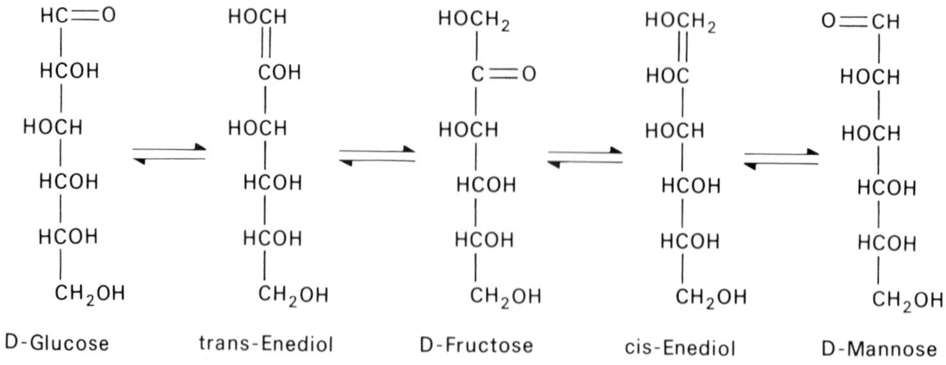

Fig. 3.78. The epimeric relationship between D-glucose, D-fructose and D-mannose.

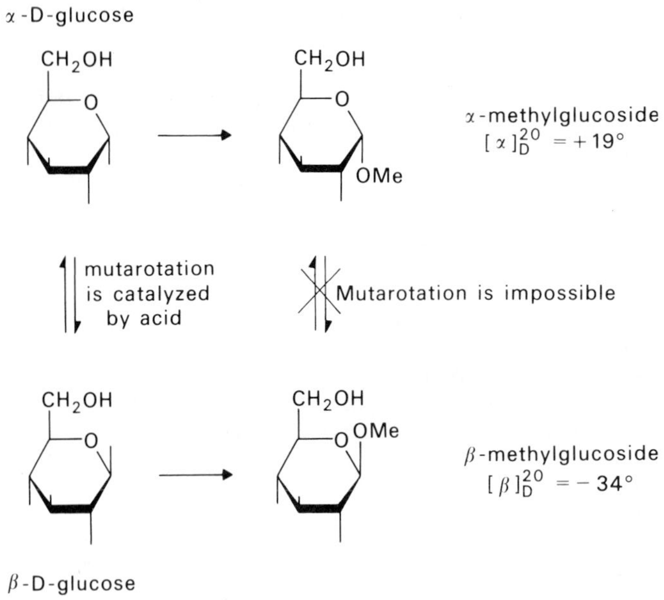

α-D-glucose

α-methylglucoside
$[\alpha]_D^{20} = +19°$

mutarotation is catalyzed by acid

Mutarotation is impossible

β-methylglucoside
$[\beta]_D^{20} = -34°$

β-D-glucose

Fig. 3.80. The formation of α and β-methylglucosides.

N-glycosides are derivatives of sugars in which the carbon of the hemiacetal (or hemiketal) linkage is joined to an alkyl or aryl group via a nitrogen atom.

Substances containing glycosidic links are widespread throughout the living world, and the most abundant of these are the oligo- and polysaccharides which are O-glycosides in which the substituted group is another sugar.

Hemiacetal formation is reversible (thereby making mutarotation possible) whereas acetal formation is irreversible (i.e. it is not an equilibrium reaction). Emil Fischer found that when a solution of D-glucose was warmed with methanol and hydrochloric acid a mixture of α- and β-methyl glucosides was formed (Fig. 3.80). Although a new asymmetric centre is created, the anomeric glucosides cannot interconvert by mutarotation.

Natural glycosides were known long before Emil Fischer had prepared such alkyl glycosides. In 1837, Justus von Liebig and Friedrich Wöhler described one of the earliest-observed instances of enzyme action. They demonstrated that an extract of bitter almonds called *emulsin*, now known to be a mixture of glycosidases (enzymes which split glycosidic bonds), would hydrolyze *amygdalin* ('oil of bitter almonds'). Naturally, the enzyme and its substrate are found in differ-ent cells. Hydrolysis converts amygdalin to one mole each of benzaldehyde and hydrogen cyanide and two moles of glucose. The familiar almond smell of crushed laurel leaves is due to hydrolysis of this kind with release of hydrogen cyanide.

The sugar residue in most glycosides is glucose but other monosaccharides such as L-rhamnose, D-fucose and D-galactose are sometimes present. The sugar is almost always present as the β-anomer.

Another simple O-glycoside is vanillin, the flavouring agent.

The *cardiac glycosides* are of considerable medical importance because of their stimulatory action on the heart. Many of these substances have a deoxy-sugar as one of the component sugars while the aglycone is of the steroid type. The general structure of a cardiac glycoside is as follows:

Aglycone−(deoxy sugar)n−(glucose)m
(where n and m are small numbers).

SUBSTITUTIONS

Sugar esters
In living organisms, the most important esters are those in which the sugar is esterified with phosphoric acid. In 1905 Sir Arthur Harden

(1865–1940) noticed that although yeast extract broke down glucose and produced carbon dioxide quite rapidly at first, the level of activity decreased after some time. Harden found that addition of phosphate to the solution restored the original rate of carbon dioxide production. This was due to the incorporation of phosphate into the sugar ester called fructose 1,6 diphosphate, an intermediate in glycolysis (p. 183). Later it was realized that phosphate esters play many essential roles in biochemistry; they are intermediates in the synthesis and degradation of starch, glycogen and sucrose; function as substrates in the glycolysis fermentation pathways; and are involved in the photosynthetic incorporation of carbon dioxide in plants, and in most oxidative biological processes. Phosphate esters also occur as constituents of nucleic acids, and of coenzymes related to vitamins of the B complex (e.g. NAD, NADP, FAD and coenzyme A).

During the first half of the 20th century there was a growing awareness of the importance of sugar phosphate esters in biochemistry. In 1941, Fritz Lipmann (1899–   ) introduced the concept of the 'high energy' phosphate bond. Lipmann found that certain types of biological compounds, such as anhydrides, had a higher free energy of hydrolysis than normal esters. The most familiar example of this type is adenosine triphosphate (ATP).

ATP is an N-glycoside of ribose in which the primary alcohol group on carbon-5 is esterified by a triphosphate unit. Within this unit there are two phosphoanhydride bonds (Fig. 3.81).

High energy bonds are defined as those bonds with free energy of hydrolysis values greater than about 30 kJ/mol. This energy is not the energy required to break bonds but is the net difference in energy between reactants and products. High energy phosphate compounds such as ATP may therefore be regarded as possessing stores of potential energy locked up in chemical form, which can be tapped and used for driving energy-requiring biochemical mechanisms.

Table 3.13 lists the phosphorylated compounds important in the conservation and release of energy throughout the body.

Table 3.13. Important phosphorylated compounds in the body and their $\Delta G^{\circ\prime}$ values.

Compound	$\Delta G^{\circ\prime}$ kJ/mol
Adenosine triphosphate (ATP)	− 31
Adenosine diphosphate (ADP)	− 27
Phosphoenol pyruvate (PEP)	− 62
Carbamyl phosphate	− 51
Creatine phosphate	− 43
Acetyl phosphate	− 43
Glucose 1-phosphate	− 21
Glucose 6-phosphate	− 14

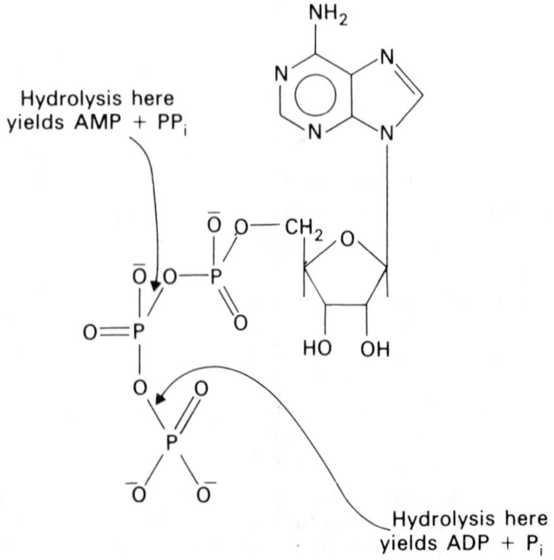

Fig. 3.81. Adenosine triphosphate.

POLYSACCHARIDES AND OLIGOSACCHARIDES

Life processes, when observed at the molecular level, are characterized by the making and breaking of carbon–carbon bonds. On a world-wide ecological scale, this perpetual activity manifests itself in the carbon cycle. Each year, as part of this cycle, green plants on land and phytoplankton in the oceans together absorb approximately 8×10^{10} tons of carbon dioxide and use it as their sole carbon source in the synthesis of the four major groups of macromolecules typical of living organisms—the proteins, lipids, polysaccharides and nucleic acids. Numerically, the greater part of this organic material is accounted for by the polysaccharides.

The carbohydrate polymers are divided into two major groups—the *homoglycans* and the *heteroglycans* ('glycan' is another term for polysaccharide, derived from the Greek word 'glykys' meaning sweet). The prefix *gly* is a generic term implying any sugar and the suffix *an* denotes a polymer). The homoglycans contain only a single type of monosaccharide repeating unit while the heteroglycans contain at least two types within the polymer chain.

It is worth emphasizing again that all the biopolymers share a common feature in that they are all condensation polymers formed from monomers with the elimination of a molecule of water.

Sugars polymerize via condensation reactions between two hydroxyl groups. In any glycosidic bond, at least one of these hydroxyl groups is attached to the aldo- or ketocarbon of one of the sugars whilst the other hydroxyl group can belong to any of the available carbons of the second sugar. Such a linkage is termed O-glycosidic (p. 128), and polysaccharides are, therefore, O-glycosides. The various possibilities of O-glycosidic linkage between two glucose molecules are indicated below (Fig. 3.82).

In Fig. 3.82 the arrows point away from the hemiacetal carbon: when both hemiacetal C-1 atoms are involved no arrow is used.

When the hemiacetal (incipient aldehydic) group on the C-1 of the glucose molecule I is linked by condensation to any hydroxyl group in glucose molecule II, it loses its mutarotation and reducing properties. When the condensation reaction involves either the C-2, C-3, C-4, or C-6 of glucose molecule II then the hemiacetal group on the C-1 of this second glucose molecule is still free in the disaccharide formed. Hence these disaccharides will be able to mutarotate and show reducing properties. However, when the C-1 of glucose molecule I condenses with the C-1 of glucose molecule II then the resulting disaccharide will possess none of the properties originally associated with each monomer.

These considerations apply equally to sugars linked by beta linkages, and indeed to polymerization of any sugar molecules.

Disaccharides are therefore either reducing or non-reducing sugars, depending on the linkages involved, and specific examples of both types are given below.

The type of linkage between consecutive sugar residues in a polymer affects not only its resultant chemical properties but also its structural characteristics. The glycosidic bond partly determines the intrinsic stiffness of a polymer because the constituent monosaccharide residues exist in ring form. The only rotational possibility along the polysaccharide backbone is that about the glycosidic bond. Two examples are shown overleaf (Fig. 3.83).

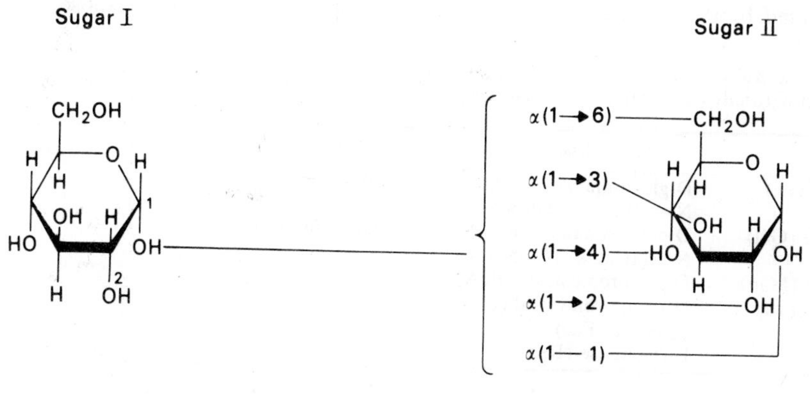

Sugar I

Sugar II

Fig. 3.82. Types of O-glycosidic linkages.

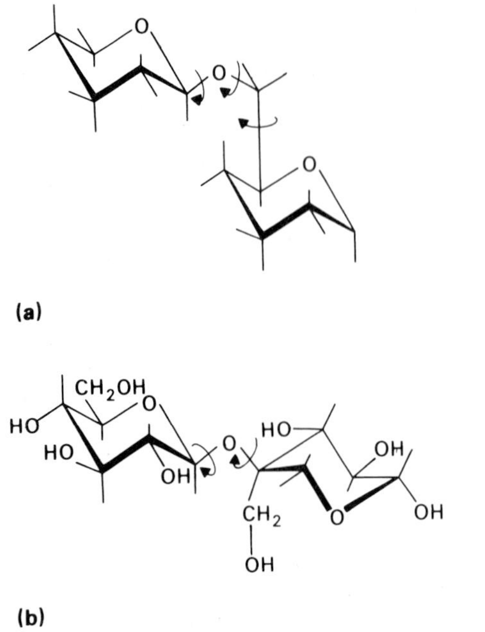

(a)

(b)

Fig. 3.83. Rotational possibilities about glycosidic linkages in polysaccharides (a) about $1 \rightarrow 6$ linkages (b) about $1 \rightarrow 4$ linkages.

Three key factors determine polysaccharide structure and function:

1 The nature and number of the constituent monosaccharides involved.

2 The identity of the specific carbon atoms involved in the carbon–carbon linkage points joining the constituent monosaccharides.

3 The stereochemistry of the linkages between the constituent monosaccharides.

Polysaccharide diversity is dictated by variations arising from these three key factors. The influence of factor 1 is particularly important in the larger polysaccharides. Factors 2 and 3 influences are well illustrated by the disaccharides.

Oligosaccharides are frequently described specifically in terms of the number of component monosaccharides, e.g. di-, tri-, tetra-, penta-, hexa-, hepta-, octa-, nona-, and decasaccharide. It is daunting to consider the number of different polysaccharides (homoglycans) that can, *in theory*, be formed from a single type of monosaccharide allowing for the permutations arising from these three factors. As there are some 100 naturally occurring monosaccharides, the potential list of different heteroglycans is astronomical. The fact that the number of glycans which actually occur in nature is relatively small is due to the restrictions on the number of molecular organizations allowable. There is no direct genetic coding for sugar synthesis and control is effected by the synthesis of relatively few specific enzymes which direct glycan synthesis in a strictly limited manner. These restrictive features have the following effects:

1 Of the naturally occurring monosaccharides, only a few occur in natural polysaccharides and they tend to be arranged systematically. These sugars include four hexoses, seven modified hexoses and two pentoses (Table 3.14).

2 A specific mode of linkage is generally uniformly repeated throughout the chain and similarly a specific stereochemistry is usually retained throughout a given polymer.

3 Most glycans are constructed from *aldose* sugar units. D-fructose is the only ketose commonly utilized in glycans. Examples of the latter are the disaccharide *sucrose*, and the fructans *inulin* and *levan*.

4 The most abundant polysaccharides are the homoglycans which are comprised of a single type of sugar monomer unit.

5 Most of the important heteroglycans contain a disaccharide repeating unit.

Some of the symbols used to indicate monosaccharide units and their residues in polysaccharides are given below in Table 3.14. Other symbols include p and f for the pyranose and

Table 3.14. Naturally occurring monosaccharides that are found in naturally occurring polysaccharides.

Hexoses	Modified hexoses	Pentoses
D-glucose (Glc)	D-glucosamine (usually N-acetylated) (GlcNAc)	D-xylose (Xyl)
D-galactose (Gal)	D-galactosamine (usually N-acetylated) (GalNAc)	L-arabinose (Ara)
D-mannose (Man)	D-glucuronic acid (GlcA)	
D-fructose (Fru)	D-mannuronic acid (ManA)	
	L-fucose (Fuc)	
	L-rhamnose (Rha)	

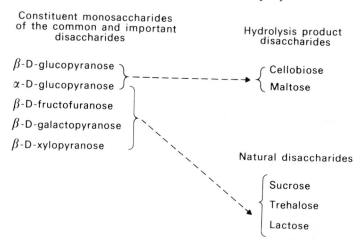

Constituent monosaccharides
of the common and important
disaccharides

Hydrolysis product
disaccharides

β-D-glucopyranose

α-D-glucopyranose

β-D-fructofuranose

β-D-galactopyranose

β-D-xylopyranose

Cellobiose

Maltose

Natural disaccharides

Sucrose

Trehalose

Lactose

Fig. 3.84. The six biologically most important disaccharides.

furanose forms and the use of arrows to indicate the direction of the glycosidic link. Thus in a polymer with a (1→4) link for example, the arrow points away from the carbon-1 which is therefore the hemiacetal carbon atom of the glycosidic link, either of the α or β form.

The disaccharides

There are some five common and important disaccharides. Three of these occur naturally and two are encountered as hydrolysis products of larger polysaccharides. These five disaccharides are formed by selection from 4 monosaccharide monomers: glucose, fructose, galactose and xylose (Fig. 3.84).

Of these disaccharides, maltose, cellobiose and trehalose contain only glucose units and differ from each other solely in terms of positional attachment and stereochemistry.

Maltose (Fig. 3.85), which can be produced by the enzymic degradation of starch, is characterized by an α (1→4) link. It therefore reduces Fehling's solution (p. 123) and exhibits mutarotation (p. 120).

(1→4)α-D-glucosidic linkage

CH₂OH   CH₂OH   Reducing group

OH   OH   H, OH

HO

OH   OH

Maltose or
O-α-D-Glcp-(1→4)-α-D-Glcp

Fig. 3.85. Structure of maltose.

The same properties are shown by a variant of maltose called *isomaltose* (Fig. 3.86), which contains glucose molecules joined via an α (1→6) link. This is one product of α-amylase hydrolysis of amylopectin.

CH₂OH   (1→6)α-D-glucosidic linkage

O

OH

HO   O—CH₂

OH

Reducing group

O

OH   H,OH

HO

OH

Isomaltose or
O-α-Glcp-(1→6)-α-D-Glcp

Fig. 3.86. Structure of isomaltose.

Cellobiose is produced in the acid hydrolysis of cellulose. It differs from maltose only in that the glucose molecules are joined by a β-link and not an α-linkage (Fig. 3.93).

Man and the other vertebrates possess enzymes which split α-linked but not β-linked glucose molecules. Therefore cellobiose is nutritionally useless in an animal diet, whereas maltose is readily digested. (Ruminant animals like cows, which chew the cud, have microorganisms in their gut which are capable of hydrolysing the β-links in cellulose to form glucose.)

The other two common disaccharides do not contain a single monosaccharide type, *lactose*

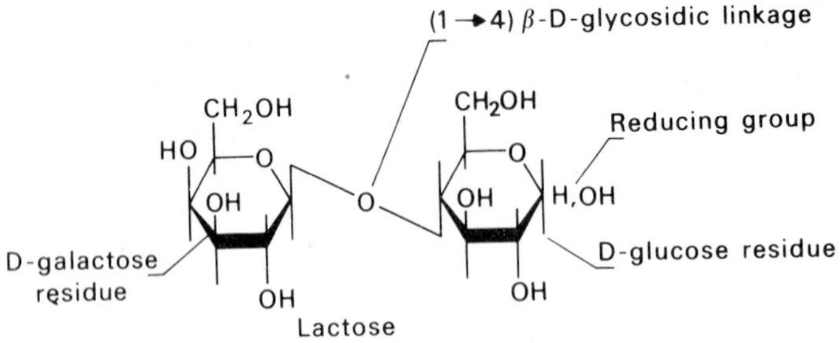

(1 → 4) β-D-glycosidic linkage

Reducing group

D-galactose residue

D-glucose residue

Lactose

O- β -D-Galp-(1→ 4)- β -D-Glcp

Fig. 3.87. Structure of lactose.

(Fig. 3.87), consists of D-glucose glycosidically linked to D-galactose and from the formula it is clear that lactose is a β-galactoside and not a glucoside. Lactose may be hydrolysed by β-galactosidase. Some people have an hereditary lack of this enzyme and show a 'lactose intolerance': they cannot drink milk, a major source of the sugar, without bringing upon themselves serious metabolic disturbance.

Commercially, *sucrose* (Fig. 3.88) is the most important of the simple disaccharide carbohydrates. The α-D-glucose and β-D-fructose are joined in a (2→1) linkage.

Since fructose is a 2-keto sugar, this means that both hemiacetal groups are involved in the linkage and sucrose is therefore non-reducing and does not mutarotate. It is important to note that fructose is in the furanose ring form when linked to other monosaccharides, as in sucrose and the levan polymers but as a free monosaccharide, fructose adopts the pyranose ring configuration.

Sucrose is indicted as the 'arch criminal' in the initiation and development of the disease dental caries, where two of its important roles are thought to be:

1   As an energy source for cariogenic (caries-

producing) bacteria. The resultant fermentation products are organic acids which can dissolve tooth enamel.

2   Utilization by cariogenic bacteria in the synthesis of *dextrans* (p. 137) important in dental plaque formation.

Storage polysaccharides

The polysaccharides have been classified above chemically as homoglycans or heteroglycans. However, they can also be classified functionally as storage or structural carbohydrates.

Within plants and animals, storage polysaccharides provide a ready source of monosaccharides which can be enzymically released when required for metabolic purposes. In times of positive sugar surplus, monosaccharide units are stored by enzymically joining them to the ends of existing polysaccharide chains. In general, large polymers make good storage materials since they tend to be insoluble, and even in solution they make only a minimal contribution to the osmotic pressure of the cell. And their accumulation in the cell does not, therefore, result in hypertonicity. The animal storage polysaccharide is glycogen, which is found prin-

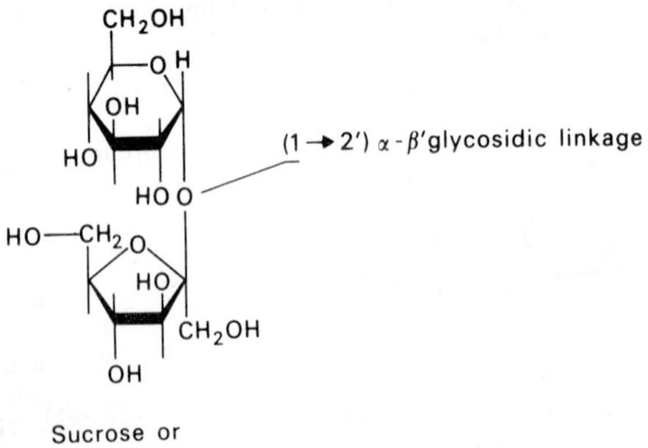

(1 → 2') α - β'glycosidic linkage

Sucrose or

O- β -D-Fmf (2 →1)- α -D-Glcp

Fig. 3.88. Structure of sucrose.

Table 3.15. Principal characteristics of the homoglucans.

Homoglucan	Constituent monosaccharide	Type of Linkage	Comments
Amylose	α-D-glucopyranose	(1——➤4)	Unbranched
Amylopectin	α-D-glucopyranose	(1——➤4) (1——➤6)	Branched: average chain length is 20–25 residues: distance between branch points on a chain is 5–8 residues.
Glycogen	α-D-glucopyranose	(1——➤4) (1——➤6)	Branched: average chain length is 10–14 residues: distance between the two branch points on a chain is 3–4 residues.
Dextrans	α-D-glucopyranose	(1——➤6) (1——➤3) Occasionally (1——➤4) and (1——➤2) links occur as well.	Branched: considerable variation occurs according to the species of microorganism responsible for synthesis of the dextran: the (1——➤6) link predominates.
Cellulose	β-D-glucopyranose	(1——➤4)	Unbranched

cipally in the liver and muscle. In plants the most abundant storage material is starch which is deposited in the cytoplasm in the form of granules. Other storage glycans of plants and microorganisms include mannans, arabinans, dextrans and fructans.

Most of the important storage polysaccharides are homoglucans. This group of polymers is constructed entirely from glucose molecules and includes four storage glucans, which are glycogen, amylose, amylopectin and dextran, and cellulose—which is a solely structural carbohydrate. Their structural features are summarized in Table 3.15 where it is clear that the storage glucans are characterized by α-linkages in contrast to cellulose, a structural homoglucan which contains β-linkages.

GLYCOGEN

Glycogen, sometimes called 'animal starch', is the reserve carbohydrate of animals and has been known since 1856 when Claude Bernard (1813–1878) discovered this starch-like substance in liver and showed that it was made of 'blood sugar'.

Glycogen is a highly branched polymer formed entirely from α-D-glucose units and contains both $\alpha(1\rightarrow4)$ and $\beta(1\rightarrow6)$ linkages. The diagrammatic representation of glycogen (Fig. 3.89) was proposed by W. J. Whelan and co-workers. Straight lines represent chains of $(1\rightarrow4)$-linked α-D-glucose residues, and arrowheads, $(1\rightarrow6)$-α-D-glucosidic, interchain linkages. Each chain consists of about 10–14

residues. The solid dot indicates the non-reducing end of the chain.

STARCH

The main plant storage carbohydrate is starch, which is not a single substance but is a mixture of two glucose polymers, amylose and amylopectin. *Amylose* is a linear or unbranched macromolecule which contains some 50–1500 glucose molecules all joined by $\alpha(1\rightarrow4)$ linkages. These molecules therefore have molecular weights ranging from about 10 000–300 000.

The stereochemistry dictated by these $\alpha(1\rightarrow4)$ linkages imposes limitations on the type of conformation which the amylose macromolecules adopt, and various studies have

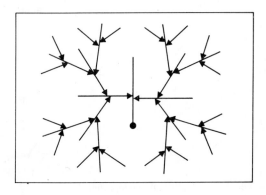

Fig. 3.89. Diagrammatic representation of glycogen structure (Whelan).

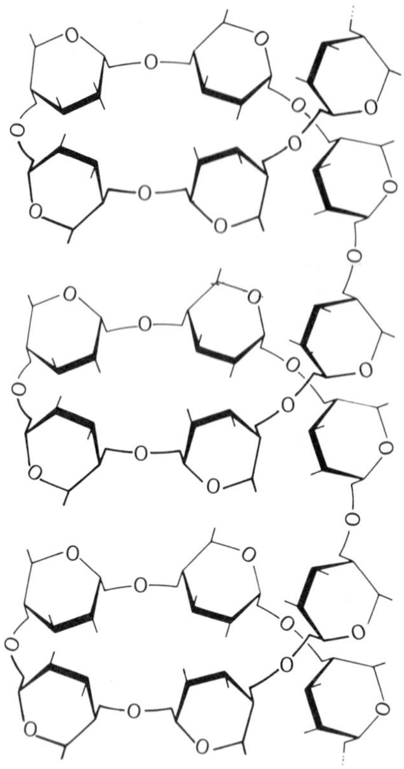

Fig. 3.90. Helical structure of amylose.

indicated that in solution amylose exists predominantly as a wormlike helical chain, a portion of which is depicted in Fig. 3.90.

The other component of starch, *amylopectin* (Fig. 3.91), is a polymer very similar to glycogen in structure but not so highly branched. Thus it also contains $\alpha(1\rightarrow4)$ and $\alpha(1\rightarrow6)$ linkages but the branch points (the $\alpha(1\rightarrow6)$ links) only occur about every 20 residues.

As amylose and amylopectin have only one hemiacetal group per molecule, therefore, like all large polysaccharides, they have virtually no measureable reducing action.

A characteristic reaction of starch solutions is the intense blue colouration that results on addition of iodine. It is the amylose component which is mainly responsible for this phenomenon. Iodine molecules become complexed within the amylose helices and cause a marked change in the absorption spectrum of the solution. Similar complexes can be formed with other α-linked glucans but the amylopectin–iodine complex is a much lighter blue–violet colour while the glycogen–iodine complex is reddish–brown. As long ago as 1864, the German physiologist Julius Sachs used this test for starch in a simple but classic experiment. He took a plant and covered part of one of its leaves. After exposing the whole plant to light for a few hours, he placed the leaf in iodine vapour. The covered portion of the leaf showed no change but the exposed area turned an intense blue colour thus demonstrating the presence of starch as one of the products of photosynthesis (p. 228).

The enzymic breakdown of starch in digestion is discussed in Chapter 13 (p. 609).

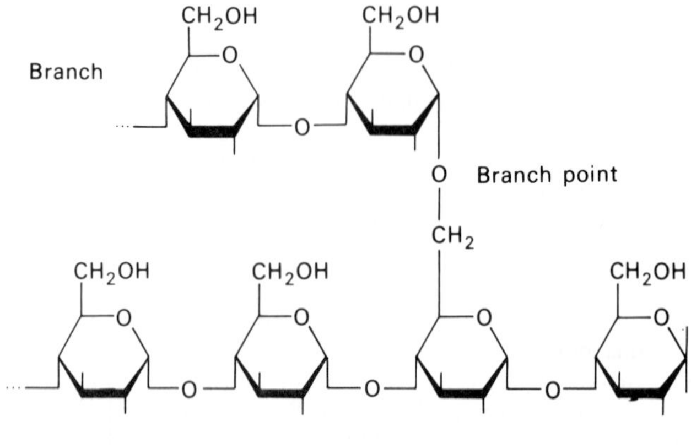

Fig. 3.91. Structure of amylopectin.

DEXTRANS

The dextrans are synthesized extra-cellularly (and exclusively, so far as is known) by bacteria belonging to the family *Lactobacillaceae* and in particular by species within the genera Lactobacillus, Leuconostoc and Streptococcus. These polysaccharides are branched D-glucans which contain predominantly (1→6)-linked α-D-glucopyranose residues. The secondary linkages (or branch points) are usually (1→3) links but (1→2) and (1→4) linkages also occur.

Dextran preparations that have been examined so far have been found to contain between 5–33% of branching residues. The proportions of the three types of secondary linkage that occur in any particular dextran depend on the species of microorganism responsible for its synthesis.

As in amylose, amylopectin and glycogen, all residues in the macromolecule are joined by α-D-glucopyranosidic linkages. Most dextrans are synthesized by bacteria using sucrose as a carbon source. Biosynthesis occurs extra-cellularly via a secreted enzyme, *dextran sucrase* (*a transglycosylase*). This enzyme exclusively catalyses the synthesis of chains of (1→6)-linked α-D-glucopyranosyl residues building them up by transferring the glucose residues from sucrose molecules (Fig. 3.92).

The synthesis of dextrans from sucrose is of special interest to dental science because these extra-cellular bacterial polysaccharides are

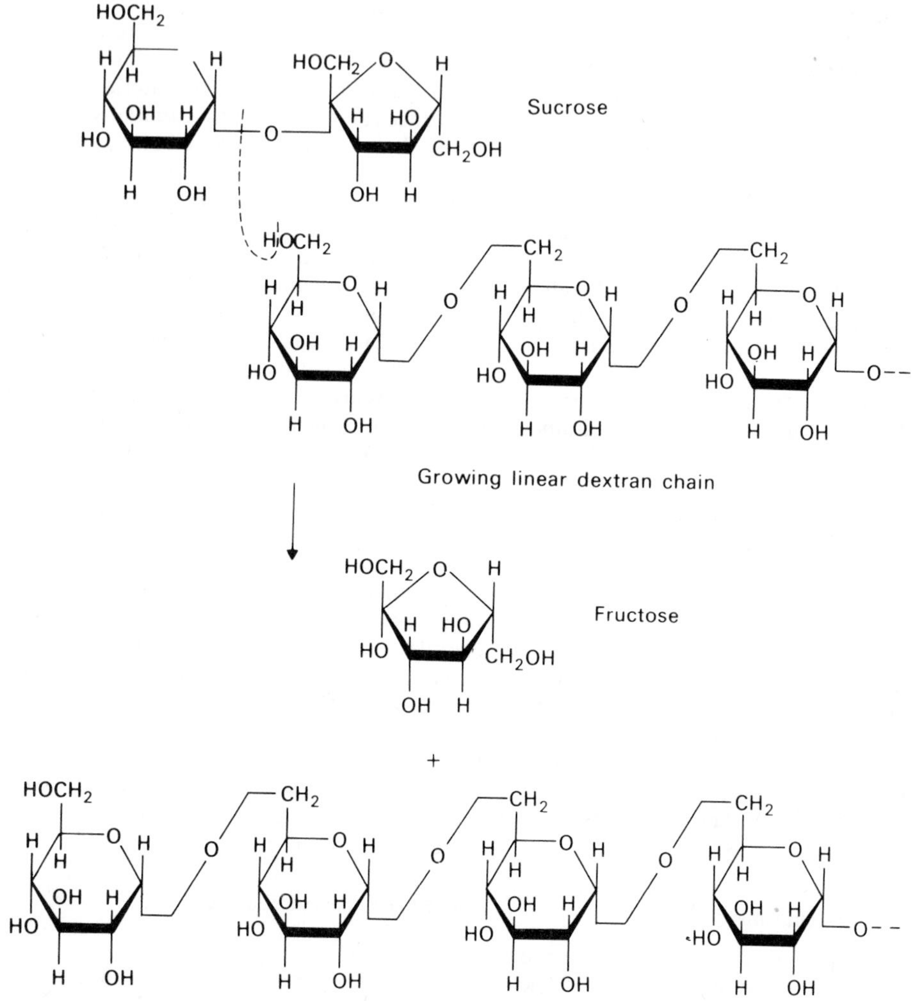

Fig. 3.92. Synthesis of dextran.

believed to play a significant role in the development of dental caries—the microbial disease that breaks down tooth enamel and dentine. There is now overwhelming evidence to indict sucrose as the dietary agent which, in association with bacteria, initiates tooth decay: part of this cariogenicity of sucrose appears to be related to its ability to act as a substrate for the synthesis of these dextran polysaccharides. Evidence suggests that the formation of dextrans in the oral cavity encourages the colonization of cariogenic bacteria and their adhesion on the tooth surface. This process occurs within the accumulation of material known as dental plaque, which consists of about 50–60% bacteria, 30–40% salivary glycoprotein and some 10% extracellular, bacterial polysaccharide—notably the dextrans with smaller amounts of the fructose polymers, the levans. Dextrans and levans also provide a source of reserve carbohydrate which can eventually be broken down to fermentable sugars. These sugars can be used by oral bacteria to produce the organic acids believed to cause the carious lesions. The biochemistry of dental caries is discussed in detail in Volume 3.

Commercial applications of dextrans include their use in pharmaceutical and cosmetic products, in photographic processes, as food additives (for example, as stabilizers in ice-cream) and even as water-loss inhibitors in oil-well drilling muds.

Clinically, dextran fractions of well-defined molecular weight are used as blood-plasma substitutes.

Modified dextrans are also used extensively in the separation technique known as molecular exclusion or gel filtration chromatography (p. 62).

FRUCTANS: LEVAN AND INULIN

Another group of storage polysaccharides, widely distributed in plants, are the *fructans*. Two examples are *levan* and *inulin*. Levan is found in plants but is also synthesized by microorganisms including some of the cariogenic bacteria. Levans are branched β-fructans with $(2\rightarrow6)$ links and $(2\rightarrow1)$ linked branch points.

Structural polysaccharides

The structural carbohydrates are so named because they feature as components of the biological support structures—the connective tissues. Such structures vary considerably in

form throughout the living world but the general plan is that of a fibrous substance embedded in an amorphous support matrix (the ground substance). The fibrous component resists tension whilst the matrix resists compression. During the evolution of plant and animal structures a variety of substances have been developed for both the fibrous phase and the matrix.

Most animal connective tissues contain collagen as the fibrous protein component and for the matrix material use a protein–polysaccharide (proteoglycan) complex, of which about 90% is carbohydrate in the form of various heteroglycans. In contrast most plants use cellulose as the fibrous component and for the support matrix a group of glycans known as the *pectic* substances.

The nature of the matrix is the more important in determining the mechanical properties of various plant and animal support structures than is the fibrous phase. Natural selection has produced a large array of matrix materials, whose properties can be altered by variations of their chemical structure. The overall structural plan tends to remain the same however, as is shown in a comparison between the *periodontium* (a set of tissues involved in tooth support, Book 2) and the seed mucilage of the mustard plant. The periodontium contains collagen fibres enmeshed within a protein–polysaccharide matrix, whereas seed mucilage consists of cellulose fibres dispersed in an exclusively polysaccharide matrix. The glycans involved are quite different in these two systems, which illustrates the principle that life forms widely separated from an evolutionary viewpoint can contain structural units with similar architecture and mechanical properties, even though constructed of different chemical components.

Some important glycans involved in biological support structures are the gel-forming polysaccharides from seaweeds. Apart from their intrinsic interest as examples of how widely different organisms have solved similar problems, namely that of withstanding stresses and strains, these substances when extracted have valuable commercial and scientific applications. Alginates and agaroses are used as dental impression materials in restorative dentistry.

The fibrous polysaccharides

CELLULOSE

Of all the structural materials in plant cell walls cellulose is the best known, for it is the most abundant polysaccharide in the plant world. Cel-

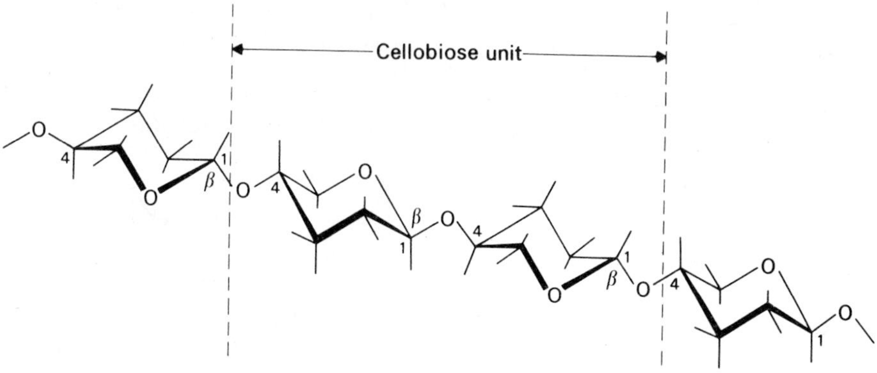

Fig. 3.93. Structure of cellulose.

lulose is a linear β-D-glucan in which glucose units are linked by $(1\rightarrow4)$-β-glycosidic bonds (Fig. 3.93). Groups of about 40 of these unbranched macromolecules aggregate to form fibrils which are stabilized by extensive inter-molecular hydrogen bonding. This bonding occurs between the hydrogen atom of a hydroxyl group on one glucose residue and the oxygen bridge in a glucose residue within an adjacent chain. It is this hydrogen bonding which is responsible for cellulose being a relatively inert material. Cellulose is quite insoluble in water in spite of its large number of hydroxyl groups because the interactions between the cellulose molecules themselves are stronger than those between the individual cellulose molecules and water molecules. The resultant close-packing of the chain also means that *cellulase* enzymes can-not easily approach the glycosidic bonds within the fibril: for this reason natural dissolution of cellulose is often a slow process. The straight (non-helical) chains found in cellulose result directly from the $1\rightarrow4\beta$ links between the glucose molecules. Unlike starch cellulose does not give a blue colour with iodine. Partial acid hydrolysis of cellulose releases the reducing disaccharide cellobiose (p. 133).

CHITIN

Chitin is a modified homoglucan consisting of an unbranched chain of β-linked N-acetyl-D-glucosamine residues. It differs from cellulose only in having an acetyl-substituted amine group attached to the second carbon atom of each glucose residue. Chitin is a tough, inert polymer which forms the major structural com-ponent in the exoskeletons of invertebrates such as insects and crustacea. It also occurs in some bacteria, yeasts and fungi. Often, inorganic mat-erial such as calcium carbonate is found to be incorporated into the polysaccharide network. The resulting complex is highly resistant to enzymic and chemical attack.

PEPTIDOGLYCAN

This is the main contributor to the rigidity of the cell wall in most bacteria. Peptidoglycan con-tains two types of modified glucose residues and is therefore in effect a heteroglycan. It is con-structed from chains of the amino sugar N-acetyl glucosamine alternating with its 3-O-D-lactyl derivative which is called N-acetyl muramic acid. These sugars are joined by β-$(1\rightarrow4)$ links (Figs. 3.94 & 3.95a).

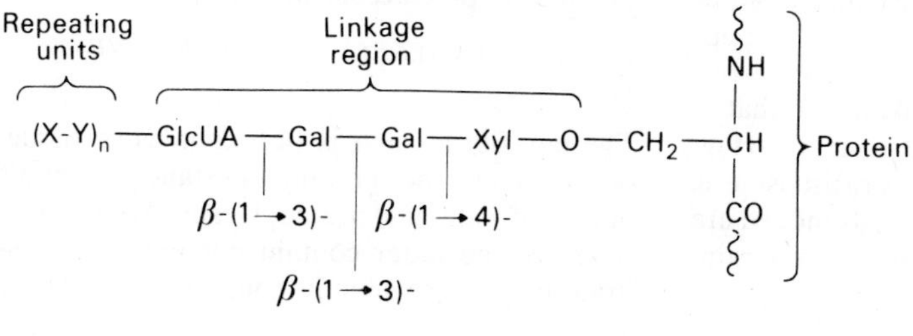

Fig. 3.94. Three various linkages in proteoglycans.

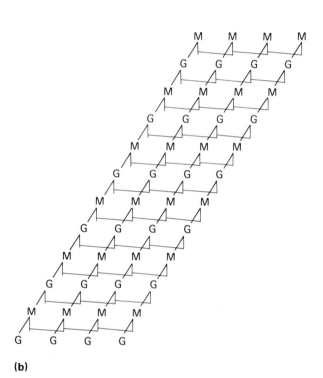

Basic unit

CH₃CHCONH peptide

(M)
MurNAc

N-acetylglucosamine
(G)
GlcNAc

(a)

(b)

Fig. 3.95. (a) Disaccharide unit of peptidoglycan. (b) Diagrammatic representation of peptidoglycan structure (M=muramic acid residue; G=glucosamine residue).

The N-acetyl muramic acid residues in adjacent chains are linked together by short peptides. In this way a macromolecular framework is set up with a role that can be likened to that of the wire netting in reinforced concrete (Fig. 3.95b). The resultant cell wall may resist osmotic pressures of up to 25 atmospheres as indeed are generated within the protoplast of a Gram-positive coccus.

The matrix polysaccharides: proteoglycans

GROUND SUBSTANCE OF CONNECTIVE TISSUE

The non-fibrous matrix of a connective tissue, often called the ground substance, consists mainly of water and proteoglycans. As the name suggests, the latter contain not only carbohydrate but also covalently bound protein. There are two main groups of carbohydrate-protein complexes: the glycoproteins and the proteoglycans. In both the carbohydrate moiety is present as a heteroglycan. The *glycoproteins* usually contain a relatively small proportion of carbohydrate and have little or no repeating structure. In contrast, the *proteoglycans* have a protein content which is usually less than 10%, and most of their carbohydrate is present as a repeating disaccharide unit.

Proteoglycans occur almost everywhere in mammalian tissues, though it is still a matter for speculation whether they function in other ways than maintaining the structural integrity of tissues.

The general plan underlying organic support tissues, that of a fibrous polymer embedded in an amorphous support matrix, was illustrated above by the tooth peridontium and the mucilage of the mustard seed. Cartilage provides another well documented example of such a system. Water ($\approx 70\%$), proteoglycan and collagen are the main extracellular components in cartilage. Collagen provides the fibrous network within which meshes of proteoglycan macromolecules are trapped. The strong affinity for water of these macromolecules is such that their presence within the matrix prevents the free flow of water when an external force is applied. In this way, collagen, proteoglycan and water together form a system able to withstand compressive forces: this is, therefore, well suited to the load-bearing functions of cartilage. Factors such as the concentration, shape and degree of entanglement of the proteoglycan macromolecules all influence these matrix properties.

THE GLYCOSAMINOGLYCANS (GAGs)

Proteoglycan molecules are constructed in the form of a central protein core to which are attached laterally a number of long chains of carbohydrate known as glycosaminoglycans (GAGs). These GAGs used to be referred to as mucopolysaccharide chains—or as the acid mucopolysaccharides.

Eight different types of GAGs are recognized at present (Table 3.16). All are constructed from a repeating disaccharide unit which contains a residue of an N-acetylated or N-sulphated hexosamine. Additionally, all glycosaminoglycans carry acidic groups which are ionized at physiological pH. These are of three kinds.

1 The *carboxyl group*

$$-C\underset{O}{\overset{O^-}{\lessgtr}}$$

is found in the carbon-6 position and is part of a uronic acid residue.

2 The *ester sulphate group*

$$(-O-\overset{\overset{O}{\|}}{\underset{\underset{O}{\|}}{S}}-O^-)$$

is present at either carbon-4 or carbon-6 and occasionally (in animals other than mammals) in both positions.

3 The *sulphamino group*

$$(-N-\overset{\overset{O}{\|}}{\underset{\underset{O}{\|}}{S}}-O^-)$$

present at carbon-2, is found only in heparin and heparan sulphates.

The distribution of acidic groups and the composition of the disaccharide repeating units—$[X-Y]_n$—is shown for the most important naturally-occurring glysosaminoglycans in Table 3.16. A hexosamine can be either N-acetylated or N-sulphated but does not carry both groups. Apart from heparin and heparan sulphate, all the sugars in these glycosaminoglycans are joined by β-linkages. This is a characteristic feature of the structural glycans (cf. cellulose, chitin and peptidoglycan).

Glycosaminoglycans are easily freed from their covalently bound protein by use of proteolytic enzymes such as papain and trypsin. Their schematic structure is as follows:

(Disaccharide repeat units $(X-Y)_n$)	–	(GAG/core linkage region)	–	Protein core)

In writing GAG structures it is a convention that the non-reducing terminal sugar monomer is written on the left, and the reducing terminal sugar residue is written on the right.

The two isomeric forms of *chondroitin sulphate*, chondroitin $4-SO_4$ and chondroitin $6-SO_4$, are the predominant glycosaminoglycans of cartilage. They also occur in bone, skin, cornea and dental pulp. A desulphated form, *chondroitin* is found in the cornea.

Keratan sulphate occurs notably in the nucleus pulposus and the cornea. The linkage region structure of keratan sulphate varies according to source—one type in corneal and another in

Table 3.16. Composition of glycosaminoglycans.

Glycosamino-glycan	Component mono-saccharides of repeating dis-accharide units (X and Y)	Structure of repeating disaccharide unit	O-sulphate groups	N-sulphate groups
Chondroitin	N-acetyl D-galactosamine and D-glucuronic acid	$\beta(1\rightarrow3)$ $\beta(1\rightarrow4)$		
Chondroitin 4-sulphate	N-acetyl D-galactosamine 4-sulphate *and* D-glucuronic acid	$\beta(1\rightarrow3)$ $\beta(1\rightarrow4)$	+ (on carbon–4)	–
Chondroitin 6-sulphate	N-acetyl D-galactosamine 6-sulphate *and* D-glucuronic acid	$\beta(1\rightarrow4)$ $\beta(1\rightarrow4)$	+ (on carbon–6)	–
Keratan sulphate	N-acetyl D-glucosamine *and* D-galactose	$\beta(1\rightarrow3)$ $\beta(1\rightarrow4)$	+ (on carbon–6 but may occur on carbon–4)	–
Hyaluronic acid	N-acetyl D-glucosamine *and* D-glucuronic acid	$\beta(1\rightarrow3)$ $\beta(1\rightarrow4)$	–	–
Dermatan sulphate	N-acetyl D-galactosamine *and* L-iduronic acid *or* D-glucuronic acid	$\beta(1\rightarrow3)$ $\beta(1\rightarrow4)$	+ (on carbon–4 or carbon–6)	–
Heparan sulphate	D-glucosamine *and* D-glucuronic acid *or* L-iduronic acid	$\alpha(1\rightarrow4)$ $\alpha(1\rightarrow4)$	+ (on carbon–4 and/or carbon–6)	+ (on carbon –2)
Heparin	D-glucosamine *and* D-glucuronic acid *or* L-iduronic acid	$\alpha(1\rightarrow4)$ $\alpha(1\rightarrow4)$	+ (on carbon–4 and/or carbon–6 and/or carbon–2)	+ (on carbon –2)

These are the two principal repeating disaccharide units found in heparin and heparan sulphate skeletal tissues. The proportion of keratan sulphate in human costal cartilage increases with age. It is absent in the embryo and during early growth but rises in concentration from the first to the fourth decade of life to a plateau value of about 55% of the total glycosaminoglycan content of the tissue.

Hyaluronic acid is found in high concentration in vitreous humour and is characteristic of synovial fluid where it acts as a lubricant. It is an extremely large molecule with a chain which may contain 100–20 000 disaccharide units. There is some evidence that hyaluronic acid may be important in tissue differentiation.

Dermatan sulphate is found in skin, tendon, blood vessels and heart valves.

Heparin and *heparan sulphate* contain both α and β-linkages and are distinct from other glycosaminoglycans in that they contain a mixture of repeating units of which the two predominant ones are shown in Table 3.16. Heparin has anticoagulant and lipid-clearing activities and is unique in that it is stored intracellularly in granules in the mast cells, predominantly within the capsule surrounding the liver. Heparan sulphate occurs at many sites, including blood vessel walls and the central nervous system.

PROTEOGLYCAN STRUCTURE

The most intensely studied proteoglycans have been those in cartilage. It is likely that the proteoglycans in oral tissues such as the dental pulp and periodontium closely resemble those from cartilage though this supposition must await confirmation. Some work has been carried out on the glycosaminoglycan moieties of proteoglycans from these sources but little on the intact macromolecules.

The major glycosaminoglycan of cartilage is *chondroitin sulphate*. Each chain contains some 25–30 disaccharide repeating units and has a molecular weight of 15 000–20 000. The chains tend to occur in pairs or 'doublets', each chain being separated by less than 10 amino acids, while the doublets are separated by about 35 amino acids. The whole glycosaminoglycan is flexible in so far that each sugar residue can move relative to its neighbouring residues as a result of rotations about the glycosidic bonds. An identical sequence of sugar residues link the glycosaminoglycan moiety to protein for chondroitin 4-sulphate, chondroitin 6-sulphate, dermatan sulphate and heparin (Fig. 3.94).

Each xylose is glycosidically linked to the hydroxyl group of the amino acid serine. In cartilage, chondroitin sulphate and keratan sulphate are linked to the same protein core though keratan sulphate is the smaller chain and the linkage sequence is different.

The size of the macromolecule varies with source. This probably relates to the fact that proteoglycan macromolecules are both *polydisperse* (i.e. they exhibit a wide range of molecular weights), and *heterogeneous* (which means that they differ slightly in their chemical composition, as for example in the degree of sulphation). Recent research work suggests that in a cartilage proteoglycan the protein core (molecular weight 200 000) bears some 25–30 chondroitin sulphate chains. Additionally it holds about 60 shorter chains of keratan sulphate which have an average molecular weight of about 9000. Carrying up to 1000 charged group sites (with contributions from ester sulphate and carboxyl groups) the overall molecular weight of this proteoglycan is about 1.3 million. In its extended form the macromolecule may be pictured as resembling a test-tube brush (Fig. 3.96) but it is possible that in solution it may adopt a more spherical conformation. There is considerable evidence that some proteoglycan macromolecules *in vivo* are linked together to form large aggregates with molecular weights exceeding 50 million.

In summary, proteoglycans are large, flexible, multi-charged macromolecules. What kind of properties do such macromolecules confer upon the systems which contain them? The answer hinges upon the key structural features particularly associated with proteoglycans—namely their large size and extremely large number of charged sites.

BIOLOGICAL ROLES OF PROTEOGLYCANS

In solution, large, flexible molecules tend to occupy much more space than might be imagined from looking at a static molecular model. The actual molecules are also subject to Brownian motion, and this movement, in association with the enormous number of conformational possibilities available to the large molecule, results in proteoglycans effectively occupying a relatively large volume of solution. This space or volume occupied by a molecule in solution is termed its *molecular domain* and is, from a functional point of view, more important than the mere size of the molecule.

Hyaluronic acid, the largest glycosaminoglycan known, has a domain so large that a single

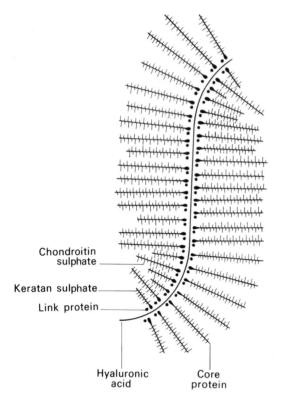

Chondroitin
sulphate

Keratan sulphate

Link protein

Hyaluronic
acid

Core
protein

Fig. 3.96. Tentative model of a proteoglycan aggregate in cartilage.

molecule occupies a sphere of diameter of one micrometre and at a concentration of 0.2 mg/ml, hyaluronic acid occupies the whole solution without any overlapping of domains (Fig. 3.97). In some tissues, proteoglycan constitutes up to some 13% of the wet weight of the matrix and the molecules form a continuous three-dimensional network of entangled polysaccharide chains. For the simple reason that two objects cannot occupy the same space at the same time, this network reduces the space available for other molecules in the system. Other molecules will be excluded, therefore, from the proteoglycan domains as a result of this *excluded volume effect*.

The effect is also partly determined by the size of the molecules attempting to enter the matrix.

Above a certain concentration the osmotic pressure of a proteoglycan solution is greater than can be accounted for in terms of the number of molecules present. In effect a single proteoglycan macromolecule acts as if it was several independent particles, each contributing to the osmotic pressure.

In some matrices, proteoglycan restricts the flow of water some fifty-fold, and this hydrodynamic damping is thought to be important in determining the mechanical properties of structures such as the intervertebral disc, heart valves, and the periodontium. This dynamic (as opposed to equilibrium) exclusion of molecules from a macromolecular domain is known as the sieve effect.

Fig. 3.97. Schematic demonstration of the volume occupied by a hyaluronic acid molecule. For comparison some other macromolecules are shown.

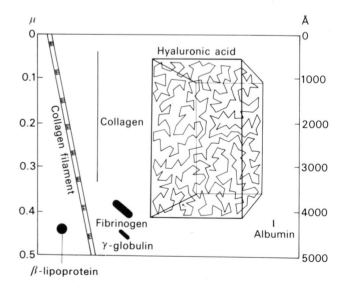

μ

0

0.1

0.2

0.3

0.4

0.5

Å

0

1000

2000

3000

4000

5000

Hyaluronic acid

Collagen filament

Collagen

Fibrinogen

γ-globulin

Albumin

β-lipoprotein

PROTEOGLYCANS AND THE DONNAN EFFECT IN CONNECTIVE TISSUES

In 1911 F. G. Donnan published the important theory which described the consequences arising when an ion or charged particle is restricted in its movements in any way (p. 995). Proteoglycan molecules with their multiple charged sites enmeshed within a network of collagen fibres (as in cartilage) is such a restricted system. Such a polyelectrolyte (i.e. a polymer containing charged groups) in a restricted zone (as within a semipermeable membrane) and in the presence of a diffusible electrolyte, will develop at equilibrium an uneven distribution of the diffusible ions. Ions of opposite charge to those on the polymer will tend to be excluded from the vicinity of the polymer, whilst ions of similar charge will tend to accumulate in that region. The degree of redistribution is directly proportional to the concentration of polyelectrolyte and inversely proportional to the concentration of diffusable ions.

Experimental evidence shows that there is a redistribution of Na^+ and Cl^- ions in cartilage slices which have been left to equilibrate in a solution of 0.15M sodium chloride and the distribution is typical of a Donnan equilibrium effect. When considering divalent cations such as Ca^{2+}, this is even more dramatic, because the accumulation ratio varies with the square of the ion valency. It has been estimated that in 0.1 M calcium chloride some 70% of calcium ions are bound to proteoglycan. This binding and exchange of calcium by the acidic groups on the glycosaminoglycans may play an important role in calcification (p. 389).

METACHROMATIC STAINING

Another phenomenon associated with the high charge density on glycosaminoglycans is the metachromatic staining reaction which proteoglycans give with histological stains such as azure A and toluidine blue. If toluidine blue is added to a proteoglycan, the blue colour changes to purple: addition of salt restores the original colour. Toluidine blue has a positively charged planar aromatic ring structure. As a cation it is electrostatically attracted to the anionic groups on the proteoglycan and large numbers of the flat dye molecules 'stack down' on top of each other with their aromatic rings aligned in parallel. This proximity of the rings causes a subtle temporary change in the electronic structure of the molecules so that light of a different wavelength is absorbed, thereby accounting for the colour change—the so-called *metachromatic shift*. With addition of salt, the Na^+ ions compete with the dye molecules for the anionic sites causing disruption of the stacking process.

THE LIPIDS

Lipids or fats are a chemically diverse group of biological substances grouped together on the basis of their common solubility in non-polar solvents, such as diethyl ether, chloroform and benzene, and their relative insolubility in water and other polar solvents. The chemical structures and the molecular shapes and sizes of the different types of lipids vary widely but the major components of many of their molecules are long chain non-polar saturated aliphatic (alkane) molecular groupings; in addition unsaturated (alkene) aliphatic chains may be present. These components of the lipid molecules are the *saturated* and *unsaturated fatty acids* respectively (Fig. 3.98 a and b). A structure which is the major component in another group of lipids is the saturated carbon ring-complex *perhydrocyclopentanophenanthrene* which occurs in the steroid compounds and the related bile salts (Fig. 3.98c).

Though most of these lipid structures are relatively large molecules, individually they do not approach the large molecular weights found in the protein and carbohydrate molecules discussed previously. However, since several lipids have the property of aggregating to form large micellar complexes and membrane structures, it is on this basis that lipids can be loosely categorized as compounds capable of forming structures of macromolecular dimensions.

The lipids form a major food store in animals and many plants, and in a normal adult human some 10 kg of lipid is stored as triglycerides in the fat stores, which can be rapidly mobilized for the production of energy. Lipids also serve to insulate and protect, as with whale blubber, human abdominal adipose tissue and the oil of sea birds' feathers. Lipids are also major structural components of cell membranes, and some lipids have specialized roles as hormones and vitamins. They are of considerable economic importance both as food and as raw material for a wide range of industrial processes and products.

Because of their diversity it is not possible to produce a simple logical sub-classification of lipids in terms of structure which would help us

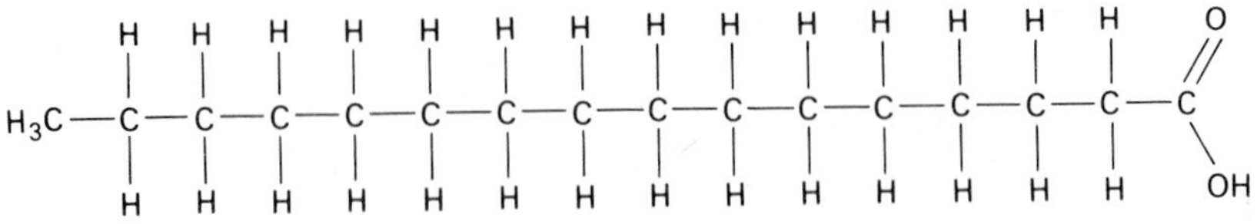

(a)   Palmitic acid (saturated)

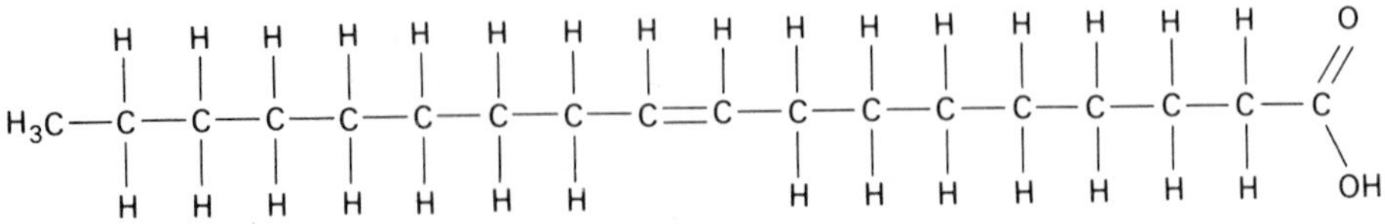

(b)   Oleic acid (unsaturated)

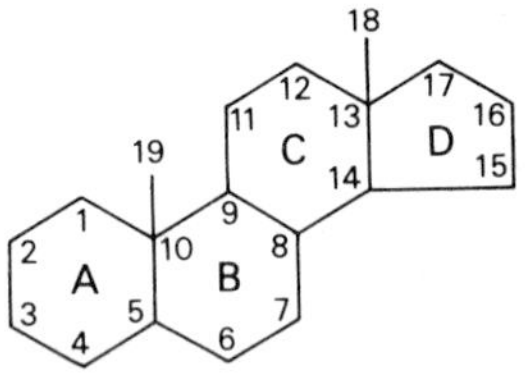

(c)   Perhydrocyclopentanophenanthrene

Fig. 3.98. Hydrocarbon components of lipids. (a)
Palmitic acid (saturated). (b) Oleic acid (unsaturated).
(c) Perhydrocyclopentanophenanthrene.

to remember and describe their various properties on a rational basis. The following lists the
main groups of lipid compounds: fatty acids;
neutral fats; glycolipids; phospho lipids; aliphatic alcohols and waxes; carotenoids; steroids; fat
soluble vitamins; and prostaglandins. Many
lipids may be classified under more than one of
these headings.

Lipid compounds, as a group, contain a very
high proportion of hydrophobic groupings.
These essentially non-polar hydrophobic groups
have little affinity for charged polar solvents
such as water and will not dissolve in them. This
is because the charged water molecules have a
greater attraction for one another than for the
non-polar molecules. These non-polar
molecules, or parts of molecules, more readily
mix with molecules chemically similar to themselves, such as the non-polar solvents. The main

non-polar groups in lipid molecules are the long
hydrocarbon chains of the fatty acid components
and the hydrocarbon ring structures of steroid
structures. Lipids can also contain polar groups,
such as charged phosphate or carboxyl groups,
which are hydrophilic in character: however, as
the major portion of lipid molecules is non-polar
the hydrophilic groups confer only a small
degree of water solubility on the molecule.

The physical and chemical properties of
lipids depend upon the size and shape of their
hydrocarbon components, the presence of double bonds, and of reactive groups such as carboxyl, hydroxyl, phosphate and ethanolamine.
The structure–function relationships of compounds, already discussed for other macromolecules, is also well illustrated by the lipids
and will be discussed in more detail as individual
lipid structures are considered.

Table 3.17. The characteristics of fatty acids.

Common name	Number of carbon atoms and double bonds	Formula	Solubility g/100 cm^3 water	m.p. °C.	Systematic name
Saturated					
Acetic acid	C2:0	CH_3COOH		+16.5	n-Ethanoic acid
Propionic acid	C3:0	CH_3CH_2COOH		−22	n-Propanoic acid
Butyric acid	C4:0	$CH_3(CH_2)_2COOH$		− 7.9	n-Butanoic acid
Capric acid	C10:0	$CH_3(CH_2)_8COOH$	5.62	31.6	n-Decanoic acid
Myristic acid	C14:0	$CH_3(CH_2)_{12}COOH$	1.0	54.1	n-Tetradecanoic acid
Palmitic acid	C16:0	$CH_3(CH_2)_{14}COOH$	Insol.	62.7	n-Hexadecanoic acid
Stearic acid	C18:0	$CH_3(CH_2)_{16}COOH$	do.	69.6	n-Octadecanoic acid
Arachidic acid	C20:0	$CH_3(CH_2)_{18}COOH$	do.	75.4	n-Eicosanoic acid
Unsaturated					
Palmitoleic acid	C16:1	$CH_3(CH_2)_5CH=CH(CH_2)_7COOH$	do.	1.0	cis-Δ-9-Hexadecenoic acid
Oleic acid	C18:1	$CH_3(CH_2)_7CH=CH(CH_2)_7COOH$	do.	10.5	cis-Δ-9-Octadecenoic acid
Linoleic acid	C18:2	$CH_3(CH_2)_4CH=CHCH_2CH=CH(CH_2)_7COOH$	do.	− 5.0	all cis-Δ-9,12-Octadecadienoic acid
α-Linolenic acid	C18:3	$CH_3CH_2(CH=CH-CH_2)_3(CH_2)_6COOH$	do.		all cis-Δ-9,12,15-Octadecatrienoic acid
γ-Linolenic acid	C18:3	$CH_3(CH_2)_4(CH=CH-CH_2)_3(CH_2)_3COOH$	do.	−10.0	all cis-Δ-6,9,12-Octadecatrienoic acid
Arachidonic acid	C20:4	$CH_3(CH_2)_4(CH=CH-CH_2)_4(CH_2)_2COOH$	do.	−49.5	all cis-Δ-5,8,11,14-Eicosatetraenoic acid
Ricinoleic acid	C18:0 (OH)	$CH_3(CH_2)_5CHCH_2CH=CH(CH_2)_7COOH$ OH	do.	5.5	12 OH.cis-Δ-9-Octadecenoic acid

FATTY ACIDS

Those occurring naturally are usually straight chain mono-carboxylic aliphatic acids of the general formula RCOOH where R is any aliphatic group. Examples are the saturated palmitic acid and the unsaturated oleic acid (Fig. 3.98a and b).

They usually have an even number of carbon atoms with all 4 valencies satisfied, though some ethylene double bond structures do occur. Only very small amounts of the free fatty acids are found in mammals.

Table 3.17 lists some of the more common fatty acids and their structures.

Properties of the fatty acids

A fatty acid RCOOH may be considered as made up of two functional parts, the reactive acidic −COOH group and the inert aliphatic carbon chain R. The observed physical and chemical properties of the fatty acids are the result of respective contributions of these two parts of their molecules.

The carboxyl group (−COOH) dissociates in water to give hydrogen and carboxylate ions:

$$RCOOH \rightleftharpoons RCOO^- + H^+$$

The dissociation of the higher fatty acids (pK=4.87) is not all that weaker than acetic acid (pKa=4.75), though there are great differences in their solubilities (Table 3.17).

Fatty acids react with bases, such as sodium hydroxide, to give salts, which are relatively soluble:

$$RCOOH + NaOH \rightleftharpoons RCOONa + H_2O$$

Thus sodium stearate, a major constituent of household soap, is readily soluble in water and acts as a lipid solvent by forming a stable emulsion in water, which accounts for its grease-dissolving properties in aqueous solution (see below, also Fig. 3.110). Some fatty acid salts, such as those formed with calcium, are insoluble in water, which accounts for the poor suds-forming properties of hard water areas.

Fatty acids can form esters with alcohols, e.g.

Such esters are of considerable biological importance as they form the bulk of all naturally occurring lipids. The most common compounds are the esters formed between fatty acids and the trihydric alcohol-glycerol (Fig. 3.99). R_1, R_2 and R_3 may be the same or different aliphatic groups.

Esters formed with alcohols other than glycerol constitute the waxes, where the alcohol may be either a long chain aliphatic or an alicyclic compound, an example of the latter is cholesterol (Fig. 3.107).

The chain length and degree of unsaturation of the non-polar aliphatic chain affects the physical properties of the fatty acid. Thus the melting point increases with the length of the chain (Table 3.17). The greater the chain length, the greater the overall hydrophobic properties of the molecule. Thus stearic acid (18 saturated carbon atoms) is virtually insoluble in water whereas acetic (2C) is completely miscible. Butyric acid (4C) is slightly soluble (Table 3.17).

These hydrophobic properties of the fatty acids also operate when they are incorporated into lipid structures, such as the triglycerides. Indeed the physicochemical properties of the triglycerides in general are predominantly determined by the nature of their constituent fatty acids.

The number and position of the double bonds in the unsaturated fatty acids also affects their physical and chemical properties. For example the melting point is much lower when double bonds are present compared with the melting point of the saturated acid with the same number of carbon atoms (Table 3.17, cf m.p. of stearic, oleic, linoleic acids).

When more than one double bond is found in a naturally occurring fatty acid it is usually part of a non-conjugated double bond system, as in linoleic acid:

$$-CH=CH-CH_2-CH=CH-$$

A methylene group separates the two double bonds.

The presence of double bonds in the chain also makes the molecule asymmetric and geometric isomerism occurs making cis or trans isomers possible (p. 988). Most naturally occurring unsaturated fatty acids are cis isomers (Fig. 3.100).

$$CH_3\overset{O}{\underset{\|}{C}}-OH \quad + \quad CH_3OH \quad \rightleftharpoons \quad CH_3\overset{O}{\underset{\|}{C}}-O-CH_3 + H_2O$$

Acetic acid   Methyl alcohol   Methyl acetate

CH₂—O—C—R₁ formulas...

$\overset{1}{CH_2OH}$				
$\overset{2}{CHOH}$				
$\overset{3}{CH_2CH}$				

Glycerol

CH_2—O—C—R₁
‖
O

CHOH

CH_2OH

1-Monoacylglycerol

CH_2—O—C—R₁
‖
O

CH —O—C—R₂
‖
O

CH_2OH

1,2-Diacylglycerol

CH_2—O—C—R₁
‖
O

CH —O—C—R₂
‖
O

CH_2—O—C—R₃
‖
O

Triacylglycerol
(neutral fat)

Fig. 3.99. Glyceryl esters.

The position of the double bonds in the fatty acid chain is indicated by numbering either from the methyl end of the R group or from the carboxyl end of the chain. When numbering from the methyl end, the carbon atom with the double bond is referred to as the ω carbon atom, when numbering from the carboxyl end it is referred to as the Δ carbon atom, i.e.

Oleic acid

$\omega 9$

$CH_3(CH_2)_7 CH = CH(CH_2)_7 COOH$

$\Delta 9$

Linoleic acid

$\omega 6.9$

$CH_3(CH_2)_4 CH = CHCH_2 CH = CH(CH_2)_7 COOH$

$\Delta 9.12$

Thus oleic acid is an 18C fatty acid with a single double bond at ω 9 (or $\Delta 9$) and linoleic acid is an 18C straight chain fatty acid containing two unsaturated double bonds in the ω 6.9 (or Δ 9.12) positions.

In terms of function the fatty acids operate mainly as compounds storing reserves of energy in chemical form and as non-polar compounds which form esters of varied compositions for utilization in structural components of cells, mainly in biomembrane structures.

Essential fatty acids (EFAs)

The essential fatty acids (EFAs) are required in the diet of animals because they cannot manufacture them for themselves. In this sense the EFAs may be regarded as vitamins because like them (p. 234) they cannot be synthesized, yet

are essential for normal function. The three essential fatty acids are:

1 *Linoleic acid*, containing eighteen carbon atoms and two unsaturated double bonds.

2 *γ-Linolenic acid*, containing eighteen carbon atoms and three unsaturated double bonds.

3 *Arachidonic acid*, containing twenty carbon atoms and four unsaturated double bonds. However animals can synthesize arachidonic acid and γ linolenic acid from linoleic acid.

The essential fatty acids cannot be synthesized by body tissues because there is no enzyme system for the insertion of a double bond in the ω 6

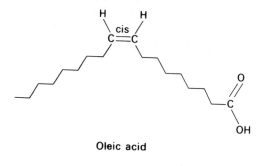

Oleic acid

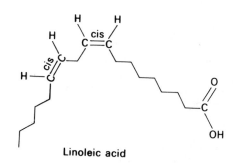

Linoleic acid

Fig. 3.100. Cis-isomerism in oleic and linoleic acids.

position, and it is the presence of this double bond on the sixth carbon atom from the methyl end of the fatty acid molecule, which confers upon them their essential fatty acid property. The three EFAs have their double bonds positioned as follows:

Linoleic acid ω 6, 9.
γ linolenic acid ω 6, 9, 12.
Arachidonic acid ω 6, 9, 12, 15.

The EFAs form a high proportion of the fatty acids in phospholipids, which are components of cell membranes (Fig. 3.103) and the absence of essential fatty acids in the diet has been shown to result in a weakening and disruption of these membranes. Phospholipids also appear to be involved in calcium transport and the calcification mechanisms involved in tooth and bone formation. An absence of essential fatty acids disrupts the calcification process, resulting in poor calcification of bones and teeth, and a possible increase in caries susceptibility (in rats).

The daily requirement of essential fatty acids for an adult human is approximately 10 g and is ultimately derived from plants which are able to synthesize them.

NEUTRAL FATS

These are fatty acid esters of glycerol. When all three hydroxy groups of the glycerol form esters with fatty acids a triacylglyceride (or neutral fat) is formed. Quantitatively these are the most important lipid components of the diet:

$$
\begin{array}{l}
{}_1\,CH_2 - O - C - R_1 \\
\qquad\qquad\quad \| \\
\qquad\qquad\quad O \\
\\
{}_2\,CH \;- O - C - R_2 \\
\qquad\qquad\quad \| \\
\qquad\qquad\quad O \\
\\
{}_3\,CH_2 - O - C - R_3 \\
\qquad\qquad\quad \| \\
\qquad\qquad\quad O
\end{array}
$$

Triacylglyceride

The carbons of the glycerol molecule are numbered 1, 2 and 3 respectively and the three fatty acid components, R_1, R_2 and R_3, may be the same or different from each other. The naturally occurring glycerol esters are mainly triglycerides with two or three different fatty acids, the most common being palmitic acid (C16:0), stearic acid (C18:0) and oleic acid (C18:1(ω9)) in animals. Triglycerides are the form in which fatty

acids are stored in the body, the fatty acids forming some 95% of the compound by weight and hence constituting the main energy store. When triglycerides are mobilized for production of energy, the fatty acids are first removed by hydrolysis and then broken down stepwise (β-oxidation, p. 205) to form acetyl SCoA (CH₃COSCoA) molecules which enter the tricarboxylic acid cycle (p. 195) to produce energy. The glycerol part of the neutral fat molecule may be metabolized either to synthesize glucose (p. 187) or release energy. The composition of the triglycerides stored in the body varies with the species, diet, environment and location within the body. In a particular species variations in the diet will alter lipid metabolism, producing changes in the ratios of fatty acids in the tissue glycerides. Thus rats maintained on a high sucrose diet, as compared with a high starch diet, have an increased level of liver lipogenesis, producing a fall in the proportion of palmitic acid and an increase in stearic and oleic acid in the tissues. The fat of cattle hooves has a lower melting point than body fat and remains liquid at lower temperatures, due to the higher proportion of unsaturated fatty acids present. Absence of EFAs from the diet results in their absence from the tissue glycerides.

THE GLYCOLIPIDS

This group of compounds consists of glycerides where a carbohydrate replaces one or more of the fatty acid components. They are constituents of cell membranes, one example being monogalactosyl diglyceride (Fig. 3.101).

Another group of compounds loosely classified under the heading of glycolipids are the *cerebrosides* (Fig. 3.102b). These compounds are not glycerides but compounds of *sphingosine* (Fig. 3.102a) joined by an ether linkage to a hexose sugar, usually galactose: they occur in the brain.

THE PHOSPHOLIPIDS

Like the neutral fats, the phospholipids are also glycerides, but in contrast contain phosphorus and usually an alcohol as well. They may be considered as derivatives of glycerol phosphate where phosphoric acid forms an ester linkage with one of the alcoholic OH groups of glycerol

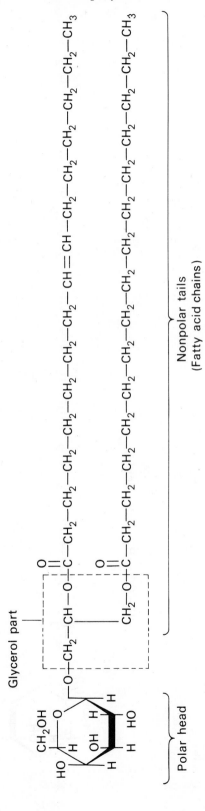

Fig. 3.101. A glycolipid structure: monogalactosyl diglyceride.

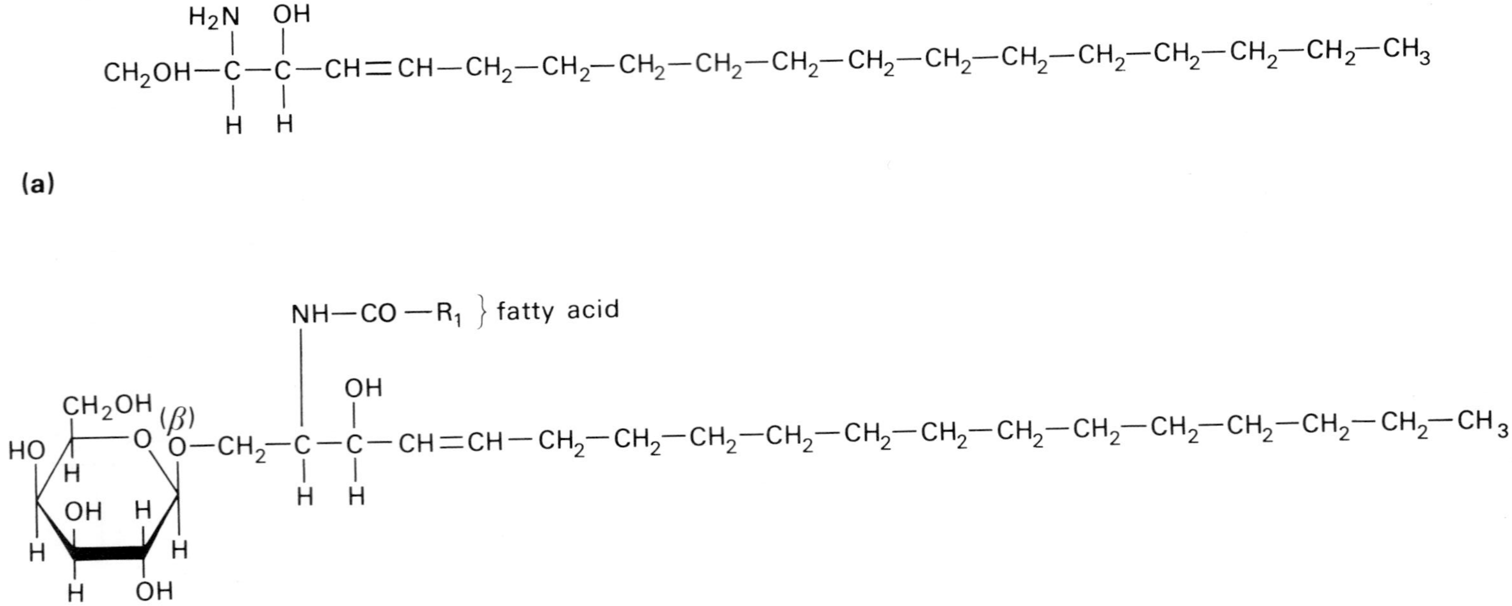

$$H_2N \quad OH$$

$$CH_2OH-\overset{|}{\underset{H}{C}}-\overset{|}{\underset{H}{C}}-CH=CH-CH_2-CH_2-CH_2-CH_2-CH_2-CH_2-CH_2-CH_2-CH_2-CH_2-CH_3$$

(a)

$$NH-CO-R_1 \left.\right\} \text{fatty acid}$$

$$OH$$

$$CH_2OH \, (\beta)$$

(b)

Fig. 3.102. (a) Sphingosine (4-sphingonine). (b) Cerebroside structure (a galactocerebroside).

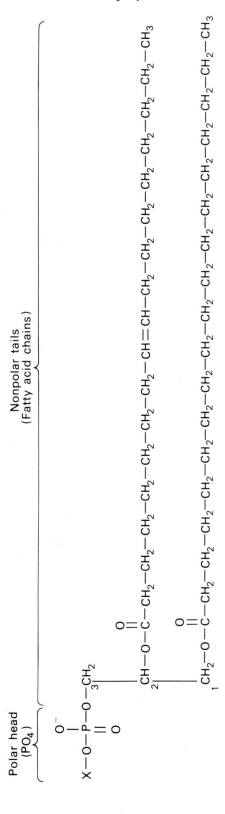

Fig. 3.103. Phospholipid structure.

to give phosphatidic acid. They are also referred to as phosphatides (Fig. 3.103).

Phospholipids are major components of cell membranes. They are not normally found elsewhere in the tissues, though the organic matrix of enamel and dentine contain approximately 35% and 2% lipid respectively, 30% of which is phospholipid. Since these phospholipids in enamel and dentine are closely associated with hydroxyapatite crystals, it has been suggested that they may be involved in the calcification process.

Phospholipids are polar compounds with non-polar hydrocarbon tails. It is this structure which enables them to form membranes, as described below.

The alcohols are attached to the OH group of the phosphate by an ester linkage.

The most common phospholipids are *phosphatidyl choline* (lecithin), *phosphatidyl ethanolamine*, *phosphatidyl serine, phosphatidyl inositol* and *diphosphatidyl glycerol* (cardiolipin) (Fig. 3.104).

The fatty acid components in these com-

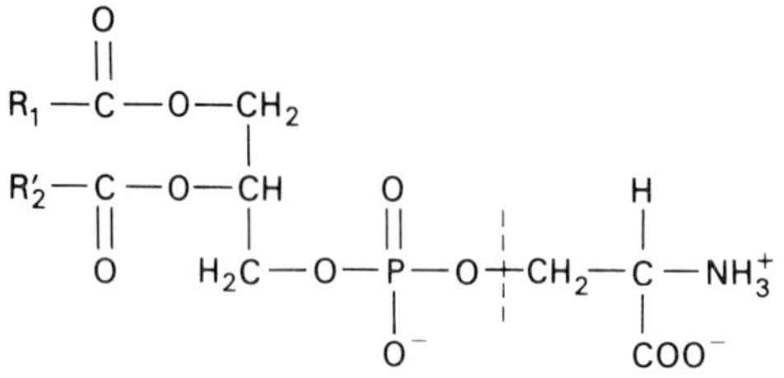

Phosphatidyl serine

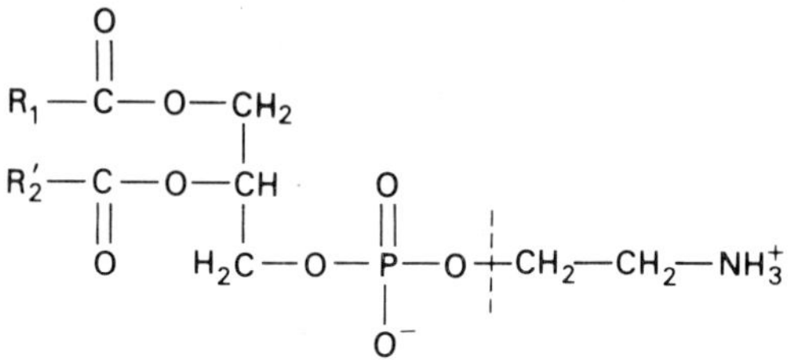

Phosphatidyl ethanolamine

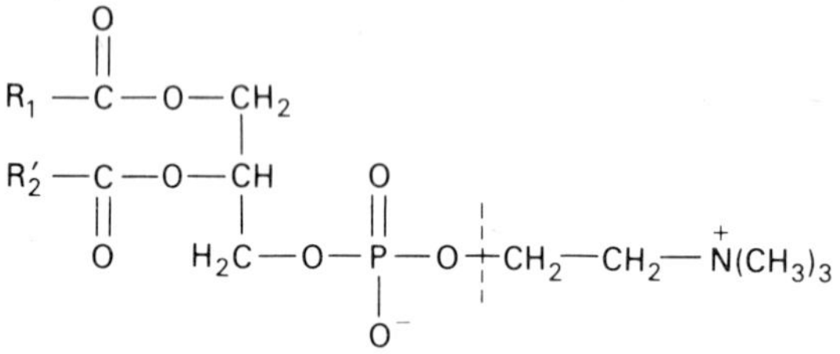

Phosphatidyl choline
(lecithin)

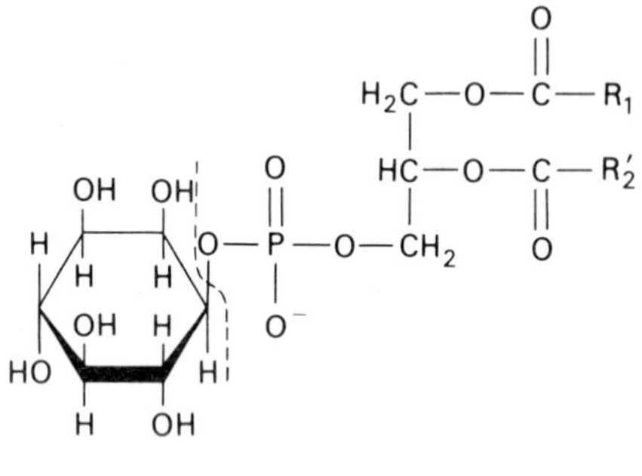

Phosphatidyl inositol

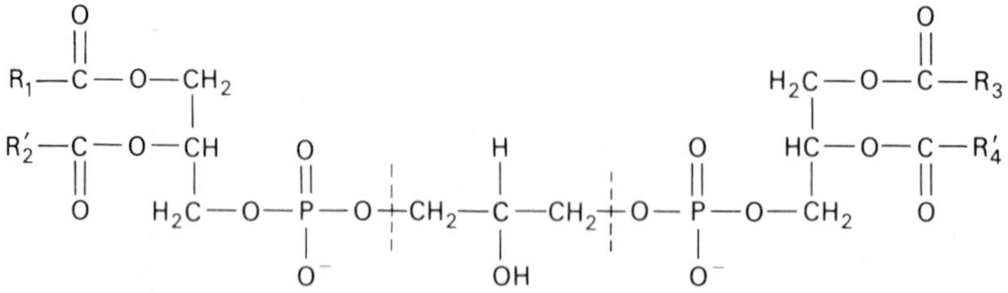

Diphosphatidyl glycerol
(cardiolipin)

Fig. 3.104. Structures of common phospholipids.

pounds are indicated by the symbols R_1, R_2, R_3 and R_4, and in animals these are mainly palmitic (C 16:0), stearic (C 18:0), oleic (C 18:1), linoleic (C 18:2) and arachidonic C20:4) acids. In animal tissues the fatty acid (R_1) on the α (1) carbon atom of glycerol tends to be saturated and that on the β (2) carbon (R_2) is usually unsaturated.

Sphingolipids are also classified as phospholipids but with long chain unsaturated amino alcohols, the *sphingosines*, instead of glycerol, as the component which combines with the fatty acids and phosphoric acid. Sphingosine (Fig. 3.102a) is a base and links to one fatty acid molecule by an amide-type linkage. The phosphate combines with one of the sphingosine alcoholic groups in an ester linkage. The structure of *sphingomyelin* (sphingosine phosphoryl choline) is shown in Fig. 3.105 where the esterification is with phosphoryl choline.

Sphingolipids are polar compounds found in considerable quantities in plant and animal membranes, particularly in nerve and brain tissues. They are currently thought to play a role in nerve fibre insulation, preventing short circuiting of nerve electrical impulse transmission.

There are a number of genetic disorders in man which result in the accumulation of certain phospholipids in the tissues. An example is Niemann–Pick disease where there is accumulation of sphingomyelin in brain and nerve tissue producing mental retardation. The accumulation is due to an inborn error of metabolism (p. 271), the absence of the enzyme sphingomyelinase in the lysosomes, which catalyses hydrolysis of sphingomyelin. There is no cure for this condition.

ALIPHATIC ALCOHOLS AND WAXES

The waxes are usually esters formed between long-chain fatty acids and long-chain primary alcohols. They occur in nature as protective coatings on fruit, leaves, fur and feathers. Examples are beeswax, which is mainly the palmitic acid ester of cetyl alcohol ($C_{16}H_{33}OH$), and lanolin (sheep wool wax) which is a long-chain fatty acid ester of cholesterol.

THE CAROTENOIDS

Terpenes include such diverse compounds as latex, camphor, and the carotenoids. They are grouped together on the basis of containing the repeating five carbon *isoprene* structure, i.e.

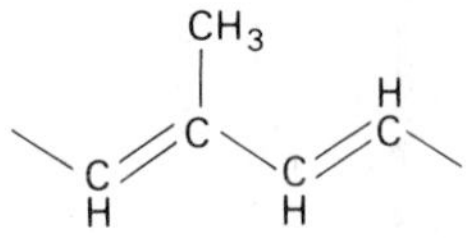

The most common carotenoid is β-carotene, a C-40 hydrocarbon which cleaves oxidatively to form two molecules of vitamin A (retinol) (shown in Fig. 3.106), important in the biochemistry of vision (p. 963).

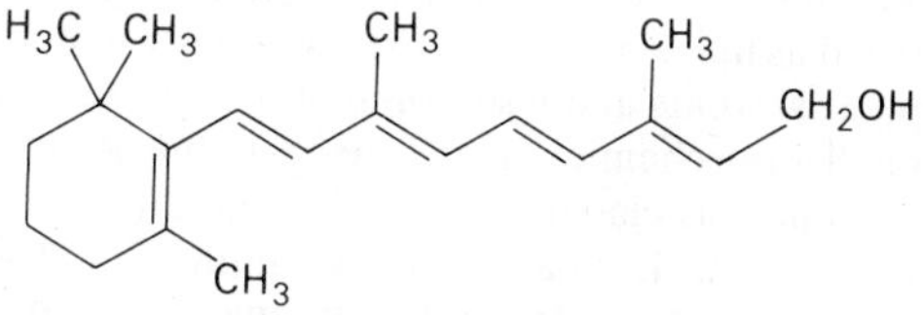

Fig. 3.106. Vitamin A (all trans-retinol).

STEROIDS

The steroids are a group of substances related to cholesterol and include the sex hormones, such as progesterone and testosterone, the bile acids and vitamin D. Cholesterol (Fig. 3.107) is a component of some cell membranes.

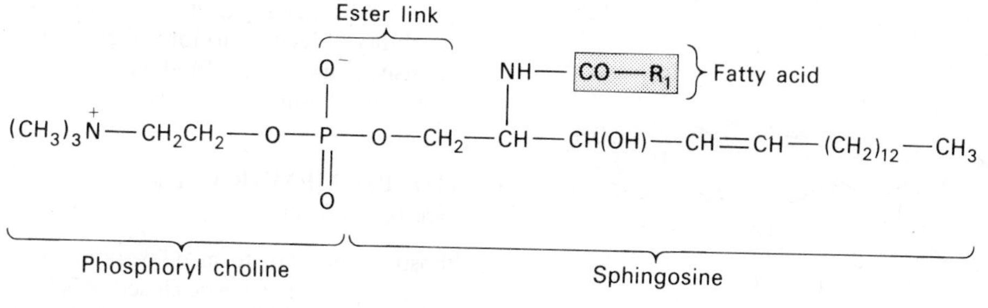

Fig. 3.105. Sphingomyelin structure.

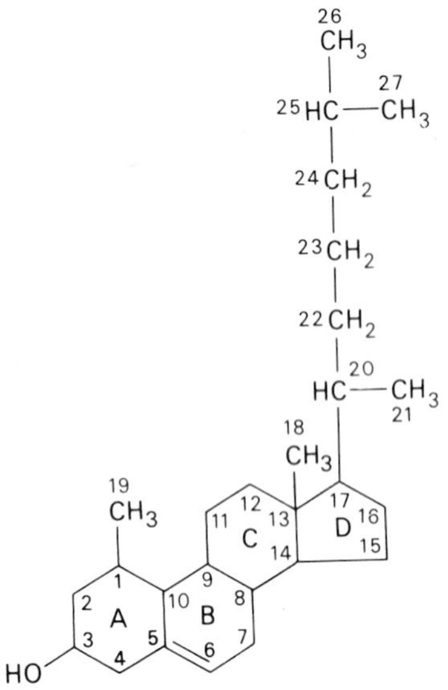

Fig. 3.107. The structure of cholesterol.

THE FAT SOLUBLE VITAMINS

Vitamins A, D, E and K are collectively classified as lipids because of their solubility in non-polar solvents and insolubility in water, but are of diverse chemical structure. Vitamin A as a terpene was classified as a carotenoid (p. 155) and vitamin D as a steroid. Vitamins E and K are tocopherol and naphthoquinone compounds respectively.

PROSTAGLANDINS

These compounds are oxygenated derivatives of unsaturated fatty acids and have a hormonal action stimulating smooth muscle. They are derived from essential polyunsaturated fatty acids, such as arachidonic acid. An example is prostaglandin E₂ (PGE₂) (Fig. 3.108).

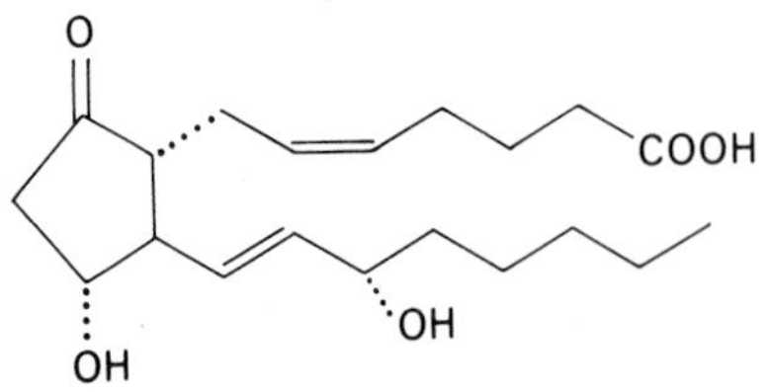

Fig. 3.108. The structure of prostaglandin E₂ (PGE₂).

The essential fatty acids (EFA) give rise to these biologically active prostaglandins (p. 236). Whether the function of EFAs in cells is due entirely to the formation and function of prostaglandins is not certain. The biological properties of the E prostaglandins have been extensively investigated: they cause such diverse effects as leucocyte migration, release of noradrenaline from nerve endings and release of calcium from bones (see p. 799).

GENERAL PROPERTIES OF THE LIPIDS

Polar and non-polar lipids behave very differently from one another in water. When non-polar lipids such as triacylglycerides are mixed with water, an unstable emulsion is formed which rapidly separates into two phases on standing. However when polar lipids such as phospholipids are mixed with water, a small amount dissolves, but the major portion forms either into structures known as micelles or into monolayers at air-water interfaces. *Micelles* are aggregates of lipid molecules so orientated that the hydrophilic part of their molecules constitute the outer surface of the structure which is exposed to the water molecules surrounding them, with the hydrophobic parts of the molecules arranged inside the micelles to give an internal hydrophobic phase (Fig. 3.109).

These water-soluble structures tend to be very stable and are similar to the micelles formed by soaps (the alkali metal salts of fatty acids) such as sodium stearate, where the polar carboxyl group forms the hydrophilic head of the molecule. The aliphatic hydrocarbon chains extending inwards to form the internal hydrophobic phase are able to dissolve other hydrophobic molecules and form stable emulsion droplets (Fig. 3.110).

This is the basis of soap and detergent action whereby water-soluble substances can dissolve large molecules of hydrophobic greasy substances. Micelles are fairly stable structures and the ability of lecithin to form these structures is extensively used in the food industry to stabilize emulsions of non-polar lipids in aqueous media.

THE BIOMEMBRANES

(See pp. 165-7).

Phospholipids can form bilayers in water (Fig. 3.111a), and these can be closed vesicles or liposomes (Fig. 3.111b), the membranes formed

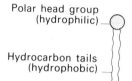

Polar head group
(hydrophilic)

Hydrocarbon tails
(hydrophobic)

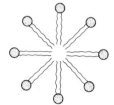

Fig. 3.109. Micelle formation. (a) Symbol for a phospholipid or glycolipid molecule. (b) Diagram of a section of a micelle formed from phospholipid molecules.

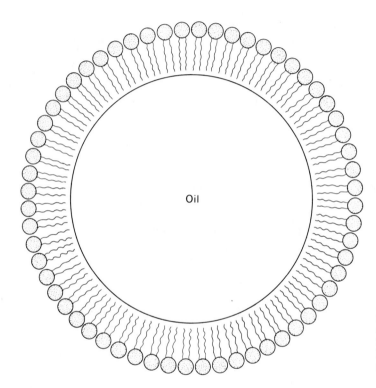

Oil

Fig. 3.110. Emulsion droplet with polar lipids serving as emulsifying agents (cross section through droplet). This is also the basis for soap and detergent action.

Water

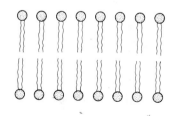

(a)

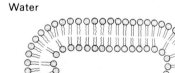

(b)

Fig. 3.111. (a) Diagram of a section of a unit bilayer membrane formed of phospholipid molecules. (b) Cross-section through a liposome. The phospholipid bilayer forms a completely closed vesicle.

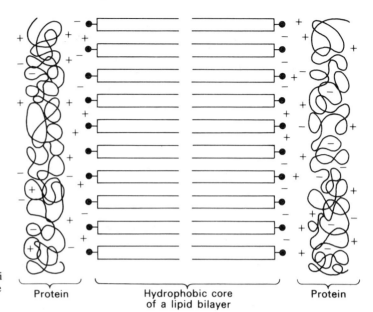

Fig. 3.112. The Davson-Danielli unit-bilayer model of membrane structure.

Protein   Hydrophobic core of a lipid bilayer   Protein

being very similar to the natural biomembranes. Indeed this phospholipid unit bilayer is the basis of a model of biomembrane structure originally proposed by Danielli and Davson in 1935. This envisages the phospholipid bilayer as sandwiched between two outer protein surface layers (Fig. 3.112).

An alternative concept is the *fluid-mosaic model* proposed by Singer and Nicolson in 1972, which envisages the phospholipid bilayer with embedded globular proteins (Fig. 3.113).

This differs from the Danielli and Davson model in that the biomembrane protein components are conceived as either partially or totally traversing the bilayer rather than being confined to its two hydrophilic surfaces. The fluid-mosaic model is more consistent with the known properties of biomembranes.

All cells are bounded by such membranes, as are various organelles within the cell. These membranes serve as barriers between different locations within the cell, and for separating it

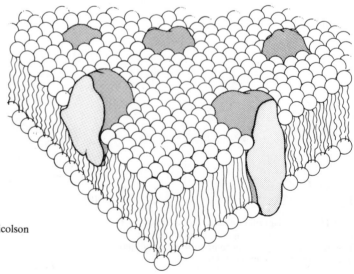

Fig. 3.113. The Singer–Nicolson fluid mosaic model for membrane structure.

from its surroundings: they also form the physical structures with which various enzyme and transport systems are associated. Membrane bound *matrix vesicles* (p. 393), which are thought to play an important role in tissue mineralization, also have a phospholipid bilayer membrane.

In summary therefore the group of compounds together classified as lipids are in fact very diverse both chemically and in their biological functions; ranging from simple fatty acids acting as a chemical energy store, through steroids with hormonal and vitamin activities, to complex phospholipids forming structural components of cell membranes. The single common property uniting them under the heading of lipids is their solubility in non-polar solvents.

FURTHER READING

The proteins

McCONNELL I. (1981) *The Immune System; A course on the molecular and cellular basis of immunity* (2nd Edition). Blackwell Scientific Publications, Oxford.
McLEAN N. (1979) *Haemoglobin*, Studies in Biology, Vol. 93. Edward Arnold, London.
RAMACHANDRAN G. N. & REDDI A. H. (1976) *Biochemistry of Collagen*. Plenum Press, New York.
ROITT I. M. & LEHNER T. (1980) *Immunology of Oral Disease*. Blackwell Scientific Publications, Oxford.
WOODHEAD-GALLOWAY J. (1980) *Collagen: the Anatomy of a protein*, Studies in Biology, Vol. 117. Edward Arnold, London.

The enzymes

BERNHARD S. (1968) *The Structure and Function of Enzymes*. W. A. Benjamin, Menlow Park, California.
BOYER P. D. (1970) *The Enzymes*, Vols. I and II. Academic Press, London.
FERDINAND W. (1976) *The Enzyme Molecule*. John Wiley & Sons, Chichester.
WYNN C. H. (1980) *Structure and Function of Enzymes*, Studies in Biology, Vol. 42. Edward Arnold, London.

Nucleic acids

CLARK B.F.C. (1977) *The Genetic Code*, Studies in Biology, Vol. 83. Edward Arnold, London.
DAVIDSON J.N. (1976) Revised by Adams, Burden, Campbell & Smellie. *The Biochemistry of the Nucleic Acids* (8th Edition). Chapman & Hall, London.
OLBY R. (1974) *The Path to the Double Helix*. Macmillan, London.

Carbohydrates

BARKER R. (1971) *Organic Chemistry of Biological Compounds*, Chapter 4. Prentice-Hall, Englewood Cliffs, New Jersey.
REES D.A. (1977) *Polysaccharide Shapes*, Outline Studies in Biology. Chapman & Hall, London.

Lipids

GURR M.I. & JAMES A.T. (1980) *Lipid Biochemistry* (3rd Edition). Chapman & Hall, London.

CHAPTER 4

The Cell and its Metabolism

CELL STRUCTURE

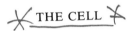
THE CELL

The nature of cells

A cell is a microscopic unit of protoplasm surrounded by a membrane and containing, or having at some stage contained, a centre of metabolic control known as a nucleus. Protoplasm is living matter and as such is composed of a complex array of molecules showing a high level of organization. Living things are recognizably 'alive' because of the complexity of this organization, not because of the materials of which they are made. In a universe where there is an ever-increasing dissipation of energy, together with an ever-increasing tendency towards disorder, living matter has the extraordinary property of locally reversing this trend, for it increases orderliness. Within the confines of the plasma membrane, the boundary between the cell and its environment, order reigns while the cell remains alive.

Development of different cell types

The cells of the body can be classified according to their structure and activities. Before considering the structure of a typical cell, it will be useful to consider how this diversity of form and function develops.

Regardless of their differences, all the cells of a human being develop from a single cell, the zygote or fertilized human egg. This is one of the largest human cells. It is roughly spherical and about 30 μm in diameter (1 μm = 10^{-6}m). It divides repeatedly by mitosis (p. 258), that is, in such a way that each of the two cells formed at a division contain the same genetic information—in the form of chromosome copies —that the parent cell contained. There are, however, differences in the local environment of the nuclei containing these copies. These differ-ences are caused initially by a lack of homogeneity in the cytoplasm (the protoplasm surrounding the nucleus) of the original zygote. This means that at each division cytoplasmic segregation occurs; different cells get different types of cytoplasm. The cells begin to behave differently, possibly as a result of environmental differences. Chemical differentiation occurs; different genes are activated in different cells with the result that different enzymes are produced, different activities become possible, and hence the cells behave differently. The various cell types begin to divide at different rates, and to move in different directions at different speeds. All these activities are, however, coordinated, and result in an embryo taking 'shape'. Gradually the cells begin to look different under the microscope and it is possible to classify them into different groups on the basis of morphological criteria. Cellular differentiation is said to have occurred. The next step is histogenesis, the development of tissues; cells of similar types group together and collaborate to perform specific functions. Muscle, nerve and epithelia are examples of tissues. This is followed by organogenesis, the grouping of tissues to form composite structures such as the liver, heart and lungs.

Histological and cytological techniques

In cytology, where interest lies in the various parts or organelles of the cell, light microscopy is often inadequate. The limit of resolution of a light microscope fitted with an oil immersion lens is about 0.2 μm. Since most organelles are smaller than this, other methods have to be used to visualize them. The absolute limit of any magnifying system is ultimately determined by the wavelength of the source of illumination. Objects which are closer together than half the wavelength cannot be distinguished as being separate. The wavelength of a beam of electrons is much shorter than that of a beam of light and so the electron microscope, whose resolving power is about 1 nm ($10^{-3}\mu$m), is used to visualize the components of individual cells.

The two techniques most widely used in histology and cytology are light and electron microscopy. The following section summarizes the principles of these techniques.

Light microscopy

Before a sample of human material can be examined with a conventional light microscope, a number of preliminary steps are necessary.

1   The sample must be 'fixed' either chemically or by freezing so that it does not decay before it can be examined.

2   It generally has to be cut into thin sections of uniform thickness through which light can pass. Tissue usually has to be embedded in a more rigid block of sectionable material such as paraffin wax. Sections are then mounted on glass slides.

3   Because the absorption of light by the various parts of the section is very similar, they are usually indistinguishable unless they are stained selectively. Staining involves the treatment of the tissue with a large variety of natural or synthetic dyestuffs. The most common combination is haematoxylin and eosin (H & E). Haematoxylin stains acidic parts of tissues blue (e.g. nuclei) and eosin (which is acidic) stains other parts pink.

HISTOCHEMISTRY

The routine histological staining techniques have the disadvantage that their mode of action is obscure. In histochemistry, however, the reactions have generally been well worked out to identify and locate a wide variety of enzymes and cellular inclusions such as secretory granules. The localization of the enzyme acid phosphatase will be considered briefly as an example. This enzyme is characteristically present in lysosomes (p. 30). To detect it, tissue sections are prepared in such a way that the enzyme remains active. When they are incubated in a solution of sodium β–glycerophosphate, the acid phosphatase 'breaks off' the inorganic phosphate. This phosphate is then combined with lead ions to produce insoluble lead phosphate which precipitates out of the solution at the spot where it forms. The colourless lead phosphate is then converted to lead sulphide, a dark brown salt which can be identified within the tissue by standard light microscopy.

AUTORADIOGRAPHY

The biosynthesis of many large molecules can often be studied by autoradiography. This makes use of techniques in which one of these molecules has been 'labelled' by incorporating a radioactive element, usually ^{14}C or ^{3}H, into a precursor used in cellular synthesis: for example, ^{3}H or ^{14}C labelled thymidine for DNA formation or glycine for protein synthesis. It is assumed that the cell treats the labelled molecule in exactly the same way as its non-radioactive counterpart. Sometimes the labelled substance is injected directly into the animal and at others it is made available to tissues or cells *in vitro*. In both cases a suitable time interval is allowed for the precursors to enter and be used by the cells. The material is then fixed, sectioned and mounted on glass slides. It is then coated with an emulsion of silver halide in gelatin and left in the dark for a few weeks. During this time the radioactive atoms in the labelled molecules (which have been incorporated by the cells) gradually disintegrate; the radiation particles leaving them pass through the emulsion and energize some of the silver salts so that when the emulsion is developed and fixed, black grains of silver are left behind over the sites of radioactivity. The processing of the autoradiograph is virtually the same as the processing of a photographic plate. The tissue section, which is trapped between the glass slide and the developed emulsion, can now be stained in a routine manner and viewed under the microscope. The silver grains in the overlying emulsion betray the positions of the labelled molecules.

Autoradiography has many uses, for example to trace the path a molecule takes through a cell. This is done by feeding the radioactive molecules to the cells and later killing and fixing samples at various intervals. Autoradiographs locate the position of the radioactive precursor at each time, enabling one to trace its pathway through the different compartments of the cells. For the fine details of the pathway, electron microscopy is used.

SPECIALIZED TYPES OF LIGHT MICROSCOPY

As well as the simple light microscopes used for general purposes in research and teaching laboratories, other specialized types are available.

Phase contrast microscopy

This technique is extremely useful for examining living unstained cells, a valueless exercise with the standard light microscope, as most unstained cells appear transparent. Because the optical density of the various organelles of a cell is about the same, the amplitude (intensity) of light is uniformly reduced. The phase of the light waves, however, is changed differentially. Some parts of the cell slow down the light more than others because of differences in their refractive indices. A phase contrast microscope alters changes in phase to changes in amplitude with the result that organelles can be distinguised because some now appear darker than others. For details of the optics of phase contrast the reader should consult a textbook on microscopy. Fig. 4.1 shows a living fibroblast photographed with a phase contrast microscope.

Polarizing microscopy

This is used to detect regions of cells or tissues where the molecular constituents are arranged in a highly ordered, repeated sequence which produces birefringence. The specimen is placed between crossed polars with the result that areas of it in which the plane of polarization has been rotated by the birefringence of the specimen appear brighter than the black background. Fig. 4.2 shows a transverse section of compact bone photographed using a polarizing microscope.

Fluorescence microscopy

Certain otherwise invisible substances either within, or secreted by, cells can be made to fluoresce and thus become detectable by light microscopy. One common application of this technique is immunofluorescence. This is used to identify and locate specific proteins in tissue sections.

A pure sample of the protein to be detected is injected into an animal which reacts by producing antibodies (p. 679) to it. The antibody is present in the animal's serum and can be obtained and purified as an antiserum. This antibody is then combined chemically with a fluorescent dye. If cells or frozen sections con-

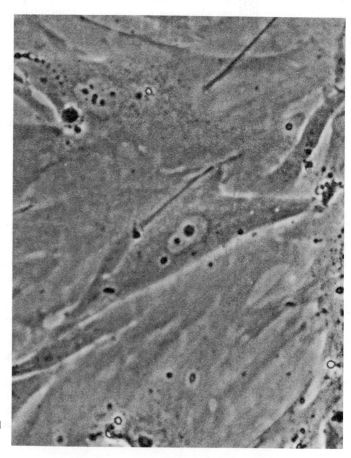

Fig. 4.1. Living fibroblast by phase contrast. (Photomicrograph provided by Miss M. Morris.)

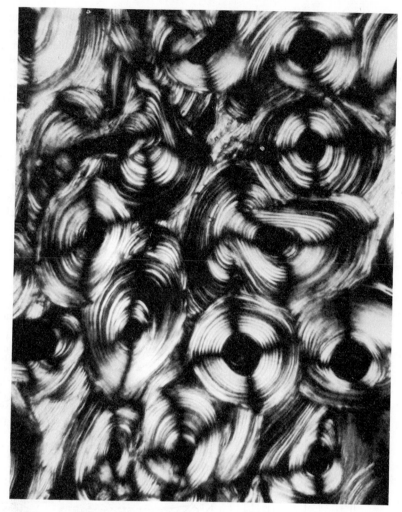

Fig. 4.2. Compact bone by polarizing microscope. (Photomicrograph provided by Mr K. Fitzpatrick.)

taining the original specific protein (antigen) are treated with the specific antibody/dye complex, strong bonds form between the protein and the complex. Any uncombined complex is washed off and the site of the fluorescent dye/antibody/antigen is revealed under ultraviolet light which causes the dye to fluoresce.

Electron microscopy

As with light microscopy, special procedures are necessary to prepare the cells or tissues for examination. To appreciate the need for the various stages in processing, it is helpful to know something of the principles of electron microscopy.

An electron microscope is basically very similar to a light microscope, except that visible light is replaced by an electron beam, and glass lenses by magnetic or electrostatic 'lenses' which focus the electrons in a similar way to that in which glass lenses focus light. As with the light microscope, the illuminating beam passes through a condenser, the specimen, an objective lens, and a projector lens (the last being equivalent to the eyepiece of the light microscope). It finally forms an image on a fluorescent screen, rather like a television screen.

In electron microscopy, fixation and staining are partly combined. Both fixatives and 'stains' contain electron dense substances, such as osmium, which are taken up by membranes which thus appear dark on the fluorescent viewing screen.

The electron beam can only travel through thin specimens; sections used have to be of the order of 0.01–0.5 μm, as compared with the 1–10 μm for light microscopy. Such delicate slices can only be cut from very hard blocks with the sharpest of knives. Polymerized resin blocks and either diamond or glass knives are used.

One of the most important advances in electron microscopy in recent years has been the advent of scanning techniques. Since only the surface is examined the specimen does not have to be thin. In a scanning electron microscope, a narrow beam of electrons is moved to and fro over the surface of the specimen. The reflected electrons are collected, their spacing magnified and they are then cast on to a viewing screen to produce an enlarged image of the surface of the object.

A few words of caution regarding the interpretation of light and electron microscope images seem appropriate at this stage. It is essential to remember that all processing prior to light or electron microscopy inevitably creates changes, or artefacts, in the tissue. It may swell or shrink;

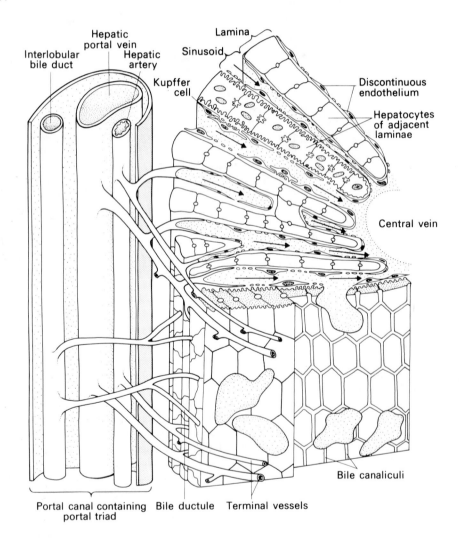

Fig. 4.3. Arrangement of hepatocytes in liver.

⟶ Arrows in sinusoids indicate direction of blood flow

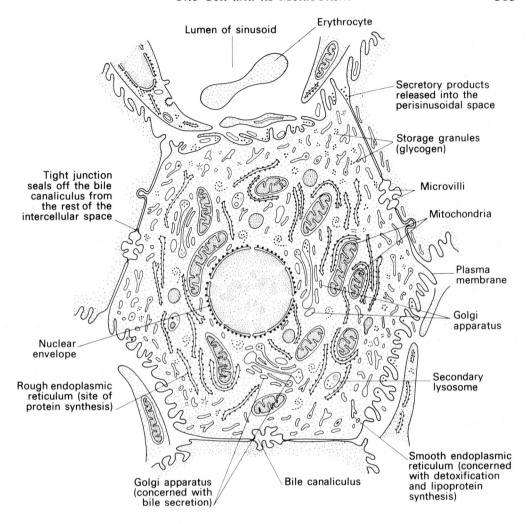

Fig. 4.4. A hepatocyte showing major ultrastructural features.

some parts may be distorted and/or show necrosis (post-mortem changes); it may have been scratched by a rough microtome blade.

CELL ULTRASTRUCTURE

It is necessary to know what a relatively unspecialized cell is like. A liver cell (hepatocyte) has been chosen because it contains virtually every type of known organelle. Fig. 4.3 shows the arrangement of hepatocytes in the liver; and Fig. 4.4 is a diagram summarizing the major structural features of a typical hepatocyte.

A cell such as a hepatocyte is bounded by a plasma membrane; it contains a nucleus and a variety of cytoplasmic organelles embedded in hyaloplasm. An organelle is a part of a cell which is specialized to perform a specific function or group of functions.

Table 4.1 lists the components of a typical cell. Some of the structures required by more specialized cells will be considered later.

Cell boundary

This comprises the plasma membrane, the outer limit of the protoplasm, together with the glycocalyx or cell coat which is secreted by it.

Table 4.1. Components of a typical cell

Cell Boundary	Nuclear compartment	Cytoplasmic compartment
Plasma membrane	Nuclear envelope	Ribosomes
Glycocalyx	Nuclear sap	Endoplasmic reticulum
	Chromatin	a) rough (granular)
	Nucleolus	b) smooth (agranular)
		Golgi apparatus
		Lysosomes
		Peroxisomes
		Mitochondria
		Microfilaments
		Microtubules
		Centrioles

PLASMA MEMBRANE

This is the interface between living matter and the extracellular environment. Even before the plasma membrane was first identified (it is only about 7 nm thick and cannot be distinguished from the underlying hyaloplasm by standard light microscopy), its presence was inferred from the attributes of the cell. Since a cell can regulate its composition and maintain its orderliness in a disordered environment it must have a limiting layer at which regulation occurs. The restriction of protoplasmic flow to the confines of the cell and the release of protoplasm when the surface is damaged also suggested the presence of such a layer.

Early studies on the entry of fat-soluble substances into cells led to the belief that the limiting membrane was made of lipid arranged as a bimolecular leaflet (Fig. 4.5a). It was then found that protein was associated with the lipid and a new model was proposed for the structure of the plasma membrane, as the limiting layer was now called; Danielli and Davson (1935) suggested that there is a layer of protein on either side of the lipid leaflet (Fig. 4.5b). With the advent of electron microscopy it was revealed that all plasma membranes look very much alike, and so a basic 'unit membrane' structure was proposed (Fig. 4.5c).

Further progress in electron microscopy has shown that all cell membranes are not alike. Surface views of membranes have shown that they have a patchy, mosaic-like appearance. The patches may represent surface proteins, many of which are enzymatic, while the regions between the patches are thought to be exposed lipid molecules. In cells like the hepatocytes, some regions specialize in secretion and others in absorption. The different regions have different enzymes associated with them, and this affects their appearance as well as their action. Changes in the conformation of the proteins can change the permeability of the membranes, opening or closing 'gates' through which metabolites may pass. The plasma membrane is a mosaic—a dynamic mosaic. If the cell is to regulate its internal composition in response to a changing external environment, then it must be able to modify its membrane structure and permeability as the occasion demands.

GLYCOCALYX

This is a layer of glycoprotein found on the outer surface of the plasma membrane of all cells. It is manufactured by the cell. Little is known yet about its functions, but it is thought to be important in giving the cell an electrostatic charge which affects its ability to make contact with other cells. When neoplastic transformations occur, the composition of the glycocalyx and the surface charge of the cells both alter; this may reduce cell adhesion and be a factor which allows some malignant cells to break away from a primary tumour and establish secondary tumours at new sites. The glycocalyx or cell coat is also thought to be the structure which enables a cell to recognize another of the same organism.

Nuclear compartment

This is the part of the cell enclosed within the nuclear envelope. It includes most of the DNA

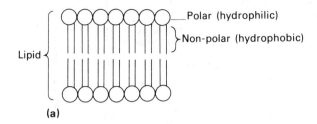

(a)

Polar (hydrophilic)

Non-polar (hydrophobic)

Lipid

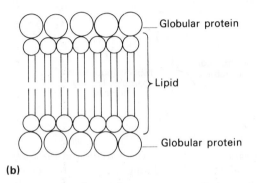

Globular protein

Lipid

Globular protein

(b)

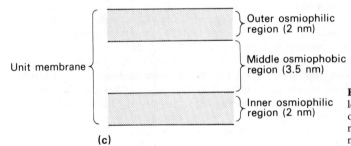

Unit membrane

Outer osmiophilic region (2 nm)

Middle osmiophobic region (3.5 nm)

Inner osmiophilic region (2 nm)

(c)

Fig. 4.5. (a) A lipid bimolecular leaflet. (b) Danielli and Davson model of membrane structure. (c) The 'unit membrane' as revealed by electron microscopy.

of the cell, together with enzymes, metabolites, DNA-associated proteins, and nuclear RNA, all of which are suspended in a colloidal proteinaceous fluid, the nuclear sap. As the DNA contains the information needed for protein manufacture, and because all enzymes are proteins, the metabolism of the cell is ultimately under nuclear control. Most human cells contain a single nucleus, but some of the larger ones, such as osteoclasts (p. 367) and skeletal muscle fibres (p. 325) are multinucleate. Mature circulating erythrocytes are anucleate. Before they are released into the blood stream they have a

nucleus and it is at that stage that the information they require for protein sythesis is transcribed into messenger RNA.

NUCLEAR ENVELOPE

This is a flattened, roughly spherical sac which separates the nuclear and cytoplasmic compartments of the cell. It retains the genetic material within the nuclear compartment while permitting the passage of metabolites. It is probably derived from the endoplasmic reticulum (p. 169) and is continuous with it at many places. One of

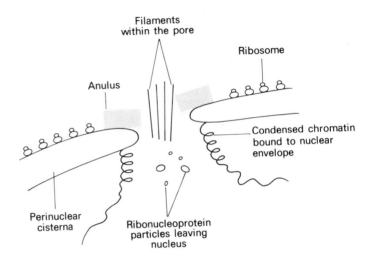

Fig. 4.6. Diagrammatic section of nuclear envelope passing through a nuclear pore.

the clearest indications of this derivation is seen during mitosis: at telophase, cisternae of endoplasmic reticulum collect around the two separate groups of chromosomes and transform into nuclear envelopes. It is interesting that most bacteria do not have an endoplasmic reticulum and also lack a nuclear envelope.

It has been shown by electron microscopy that the nuclear envelope consists of two concentric membranes, separated by a space of 10–15 nm. The outer membrane is studded with ribosomes. Small, circular, nuclear pores, about 60 nm in diameter and separated from each other by about 150 nm, are distributed regularly over the envelope, the inner and outer membranes of which fuse at the edge of each pore (Fig. 4.6). The inner wall of the envelope has nuclear chromatin tightly bound to it so that the material carrying the genetic code is effectively anchored within the confines of the porous nuclear envelope.

CHROMATIN

This is a thread-like association of DNA, protein, RNA and possibly some lipid. It is called 'chromatin' because of its strong staining properties (its acidic components cause it to react with basic stains such as haematoxylin). During nuclear division, the threads of chromatin coil up to form rod-like structures called chromosomes. Between nuclear divisions (interphase) the chromatin takes on a different form, appearing as flakes and filaments suspended in nuclear sap.

This variation in the form of the chromatin during the life of the cell is a reflection of the variation in its activity. The units of DNA (genes) which dictate the structure of the proteins that a cell manufactures are arranged in a line along the chromatin threads. During nuclear division, virtually all the genes are inactive, in the sense that they are not being transcribed into messenger RNA (p. 245), an essential preliminary to the manufacture of specific proteins by the cell. When genes are inactive, their DNA is masked by histones and the chromatin containing them is tightly coiled. During interphase the DNA of specific genes is transcribed, and in these regions the chromatin uncoils and the masking histones are removed. When this occurs the chromatin loses its affinity for basic stains and heavy metals and thus becomes difficult to detect by either light or electron microscopy.

The uncoiled, active sections of the chromatin and the tightly coiled regions comprise the 'extended' and 'condensed' chromatin respectively. At interphase the chromosomes do not fragment, as their microscopical appearance might suggest, but when various genes are activated and become transcribed the sections of the chromosome carrying these genes uncoil and lose their affinity for stains; the intervening regions of each chromosome remain inactive, coiled and stainable, and thus appear to be discontinuous although in reality they are connected by extended chromatin.

In a hepatocyte at interphase the condensed, inactive chromatin is found at three sites:

attached to the inner aspect of the nuclear envelope, scattered in the nuclear sap between the envelope and the nucleolus, and surrounding the nucleolus (Fig. 4.4).

The nuclei of the cells of females also contain a distinctive type of chromatin called sex chromatin. This is a dense mass of basophilic material which usually lies close to the nuclear envelope and which is known as a Barr body since it was first described by Barr and Bertram in 1949. A Barr body is an X-chromosome (p. 000) which remains tightly coiled throughout interphase. In addition to the usual complement of 44 autosomes common to the somatic cells of both sexes, normal females have two X-chromosomes while normal males have one X and one Y chromosome. Although the X and Y chromosomes are generally called sex chromosomes, the X chromosome carries over 50 genes unconnected with sex and in both males and females some of the genes of one X-chromosome are active and therefore uncoiled and extended. Sex chromatin can be seen readily in leucocytes and in smears obtained from the oral mucosa.

NUCLEOLUS

This is a basophilic, roughly spherical structure found within the nucleus. Several nucleoli may be present in each nucleus and each is associated with part of a chromosome called a nucleolar organizer. A loop of DNA which extends from the organizer into the nucleolus is thought to contain the genetic information needed for the synthesis of the remainder of the nucleolus. Surrounding the DNA loop are fibrils and granules of ribonucleoprotein. The fibrils are precursors of the granules, and both are precursors of the cytoplasmic ribosomes (p. 169). Ribosomes play an essential role in protein sythesis and it is interesting to note that cells which are active in protein synthesis have more nucleolar material than those that are not. Particles of ribonucleoprotein which have been fixed in the act of passing through pores in the nuclear envelope are assumed to have been produced in the nucleolus.

Nucleoli disappear at the beginning of mitosis (prophase). The loop of DNA is retracted and coils up within the rest of the chromosome, and the fibrils and granules of ribonucleoprotein disperse into the nuclear sap. When gene activation begins again at the end of mitosis (telophase) a loop of DNA extends from the nucleolar organizer and shortly afterwards the rest of the nucleolus appears, having presumably been manufactured with the aid of the instructions coded in the loop of DNA.

Cytoplasmic compartment

RIBOSOMES

From a functional point of view, these are the 'engines' used by the cell for assembling amino acids in a definite predetermined sequence to produce polypeptide chains (p 243). Ribosomes are coiled strands of RNA with which proteins are associated. They are at present in almost all the cells of every organism, generally in large numbers; even a small bacterium may contain 10,000 ribosomes, while a hepatocyte may have several million—one millilitre of liver homogenate contains about 2×10^{13} ribosomes. If the protein being made is destined to become part of the cell, then most of the ribosomes are 'free', that is, not attached to membranes within the cell. If, however, the protein is to be secreted from the cell, then the ribosomes are generally bound to the surface of the endoplasmic reticulum, giving it a 'rough' or granular appearance (see below). Although most of the ribosomes are cytoplasmic in position, many are also present in the nucleus, especially in the nucleolus, where they are synthesized.

ENDOPLASMIC RETICULUM

This is a system of membranes which form interconnecting cisternae (flattened sacs), vesicles and tubules, the whole comprising a network or 'reticulum' extending from the nuclear envelope to the plasma membrane. The interconnections are temporary, making and breaking as the various organelles move around the cell. It is called an 'endoplasmic' reticulum because when it was first described it seemed to be most concentrated in the inner part of the cytoplasm, the so-called endoplasm. It can be subdivided into rough and smooth endoplasmic reticulum. The former is studded with ribosomes while the latter is ribosome-free. The nuclear envelope, although a derivative of the endoplasmic reticulum, is unusual in that the cisternae of which it is composed have a 'rough' cytoplasmic surface and a 'smooth' nucleoplasmic surface (p. 168).

Rough endoplasmic reticulum

This is best developed in cells which export protein. It consists of large interconnecting cisternae, often arranged so that the sacs lie parallel to each other (Fig. 4.4). The ribosomes are disposed in spiral patterns on its outer surface. The ribosomes are attached to the membranes by their larger subunits (Fig. 4.6). As the polypeptide chains are synthesized, they emerge through the central hole in the large subunit of the ribosome, and pass immediately through the supporting membrane into the cavity of the cisterna.

The rough endoplasmic reticulum can give rise to smooth endoplasmic reticulum and can also transform into nuclear envelope material during telophase (p. 260).

Smooth endoplasmic reticulum
This generally takes the form of a series of tubules and vesicles. Unlike the rough endoplasmic reticulum, it rarely forms parallel cisternae and, by definition, never has attached ribosomes; it is therefore not involved in protein synthesis. The enzymes incorporated into its membranes enable it to synthesize other substances, the nature of which depends on the type of cell.

GOLGI APPARATUS

Electron microscopy has established that the Golgi apparatus is an organelle and has shown it to consist of a stack of 3–12 disc-shaped, concavo-convex saccules, collectively forming a structure rather like a pile of saucers (Fig. 4.7). The position of the Golgi apparatus varies according to the type of cell; in epithelial cells it usually lies at the end furthest from the basement membrane, while in neurons and plasma cells it lies close to the nucleus. It is particularly well developed in phagocytic and secretory cells.

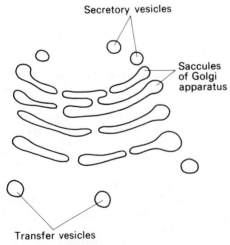

Secretory vesicles

Saccules of Golgi apparatus

Transfer vesicles

Fig. 4.7. Golgi apparatus.

The origin of the Golgi apparatus is somewhat uncertain, but it is probably formed from transfer vesicles which bud from the endoplasmic reticulum and fuse together to form new saccules at the bottom of the pile. Materials present within the endoplasmic reticulum, proteins for example, are transported to the Golgi apparatus in such vesicles, and may be modified chemically within it. Certainly, carbohydrates are added to proteins within the Golgi apparatus and there is also evidence that lipids may be incorporated there. The enzymes needed for these processes are bound to the membranes of the saccules.

LYSOSOMES

The term 'lysosome' was introduced in 1955 to describe what was then a hypothetical organelle which had been detected biochemically in liver homogenates and was considered to be a collection of hydrolytic enzymes surrounded by a membrane. A combination of electron microscopy and enzyme histochemistry showed lysosomes to be particles of 0.2–0.8 μm. In hepatocytes they are situated near the plasma membranes and contain hydrolytic enzymes.

So far more than a dozen hydrolytic enzymes have been identified in lysosomes of different types. Between them, they are capable of digesting virtually all the macromolecular components of the cell. Normally their segregation within the lysosomal membrane is sufficient to protect the rest of the cell from their action, but anything that destabilizes the lysosomal membranes can cause autolysis; cells die, tissues and organs are injured, and the body responds by producing scar tissue.

One of the lysosomal enzymes, acid phosphatase, can be readily identified in suitably prepared sections at the electron microscope level of magnification, and any membrane-bound structure in which this enzyme is detected is defined as a lysosome. Applying this definition, lysosomes show considerable polymorphism.

Some years ago a new role was proposed for lysosomes in the normal acitivity of the cell, that of triggering transcription in the nucleus in response to changes at the plasma membrane. This possible function was proposed by Clara Szego in 1974 and is based on evidence which includes changes observed in the lysosomal distribution in cells which secrete specific proteins when exposed to certain hormones. Lysosomes were 'labelled' with fluorescent dyes so that their movement around the cell could be followed photographically. Before exposing the cell to a stimulating concentration of hormone the lysosomes were mainly positioned near the plasma membrane, but within seconds of adding the hormone they moved towards the nucleus, and within minutes fused with it. It has been suggested that they release proteolytic hormones into the nucleus which help remove the masking proteins which inhibit transcription. Presumably, if this hypothesis is correct, mechanisms must exist for protecting the genome from hydrolysis.

PEROXISOMES OR MICROBODIES

These are membrane-bound particles rich in oxidative enzymes such as peroxidase and catalase. Their contents often appear in crystalline form in electron micrographs. They have an average diameter of about 0.6 μm and, as well as being in the same size range as lysosomes, develop in a similar manner. However, unlike lysosomes, which function by hydrolysis in intracellular digestion, peroxisomes are concerned with the oxidation of certain substances and the decomposition of the product, hydrogen peroxide, to water and oxygen. The packaging within membranes of the enzymes which generate potentially dangerous metabolites such as hydrogen peroxide protects the cell from their effects.

MITOCHONDRIA

These are the 'power-houses' of the cell, where energy-rich substances such as fats, carbohydrates and amino acids are oxidized and where the energy released is trapped as adenosine triphosphate (ATP). The enzymes required for these processes, and the cytochromes needed for electron transport, are all found within these membrane-bound organelles.

When examined by light microscopy the mitochondria resemble filaments or granules, and this is why they were given the name (mitos = thread, chondros = granule). They are difficult to distinguish in living cells unless phase contrast microscopy or vital staining are used. The vital stain generally used to reveal mitochondria is Janus green.

Most mitochondria are about 0.5 μm wide but of variable length up to a maximum of 7 μm. Their size and shape varies from cell to cell but is fairly constant in cells of the same type or with similar functions. In hepatocytes, for example, they are generally filamentous, about 0.5 μm wide and from about 3–5 μm long.

The distribution of the mitochondria seems to be related to their function as suppliers of energy in a readily available form: they tend to gather in regions of a cell which use more energy than others.

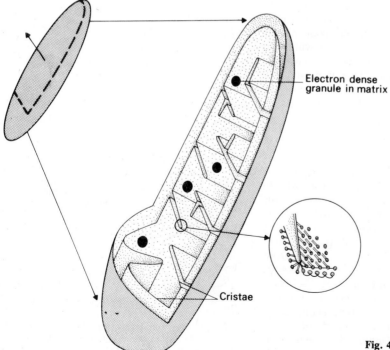

Electron dense granule in matrix

Cristae

Fig. 4.8. Basic structure of a mitochondrion.

The electron microscope shows that mitochondria are partitioned by an intricate array of membranes. The basic structure of a mitochondrion is shown diagrammatically in Fig. 4.8. Each mitochondrion consists of two membranes, the outer smooth and the inner folded. There are thus two compartments in each mitchochondrion; one lies between the outer limiting membrane and the inner membrane; the second and larger lies between the folds or cristae and contains the mitochondrial matrix. The matrix often contains electron dense granules which act as chelation (binding) sites for divalent cations such as calcium and magnesium.

Mitochondria are biochemically very complex: for them to function adequately some 70 enzymes and 14 coenzymes need to collaborate in an orderly fashion, and this orderliness is made possible by their arrangement on and in the various compartments and membranes of the mitochondria. The main function of the mitochondria is that of aerobic glycolysis, or biological oxidation. The folded inner membrane contains the enzymes necessary for the respiratory chain to function. The respiratory chain is the main energy transforming system of the mitochondrion. It is said to be coupled to phosphorylation because at three points along it the energy released is used to form ATP from ADP and phosphate.

In many ways mitochondria behave independently of the rest of the cell. They contain their own DNA and ribosomes, and can synthesize their own proteins if supplied with amino acids. Before they divide their DNA is presumably copied, providing an example of cytoplasmic (rather than nuclear) inheritance.

MICROFILAMENTS

These are thin strands of electron dense material contained in the cytoplasm of most cells. In many cells they appear to be arranged at random but in others, for example in muscle cells (p. 328) and in the microvilli which extend from the surface of some absorptive cells (p. 600), they are arranged in parallel arrays. There is a growing body of evidence to suggest that they are actomyosin-like protein complexes. For example, the metabolic inhibitor cytochalasin B is known to combine with muscle actin; it also combines with microfilaments in cells other than muscle, and in doing so inhibits phagocytosis and pinocytosis (the ingestion of solids and liquids,

respectively, at the cell surface), exocytosis (the extrusion of substances from the cell surface), cytokinesis (cell cleavage), and various other cell activities associated with or involving changes in the properties of the plasma membrane. It is therefore possible that these activities are brought about by microfilaments containing actin or some actin-like protein. Recently this hypothesis has gained support because fluorescent antibody techniques have demonstrated actin-containing complexes in a wide range of cell types. Individual microfilaments are about 8–12 nm in diameter and so can only be seen by electron microscopy.

In cells such as fibroblasts, which are capable of independent amoeboid movement, the microfilaments probably slide over each other and produce localized contractions similar to those in muscle cells (p. 329). They may also give mechanical support to cells, acting as a cytoskeleton; this is probably the role they play in epithelial cells where they are grouped together to form tonofibrils converging on the desmosomes which join such cells together (p. 174). As analytical techniques improve it will probably be found that the microfilaments are a heterogeneous population which can be subdivided into different types with different functions.

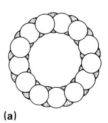

(a)

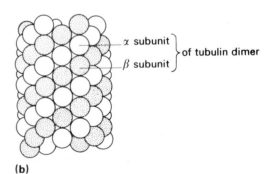

α subunit ⎱
β subunit ⎰ of tubulin dimer

(b)

Fig. 4.9. Microtubule structure. (a) Transverse section. (b) Surface view. (From Bryan J. (1974) *Federation Proceedings* **33**, 156.)

MICROTUBULES

These are hollow structures usually about 23 nm in diameter and of variable length, up to an enormous 70 μm in sperm flagella. Because of their thinness they can only be seen with the aid of the electron microscope and then only after special preparative procedures. They are formed from recurring molecules of tubulin, a globular protein consisting of two subunits, termed α and β. The tubule is built of alternating helices of the two subunits, as shown in Fig. 4.9.

Microtubules have a variety of functions: they can contract to aid cell mobility; they act as a cytoskeleton, giving support to the cell; they may also act as a 'microcirculatory system', providing pathways along which small molecules are guided. They form the mitotic spindle (p. 261), where they actively push the centrioles apart and separate the members of each chromatid pair. They are present in centrioles, basal granules, cilia and flagella (p. 173), and in the ruffled membranes of motile cells such as fibroblasts; in all these sites they are thought to cause or control movement. In the axons of neurons they are constantly being formed and broken down, and this turnover seems to be important in maintaining axonal flow.

CENTRIOLES

These are cylindrical structures about 1 μm long and 0.25 μm wide. They are generally arranged in pairs at right angles to each other in a clear area of cytoplasm termed the centrosome, which, as its name implies, ideally lies at the geometrical centre of the cell: wherever this is possible, for example in leucocytes with a horseshoe-shaped nucleus, this does, in fact, occur but generally the 'centrosome' is displaced by either the nucleus or some cytoplasmic product to an excentric position.

Centrioles are thought to regulate the organization of microtubules in the cytoplasm, and to play an important part in the formation of the spindle during cell division. It has been suggested that a cell at interphase contains two pairs of centrioles, each pair consisting of a 'parent' centriole with a 'daughter', whose formation it has induced, lying at right angles to it. During prophase the parent and daughter pairs migrate to opposite poles of the cell and induce the formation of the microtubules of the spindle between them.

Specialized structures

In the preceding section, the components of rather unspecialized cells such as hepatocytes were described. A few of the more common specialized structures found in some other cells are considered below.

CILIA, FLAGELLA AND KINETOSOMES

Cilia and flagella are motile, rod-like extensions of the surfaces of certain cells. They contain microtubules arranged in a universally similar pattern and terminate within the surface cytoplasm in structures called kinetosomes (or basal granules, basal bodies, or blepharoplasts). If the cells are free to move, then the beating of the cilia or flagella causes them to do so, but if they are linked to adjacent cells and so cannot move, then the beating causes a current in the extracellular fluid in which they are bathed and which therefore moves over them.

If a cell has many small extensions of this type, then they are by definition cilia, but if it has only a few long extensions they are termed flagella. Cilia are to be found on the free surface of the epithelium lining most of the respiratory tract, the ventricles of the brain, the central canal of the spinal cord, parts of the reproductive tract, and parts of the pleural and peritoneal cavities, while modified cilia are found on various sensory cells, for example, the photoreceptors of the retina. In man only spermatozoa are flagellated, each having a single flagellum some 70 μm in length.

The kinetosome has a structure similar to that of a single centriole (Fig. 4.10). It is about 0.5 μm long and 0.15 μm wide, and it serves to transfer ATP and possibly other materials to the shaft of the cilium or flagellum.

The movement of a cilium can be conveniently divided into a downward effective stroke and an upward recovery stroke. In the former, the

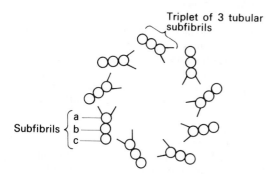

Triplet of 3 tubular subfibrils

Subfibrils { a b c

Fig. 4.10. Transverse section through a centriole.

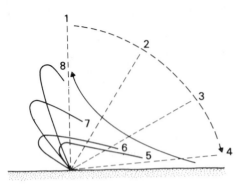

Fig. 4.11. Stages in the effective (1–4) and recovery (5–8) strokes of a beating cilium.

cilium is held stiffly and bends only at its base, while in the latter it becomes flaccid and a wave of movement passes along it from its base to its tip as it returns to the upright position (Fig. 4.11).

Microtubules do not contract, but slide over each other, in a manner reminiscent of the sliding-filament model of muscle contraction (p. 329) and, as with muscle, the energy is provided by ATP.

MICROVILLI

These are solid, finger-like extensions which massively increase the surface area of cells specialized for absorption. They are usually about 0.1 μm wide and up to 5 μm long. In some cells they are all the same length, constituting a striated border, for example in the epithelial cells covering the villi of the small intestine. In other situations they are more irregular and constitute a brush border.

Each microvillus is covered by a plasma membrane and glycocalyx and contains microfilaments embedded in a matrix of hyaloplasm. The plasma membrane covering the microvilli contains enzymes concerned with the active transport of substances into the cell.

INTERCELLULAR JUNCTIONS

There is a tendency for cells of similar type to adhere together. When, for example, liver cells and kidney cells are mixed in tissue culture, they segregate into the two tissue types. This selective adhesion is thought to be due to the antigenic properties of the glycocalyx. When the cells are

examined by electron microscopy it is found that a gap of about 20 nm generally separates the membranes of adjacent cells, although at certain points there are specialized junctions where this gap is reduced.

The specialized junctions found between cells can be subdivided into tight junctions (zonulae occludentes), gap junctions (nexuses), adhesive zones (zonulae adherentes) and desmosomes (maculae adherentes).

Tight junctions

Here the plasma membranes of adjacent cells fuse completely, eliminating the 20 nm space usually occupied by the glyocalyx. When such junctions are found between epithelial cells they extend as a band or belt around the whole periphery of the cell (Fig. 4.12). Tight junctions stop materials diffusing through the intracellular spaces, which are effectively sealed or occluded, and help to link the cells together firmly. They also have the important function of allowing ionic continuity between the cells they link, so that it is possible for electrotonic currents to pass unimpeded from cell to cell. Small molecules may also be able to pass across the tight junctions thereby allowing intercellular communication.

Gap junctions

Here there is a gap of about 3 nm between the adjacent membranes which is sufficient to allow colloids to pass between the cells. Gap junctions are spots, rather than continuous bands, on the surface of the cell. This arrangement allows materials to pass through the intercellular spaces. They are found between hepatocytes, smooth muscle cells and cardiac muscle cells and in the central nervous system. As with tight junctions, they probably allow ionic and molecular movement between the cells they link.

Adhesive zones

These are continuous bands which circle some cells (epithelia, for example): the cytoplasm just below the adjacent plasma membranes contains an electron-dense material by which the adhesive zone is recognized. The usual 20 nm space separates the adjacent plasma membranes and presumably contains cell coat material (Fig. 4.12).

Desmosomes

These junctions appear to be the most complex. Each is a discontinuous patch on the adjacent surfaces of two cells which serves to link them

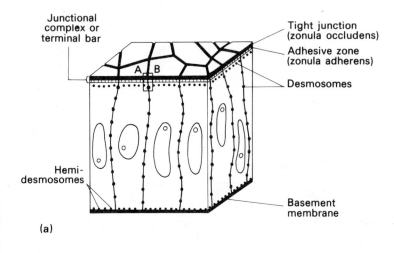

(a)

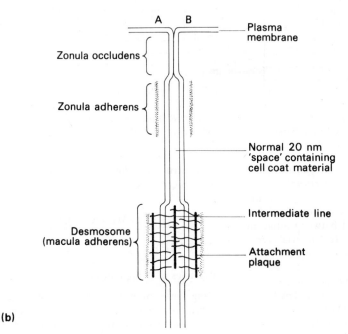

(b)

Fig. 4.12. Intracellular junctions. (a) A portion of columnar epithelium showing their positions. (b) Ultra-structure of a junctional complex.

together mechanically, rather in the way in which a press-stud links together two pieces of cloth. The linkages are very strong and when fixation causes cells to contract, desmosomes often hold while other junctions rupture. For this very reason the so-called 'prickle cells' of the epidermis (p. 407) take on their spiky shape in skin fixed for histological examination.

At desmosomes the intercellular gap between adjacent cell membranes is about 25 nm, but it is bridged by filaments of fibrillar proteins each about 5 nm wide. Each filament seems to pene-

trate the membrane of one or other of the cells involved and to overlap filaments from the other cell in the middle of the intercellular space (Fig. 4.12).

Where an epithelial cell rests on a basement membrane it is common to find hemi-demosomes, that is, half-demosomes. These consist of a disc of modified plasma membrane pierced by proteinaceous fibrils, and the adjacent glycocalyx, the latter making contact with the basement membrane and presumably attaching the cell firmly to it.

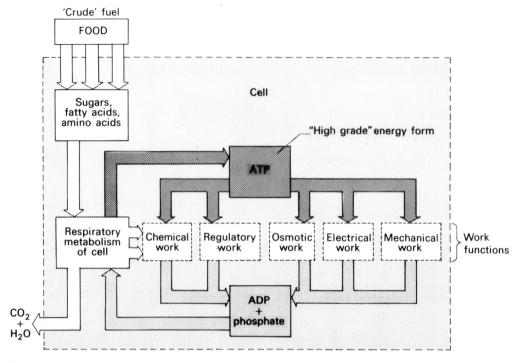

Fig. 4.13. Energy sources, its release and the work functions in the cell. (After Loewy A.G. & Siekevitz P. (1976) *Cell Structure and Function*, 2nd edn. Eastbourne, Holt, Rinehart & Winston.)

Often the various intercelluar junctions are combined to form a *junctional complex* (Fig. 4.12a). In some situations, for example, in the epithelium lining the intestine, it is essential that there should be a tight seal between adjacent cells to stop potentially harmful materials crossing the epithelial barrier and entering the body. Electron microscopy has shown that this seal is a junctional complex consisting of (a) a tight junction just below the microvilli, followed by (b) an adhesive zone, followed by (c) a series of desmosomes (Fig. 4.12b). The tight junction and adhesive zone are both zonulae, that is, belts or bands which completely encircle each cell, sealing it to its neighbour. Material can only enter the body by passing through the selectively permeable plasma membranes of the epithelial cells rather than by infiltrating between the cells. At the place where the greatest strength and the tightest seal is required, the free borders of the cells, the plasma membranes are fused.

Virtually all that is known of the connections between cells has been gained from their examination after fixation and processing for electron microscopy. The continuous movement of cells grown in tissue culture suggests that connections between individual cells must generally be temporary structures, forming and breaking as and where required.

CELL METABOLISM

OVERVIEW

Properties of living matter

Living matter or protoplasm is difficult to define in absolute terms. Nevertheless living organisms are characterized by the possession of the distinctive properties of growth, locomotion, sensitivity, reproduction and selfmaintenance and repair processes. The essential 'spark' that distinguishes living from inanimate matter is still only dimly understood, but the fabric structures of organisms, and the mechanisms whereby the essential qualities of life are operated and maintained are increasingly becoming comprehended at the molecular level. Most of the life's underlying metabolic reactions proceed at greater speeds and at lower temperatures than comparable laboratory reactions, because of the numerous enzyme-catalysed steps involved. Intricate networks of multi-enzyme metabolic pathways and cycles govern the processes of living matter.

The cell as the unit of life

The cell may be regarded as the module of life, a fundamental unit of biological activity possessing the characteristic properties of life. Much knowledge of the chemistry of living matter has come from studies on individual cells—both the prokaryote (bacterial) cells and the eukaryote (plants and animal) cells.

A cell, a tissue, or as complex an organism as man—each is essentially a machine doing work (Fig. 4.13) in various forms such as:

1 *Mechanical work*: movement as involved with muscles in walking and lifting.

2 *Electrical work*: as involved with the transmission of signals in the nervous system.

3 *Osmotic work*: as with the transport of ions or molecules against an osmotic gradient across cell and cell organelle membranes.

4 *Chemical work*: as in the various steps in the synthesis and disposal of biomolecules which involve energy-requiring steps.

5 *Regulatory work*: the mechanisms whereby the total complex of reactions and products is regulated overall, and held in a self-contained and balanced harmony—indeed another attribute of living matter only now beginning to be understood is its ability to organize and control the orderliness of its chemical reactions.

Metabolism

Each form of living matter as a machine doing work requires both energy sources to drive its various work functions and the raw materials from which to build its required materials.

Metabolism is the subject area of the chemical changes whereby the raw materials from the environment are utilized for these requirements of tapping chemical energy and the biosynthesis of the organisms' own individual biomolecules and structural macromolecules.

Metabolism is divided into two main categories—*catabolism* and *anabolism*. Catabolism is the degradative chemical changes within the cell or tissue, concerned with breaking down the more complex molecular structures of carbon to simpler forms, ultimately to CO_2 in the presence of O_2, and the associated stepwise release and capture of their locked-up chemical energy. Conversely anabolism is the area of metabolism involved with the biosynthetic mechanisms whereby complex structures are built up.

Energy and metabolism (Fig. 4.13)

Thus metabolism is closely linked to energy in all aspects of its release, capture, storage and utilization. Whether the chemical energy available is in an organism's food supply, or in its own stores (mainly as lipids and carbohydrates) it is released through the cellular processes of respiratory metabolism. By means of a series of regulated steps the 'crude fuel' stores of the lipids and carbohydrates are converted to a 'high grade fuel', predominantly ATP (adenosine triphosphate) and similar 'high-energy phosphate compounds'. A rough analogy is the utilization of the crude chemical energy of oil, converting it to the high grade energy form of electricity which is able to operate a wide range of energy-requiring processes. 'High energy' molecules like ATP are the more freely utilizable and convertible forms of energy currency in the cell, used to 'drive' not only numerous energy-requiring metabolic steps but also, directly and indirectly, all the work functions of the cells' activities.

Details of the controlled steps whereby respiratory metabolism releases chemical energy and converts it to the high grade ATP currency are described later in this chapter. The crude energy fuel—the lipids and carbohydrates, and to a lesser extent the proteins, are broken down, stepwise, to 2-carbon molecule fragments, namely the acetyl group. This forms an acetyl-S-coenzyme A complex (acetyl-S-CoA). Formation of acetyl-S-CoA from carbohydrates is via the *glycolysis* sequence of metabolic steps (p. 180) which, en route to acetyl-S-CoA releases and captures some energy as ATP. Since glycolysis also uses up some ATP in the process there is a net gain of only 2 ATP molecules per glucose molecule oxidized to pyruvate. Lipids are catabolized to the 2C acetyl fragments by the stepwise process of β-oxidation of fatty acids (p. 205).

The tricarboxylic acid (TCA) cycle

The major source of the cells' energy supply, in terms of ATP production, is via an oxidative metabolic wheel (also referred to as a 'metabolic dynamo'), usually known as the TCA cycle (tricarboxylic acid), but also sometimes referred to as the Krebs or the citric acid cycle. In essence a 2C (acetyl) fragment combines with a 4C intermediate (oxaloacetic acid) to form the 6C compound, citric acid (Fig. 4.14). One turn round the TCA metabolic wheel to bring it back to the 4C oxaloacetate intermediate involves several

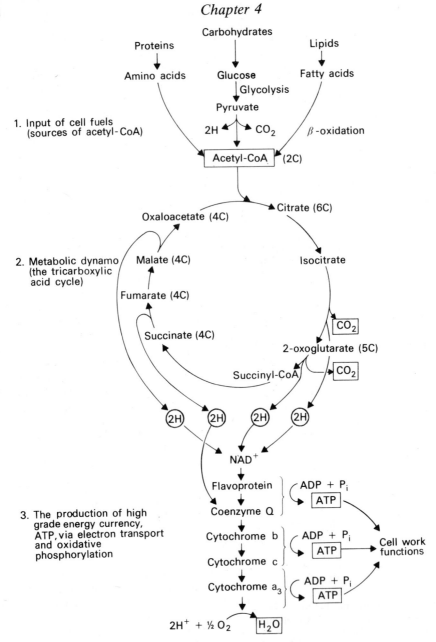

1. Input of cell fuels (sources of acetyl-CoA)

2. Metabolic dynamo (the tricarboxylic acid cycle)

3. The production of high grade energy currency, ATP, via electron transport and oxidative phosphorylation

Fig. 4.14. Flow sheet of the metabolic release of energy via the TCA cycle and the respiratory chain.

(After Lehninger A.L. (1976) *Biochemistry*, 2nd edn. New York, Worth.)

metabolic steps, which include 2 decarboxylation and 4 oxidation stages, the latter via the H carrier coenzymes NAD^+ and FAD. Chemically, the net effect is the conversion of each acetyl group 'injected' into the TCA cycle to 2 molecules of CO_2 and H_2O. From the more important energy point of view, however, each

oxidation stage in the TCA cycle is linked to molecular oxygen via a chain of respiratory pigments (flavoproteins and the cytochromes), this oxidation sequence being termed the electron transport carrier mechanism. It is this latter chain of events which is associated with ATP production, the overall process, therefore, being referred to as *oxidative phosphorylation*. The net effect of 1 turn of the TCA wheel in oxidizing 1 acetyl group is to produce 12 ATP molecules by the oxidative phosphorylation mechanism. The TCA cycle is the major source of cell CO_2 production and also the reduced coenzymes (NADH) which drives the ATP production mechanisms via the cytochrome electron transport system.

The utilization of cell energy

As stated the major purpose of tapping chemical energy stores and converting them to ATP is to use the latter to drive various energy-requiring processes involved in the cells' total activities. Throughout the text various examples of this are discussed in different contexts. In the 'Energy requiring processes' section (p. 228) details of some of the major biosynthetic mechanisms of the cell are examined. These include that most important area of the cell's synthetic activities, protein synthesis. It is here that the nub of cell life resides; in the production of the enzymes, the structural, transport and contractile proteins, the defence and hormonal proteins, the membrane proteins, and many others. Also described is the synthesis of small molecules such as the nucleosides and nucleotides and the fatty acids.

Sites of metabolic activity in the cell

Thirty to forty years ago, the cell, from a metabolic point of view, was more or less regarded as 'a bag of enzymes in solution'. Today the combination of electron microscope, centrifugation, histochemical and biochemical techniques has established that the various metabolic functions are housed or located at specific organelle sites within the cell (Fig. 3.2). The cytoplasm contains the multienzyme system of the glycolysis pathway of carbohydrate oxidation and is also involved with fatty acid activation before their stepwise β-oxidation degradation inside mitochondria. Some of the small microbodies suspended in the cytoplasm probably consist of complete multi-enzyme complexes, such as that involved in the *pyruvate oxidase* system. The mitochondria have been rightly termed the 'power houses' of the cell, because the whole of the TCA cycle and the electron transport chain is housed within them, situated on the cristae shelves of the inner-membrane (Fig. 4.8). It is here that the 'metabolic dynamo' system for ATP production

sits, and there is even evidence that the enzymes involved may be physically lined up on the cristae in the precise order of the reactions that have been elucidated from *in vitro* studies.

The rough endoplasmic reticulum is lined with the small cottage-loaf shaped ribosomes upon which the cells' protein synthetic mechanisms occur (p. 243). Thus the ribosomes are major production line or 'work bench' sites within the cell. They are approximately half RNA and half protein.

The nucleus contains the hereditary information in chemical code form (the genetic code), in the sequence of bases which constitute the DNA molecules (p. 104). At these DNA sites the messenger RNA molecules (p. 240) are made, which then travel out from the nucleus and across the cytoplasm, carrying their information to the ribosomes.

The cytoplasm also contains the transfer RNA molecules involved with the activation and transport of amino acids in the cytoplasm to the ribosome 'work benches' for assembly into protein molecules. The lysosome bodies suspended in the cell cytoplasm, house packages of hydrolytic and degradative enzymes which only appear to be released upon the death of the cell. They are involved in the post-mortem autolysis mechanisms.

Also suspended in the cytoplasm are microbodies known as the peroxisomes which are rich in *catalase* and so associated with the degradation of H_2O_2 to O_2 and H_2O. The cytoplasm also contains the enzymic mechanisms involved with the disposal of certain other waste products.

METABOLISM AND ENERGY PRODUCTION

Anaerobic carbohydrate oxidation: the breakdown of glucose: glycolysis

Glucose is a sugar converted by living organisms to a wide range of compounds and is one of the most important fuels from which tissue cells can derive energy. Use of ^{14}C-labelled glucose (a radioactive isotope of carbon) has shown that it is metabolized very rapidly, most of the label being found in expired CO_2. Smaller amounts of ^{14}C labelling are found in numerous other compounds including amino acids, sugar phosphates, fat and TCA (Krebs) cycle intermediates. Such a diversity of products formed from the breakdown of a single compound implies the existence of numerous metabolic pathways.

The glucose present in the blood of human beings is distributed almost equally between red cells and plasma. In an overnight-fasted subject, the blood glucose is normally in the range 60–90 mg/100ml of blood (3.3–5.0 mmol/dm³) measured by the glucose oxidase method. Variations occur in these reported values for normal individuals. The older analytical methods such as Benedict's reagent give higher 'glucose' values due to their measurement of other reducing substances present in blood. After a meal containing carbohydrate, or after a measured amount of glucose has been ingested (the 'glucose tolerance' test), blood glucose levels begin to rise within a few minutes and, by 30 minutes, reach 130–150 mg/100ml (7.2–8.3 mmol/dm³), although the actual level attained depends on the individual concerned. Such factors as rate of absorption and rate of metabolism cause considerable variations. However, within two hours of the carbohydrate load, the blood glucose normally returns to fasting levels. This rapid return to normal levels is due to both prompt metabolism of the ingested glucose and control mechanisms rapidly called into play in response to the elevated blood glucose level. These hormonal mechanisms are discussed elsewhere (see p. 794).

Some of the ingested glucose (or glucose derived from digestion of dietary carbohydrate) is converted rapidly in the liver to the polysaccharide glycogen, where it acts as a carbohydrate store that can be called upon at short notice should the blood glucose level become lowered as in starvation. Normally, animal liver contains 6–8% of its weight as glycogen but this is almost completely depleted after as little as 24 hours' starvation. In a normal well-fed animal, glycogen is being synthesized or catabolized continually and is said to be in a 'dynamic steady state'.

GLYCOLYSIS STAGES

As indicated, most ingested glucose is converted to carbon dioxide and water, the complete oxidation represented by the equation:

$$C_6H_{12}O_6 + 6\ O_2 = 6\ CO_2 + 6\ H_2O$$

The respiratory quotient, RQ, defined as the number of moles CO_2 produced divided by the number of moles O_2 utilized (p. 804), for glucose, therefore, equals unity. When such an oxidation is performed chemically in a bomb calorimeter, a considerable amount of energy is obtained —approximately 3010 kJ/g mol (180 g) of glucose used, but as will be seen later, it is not possible to achieve this yield of energy in living tissues. The complete catabolism of glucose to CO_2, H_2O and energy by the body tissues occurs in a series of graded stages. The first stage, in which glucose is converted to pyruvate by a number of enzymically-controlled reactions, is called *glycolysis* and this can occur anaerobically or aerobically. Under aerobic conditions pyruvate eventually forms the end products, carbon dioxide and water via the oxidative reactions of the Krebs TCA cycle and cytochrome chain (see below). Conversely, under anaerobic conditions, pyruvate is converted to lactate (Fig. 4.15).

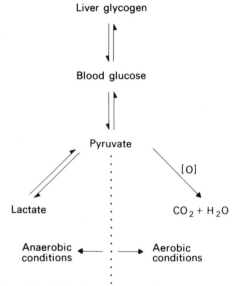

Fig. 4.15. The end products of glycolysis under aerobic and anaerobic conditions.

This difference in the final products of glycolysis, depending on whether or not oxygen is present, was discovered in the early years of the present century, when it was shown that less lactic acid is produced in a muscle preparation contracting under aerobic conditions than anaerobic. In the absence of oxygen, lactic acid production increases markedly until the muscle becomes fatigued and the contractions cease. When placed in an atmosphere of oxygen, the amounts of lactic and pyruvic acids formed decrease and contractions recommence. Muscle glycogen is converted to lactic acid but, unlike the glycogen of liver, this remains relatively con-

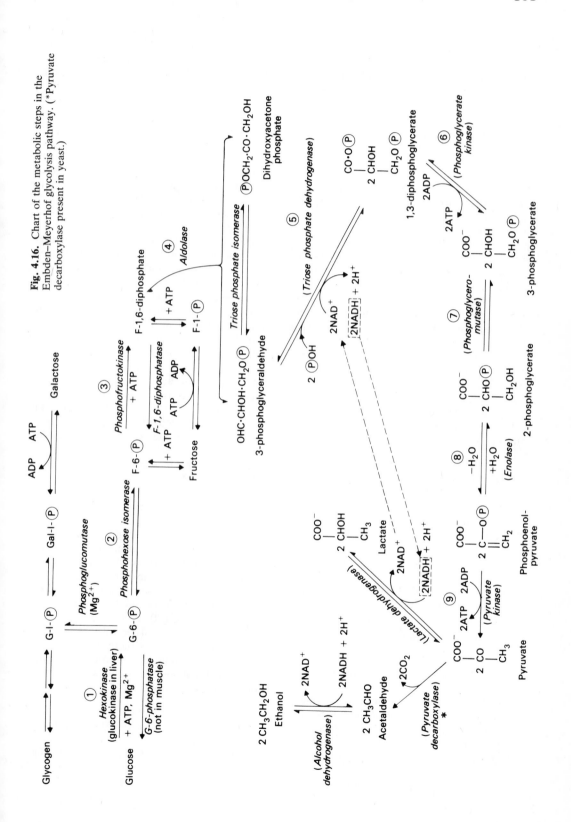

Fig. 4.16. Chart of the metabolic steps in the Embden-Meyerhof glycolysis pathway. (*Pyruvate decarboxylase present in yeast.)

stant in amount except during severe muscular exercise.

Further details of glycolysis remained obscure until the phosphate esters (p. 130) of glucose and other sugars were discovered in animal liver and muscle and in yeast. As early as 1905 it was known that the fermentation of sugar by yeast is activated by the addition of inorganic phosphate and that this is gradually converted to organic phosphates as the fermentation proceeds, eventually to ethanol. With the discovery of the enzymes it subsequently became clear that glycolysis consists of a complex series of enzymically-controlled reactions whereby glucose is converted to pyruvic and lactic acids (or more correctly pyruvate and lactate at physiological pH). This is known as the *Embden-Meyerhof* pathway and is summarized in Fig. 4.16. The steps involved are essentially similar in yeast and animal cells.

With animals, however, glucose from the blood must first enter the cells, where the cytoplasm contains the glycolytic enzymes. The membranes of liver cells are known to be permeable to glucose but this is not so for cells of other tissues, such as muscle. One important effect of insulin in controlling the rate of glucose catabolism is its ability to facilitate the transport of glucose into such cells. Once in contact with the cytoplasmic enzymes, the process of glycolysis can proceed.

1 The conversion of glucose to glucose-6-phosphate

Glucose and phosphate at physiological pH do not normally react together to any extent, because the equilibrium constant for the reaction:

$$\text{glucose} + \text{HPO}_4^{2-} \rightleftharpoons \text{glucose-6-phosphate} + \text{H}_2\text{O}$$

is exceedingly small. The reaction therefore lies far to the left-hand side. However, the equilibrium constant for the reaction:

$$\text{glucose} + \text{ATP} \xrightarrow{\text{kinase}} \text{glucose-6-phosphate} + \text{ADP}$$

is very large, so that the forward reaction is favoured in the presence of ATP and enzyme. There are two types of kinases that catalyse the reaction. One of these, *hexokinase*, is found in numerous tissues and, as its name implies, can catalyse the phosphorylation of various hexose substrates including glucose, fructose, mannose and even 2-deoxyglucose and glucosamine.

Like many of the glycolytic enzymes, hexokinase occurs in the form of isoenzymes. Three hexokinase isoenzymes occur in most tissues including erythrocytes, brain, skeletal muscle, adipose tissue, liver and heart; designated types I, II and III, they have relatively low K_m values with respect to glucose ($5 \times 10^{-6} - 2 \times 10^{-4}$M). Liver and kidney contain, in addition, a type IV hexokinase which has a much higher K_m for glucose (1.6×10^{-2} M).

Tissues which are insulin-sensitive (skeletal muscle, heart and diaphragm) contain large amounts of the type II isoenzyme. In contrast, in tissues such as brain and liver, the type I isoenzyme predominates. The cells of these tissues are freely permeable to glucose and are independent of insulin.

Hexokinase has low K_m values for both glucose and ATP and the reaction in liver is zero-order with respect to glucose. This could mean that the metabolism of glucose in liver would be independent of blood glucose level (normally approx. 5 mmols/dm³) because the concentration of glucose in liver is very similar to that in blood. However, another enzyme, *glucokinase*, which is specific for glucose occurs in liver. This is an inducible kinase which has a K_m of 10 mM, and increases in activity after a carbohydrate meal, with the activity decreasing subsequently as the blood glucose levels decrease. During fasting, glucokinase activity diminishes to zero, in-keeping with the body cells maintaining blood glucose at a relatively constant level.

For both hexokinase and glucokinase activity, Mg^{2+}ions (or Mn^{2+}) are necessary as most ATP in cells occurs as active Mg^{2+} or Mn^{2+} complexes, the form in which the ATP binds to the kinases.

Although the glucose to glucose-6-phosphate hexokinase-catalysed conversion is essentially irreversible, the reverse reaction can be accomplished by means of a specific enzyme, *glucose-6-phosphatase*. This occurs in the endoplasmic reticulum of liver cells and its activation by corticotrophin (ACTH) and glucocorticoids is important in the overall control of blood glucose level (see p. 794). As there is no glucose-6-phosphatase in muscle, the products of muscle glycogen breakdown are glucose-1-phosphate and glucose-6-phosphate.

2 Conversion of glucose-6-phosphate to fructose-6-phosphate

Glucose-6-phosphate is a key metabolite of glucose because it marks a junction of metabolic pathways for that sugar, i.e.

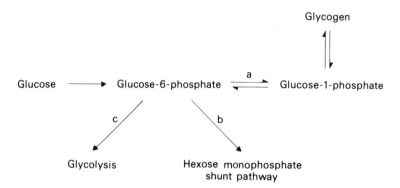

A number of possibilities exist for its further metabolism:

(a) It can be converted to glycogen via an initial isomerization to glucose-1-phosphate.

(b) It can be converted to pentose phosphates in the hexose monophosphate shunt pathway (p. 210) or

(c) It can proceed along the glycolytic pathway.

This third possibility continues by means of a reversible isomerization to fructose-6-phosphate, catalysed by *phosphohexose isomerase*.

3 Formation of fructose-1,6-diphosphate

Since fructose-6-phosphate, like glucose-6-phosphate, is a 'low-energy' phosphate compound, it does not react spontaneously with phosphate to give fructose-1,6-diphosphate. ATP is the required phosphate donor, in the presence of *phosphofructokinase* (PFK) and Mg^{2+} ions. This enzyme is present in most tissues at a lower concentration than the other enzymes of the glycolytic pathway. As it is a key enzyme, which can be controlled allosterically (p. 269), changes in its activity can, therefore, alter the whole rate of glycolysis. Increasing levels of ATP and citrate inhibit its activity while AMP, cyclic AMP, fructose-6-phosphate and (to a lesser extent) ADP activate the enzyme. Thus, in situations where ATP is being synthesized more rapidly than it is being utilized, the activity of PFK is diminished progessively and thus reduces the rate of glycolysis.

4 Cleavage of fructose-1,6-diphosphate to two fragments

Fructose-1,6-diphosphate is further metabolized by cleavage to two trioses, glyceraldehyde-3-phosphate and dihydroxyacetone phosphate. The reaction, which is reversible, is catalysed by the enzyme *aldolase*. Of the two products of the reaction, one, namely dihydroxyacetone phosphate, forms a link with glycerol metabolism because it can be reduced to glycerolphosphate by means of the activity of the NAD^+-linked *glycerol-1-phosphate dehydrogenase*. Dihydroxyacetone phosphate is not metabolized further on the glycolytic pathway but is readily converted to glyceraldehyde-3-phosphate by the action of *triose phosphate isomerase*. Dihydroxyacetone phosphate does not, therefore, accumulate in glycolysis.

5 Formation of 1,3-diphosphoglycerate

The next stage, the conversion of glyceraldehyde-3-phosphate to 1,3-diphosphoglycerate occurs in two steps involving dehydrogenation and phosphorylation. The former occurs by means of the NAD-linked *glyceraldehyde-3-phosphate dehydrogenase*, an enzyme which exists in four subunits. Sulphydryl groups are necessary in the reaction. Next phosphorylation with inorganic phosphate results in the formation of 1,3-diphosphoglycerate and regeneration of the enzyme (see overleaf).

The NADH formed in the reaction can be reoxidized in a number of ways:

1 If the oxygen supply is temporarily inadequate, pyruvate is used as substrate by the enzyme *lactate dehydrogenase*.

$$CH_3COCOO^- + NADH + H^+ \rightleftharpoons CH_3CH(OH)COO^- + NAD^+$$

Under these conditions, glycolysis is said to be anaerobic.

2 When the oxygen supply to the tissue is sufficient, as is normally so, the reduced cofactor is reoxidized through the electron-transport chain in the mitochondria.

Step 1:

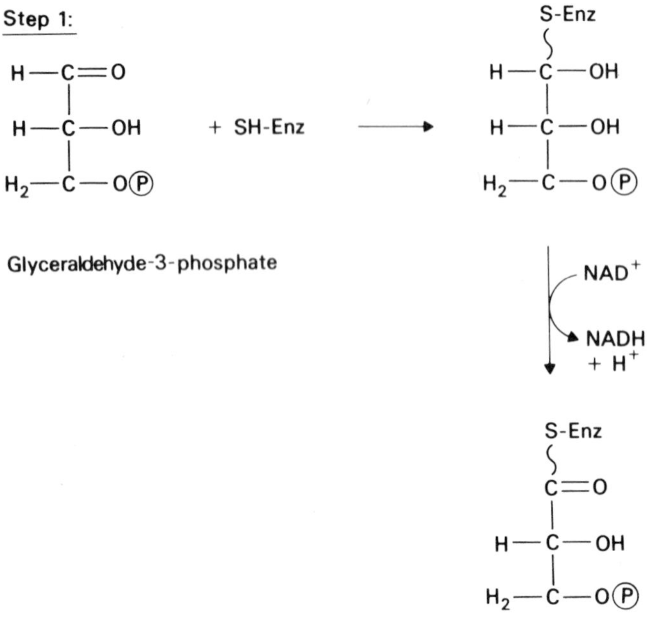

Glyceraldehyde-3-phosphate

Step 2:

1,3-diphosphoglycerate

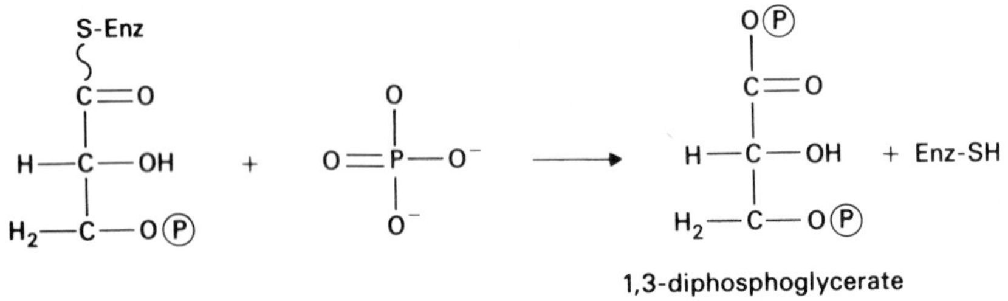

3 A third possibility links it to glycerol metabolism through the reduction of dihydroxyacetone phosphate, to glycerol-1-phosphate as described as follows:

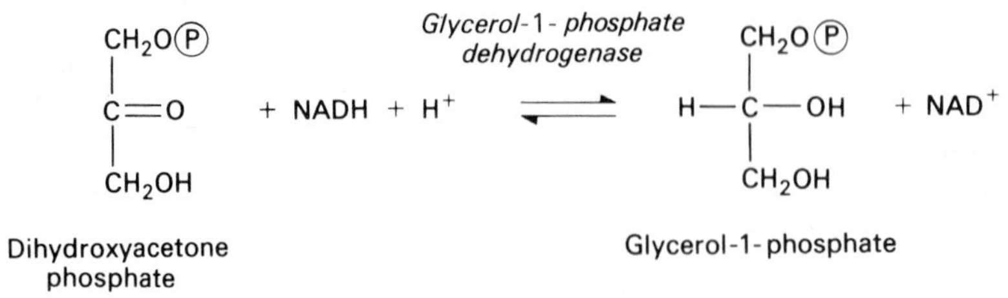

Dihydroxyacetone
phosphate

Glycerol-1-phosphate

6 Conversion of 1,3-diphosphoglycerate to 3-phosphoglycerate

Next in the glycolytic sequence is the conversion of 1,3-diphosphoglycerate to 3-phosphoglycerate

by *phosphoglycerate kinase*, in the presence of Mg^{2+} ions and ADP. *In this reaction, ATP is synthesized*—the first reaction in the glycolytic

sequence in which this occurs. The reason for this is the high negative $\Delta G_0'$ of hydrolysis of 1,3-diphosphoglycerate (49 kJ/mol), which strongly favours the forward reaction:

$$
\begin{array}{c}
O-\text{(P)} \\
| \\
C=O \\
| \\
H-C-OH \\
| \\
CH_2O\text{(P)}
\end{array}
\quad + \;\; ADP
\quad \underset{}{\overset{(\textit{Phosphoglycerate kinase})}{\rightleftharpoons}}
\quad ATP \;+\;
\begin{array}{c}
COO^- \\
| \\
H-C-OH \\
| \\
CH_2O\text{(P)}
\end{array}
$$

1,3-diphosphoglycerate   3-phosphoglycerate

The free energy (ΔG_o) concept and other thermodynamic aspects of reactions are discussed in Appendix 1 (p. 993).

Hitherto, in the glycolytic sequence ATP has been utilized in the glucose $\longrightarrow$ glucose-6-phosphate and fructose-6-phosphate $\longrightarrow$ fructose-1,6-diphosphate steps.

7 Formation of 2-phosphoglycerate

Next follows a reversible isomerization of 3-phosphoglycerate to 2-phosphoglycerate through action of the enzyme *phosphoglucomutase*.

8 Phosphoenolpyruvate (PEP) formation

The 2-phosphoglycerate formed in reaction 7 is next converted to phosphoenolpyruvate (PEP) as follows:

$$
\begin{array}{c}
COO^- \\
| \\
H-C-O\text{(P)} \\
| \\
H_2-C-OH
\end{array}
\quad \underset{\textit{Enolase}\,(Mg^{2+})}{\overset{H_2O}{\longrightarrow}}
\quad
\begin{array}{c}
COO^- \\
| \\
C-O\text{(P)} \\
|| \\
CH_2
\end{array}
$$

2-phosphoglycerate   Phosphoenolpyruvate

The enzyme involved, *enolase*, has a requirement for Mg^{2+} and is inhibited by F^- ions, due to the formation of a magnesium fluorophosphate complex.

9 Pyruvate formation

Like 1,3-diphosphoglycerate, PEP is an 'energy-rich' compound having a $\Delta G_o'$ of -53.5 kJ/mol. In the presence of *pyruvate kinase*, PEP is readily converted to enolpyruvate and this spontaneously undergoes a molecular rearrangement to form the tautomer:

This is the second important reaction in glycolysis where ATP is synthesized. The reaction is theoretically reversible, but in practice the equilibrium constant strongly favours the forward reaction. However, a by-pass is available using alternative enzymes so that the synthesis of glucose from small molecules such as pyruvate is possible (p. 188).

As indicated above, if O_2 is present pyruvate can be oxidized via the TCA cycle reactions and cytochrome chain; however if the supply of oxygen is temporarily diminished, pyruvate is then reduced to lactate by the action of *lactate dehydrogenase* (reaction 10). The properties and significance of this important enzyme are discussed below.

ENERGY YIELDS IN GLYCOLYSIS

The diagram summarizing the glycolytic sequence (Fig. 4.16) shows that for every mole of glucose metabolized, 2 moles of ATP are utilized. However, 2 moles of ATP are synthesized for every mole of glyceraldehyde-3-phosphate used in the two energy-yielding steps: 1,3-diphosphoglycerate $\longrightarrow$ 3-phosphoglycerate (6), and PEP $\longrightarrow$ enolpyruvate (9). Since two moles of glyceraldehyde-3-phosphate are formed from one mole of glucose, this means a total net yield of $(2 + 2) - 2 = 2$ ATP moles formed per mole of glucose. 1 ATP represents 29 kJ, so the net yield in glycolysis is therefore $2 \times 29 = 58$ kJ/mol glucose. Since the complete total oxidation of glucose theoretically provides 3010 kJ/mol the percentage yield through anaerobic glycolysis is extremely small, (i.e. $\dfrac{58}{3010} \times 100 = 2\%$).

$$
\begin{array}{c}
CH_2 \\
|| \\
C-O\text{(P)} \\
| \\
COO^-
\end{array}
\quad \underset{\textit{Pyruvate kinase}}{\overset{ADP\quad ATP}{\longrightarrow}}
\quad
\begin{array}{c}
CH_2 \\
|| \\
C-OH \\
| \\
COO^-
\end{array}
\quad \overset{Spontaneous}{\longrightarrow}
\quad
\begin{array}{c}
CH_3 \\
| \\
C=O \\
| \\
COO^-
\end{array}
$$

Phosphoenolpyruvate   Enolpyruvate   Pyruvate

The product of *glycogenolysis* is glucose-1-phosphate (p. 189), which is readily isomerized to glucose-6-phosphate by *phosphoglucomutase*. Hence, one less mole of ATP is used up in the conversion of glycogen to lactate, compared with the conversion directly from glucose. The total net ATP yield will therefore be $(2 \times 2) -1$ moles of ATP $= 3$ATP per mole of glycogen. This energy yield is approximately 3% of the total theoretical maximum of 3010 kJ/mol.

By far the greatest amount of cell energy is obtained through the aerobic oxidation of pyruvate to CO_2 and water via the reactions of the TCA cycle. However, in aerobic glycolysis there is the possibility of the synthesis of more ATP as a result of the re-oxidation of the NADH formed in the dehydrogenation of glyceraldehyde-3-phosphate to 1,3-diphosphoglycerate. As shown later three moles of ATP are synthesized during the oxidation of one mole of NADH in the mitochondrial electron-transport chain, and since two moles of glyceraldehyde-3-phosphate are formed from one mole of glucose the total ATP formed in this way amounts to $2 \times 3 = 6$ moles ATP/mole of glucose.

Under these circumstances, the yield is $(2 + 6) = 8$ moles ATP/mole of glucose, which equals $8 \times 29 = 232$ kJ. This represents an efficiency of

$$\frac{232}{3010} \times 100 = 8\%.$$

In the event of any temporary reduction in the energy supply, the NADH produced in the dehydrogenation of glyceraldehyde-3-phosphate is re-oxidized by the conversion of pyruvate to lactate. The theoretical energy yield from the electron-transport system will therefore be lost and the energy yield under these totally anaerobic conditions will amount to only 2 ATP per mole of glucose (or 3, in the case of glycogen as explained above).

LACTATE DEHYDROGENASE

Lactate dehydrogenase (LDH) is an enzyme of great importance from both biochemical and clinical points of view. It is a tetramer with four independent catalytic sites and can be dissociated into four inactive subunits each of molecular weight approx 34 000. There are five isoenzymes consisting of five different combinations of two different polypeptide chains which occur predominantly in skeletal muscle (M) and heart (H). These two tissues contain the pure tetramer isoenzymes, M_4 and H_4, more usually known as LD_5 and LD_1 respectively. In addition to these, three hybrid tetramer forms are found in most tissues; M_3H, M_2H_2 and MH_3, known as LD_4, LD_3 and LD_2 respectively, which exhibit properties intermediate between those of LD_1 and LD_5. All five isoenzymes catalyse the same reaction, lactate $\rightleftharpoons$ pyruvate, and each has a molecular weight of approximately 135 000 but with different net charges, due to the different relative proportions of acidic and basic amino acids present. The net negative charge decreases progres-

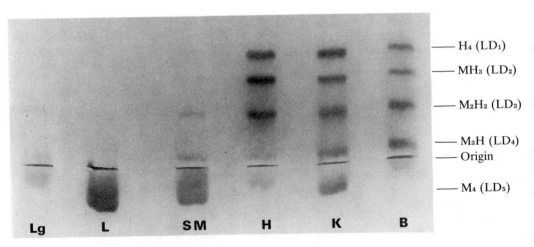

Fig. 4.17. Electrophoretic separation of LDH isoenzymes in various rat tissues. Lg = lung; L = liver; SM = skeletal muscle; H = heart; K = kidney; B = brain. (Top = +, bottom = −.)

sively from LD₁ to LD₅ and, on electrophoresis at pH 8.6, LD₁ moves fastest towards the anode, whilst LD₅ moves slightly from the origin towards the cathode.

Fig. 4.17 shows a typical separation on cellulose acetate paper of LDH isoenzymes of various rat tissues. Tissues such as heart muscle, which function under aerobic conditions, contain predominantly LD₁ and LD₂, whilst skeletal muscle contains predominantly LD₅. A suggested explanation for this difference is as follows: heart muscle requires energy continuously, and this is derived largely through the complete oxidation of pyruvate and lactate. LD₁ has a relatively low turnover with respect to pyruvate and is maximally active at only low concentrations as shown by the low K_m (0.0777mM at pH 7.4) for human LD₁. Its activity is inhibited by high pyruvate concentrations. This sensitivity of LD₁ to pyruvate ensures that this compound is not channelled to lactate formation.

In contrast, skeletal muscle requires energy intermittently, and this is derived almost entirely from glycolysis. There is therefore a high concentration of pyruvate produced, which must be reduced to lactate. The predominant isoenzyme present in muscle (LD₅) has a relatively high K_m (0.83 mM for human skeletal muscle at pH 7.4) with pyruvate as substrate, thus ensuring that this is converted efficiently to lactate. This suggestion has been questioned in the light of recent work, however, because LD₁ activity is not necessarily reduced at higher pyruvate concentrations and, in many cases, it is unlikely that sufficient pyruvate will accumulate in cardiac tissue.

The flight habits of birds are well correlated with the sensitivity of their breast muscle LDH to pyruvate. Birds such as grouse, pheasant and domestic fowl possess breast muscle LDH which is similar to that of human skeletal muscle. This is not inhibited by pyruvate so that lactate is formed readily and the muscles become easily fatigued. In contrast the storm petrel and humming bird, which can fly for long periods, have breast muscle LDH like that of human cardiac muscle. Thus, pyruvate is channelled to complete oxidation, lactate does not accumulate, and the muscles are less likely to become fatigued.

Clinical sigificance of LDH

As LDH is a cytoplasmic enzyme, it is easily lost from cells if the tissue is damaged and cell membranes are ruptured. Such a situation can occur in cardiac infarction or in infective hepatitis.

Normally, the amount of LDH in plasma is small but if damage to a particular organ ensues, the plasma LDH rises to a maximum value some 48 hours after the episode and returns to normal within about a week. It is particularly useful to subject plasma with a high LDH content to electrophoresis when the isoenzymes are separated, and it is possible to obtain an 'organ-print': A marked increase in LD₁, and to some extent LD₂, is found after myocardial infarction; in infective hepatitis, an increase in LD₅ is noticed even before jaundice is clinically apparent. The level in activities is roughly proportional to the extent of tissue damage.

PASTEUR AND CRABTREE EFFECTS

The fact that less lactate is formed from glycolysis in aerobic than in anaerobic conditions has been known for many years; glycolysis is also known to decrease when oxygen is present. The reasons for these phenomena, known as the *Pasteur effect*, are uncertain but a likely explanation is the inhibition of the activity of the *enzyme phosphofructokinase* (PFK) (p. 183). Under oxidative conditions ATP and citrate are produced as pyruvate is oxidized. Both ATP and citrate inhibit PFK allosterically, hence the rate of glycolysis will decrease and pyruvate will be oxidized completely rather than being reduced to lactate. Another possible explanation is that ADP and inorganic phosphate are utilized so extensively in oxidative phosphorylation (p. 202) that less is available for use in the ATP-producing steps of the glycolytic pathway.

The Crabtree effect describes the phenomenon of inhibition of cellular respiration by high concentrations of glucose during the incubation of certain tissues *in vitro*. The likely explanation is that metabolism of such large amounts of glucose uses up much inorganic phosphate and NADH, leading to their relative deficiency for oxidative phosphorlyation.

REVERSAL OF GLYCOLYSIS: GLUCOGENESIS AND GLUCONEOGENESIS

Although many of the reactions in the glycolytic sequence are reversible, three reactions catalysed by *hexokinase* (step 1), *phosphofructokinase* (step 3), and *pyruvate kinase* (step 9) are physiologically irreversible. These clearly impose a total blocking in three places to a synthesis of glucose and glycogen from, for example, pyruvate via a simple reversal of the Embden-Meyerhof pathway sequence. Nevertheless, the conversion of glucose-6-phosphate to glucose can be accomplished by means of *glucose-6-phosphatase* and the conversion of fructose-1,6-diphosphate to fructose-6-phosphate occurs by means of the enzyme *fructose-1,6-diphosphatase*:

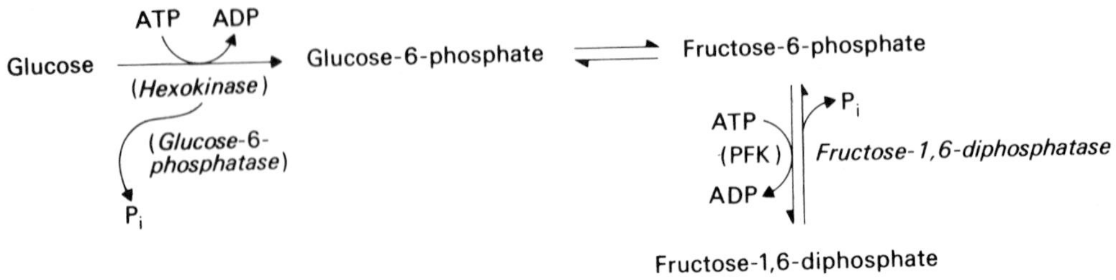

the mitochondria and there converted to oxaloacetate. Since this does not readily diffuse out of the mitochondria, it is converted to malate by means of the mitochondrial enzyme *malate dehydrogenase*, and diffuses out into the cyto-

Both phosphatases occur in liver and kidney, but glucose-6-phosphatase is absent from muscle.

The reversal of the phosphoenolpyruvate to enolpyruvate step is achieved by means of a by-pass (Fig. 4.18). The pyruvate produced from glycolysis in the cytoplasm is transported into

plasm. Here the malate is converted back to oxaloacetate through the action of the cytoplasmic *malate dehydrogenase*. The oxaloacetate so produced can then react with GTP or ITP in the presence of *phosphoenolpyruvate carboxykinase* to give phosphoenolpyruvate:

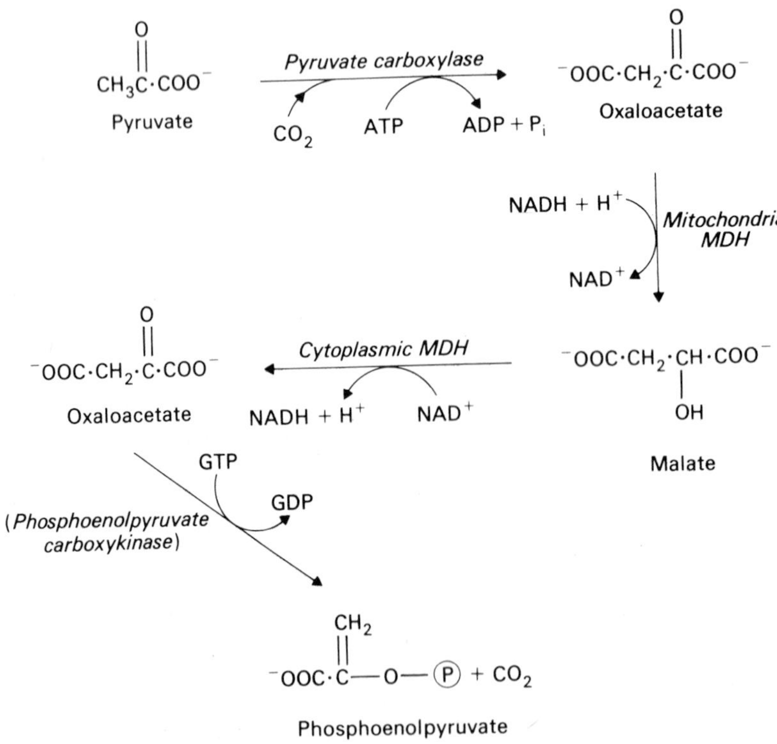

Fig. 4.18. Glucogenesis: the pyruvate → oxaloacetate → phosphenolpyruvate by-pass.

It is by means of these pathways that glucose can be formed from the products of its metabolism e.g. glycolysis intermediates, pyruvate, Krebs cycle intermediates. These overall processes leading to glucose are called *glucogenesis*. Glucose can also be formed from non-carbohydrate sources such as amino acids and glycerol, where the process is known as *gluconeogenesis*. These reactions occur particularly during starvation and, when dietary carbohydrate is in short supply, glucose can then be supplied to various tissues such as liver, brain and to the blood. The conversion of amino acids to glucose takes place by means of transamination (p. 216), with the resulting ketoacids (pyruvate, oxaloacetate or 2-oxoglutarate) are metabolized by the processes outlined above, i.e.

The breakdown and synthesis of glycogen

GLYCOGENOLYSIS

The breakdown of glycogen is called *glycogenolysis*, occurs in liver and muscle, and is a process under hormonal control (Fig. 4.19). The mechanism of its breakdown involves three enzymes:

1 *Glycogen phosphorylase*, which adds inorganic phosphate across α-1,4-linkages and then catalyses the rupture of the bonds (phosphorolysis), forming glucose-1-phosphate. Glycogen phosphorylase cannot catalyse the phosphorolysis of the three α-1,4-links adjacent to an α-1,6-branch point, possibly because of their inaccessibility. The enzyme requires activation, as described below.

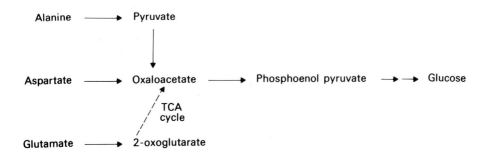

Gluconeogenesis from glycerol is through its conversion to dihydroxyacetone phosphate via 1-glycerophosphate by means of *glycerokinase* and ATP. Oxidation by the NAD-linked *glycerolphosphate-1-dehydrogenase*, forms dihydroxyacetone phosphate, which is then converted to glucose by reversal of the normal glycolysis steps:

2 A *transferase* (oligo-α-1,4$\longrightarrow$$\alpha$-1,4-glucose-transferase) which transfers the three glucose units from the branch-point to the non-reducing end of the main chain. The branch-point is thus exposed and is then hydrolysed by:

3 The *debranching enzyme* (amylo-1,6-glucosidase), forming a glucose molecule.

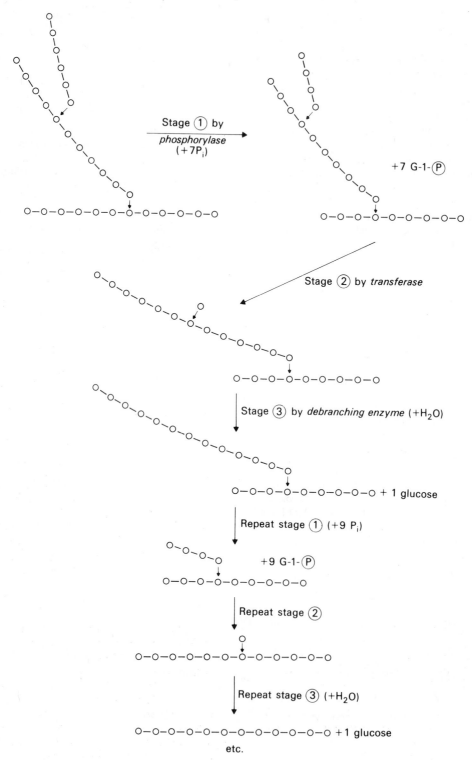

Fig. 4.19. Glycogenolysis: the sequence of the reactions involved in glycogenolysis.

As a result of these three enzymes acting in sequence, the glycogen molecule is degraded completely to glucose-1-phosphate and glucose. The former may be isomerized to glucose-6-phosphate by the enzyme *phosphoglucomutase*:

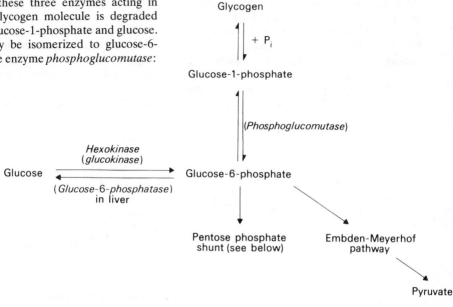

Glycogen

$\downarrow\uparrow$ + P_i

Glucose-1-phosphate

$\downarrow\uparrow$ (*Phosphoglucomutase*)

Hexokinase
(*glucokinase*)

Glucose $\rightleftarrows$ Glucose-6-phosphate

(*Glucose-6-phosphatase*)
in liver

Pentose phosphate shunt (see below)   Embden-Meyerhof pathway

Pyruvate

Adenylate cyclase
Mg^{2+}

Adenosine triphosphate
(ATP)

Cyclic-3,5'-adenosine
monophosphate (cAMP)

Fig. 4.20. The conversion of ATP to cyclic-3′,5′-adenosine monophosphate (cAMP).

Glycogenolysis activation
Glycogenolysis is accelerated by the activation of *glycogen phosphorylase* and by the hormones glucagon and adrenaline. Adrenaline is effective in both liver and muscle whilst glucagon only stimulates hepatic glycogenolysis, presumably due to lack of specific receptors in liver. The process of stimulation is a complex one and provides an example of a 'cascade' process.

Initially the hormone binds to the tissue concerned, activating the enzyme *adenylate* (or *adenyl*) *cyclase* which is a membrane-bound enzyme found in many tissues but normally inactive. This then stimulates the conversion of ATP to cyclic-3'5'-adenosine monophosphate (cAMP) (Fig. 4.20).

c-AMP is an important compound which mediates the effects of many hormones on intracellular processes (insulin is an exception). For this reason, cAMP is called the 'second messenger', the hormone itself being the 'first messenger' to the cell. Once formed cAMP can activate by phosphorylation in muscle, liver and adipose tissue, an inactive protein kinase. This activated kinase in turn brings about the phosphorylation (and activation) of an inactive *phosphorylase b kinase* in muscle and liver. Finally, this stimulates the *phosphorylase b* form (a dimer), and results in the active a form (a tetramer) (Fig. 4.21). In liver, only two molecules of ATP are required in the final phosphorylation of hepatic *glycogen phosphorylase b*, the

enzyme probably being a dimer in both the inactive and activated forms.

The *protein kinase* mentioned above is composed of two subunits which are firmly bound together in the absence of cAMP. When cAMP is formed it binds strongly with the regulatory subunit thus causing the catalytic subunit to dissociate from it and become functional. This kin-

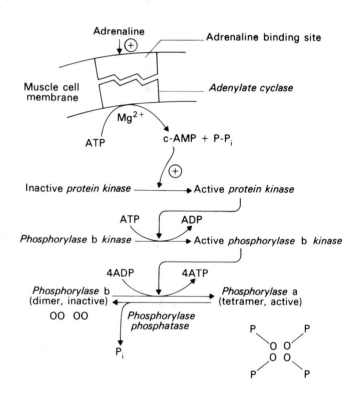

Fig. 4.21. The role of cAMP in glycogenolysis activation in skeletal muscle.

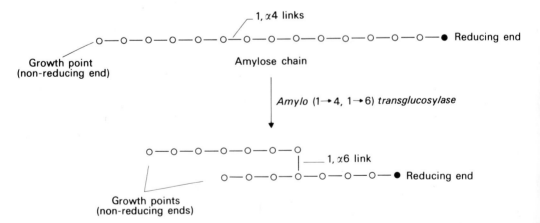

Fig. 4.22. Glycogenesis: the action of branching enzymes.

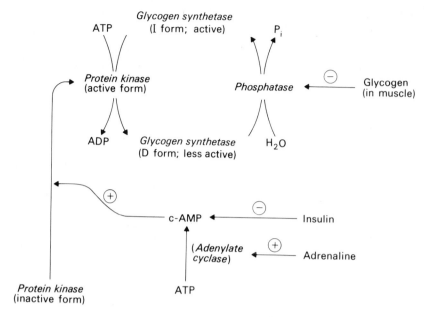

Fig. 4.23. Control of glycogenesis.

ase catalyses not only the activation of the phosphorylase b kinase but also the covalent modification of *glycogen synthetase* (Fig. 4.23) and the lipase of adipose tissue. Thus when adrenaline increases tissue levels of cAMP, glycogenolysis is increased, glycogen synthesis is depressed and fat stores are broken down.

When the need for glycogenolysis diminishes, the specific inactivation of phosphorylase a is catalysed by a *phosphorylase a phosphatase*.

GLYCOGEN SYNTHESIS (GLYCOGENESIS)

The synthesis of glycogen takes place in numerous tissues of the body but mainly in liver and muscle. The 'building blocks' are glucose-1-phosphate molecules, formed initially from glucose-6-phosphate by *phosphoglucomutase*, i.e.

The next stage involves formation of uridine diphosphate glucose (UDPG), a nucleoside phosphate which often acts as a carrier of small molecules such as glucose, galactose, glucuronic acid and mannose, in biosynthetic reactions. Glucose-1-phosphate reacts with uridine triphosphate (UTP) in the presence of *UDPG pyrophosphorylase*:

$$\text{UTP + glucose-1-phosphate} \xrightarrow{\substack{UDPG \\ pyrophosphorylase}} \text{UDPG + PP}_i$$

The glycosyl group of UDPG is transferred to the terminal glucose residue at the non-reducing end of a polyglucose chain (known as a primer). The formation of a $1\rightarrow4\alpha$-link is catalysed by the enzyme *glycogen synthetase*. The process is repeated until eight to twelve glucose units have been added to the growing chain. The formation of $1\rightarrow6\alpha$-links, however, is catalysed by

$$\text{Glucose} \xrightarrow[\substack{ATP \quad ADP}]{Hexokinase} \text{Glucose-6-phosphate} \xrightleftharpoons{Phosphoglucomutase} \text{Glucose-1-phosphate}$$

a 'branching' enzyme (*amylo(1→4, 1→6) transglycosylase*). This transfers six or seven glucose units to C-6 of the glucose unit approximately twelfth from the end. The two non-reducing ends of the molecule are both growth points for the molecule and, since the sidechains can be branched, growth results in a highly-branched polysaccharide. A 1,α6-link forms approximately every 8 glucose units in glycogen (Fig. 4.22).

Control of glycogenesis
Control of glycogenesis occurs through the action of various hormones on the key enzyme in the process, *glycogen synthetase*. This occurs in two forms: *glycogen synthetase (I)*, the 'active' form which acts independently (I form) of

fructose-6-phosphate through *hexokinase* and ATP. *Phosphofructokinase* then accelerates the further phosphorylation to fructose-1,6-diphosphate, in the presence of ATP (see Fig. 4.16).

An alternative metabolic route for fructose is its conversion first to fructose-1-phosphate by the enzyme *fructokinase*. Further phosphorylation then leads to the formation of fructose-1,6-diphosphate.

GALACTOSE

Rather more complicated reactions are required for the entry of galactose into glycolysis. It is first phosphorylated to galactose-1-phosphate by galactokinase and then the phosphate group transferred to glucose (in the form of uridine diphosphoglucose, UDPG) as follows:

$$\text{Galactose} \xrightarrow[\text{(\textit{Galactokinase})}]{\overset{\text{ATP} \qquad \text{ADP}}{\diagdown (\text{Mg}^{2+}) \diagup}} \text{Galactose-1-phosphate}$$

$$\text{Galactose-1-phosphate} + \text{UDPG} \xrightarrow{\overset{(\textit{Gal-1-phosphate uridyl}}{\textit{transferase})}} \text{Glucose-1-phosphate}$$

$$+ \text{ UDP-galactose}$$

glucose-6-phosphate levels: *glycogen synthetase (D)*, the inactive form which is dependent (D form) for activity on glucose-6-phosphate. The inactive form is converted to the active form by a phosphatase, the reverse reaction being accomplished by the protein kinase described above (Fig. 4.23). This enzyme also exists in two forms, and is activated by cAMP and adrenaline. By this means glycogen synthesis is depressed. On the other hand, insulin stimulates the process in two ways, one by direct action on the *phosphatase* and resulting in active *glycogen synthetase*, the other by reducing cAMP levels thereby reducing the activation of the kinase and indirectly increasing the amount of *glycogen synthetase(I)* present.

The metabolism of hexoses other than glucose

FRUCTOSE

The major route by which fructose enters the Embden—Meyerhof pathway is by conversion to

Finally, UDP-galactose is epimerized to UDP-glucose by *UDP-galactose-4-epimerase* which alters the configuration at C-4 of galactose.

DISORDERS OF FRUCTOSE AND GALACTOSE METABOLISM

Fructosuria
This is a rare inherited disorder of fructose metabolism in which the individual concerned has a higher than normal blood fructose level. Apart from this and fructosuria, no other symptoms are noticed. The disease is believed to be caused by a deficiency of *fructokinase*.

Galactosaemia
This is a rare inherited disorder which manifests itself early in infancy. As a result of deficiency of the enzyme, *galactose-1-phosphate uridyl transferase*, the galactose component of the lactose in milk cannot be metabolized. Blood galactose levels are therefore raised and galactose is found in the urine. Clinical manifestations include abdominal pain, diarrhoea and mental retarda-

tion, resulting in the death of the infant concerned. If a diagnosis is made promptly and galactose withdrawn from the diet, there is usually complete recovery although there may be some pre-natal damage as a result of the fetus being affected by galactose ingested by the mother.

Carbohydrate metabolism in yeast and bacteria

YEAST

The fermentation of sugar by yeast to produce alcohol and CO_2 has been known for many centuries, the overall reaction being:

$$C_6H_{12}O_6 \rightarrow 2\ CH_3CH_2OH + 2\ CO_2$$

In the early part of the present century yeast fermentation was shown to be accelerated by the presence of inorganic phosphate and, as the reaction proceeded, the inorganic phosphate was converted to organic phosphates, such as glucose-6-phosphate. The anaerobic glycolytic sequence in yeast is the same as occurs in mammalian cells (Fig. 4.16), leading to pyruvate formation. However the *pyruvate decarboxylase* present in yeast cells then forms CO_2 and acetaldehyde, which is reduced to ethanol in the presence of NADH-dependent *alcohol dehydrogenase*:

bacteria can convert glucose and polysaccharides to lactic acid and the fatty acids acetic and propionic.

Oral microorganisms such as *S. mutans* and *S. sanguis* are major components of dental plaque and can produce acid in close proximity to the enamel. This is thought to be the major means of caries initiation and development.

AEROBIC CARBOHYDRATE OXIDATION

The tricarboxylic acid cycle

This cycle of reactions is the common terminal oxidation pathway of metabolism because products of carbohydrate metabolism (pyruvate), amino acid metabolism (keto acids) and fat metabolism (acetyl CoA) can all be completely oxidized to CO_2 and water by this series of enzymatically-catalysed reactions. The cycle is referred to variously as the tricarboxylic acid cycle (TCA cycle), the citric acid cycle (a key intermediate) or the Krebs' cycle (after its discoverer, Sir Hans Krebs). It is the most important energy yielding pathway in the animal body.

In 1953, Krebs was awarded the Nobel Prize

$$CH_3COCOO^- \xleftarrow{\text{(Pyruvate decarboxylase)}} CH_3CHO \xleftarrow{\text{(Alcohol dehydrogenase)}} CH_3CH_2OH$$

$$CO_2 \qquad\qquad \underset{\substack{+\\ H^+}}{NADH} \quad NAD^+$$

The rate of fermentation by yeast varies depending on the structure of the sugar concerned. Thus, the rate for glucose is greater than that for sucrose, presumably because the latter has to be hydrolysed into its constituent monosaccharides first. Lactose is not fermented, due to the absence of the enzyme *lactase* which is required for the hydrolysis of the $1\rightarrow4\beta$-link.

BACTERIA

The reactions involved in the conversion of glucose to lacic acid (Fig. 4.16) are known to occur also in several microorganisms, the overall reaction being:

$$C_6H_{12}O_6 \longrightarrow \underset{\underset{OH}{|}}{2CH_3 \cdot CH - COOH}$$

This fact is particularly relevant to the aetiology of dental caries because various strains of oral

for his investigations into intermediary metabolism. He had shown that substances like citrate (a 6-carbon compound), and 4-carbon dicarboxylic acids, such as succinate, fumarate and malate, catalytically enhanced the rate of O_2 uptake by tissue slices and homogenates. Later workers elucidated the enzymic reactions leading from citrate to 2-oxoglutarate which was in turn converted to succinate by tissue preparations. Another significant finding was that malonate, a competitive inhibitor of the enzyme *succinate dehydrogenase* (p. 98), markedly lowered the rate of O_2 uptake by tissue slices, indicating that this enzyme was of crucial importance in respiration.

The discovery by Krebs that citrate was formed by a muscle suspension if oxaloacetate was added, was the last link in the chain of evidence that enabled him to formulate the complete cyclic scheme of reactions for the oxidation of acetate (Fig. 4.24).

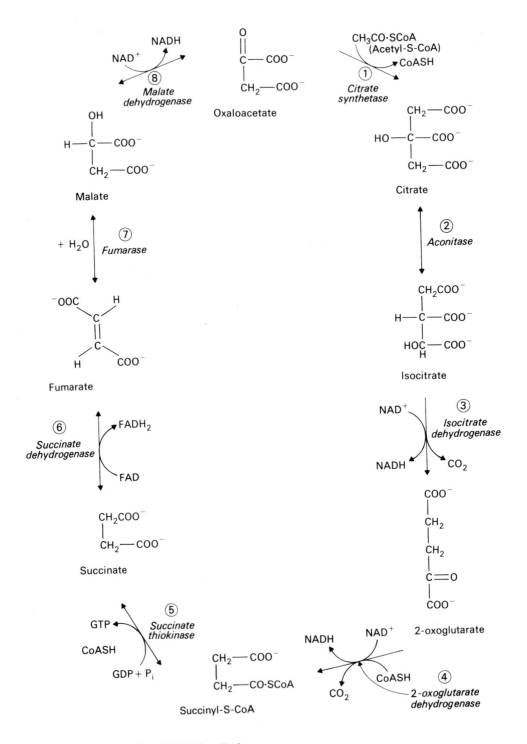

Fig. 4.24. The tricarboxylic acid (TCA) or Krebs cycle.

These TCA enzymes are located in the cell mitochondrial matrix, in close proximity to the enzymes and cytochromes of the electron transport chain (Fig. 4.26). Pyruvate freely diffuses into mitochondria from the cytoplasm, but before it enters the citric acid cycle, it is converted to the thio-ester, acetyl coenzyme A by an oxidative decarboxylation catalysed by the multi-enzyme system, *pyruvate dehydrogenase*. In this reaction, one molecule of carbon dioxide is released and the hydrogen acceptor, NAD^+ becomes reduced to NADH. Additional cofactors, thiamine pyrophosphate (TPP), lipoic acid and FAD are required, all of which are regenerated unchanged at the end of the reaction:

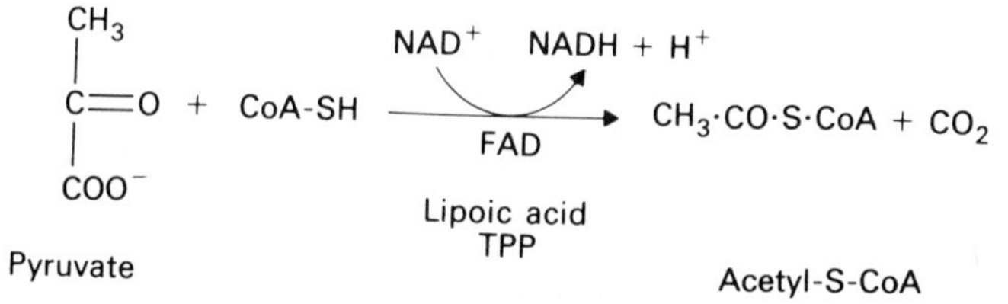

enzyme *citrate synthetase* (or condensing enzyme) to form the 6-carbon tricarboxylic acid, citrate, from which the pathway takes its popular name.

The reaction is exergonic ($\Delta G'_0 = -31.3$ kJ/mol) and proceeds predominantly in the direction of citrate formation. This is probably one of the factors which 'drives' the citric acid cycle forwards in a clockwise direction.

2 The enzyme *aconitase* (2) catalyses the isomerization of the citrate molecule to the related compound isocitrate where the OH is attached to a different C atom.

3 The first oxidation reaction (3) of the cycle involves a two-stage decarboxylation step, cata-

$$
\begin{array}{c}
CH_3 \\
| \\
C{=}O \ + \ CoA\text{-}SH \\
| \\
COO^-
\end{array}
\qquad
\xrightarrow[\substack{\text{FAD} \\ \text{Lipoic acid} \\ \text{TPP}}]{\substack{NAD^+ \quad NADH + H^+}}
\qquad
CH_3 \cdot CO \cdot S \cdot CoA \ + \ CO_2
$$

Pyruvate   Acetyl-S-CoA

The essential basis of the citric acid cycle (Fig. 4.24) is the condensation of this 2-carbon acetyl unit with a 4-carbon molecule, oxaloacetate, to form the 6-carbon compound citrate, followed by a series of oxidation and decarboxylation reactions during which the citrate is degraded in a step-wise fashion to oxaloacetate. The two carbon atoms of the acetyl group appear eventually as two molecules of carbon dioxide. Oxaloacetate is thus regenerated with each turn of the cycle, ready to combine with another unit of acetyl-S-CoA.

There are four oxidation steps (steps 3, 4, 6 & 8 in Fig. 4.24) in the cycle, three of which require NAD^+ as cofactor, which is reduced to NADH. The fourth oxidative step, the succinate dehydrogenase reaction (6), requires FAD as cofactor, which is reduced to FADH2.

THE INDIVIDUAL REACTIONS OF THE TCA CYCLE (Fig. 4.24)

1 The initial condensation step (1) between acetyl CoA and oxaloacetate is catalysed by the

lysed by the enzyme *isocitrate dehydrogenase*. This enzyme exists in two forms, one found in mitochondria, the other in the cytoplasm. The mitochondrial enzyme is specific for NAD^+ (reduced to NADH and H^+), with the C1 of the citrate molecule removed as CO2, leaving the 5-carbon compound 2-oxoglutarate (alternatively called α-ketoglutarate) as the product of the reaction. *Isocitrate dehydrogenase* is an important allosteric enzyme (p. 101), and is considered to be the rate-controlling step of the whole pathway. Its activity is markedly increased by activators such as ADP and isocitrate itself, or decreased by ATP and NADH.

The cytoplasmic enzyme differs in several respects from the mitochondrial form:
(a) it requires $NADP^+$ as cofactor,
(b) the reaction appears to proceed through the enzyme-bound intermediate, oxalosuccinate, and
(c) the enzyme does not have allosteric properties.

4 The conversion of 2-oxoglutarate to the 4-carbon compound, succinyl CoA, by the

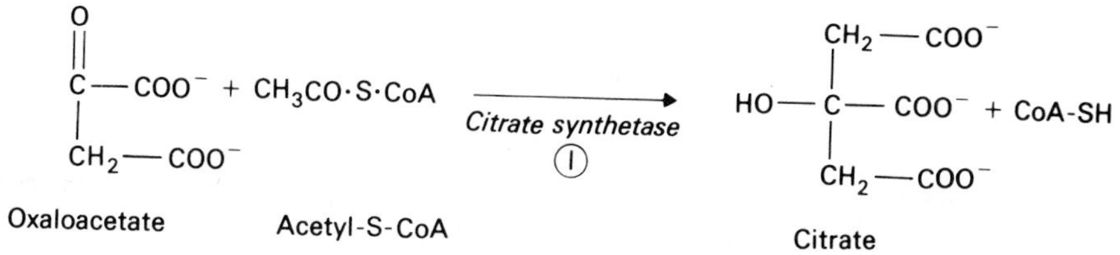

$$
\begin{array}{c}
O \\
\| \\
C\text{---}COO^- \ + \ CH_3CO \cdot S \cdot CoA \\
| \\
CH_2\text{---}COO^-
\end{array}
\qquad
\xrightarrow[\substack{\textit{Citrate synthetase} \\ \textcircled{1}}]{}
\qquad
\begin{array}{c}
CH_2\text{---}COO^- \\
| \\
HO\text{---}C\text{---}COO^- \ + \ CoA\text{-}SH \\
| \\
CH_2\text{---}COO^-
\end{array}
$$

Oxaloacetate   Acetyl-S-CoA   Citrate enzyme *2-oxoglutarate dehydrogenase* is similar to the oxidation of pyruvate to acetyl CoA. Free coenzyme is required to form a thioester with the succinyl group, one molecule of CO_2 is released and NAD^+ is reduced to NADH; TPP, lipoic acid and FAD act as essential additional cofactors:

pathway, and also by malonate.

7   The next stage is the reversible hydration of fumarate, catalysed by the enzyme *fumarase*. The addition of water occurs in a stereospecific manner so that only the L-form of malate is formed (p. 199).

8   The fourth and last oxidation is catalysed by

2-oxoglutarate   Succinyl-S-CoA

The reaction is strongly exergonic ($\Delta G'_o = -30.1$ kJ/mol), and is probably the other major factor in addition to reaction (1) determining the uni-directionality of the pathway.

5   In the next step the thio-ester bond of succinyl CoA is hydrolysed to give succinate and free coenzyme A by *succinate-thiokinase*. The reaction is coupled to the synthesis of one molecule of GTP (guanosine triphosphate) from GDP and one inorganic phosphate ion (Pi).

malate dehydrogenase and requires NAD^+ as cofactor (p. 199). The product of this reaction, *oxaloacetate* can then re-enter the cycle by condensation with another molecule of acetyl-S-CoA (reaction 1).

In summary the reactions of the pathway can be written as:

acetyl-S-CoA + 3 NAD^+ + FAD + GDP + P_i + 2H_2O

$= 2CO_2 + CoASH + 3NADH + 3H^+ + FADH_2 + GTP$

Succinyl-S-CoA   Succinate

6   The next stage, the oxidation of succinate to fumarate, is catalysed by the enzyme *succinate dehydrogenase*, a flavoprotein with a prosthetic group hydrogen acceptor, FAD.

ANAPLEROTIC REACTIONS

A sudden influx of pyruvate or acetyl-S-CoA into the TCA cycle could deplete the level of oxaloacetate required for the *citrate synthetase*

Succinate   Fumarate

The enzyme is inhibited competitively by oxaloacetate, the last intermediate of the TCA

reaction (1), and seriously slow down the cycle. As the TCA cycle is a central crossroad for all

Fumarate — Malate — Oxaloacetate

metabolism any sluggishness will affect the entire activity of the cell. This undesirable situation is prevented by a set of metabolic safety valves, collectively termed *anaplerotic ('filling up') reactions*. Their function is to ensure maintenance of an adequate supply of key TCA intermediates.

An important example in mammals is *pyruvate carboxylase*, located within the mitochondria and catalysing the first stage of glucogenesis from pyruvate (Fig. 4.18), i.e.

Pyruvate — Oxaloacetate
Pyruvate carboxylase

It is an allosteric enzyme (p. 101) with acetyl-S-CoA as its positive effector. Once oxaloacetate starts to be depleted acetyl-S-CoA from various sources begins to accumulate. This then activates *pyruvate carboxylase* allosterically and so tops-up the depleting oxaloacetate level.

Another control of TCA metabolism is via *malic enzyme* which converts pyruvate to malic acid, i.e.

Malic enzyme

This anaplerotic reaction converts excess pyruvate to malic acid and hence 'fills-up' the oxaloacetate level via reaction 8 of the TCA cycle.

The respiratory chain

The cell contains only very small amounts of the cofactors, NADH and $FADH_2$ which must, therefore, be rapidly reoxidized to NAD^+ and

FAD for the citric acid cycle to function effectively. The only reoxidative process available in the mitochondria for the regeneration of these cofactors is the electron transport chain with molecular oxygen as the final electron acceptor. Thus, in contrast to glycolysis, the citric acid cycle can only operate in the cell under aerobic conditions.

Mitochondria have been called the 'power houses' of the cell because within these subcellular structures energy available from fat oxidation, amino acid metabolism, and carbohydrate metabolism is released and captured in the more readily utilized form of ATP.

Mitochondria are bounded by two membranes, an outer smooth membrane, and an inner one which is elaborately folded back on itself to form long projections called *cristae* (Figs. 4.8 & 4.25). These provide an extremely large surface area for the processes involved in the transport of *reducing equivalents* (the hydrogen atoms and electrons, p. 204) carried along the respiratory chain. The components of this chain (the flavoproteins, coenzyme Q and cytochromes) are believed to be structurally embedded in the inner membrane, together with the enzymes and coupling factors essential for the synthesis of ATP.

The interior matrix of the mitochondria contains the enzymes of the TCA cycle and of fat

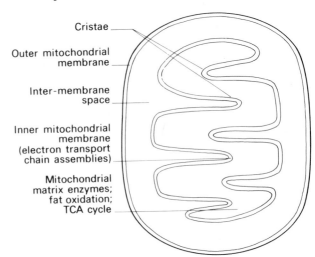

Cristae

Outer mitochondrial membrane

Inter-membrane space

Inner mitochondrial membrane (electron transport chain assemblies)

Mitochondrial matrix enzymes; fat oxidation; TCA cycle

Fig. 4.25. Diagram of mitochondrion showing enzyme system locations.

oxidation (see p. 205) together with some of the enzymes concerned with amino acid metabolism (p. 215). Reducing equivalents are rapidly transported along the respiratory chain assemblies located nearby on the walls of the cristae, to be passed finally to oxygen to form water.

There is evidence that the major components of the respiratory chain are arranged in precise functional and spatial orientations within the membrane, so that reducing equivalents and electrons can be passed directly from one electron carrier to the next along the chain.

THE CARRIERS OF THE RESPIRATORY CHAIN (Fig. 4.26)

1   Nicotinamide adenine dinucleotide (NAD^+)
Three of the oxidation steps (3, 4 and 8) of the TCA cycle involve removal of 2 hydrogen atoms from the substrate, one to the NAD^+ molecule reducing it to NADH, and the second (minus its electron), appears momentarily in solution as a proton H^+, to be absorbed by the cell's buffer systems, e.g.

Malate + NAD^+ $\overset{\text{\textcircled{8}}}{\rightarrow}$ oxaloacetate + NADH + H^+

2   Flavoprotein
The reduced cofactor NADH is reoxidized by the first membrane-bound component of the respiratory chain, the flavoprotein enzyme, *NADH dehydrogenase*. This enzyme's prosthetic group, flavin mononucleotide (FMN), accepts two hydrogen atoms during the hydrogen transfer:

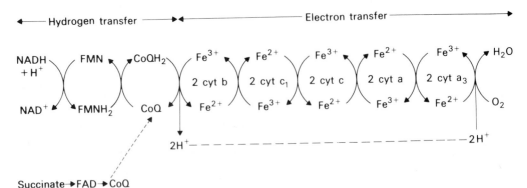

←——— Hydrogen transfer ———→◄——————————— Electron transfer ———————————→

NADH +H^+ FMN $CoQH_2$ Fe^{3+} Fe^{2+} Fe^{3+} Fe^{2+} Fe^{3+} H_2O

                    2 cyt b   2 cyt c_1 2 cyt c   2 cyt a   2 cyt a_3

NAD^+ $FMNH_2$ CoQ Fe^{2+} Fe^{3+} Fe^{2+} Fe^{3+} Fe^{2+} O_2

$2H^+$ — $2H^+$

Succinate→FAD→CoQ

Fig. 4.26. Sequence of carriers in the electron transport respiratory chain.

$$(NADH + H^+) + FMN \xrightarrow{\textit{NADH dehydrogenase}} NAD^+ + FMNH_2$$

3   Coenzyme Q (Ubiquinone)

This coenzyme (CoQ—sometimes called ubiquinone) is a lipid abundantly distributed in the inner mitochondrial membrane of many species. It exists either in reduced (quinol) or in oxidized (quinone) form, accepting pairs of hydrogen atoms from the flavoprotein in a reaction catalysed by the membrane-bound enzyme, *coenzyme Q reductase*.

$$FMNH_2 + CoQ \xrightarrow{\textit{CoQ reductase}} FMN + CoQH_2$$

4   Cytochromes

The cytochromes are a group of coloured proteins each containing a tightly bound porphyrin ring, the iron atom in the centre of each giving these proteins characteristic pink and orange colours. The porphyrin ring (Fig. 4.27) is identical to that found in haemoglobin (p. 73), but in contrast the iron atoms of the cytochromes exist in the Fe^{2+} (ferrous) or the Fe^{3+} (ferric) form, and undergo repeated oxidations and reductions, i.e.

$$Fe^{3+} + e^- \rightleftharpoons Fe^{2+}$$

Several different cytochromes (e.g. b, c, c_1, a and a_3), have been identified as carriers of electrons in the respiratory chain assembly. Cytochrome c is the only cytochrome which is soluble and readily extracted from the mitochondrial membrane; the others are deeply embedded within the structural lipids of the membrane. The last two carriers of the chain, cytochromes a and a_3, are tightly associated and collectively referred to as the *cytochrome oxidase complex*.

Cytochrome oxidase is the terminal member of the electron transport chain and catalyses the final combination of the reducing equivalents with oxygen.

SEQUENCE OF CARRIERS IN THE ELECTRON TRANSPORT CHAIN

The redox potential, E_0, of a compound represents the tendency of that molecule to donate or accept electrons from another compound. For example, if compound A reacts with the reduced form of compound B, and the reaction goes virtually to completion,

$$A + BH_2 \longrightarrow AH_2 + B$$

then A must have a higher redox potential than compound B; electrons and hydrogen atoms will flow from the more electro-negative component to the more electro-positive one.

If the carriers of the respiratory chain are arranged in the order of their increasing E_0'

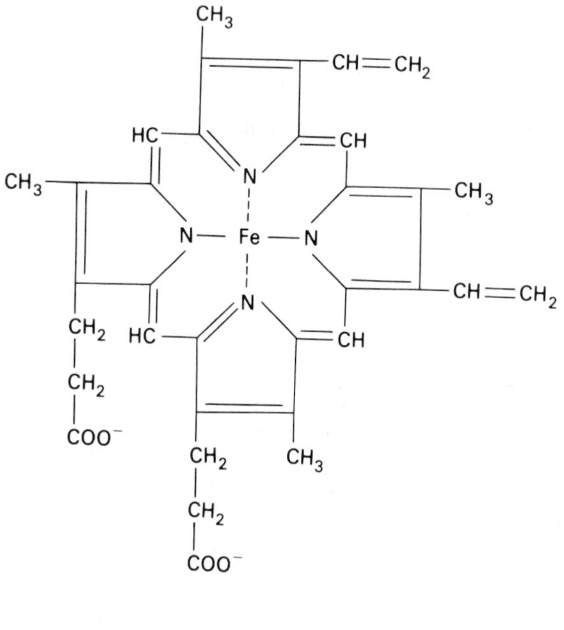

Fig. 4.27. The porphyrin ring of cytochrome b.

values (Table 4.2), the sequence mostly agrees with the relative positions suggested by experimental observations.

Table 4.2. Standard redox potentials (E'_0) of important respiratory chain components.

Oxidation/reduction system	E'_0 (volts)
Oxygen/water	+ 0.82
Cytochrome a_3 Fe^{3+}/Fe^{2+}	+ 0.50
Cytochrome a Fe^{3+}/Fe^{2+}	+ 0.29
Cytochrome c Fe^{3+}/Fe^{2+}	+ 0.26
Cytochrome c_1 Fe^{3+}/Fe^{2+}	+ 0.22
Coenzyme Q, quinone/quinol	+ 0.10
Cytochrome b Fe^{3+}/Fe^{2+}	+ 0.03
Flavoprotein $FMN/FMNH_2$	− 0.12
$NAD^+/NADH$	− 0.32
H^+/H_2	− 0.42

Fig. 4.26 shows the currently accepted arrangement of the carriers within the electron transport chain.

The two hydrogen atoms removed from the initial substrate are passed together along the chain as far as coenzyme Q. After this point the two electrons of the two hydrogen atoms are transferred along the cytochrome region of the chain, and the two protons (H^+) are released into the various buffer systems of the cell. At the end of the chain *cytochrome oxidase* catalyses the final combination of the two electrons and the two protons with oxygen to form one molecule of water.

OXIDATIVE PHOSPHORYLATION

The process described above for the transfer of hydrogen atoms and electrons down the respiratory chain, can be coupled to the production of ATP from ADP and inorganic phosphate (P_i). When a substrate such as malate is oxidized, three molecules of inorganic phosphate are

combined with ADP to form three molecules of ATP for every atom of oxygen taken up by the respiratory chain. This is referred to as a P:O ratio of 3. With a substrate such as succinate, which is oxidized by a flavoprotein-linked dehydrogenase, only two molecules of ATP are formed (Fig. 4.28), giving a P:O ratio of 2.

The $\Delta G'_0$ for oxidation-reduction reactions can be calculated using the equation $\Delta G'_0 = n.F.\Delta E'_0$, where n is the number of electrons transferred in the reaction; F is the Faraday (96.5 kJ/volt) and $\Delta E'_0$ is the difference in standard redox potential for the oxidation–reduction pair.

Such calculations show that there must be a difference of approximately 0.2 volts ($\equiv$38.6kJ) between the E'_0 values of two adjacent components of the chain if that particular site is to be involved in the synthesis of ATP from ADP.

The synthesis of ATP from ADP and P_i may be regarded as the reversal of the reaction for the hydrolysis of ATP, i.e.

$$ATP + H_2O \rightarrow ADP + P_i,$$

for which $\Delta G'_0 = -29.5$ kJ/mol

The $\Delta G'_0$ for the coupled oxidation–reduction reaction therefore must be greater than -29.5 kJ/mol to 'drive' the reaction for the synthesis of ATP to completion.

Table 4.2 shows that three pairs of redox carriers fulfil the requirement for a minimum difference of 0.2 volts between their respective E'_0 values, i.e.

1 NAD^+ and the FMN flavoprotein,
2 Cytochrome b and cytochrome c_1 and
3 Cytochrome a and cytochrome a_3

These possible sites of ATP synthesis are called sites I, II and III (see Fig. 4.28).

The P:O ratio of 2 obtained for succinate is explained in terms of the above diagram. Oxidation of succinate involves transfer of reducing equivalents directly to a flavoprotein carrier, missing out site I: thus only two molecules of

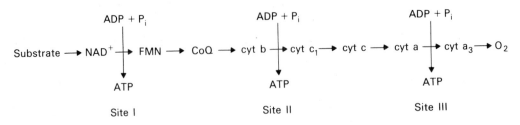

Fig. 4.28. Possible sites of ATP production in the respiratory chain.

ATP are synthesized by the respiratory chain per mole of succinate oxidized.

In intact mitochondria, the two processes of phosphorylation and oxidation are tightly coupled, so that transfer of electrons along the chain cannot occur in the absence of ADP or Pi. In general, the availability of ADP in the resting cell determines the rate of functioning of the electron transport chain. When work is performed by the cell, involving the conversion of ATP to ADP, the increased concentration of ADP speeds up the rate of the respiratory chain, which in turn restores the levels of ATP to their resting state.

In summary, the cell captures energy in a gradual, stepwise and controlled manner through many intermediate carriers, rather than in one wasteful and uncontrolled reaction.

EFFICIENCY OF ENERGY CAPTURE BY THE RESPIRATORY CHAIN

Calculations on the efficiency of the respiratory chain show that the oxidation of NADH ($E_0' = -0.32$ volts) by oxygen ($E_0' = +0.82$ volts) should yield a total free energy change of $\Delta G_0' = n \times F \times 1.14$ kJ $= 219.8$ kJ/atom of oxygen.

Taking $\Delta G_0'$ for the synthesis of ATP as 29.8 kJ/mol, then the overall efficiency of the respiratory chain is

$$\frac{3 \times 29.8}{219.8} \times 100 \ = 40.6\%.$$

However, it must be emphasized that this is purely a theoretical estimation because, in the lipid environment of the mitochondrial membrane, the energetics of the reaction for the synthesis of ATP are probably very different from the simple reversal of the hydrolysis of ATP measured in aqueous solution.

The remaining free energy not captured in the synthesis of ATP appears as heat, but this should not be thought of as 'wasted' energy as it plays an important role in maintaining the constant body temperature of warm-blooded animals.

ENERGY YIELDS FROM AEROBIC GLUCOSE METABOLISM

In working out the total energy production it should be recalled that three ATP molecules are generated for each NADH oxidized and two ATP for each $FADH_2$.

The conversion of glucose to lactate under anaerobic conditions gives a net yield of only 2 ATP molecules (p. 185). However, glycolysis under aerobic conditions forms a further 2×3 molecules of ATP from the reoxidation by the cytochrome chain of the NADH produced in the *glyceraldehyde-3-phosphate dehydrogenase* step. The aerobic glycolysis of glucose to pyruvate produces, therefore, a total of $2 + (2 \times 3) = 8$ ATP molecules (p. 186).

However, by far the major part of the metabolic energy available from glucose is released in the mitochondria during the oxidative reactions of the TCA cycle as follows:

		ATP Yield
1	Reactions involving NAD^+	
	(a) formation of acetyl CoA	
	pyruvate $\longrightarrow$ acetyl CoA	3
	(b) reactions TCA cycle proper	
	isocitrate $\longrightarrow$ 2-oxoglutarate	3
	2-oxoglutarate $\longrightarrow$ succinyl CoA	3
	malate $\longrightarrow$ 2-oxaloacetate	3
2	Reaction involving FAD	
	succinate $\longrightarrow$ fumarate	2
3	Reaction involving GTP	
	(equivalent to 1 ATP molecule)	
	succinyl CoA $\longrightarrow$ succinate	1
		—
		15

Thus, the complete oxidation of pyruvate to CO_2 and water yields 15 ATP, the last 12 produced by the TCA cycle.

Starting with one molecule of glucose, two molecules of pyruvate are produced. Thus a total of $8 + (2 \times 15) = 38$ molecules of ATP are produced by the complete aerobic oxidation of one glucose molecule.

THE MECHANISM OF 'ENERGY CAPTURE' IN OXIDATIVE PHOSPHORYLATION

It is not yet known exactly how ATP is synthesized at certain points along the respiratory chain when two electrons are transferred from one carrier to the next. The two most important hypotheses are as follows:

1 *The chemical hypothesis (or high energy intermediate, I ~ P hypothesis)*
In its original form it was proposed that a 'high

energy compound', A ~ I, was formed between the reduced form of carrier A and an intermediate I, and at the same time transferred its electrons to the oxidized form of carrier B(1). The breaking of the 'high energy bond' is used in a coupled reaction to 'drive' the phosphorylation of ADP to ATP(2), i.e.

$$A + B + I \longrightarrow A \sim I + B \quad (1)$$
$$\text{red. ox.} \qquad \text{ox.} \quad \text{red.}$$

$$A \sim I + ADP + P_i \longrightarrow I + A + ATP \quad (2)$$
$$\text{ox.} \qquad \qquad \text{ox.}$$

Later versions of the hypothesis were elaborated to account for the observations that compounds such as dinitrophenol uncoupled phosphorylation and allowed the oxidation and reduction steps of the reaction to proceed without the subsequent formation of ATP. The postulated A~ I complex was assumed to react with a second intermediate, X, to form I ~ X, this high energy intermediate then reacted with Pi to give X ~ P which in turn reacted with ADP to give ATP, i.e.

$$A \sim I + X \longrightarrow A + I \sim X$$
$$I \sim X + P_i \longrightarrow I + X \sim P$$
$$X \sim P + ADP \longrightarrow X + ATP$$

However, the hypothetical intermediates I and X have never been identified, nor has it been possible to demonstrate coupled oxidative phosphorylation in a completely soluble, membrane-free, system of carriers, as the chemical hypothesis would imply.

2   The chemi-osmotic hypothesis

The failure to demonstrate coupled oxidative phosphorylation with reconstituted, solubilized systems has led to the alternative hypothesis that the mitochondrial membrane forms an integral part of the mechanism for the formation of ATP. The inner mitochondrial membrane is impermeable to most ions and, during oxidative phosphorylation, protons are expelled to the outer surface of this membrane into the intermembrane space. This accumulation of protons on one side of the membrane would create an electrochemical potential which could then be used to drive the reversal of a membrane-bound ATPase to synthesize ATP from ADP and Pi. The essential feature of this hypothesis is that the electron carriers, the flavoproteins and cytochromes, are spatially arranged in the membrane so that protons are released only to the outer surface to generate a proton gradient. Uncoupling reagents, such as dinitrophenol,

would exert their effect by increasing the permeability of the membrane to protons, thus lowering the electrochemical potential and short-circuiting the force that couples the proton to the synthesis of ATP.

Transfer of reducing equivalents

The inner mitochondrial membrane only permits passage of certain metabolites and cofactors. Permeable substances include pyruvate, citrate, isocitrate, malate, succinate, 2-oxoglutarate, aspartate, glutamate, ATP, ADP and Ca^{2+} ion. Conversely the membrane is impermeable to substances such as oxaloacetate, acetyl CoA, $NAD^+/NADH$ and H^+ and K^+ ions.

Each turn of the TCA wheel, oxidizing an acetyl group to CO_2 and H_2O, at the same time produces three molecules of NADH and one of $FADH_2$. The H atoms so produced and carried by these coenzymes are termed the *reducing equivalents*. It is the production of these reduced coenzyme forms which is the basis of ATP generation by the oxidative phosphorylation that occurs within the respiratory chain.

Within the mitochondrion the oxidation of these reduced coenzymes via electron transfer presents no problem. However, they are also formed in the cytosol as a result of the glycolysis and the pentose shunt pathways (p. 211). If these cytosol-produced $NAD^+/NADH$ and $NADP^+/NADPH$ molecules cannot cross the inner mitochondrial membrane, how then can they become reoxidized? This is achieved by the combined action of certain TCA metabolite *translocases* which are bound to the mitochondrial membrane and provide, in effect, a shuttle mechanism for carrying the reducing equivalents across by a permeable (reduced) metabolite. An example is the oxidation–reduction pair malate:oxaloacetate which, via a specific translocase carrier system, shuttle the H reducing equivalents in the cytosol to inside the mitochondria with the effect that each cytosol NADH can be oxidized (at a distance) to three ATP molecules (the lower half of Fig. 4.29). Such translocase systems can also be linked in tandem as the whole of Fig. 4.29 illustrates, where the malate:oxaloacetate pair are linked to an aspartate:glutamate translocase system.

Another important example in animal cells is the glycerol phosphate shuttle system whereby cytosol-produced NADH can transfer its reducing equivalents to mitochondrial FAD-linked *glycerol dehydrogenase*:

$$\text{CH}_2\text{OH}$$
$$|$$
$$\text{C}=\text{O}$$
$$|$$
$$\text{CH}_2\text{OPO}_3^{2-}$$

Dihydroxyacetone phosphate

NADH + H$^+$ → NAD$^+$ (In the cytosol)

$$\text{CH}_2\text{OH}$$
$$|$$
$$\text{HO}-\text{C}-\text{H}$$
$$|$$
$$\text{CH}_2\text{OPO}_3^{2-}$$

Glycerol 3-phosphate

Mitochondrial membrane

Diffuses into the cytosol — Diffuses into mitochondria

$$\text{CH}_2\text{OH}$$
$$|$$
$$\text{C}=\text{O}$$
$$|$$
$$\text{CH}_2\text{OPO}_3^{2-}$$

FADH$_2$ → FAD (In mitochondria)

$$\text{CH}_2\text{OH}$$
$$|$$
$$\text{HO}-\text{C}-\text{H}$$
$$|$$
$$\text{CH}_2\text{OPO}_3^{2-}$$

Glycerol dehydrogenase

THE β-OXIDATION OF FATTY ACIDS

Fatty acids are a common means whereby energy can be stored in chemical form in plants and animals, usually in a combined state as triglycerides in seeds and adipose tissue in plants and animals, respectively. Fat is usually present in the forms of oil droplets and, therefore, in large molar quantities in a small volume within the cell. Fatty acids have a high calorific value. In animals fat can be stored in almost unlimited quantities when the food intake is high and it is then readily available for future use serving as the major or sole energy source during starvation. Fat is also utilized in such states as hibernation or for activities such as milk production. Other reserve energy storage compounds like starch, inulin or glycogen are relatively much more bulky for any given quantity of energy, compared with fat, as they are polar and have a high water content. Triglycerides are non-polar and contain virtually no water. In animals only small quantities of glycogen can be stored in the liver and muscles. For these various reasons fats are therefore the most convenient and efficient means of storing reserves of energy. Hazelnuts, for example, contain 60% fat and 100 g can yield 540 kcal of energy. Conversely raw potato with 19% starch will only yield 85 kcal per 100 g.

For release of the energy from these stores the triglycerides in fat stores are first hydrolysed by lipase enzymes. The fatty acids formed then enter the blood stream where they bind to serum albumin and are carried to the liver or other tissues to be metabolized. The process of breakdown commences at the carboxyl group end of each fatty acid molecule, with initial formation of an activated complex in the cytoplasm which then enters the mitochondria where the oxidative breakdown occurs. Most tissues are able to oxidize fatty acids and some, such as heart muscle, can use fatty acids as their major energy source. Fatty acids do not readily pass across the mitochondrial membrane and require linkage with carnitine to achieve this (Fig. 4.30).

The glycerol formed from the initial hydrolysis of triacyl glycerides is utilized via the glycolysis pathway either to form glucose, or, alternatively, release further energy.

During starvation, when liver glycogen is depleted and fatty acids are utilized for energy, the released glycerol is converted to glucose to maintain the blood glucose level; also the formation of acetyl-S-CoA from β-oxidation tends to inhibit breakdown of pyruvic acid and stimulate its carboxylation to oxaloacetate and hence gluconeogenesis (p. 187).

The stages of β-oxidation

This process whereby fatty acids are broken down to release energy involves the removal of

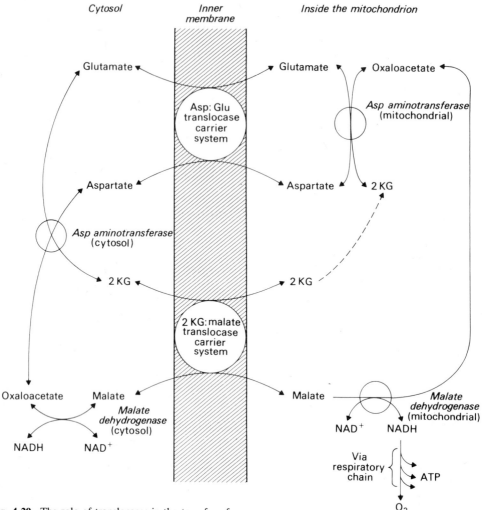

Fig. 4.29. The role of translocases in the transfer of reducing equivalents. (KG = α-ketoglutarate (2-oxyglutarate).)

'two carbon fragments' in the form of acetyl-coenzyme A (CH₃CO-S-CoA). As most of the fatty acids eaten by man have an even number of carbon atoms this results in the complete break-down of each fatty acid to acetyl-S-CoA fragments.

The first reaction in the process of β-oxidation of a fatty acid is with a molecule of coenzyme A (HS-CoA), which is an activation reaction giving a molecule of fatty acid acyl-S-CoA. This is an enzyme-catalysed reaction (*acyl-S-CoA synthetase*) requiring energy, which is provided by ATP. The fatty acid acyl group is next transferred to a carrier molecule, carnitine, which is involved in the transport of the acyl group from the outer mitochondrial membrane across to the inner and on to the interior of the mitochondrion where the subsequent reactions of β-oxidation occur. The acyl group is then transferred to a molecule of intra-mitochondrial HS-CoA to give fatty acid acyl-S-CoA and release the carnitine. The overall process is referred to as the 'carnitine fatty acid shuttle' (Fig. 4.30). The further reactions of β-oxidation then take place on the inner membrane of the mitochondrion (Fig. 4.25). The overall reaction chemistry whereby fatty acid is first activated and then carried into the mitochondria is shown in Fig. 4.30.

In the ensuing series of reactions the acyl-S-CoA is broken down to acetyl-S-CoA in the following steps:

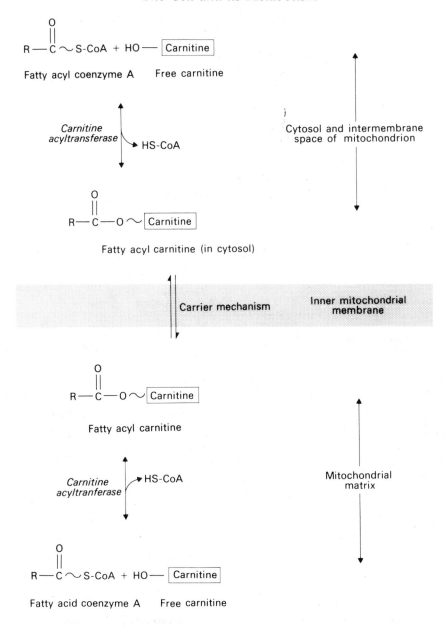

Fig. 4.30. The carnitine fatty acid shuttle system.

1 A dehydrogenation reaction to give an α–β double bond.
2 The addition of water across this double bond.
3 A further dehydrogenation reaction to produce a β-keto acyl-S-CoA compound.
4 Reaction of this β-keto complex with a molecule of HS-CoA to give acetyl-S-CoA and a molecule of acyl-S-CoA which is two carbon

atoms shorter than at the start of the series of reactions.
The reaction sequences are then repeated on this shortened molecule until the fatty acid is completely broken down to acetyl-S-CoA. Fig. 4.31 illustrates this spiralling series of reactions, each turn of the spiral removing 'two-carbon (2C)' fragments of the fatty acid chain as acetyl-S-CoA for its further oxidation and consequent energy

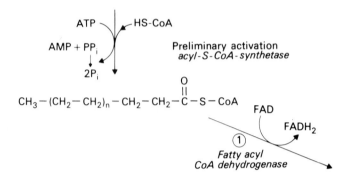

$$CH_3-(CH_2-CH_2)_n-CH_2-CH_2-COOH$$

a C_{16} fatty acid: Palmitic acid (n = 6 at start)

ATP   HS-CoA

AMP + PP$_i$ Preliminary activation
                                acyl-S-CoA-synthetase

2P$_i$

$$CH_3-(CH_2-CH_2)_n-CH_2-CH_2-\overset{\overset{\displaystyle O}{\|}}{C}-S-CoA$$ FAD

                                                        FADH$_2$

①
                                *Fatty acyl
                                CoA dehydrogenase*

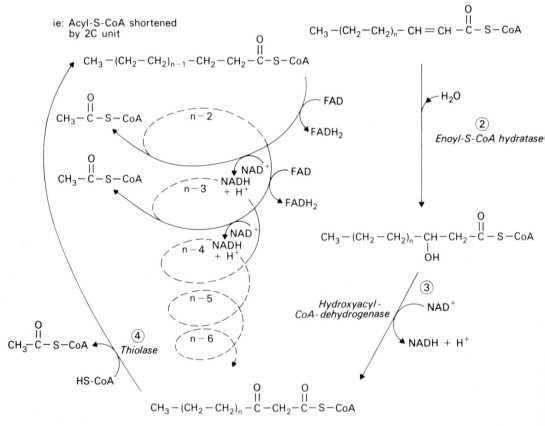

ie: Acyl-S-CoA shortened
    by 2C unit

$$CH_3-(CH_2-CH_2)_n-CH=CH-\overset{\overset{\displaystyle O}{\|}}{C}-S-CoA$$

$$CH_3-(CH_2-CH_2)_{n-1}-CH_2-CH_2-\overset{\overset{\displaystyle O}{\|}}{C}-S-CoA$$

$$CH_3-\overset{\overset{\displaystyle O}{\|}}{C}-S-CoA \qquad n-2$$ FAD

                                                            FADH$_2$ H$_2$O

$$CH_3-\overset{\overset{\displaystyle O}{\|}}{C}-S-CoA \qquad n-3$$ NAD$^+$ FAD   ②
                                        NADH   *Enoyl-S-CoA hydratase*
                                        + H$^+$ FADH$_2$

                                NAD$^+$
                        n-4   NADH
                                + H$^+$ $$CH_3-(CH_2-CH_2)_n-CH-CH_2-\overset{\overset{\displaystyle O}{\|}}{C}-S-CoA$$
                                                              |
                                                              OH
                        n-5
                                                        ③
                                        Hydroxyacyl-   NAD$^+$
              ④   n-6   *CoA-dehydrogenase*
$$CH_3-\overset{\overset{\displaystyle O}{\|}}{C}-S-CoA$$ *Thiolase*   NADH + H$^+$

HS-CoA

$$CH_3-(CH_2-CH_2)_n-\overset{\overset{\displaystyle O}{\|}}{C}-CH_2-\overset{\overset{\displaystyle O}{\|}}{C}-S-CoA$$

Fig. 4.31. The fatty acid β-oxidation spiral. (After Edelstein S.J.
(1973) *Introductory Biochemistry*. San Francisco,
Holden-Day.)

production via the tricarboxylic acid (TCA) cycle (p. 206).

ENERGY YIELDS FROM β-OXIDATION OF FATTY ACIDS

During the formation of each molecule of acetyl-S-CoA one molecule of reduced FAD plus one molecule of $NADH + H^+$ are formed, which when oxidized via oxidative phosphorylation will produce in total $(2+3) = 5$ molecules of ATP from ADP (p. 202). Each molecule of acetyl-S-CoA when its 2C acetyl group is oxidized via the tricarboxylic acid cycle produces 12 molecules of ATP (p. 203). As only one molecule of ATP is required in the initial fatty acid activation reaction regardless of its chain length it is a very efficient process. For example one molecule of palmitic acid (C16-fatty acid) completely broken down to CO_2 and H_2O will produce 129 molecules of ATP from ADP, as illustrated in Table 4.3. The overall reaction for conversion of palmitic acid to eight acetyl-S-CoA molecules is written:

Palmitic acid + ATP + 8 HS-COA + 7FAD + 7NAD$^+$ + 7H$_2$O

$$\longrightarrow$$

8 acetyl-S-CoA + AMP + PP$_i$ + 7FADH$_2$ + 7NADH + 7H$^+$

Note that the formation of AMP from ATP in the initial activation reaction is equivalent in effect to the formation of 2 ADP from 2 ATP.

Ketone body formation

Under certain conditions the liver will convert acetyl-S-CoA to free acetoacetate, which can be converted to β-OH butyrate. These compounds are then transported to other tissues where they can be metabolized to give energy via the tricarboxylic acid cycle. β-hydroxybutyrate is derived from acetoacetate which is formed from acetoacetyl-S-CoA arising (Fig. 4.32) in the last stage of β-oxidation of fatty acids before the 4C β-keto acyl-S-CoA breaks to form two molecules of acetyl-S-CoA.

Acetoacetyl-S-CoA may also be formed by condensation of two molecules of acetyl-S-CoA.

The main pathway forming acetoacetate from acetoacetyl-S-CoA is via 3-hydroxy-3-methyl glutaryl-S-CoA: the formation of acetoacetate by hydrolysis of acetoacetyl-S-CoA with water is only a minor pathway.

The extra-hepatic tissues, including the brain, are able to metabolize β-hydroxybutyrate and acetoacetate as a normal energy source via the TCA cycle, in contrast to liver. This is because these tissues contain *CoA transferase* which catalyses the formation of acetoacetyl-S-CoA from acetoacetate: acetoacetyl-S-CoA is then converted to two molecules of acetyl-S-CoA. The *CoA transferase* is absent from liver and acetoacetyl-S-CoA cannot cross the cell membrane, whereas acetoacetate can. Hence any excess acetoacetate produced is lost from the liver.

During starvation or the disturbance of carbohydrate metabolism produced by diabetes mellitus, the quantities of acetoacetate and β-hydroxybutyrate produced by the liver and released into the blood stream may be very high and can exceed the capacity of peripheral tissues to metabolize them. Together with acetone, which is formed as a spontaneous breakdown

Table 4.3. Energy yield from β-oxidation of 1 mole palmitic acid.

8 acetyl-S-CoA	$\xrightarrow{\text{TCA cycle}}$	8×12 ATP (From the 8×2–C fragments)	
7 FADH$_2$	$\xrightarrow[\text{phosphorylation}]{\text{Oxidative}}$	7×2 ATP	From the formation of each molecule of acetyl-S-CoA
7 NADH + H$^+$	$\xrightarrow[\text{phosphorylation}]{\text{Oxidative}}$	7×3 ATP	
		131 ATP	
1 AMP	$\longrightarrow$	-2 ATP	(for the AMP formed in the initial activation
Net. yield		129 ATP	

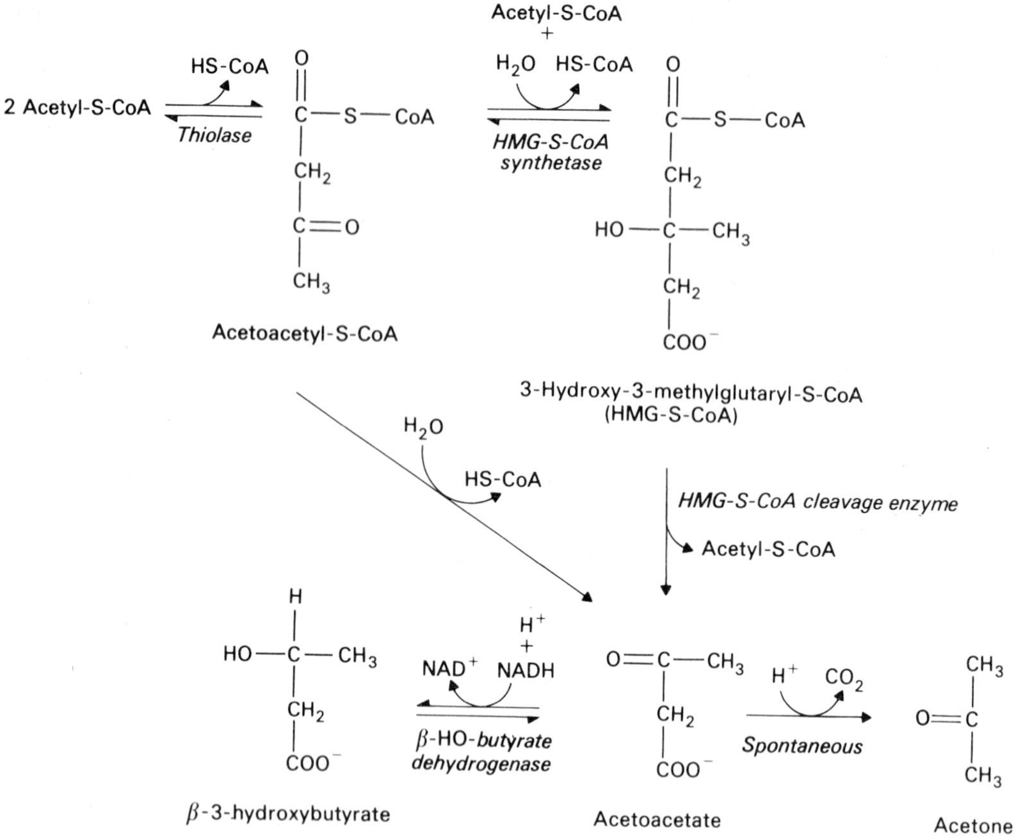

Fig. 4.32. Ketone body formation.

product of acetoacetate, the ketone bodies are lost into the urine producing ketonuria (p 808). Hence also the 'acetone' breath of diabetics.

Minor modifications of β-oxidation occur in the metabolism of unsaturated fatty acids. Fatty acids with an odd number of carbons in the chain produce a molecule of propionyl-S-CoA which is converted to succinyl-S-CoA and enters the TCA cycle for further metabolism to CO_2 and H_2O with production of ATP.

THE PENTOSE PHOSPHATE PATHWAY

General principles

Glycolysis, the TCA cycle, and β-oxidation of fats are principally concerned with the generation of metabolic energy—the production of ATP. However many energy-requiring processes such as the biosynthesis of fats, cholesterol, steroids etc., require not only ATP but also the presence of what is termed 'reducing power'. This is usually supplied by the reduced form of the nicotinamide cofactor $NADP^+$ (Fig. 4.33), which differs from NAD^+ in the presence of a phosphate ester group on the C_2 position of the ribose ring.

As a general rule, the two nicotinamide cofactors serve different metabolic functions in the cell. Energy yielding pathways convert NAD^+ to NADH which is then reoxidized by the cytochrome chain to generate ATP, whilst NADPH is restricted to reductive biosynthetic pathways, where it serves as the hydrogen and electron donating cofactor. The major source of the reduced cofactor NADPH is the *pentose phosphate pathway*, alternatively called the pentose shunt, the hexose monophosphate pathway, the phosphogluconate oxidative pathway, or just the 'alternative pathway' (Fig. 4.34).

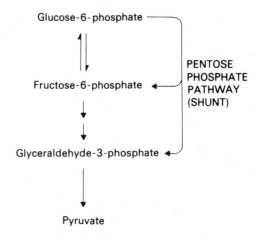

Fig. 4.33. $NADP^+$ structure.

A second important function of the shunt is to produce 5-carbon sugars, especially ribose-5-phosphate, which is required for the synthesis of the nucleic acids, DNA and RNA, and the enzyme cofactors ATP, NAD^+, FAD and co-enzyme A.

The proportion of glucose metabolized by the enzymes of the glycolysis pathway or by the shunt, depends on the relative requirements of that particular tissue for either energy, ribose units or NADPH. For instance, the activity of the shunt pathway is very low in skeletal muscle which has a predominantly glycolytic pattern of glucose metabolism to provide rapid bursts of energy for muscle contraction. In contrast, adipose tissue, liver, adrenal, testis and ovary have relatively high concentrations of the enzymes of the shunt pathway, since these tissues are very active in the synthesis of fatty acids or steroids.

The shunt pathway is also important in red blood cells where it generates NADPH for the *glutathione reductase* system necessary for the stability of haemoglobin. The pentose shunt name derives from the fact that the pathway begins with the same intermediate as the glycolysis pathway, namely glucose-6-phosphate, but by the various interconversions catalysed by the enzymes of the pentose pathway, it leads to the formation of fructose-6-phosphate and glyceraldehyde-3-phosphate, which can then be further metabolized by the glycolytic enzymes.

Glycolysis and the shunt are thus linked by common intermediates and, since both series of reactions take place in the cytoplasm of the cell, the activities of the two pathways may well be closely coordinated.

The metabolic steps

1 The pathway begins with the oxidation of glucose-6-phosphate at the C1 position by the enzyme *glucose-6-phosphate dehydrogenase* (G6PD) which is highly specific for $NADP^+$. This is the first of the two important steps of the shunt that produce NADPH, and is tightly controlled by the reduced cofactor competitively

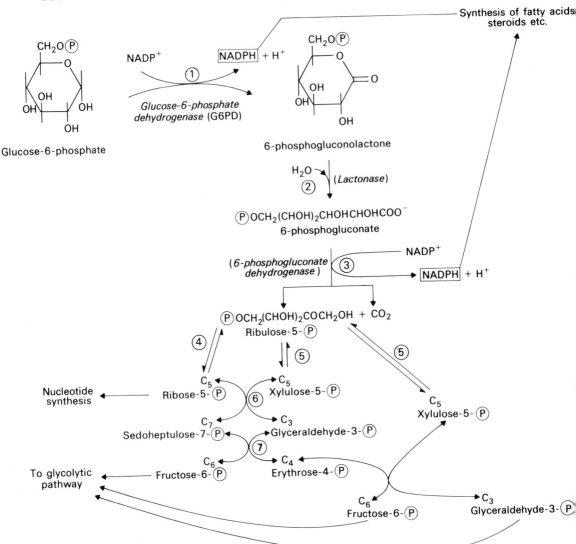

Fig. 4.34. Pentose phosphate pathway reactions.

inhibiting G6PD. When NADPH:NADP$^+$ is 10, the inhibition is approximately 90%.

2　The product of the reaction, 6-phosphogluconolactone, is then hydrolysed by a *lactonase* enzyme to give the carboxylic acid 6-phosphogluconate: this is an irreversible reaction and is the 'committing step' in the shunt pathway.

3　The next step ③ is an oxidative decarboxylation, catalysed by an NADP$^+$ specific enzyme *6-phosphogluconate dehydro-genase*, to give CO$_2$ and ribulose-5-phosphate.

4　The ribulose-5-phosphate is then isomerized to the aldosugar ribose-5-phosphate, by the enzyme *pentose phosphate isomerase*.

If the tissue requires the ribose units for nucleic acid synthesis or cofactor production, then this isomerization will be the last enzyme step that is necessary to convert glucose molecules into ribose-5-phosphate.

However, if the pathway is functioning in adipose tissue or liver where there may be a

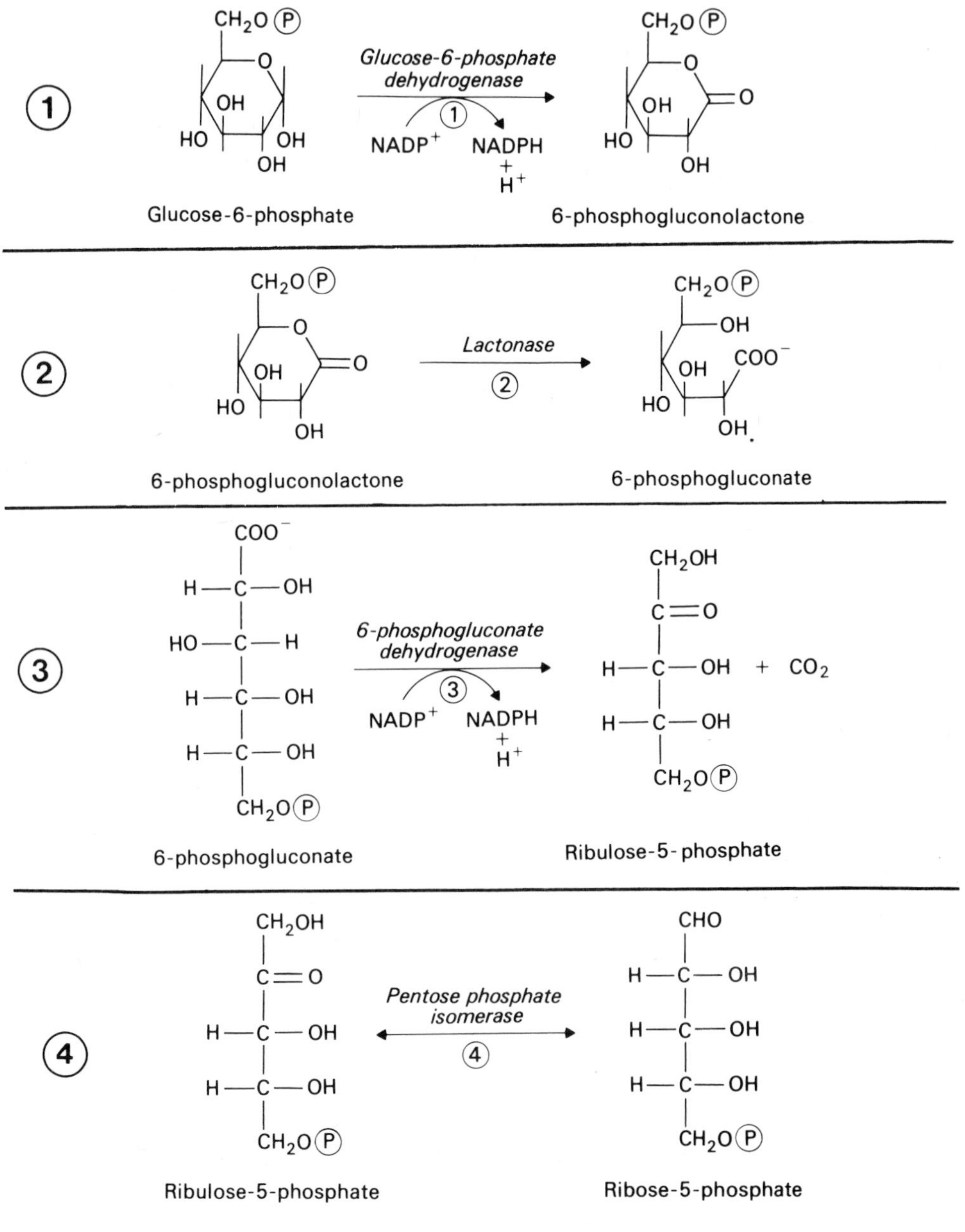

(1)

CH$_2$O Ⓟ

Glucose-6-phosphate dehydrogenase → ①

NADP$^+$ → NADPH + H$^+$

Glucose-6-phosphate

CH$_2$O Ⓟ

6-phosphogluconolactone

(2)

CH$_2$O Ⓟ

Lactonase → ②

6-phosphogluconolactone

CH$_2$O Ⓟ

6-phosphogluconate

(3)

COO$^-$

H—C—OH

HO—C—H

H—C—OH

H—C—OH

CH$_2$O Ⓟ

6-phosphogluconate

6-phosphogluconate dehydrogenase → ③

NADP$^+$ → NADPH + H$^+$

CH$_2$OH

C=O

H—C—OH + CO$_2$

H—C—OH

CH$_2$O Ⓟ

Ribulose-5-phosphate

(4)

CH$_2$OH

C=O

H—C—OH

H—C—OH

CH$_2$O Ⓟ

Ribulose-5-phosphate

Pentose phosphate isomerase ⇌ ④

CHO

H—C—OH

H—C—OH

H—C—OH

CH$_2$O Ⓟ

Ribose-5-phosphate

greater requirement for NADPH than for ribose-5-phosphate, the pentose sugar units can be converted back to hexose units (fructose-6-phosphate) which are then either oxidized by glycolysis to yield energy, or isomerized back to glucose-6-phosphate to re-enter the shunt pathway to produce more NADPH.

This reverse interconversion of pentose to hexose sugars is catalysed by the combined action of two enzymes, *transketolase* (TK) ⑥ and *transaldolase* (TA) ⑦ .

Transketolase, with its prosthetic group thiamine pyrophosphate (TPP), transfers a 2-carbon unit from a ketosugar to an aldosugar.

Transaldolase transfers a 3-carbon unit from a ketosugar to an aldosugar acceptor molecule. The ribulose-5-phosphate produced in the first part of the shunt is converted by *pentose phosphate isomerase* ④ to ribose-5-phosphate and by *pentose phosphate epimerase* ⑤ to xylulose-5-phosphate.

⑤

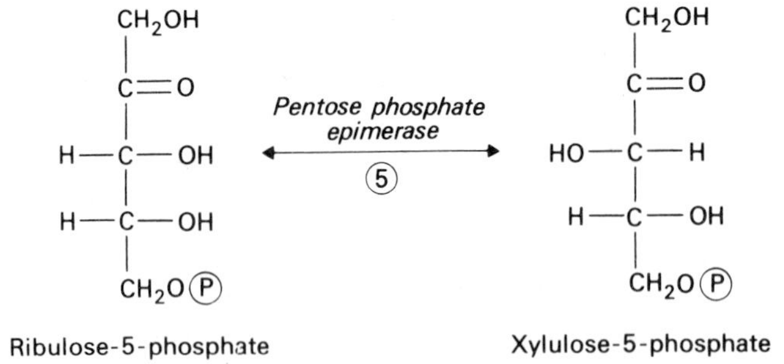

$$
\begin{array}{ccc}
\text{CH}_2\text{OH} & & \text{CH}_2\text{OH} \\
| & & | \\
\text{C}=\text{O} & & \text{C}=\text{O} \\
| & \xleftrightarrow{\text{Pentose phosphate}} & | \\
\text{H}-\text{C}-\text{OH} & \text{epimerase} & \text{HO}-\text{C}-\text{H} \\
| & ⑤ & | \\
\text{H}-\text{C}-\text{OH} & & \text{H}-\text{C}-\text{OH} \\
| & & | \\
\text{CH}_2\text{O}\;Ⓟ & & \text{CH}_2\text{O}\;Ⓟ \\
\end{array}
$$

Ribulose-5-phosphate   Xylulose-5-phosphate

---

⑥

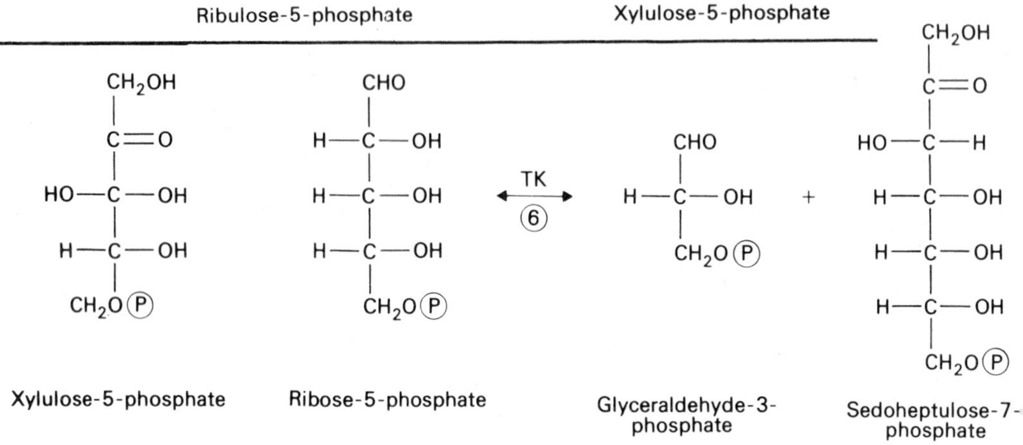

$$
\begin{array}{ccccc}
\text{CH}_2\text{OH} & \text{CHO} & & \text{CHO} & \text{CH}_2\text{OH} \\
| & | & & | & | \\
\text{C}=\text{O} & \text{H}-\text{C}-\text{OH} & & \text{H}-\text{C}-\text{OH} & \text{C}=\text{O} \\
| & | & \xleftrightarrow{\text{TK}} & | & | \\
\text{HO}-\text{C}-\text{OH} & \text{H}-\text{C}-\text{OH} & ⑥ & \text{CH}_2\text{O}\;Ⓟ & \text{HO}-\text{C}-\text{H} \\
| & | & & + & | \\
\text{H}-\text{C}-\text{OH} & \text{H}-\text{C}-\text{OH} & & & \text{H}-\text{C}-\text{OH} \\
| & | & & & | \\
\text{CH}_2\text{O}\;Ⓟ & \text{CH}_2\text{O}\;Ⓟ & & & \text{H}-\text{C}-\text{OH} \\
& & & & | \\
& & & & \text{CH}_2\text{O}\;Ⓟ
\end{array}
$$

Xylulose-5-phosphate   Ribose-5-phosphate   Glyceraldehyde-3-phosphate   Sedoheptulose-7-phosphate

---

⑦

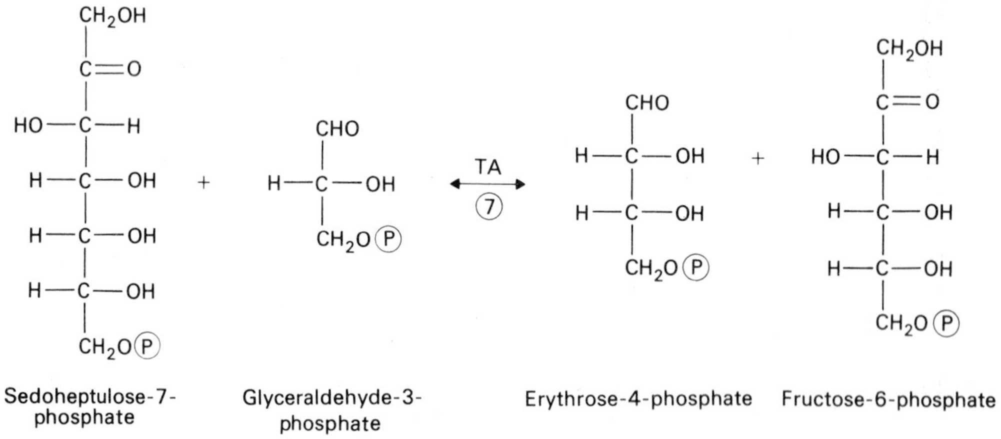

$$
\begin{array}{ccccc}
\text{CH}_2\text{OH} & & & \text{CHO} & \text{CH}_2\text{OH} \\
| & & & | & | \\
\text{C}=\text{O} & & & \text{H}-\text{C}-\text{OH} & \text{C}=\text{O} \\
| & \text{CHO} & & | & | \\
\text{HO}-\text{C}-\text{H} & | & \xleftrightarrow{\text{TA}} & \text{H}-\text{C}-\text{OH} & \text{HO}-\text{C}-\text{H} \\
| & \text{H}-\text{C}-\text{OH} & ⑦ & | & | \\
\text{H}-\text{C}-\text{OH} & | & & \text{CH}_2\text{O}\;Ⓟ & \text{H}-\text{C}-\text{OH} \\
| & \text{CH}_2\text{O}\;Ⓟ & & + & | \\
\text{H}-\text{C}-\text{OH} & & & & \text{H}-\text{C}-\text{OH} \\
| & & & & | \\
\text{H}-\text{C}-\text{OH} & & & & \text{CH}_2\text{O}\;Ⓟ \\
| & & & & \\
\text{CH}_2\text{O}\;Ⓟ & & & & \\
\end{array}
$$

Sedoheptulose-7-phosphate   Glyceraldehyde-3-phosphate   Erythrose-4-phosphate   Fructose-6-phosphate

Then, in the presence of *transketolase* (TK), a 2-carbon unit transferred from the xylulose-5-phosphate (a ketosugar) to the ribose-5-phosphate (an aldosugar) to form glyceraldehyde-3-phosphate and sedoheptulose-7-phosphate respectively, i.e. ⑥

The subsequent action of the *transaldolase* (CTA) enzyme transfers a 3-C unit from sedoheptulose-7-phosphate to glyceraldehyde-3-phosphate to form erythrose-4-phosphate and fructose-6-phosphate, i.e. ⑦

The fructose-6-phosphate can then be metabolized by the glycolysis pathway.

Glucose-6-phosphate dehydrogenase (G6PD) deficiency

When the antimalarial drugs pamaquine and primaquine became widely used in the 1920s, it was found that certain individuals, who had previously shown no history of anaemia, underwent severe anaemic crises within a few days of drug therapy, with symptoms of jaundice, dark urine and rapid destruction of the red blood cells. On further investigation it was found that these patients had very low levels of *glucose-6-phosphate dehydrogenase* in their red blood cells (less than 1/10 of the levels in normal individuals) and that this deficiency of the G6PD enzyme was a genetically inherited condition. This partial block of the pentose shunt pathway results in a decreased rate of production of NADPH, required in the red blood cells for the formation of reduced glutathione which plays an important role in maintaining the normal red cell structure.

Glucose-6-phosphate dehydrogenase deficiency is relatively common in certain areas of the world, particularly West Africa, the Mediterranean, S.E. Asia, and among black Americans who originated from West and Central Africa.

THE FATE OF NITROGEN IN THE BODY: AMINO ACID CATABOLISM AND UREA FORMATION

Various aspects of amino acid metabolism are considered in the text, i.e.

1 In their derivation from the digestion of food stuffs (p. 624).

2 As the 'building-brick' biomolecules utilized in protein synthesis (p. 238).

3 In their role as linkage points connecting nitrogen metabolism to carbohydrate and lipid metabolism via the TCA cycle (p. 226).

4 In their involvement in providing the carbon skeletons for purines and pyrimidines and other small biomolecules (p. 236).

5 In the metabolism of aromatic amino acids and associated genetic disorders (p. 274).

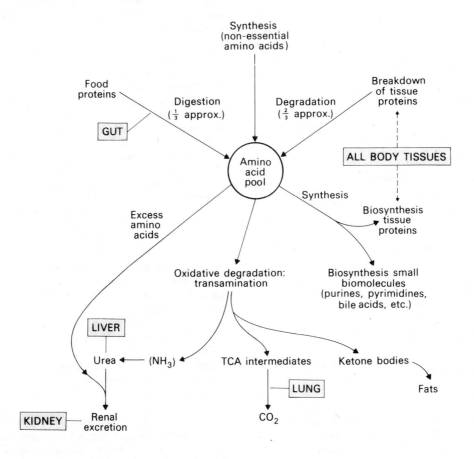

Fig. 4.35. Interrelationships between the amino acid pool and general tissue metabolism.

In this section the metabolic sequences of events leading to the removal of waste nitrogen as urea, and examples of amino acid metabolic pathways leading to formation of certain key intermediates of the TCA cycle and other metabolic sequences are described. Also considered are genetic defects in urea cycle metabolic steps, as the cause of certain grave, though fortunately rare, human conditions.

The major utilization of the amino acids in the body is in protein synthesis, which accounts for some 75% of their total metabolism. This is largely due to the constant recycling of amino acids formed from destruction of 'old' body proteins and their use for the synthesis of their replacements. It is estimated that in the adult human about 140 g/day amino acids enter the amino acid pool from the turnover of tissue protein alone: this constitutes about two-thirds of the total pool, the remaining one-third deriving from food proteins.

Amino acids are also an important source of energy supply in the body. The average human adult derives 15–20% of the total energy requirement from amino acid oxidations.

Fig. 4.35 summarizes the various major areas of amino acid metabolism and their interrelationships via the amino acid pool.

The various aspects of amino acid metabolism are categorized under the following headings.

Transamination
Deamination (oxidative and nonoxidative)
Removal of ammonia
    Formation of glutamate
    Formation of glutamine
    Formation of urea
Biochemistry of certain liver disorders
One-carbon group transfers
    Transmethylation
    Transcarboxylation
    Transamidation
    Decarboxylation
Glucogenic and ketogenic amino acid

Transamination

Transamination involves—as the name implies —the transfer of an amino group. The reaction is catalysed by enzymes called *transaminases* (or *aminotransferases*), and involves the reversible transfer of an amino group from one amino acid (AAI) to a recipient α-keto (or 2-oxo) acid (KA2) which as a result becomes an amino acid

(AA2). The amino acid donating the NH_2 group (AAI) becomes a keto acid (KAI).

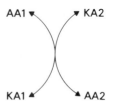

Transamination occurs most predominantly in the liver although it is found at varying levels in other tissues.

An example is the reaction between the amino acid alanine and the keto-acid, α-keto glutaric acid (2-oxoglutaric acid) catalysed by the enzyme *alanine-glutamate aminotransferase*, the name derived by placing the name of the amino acid donating the amino group first (alternative names are *alanine-ketoglutarate transaminase*, or simply *alanine transaminase*). The removal of the amino group from alanine converts it to the corresponding α-keto acid, pyruvic acid, as shown in Fig. 4.36.

The acquisition of the amino group by α-keto glutaric acid converts it to its corresponding amino acid, glutamic acid. The transamination reaction is reversible, with the amino group of glutamate transferring to pyruvate to form alanine and itself reverting to α-keto glutarate.

Transamination therefore involves a coupled reaction between two amino acid–keto acid pairs. The equilibrium constant in most cases is around 1, so that at equilibrium equal amounts of each participant are present. Movement of the reaction in either direction will, therefore, depend upon the removal of one or more participants.

Specific transaminases exist for all the amino acids—with the possible exceptions of lysine, threonine, proline and hydroxyproline. However, only three keto acids (pyruvate, α-ketoglutarate, oxaloacetate) act as amino group recipients which classifies the three broad groups of transaminases: within these are specific enzymes for each AA-KA pair.

The transfer of the amino groups is not directly from amino acid to keto acid molecule but involves an intermediary prosthetic group coenzyme carrier molecule, pyridoxal phosphate (Fig. 4.37).

Figure 4.37 is a simplification of the carrier mechanism involved. In fact AAI first reacts with the pyridoxal phosphate–enzyme complex to form a Schiff base aldimine structure. This undergoes a molecular rearrangement, then hydrolysis

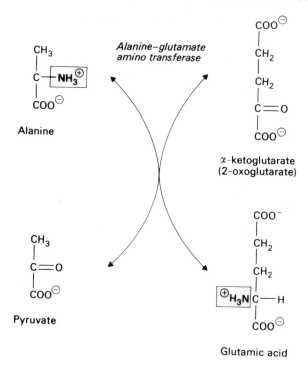

Fig. 4.36. Transfer of amino acid group from alanine to 2-oxoglutarate by alanine–glutamate amino transferase.

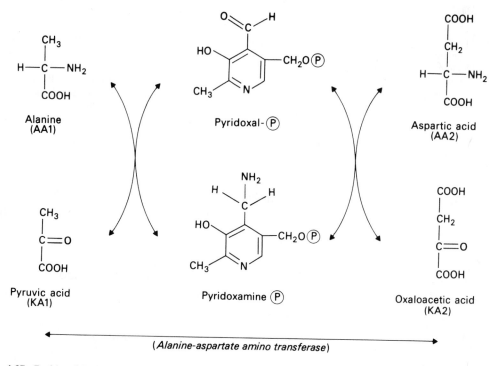

Fig. 4.37. Pyridoxal-P/ Pyridoxamine-P coenzyme system as amino group carrier for an aminotransferase.

to release KAI and the pyridoxamine phosphate–enzyme complex. This in turn reacts with KA2 to form AA2, regenerating the pyridoxal phosphate–enzyme complex in the process.

The clinical relationships between vitamin B6 and this coenzyme and related vitamin deficiency symptoms are indicated elsewhere (p. 814). The underlying metabolic causes of such symptoms are due to the effects on the activities of the various pyridoxal-dependent enzymes (Table 4.4).

Transamination plays two important roles in amino acid metabolism.

1 It provides a mechanism whereby a large number of amino acids may be interconverted: this is important should any one or more come to be in short supply.

2 It serves to channel the metabolism of the amino groups of all amino acids through glutamic acid. This is important because the oxidative deamination of glutamic acid by *glutamic dehydrogenase* provides the major outlet route for ammonia formed in catabolism of all amino acids. The enzyme occurs in the mitochondria of most, if not all, tissues.

Table 4.4. Examples of enzyme reactions requiring pyridoxal phosphate.

1 Those removing or replacing substituents on a α-carbon atom
    Transaminases (aminotransferases)
    Amino acid oxidases
    Amino Acid decarboxylases
    Serine and threonine deaminases

2 Those removing or replacing substituents on a β-carbon atom
    Tryptophanase
    Tryptophan synthetase
    Aspartate-β-decarboxylase

3 Those removing or replacing substituents on a γ-carbon atom
    Homoserine dehydrase
    Threonine synthetase
    Cystathionine synthetase

Deamination

Transamination is one major means of removing NH_2 groups from amino acids. Deamination provides the other and can be oxidative or non-oxidative. Both occur to a large extent in liver cells (p. 624).

Oxidative deamination of amino acids is achieved with the aid of two types of oxidative enzymes—the *dehydrogenases* and the *oxidases*.

Reference has been made above to the key role of *glutamic dehydrogenase* in its catalysis of the major outlet for directing metabolically-formed ammonia to urea formation. In this reaction NAD is required as coenzyme (Fig. 4.38).

Because all amino acids can, via transamination pathways, funnel their amino groups through to glutamate, the above reaction is the key step leading to the transport of waste nitrogen to the urea cycle for disposal. In effect *glutamic dehydrogenase* acts, at one step removed, as a dehydrogenase for all the amino acids. The overall sequence of this series of events in liver is shown in Fig. 4.39.

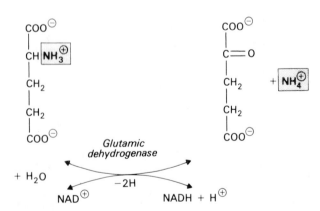

Fig. 4.38. The action of glutamic dehydrogenase.

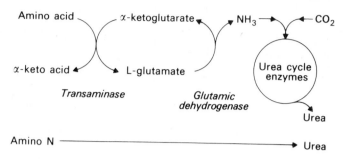

Fig. 4.39. The role of transaminase and glutamic dehydrogenase enzymes funelling amino acid catabolism to ammonia and urea formation.

An important feature of liver *glutamic dehydrogenase* is that its activity is regulated by allosteric modifiers (p. 269) which either inhibit (ATP, GTP, NADP) or activate it (ADP). The flow of nitrogen towards urea formation is therefore subject to metabolic control and regulation.

The amino acid oxidases in mammalian liver and kidney are flavoprotein enzymes in which the reduced coenzyme FMNH₂ (flavin mononucleotide) is directly reoxidized by molecular oxygen so forming hydrogen peroxide which in turn is removed by the liver *catalase* (Fig. 4.40).

Both L and D amino acid oxidases are found in mammalian renal and liver tissues: the physiological significance of the D isomer enzyme is uncertain.

There are also non-oxidative deamination mechanisms for removing amino groups from amino acids. These deaminase enzyme systems involve only relatively few amino acids, e.g. threonine, serine, homoserine, cysteine. The

enzymes are more correctly called *dehydratases* because of the initial removal of a molecule of H_2O (even though one is later added back) in the reaction (Fig. 4.41).

Removal of ammonia

The ammonia produced in the catabolism of amino acids by the various reactions described above cannot be allowed to accumulate in animal tissues or fluids to any significant level without dire consequences. Ammonia (more correctly in its dissolved form as ammonium ion (NH_4^+)), is highly toxic to the animal, even quite small amounts producing symptoms of tremor, slurred speech, blurred vision and even coma or death. The animal body has evolved various mechanisms for the rapid removal of ammonia to non-toxic forms.

In mammals a major method of ammonia disposal is by means of urea formation in the liver. However it is also necessary to have additional means of controlling its level to below toxic limits

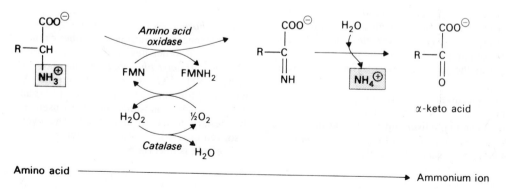

Fig. 4.40. Amino acid oxidase removal of amino acid NH₂ groups.

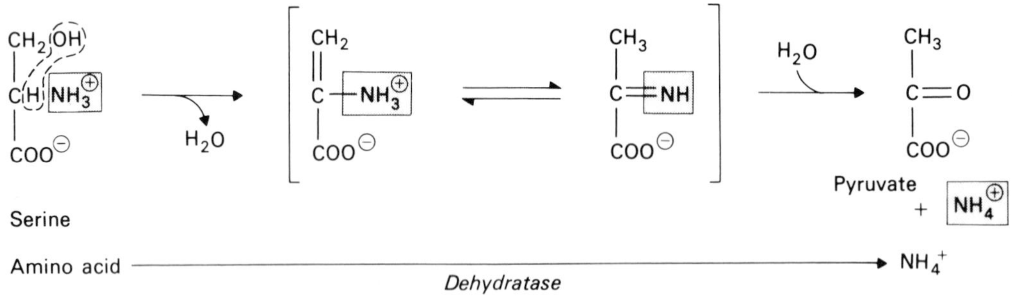

Fig. 4.41. Dehydratase removal of amino acid NH₂ groups.

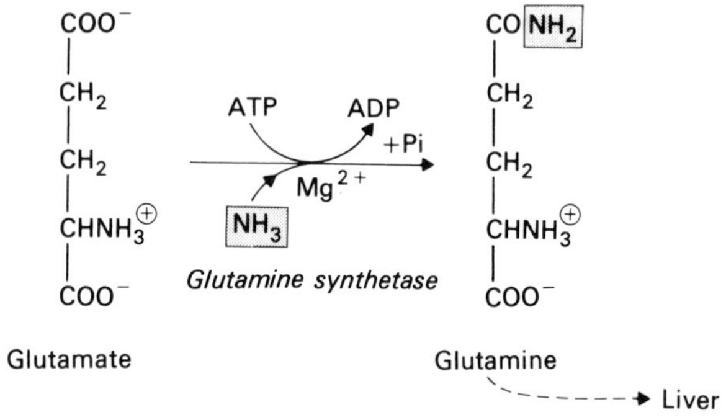

Fig. 4.42. Formation of glutamine by glutamic synthetase.

in other tissues and transporting it in non-toxic forms.

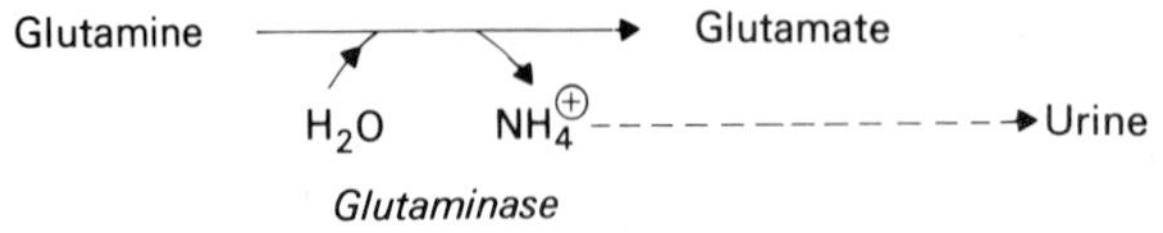

Glutamine formation is the prime means of ammonia removal in animal brain tissue.

FORMATION OF GLUTAMATE

One method already discussed is the *glutamic dehydrogenase system* which being reversible can mop up NH₃ by combining it with α-ketoglutarate to form L-glutamate which is non-toxic. This is a major route for either the excretion or recycling of ammonia, formation of other amino acids by transamination as in the reactions.

FORMATION OF GLUTAMINE

Another method of NH₄ removal is through formation of glutamine from glutamate by means of the enzyme *glutamine synthetase*, catalysing an energy-requiring biosynthetic step. Its activity is high in the mitochondria of kidney cells (Fig. 4.42).

This formation of glutamine provides a temporary non-toxic storage form for ammonia either for transit to the liver and removal as urea, or to the kidney where it is hydrolysed by *glutaminase* to NH₄⁺ for excretion directly in the urine, i.e.

FORMATION OF UREA

This major path for removing ammonia occurs in the liver by means of a metabolic wheel called either the 'ornithine-urea' cycle or the 'Krebs-Henseleit' cycle, after its discoverers. The overall cycle of events is shown in Fig. 4.43. It is convenient to consider the sequence involved in the form of five steps.

Step 1 Formation of carbamyl phosphate
This is an energy-requiring biosynthetic reaction using 2ATP molecules and is catalysed by the enzyme *carbamyl phosphate synthetase*. 1 mole each of NH₃, CO₂ and PO₄³⁻ (from one ATP molecule) combine to form carbamyl phosphate. Two high energy phosphate bonds are used in the synthesis of the two covalent bonds. The reaction also requires Mg²⁺ and N-acetyl glutamate, whose role is uncertain.

Carbamyl phosphate

Carbamyl phosphate synthetase

Step 2 *Formation of citrulline*

The enzyme *L-ornithine transcarbamylase* in liver mitochondria catalyses transfer of the carbamyl group to ornithine to form citrulline and PO_4^{3-}.

Step 3 *Formation of argino-succinate*

The enzyme in step 3, *arginosuccinate synthetase*, requires Mg^{2+} and ATP to drive the reaction which joins citrulline with exogenous aspartate from the TCA cycle to form arginosuccinate. Scission and the removal of the PPi as $2\ PO_4^{3-}$, 'drives' urea synthesis.

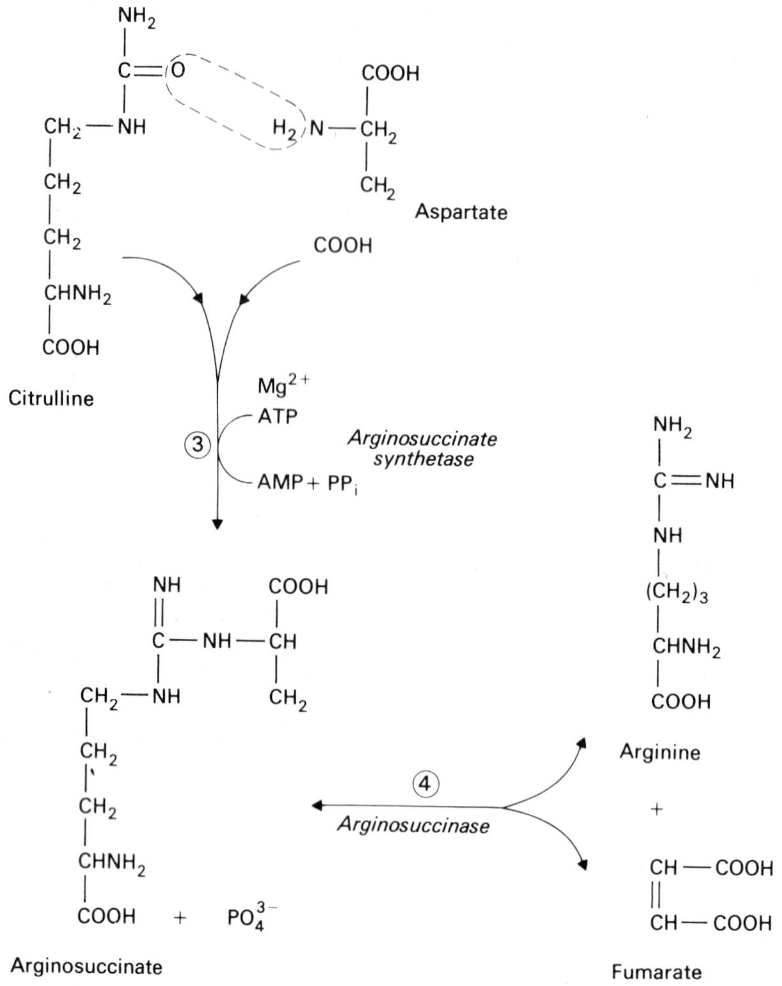

The chemical structures for the urea cycle Step 4, showing Citrulline reacting with Aspartate via Arginosuccinate synthetase (step 3, with Mg²⁺, ATP, AMP+PPᵢ) to form Arginosuccinate, which is cleaved by Arginosuccinase (step 4) to Arginine and Fumarate.

Citrulline

Aspartate

Mg^{2+}

ATP

(3)

Arginosuccinate synthetase

AMP + PPᵢ

Arginine

(4)

Arginosuccinase

+

Arginosuccinate   + PO_4^{3-}

Fumarate

Step 4   Formation of arginine

The enzyme *arginosuccinase* catalyses the reversible cleavage of arginosuccinate to arginine and fumarate. The fumarate can be converted to oxaloacetate via the TCA cycle, whose transamination then regenerates the aspartate, which it tapped from the TCA cycle earlier in step 3.

Step 5   Formation of urea

Hydrolysis of arginine by *arginase* splits off urea and regenerates ornithine for re-entry into reaction 2 in combination with a freshly formed molecule of carbamyl phosphate to repeat the urea cycle.

Steps 1 and 2 occur in the liver cell mitochondria, the others in the cytosol.

In summary the overall reaction is:

$$NH_4 + CO_2 + 4\ ATP + aspartate \longrightarrow$$
$$urea + fumarate + 4\ ADP + 4\ Pi$$

The urea so formed is excreted in the urine as the major end product in mammals for disposing of waste nitrogen. The average human adult excretes 25–30 g a day and this constitutes 90% of the total N excreted. Ammonium ion may account for 3–4% of urine nitrogen and its excretion is important in maintaining the acid–base balance of the body (see p. 746).

Biochemistry of liver disorders

With only very small levels of ammonia in tissues and body fluids producing such major adverse toxic effects it is to be expected that functional or inherited defects of the liver metabolism can have serious consequences. Degeneration of the

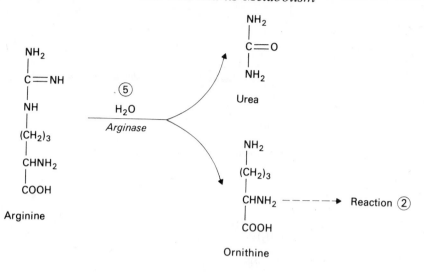

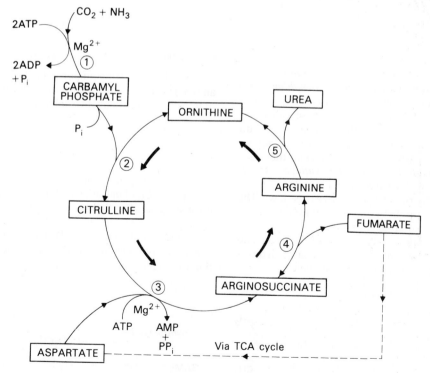

liver, due to many causes, but most commonly from excessive intake of alcohol, leads to hepatic cirrhosis which if severe enough causes the ammonium ion concentration to rise sufficiently to cause coma. Administration of glutamate or ornithine to bolster the rate of ammonia removal (via glutamine and urea formation

respectively), has been used with some success but the best way is to reduce the protein food intake and hence NH_4^+ production. Unfortunately, the latter method involves attendant dangers associated with a protein deficient diet.

Genetic defects causing low levels of activity in each of the five enzymes involved in the urea

Fig. 4.43. The Krebs–Henseleit ornithine–citrulline–arginine urea cycle. One nitrogen atom in urea derives from NH_4, the other from aspartate.

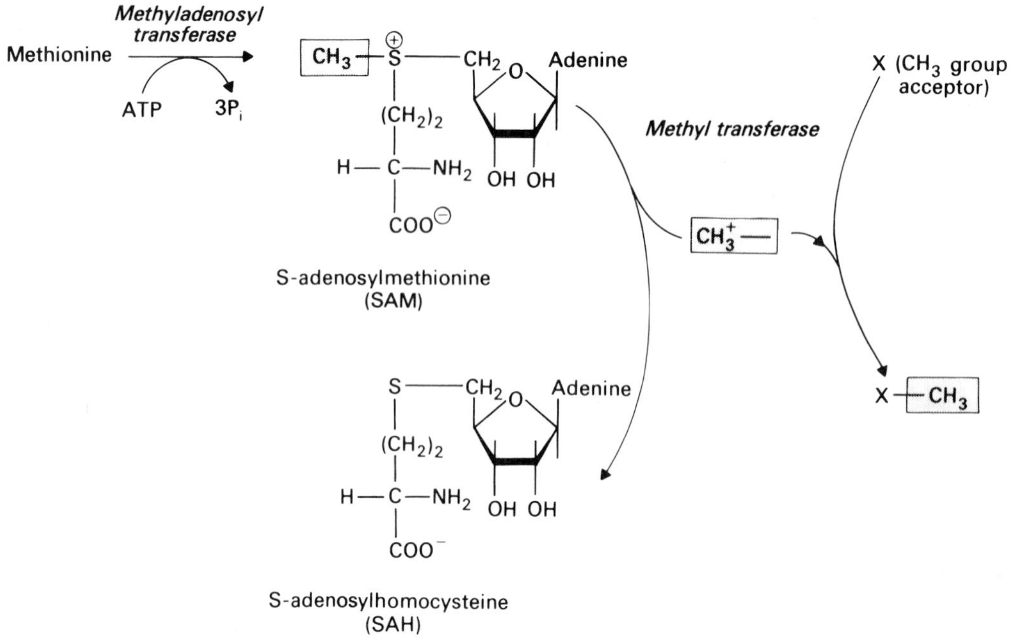

Fig. 4.44. Mechanism of transmethylation.

cycle are known in humans—usually in children and fortunately very rare. *Hyperammonaemia* is characterized by deficiencies in *ornithine transcarbamylase* (reaction 2) and *carbamyl phosphatesynthetase* (reaction 1). These can cause increased NH_4^+ levels in the urine and liver with clinical symptoms of protein-induced vomiting, coma and spasticity. In *citrullinaemia* there is a deficiency in *arginosuccinate synthetase* (reaction 3) and in *arginosuccinic aciduria* the *arginosuccinase* enzyme activity is low. The symptoms for both these conditions may be those of general ammonia intoxication (vomiting and stupor) with mental retardation and convulsive seizures. As with hepatic cirrhosis control measures are largely dietary.

One carbon group removal or transfer

Included here are some important categories of amino acid metabolism which involve removal or transfer of a 1C fragment from their molecules.

TRANSMETHYLATION

The S-containing methionine, an essential amino acid (p. 227), is of major importance in metabolism as a source of methyl groups. For this purpose it requires, first, an activation to the form S-adenosyl methionine (SAM), Fig. 4.44.

An example is choline formation by methylation of ethanolamine:

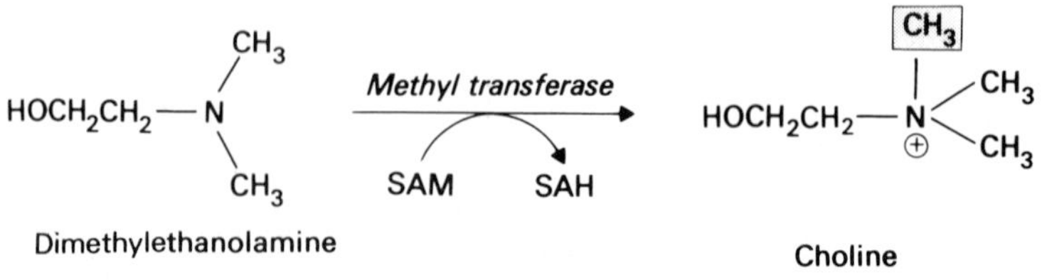

Dimethylethanolamine   Choline

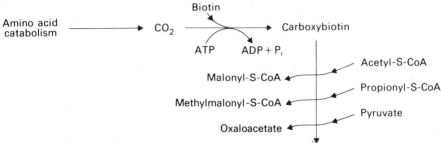

Fig. 4.45. Transcarboxylation reactions.

Phosphatidyl choline, an important phospholipid in cell membranes (p. 46), is formed by 3 successive SAM/SAH methylations of phosphatidyl ethanolamine. Creatine, important as its phosphocreatine derivative in muscle activity (p. 340), is similarly formed by the *methyltransferase*-catalysed methylation of guadinoacetic acid (Fig. 4.46).

ONE CARBON GROUP TRANSFER VIA TETRAHYDROFOLATE

Several amino acids form '1C fragments' metabolically, e.g. serine, glycine, histidine and tryptophan. The transfer of these and formyl 1C fragments is via a coenzyme carrier intermediary, tetrahydrofolate, derived from the vitamin folic acid (p. 816). Examples are the conversion of homocysteine (4C) to methionine (5C) and glycine (2C) to serine (3C). Such 1C fragment metabolism is also involved in purine and pyrimidine nucleotide synthesis (p. 236). Cobalamin, a vitamin B_{12} derivative (p. 814), is also an important coenzyme in 1C metabolism.

TRANSCARBOXYLATION

Another type of 1C fragment metabolism involves carboxyl groups. CO_2 formed by oxidation of amino acids via TCA cycle intermediates, or

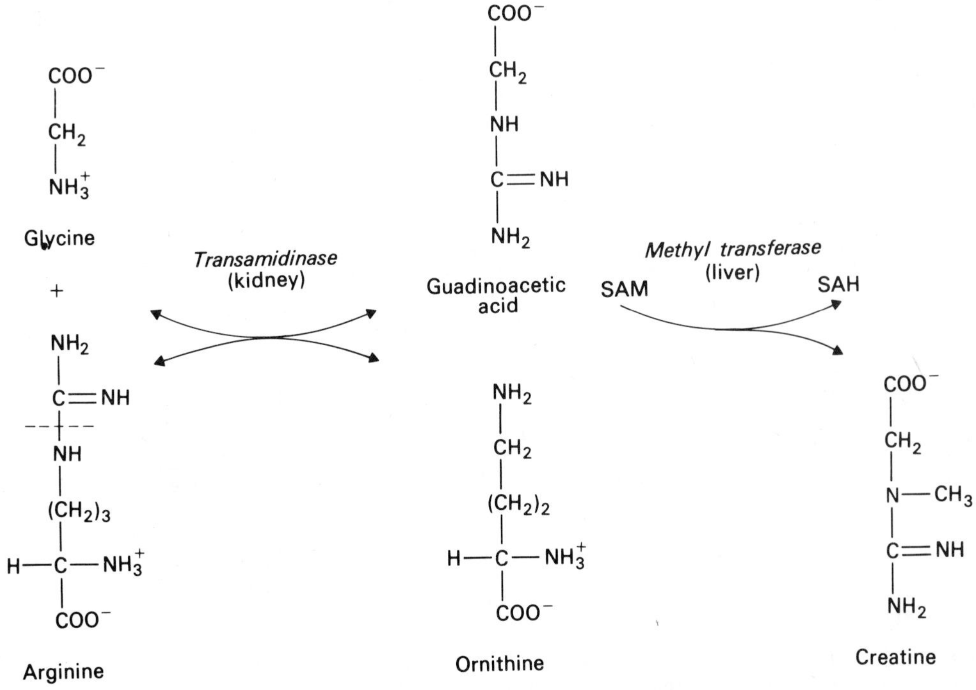

Fig. 4.46. Transamidination and transmethylation in biosynthesis of creatine.

from direct decarboxylation (see below), is fixed by biotin to form carboxybiotin. This reaction requires ATP and a specific carboxylase enzyme (Fig. 4.45, p. 815).

These reactions therefore serve to recycle the degradation products of the carbon chains of amino acids, directing them into useful pathways as in the synthesis of malonyl CoA, methyl malonyl CoA and oxaloacetate.

TRANSAMIDINATION

Transamidination enzymes transfer an amidine group, and such a reaction is an important step in the formation of creatine already referred to in the context of transmethylation (Fig. 4.46).

This is one of the rare known examples of negative feedback repression (p. 269) demonstrable in mammals. When rats and other experimental animals are fed creatine the level of renal transamidinase falls dramatically.

DECARBOXYLATION
(see also pp. 197, 813)

The amino acid *decarboxylase* enzymes are widely distributed in tissues. They catalyse removal of the amino acid carboxyl groups as CO_2, leaving behind the corresponding amines. They are pyridoxal phosphate requiring enzymes (Table 4.4), except possibly *histidine decarboxylase*. Through their action several

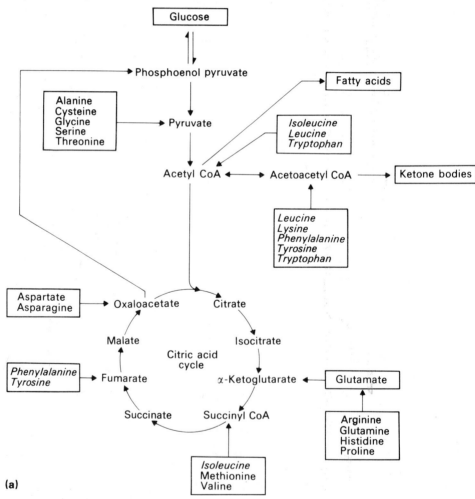

(a)

Fig. 4.47. (a) Metabolic fates of the carbon skeletons deriving from amino acid catabolism. The ketogenic amino acids are italicized: only leucine and lysine are exclusively ketogenic.

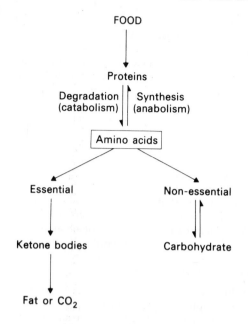

FOOD

↓

Proteins

Degradation (catabolism) / Synthesis (anabolism)

Amino acids

Essential / Non-essential

Ketone bodies / Carbohydrate

Fat or CO_2

Fig. 4.47. (b) Fat and carbohydrate formation from the ketogenic essential amino acids and the glucogenic non-essential amino acids.

biologically active amines are formed such as histamine, tyramine and serotonin (5-hydroxytryptamine).

Histamine is liberated in traumatic shock and in allergic reactions. It is a vasodilator which in excess can cause vascular collapse. Serotonin is a potent vasoconstrictor.

GABA (γ-aminobutyric acid) is formed by decarboxylation of glutamate and is in high concentration in brain where it is thought to inhibit synaptic transmission (pp. 289, 814).

Are there glycogenic and ketogenic amino acids?

After removal or transfer of the NH_2 groups of amino acids by the various reactions described, or the removal of other fragments as in 1C fragment metabolism, the disposal of their remaining carbon skeletons is mainly via the TCA cycle. The individual degradative metabolic pathways for each amino acid differ widely and are too involved and complex to consider separately in detail here. Their ultimate points of entry into the TCA cycle or ketone body formation are summarized in Fig. 4.47a.

Those amino acids whose residual keto acid skeletons can enter the TCA cycle and ultimately form glucose via gluconeogenesis are called glucogenic amino acids. Those whose metabolic pathways lead to ketone bodies are called ketogenic. The majority are glucogenic, three are glucogenic and ketogenic according to conditions, and two, leucine and lysine, are exclusively ketogenic (Table 4.5).

However, this oft-quoted and archaic division is questionable. Although the 'glucogenic' amino acids can clearly lead to net glucose formation they, via pyruvate, can also be metabolized to fatty acids and ketone bodies. In this sense all the glucogenic amino acids can also be regarded as ketogenic, and the division into the two classes becomes therefore somewhat confusing. At best it serves to indicate the amino acids which are more readily and efficiently incorporated in one or other direction.

All the ketogenic amino acids belong to the essential amino acid group (p. 807), and all the non-essential amino acids are glucogenic. This is

Table 4.5. The glycogenic, ketogenic and essential amino acids.

Glycogenic		Glycogenic and ketogenic	Ketogenic	Essential (in adults)
Alanine	Hydroxyproline	Isoleucine	Leucine	Histidine*
Arginine*	Methionine	Phenylalanine	Lysine	Isoleucine
Aspartic acid	Proline	Tyrosine		Leucine
Asparagine	Serine	Tryptophan		Lysine
Cystine-cysteine	Threonine			Methionine
Glutamic acid	Valine			Phenylalanine
Glutamine				Threonine
Glycine				Tryptophan
Histidine				Valine

*Essential in children.

because the latter can synthesize glucose via metabolic pathways that are reversible. Conversely the essential amino acids synthesize fats via ketone body pathways which are not reversible (Fig. 4.47b).

A corollary of this is that fats differ from carbohydrates in that they cannot contribute to amino acid synthesis.

The metabolism of phenylalanine and tyrosine

Some important features of the metabolic pathways involving these aromatic amino acids are discussed in the context of related inborn errors of metabolism (p. 274).

ENERGY REQUIRING PROCESSES

Photosynthesis is the means whereby light energy from the sun is used to build up the biomolecular structures of the plant world from carbon dioxide and water. The products are then utilized by the animal world for release and capture of their own biomolecular and energy requirements.

Turning from the plant world to our own, there are numerous important sequences of events in animal metabolism which, like photosynthesis, are essentially energy-requiring (endergonic or endogonic) in their overall nature. These use the energy-rich 'currency' molecules such as ATP and GTP to drive the reactions concerned. These high energy phosphate compound 'banks' are formed by various energy yielding (exergonic) metabolic sequences such as those examined in the preceding section on metabolism and energy production.

Fatty acid and glyceride biosynthesis are endergonic processes. Other examples of endergonic synthesis mechanisms in the formation of small molecules are the purines and pyrimidines, which are important in the structure of various coenzymes as well as in DNA and RNA.

The biological mechanism of protein biosynthesis defied analysis until the structure of DNA and RNA had been solved. Then followed the elucidation of the mechanisms whereby genetic information was carried from the nucleus to the ribosome sites, and how the amino acids, first activated by ATP, were then lined up in correct sequence to make specific proteins. These discoveries constitute some of the great achievements of post-war biochemistry. There are other aspects of protein formation which are post-ribosomal events and these are well illustrated

by the example of collagen biosynthesis, the latter also serving to describe the biochemical basis of several genetically determined collagen diseases. Further examples of genetically determined metabolic disorders are also found in the texts on glycogen, amino acid metabolism and urea formation in this chapter. The biosynthesis of glycogen was more conveniently discussed earlier (p. 191) in association with the section on glycogen breakdown, but its synthesis should also be considered in the context of this section, as it illustrates one more endergonic process.

The transport of molecules and ions in biological systems also often requires energy utilization, when the mechanisms involved are collectively termed 'active transport'.

Photosynthesis

A brief consideration of the means whereby plants capture energy and build up potential food and energy stores is important for two major reasons. Firstly the ultimate source of food, with its essential nutrients and chemically locked-up energy forms, is the plant world, whether we be carnivores, herbivores or omnivores. Photosynthesis is therefore the fundamental energy-capturing and storing mechanism on this planet upon which most other life-forms depend. Secondly, the metabolic steps and sequences involved illustrate and underline the essential unity of life in biochemical terms. It will be observed that the carbohydrate components involved (e.g. glyceraldehyde, glucose, fructose, etc.), the H carrier cofactors (e.g. $NADP^+$), the 'high energy compounds' (ATP) and the chemical changes involving them, are essentially common in principle to both plant and animal kingdoms. Their fundamental metabolism is remarkably similar in many ways. As will be apparent even the connection between photosynthesis and dental caries is not that remote!

The development of animal life, dependent for its energy requirements on the oxidation by oxygen of complex organic molecules, was only possible following the evolution of plant life. Plants developed a system for utilizing light energy provided by the sun to synthesize organic carbon compounds such as carbohydrates using carbon dioxide and water as starting materials, and releasing free oxygen into the atmosphere. The overall reaction is represented as follows:

$$CO_2 + H_2O \xrightarrow{\text{light energy}} [CH_2O]_n + O_2$$

All the oxygen in the atmosphere (21%) has ultimately originated from decomposition of water during photosynthesis. This oxygen is available for respiration in both plants and animals converting carbohydrates and other compounds to CO_2 and H_2O, releasing energy, thus maintaining a continuous carbon and oxygen cycle and making energy available for living systems to function.

Man is able to make use of a number of other sources of energy in the form of coal and oil, previously fixed by photosynthesis before microbial action and/or fossilization. It is these stores of solar energy built up over millions of years which have enabled man to reach his present high state of technology.

The photosynthetic process divides into two parts, The first involves the capture of light energy by means of light absorbing pigments and results in the formation of reduced $NADP^+$ by breakdown of water to give oxygen, with the formation of ATP. The second stage involves utilization of energy from the energy-rich $NADPH + H^+$ and ATP, by a reduction of CO_2 to form, ultimately, glucose. The first reaction is

the synthesis of glucose and fructose polymers (dextrans and levans p. 137), which are formed extracellularly and whose cohesive and adhesive properties help attach oral microorganisms to the tooth surface and also build up dental plaque. The streptococci and other bacteria present in the plaque are also able to ferment glucose and fructose to organic acids, which initiate the caries process by dissolution of the enamel hydroxyapatite. This energy, in the form of acid, which is able to destroy the enamel structure, therefore derives ultimately from the light energy used to make sucrose via photosynthesis.

CHLOROPLASTS: THE LIGHT AND DARK REACTIONS

The photosynthetic reactions occurring in higher plants are carried out in the chloroplasts. These organelles are highly membranous structures, the membranes containing the photosynthetic pigments responsible for the initial light reaction.

The overall light and dark reactions can be represented diagrammatically:

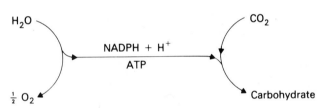

usually referred to as the *light reaction* and the second, not requiring light, as the *dark reaction*.

In considering the importance of the photosynthetic process in terms of its relevance to dentistry, some details of sucrose metabolism are of interest. Higher plants are able to synthesize glucose and fructose from CO_2 and H_2O utilizing $NADPH + H^+$ and ATP as the intermediate energy source originally derived from sunlight. These two sugars are highly ordered structures with a high energy content. A further energy-requiring reaction joins these two sugars by a glycosidic bond to form the disaccharide sucrose, and the sucrose consumed by man is considered to be the major dietary factor responsible for initiating dental caries. One of the main reasons for its cariogenicity is that certain oral streptococci are able to catabolize sucrose, so releasing the energy present in the disaccharide. Some of this energy can be utilized in

The formation of ATP is coupled to the flow of electrons from H_2O to reduce $NADP^+$ to $NADPH + H^+$.

Electron transfer takes place through a series of electron carriers (cytochromes) similar to the electron transport system in mitochondria, though in the opposite direction with the formation of reduced $NADP^+$ and ATP instead of H_2O and ATP. This requires the input of energy into the system to drive the reaction against the potential gradient, and this energy is supplied by light. The potential gradient produced by the flow of electrons between biological electron carriers is known as the redox potential with a range between $+0.8$ and -0.4 electron volts.

Photosynthetic phosphorylation produces ATP from ADP and inorganic phosphate (Pi), together with molecular oxygen from H_2O, and formation of $NADPH + H^+$ from $NADP^+$.

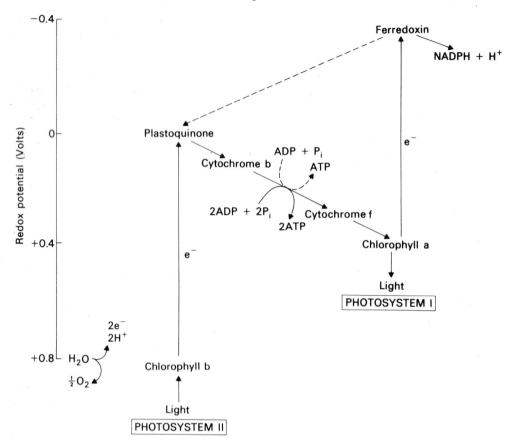

Fig. 4.48. The light reaction in photosythesis.

These reactions occur by means of an electron transport system referred to as the 'Z' scheme (Fig. 4.48). This is non-cyclic photo-induced electron transport. Cyclic photo-induced electron flow occurs in Photosystem I alone, with ATP production but no reduced $NADP^+$ formation.

The overall reaction is expressed:

$$NADP^+ + H_2O + 2ADP + P_i \xrightarrow{\text{Light}} NADPH + H^+ + \tfrac{1}{2}O_2 + 2ATP$$

The formation of ATP is coupled to the transfer of electrons from cytochrome b to cytochrome f. The energy stored in $NADPH + H^+$ and ATP can then be utilized in the dark reaction to reduce CO_2 to carbohydrate.

As shown in Fig. 4.48 two light reactions occur when energy enters the system to raise the energy from a redox potential of $+0.8$ volts in H_2O to -0.34 volts in $NADPH + H^+$. These two systems known as Photosystem I and Photosystem II, involve two types of chloro phyll—chlorophyll a or I, with a light absorption maximum in the blue-green wavelength and chlorophyll b or II, with an absoption maximum in the yellow-green wavelength.

The dark reaction, wherein CO_2 is reduced to carbohydrate, requires the presence of 2 $NADPH + H^+$ and 3 ATP per molecule of CO_2 and is also referred to as CO_2 fixation (or the Calvin cycle after Melvin Calvin, under whose direction most of the work was carried out). This cycle involves a series of reactions similar to those of the pentose phosphate pathway (p. 212) and glycolysis (p. 181) in which reactions of triose, tetrose, pentose, hexose and heptose sugars are interrelated. The initial reaction involves the addition of CO_2 to ribulose-1,5-diphosphate

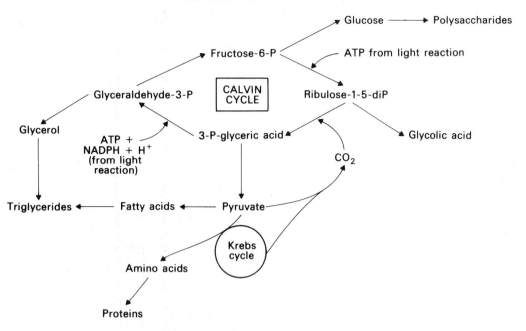

Fig. 4.49. The dark reaction (Calvin cycle) in photosynthesis.

with the formation of two molecules of 3-phosphoglyceric acid.

The conversion of 3-phosphoglyceric acid to glyceraldehyde-3-phosphate involves utilization of ATP energy and reduction of the carboxyl group to an aldehyde; thus the energy trapped by the photosynthetic reactions in the form of ATP and NADPH + H$^+$ has been transferred to a triose sugar. Subsequent reactions involve regeneration of CO_2 and ribulose-1,5-diphosphate and the conversion of glyceraldehyde-3-phosphate to carbohydrates, fats and amino acids. Some of these interrelationships are illustrated in Fig. 4.49.

The overall efficiency of plants in capturing light energy is only about 2%·

The biosynthesis of small molecules

THE FATTY ACIDS

The β-oxidation breakdown of fatty acids (p. 205) is not a reversible process whereby fatty acids can be synthesized. Their synthesis involves addition of a 2C unit to a 3C unit; with subsequent loss of CO_2, to form a 4C unit. In effect fatty acids are thus built up by successive condensations of 2C units. This distinctly different process (Fig. 4.50) occurs in the cytoplasm.

The 3C compound involved in the reaction is malonyl-S-CoA, formed by carboxylation of acetyl-S-CoA. This formation of malonyl-S-CoA involves addition of CO_2 (from bicarbonate), to acetyl-S-CoA in the presence of ATP, and is catalysed by the enzyme *acetyl coenzyme A carboxylase* which requires biotin as cofactor (p. 815). In the presence of an acyl carrier protein (ACP-SH) the 3C malonyl-S-CoA formed reacts with a molecule of acetyl-S-CoA (the 2C unit), to form a 'starter' molecule for the subsequent build up of fatty acids with an even number of carbon atoms. This 5C starter compound is then decarboxylated, in the presence of NADPH, to give 4C butyryl-S-CoA which then reacts with a further molecule of malonyl-S-CoA to produce, after removal of CO_2, a 6C fatty acid. Repetition of this mechanism leads eventually to the formation of the commonly occurring saturated fatty acids such as palmitic acid (16C) and stearic acid (18C).

The group of enzymes catalysing these reactions is known collectively as the '*fatty acid synthetase complex*'.

The formation of unsaturated fatty acids in most organisms is by oxidation of the already formed saturated fatty acids, and involves O_2, and NADPH. Double bond formation (desaturation) occurs most readily at the $\omega 9$ position (e.g. oleic acid; p. 149): only plants have the

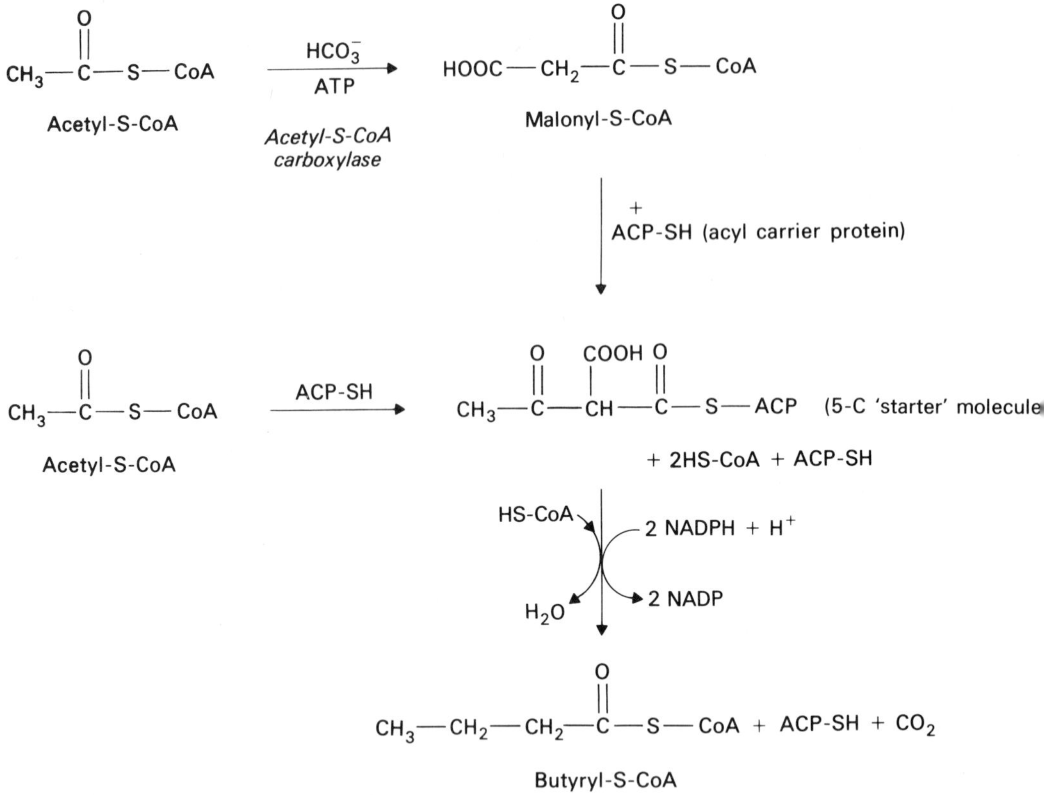

Fig. 4.50. The biosynthesis of fatty acids.

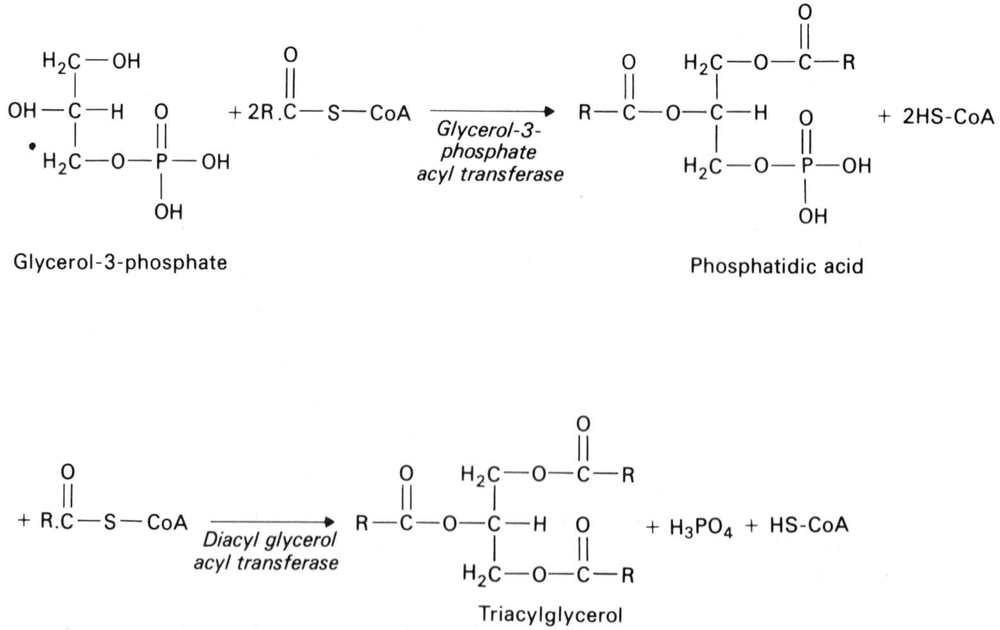

Fig. 4.51. Triglyceride biosynthesis.

ability to insert a double bond in the $\omega6$ position to produce the essential fatty acid linoleic (18:2).

Triglyceride synthesis (Fig. 4.51)

Triglyceride synthesis is mainly via the glycerol phosphate pathway. Fatty acids are first activated by reaction with acetyl-S-CoA, and two of these thiolester fatty acyl-S-CoA molecules (R.CO-S-CoA) react with glycerol-3-phosphate to give phosphatidic acid, a phosphorylated diglyceride. Next this is dephosphorylated and reacts with a third fatty acyl-S-CoA molecule to give the triglyceride.

Glycerol-3-phosphate is formed by reduction of dihydroxyacetone phosphate, an intermediate in the Embden–Meyerhof glycolysis pathway (Fig. 4.16).

Phospholipid synthesis (Fig. 4.52)

The simplest phospholipid is the glycerophospholipid phosphatidic acid, which also serves as the starting material for the synthesis of the other glycerophospholipids. In phosphatidyl choline (lecithin), choline is bound in an ester linkage to the phosphate group of phosphatidic acid. In its biosynthesis choline (p. 224) is first phosphorylated with ATP by the enzyme *choline kinase*. The phosphorylcholine (PC) so formed is then activated by cytidine triphosphate (CTP) when *PC-cytidyl transferase* enzyme forms cytidine diphosphoryl (CDP)-choline, which then reacts with the phosphatidic acid to yield phosphatidyl choline with release of cytidine monophosphate (CMP).

The sphingophospholipids contain sphingosine as the alcohol instead of glycerol, and one fatty acyl chain only. The main biosynthetic reaction also involves cytidine triphosphate

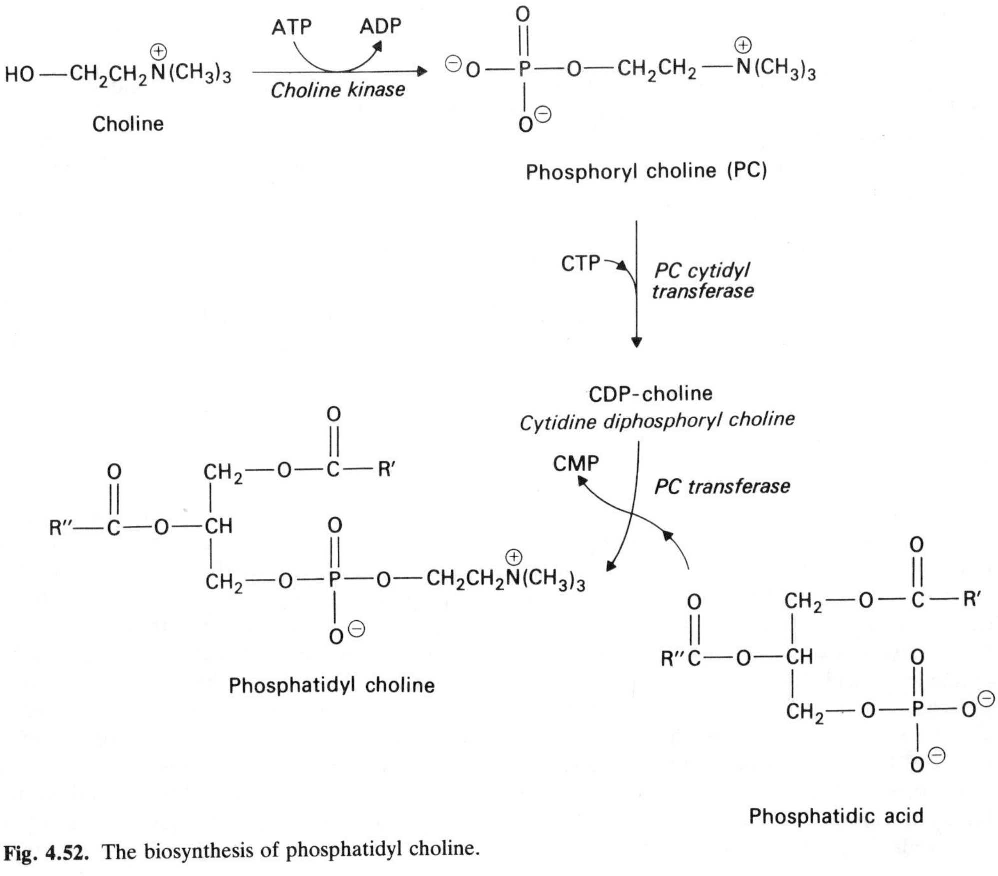

Fig. 4.52. The biosynthesis of phosphatidyl choline.

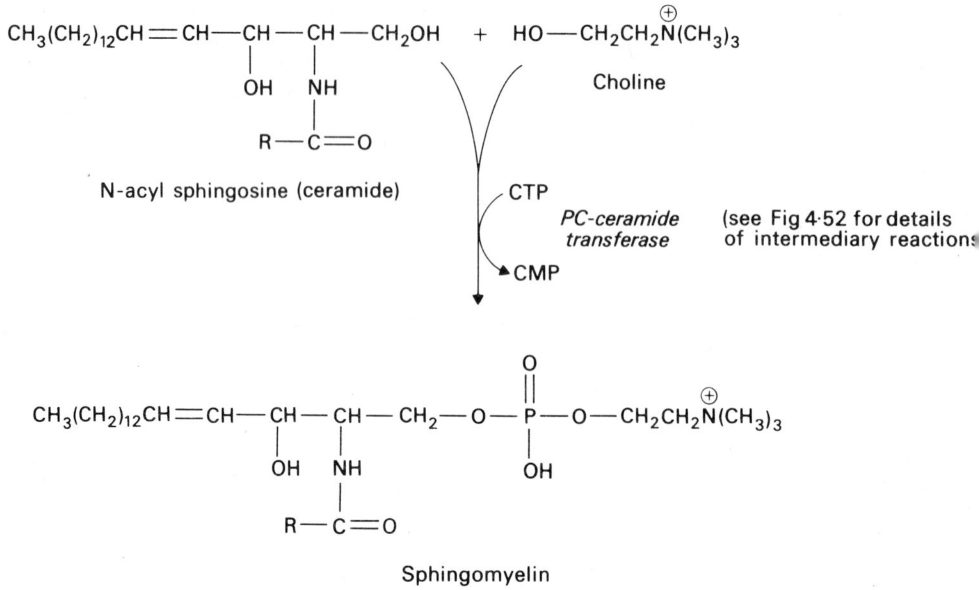

$$CH_3(CH_2)_{12}CH=CH-CH-CH-CH_2OH \quad + \quad HO-CH_2CH_2\overset{\oplus}{N}(CH_3)_3$$

with OH and NH substituents on the CH groups, and R—C=O attached to NH.

N-acyl sphingosine (ceramide)

Choline

CTP

PC-ceramide
transferase

(see Fig 4·52 for details
of intermediary reactions)

CMP

$$CH_3(CH_2)_{12}CH=CH-CH-CH-CH_2-O-\overset{\overset{\displaystyle O}{\|}}{\underset{\underset{\displaystyle OH}{|}}{P}}-O-CH_2CH_2\overset{\oplus}{N}(CH_3)_3$$

with OH and NH substituents, and R—C=O attached to NH.

Sphingomyelin

Fig. 4.53. The biosynthesis of sphingomyelin.

(CTP) acting in a similar way to phosphatidyl choline synthesis but with ceramide as the phosphorylcholine (PC) acceptor (Fig. 4.53). Recently an additional biosynthetic pathway has been found:

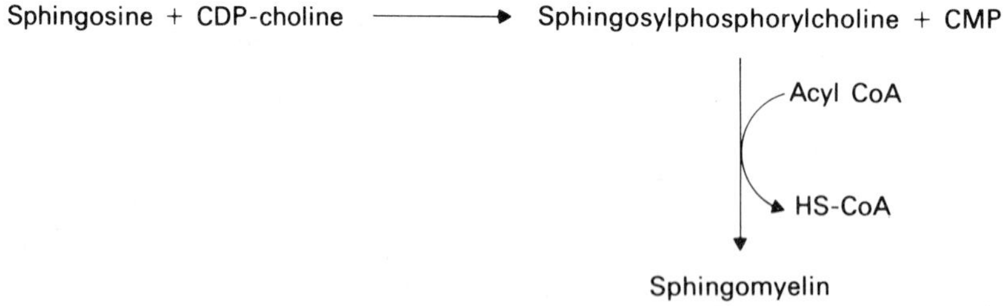

Sphingosine + CDP-choline $\longrightarrow$ Sphingosylphosphorylcholine + CMP

Acyl CoA

HS-CoA

Sphingomyelin

ture of linoleic acid and arachidonic acid i shown in Table 3.17 (p. 147).

The symptoms of EFA deficiency are divers and appear within three or four weeks of placing weanling rats on a deficient diet. Major symp

Essential fatty acids

The importance of fatty acids in the diet of animals was not realised until 1929 when Burr and Burr showed that a fat-free diet fed to rats produced acute deficiency symptoms which could be relieved by administering linoleic or arachidonic acid. First called vitamin F, these fatty acids were later termed the essential fatty acids (EFAs) and others have since been found to have EFA activity. The common feature between them is the position of specific double bonds on carbon atoms 6 and 9, counting from the terminal methyl group (i.e. $\omega 6,9$). The struc-

toms are poor growth which stops completely a three to four months, scaly skin resulting in water loss, swelling of the tip of the tail which may become necrotic, swelling of the feet, loss o hair and a general failure to thrive. The animal become sterile and many cell and tissue change occur: liver mitochondria become swollen periodontal tissues become inflamed, there is associated bone resorption, and malformation in enamel and dentine occur with an increase in caries incidence reported. Lipid metabolism i altered to give increased triglyceride synthesi and alterations in the fatty acid composition o phospholipids. All these symptoms are pre-. vented or reversed by administration of linoleic or arachidonic acid. Some EFA deficiency effects occur in a variety of animals including man, though no well documented deficiency-state symptoms have been described in humans.

Linoleic acid is produced by plants and is a major component of many seed oils. Arachidonic acid is only found in animal tissues and is derived from linoleic acid via γ-linolenic acid. Animals are unable to synthesize linoleic acid because they lack the enzyme for introduc-

tion of a double bond between carbon atoms Δ12 and 13 (or ω6 and 7: see p. 149).

The metabolic pathway for conversion of linoleic acid to arachidonic acid in animals which occurs in the liver is as follows:

$$\text{Linoleic} \longrightarrow \text{γLinolenic}$$
$$(\omega 6,9; \text{C18:2}) \qquad (\omega 6,9,12; \text{C18:3})$$
$$\downarrow$$
$$\text{Arachidonic} \longleftarrow \text{Dihomo-γlinolenic}$$
$$(\omega 6,9,12,15; \text{C20:4}) \qquad (\omega 6,9,12; \text{C20:3})$$

The mechanism is shown in Fig. 4.54

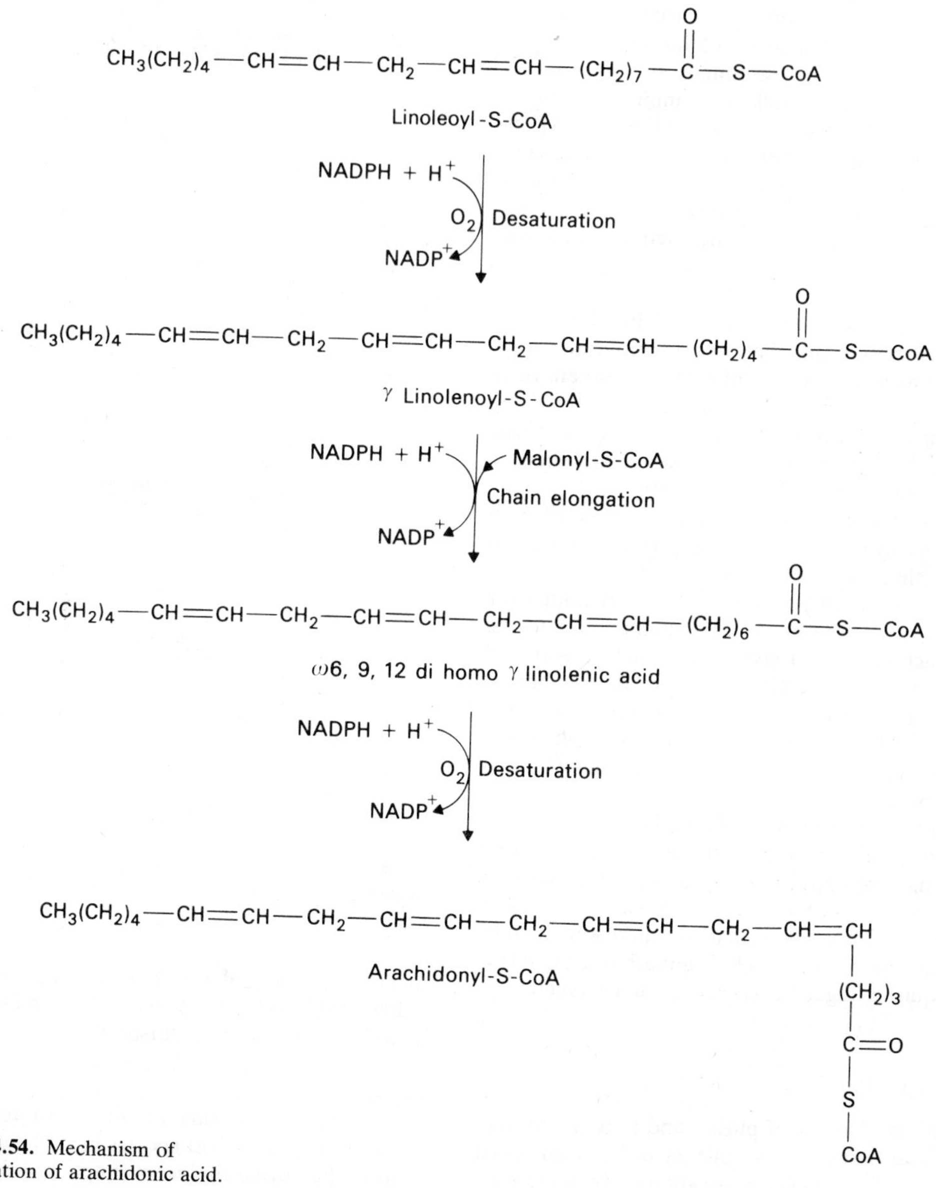

Fig. 4.54. Mechanism of formation of arachidonic acid.

The detailed function of EFAs is still uncertain but in animals they appear to have at least two roles. Firstly linoleic acid, as a component of many phospholipids, notably phosphatidyl ethanolamine, is important in cell membrane structures (p. 156). In the EFA deficiency state the linoleic acid is replaced by fatty acids such as stearic and oleic acids, altering the properties of the phospholipids and so weakening the membranes. Liver mitochondria in EFA deficient rats swell and are readily disrupted. This may explain other symptoms such as scaly skin and tissue swelling.

A second function of essential fatty acids in animals is as precursors of the prostaglandins These compounds stimulate smooth muscle, increase platelet stickiness, inhibit release of fatty acids from adipose tissue, affect blood pressure and capillary permeability, release calcium from bones and noradrenalin from nerve endings. Disturbance of prostaglandin formation may explain many EFA deficiency symptoms.

Prostaglandins
Prostaglandins are elevated in fever and inflammation and fall when antipyretic drugs such as aspirin are administered. The enzymes synthesizing prostaglandins are inhibited by aspirin and it is thought therefore that its pharmacological effect may be due to inhibition of prostaglandin synthesis (p. 800).

The formation of prostaglandin from EFAs is primarily dependent on the presence of the $\omega 6$ double bond.

There are three classes of prostaglandin, each with two double bonds less than their precursors. Arachidonic acid gives rise to the E_2 series of prostaglandins (PGE_2) with two double bonds. The PGE_1 and PGE_3 series have one and three double bonds and are derived from di-homo-γ-linolenic acid and eicosapentanoic acid (C20:5) respectively.

Fig. 4.55 shows the PGE_2 biosynthesis. The ability of the arachidonic acid chain to fold brings the appropriate groups into position to allow ring closure; the enzymes responsible for the reaction are present in the microsomes, and a reducing cofactor such as glutathione (GSH) is required, together with molecular oxygen.

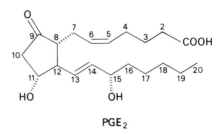

Fig. 4.55. Synthesis of prostaglandin PGE_2.

to the formation of the final nucleotides, the individual bases are built up in a *de novo* fashion attached to a ribose precursor.

THE PURINE AND PYRIMIDINE NUCLEOTIDES

The mechanism of purine and pyrimidine nucleotide biosynthesis appears to be a universal process in both plants and animals. In both, prior

Purines
Only a few organisms require a preformed source of purines: most species have the ability to form the purine ring from simple precursors.

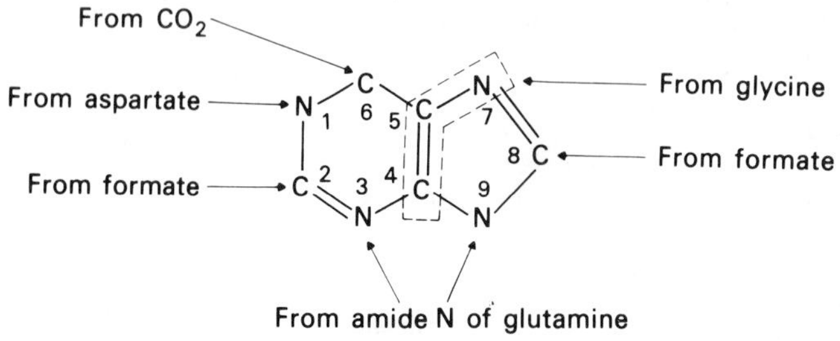

Fig. 4.56. Origin of atoms present in the purine nucleus.

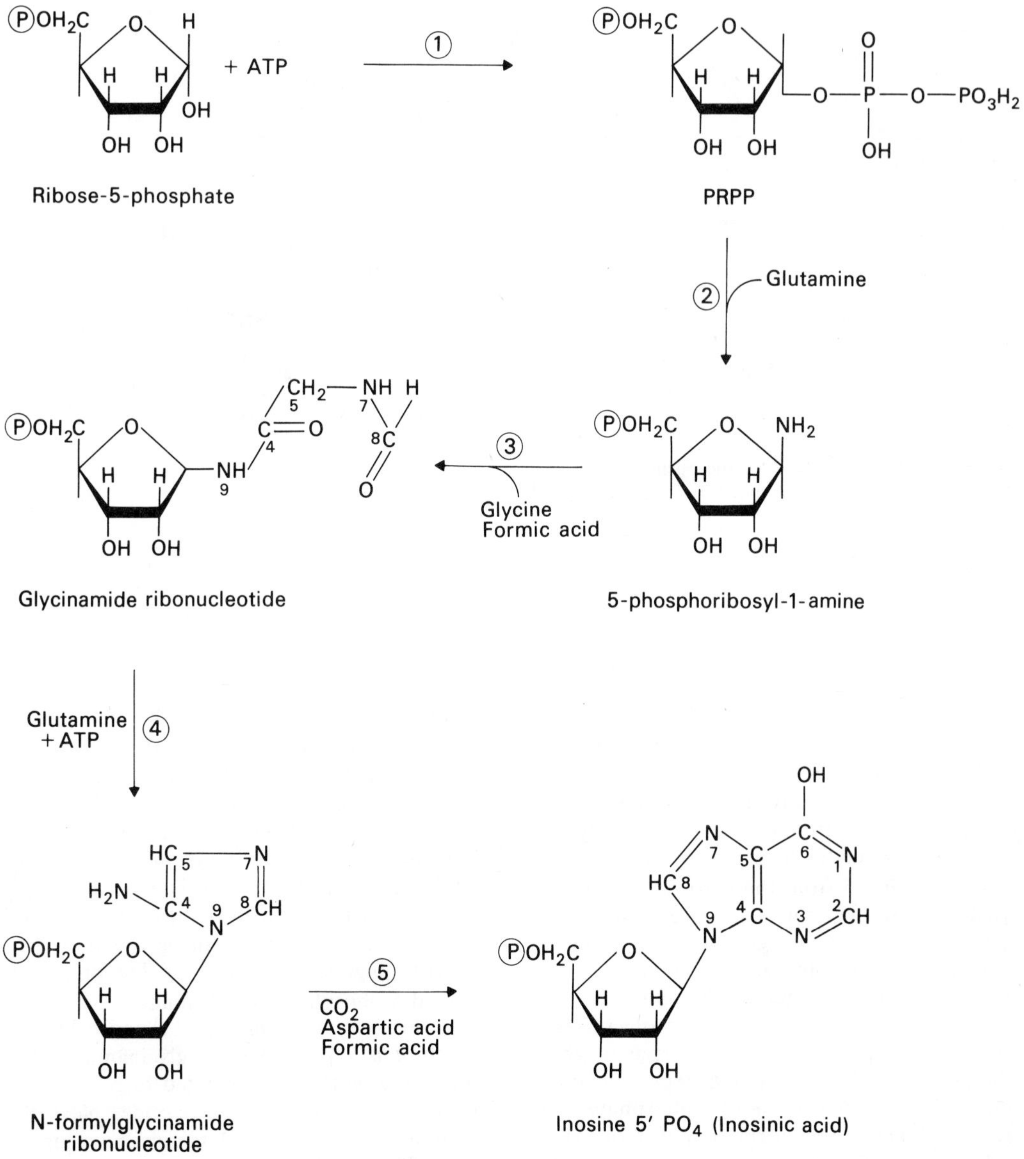

Fig. 4.57. The biosynthesis of the purine ring I. The formation of inosine 5′ phosphate from precursors.

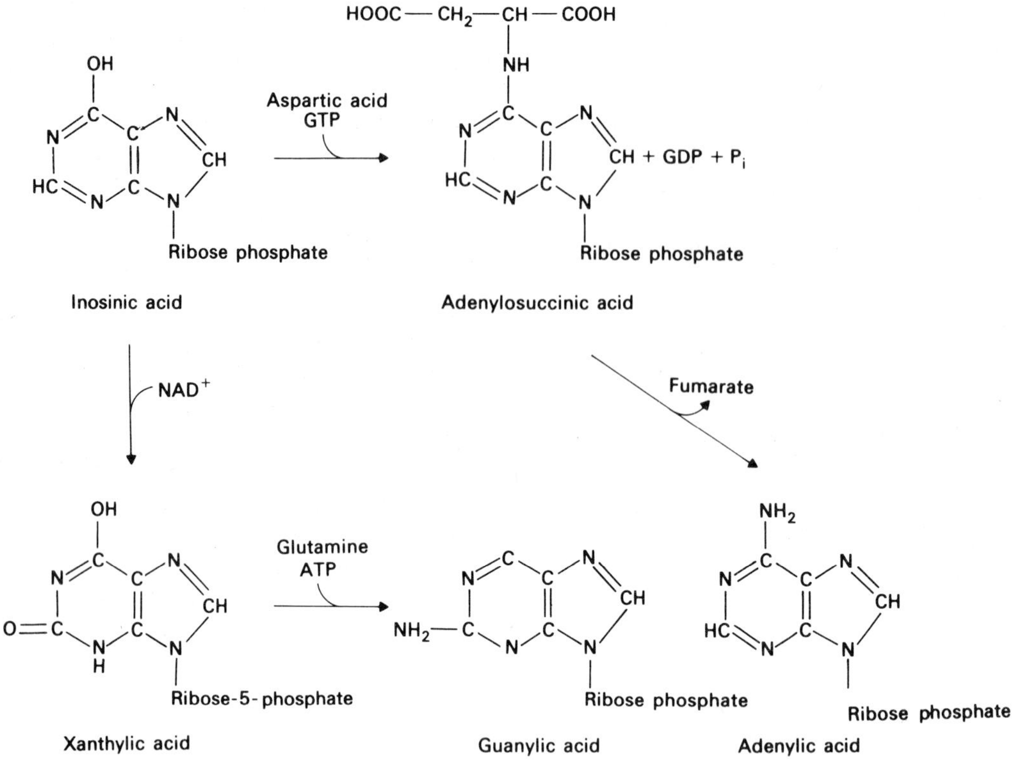

Fig. 4.58. The biosynthesis of the purine ring. The conversion of inosinic acid to adenylic acid and guanylic acid.

The origin of the individual atoms of the purine nucleus was established by use of classical isotope incorporation studies (Fig. 4.56).

Carbons 2 and 8 derive from formate, or from 1-C units arising from either serine or glycine. Carbon 6 originates from carbon dioxide, and carbons 4 and 5 from the carboxyl and methylene carbons of glycine respectively. Nitrogen 7 arises from glycine nitrogen. Nitrogen 1 derives from aspartic acid and nitrogens 3 and 9 come from the amide nitrogen of glutamine.

The biosynthetic process consists of a series of successive enzyme-catalysed reactions in which the purine ring is built up in a stepwise manner on the C-1 position of ribose-5-phosphate, thus leading directly to the formation of purine ribonucleotides appear as intermediates in the sequence. A key nucleotide, inosinic acid, is formed, which is the reactive form from which the subsequent purine nucleotides are derived. sequent purine nucleotides are derived.

In the early part of the synthetic sequence 5-phosphoribosyl-1-pyrophosphate (PRPP) is formed by phosphorylation of ribose-5-phosphate (Fig. 4.57, reaction 1). Next the amine group of glutamine is enzymically transferred to carbon 1 of the ribose ring of PRPP giving rise to the eventual nitrogen 9 of the purine ring (Fig. 4.57, reaction 2). The product is termed 5-phosphoribosyl-1-amine.

In the next reaction (3), the entire glycine structure is added to yield glycinamide ribonucleotide which is formylated to produce N-formyl glycinamide ribonucleotide. Next the addition of a further glutamine nitrogen in an ATP-requiring reaction (4) produces N-formylglyciniamidine ribonucleotide. In a further complex series of enzymically controlled

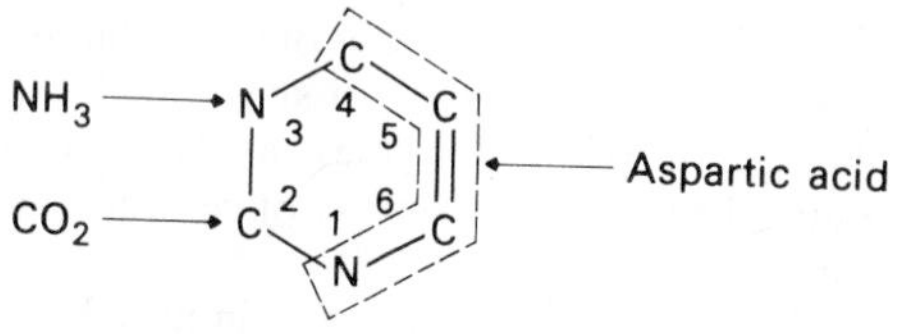

Fig. 4.59. Origin of the atoms present in the pyrimidine nucleus.

reactions (5) carbon 6, nitrogen 1 and carbon 2 are formed from carbon dioxide, aspartic acid and formate respectively and lead to the formation of inosine-5-phosphate (inosinic acid).

Inosinic acid undergoes a series of conversions to give rise to adenylic acid and guanylic acid. In the former instance inosine-5-phosphate reacts with guanosine triphosphate (GTP) and aspartic acid to give adenyl succinic acid which subsequently undergoes a non-hydrolytic cleavage to

yield adenylic acid and fumaric acid (Fig. 4.58).

The conversion of inosine-5-phosphate to guanylic acid proceeds via an initial oxidation to xanthylic acid followed by amination in the presence of glutamine and ATP (Fig. 4.58).

The deoxyribonucleotides of the above derivatives are formed by a reduction of the hydroxyl group of carbon-1 of the ribose sugar. The reactions involve Vitamin B_2 and occur at the nucleotide level.

Pyrimidines

A main distinction between the metabolic routes leading to the formation of purine and pyrimidine nucleotides is the timing in the synthetic sequence of the introduction of the N-glycosidic linkage between the sugar and the nitrogenous base. In contrast to purine synthesis the complete pyrimidine nucleus is synthesized prior to its attachment to 5-phosphoribosyl-1-pyrophosphate (PRPP). The key intermediate involved in the forma-

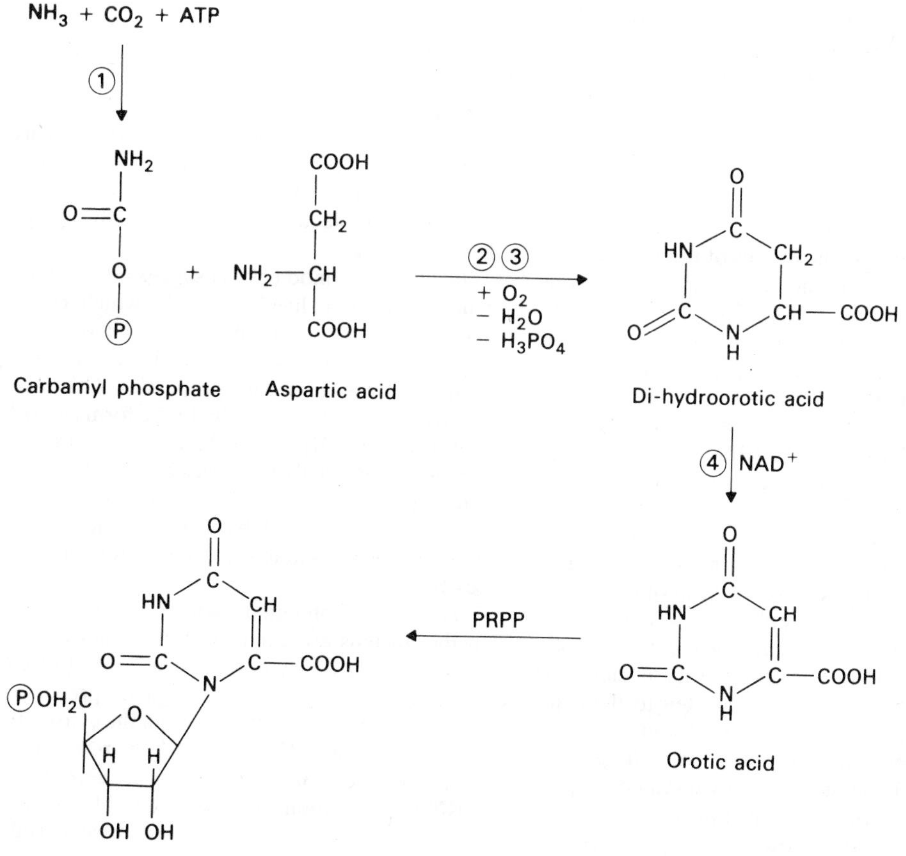

Fig. 4.60. The biosynthesis of pyrimidines. The formation of orotidylic acid from carbamyl phosphate.

tion of the N-glycosidic linkage is orotic acid which contains the pyrimidine nucleus.

Studies with isotopic precursors have shown that the pyrimidine nucleus is formed from simple precursors as shown in the structure below (Fig. 4.59).

The initial step in the formation of the pyrimidine nucleus is the formation of carbamyl phosphate from ammonia, carbon dioxide and ATP (Fig. 4.60, reaction 1). The carbamyl phosphate then reacts with L-aspartic acid to produce N-carbamylaspartic acid under the control of the enzyme *aspartate transcarbamylase* (2). The structure of the pyrimidine ring is effected by ring closure of the N-carbamylaspartic acid following the removal of a water to give dihydroorotic acid (reaction 3), which is subsequently oxidized (4) to the key precursor of pyrimidines, orotic acid.

The pyrimidine nucleotide is formed by the coupling of orotic acid with PRPP to produce orotidine-5-phosphate (orotidylic acid).

Orotidine-5-phosphate is decarboxylated to yield uridine 5 phosphate. The only known pathway for the formation of a cytidine nucleotide involves the ATP-controlled amination of uridine-5-phosphate to produce cytidine triphosphate.

Biosynthesis of proteins

Before describing the details of the mechanisms of protein synthesis the properties and functions of the different RNA structures (mRNA, tRNA, sRNA) (p. 105) will be examined in relation to the role they play individually in translating the genetic information into tangible structural features and metabolic activities in the cell. As discussed (p. 102) the genetic information is locked up in a chemically coded form in each nuclear DNA molecule and it is the ordered arrangement of the purine and pyrimidine bases along the DNA strands which constitute the variables that are the basis of the chemically determined genetic code. These coded genetic instructions in the nuclear DNA molecules are 'read' (transcribed) in the nucleus and the messages received transported to the cytoplasm where they are translated and expressed physically by exactly ordering (directly and indirectly) the synthesis of vast numbers of proteins—the enzymes, structure proteins, immunoglobulins, transport proteins, etc.

The DNA coded information is therefore expressed in:

1   A direction of the synthesis of the architectural components of cells and tissues,
2   Formation of the enzymes involved in the myriads of biological reactions of cell metabolism and
3   The synthesis—directly or indirectly—of numerous biomolecules.

Thus the sum total of the organism's activity is determined and controlled by nuclear information directing protein synthesis (p. 271).

The detailed decription of how this is achieved and the exact chemical nature of the genetic code is largely based on investigations made on bacterial (prokaryote) cells. The results of such work are not necessarily applicable to understanding the activities of the multi-chromosomal nucleated cells of higher eukaryote organisms such as trees or mammals. Nevertheless the essential unity of biochemistry throughout life processes does suggest that such data provide a substantial basis for understanding the same processes in higher life forms.

MESSENGER RNA (mRNA)

The copying of a DNA molecule to form mRNA is called transcription (p. 107). This phase of nucleotide activity is the first of the events by which the genetic information stored in the DNA molecule is transferred to the cytoplasm of the cell.

Jacob and Monod (1961) suggested the existence of a short-lived molecule which could physically carry information between the nucleus and the cytoplasm and which by definition would possess messenger properties. This then acted as a template and code for the formation of one or more polypeptide chains during protein synthesis. Originally there was only circumstantial evidence for the existence of such a messenger RNA (mRNA), but later specific mRNA moleules were isolated and characterized successfully.

The mRNA precursor molecules synthesized in the nucleus are extensively modified before they leave for the cytoplasm as mRNA. Indeed only a fraction of the original precursor molecules are transported through the cytosol to the ribosome site. The reason for the removal of large sections of intervening sequences in mRNA maturation, and the roles of the discarded sequences is uncertain at present (but see p. 246).

A complicating factor in purification of

mRNA is that the half-life for mRNA in bacterial cells is only about 2 minutes, due to their degradation by RNA *depolymerases*. The liberated nucleotides found are used for resynthesis—a process important to the economy of the cell in adapting to rapidly changing environmental influences.

The region of a mRNA chain which codes for the complete synthesis of a particular polypeptide chain of a protein molecule is termed a *cistron*. Certain mRNAs carry the information for more than one polypeptide and are therefore called polycistrons.

TRANSFER RNA (tRNA)

Transfer RNA molecules are specifically used in the recognition and transfer of amino acids from the cytoplasmic amino acid pool to the sites of protein synthesis on the ribosomes. There is a different and specific tRNA for each amino acid coded for in the DNA molecule.

Transfer RNAs are relatively small molecules composed of about 75–93 nucleotide units, and with molecular weights in the range 23 000–30 000. Although each tRNA molecule is specific for a particular amino acid some amino acids may have more than one tRNA. For example *E. coli* possesses five tRNA molecules specific for leucine. Transfer RNAs are characterized by the presence of a small quantity of unusual nucleotides which may comprise up to 10% of the total structure. Examples of these bases are 5-methylcytosine, 5-hydroxymethylcytosine, pseudouridylic acid and ribothymidylic acid.

A feature of all tRNAs so far studied is the occurrence of a strict order of terminal nucleotides. At their 3'-end all tRNAs have the trinucleotide sequence cytosine–cytosine–adenine. This is the site of attachment for the particular amino acids involved. The 2' and 3'-hydroxyl groups of the terminal adenine nucleotide remain unsubstituted and are essential for binding the amino acid. The 5'-end of all tRNA polynucleotides terminates in guanine which contains an extra phosphate group on its 5'-hydroxyl position.

In view of these identical terminal sequences in all tRNAs other structural features of the molecules must explain their individual specificities shown for particular amino acids and also their recognition of each tRNA-amino acid complex in the protein synthesis mechanism.

To this end there is evidence that tRNAs each possess a highly ordered 3-dimensional cloverleaf type configuration (Fig. 4.61) which includes a certain sequence of bases quite specific to each tRNA. Base sequence studies show that each tRNA contains its own characteristic triplet base sequence important for recognition of its template site during polypeptide formation. This base triplet sequence is termed the *anticodon* region and its role is important to the later discussion on protein synthesis. Moreover one further recognition site must be present in the molecule to find the correct aminoacyl synthetase enzymes necessary for linking the specific amino acid to the tRNA structure.

Double helical regions exist in tRNA where complementary base pairs form hydrogen bonding. The importance of this configuration to biological activity is indicated from the observation that unfolded tRNA is unable to accept amino acids.

The presence of the minor bases in tRNA is now seen to be important in establishing the configuration of these molecules. Certain of these bases have been described (p. 102). others include inosine and the sulphur-containing base, thiouridine., These bases are unable to form hydrogen-bonded complementary pairs and may explain one fascinating feature which has characterized each tRNA molecule isolated to date. Although the base sequence of the tRNAs differ markedly in composition each is potentially capable of existing in a clover-leaf structure which contains four spatial arms. In the larger tRNA molecules a fifth arm may exist. The formation of spatial arms of the tRNA is thought to be due to the presence of the unusual bases in the molecule preventing pairing and so exposing parts of the nucleotide chain.

RIBOSOMAL RNA(rRNA) AND RIBOSOME STRUCTURE

Ribosomes are composed of rRNA and protein. The ratio of rRNA to protein in eukaryotic cells is approximately 1:1 whereas in *E. coli* the ratio is nearer 2:1. In eukaryotic cells the ribosomes are generally associated with the endoplasmic reticulum: in *E. coli* most of the ribosomes are free in the cytoplasm where they comprise almost 25% of the total cell mass. In most instances ribosomes are arranged like beads, being attached to a mRNA thread. Ribosomes arranged in this way are called polyribosomes or polysomes.

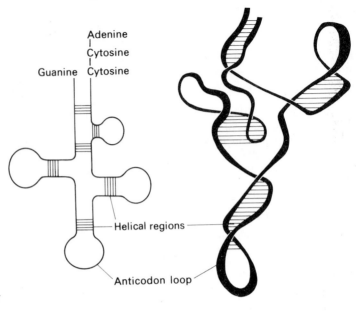

Adenine
Cytosine
Guanine Cytosine

Helical regions

Anticodon loop

Fig. 4.61. Structures of transfer RNA showing (a) the clover-leafed model, and (b) its suggested spatial structure.

(a)   **(b)**

Electron microscopy of the ribosomes isolated from the cells of many organisms showed that each ribosome was constructed of two subunits differing in size and sedimentation coefficients. The intact ribosome unit from *E. coli* has a sedimentation coefficient of 70S while the separated subunits have coefficients of 50S (large subunit) and 30S (small subunit) respectively. Three sizes of rRNA are found in these subunits. The 50S component possesses rRNA molecules of 23S and 5S sedimentation values while the small subunit contains 16S rRNA. Ribosomes are stable and undissociated at relatively high concentrations of magnesium ions but readily dissociate into the two subunits when the magnesium ion concentration is lowered. The overall architecture of the intact ribosome has been compared to a cottage-loaf with the 30S unit placed on the upper part of the structure.

The role of ribosomal RNA in the ribosome is still uncertain. Current opinion favours the view that it functions in orientating the ribosomal structure during peptide synthesis and in some way must interact with the mRNA molecules during its association with the ribosome.

GENETIC CODE

How is the actual genetic information locked up in a polynucleotide examined, understood, and the message translated into the production of a polypeptide?

The story of this investigation constitutes one of the most exciting pieces of biological detective work achieved by modern science. One major problem was how the four bases present in DNA (adenine, guanine, thymine and cytosine) could code for each of the 20 different amino acids normally present in proteins. From a permutation and combination standpoint if one base codes for one amino acid then theoretically only four amino acids will be coded for. If two bases together coded for one amino acid then only a maximum of 16 (4^2) amino acids could be specified, as 4^2 is the total number of possible ways two bases can be chosen from a pool of four different bases. The minimum number of bases required for the coding of one amino acid must therefore be three. 64 is the total number of ways three can be selected from four different bases ($4^3=64$), a figure large enough to allow coding for all of the 20 amino acids. Experimental evidence that the code was arranged in such triplet form was provided by Francis Crick (1966) using mutants of the virus, T4 bacteriophage. His evidence proved that the code functioned as a series of base triplets of purines and/or pyrimidine combination, arranged alongside each other and not overlapping. Each triplet of bases is termed a *codon* and the evidence for

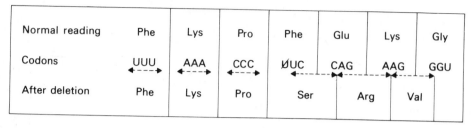

Fig. 4.62. Evidence for triplet codons. The triplets normally give rise to the amino acid sequence shown above. Deletion of a single base alters the triplet sequencing to produce the amino acid pattern shown on the lower line.

their presence is shown diagrammatically in Fig. 4.62.

The code is called *degenerate* because more than one codon exists for each amino acid. With 64 possible combinations of the 4 nucleotide bases and only 20 amino acids needed to be coded for, then either 44 triplet codes have no role to play or there must be more than one triplet code for some or all of the amino acids. This latter possibility (a degenerate code) occurs, supported by such experimental evidence as the fact that several tRNAs exist for each amino acid.

The solution to the problem of the spelling of a code with respect to the amino acids, was initiated by Nirenberg who used *E. coli* extracts freed of DNA by treatment with deoxyribonuclease, but still containing all the necessary ingredients to carry out protein synthesis. Addition of a synthetic messenger RNA to this system in the form of polyuridylic acid (poly U) greatly increased the incorportation of ^{14}C-phenylalanine into a polypeptide which was then found to be a polyphenylalanine. Of 18 amino acids tested in this poly U system only phenylalanine was incorporated into the polypeptide formed, thus establishing that one of the codons for phenylalanine was UUU. Similar studies indicated that polyadenylic acid coded for polylysine and polycytidylic acid coded for polyproline establishing that AAA and CCC were codons for lysine and proline respectively.

Use of synthetic heteropolynucleotides by Nirenberg and Leder in 1964 provided further information on the spelling of the code. These workers were able to synthesize a mRNA from uracil and guanine present in the ratio 2:1. Fragmentation of the polynucleotide formed into three-base sequences led to the isolation of a number of combinations of U and G including three triplets composed of UUG, UGU, and GUU. Using their *E. coli* synthetic system they showed that GUU coded for valine. It was next shown that a synthetic mRNA composed of the base sequence UCUCUCUC led to the alternate incorporation of serine and leucine. A reading of the code as non-overlapping triplets indicated that UCU and CUC must code for serine and leucine respectively.

In this way a whole dictionary has been compiled of the codes (codons) for each amino acid (Table 4.6). Present evidence indicates that the code is universal in operation, in the sense that the same codons operate throughout all forms of living matter. Thus in cell-free extracts of many microorganisms, and from the tissues of higher plants and animals the addition of poly U stimulates the incorporation of phenylalanine into proteins. Further evidence for the universality of the code stems from studies on homologous proteins isolated from many distantly related species. Studies on cytochrome c for example indicate that large portions of the primary protein sequence are identical for a wide variety of organisms.

THE RIBOSOMAL EVENTS OF PROTEIN SYNTHESIS (Fig. 4.63)

First the amino acids taking part in the synthetic process are carried to the ribosomal surface by their respective tRNA molecules. As described, the linkage of the amino acids to their respective tRNA molecules occurs at the 3′ terminal adenosine and is a covalent bond formed between the α-carbon carboxyl group of the amino acid and the terminal ribose component of the tRNA. The 'high energy' bond linking the amino acid to its tRNA forms an activated precursor. This energy is utilized for the formation of

Table 4.6. The genetic code.

Amino acids		DNA codons
Alanine	(Ala)	CGA, CGG, CGT, CGC
Arginine	(Arg)	GCA, GCG, GLT, GCC, TCT, TCC
Asparagine	(Asn)	TTA, TTG
Aspartic acid	(Asp)	CTA, CTG
Cysteine	(Cys)	ACA, ACG
Histidine	(His)	GTA, GTG
Isoleucine	(Ile)	TAA, TAG, TAT
Glutamic acid	(Glu)	CTT, CTC
Glutamine	(Gln)	GTT, GTC
Glycine	(Gly)	CCA, CCG, CCT, CCC
Leucine	(Leu)	GAA, GAG, GAT, GAC, AAT, AAG
Lysine	(Lys)	TTT, TTC
Methionine	(Met)	TAC
Phenylalanine	(Phe)	AAA, AAG
Proline	(Pro)	GGA, GGG, GGT, GGC
Serine	(Ser)	AGA, AGG, AGT, AGC, TCA, TCG
Threonine	(Thr)	TGA, TGG, TGT, TGC
Tryptophan	(Tp)	ACC
Tyrosine	(Tyr)	ATA, ATG
Valine	(Val)	CAA, CAG, CAT, CAC

A = Adenine, G = Guanine, T = Thymine, C = Cytosine

The three remaining possible combination of bases, ACT, ATT and ATC, are the coded instructions to terminate synthesis of a polypeptide chain.

A few amino acids (e.g. hydroxyproline, hydroxylysine and γ-carboxyglutamic acid) are not incorporated directly into proteins during translation, but are formed by subsequent modification of amino acids which are incorporated in the usual way (p. 248).

the lower-energy peptide bond and comes initially from the pyrophosphate linkage (P~P) in ATP. Under the control of enzymes, the *amino-acyl synthetases*, the amino acids are activated to form amino acid adenylates in which the amino acid is combined with adenosine monophosphate (AA~AMP). The same *amino-acyl synthetases* transfer the amino acids from the adenylate complex to the respective tRNA. The overall reaction is as follows:

$$\text{Amino acid (AA)} + \text{ATP} \rightarrow \text{AA} \sim \text{AMP} + \text{PPi} .$$

amino-acyl synthetase

$$\text{AA} \sim \text{AMP} + \text{tRNA} \rightarrow \text{AA} \sim \text{tRNA} + \text{AMP}$$

The *amino-acyl synthetases* possess two recognition sites, one involved in binding a specific amino acid prior to activation and another for recognition of relevant tRNA.

In this activated form the amino acid–tRNA complex arrives at the ribosomal surface. The function of the ribosome is to correctly orientate the amino acid tRNA molecules for the translation of the genetic code, and it must necessarily also align the template mRNA and the emerging polypeptide chain. As discussed earlier ribosomes do not occur singly but as polysomes joined by a common thread of mRNA which is attached in a central groove of the smaller 30S ribosomal unit.

Polypeptide chain growth begins at the N-terminal end. In all bacterial systems studied the initiator amino acid is a specially adapted amino acid called N-formylmethionine . The methionine is formylated during attachment to tRNA and this blocking of its amino group prevents its utilization in the polypeptide chain. The formyl group is presumably then removed once the newly-synthesized polypeptide chain emerges, since N-formyl methionine has not been detected as a protein constituent. It is probable that an *amino peptidase* cleaves the intact formylated amino acid. Studies have also shown that an AUG triplet codes for N-formyl methionine, a feature which functions essen-

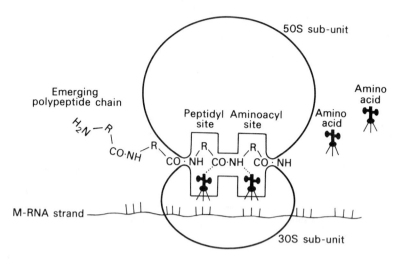

Fig. 4.63. Polypeptide synthesis at a ribosomal level. Amino acid-tRNA complexes arrive at the ribosome and take up their respective positions at the peptidyl and aminoacyl sites as determined by the mRNA anticodon triplet. The peptide bond is 'forged' between the two sites by the enzyme *peptidyl transferase* and the polypeptide chain emerges from the peptidyl site as the ribosome moves along the mRNA molecule.

tially as the capital letter beginning the sentence which spells out the genetic code to be read for a protein chain synthesis.

Chain initiation begins proper with the formation of a complex between N-formylmethionine, mRNA and the smaller 30S ribosomal subunit. The 50S unit then joins and forms the 70S ribosome. The N-formylmethionine does not join in the presence of the 50S unit, presumably a safeguard against commencing protein synthesis at a place other than the correct starting point. The 70S ribosomal particle contains two cavities or grooves termed the P (peptidyl) and A (aminoacyl) sites. Each cavity is bounded by the 30S and 50S ribosomal units and a specific mRNA codon. The AA ~ tRNA complexes fit perfectly into the cavities where their three base anticodon region recognises its specific codon triplet on the mRNA molecule.

Once the N-formylmethionine tRNA complex is fixed in the 'P' site from which the newly-synthesized protein chain will emerge, a second AA ~ tRNA unit locates on the 'A' site. Under the action of the enzyme *peptidyl transferase* a peptide bond is formed between the 'P' site carboxyl group and the 'A' site amino group. The binding of the second AA ~ tRNA complex to the 'A' site is a complicated operation. A protein transfer factor (TFI) is required, which reacts with guanosine triphosphate (GTP). A TFI-GTP complex is released and the terminal ~ Ⓟ

of the GTP is employed as an extra energy source in synthesis of the peptide bond between the 'P' and 'A' site amino acids.

After peptide bond formation the 'P' site tRNA is enzymically removed and released from the system. In order that protein synthesis may continue the 'A' site must now be vacated for receipt of a further AA-tRNA complex. This is achieved by the process termed translocation and occurs as the ribosome migrates relative to the mRNA molecule. This 'translocation' of the peptidyl-tRNA from the 'A' site to the 'P' site is also a complicated process requiring a transfer factor II and GTP. One high-energy-P is hydrolysed for each translocation step.

The model for the above stages is shown in Fig. 4.63. The newly-formed protein chain emerges via the 'P' site end of the groove, as do the released tRNA molecules which are then free to return to the cytoplasm for conveyance of further amino acids to the ribosomal surface for their incorporation.

Polypeptide chain formation ceases when a mRNA termination code (UGA, UAA, UAG) reaches the 'A' site and signals that peptide formation is to stop. This is brought about with the aid of *protein release factors* which break the bond joining the carboxyl end of the polypeptide chain so far formed with the last tRNA that arrived.

In 1977 recombinant-DNA technology estab-

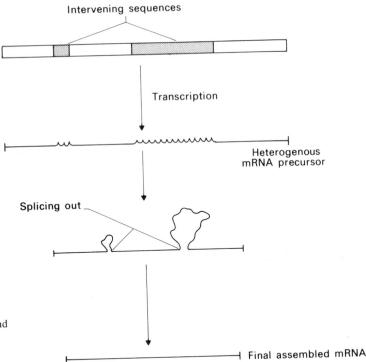

Fig. 4.64. The transcription and splicing out of intervening sequences in β-globin mRNA production.

lished that mammalian genes coding for globin polypeptides were composed of several gene segments, separated from each other by 'intervening sequences' of DNA, which do not code for amino acids.

The entire gene, with these intervening sequences, is transcribed within the cell nucleus, and the resultant 'heterogeneous RNA' is then processed by splicing out the intervening sequences to yield the messenger RNA. This then leaves the nucleus and is translated into β-globin protein on polysomes in the usual way (Fig. 4.64). Many other examples of intervening sequences have now been observed, not only in mammals, but also in birds, yeasts and viruses. The existence of the intervening sequences is established but their biological role remains a mystery.

Another recent observation is that in some viruses the genetic code is overlapping. By 'reading' the viral genome in different triplet reading frames, some organisms are able to produce different proteins from effectively the same stretch of DNA.

The biosynthesis of collagen

The fundamental mechanism of protein synthesis on the ribosomes has now been examined. This showed how the genetic information locked up in the purine–pyrimidine base triplet code was interpreted and carried by messenger RNA to the ribosome sites where the individual transfer RNAs brought their activated amino acids to be joined in the specific primary sequence structures as dictated by the genetic code message.

However, the story of protein biosynthesis does not end there—there are many subsequent modifications, orientations and cross-linking mechanisms, collectively termed the post-ribosomal events, which are not coded for in the primary message, yet contribute to the form the proteins take up in their secondary, tertiary and quaternary structures. Genetic information still directs these post-ribosomal changes but, in the indirect sense that they are brought about via other paths, usually involving enzymes which will of course have been synthesized quite separately and on the basis of quite different genetic messages.

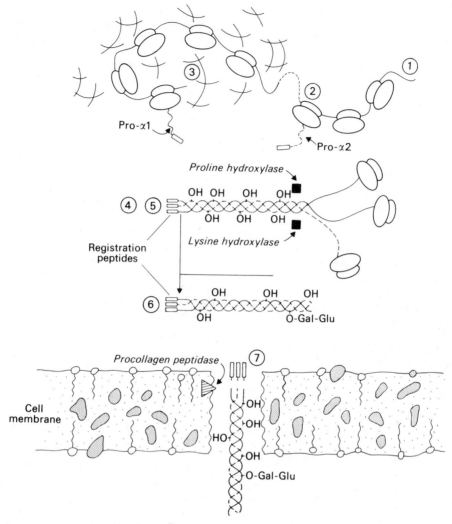

Fig. 4.65. Collagen biosynthesis I : intracellular events. (1) Synthesis of specific mRNA for collagen. (2) Translation of message by ribosomes. (3) Clustering of polysomes and association with endoplasmic reticulum. (4) Recognition and alignment of α-chains by N_t registration peptides. (5) Coiling of chains and hydroxylation of specific proline and lysine residues. (6) Glycosylation of specific hydroxylsine residues. (7) Extrusion of the completed molecule. (Carbon terminal (C_t) extensions not shown.)

The biosynthesis of collagen is a useful model for illustration of post-ribosomal stages in protein synthesis and also provides a basis for an understanding of various collagen-related genetic disorders.

Before embarking on this study of collagen biosynthesis it is essential that there is a thorough knowledge of the main features of collagen composition and structure (p. 64).

The biosynthesis of collagen is divided into two major sequences of events—first the *intracellular* events, followed by the *extracellular* stages of completion.

INTRACELLULAR EVENTS (Fig. 4.65)

These are subdivided into the following stages:
1 Formation of procollagen α-chains by polyribosome clusters.
2 Orientation of α-chains by registration peptides.

3   Hydroxylation of specific proline and lysine residues.

4   Glycosylation of some hydroxylsine residues.

1   Formation of procollagen

Because the fundamental collagen molecule is the tropocollagen subunit and because of its size —it is the longest protein molecule known— single ribosomes are not large enough to individually accommodate all the genetic information brought by the mRNA molecules directing the formation of the over 1000 residue long α-chains of collagen.

Consequently collagen is made by a continuous assembly line process which employs groups of ribosomes in polyribosome clusters. There are separate mRNAs for the α_1 chains and α_2 chains respectively which means that two different structural genes control the biosynthesis of the collagen (type I) found in bone, dentine, skin, tendon etc.

These polyribosome clusters line the endoplasmic reticulum and up to 60 may be linked together. The procollagen α (or pro-α) chains formed then pass down the cisternae of the endoplasmic reticulum, but these procollagen molecules contain no hydroxyproline (Hyp) or hydroxylysine (Hyl). This is because there is no triplet code for these two amino acids—only for proline and lysine: the formation of their hydroxy derivatives at specific positions on the α-chains is a post-ribosomal event brought about by the specific enzyme reactions described below.

The pro-α chains are formed at the rate of about 200 residues each minute, and it takes about 6 minutes to form one pro-α chain as these pro-α chains are 210 residues longer than the final α chains found in the tropocollagen molecules. A pro-α_1 chain is 1250 residues in length (mw 115 000) compared with the 1040 residue-long α_1 chain (mw 95 000).

Since there is evidence that triple helix formation occurs within 6 minutes this must mean that coiling of the three α chains begins sometime before the pro-α chain formation is complete.

2   Orientation of α-chains by registration peptides

Additional residues at the N terminal end of the pro-α_1 chains (they are the first formed, as protein synthesis starts at the N terminal end) and the corresponding regions of the α_2 chains are called the registration peptide regions of the procollagen because it is thought that they assist from the earliest stages of protein synthesis in holding the 3 polypeptide chains in correct register to each other.

These registration peptides (which are removed later) contain cysteine residues and it is thought that disulphide link bridges play a role in this orientation. This early orientation and 'recognition' mechanism provides the means whereby the 3 chains subsequently coil together into a tropocollagen 'super-helix' which forms spontaneously. Pro-α chains also bear C_t peptide extensions with disulphide links.

3   Hydroxylation of specific proline and lysine residues

As indicated the absence of specific codons for Hyp and Hyl means that their residues must be formed *in situ* by hydroxylation of Pro and Lys residues present in the pro-α chains at some time after polypeptide synthesis at the ribosome site. This occurs through the action of two enzymes, a *proline hydroxylase* and a *lysine hydroxylase*.

Both enzymes require the following to be present:

   (a) Molecular O_2 (the O for the OH comes from O_2, not H_2O)
   (b) Ferrous ion, Fe^{2+}
   (c) Ascorbic acid (vitamin C)
   (d) α-ketoglutaric acid (there is a stoichiometric relationship between pro-α chain hydroxylation and the decarboxylation of α KG to succinate + CO_2).

The need for ascorbic acid (vitamin C) as an essential redox molecule is the biochemical basis of the vitamin C deficiency disease, scurvy. Lack of vitamin C leads to imperfectly hydroxylated collagen molecules. This will result in poorly crosslinked collagen because of a resultant insufficiency of Hyl residues that are involved in such linkages (p. 69).

One of the manifestations of scurvy is fragile and bleeding gums, reflecting the defective collagen structural component of the tissue, as illustrated in this graphic contemporary account given by a French sea captain in the 16th century:

> 'Their mouths became stinking, their gums so rotten that all the flesh did fall off, even to the roots of the teeth which did also almost all fall out'.

Not only the gingival tissues are affected, but all the connective tissues—there is a general debility, loss of strength and inability to stand properly. The skin too becomes fragile, easily bruised and spotted. As is well known this condition, which particularly affected sailors on long sea voyages without ready access to fresh fruit and vegetables, was eventually prevented in the British Royal Navy in the 18th century by adoption of the policy of carrying stores of limes and lemons on long voyages. It is said this is the origin of the nick name 'limeys' given to the British by the Americans.

The factors that determine which specific Pro and Lys residues become hydroxylated are not clearly understood. However, ultimately nearly 50% of Pro residues are hydroxylated and this certainly happens before triple helix formation starts and before procollagen synthesis completes.

4 Glycosylation of hydroxylysine residues

Either galactose direct, or a glucosidyl-galactose unit, are linked via β-2,O-glycosidic links to a few Hyl residues in collagen, the numbers varying between tissues and species.

Again two enzymes are involved, a *UDP galactotransferase* to link the Gal to the Hyl residues and a *UDP glucotransferase* to link a glucose molecule to a galactose residue. Both are metalloenzymes requiring Mn^{2+}.

This also starts before procollagen synthesis is completed but clearly must follow hydroxylation of Lys residues, and is probably completed after triple helix formation.

EXTRACELLULAR EVENTS (Fig. 4.66)

These are subdivided into the following stages, which follow in time the four preceding intracellular events.

5 Removal of registration peptides
6 Formation of intramolecular crosslinks.
7 Formation of intermolecular crosslinks
   (a) intrafilamentous
   (b) interfilamentous

5 Removal of registration peptides

As explained the final hydroxylated α_1 and α_2 chains in tropocollogen are shorter than the corresponding pro-α chains by some 200 or more residues. Both the C_t peptide extension and N_t peptide used in orientating the 3 α-chains in preparation for the triple helix conformation are subsequently removed after extrusion from the cell each by a specific *procollagen peptidase* whose exact location is uncertain. Whether membrane-bound or extracellular the removal of the

C_t and N_t peptides occurs some 20 minutes after extrusion of the pro-α chains from the cell. This removal promotes fibril formation, also negatively controlled by a feed-back inhibition by the cleaved peptides on collagen synthesis.

6 Formation of intramolecular crosslinks

Description of the various Lys and Hyl aldol cross-links has been given earlier (p. 69). Here it is necessary only to add that the conversion of the sidechain terminal ϵ-NH_2 group of lysine to an aldehyde (CHO) group is catalysed by a metalloenzyme *lysine (amino) oxidase*; this requires Cu^{2+} for activation and attacks only very few residues—such as the Lys in position 9 on α_1 chains, and 5 on α_2 chains. These are in the N-terminal telopeptide region where a single aldol type intramolecular cross-link occurs between the α_1 and α_2 chains within the tropocollagen subunit.

Lathyrism. This is a condition characterized by spine deformation, bone demineralization and joint dislocation. The tissues are gelatinous and pull apart readily, and weak acetic acid or NaCl extracts of the collagenous tissues yield 5–10 times the normal content of soluble tropocollagen. It can be induced experimentally by feeding sweet peas to rats and the active principle involved is β-amino proprionitrile ($H_2N-CH_2-CH_2-C\equiv N$) which inhibits the enzyme *lysine oxidase*. Thus the symptoms of the condition reflect lack of crosslink formation involving the aldehyde derivatives of lysyl residue sidechains.

Copper deficiency. As lysyl oxidase is a Cu^{2+} dependent metalloenzyme, copper deficient diets will cause symptoms similar to lathyrism.

7 Intermolecular cross-links

(a) *Intrafilament.* These are the cross-links involved in the lateral alignment of tropocollagen subunits to produce the quarter-staggering arrays (Fig. 3.29) and the primary filaments.

(b) *Interfilament.* These form between the primary filaments, which form into the collagen fibrils (Fig. 4.66).

These intermolecular links involve predominantly the formation of Schiff-base type aldimine condensation reactions and there are four possibilities (p. 71). These cross-links characterize both intra- and interfilament connections and again, arise predominantly in the telopeptide

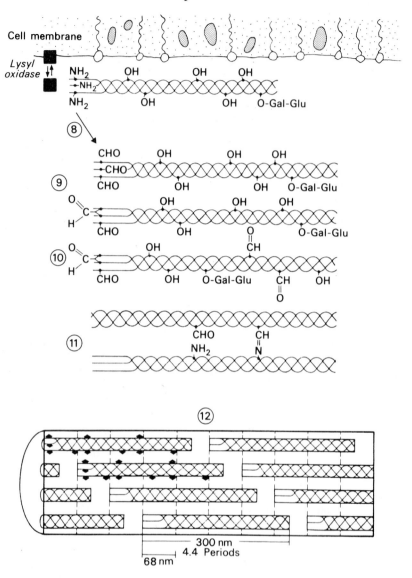

Fig. 4.66. Collagen biosynthesis II : extracellular events. (8) Biosynthesis of aldehydes near the N-terminal region. (9) Aldol condensation leading to formation of intramolecular cross-links. (10) Appearance of aldehydes in the helical region of collagen. (11) Formation of intermolecular cross-links (Schiff bases). (12) Staggering of collagen molecules within a fibre to generate the 68 nm periodicity (in the dry state). Arrows indicate the potential sites for intermolecular crosslinking (for rat skin collagen).

regions (Summary in Fig. 4.66). With progressive maturation and the age-associated changes in collagen it seems probable that increasing numbers of intermolecular cross-links should form along the whole length of tropocollagen molecules, but the evidence for this is sparse and contradictory at present.

Fig. 4.67 summarizes the above features of collagen biosynthesis in the context of cell structure (pp. 357–399).

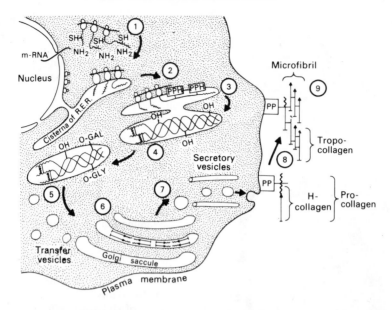

Fig. 4.67. Summary of collagen biosynthesis features in the context of cell structure. (1) Assembly of polypeptide chains by ribosomes using coded information of mRNA molecules. (2) Passage of polypeptide chains into granular endoplasmic reticulum. (3) Hydroxylation of specific lysine and proline residues by membrane-bound enzymes (PPH). (4) Alignment and coiling of polypeptide chains (α-units) to form triple helices. Note presence of terminal non-helical registration peptides. (5) Glycosylation of specific hydroxylysine residues completes the synthesis of the procollagen molecule. (6) Transport of procollagen in transfer vesicles to Golgi apparatus. (7) Transport from Golgi apparatus to plasma membrane in secretory vesicles, using microtubules as transport conduits. (8) Removal of registration peptides by enzymes (PP) to form tropocollagen. (9) Linking of tropocollagen units to form collagen microfibrils.

THE BIOCHEMICAL BASIS OF SOME GENETICALLY DETERMINED COLLAGEN DISORDERS

Knowledge of the collagen biosynthetic mechanism explains certain genetically-determined disorders on a biochemical basis.

Marfan's syndrome
This connective tissue disease is characterized by weak tendons and ligaments, 'double joints' and heart valve defects. The skins of such patients have much greater than normal amounts of soluble tropocollagen implying impaired cross-linking of tropocollagen units into insoluble quarter-staggered arrays and protofilaments. The collagen-forming cells of these individuals show a significant lack of the *lysine oxidase* enzyme needed to form the aldehyde derivatives of Lys and Hyl side-arms involved in formation of both aldol type intramolecular (aldol condensation) cross-links and the Schiff base aldimine type intermolecular crosslinks.

Scleroderma
Sufferers from this ailment show excessive amounts of collagen in the dermis, oesophagus and in cardiac and striated muscle. The explanation offered is that there is some defect in the 'feed-back' information system telling cells when to switch off collagen synthesis. The treatment involves giving patients compounds such as β-amino proprionitrile, the lathyritic agent, which blocks collagen cross-linking, thus (hopefully!) limiting the excessive overproduction of mature insoluble collagen fibres.

Homocystinuria
Clinically this condition resembles Marfan's syndrome but interestingly the genetic defect involved is not directly related to any stage of collagen biosynthesis. It involves a genetic lesion leading to lack of synthesis of the enzyme *cystathionine synthetase*. This defect leads to accumulation of homocysteine in the tissues which blocks aldehyde groups and so interferes with collagen crosslinking mechanisms.

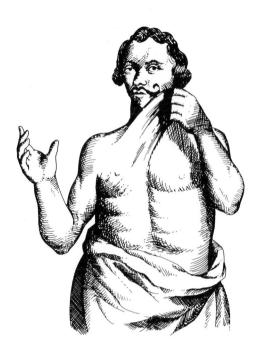

Fig 4.68. An early case of Ehlers-Danlos syndrome (1657). '...we saw in our hospital a certain young Spaniard, 23 years of age, by the name of George Albes, who with his left hand grasped the skin over his humerus and right breast and stretched it until it was quite close to his mouth. With each hand he first pulled the skin of his chin downwards like a beard to his chest, hence he lifted it upward to the vertex of his head so as to cover each eye with it. As soon s he removed his hand the skin contracted to reassume its proper smoothness. It has, so far, not been possible to learn the cause.' (After McKusick V.A. (1972) *Heritable disorders of connective tissue*, 4th edn. Philadelphia, C. V. Mosby.)

Dermatosporaxis

This is a disease of cattle and sheep characterized by fragility of the skin and due to a recessive gene. There is a lack of order in the packing arrangements of the fibrils and filaments and tissue extracts show the presence of extra peptide segments of the N-terminal ends of α-chains, which also contain cysteine. A significant proportion of pro-α_1 and pro-α_2 chains are found in the collagen of these animals. Their collagenous tissues lack the enzyme *procollagen peptidase* which clearly explains the histological features: the lack of ability to remove the registration peptides results in extrusion of collagen subunits incapable of forming into protofibrils and filaments.

Ehlers–Danlos syndrome

There are 7 types of this genetically determined collagen disease, characterized by fragility of the skin and hypermobile joints and the macabre ability to pull up great handfuls of skin (Fig. 4.68).

Examination of the tissues of patients of type VI category shows a considerable deficiency of hydroxylysine. This is due to a genetically determined lack of the enzyme *lysine hydroxylase* (the *proline hydroxylase* is present in normal amounts). The consequence is the virtual absence of Hyl, which effectively eliminates the formation of cross-links involving this amino acid residue. In contrast the Ehlers–Danlos type VII condition is due to a genetically determined deficiency of *procollagen peptidase* activity and is, therefore, the human equivalent of cattle dermatosporaxis.

Active transport

Last but by no means least in the selected examples of energy-requiring processes are the various movements of biomolecules and ions across cell membranes against concentration gradients. In the kidney 70% of metabolic energy is utilized for this purpose alone.

Such active transport mechanisms use energy-rich compounds such as ATP and are involved in a wide range of functions, for example: the maintenance of optimal cellular concentrations of important inorganic electrolytes such as Na^+ and K^+ (p. 419); modification of salivary components (p. 548); absorption of dietary sugar and amino acid molecules from the gut (p. 611); relaxation of muscle (p. 341); and transport of 'reducing equivalents' across mitochondrial membranes (p. 204). Such processes are often referred to as 'pumps'.

The common features of such active transport pumps are:
1 They operate against a concentration gradient.
2 They are dependent upon a metabolic energy source.
3 They are usually unidirectional, i.e. they

move a substance across a membrane in one direction only.

4 The free energy of the system increases.

Such active transport activities involve *mediators* which facilitate the movement of the molecules and ions involved. The translocases in the transport of reducing equivalents are one example (p. 204); another is the transport of amino acids across the gut wall and kidney cell membranes, which involve specific protein, transport carrier molecules linked to Na^+. At least 5 transport processes specific to amino acid types are thought to be involved. Human genetic mutations are known which result in the formation of defective amino acid transport proteins in much the same way as HbS is defective in sickle-cell anaemia (p. 74). The inherited condition, Hartnup's disease, is due to the absence of the transport protein needed for certain neutral and aromatic amino acids. Sufferers excrete 5–20 times the levels of Ala, Ser, Thr, Leu, Ile, Val, Phe, Try and Trp, and there is associated mental retardation. The effect on tryptophan transport causes pellagra-like symptoms (p. 814) because of the involvement of the amino acid in niacin biosynthesis.

Such examples illustrate other characteristics of active transport systems in that they possess a degree of specificity to the substance(s) transported, and they can often be specifically inhibited. However, these two latter properties are not unique to active transport systems, but are common with the processes of *facilitated diffusion* which also use specific carrier molecules as mediators, but are not energy-requiring. For this reason these are termed *passive* transport systems: though exhibiting specificity they only move their transported molecules down a concentration gradient, and when equilibrium is attained there are equal concentrations each side of the membrane. Also the free-energy in passive systems decreases, in contrast to active transport.

Both systems, active and passive transport, exhibit saturation kinetics, with the transport systems capable of becoming saturated in the presence of an excess of substances being transported. This is very similar to saturation of the active sites of enzymes by excess substrate concentration, and the similarity of transport kinetics to Michaelis–Menten enzyme kinetics (p. 95) suggest that, likewise, membrane transport systems involve specific sites.

Both the active and passive (mediated) transport systems are to be distinguished from simple biological diffusion processes of ion and molecule movements. The latter are not facilitated by carrier molecules and their rate of movement is directly dependent on substance concentration and temperature effects. No saturation kinetics, specificity, or inhibition effects are observed.

CELL GROWTH AND DIVISION

Growth is a characteristic property of living matter. It can be defined as an increase in size brought about by the synthesis of protoplasm and/or apoplastic substances, the latter being non-living materials which are produced by cells and which are a functional part of all tissues. Collagen fibres, and the matrices of bone, cartilage, dentine and enamel are examples of apoplastic substances.

If life is to continue, then growth must be controlled. This is true at every level of organization, from the organelle, through the cell, tissue, organ and individual, up to the entire population of a species. At the upper end of the scale, growth control is an unsolved problem. The human population is growing at a pace which threatens to outstrip the growth of the materials needed for survival. Unless intrinsic controls are applied, then extrinsic factors, such as food shortage, will limit our growth for us, and the Darwinian principle, the survival of the fittest, will apply. Lower down the scale intrinsic controls generally operate. In the case of a multicellular organism such as man the survival of the individual is only possible if the individual cells cooperate: their growth must be regulated in the interests of the whole organism. The fact that so many fertilized ova succeed in developing into normal healthy adults shows that mechanisms controlling cell growth, division and differentiation must exist. Once the optimum number of each cell type has been reached, and the optimum amount of the various apoplastic substances produced, then growth ceases. From that time on there is just enough synthesis and cell division to compensate for tissue loss.

An excellent example of the precision of this control is found in the repair of the epidermis. If it is injured and cells are lost from it, then the healthy epidermal cells around the lesion grow and divide faster than usual until the defect is made good. If the rate of replacement is too slow, then the skin can become chronically ulcerated; if it is too fast, then an epithelial tumour may form.

In most cases the control mechanisms work perfectly, but occasionally things go wrong. In a fetus, this may lead to malformation; in a child or adult, it may even lead to cancer. It is perhaps because things do sometimes go wrong that there is so much interest in the control of cell growth and division, one of the most challenging and exciting fields of current biological research.

Yin-Yang hypothesis of growth control

Early in the 1970s a new hypothesis was put forward in an attempt to reconcile and explain the results of the many research groups then studying cell growth, division and differentiation. It has been described as the Yin-Yang hypothesis because it involves the activity of two opposed but complementary substances, cyclic AMP and cyclic GMP, which were likened to the two opposed but complementary forces of oriental philosophy, Yin and Yang.

Cells can respond to changes in their environment either by growing and dividing or by differentiating. According to the Yin-Yang hypothesis, these changes are monitored at the plasma membrane and translated into simple chemical signals, namely changes in the levels of cAMP and cGMP, the relative concentrations of which determine how each cell subsequently behaves (Fig. 4.69).

Suppose, for example, that the hormone insulin is added to a culture of embryonic cells which has stopped growing. It interacts with receptors in their plasma membranes and sets off a number of biochemical processes collectively known as the growth programme. The hormone acts as a messenger, and the changes it produces at the plasma membrane result in a reduction in the amount of cAMP present in the cells, following which they are again able to grow and divide. Other hormones can raise the cAMP level by activating the enzyme *adenylate cyclase* which catalyses the synthesis of cAMP from its precursor ATP (Fig. 4.70). Cells in which the cAMP level is high stop growing and start to synthesize the specific luxury molecules that mark their differentiation.

The way in which cAMP operates is not yet fully understood, but it seems likely that it activates specific *protein kinases* which in turn catalyse some synthetic processes and inhibit others (Fig. 4.71) with the result that the entire growth programme is switched off. Reduction in the amount of intracellular cAMP is not sufficient to

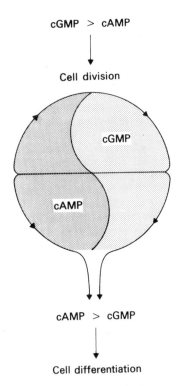

Fig. 4.69. The Yin-Yang hypothesis.

switch the growth programme on again. Another mediator is required, namely cGMP. When insulin is added to a nongrowing culture of embryonic cells, not only does the cAMP level fall, but the cGMP level rises; this is because the enzyme *guanylate cyclase* is activated and this catalyses the synthesis of cGMP from its precursor GTP. As with cAMP, the mode of operation of cGMP is still unclear. It may activate other protein kinases which this time switch the growth programme on.

Growth regulation by negative feedback

Various attempts have been made to explain the phenomenon of the regulation of cell growth and division in terms of negative feedback. The model proposed in 1957 by Weiss and Kavanau is among the more concise and useful. They suggested that each tissue and organ consisted of two functionally different components: a generative cell mass capable of growth and division, and a differentiated cell mass derived from it. The differentiated cells fulfil the functions of the particular tissue or organ and also produce an inhibitor which, by negative feedback,

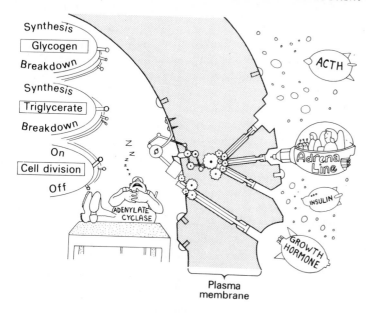

Plasma membrane

Fig. 4.70. The second messenger about to be galvanized into action by a messenger from the outside. (After J. B. Finean, R. Coleman and R. H. Michell (1974) *Membranes and their cellular functions*, 1st edition. Blackwell Scientific Publications, Oxford.)

reduces the rate of growth and division of the generative cells. The degree of inhibition is directly proportional to the amount of inhibitor produced. If the number of differentiated cells falls because of injury, for example, then the amount of inhibitor produced will fall, and with it the degree of inhibition. The generative cells then respond by growing and dividing at an increased rate. Many of the new cells formed differentiate and begin to produce inhibitor. Once the optimum number of differentiated cells has been reached, then the level of inhibitor will be such that the rate of cell growth and division returns to the normal level. This model of growth control is shown diagrammatically in Fig. 4.72.

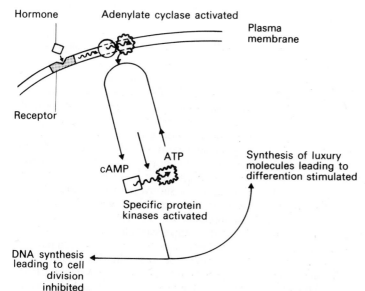

Fig. 4.71. Possible effects of high levels of cyclic AMP on cell activity.

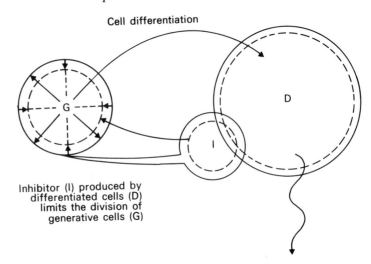

Cell differentiation

D

I

G

Inhibitor (I) produced by
differentiated cells (D)
limits the division of
generative cells (G)

Cell death reduces the number of
inhibitor-producing cells and is
compensated for by more cell
division

Excretion of remains of dead cells

Fig. 4.72. Growth regulation
with negative feedback
(Weiss–Kavanau model).

CHALONES

The Weiss and Kavanau model of growth control by negative feedback was given considerable support by the work of Iverson, Bullough and others. Bullough suggested that the term chalone be used for the inhibitor, deriving it from the Greek work meaning 'slow down'. Chalones have now been extracted from the tissues of many animals and they all have the following characteristics.

1　They are cell or tissue specific, that is, they only inhibit the growth of the cell or tissue type from which they were extracted.

2　They are species non-specific, that is, they can act as inhibitors in other animal species. Chalones extracted from rat, mouse and even cod epidermis have been shown to inhibit the growth and division of human epidermal cells.

3　Their effects are reversible. Growth and division proceed normally once the chalone has been withdrawn.

4　They are all low molecular weight glycoproteins.

Some cells pay no heed to the growth regulating instructions of the chalones but grow in an uncontrolled way producing tumours. It is now known that tumours contain the chalone of the original tissue, and that the serum of tumour-bearing animals has a higher chalone content than normal, presumably because the tumour cells are producing chalone but the generative cell mass within the tumour is not responding to it. The problem is permeability. All the experimental evidence available so far suggests that tumour cells leak; chalones reach and enter them, but cannot be retained for long enough to act.

The cell cycle

A single cell cannot grow indefinitely. Eventually it reaches a limiting volume. It then stops growing and may divide. The limiting volume is determined to a large degree by the shape of the cell. What is particularly important is the ratio between its surface area and its volume. All essential metabolites must enter the cell through the plasma membrane at its surface, and all toxic waste products must leave by the same route. For the cell to survive, its surface area must be large enough to cope with the exchange requirements of the volume of protoplasm covered. A spherical cell has a smaller surface area:volume ratio than, for example, a flattened or elongated cell, so the limiting volume for the former cell type is smaller than that for the latter. When a cell divides into two daughter cells, the volume of each falls below the limit and both can grow until that limit is once again reached.

With very few exceptions (red blood cells and platelets) all human cells contain a nucleus, within which the genetic material is housed. Division of the cell must be preceded by duplication of this material and the distribution of a complete set of it to each daughter cell, if they are to continue to function normally. In somatic cells the distribution period is called *mitosis*, and the intervening period between this and the next mitosis *interphase*, while the process as a whole, being repetitive, is termed the *cell cycle*. It can vary in length from a few hours to many days, depending on the environmental conditions and the cell type.

The cell cycle can be subdivided into four phases: G_1, S, G_2 and M (Fig. 4.73). Immediately after one mitosis ends, there is a variable period called G_1, the first 'gap' in the cycle and the beginning of interphase. It precedes DNA synthesis, and during it the cell is diploid. During G_1 the materials needed for the duplication of the genetic material of the cell are assembled. Next comes the S or 'synthetic' phase, when the DNA is copied and associated with new nucleoproteins. It lasts about six hours and by the time it ends each chromosome is represented by two chromatids; chromatin replication is complete, and the cell is now tetraploid. G_2, the second 'gap' in the cycle, follows, and during it the enzymes and other requirements needed for mitosis are assembled. This may take approximately 2–4 hours, after which the final phase, mitosis or M, begins. During mitosis, which lasts for about one hour, the nuclear membrane of the parent cell breaks down, the tetraploid genetic material separates into two complete diploid sets as the members of each chromatid pair move apart, and a new nuclear membrane forms around each set, so that the cell now contains two nuclei. The cell then divides to from two daughter units, each containing one of the two nuclei. The resulting daughter cells react to the local conditions in which they find themselves in one of the following ways. They may rejoin the cell cycle, passing immediately into interphase; they may leave it but retain the capacity to divide, in which case they are said to have entered the G_0 state; or they may leave it, differentiate, lose the capacity to divide, age and eventually die. Cells which have entered the G_0 state can, under the stimulation of certain mitogenic control factors such as specific hormones, re-enter the cycle once more. They may, however, leave the G_0 state by differentiating (Fig. 4.74).

Any cell capable of dividing mitotically can be affected by mitogenic control factors of some type or other, even tumour cells. These factors may be general, for example, temperature, availability of nutrients, presence of toxic agents, which affect all dividing cells indiscriminately, or they may be specific, for example, the chalones. The mode of action of the latter always seems to involve the mediation of the cyclic nucleotides cAMP and cGMP (p. 254), but their time of action varies with the chalone. Some act at G_1, inhibiting entry into S, the phase of DNA synthesis; others act at G_2 and block mitosis temporarily; yet others act immediately after mitosis, reducing the number of cells which enter G_1 and, in consequence, increasing the numbers of those which either enter the quiescent state G_0 or of those which differentiate, age and eventually die. It should be remembered that, although

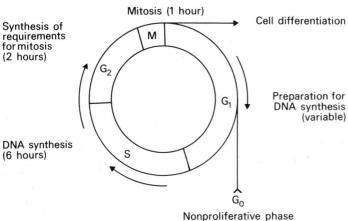

Fig. 4.73. The cell cycle.

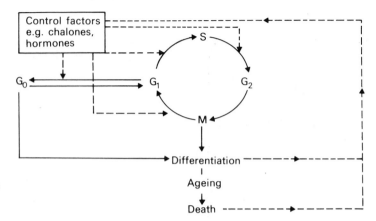

Fig. 4.74. Stages in the cell cycle
which are sensitive to specific
mitogenic control factors.

important, chalones need the backing of other
agents if they are to control cell division and
growth. As Iverson is reported to have said:
'Perhaps they play first violin in the symphony
orchestra of growth regulation'.

Mitosis: The division of somatic cells

Cell division is essential for the growth and
maintenance of most multicellular organisms.
Somatic cells differentiate, age, die and are generally replaced by the proliferation and differentiation of other cells. Failure of replacement
leads to the death of the organism. Ideally, the
replacement cells should have exactly the same
genetic composition as the cells they replace. For
this to be achieved, mechanisms must exist for
the exact duplication of the nuclear DNA of the
parent cell and for the precise segregation of
each strand of the original DNA from the duplicate material so that each of the two daughter
cells into which the parent cell divides receives a
complete set of genetic instructions. Duplication
takes place during the S phase of the cell cycle (p.
257), and segregation during mitosis.

STAGES IN MITOSIS

Mitosis begins at the end of the G_2 phase of the
cell cycle (p. 257). It generally takes about one
hour in homoeothermic animals. Although a
continuous process, it is traditionally divided
into stages to aid description. It begins with
karyokinesis, division of the nucleus, and ends
with cytokinesis, division of the cytoplasm. Usually karyokinesis and cytokinesis overlap, the
latter beginning before the former is complete.
Karyokinesis is further subdivided into four

stages: *prophase, metaphase, anaphase* and *telophase.*

Before mitosis begins the genetic material of
the parent somatic cell is duplicated. For most of
its life the parent cell is diploid, but during the
interval between the completion of duplication
and the completion of mitosis it is tetraploid,
that is, it contains twice the usual diploid number
of chromosomes and therefore twice the usual
amount of nuclear DNA (Fig. 4.75). Each original chromosome of the parent cell has a duplicate lying next to it, the two being referred to a
sister chromatids.

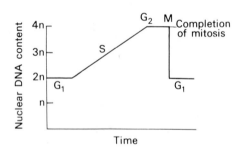

Fig. 4.75. Variation in DNA content during the life
cycle of a somatic cell.

Karyokinesis
Prophase (Fig. 4.76). The first indication that
this, the first stage of karyokinesis, is beginning
is that the parent cell rounds up. The chromosomes, which are virtually invisible during interphase in living cells, and which do not appear as
discrete entities in stained preparations, become
readily demonstrable. They appear first as deli-
cated coiled threads lying within the confines of
the nuclear membrane. Close examination shows

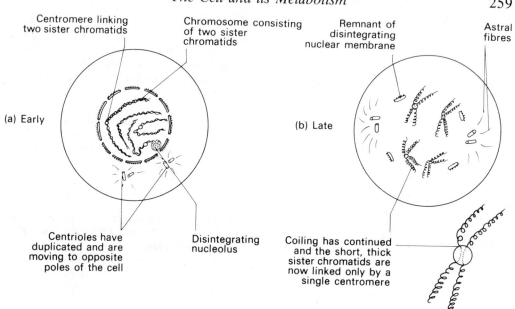

Centromere linking two sister chromatids

Chromosome consisting of two sister chromatids

Remnant of disintegrating nuclear membrane

Astral fibres

(a) Early

(b) Late

Centrioles have duplicated and are moving to opposite poles of the cell

Disintegrating nucleolus

Coiling has continued and the short, thick sister chromatids are now linked only by a single centromere

Fig. 4.76. Prophase, (a) early, (b) late.

that each 'chromosome' is a double structure. Each is really two chromosomes lying side by side, one a duplicate of the other and produced during the S phase of interphase. To avoid terminological confusion the two members of each chromosome pair will be termed sister chromatids. Sister chromatids are linked firmly together by a single small, clear, circular region called a centromere.

As prophase progresses the chromatids coil up, with the result that they appear shorter and thicker. By the end of prophase they are only 5–10% of the length they were when mitosis began. They now move out towards the nuclear membrane, leaving behind a region of clear nuclear sap in the centre of the nucleus.

Meanwhile the nucleoli break up, the centrioles duplicate, and each of the resulting two pairs of centrioles migrates to opposite poles of the cell.

The final act of prophase is the disintegration of the nuclear membrane.

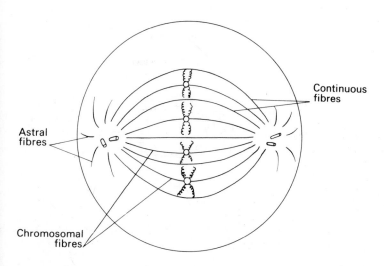

Continuous fibres

Astral fibres

Chromosomal fibres

Fig. 4.77. Metaphase.

Others form chromosomal fibres which extend from one of the poles and terminate in contact with the centromere of a pair of sister chromatids, while others, the astral fibres, radiate out from the centrioles and appear to end freely in the hyaloplasm. When the spindle is complete each pair of sister chromatids has two chromosomal fibres attached to it. These fibres extend to the opposite poles of the spindle and as they end on the centromere the pair of chromatids is suspended between them. All the chromosomal fibres are of similar length and so the chromatid pairs come to lie in the equatorial plane of the spindle.

The end of metaphase is marked by a moment of stillness. The chromatid pairs are lined up in the equatorial plane, linked to the poles of the spindle by the chromosomal fibres, but they are held firmly together as pairs by the centromeres, and these must divide before they can move apart.

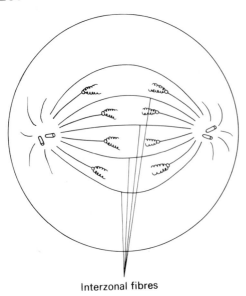

Interzonal fibres

Fig. 4.78. Anaphase.

Metaphase (Fig. 4.77). This begins with the organization of the mitotic spindle. This is the structure which controls the key action of mitosis, the separation of the sister chromatids. Subunit polymerization results in the formation of microtubules around the centriole pairs which by now lie at opposite poles of the cell with the chromatids lying in pairs between them. Some of the microtubules form fibres extending from pole to pole, the continuous fibres of the spindle.

Anaphase (Fig. 4.78). This, the stage when the sister chromatids separate, is initiated by the division of the centromeres, a division which takes place simultaneously in all the chromatid pairs. The daughter centromeres, each attached to a chromosomal fibre, are pulled or pushed apart and migrate to the opposite poles of the spindle, pulling the chromatids after them. The centromeres always lead, and the 'arms' of the chromatids trail out behind them.

It is not yet clear by what mechanism the sister chromatids are drawn apart at anaphase. Their

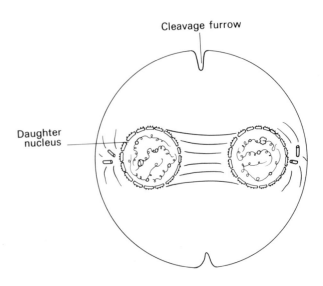

Cleavage furrow

Daughter nucleus

Fig. 4.79. Telophase and the beginning of cytokinesis.

own role is certainly passive; the difficulty lies in the nature and mode of action of the mitotic force which acts upon them. This seems to operate through the microtubules which group into bundles to form the spindle fibres. It is not yet known whether the chromosomal fibres actively shorten, thus pulling the chromatids apart, or whether the elongation of the equatorial region of the continuous fibres pushes the chromatids apart.

Shortening, if it occurs, could be due to loss of microtubular subunits from the polar end of the chromosomal fibres and the consequent pulling in of the remainder of the fibres. Elongation could be caused either by the addition of extra subunits to the middle of the continuous fibres, or by the sliding of the microtubules which comprise these fibres over each other. Whatever the mechanism the end result is that the sister chromatids move apart and gather at the oppo-

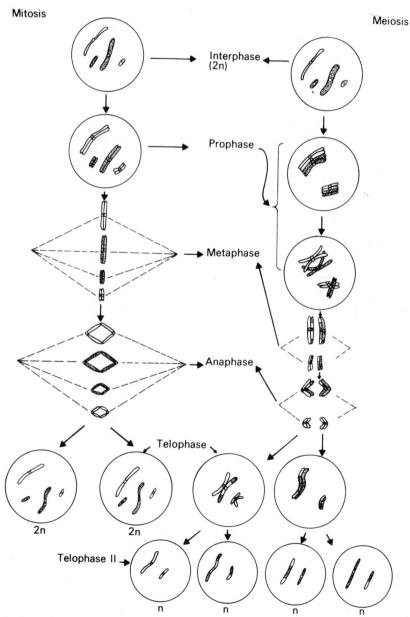

Fig. 4.80. Comparison of mitosis and meiosis.

site ends of the mitotic spindle. Once they separate they are referred to as chromosomes. The region of the spindle between the two groups of separating chromosomes appears to be under tension, and its constituent microtubules are now referred to as interzonal fibres.

Telophase (Fig. 4.79). This begins when the chromosomes have reached their destination, the poles of the spindle. The chromosomes begin to uncoil and lengthen, becoming less readily detectable as they do so. Nucleoli reappear at the sites of the nuclear organizers (p. 169), and a nuclear membrane forms around each of the two groups of chromosomes. Once this has been accomplished karyokinesis is at an end; the cell now contains two genetically identical nuclei.

Cytokinesis

While telophase is still in progress cytokinesis usually begins. The cytoplasm becomes constricted midway between the two developing nuclei, forming a cleavage furrow which extends inwards until it reaches the bundle of interzonal fibres which marks the position of the mitotic spindle. These form a slender, temporary bridge between the two daughter cells—a bridge which soon snaps, separating the daughter cells completely.

There are several current theories as to the mechanism of cytokinesis. Amoeboid movement may pull the daughter cells apart, there may be a contractile equatorial ring in the cortical cytoplasm, or the radiating astral fibres at the poles of the spindle may push against the cell membrane and somehow trigger cleavage. The actual mechanism remains to be resolved.

SUMMARY

To summarize, mitosis is the process which allows for the formation of two genetically identical cells from a single diploid parent cell. It is subdivided, for the sake of descriptive convenience, into karyokinesis (division of the nucleus) and cytokinesis (division of the cytoplasm), karyokinesis being further subdivided into prophase, metaphase, anaphase and telophase. The end result is the perfect copying of the genetic instructions of the parent cell and the segregation of a complete set of instructions into each of two separate cells which may divide or differentiate as the occasion demands. The process is shown diagrammatically and compared with meiosis in Fig. 4.80.

CONTROL OF METABOLISM

Several examples of biochemical control mechanisms have already been given in the text, for example in relation to glycolysis, glucogenesis, pentose phosphate pathways, amino acid metabolism and purine and pyrimidine biosynthesis. These should be referred to in the context of this section with others listed under control mechanisms in the index.

The purpose of this section is to group the various types of control mechanisms into a general classification to which they can be referred. In addition a detailed account is given of the proposed mechanisms for control of metabolism at the transcription and translation levels of protein synthesis. Much of this derives from now classic studies on bacterial metabolism, which provided the foundation upon which an understanding of control mechanisms in higher organism is being built.

Control mechanisms are divided broadly into two major categories:

Control of the amount of enzyme present (coarse control)

This can be regulated by stimulation of biosynthesis of the enzyme, or adversely by acceleration of its proteolytic degradation.

Controls of this nature can operate therefore:

1   (a) at the transcription level
    (b) at the translation level
2   At the enzyme degradation level.

Post-translational controls of the activity of enzymes (fine control)

These control metabolism by a positive (activation) or negative (inhibition) effect on enzyme activity.

1   *Substrate control.* The simplest examples in this category are via substrate concentration effects, as dictated by the Michaelis–Menten equation kinetics (p. 94).
2   *Allosteric controls.* Enzymes are inhibited or activated by small molecules which are not necessarily reactants of the catalysed reaction involved. Such small molecules do not affect the enzyme function at the active site but modify its activity by binding elsewhere to the molecule altering, for example, the structural conformation to modify the enzymes' catalytic powers.

Stages of gene expression		Possible control mechanisms

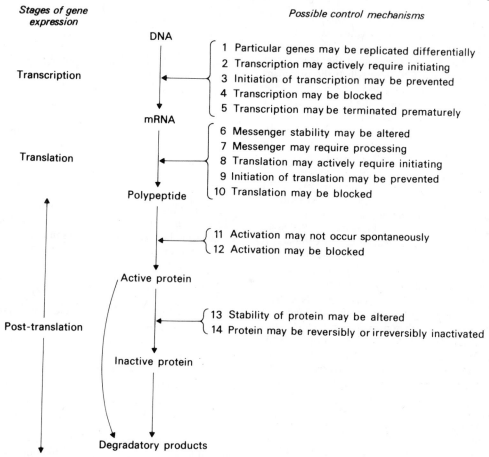

Fig. 4.81. Gene expression and some possible ways of controlling it.

Many examples are given in the text and index under 'allosteric control mechanisms'.

3 *Covalent modification.* Here enzyme activation or inhibition is effected by breaking or forming of covalent bonds. Examples are activation of the zymogen forms of proteolytic digestive enzymes, as in the conversion of inactive trypsinogen to active trypsin by removal of a peptide 'keeper' (p. 610). Another is the phosphorylation and dephosphorylation of enzymes involved in glycogen breakdown (p. 191) and synthesis (p. 192).

Some examples of genetic disorders of metabolism are briefly reviewed in this chapter in the context of metabolism and control of metabolism which has gone wrong as a result of genetic mutations, identified as affecting specific stages in metabolism.

The control of gene expression (Fig. 4.81)

As described previously, most of the genetic information of an organism is stored in the nucleotide base sequence of DNA. In this form it is easily replicated, but has little direct influence on the cell's structure and function. However, much of this genetic information is used during protein synthesis to specify the order of assembly of amino-acids into polypeptides and it is these assemblies, in the form of enzymes and structural proteins etc., which determine a particular cell's various characteristics. Cells are very selective in their use of the genetic information they contain, and the presence in a cell of a DNA sequence coding for the amino acid sequence of a particular polypeptide by no means guarantees that the cell will actually synthesize it. For example a zygote of an organism (the product of fusion of two gametes—the fertilized egg in animals) must contain the genetic information for the specification of the amino acid sequence of every protein which the organism will make during its lifetime; yet most of these proteins are not made by the fertilized egg and indeed many may not be made until late in the organism's development; nor is gene expression controlled only in a developmental context. In many organisms, especially microorganisms, the activities of certain biosynthetic enzymes cannot be detected when their products are present in excess and many degradatory enzymes cannot be detected unless their substrate is present in excess. Much of our present knowledge of the molecular basis of the control of gene expression is derived from such studies on metabolic control in microorganisms and developmental gene control may well be achieved by similar mechanisms.

Gene expression, in which a DNA base sequence specifies the amino-acid sequence of a polypeptide, which in turn gives rise to an active functional protein, is a complex process which can be controlled in many ways. Figure 4.81 summarizes the principal stages of gene expression and lists ways, at different stages, by which the process might be controlled. Gene expression may not be controlled in all the ways listed but there is evidence that a number are utilized. For example protein synthesis can be regulated at the stage the mRNA code is transcribed from the DNA code and at the translational level, where initiation and rate of synthesis of the protein chains can be controlled.

DETECTING MECHANISMS OF GENE CONTROL

In general, changes in gene expression are monitored by observing changes in the amount of active enzyme present compared with total protein. Changes in the rate of gene expression are easily observed in microorganisms when the gene concerned specifies an enzyme involved in the biosynthesis or degradation of a particular metabolite. For example tryptophan added to a growing culture of the bacteria *E. coli* produces a fall in the relative amounts of the enzymes involved in tryptophan biosynthesis.

Another example is found when a culture of *E. coli* is transferred from medium in which glucose is the carbon source to one where the disaccharide lactose is the carbon source. Upon transfer the enzyme activities required for the utilization of lactose (e.g. *β-galactosidase*), which were not detectable in the glucose-grown culture, begin to be detected (Fig. 4.82).

If the mechanism causing these changing patterns of enzyme activity was due to alterations in the activity of enzymes already synthesized and present, then gene expression could be said to be controlled at the post-translational level. Alternatively the appearance or disappearance of an enzyme activity may be due to an alteration in the rate of synthesis of that enzyme, i.e. at the level of transcription or translation. Post-translational control, involving reversible enzyme activation or inhibition, can often be detected *in vitro*. An example is *aspartate transcarbamoylase*, an enzyme in pyrimidine biosynthesis inhibited by cytidine triphosphate, one of the products of the biosynthetic pathway of which it is a part.

It is less easy to establish when changes in levels in enzyme activity are due to alterations in the rate of enzyme synthesis. One approach is to add a radioactive amino acid to the culture, at the same time altering the environmental conditions and so labelling protein synthesized after the switch. In this way it was shown that the increase in the *β-galactosidase* levels which followed the above substitution of lactose for glucose as carbon source for an *E. coli* culture, was due to an enzyme synthesis effect which occurred after the environmental change was made. The other possibility, that in the glucose-grown culture there was inactive *β-galactosidase* already present, activated subsequently by the addition of its substrate, lactose, could therefore be eliminated. Control at the transcription level was operating. How did this function?

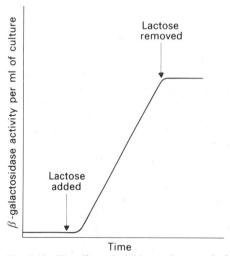

Fig. 4.82. The effect of addition and removal of lactose to an *E. coli* culture.

THE JACOB–MONOD OPERON MODEL OF
LACTOSE METABOLISM AT THE
TRANSCRIPTION LEVEL

The enzymes involved in lactose metabolism
Lactose metabolism in *E. coli* was the first gene
control mechanism to be understood in detail
and remains one of the best understood examples of gene control at the level of transcription.
The elucidation of the molecular mechanisms
involved resulted mainly from the pioneer work
of two French scientists at the Institut Pasteur,
Francois Jacob and Jacques Monod.

To be used as a carbon source, the disaccharide sugar lactose has first to enter the cell,
where its passage across the cell membrane is
dependent on a transport protein, or permease.
This *lactose permease*, which also transports a
number of other related galactosides, is coded
for by a specific gene (the *lac* y gene) and mutations in this gene (designated *lac* y⁻) result in
cells unable to take up lactose. Once in the cell,
the enzyme *β-galactosidase* hydrolyses lactose to
its component monosaccharides, galactose and
glucose. Each *E. coli* cell grown in the absence of
lactose only contains some ten molecules of the
enzyme but the presence of the substrate induces
production of several thousands of *β-
galactosidase* molecules per cell: this process
is called induced enzyme synthesis.

The inducible enzyme is coded for by a structural gene (*lac* z). A structural gene is defined as
a gene which codes for the amino acid sequence
of a particular polypeptide—in this case
β-galactosidase, which is situated within the
DNA genetic material of *E. coli* immediately
adjacent to the *lac* y structural gene. A further
structural gene, (*lac* a), is located adjacent to the
lac z and *lac* y genes and this *lac* a gene is responsible for synthesis of the enzyme *thiogalactoside
transacetylase*. The exact physiological role for
this enzyme has not yet been established, as
mutants lacking *thiogalactoside transacetylase*
activity do not have a growth pattern different
from the wild-type.

These 3 adjacent structural genes on the
chromosome, (*lac* z, y and a) are responsible for
the formation of the *β-galactosidase, permease*,
and the *transacetylase* respectively. All 3
respond in concert to addition of lactose to the
environment.

Thus *E. coli* growing on carbon sources such
as glucose, makes only very small amounts of
β-galactosidase, permease and *thiogalactoside
transacetylase*, but all three begin to be synthesized when lactose is added to the culture. The
use of antibiotics which inhibited protein synth-

esis at the level of either transcription or translation, and of assays which specifically detect the
messenger RNA from the *lac* y, z and a genes,
showed control was exerted at the level of transcription. Thus in the absence of lactose not only
the enzyme products of the *lac* z, y and a genes
were absent, but also their associated messenger
RNA.

The repressor
The *lac* z, y and a genes can be induced to
become active, not only by the presence of lactose, but also by certain lactose analogues. For
example, some lactose analogues, such as
phenyl-β-D-galactoside, though excellent sub-
trates for *β-galactosidase*, are not very effective
in inducing enzyme synthesis; in contrast
isopropyl-β-D-thiogalactoside induces enzyme
synthesis very well, but is not a substrate for
β-galactosidase. Such observations led Jacob
and Monod to suggest that the cell might
contain some other substance, distinct from
β-galactosidase, which was responsible for
recognising lactose or related compounds and,
in their presence, allow the transcription of
the *lac* z, y and a genes. If such a 'recognition'
substance in fact existed, it might then be
possible to select mutations which affected its
structure. Such mutations should not affect
the activities of *β-galactosidase, galactoside
permease* or *thiogalactoside transacetylase*
directly, but might alter the control of their
synthesis.

A mutant organism was selected in which
the synthesis of *β-galactosidase, permease* and
transacetylase occurred even in the absence of
an inducing substrate. Strains carrying such
mutations are said to be constitutive mutants,
because they behave as though the *β-
galactosidase* were a constitutive rather than an
inducible enzyme. Genetic analysis of such constitutive mutants showed that mutations in two
genes could result in constitutive synthesis of
β-galactosidase. These genes, designated *lac* i
and *lac* o, were found to be located close to the
lac z, y and a genes, with a gene order along the
chromosome of *lac* i-o-z-y-a: *lac* i constitutive
mutants are designated *lac* i⁻ and *lac* o constitutive mutants as *lac* oᶜ.

Further studies established that the *lac* i gene
product had a negative role in preventing *lac* z, y
and a gene expression, and also showed that this
product diffused freely into the cytoplasm.
Because such genes act to modify the rate of
transcription of structural genes they are called
regulatory genes. Jacob and Monod proposed

that the *lac* i regulatory gene product, which they designated a *repressor*, was a diffusible substance whose function was to prevent *lac* gene expression in the absence of an inducing galactoside. In the presence of an inducing galactoside the repressor was no longer active and the *lac* z, y and a genes could be expressed, and their gene products, the 3 enzymes involved in lactose metabolism, formed.

The operator site
Further investigations indicated that the *lac* o gene did not make a diffusible product, but instead was more likely to be a site, termed *the operator*, whereby the repressor recognized the

lac structural genes binding tightly to it and so preventing transcription. Thus the repressor acts on the operator to switch off the activity of various groups of structural genes.

The lactose operon model (Fig. 4.83)
In summary the regulation of enzyme synthesis as proposed by Jacob and Monod envisages several structural genes on a strand of chromosomal DNA. Immediately in front of these, reading from left to right, is the operator gene which controls whether the structural genes are copied by the enzyme RNA polymerase. A group of genes sharing a common operator gene is called collectively an *operon*. In the lactose metabolism

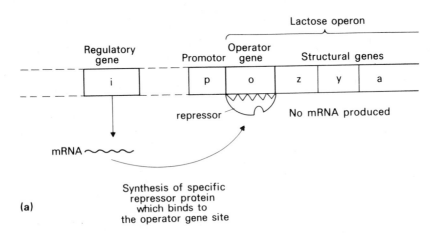

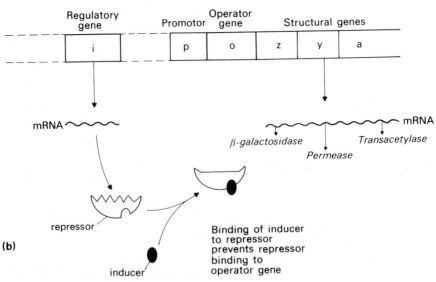

Fig. 4.83. The lactose operon model. (a). Repression of genes. (b) Derepressed state. (After Stryer L. (1981) *Biochemistry*, 2nd edn. San Francisco, W. H. Freeman.)

system, the *lac* o, z, y and a genes together constitute the *lac operon* represented diagrammatically in Fig. 4.83.

The third gene, *the regulator gene*, can be located next to the operator gene although its position is not crucial to its function (see below). This regulator gene produces mRNA which codes for the synthesis of a specific repressor protein, which has one site that binds to the operator site and switches off the activities of the various structural genes as long as inducing substrate is absent. The action of the inducers of enzyme synthesis is to bind to a second site on the repressor molecule, so causing a small change in its conformation and preventing the binding of the repressor to the operator gene. The repressor is thereby removed from this segment of DNA, thus allowing copying of the adjacent structural genes to proceed.

The repressor protein was subsequently isolated and shown to be a tetramer with each identical subunit of molecular weight 37 000. The amino acid sequence has been worked out and it has been demonstrated that each subunit has one binding site for an inducer. Once isolation of the repressor was achieved, the way was paved for the execution of a series of experiments, confirming Jacob and Monod's model. The repressor was shown to bind specifically to *E. coli* DNA in the region of the *lac* o gene, but only in the absence of inducing galactosides. A correlation was established between the efficacy of induction by a galactoside *in vivo*, and the tightness of its binding to repressor *in vitro*. Finally, a system was devised in which β-galactosidase was synthesized *in vitro*, using the *lac* region DNA as a template. In the presence of repressor and absence of an inducing galactoside no β-galactosidase synthesis occurred, but when a suitable galactoside was added repression was lifted and synthesis begun.

An ingenious analogy to the control of the *lac* genes described above has been put forward by Jacob and Monod. The *lac* i gene (a regulatory gene) is compared to a radio transmitter broadcasting the message 'do not drop bombs' (the repressor) to an aircraft. The *lac* o gene (the operator site) is represented by the radio receiver within an aeroplane carrying bombs, with the act of dropping bombs representing the activity of the *lac* z, y and a genes. If the instructions given to the pilot are that his bombs are to be dropped immediately he ceases to receive instructions to the contrary, there will be three ways in which he will come to drop his bombs.

Firstly a decision can be taken to stop broadcasting the 'do not drop bombs' message. This would represent the normal method of achieving bomb release, and correspond to the inactivation of repressor by an inducing galactoside. However, a transmitter breakdown could also result in bomb release. This would correspond to a *lac* i⁻ constitutive mutation. If duplicate transmitters were provided however, a breakdown of one would still leave the other transmitter functioning and hence no premature bomb release would occur. This parallels the situation in diploid cells where a *lac* i⁻ gene mutation is recessive. Finally, a receiver fault, corresponding to a *lac* o operator site mutation, (i.e. *lac* oᶜ) would also result in premature bomb release. Here however if there were two aeroplanes, each with their own receiver, a receiver failure in one would not influence the other to drop its bombs prematurely, nor would the aeroplane whose receiver had stopped working be prevented from dropping its bombs by the still working receiver in the other aeroplane. This is exactly equivalent to the properties of the *lac* o gene, which can only influence the expression of the *lac* z, y and a genes adjacent to it on the same piece of DNA.

The role of cyclic AMP in transcription of operons

The presence or absence of inducing galactosides such as lactose is not the only environmental factor to affect the expression of the *lac* operon. In the presence of glucose, or other good carbon sources, little induction of the *lac* operon occurs even if a suitable inducing galactoside is present. A number of other potential gene products involved in the breakdown of carbon-containing metabolites, are not produced when an alternative better source of carbon is present. This situation ensures that, when an adequate source of carbon such as glucose is already available, energy is not wasted in the breakdown of other metabolites which are poorer sources of carbon.

This whole phenomenon, first known as the glucose effect, but now termed carbon catabolite repression, remained a mystery for some time. Then it was observed that levels of the nucleotide, 3′5′ cyclic AMP (p. 192) were much lower in *E. coli* cells grown on glucose than in cells grown on poorer carbon sources such as glycerol and lactose. Also carbon catabolite repression of the *lac* operon was reversed by addition of cyclic AMP to glucose-grown cultures.

These and other studies using mutant strains

of *E. coli* indicated that cAMP was used by the micro-organism to monitor its carbon status. When an adequate carbon supply such as glucose is present, cAMP levels are low but when there is insufficient carbon, cAMP levels are high: somehow glucose and its derivatives inhibit cAMP synthesis.

Strains unable to synthesize cAMP, resulting from mutation in the gene specifying adenylate cyclase (i.e. cya⁻ mutants), therefore mimicked the conditions of carbon sufficiency and exhibited carbon catabolite repression.

In a second class of *E. coli* mutants the carbon catabolite repression could not be reversed by addition of an exogenous supply of cyclic AMP. Mutants of this class, designated crp⁻, lack the crp gene product which interacts with cAMP, and in its presence allowed the expression of genes which are subject to carbon catabolite repression. crp⁻ mutants, lacking this product, are unable to express any of these genes. The crp gene product has been isolated and found to be a protein dimer of molecular weight 45 000, which binds cAMP. The crp protein in the presence of cAMP binds to the DNA of the *lac* region close to the operator.

The promoter

Further *in vitro* studies showed that the binding of the crp gene product to the DNA was necessary in order that transcriptase (DNA polymerase) could itself bind to the DNA. The region of the DNA where crp protein, and transcriptase bind lies between the site of the *lac* i regulatory gene and the *lac* o operator gene, and is termed the *promoter region* (p; Fig. 4.83). It is a relatively short DNA section, less than 100 nucleotides in length.

All genes coding for proteins are associated with promoters. If the gene is a member of an operon, then it shares a promoter with the other genes in the operon, but for many genes which are not found in operons, each gene has its own promoter.

Fig. 4.83 summarizes the present state of knowledge of how control of the *lac* operon is achieved.

OTHER SYSTEMS INVOLVING
TRANSCRIPTIONAL CONTROL

The *E. coli lac* system involves two different methods of controlling gene expression at the level of transcription. First the *lac* repressor acts negatively to prevent the initiation of transcription. Secondly the crp gene product acts positively, being required for the binding of transcriptase to the promoter. Few other gene systems have been studied in such detail but positive and negative control systems do occur in other organisms, both prokaryotic and eukaryotic, though it is not always known whether or not control is at the level of transcription. However, there is evidence that the two mechanisms found in the *lac* system are by no means the only way of achieving transcriptional control.

For example, the control of arabinose metabolism in *E. coli* is due to the regulatory gene product having positive and negative roles in the control of transcription. It binds to the DNA in the absence of arabinose to prevent transcription, and in its presence to promote transcription.

Recent developments show that the distinction between proteins having regulatory roles and those having catalytic or structural roles, is not as always clear cut as was at first thought. In a number of systems an enzyme has been found to have in addition to its catalytic role a regulatory role. For example *glutamine synthetase* in *E. coli*, is directly involved in the mediation of the repression of a number of enzymes involved in the breakdown of nitrogen containing metabolites when ammonium ion is plentiful. The precise mechanism has not yet been established, but it is known that a regulatory effect is exerted at the level of transcription. Similar effects are likely in higher organisms though difficult to establish unequivocally.

CONTROL OF GENE ACTIVITY AT THE LEVEL OF TRANSLATION

There are many observations in both prokaryotic and eukaryotic organisms which suggest that gene expression can be controlled at the level of translation. One of the most studied examples involves the maturation of certain small *E. coli* viruses which have RNA rather than DNA as their genetic material. Because of this, if control of gene expression is to be achieved at all it cannot, of course, be at the level of transcription. These viruses do show controlled gene expression and this is achieved by interaction of proteins with the RNA, so as to prevent it being translated into polypeptides. Whilst such viruses do therefore provide evidence that the process of messenger RNA translation can be controlled, they can hardly be regarded as satisfactory models for other systems of translational control. Further studies are needed to establish how widespread translational control is, and how it is achieved.

The control of gene expression in higher organisms

In eukaryotes control of protein concentration is more complicated and more difficult to evaluate than in prokaryotes. However, there is some evidence for control at the level of transcription, mRNA processing, and at translation levels. Changes in rates of protein degradation have also been shown to occur for a number of animal enzymes, although a change in the amount is often achieved by an increase or decrease in the rate of its synthesis.

An increased translation of haemoglobin mRNA, brought about by haem in reticulocytes, is an example of such translational control. Certainly hormones are important effectors in modulating the rates of transcription and/or translation of proteins: an example is the presence of cortisol or glucagon inducing synthesis of three key enzymes in gluconeogenesis, whereas insulin induces synthesis of three key enzymes in glycolysis (p. 794). The role of cAMP controlling animal metabolism via effects on mRNA and protein synthesis is cited below.

Regulation of enzyme action: the post-translational fine control of gene activity

The preceding section has examined how gene expression at the transcription and translation stages of enzyme synthesis can be controlled and modified by environmental conditions. Another way in which gene expression can be controlled is at the post-translational stage, by the modification of the activities of already formed enzymes due to changes in the cell environment. This control of gene action by the modification of the activity of already synthesized proteins, has been studied for many years and in a wide range of organisms. As a result, many such control systems are well understood in molecular terms.

Feedback inhibition

The activity of enzymes is modified both by inhibitors and activators. The enzymes of many biosynthetic pathways as well as having their synthesis repressed when the pathway's end product is present in excess, are also subject to direct inhibition by the end product. In general no more than the first enzyme in the pathway is subject to such direct feedback inhibition in this way, though synthesis of all the enzymes in the pathway may be repressed. Feedback inhibition therefore serves as a quick acting control which leads to the conservation of cell metabolites by preventing further flow through the pathway. In comparison repression, although slower acting, can lead to greater economics because enzymes no longer required are not synthesized. The simplest form of end-product inhibition involves the inhibition by some metabolite of the first enzyme uniquely involved in the biosynthesis of the metabolite. Many metabolites share biosynthetic steps with others, and with such branched pathways, quite complex patterns of feedback inhibition are found.

Allosteric enzymes

Although inhibition of enzyme activity is the most commonly found form of regulation, involving the modification of enzyme activity by the reversible binding of a substance, comparable examples involving enzyme activation are known. A well characterized example is the activation of protein kinase by cAMP in mammals (p. 191). The role of cyclic AMP in mammalian tissues is discussed in greater detail on pp. 270–271.

In the majority of examples involving the modification of enzyme activity, the substance bound, whether activator or inhibitor, bears little structural relationship to the substrates or the enzyme. It is argued that the enzyme must have binding sites for the recognition of the inhibitor or activator, as well as the usual substrate binding sites. For this reason, this class of regulatory enzymes has been termed *allosteric* (p. 101). In many cases, allosteric enzymes consist of more than one type of polypeptide subunit. One type of subunit has the catalytic activity of the enzyme, while another binds the inhibitor or activator. The regulatory subunit can influence the activity of the catalytic subunit in a number of ways. For example the catalytic subunit of protein kinase is inactive when bound to the regulatory subunit. The binding of cAMP to the regulatory subunit causes it to dissociate from the catalytic subunit, which now becomes active. Not all allosteric enzymes work in this way, and at least in the case of threonine deaminase in *E. coli*, it appears that the same polypeptide forms both catalytic and regulatory sites.

Many examples of allosteric control in animal metabolism are given in the text and should be referred to via the index.

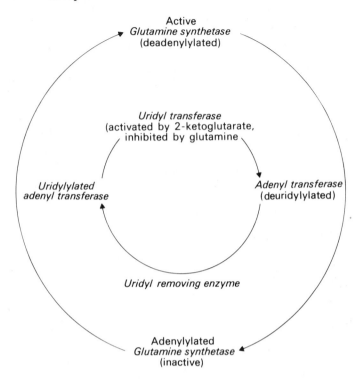

Fig. 4.84. The control of glutamine synthetase activity by chemical modification.

The regulation of enzyme activity by chemical modification

In addition to enzyme activity regulated by reversible binding of metabolites, there are a number of examples known where the activity of an enzyme is altered as a result of chemical modification. This modification is brought about by the action of another enzyme, and usually involves the addition and removal of phosphate or adenyl residues. For example, the activity of *glutamine synthetase* can be modified in this way (Fig. 4.84). The enzyme, in its adenylylated form, is less active than when adenyl residues are absent. There are two modifying enzymes, *adenyl transferase* and the *deadenylating enzyme*. The activity of both these modifying enzymes are themselves subject to modification, however in this case reversible inhibition and activation is involved. Glutamine activates adenyl transferase and inhibits the deadenylating enzyme whilst α-ketoglutarate and uridine monophosphate levels are high. As well as being regulated by chemical modification, glutamine synthetase in *E. coli* is also subject to feedback inhibition, and in addition its synthesis is regulated. This complex pattern of regulation no doubt reflects the central role of this enzyme in the metabolism of *E. coli*.

The best characterized examples in mammals of the chemical modification of enzymes (by phosphorylation) involve the enzymes interconverting glucose and glycogen.

The role of cAMP in animals

Many hormones, including glucagon, adrenaline, TSH, ACTH, and parathormone, have some of their actions mediated through cAMP. After binding to the cell membrane, the hormones activate the enzyme *adenyl cyclase*, which is associated with many tissue cell membranes, possibly as part of the receptor.

The conversion of ATP to cAMP by adenyl cyclase has been described earlier (p. 191), with the consideration that the hormone (the 'first messenger' to the cell), activated cAMP as the 'second messenger'.

The cyclic nucleotide has several functions.
1 Alteration of membrane permeability and passage of Ca^{2+} from the membrane into the cell cytoplasm. Normally, the intracellular Ca^{2+} concentration is very much less than the extracellular, the situation maintained by the action of an energy-requiring (ATP) pump sited in the cell membrane. Ca^{2+} ions are required by many enzymes activated by the binding of a

hormone to the cell receptor, e.g. glucagon in liver cells (see p. 420).

2 Phosphorylation of proteins. The protein kinases in the cytoplasm of the cells of various tissues are inactive until cAMP binds to them. The activated kinase can then catalyse phosphorylation of enzymes in the presence of ATP, as occurs in the activation of the phosphorylase b kinase of liver, involved in glycogenolysis (p. 191).

3 Action of ACTH in adrenal cortical cells. The effects of ACTH are mediated through cAMP and protein kinase in adrenal cells that stimulate ribosomal phosphorylation in the presence of ATP. This cAMP-activated kinase catalyses the synthesis of what is termed 'labile' protein. The function of this is to stimulate the translocation of cholesterol from the cytoplasm into the mitochondria of adrenal cells. The first enzyme-catalysed steps in corticosteroid biosynthesis can then occur (p. 780).

Effects of hormones on mRNA and protein synthesis

Synthesis of mRNA and protein can be affected by the action of many hormones, as shown by the use of antibiotics such as puromycin and actinomycin D. Puromycin is similar in structure to the tRNA for tyrosine and binds to ribosomes and is built into the polypeptide chain. Short polypeptide chains, with puromycin at the end of each, are released subsequently; and protein synthesis is thereby inhibited. In contrast, actinomycin D inhibits mRNA synthesis by binding to DNA and pairing specifically with guanine. This then prevents DNA from acting as a template for RNA synthesis.

In this brief account, three examples can be given illustrating the effects of these antibodies. If actinomycin D is administered to animals prior to administration of parathormone, the expected hypercalcaemic effects (see p. 763) are abolished. A similar situation holds in the case of 1,25-dihydroxycholecalciferol because its effects on calcium absorption from the intestine and from kidney tubules are abolished by the action of actinomycin D. In the case of cortisone, puromycin blocks its stimulatory effects on liver enzymes involved in gluconeogenesis.

Genetic disorders of metabolism

For the purpose of this section the salient points of protein synthesis (p. 238) are recalled and summarized as follows:

1 The bulk of human cell genetic information is contained in the deoxyribonucleic acid (DNA) of chromosomes.

2 This chromosomal DNA has two key functions:

(a) to transmit information from parent to daughter cells during division, and

(b) to govern protein synthesis.

3 DNA is composed of long linear arrays of the four nucleotide bases: adenine, thymine, guanine and cytosine.

4 Fidelity in DNA replication is ensured by the base-pairing mechanism of adenine–thymine and guanine–cytosine. Amino acid sequence in proteins is dictated by the nucleotide base sequence of DNA—the genetic code (Table 4.6).

5 During the process of transcription the information in DNA is transmitted to messenger ribonucleic acid (mRNA), which subsequently passes from the nucleus to the cytoplasm of the cell where it associates with ribosomes to form polysomes.

6 The ribosomes are sites of translation of the nucleic acid message written in the language of amino acids.

7 A particular protein function is determined by the specific amino acid sequence dictated by its genetic code.

8 A single amino acid is coded for by three consecutive nucleotide bases in DNA known as a codon (see Table 4.6, p. 244).

9 Specific transfer RNA molecules exist for each of the twenty different amino acids and these have the function of recognising, transporting and attaching amino acids to the growing polypeptide chain of the protein.

The whole sequence of events is summarized with an example in Figure 4.85.

THE BIOCHEMISTRY OF MUTATION

Errors in replication, transcription and translation

Accidental 'copy errors' in DNA replication occur about once in every 10^5 replications. Mistakes can occur not only in replication but also in transcription or translation. For example it has been calculated that the isoleucyl transfer RNA *synthetase* enzyme picks up a valine residue in error about once in a hundred times. The cell possesses an editing mechanism which reduces the number of times that valine is incorporated into a protein instead of isoleucine to about one in 3000 times.

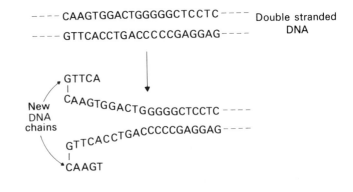

1 *Replication*

2 *Transcription*

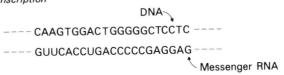

3 *Translation*

Messenger RNA

GUU CAC CUG ACC CCC GAG GAG

Val — His — Leu — Thr — Pro — Glu — Glu

Growing polypeptide chain

Fig. 4.85. Protein synthesis summary. *Note*: In RNA uracil replaces thymine bases in DNA.

Mutagenic agents

Mistakes in DNA can also be induced by irradiation. Ultraviolet light can cause certain adjacent nucleotide bases to become covalently linked. These errors are normally repaired by the enzyme *DNA polymerase*, but a few individuals lack this enzyme and consequently suffer from a rare inherited disease which carries an increased risk of developing skin cancer (xeroderma pigmentosa).

Other causes of a sudden alteration of DNA include mutagenic chemicals and ionizing radiation. The latter is the reason why it is sometimes insisted that patients wear a protective lead apron when dental X-rays are being taken. Whilst the majority of mutations are usually either deleterious or neutral in effect, very occasionally they are beneficial. According to the most generally accepted view, evolutionary advance has occurred as a result of the occasional emergence of mutant proteins which have improved functional properties compared with those of the wild-type parental cells from which they derived.

TYPES OF MUTATION

Point mutations involve either substitution or else deletion or insertion of nucleotide bases in DNA.

Substitution mutations

Substitution of a new 'wrong' nucleotide base in DNA in place of a 'correct' base has three possible consequences for protein synthesis.
1 No change may occur in the amino acid incorporated into the protein. Because of the 'degeneracy' of the genetic code (p. 243) a change in the third base of a codon will not necessarily entail an amino acid change. For example alanine is coded for by four codons of the type CGX, where X may be A, G, T, or C (see Table 4.6).

2 Incorporation of a single 'wrong' amino acid may occur. For example if the DNA codon CTC is changed to CAC, the amino acid incorporated into protein will be valine instead of glutamic acid. Otherwise the primary structure of the protein will be unaffected by this change.

3 Early or late termination of a polypeptide chain may occur. The normal signal given by DNA to stop adding amino acids to a polypeptide chain is coded by specific 'chain end' codons (ACT, ATT or ATC). If other codons mutate to these, or if these codons mutate to others, then early or late termination of polypeptide synthesis occurs. For example if CTC is changed to ATC, polypeptide chain synthesis will terminate, instead of glumatic acid being incorporated, and peptide chain synthesis continued.

Frame-shift mutations

The deletion or insertion of nucleotide bases into DNA is known as a frame-shift mutation. This will alter the way in which the whole message is read from the point of occurrence of the mutation onwards. Consequently multiple amino acid incorporation changes will occur onwards from the site of deletion or insertion. Also, termination of the polypeptide chain will be either late or early. For example, if a thymine base is deleted from the following DNA sequence as shown below:

TGTAGATTTATGGCAATTCGACCTCGGGTCCACT...

    ↑

    delete

the corresponding sequence of amino acids will change from ...thr-ser-lys-tyr-arg-STOP! to ...thr-ser-asn-thr-val-lys-leu-glu-pro-arg-STOP!

This type of mutation has been detected in a mutant haemoglobin, Haemoglobin Wayne. This is caused by a frame-shift mutation near the −COOH terminus of the α-globin chain. The third base of a lysine codon appears to have been deleted from DNA so that the first base of the following codon now takes its place. The net result is that not only are three 'wrong' amino acids incorporated into the polypeptide chain but also the normal 'chain terminate' message is not read, and five additional amino acids occur in the protein.

MUTATIONS AND GENETIC DISORDERS

General considerations

As described above, mutations may result in a change in the amino acid sequence of a protein. While this is by definition a change in primary protein structure, it does not necessarily entail a change in protein function. Many mutations described as neutral have no significant consequences for protein function. It is probable that many such mutations at present remain undetected, because if virtually any protein is examined in a large number of individuals rare variants are usually discovered. Approximately one-third of all amino acid substitutions result in a charge difference enabling mutant and wild-type proteins to be separated by electrophoresis. The remaining two-thirds of amino acid substitutions are more difficult to detect.

When a mutation does lead to a change in protein function, then there may be a genetic disorder of metabolism. These inherited diseases may be classified into two groups:

1 Those arising from a single rare random change in the DNA nucleotide sequence, resulting in the absence or change in structure and function of a single important protein.

2 Those arising from an accumulation of random DNA nucleotide changes, resulting in absence of, or change in, structure and function of a few or several less important proteins, and leading to a pattern of inheritance described as polygenic.

Changes in physiologically important proteins

Non-enzymic proteins. See for example Haemoglobin Wayne above and HbS in sickle cell anaemia (p. 74).

Enzymic. Enzyme molecules have an active site (p. 85) composed of a few key amino acids, involved in substrate binding and catalysis. Frequently there is in addition an allosteric site (p. 101) where either activators or inhibitors can bind and modify enzymic activity exercising a control of metabolism. Some enzymes cannot function unless cofactors or enzymes (p. 88) are attached at yet other positions on their molecules. Thus substituting one amino acid for another at a single position can have varied consequences in an enzyme composed of over a hundred amino acids. A change in just one amino acid at the active site can abolish enzyme activity altogether. At another site a similar change might render the molecule more susceptible to proteolytic digestion, decreasing its biological life and resulting in lowered enzyme activity. A change at a third site may have no effect at all directly on enzymic activity. This type of neutral mutation gives rise to the class of polymorphic enzymes known as genetic variants or isoenzymes.

Numerous genetic disorders of metabolism are now believed to arise from deficiencies in

OVERFLOW AMINOACIDURIA

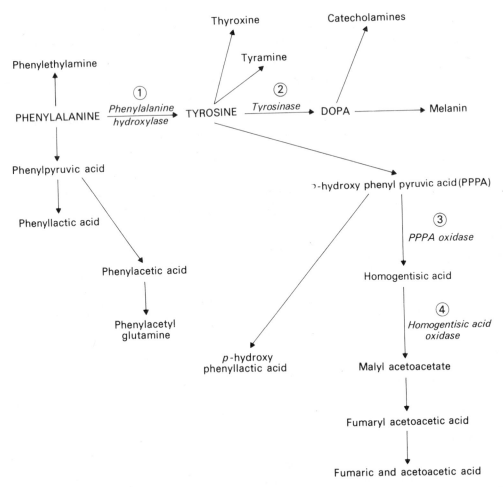

Fig. 4.86. Inborn errors of aromatic amino acid metabolism. (1) Deficient in phenylketonuria. (2) Deficient in albinism. (3) Deficient in tyrosinaemia. (4) Deficient in alkaptonuria.

production levels of specific enzymes. Consider a substrate A, metabolized in a tissue by a series of enzymes to form the end product D, i.e.

$$A \longrightarrow B \longrightarrow C \longrightarrow D$$
$$A\text{-ase} \quad B\text{-ase} \quad C\text{-ase}$$

Individuals with a genetic defect causing absence of enzyme C-ase activity will accumulate a high level of the intermediate substrate C, with a resultant low level of D compared to a normal individual. A further result of the block may be a pile-up of B and A in tissues and their urine.

Examples of genetic disorders of this type are found in the human metabolism of the amino acid phenylalanine which for normal humans is summarized on Fig. 4.86.

The enzymes catalysing four key metabolic steps are:

1   *Phenylalanine hydroxylase*
2   *Tyrosinase*
3   *PPPA oxidase*
4   *Homogentisic acid oxidase*

A genetically determined impaired formation of enzyme 4 in this pathway occurs in approximately one individual in 1 000 000 and causes the condition *alkaptonuria*. Excessive amounts of homogentisic acid are excreted in the urine which if left to stand turns black as the homogentisic acid is slowly oxidized—one of the clinical symptoms of the disorder.

A more serious disorder is *phenylketonuria* (PKU) caused by absence of enzyme 1. This affects approximately one in 25 000 of the population and if not treated leads to severe mental retardation. The pathological changes in brain and skin of PKU sufferers are due to the toxic accumulation of phenylalanine and its metabolites in these tissues. Phenylalanine, phenyl lactic acid and phenyl pyruvic acid are excreted, the latter causing the urine's characteristic mousy odour. The changes can be prevented if a diet very low in phenylalanine is instituted early in the life of the baby. Other genetic disorders associated with the same pathway are *albinism* caused by lack of enzyme 2 which blocks melanin formation, affecting one in 20 000 of the population. Loss of *PPPA oxidase* (enzyme 3) causes *tyrosinaemia* with an associated increase in plasma and urine tyrosine and excretion of p-hydroxy phenyl pyruvic acid.

Another inherited disorder which was discovered from a survey of the urinary metabolites of mentally retarded children in 1962 is *homocystinuria*. The high urinary levels of homocystine, from which the disease receives its name, were found to be due to the absence of the enzyme *cystathionine synthetase*. This enzyme normally converts homocystine to cystathionine on the metabolic pathway from methionine to cysteine:

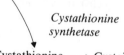

Methionine $\longrightarrow$ Homocysteine $\longrightarrow$ Homocystine

Cystathionine synthetase

Cystathionine $\longrightarrow$ Cysteine

Exactly why accumulation of homocystine produces mental retardation and a range of other disorders is not yet known. It also has an indirect effect on collagen biosynthesis at the post-ribosomal stage (p. 251).

FURTHER READING

Metabolism and energy production

LARNER J. (1971) *Intermediary metabolism and its regulation*. Prentice-Hall, Englewood Cliffs, New Jersey.

LEHNINGER A.L. (1965) *Bioenergetics*. Benjamin, Menlow Park, California.

McMURRAY W.C. (1977) *Essentials of Human Metabolism*. Harper and Rowe, New York.

NEWSHOLME E.A. & START C. (1973) *Regulation in Metabolism*. John Wiley and Sons, Chichester.

RACKER E. (1965) *Mechanisms in Bioenergetics*. Academic Press, New York.

RACKER E. (1976) *A New Look at Mechanisms in Bioenergetics*. Academic Press, New York.

Energy requiring processes

CLARK B.F.C. (1977) *The Genetic Code*, Studies in Biology, Vol. 83. Edward Arnold, London.

GURR M.I. & JAMES R.T. (1980) *Lipid Biochemistry* (3rd Edition). Chapman and Hall, London.

PROCKOP *et al* (1979) The biosynthesis of collagen and its disorders. *New England Journal of Medicine*, **301**, pp. 13 & 77.

SMITH A.E. (1976) *Protein Biosynthesis*, Outline Studies in Biology. Chapman and Hall, London.

Control of metabolism

CLOWES R. (1967) *The Structure of Life*. Penguin Books, Harmondsworth.

COHEN P. (1976) *Control of Enzyme Activity*, Outline Studies in Biology. Chapman and Hall, London.

COVE D.J. (1975) *Genetics*. Cambridge University Press, Cambridge.

JOHNSON H.F. (1975) *The Eighth Day of Creation*. Jonathan Cape, London.

LARNER J. (1971) *Intermediary Metabolism and its Regulation*. Prentice-Hall, Englewood Cliffs, New Jersey.

NEWSHOLME E.A. & START C. (1973) *Regulation in Metabolism*. John Wiley & Sons, Chichester.

WATSON J.D. (1976) *The Molecular Biology of the Gene*. Benjamin, Menlow Park, California.

WOODS R.A. (1975) *Biochemical Genetics*, Outline Studies in Biology, Chapman and Hall, London.

CHAPTER 5

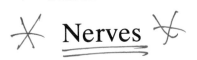

Nerves

THE STRUCTURE AND DEVELOPMENT OF NEURONS

The vertebrate nervous system can be sub-divided into an axial block of nervous tissue, lying within the bones of the skull and vertebral column, and called the Central Nervous System (which may conveniently be abbreviated to CNS), and the Peripheral Nervous System (PNS), consisting of elongated cytoplasmic processes which pass out into the tissues of the trunk and limbs from centrally located nerve cell bodies.

Nervous tissue is composed of nerve cells or neurons, and populations of satellite cells called macroglia: the latter may be either astrocytes or oligodendrocytes (CNS) or Schwann cells (PNS). Nervous activity is involved in the perception of and reaction to any form of external stimulus. The nervous system can accordingly be divided into sensory and motor components. Sensory fibres bring information from specialized peripheral receptors into the CNS, and are thus termed afferent fibres, while impulses initiating, or inhibiting muscular activity travel via efferent motor fibres. A distinction is conventionally made between the somatic nervous system of motor and sensory fibres innervating striated muscle, skin, joint capsules and tendons, and the autonomic or visceral nervous system, innervating smooth muscle, glands and myocardium.

The vertebrate neuron is a mononucleate, diploid cell covered by an excitable plasma membrane. Physiological, morphological and biochemical studies have revealed that the latter is specialized for the reception and conduction of frequency-coded stimuli which continuously converge upon each neuron from central and peripheral sources.

The shapes and sizes of neurons differ widely not only between species, but also between different sites within an individual nervous system. Irrespective of shape, however, it is helpful to subdivide any neuron into a cell body, the soma or perikaryon, and a population of cytoplasmic extensions from the soma, known collectively as neurites, which may be further subdivided into an axon, usually single, and dendrites, generally multiple (Fig. 5.1). A functional and topographical polarization of these neuronal components has long been acknowledged: an axon is defined as an impulse-generating neurite which conveys somatofugal (fleeing from the soma) information, while dendrites are usually non impulse-generating structures bearing somatopetal (seeking the soma) information. The number of dendrites, though variable, is frequently large: the manner in which they branch (dendritic tree) about a parent soma is often a characteristic by which a suitably stained neuron may be recognized under the light microscope (Fig. 5.1). While in some small neurons this arrangement is simple, the dendrites of large neurons branch many times (e.g. cerebellar Purkinje cells) thereby effectively increasing the surface area of neuronal plasma membrane available for the reception of afferent stimuli.

Classification

Neurons can be classified in a number of different ways, using morphological, pharmacological or physiological criteria. Probably the commonest distinctions are those made by light microscopy, either on the basis of the arrangement of neurites about their somata (unipolar, bipolar or multipolar) (Fig. 5.2), or according to the shape of the dendritic field of a neuron (fusiform, stellate or pyramidal).

The different types of neurons are illustrated in Figs. 5.1 and 5.2. Unipolar neurons are found in the dorsal root ganglia; bipolar neurons are seen in the retina; and multipolar neurons are the most numerous cells in the CNS.

Neurons with spindle-shaped somata from which dendrites emerge at one or both poles are termed fusiform cells; pyramidal neurons such

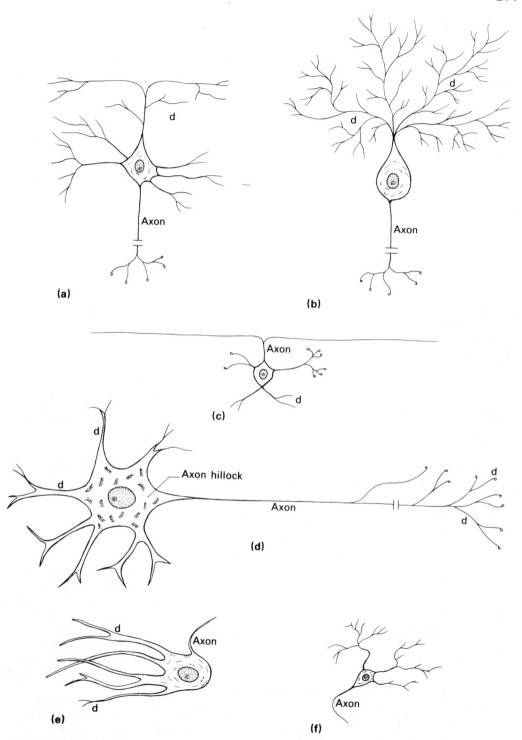

Fig. 5.1. Appearance of different nerve cells. (a) Pyramidal cell of the cerebral cortex. (b) Purkinje cell of the cerebellar cortex. (c) Granule cell of the cerebellar cortex. (d) Anterior horn cell of the spinal cord. (e) Sympathetic neuron of the stellate ganglion. (f) Small neuron of spinal trigeminal nucleus (d = dendrite).

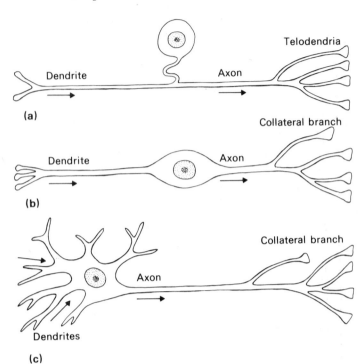

Fig. 5.2. Classification of neurons on basis of arrangement of neurites about their somata. (a) Unipolar neuron. (b) Bipolar neuron. (c) Multipolar neuron.

as those of the cerebral cortex possess conical somata from which basal and apical dendrites emerge; the dendrites of stellate cells extend ·more or less symmetrically in all directions away from the somata.

Although such schemes are useful for descriptive analyses, it is important to remember that a similarity in the shapes of neurons from different sites does not necessarily imply that they have the same functions. However, a basic and important subdivision reflects differences in phylogeny, ontogeny, 'plasticity', function and structure, between what are known as Golgi type I and Golgi type II neurons. Golgi type I neurons, also called macroneurons, principal neurons or Class I neurons, have long axons which make the primary connections between different regions within the nervous system. Golgi type II neurons, also known as short-axon cells, microneurons, intrinsic neurons, interneurons or Class II neurons, have either a very short axon terminating in the vicinity of the parent soma and overlapping its own dendritic field, or may have no recognizable axon (e.g. granule cells of the olfactory bulb and amacrine cells of the retina). Short-axon neurons are involved exclusively in localized, integrative activity and often function as inhibitors.

Physiological criteria coupled with measurements of total fibre diameter have long been used to divide peripheral nerve fibres into three major groups (A, B and C) and various subgroups. Groups A and B are composed of myelinated fibres, while group C contains only unmyelinated fibres. The functional significance, size and conduction velocities of the main groups are summarized in Table 5.1.

Soma

One of the striking features of light microscope preparations of the nervous system is the often intense basophilia of somal cytoplasm displayed by many neurons. This basophilic material, called the Nissl substance or Nissl body, is rough endoplasmic reticulum. The presence of this in considerable quantities reflects the continuous, large-scale protein synthesis carried on by neuronal somata.

Somal cytoplasm contains other populations of membrane-bound sacs, notably components of the smooth endoplasmic reticulum and Golgi apparatus. In some cells, the distribution of the smooth is as characteristic as is that of the rough endoplasmic reticulum. The Golgi apparatus appears to be widely dispersed throughout the

Table 5.1. Classification of nerve fibres.

Group	Sub-group		Functional significance	Size (μm)	Speed (m/s)
A	Motor	α	Extrafusal skeletal muscle	12–20	50–100
		γ	Intrafusal skeletal muscle	2–10	10–45
	Sensory	I	Muscle spindles and tendon organs	5–20	20–100
		II	Muscle spindles, touch and pressure receptors	5–15	20–90
		III	Temperature, touch and pain receptors	1–7	12–30
B	Motor		Preganglionic fibres	<3	3–15
C	Motor		Postganglionic autonomic fibres		
	Sensory		Autonomic and somatic (mostly 'pain' fibres)	0.1–1.5	0.2–1.6
			Olfactory fibres		

cytoplasm as a circumnuclear network, extending into dendrites but not axons. Experimental data suggest that the Golgi apparatus has the properties of a 'gate' which exerts some sort of control over the type of material exported into the axon from the soma. Lysosomes, mitochondria and centrioles are frequently observed in the Golgi region.

Subsurface cisternae, which are flattened vesicles closely applied to the inner aspect of the plasma membrane of the soma and dendrites as the latter approach the cell body, have been described: it has been suggested that they are associated with the uptake of material from the extracellular space.

Other typical somal organelles are lysosomes, which are visible in phase-contrast preparations of unstained tissue, mitochondria, microtubules and microfilaments, and, particularly in older neurons, lipofuscin granules. Pigment granules are characteristic in certain parts of the brain, and in some sites are visible on naked eye inspection of cut sections, as for example in the substantia nigra. Certain of the pigments have been related to the catecholamine-synthesizing ability of the cell in which they are found.

The nucleus is usually large, euchromatic and possesses at least one large and conspicuous nucleolus, whose diameter can be 1/3–1/4 that of the nucleus. The size and shape are variable. In some smaller neurons the nucleus may almost fill the cell body and appear surrounded by a narrow rim of cytoplasm. Some nuclei are spherical, but many others have complex and irregular profiles: the indentations in these nuclear surfaces usually contain basophilic material.

Dendrites

Dendrites (apart from the peripheral processes of dorsal root ganglion cells) contain the same complement of organelles as is found in the soma. Unlike the soma and its axon, dendrites are never ensheathed by multiple layers of satellite cell plasma membranes.

As can be seen in Golgi preparations, dendrites are not smooth-walled tubes like axons, but are covered with numerous small protrusions called dendritic spines or gemmules which range in shape from short, squat structures to the more usual narrow extensions of dendritic cytoplasm, 1–2 μm long with terminal expansions. Dendritic spines such as those found on the apical and basal dendrites of cortical Purkinje cells, have been intensively studied both histologically and physiologically. They provide a mechanism for enormously increasing the surface area of a neuron that is available for the formation of synaptic contacts with other dendrites, somata or axons. Probably the most conspicuous element of mammalian cortical dendritic spines is the spine apparatus: this consists of two or more parallel and flattened sacs separated by electron dense plates. The significance of this structure is not known.

Axon

In large multipolar neurons, an axon leaves its soma at the axon hillock, a region of somal cytoplasm characterized by a paucity of ribosomes, which results in a loss of basophilia, and by bundles of microtubules. The axon hillock is less easily defined in small neurons. In myelinated nerve fibres (see later) there is a short interval between the axon hillock and the beginning of the myelin sheath which is called the initial segment (Fig. 5.3). It has been suggested that a condensation of granular electron dense material beneath the plasma membrane of the initial segment is somehow associated with the generation of an action potential.

synapse may be distinguished ultrastructurally and pharmacologically on the basis of the shape and content of the vesicles in the pre-synaptic bouton (e.g., whether flattened, spherical, noradrenergic or neurosecretory) and on the patterns of pre- and postsynaptic cytoplasmic densities (Fig. 5.4). Somatic axons in the PNS ramify terminally as fine telodendria which effect functional contact with muscle fibres at either 'en plaque' (α-motoneurons on to extrafusal fibres) or 'en grappe' (γ-motoneurons on to intrafusal fibres) neuromuscular junctions. Autonomic efferent axons end in fine sprays of varicose unmyelinated branches lying in shallow grooves on the surface of smooth muscle cells in blood vessels, glands, etc.

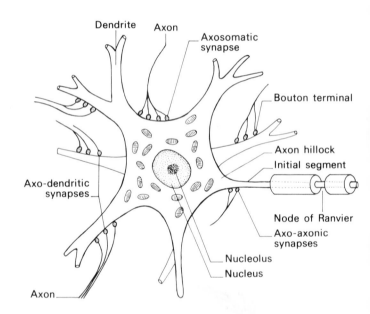

Fig. 5.3. Representation of a single neuron with axon, dendrites and three different arrangements of synapses.

While the axon is typically single at its origin, it usually branches at one or several points along its length. Axons and their collateral branches contained within the CNS make specialized functional contacts, synapses (Fig. 5.4), with sites on the plasma membranes of other axons, somata or dendrites (Fig. 5.3). At the synapse, the axon swells into a characteristic enlargement or bouton: where this occurs at the end of an axon, the swelling is known as a bouton terminal, while those found along the length of an axon are boutons de passage. Various different types of

All axons consist of axoplasm, bounded by plasma membrane continuous with that covering the somata and dendrites and here called the axolemma. The axolemma is separated from the plasma membrane of the investing layer of Schwann cells by a 10–20 nm peri-axonal space. Axoplasm contains mitochondria, microtubules, microfilaments and smooth endoplasmic reticulum.

Autonomic efferent axons and neurosecretory axons contain varieties of vesicles, some of them with dense cores.

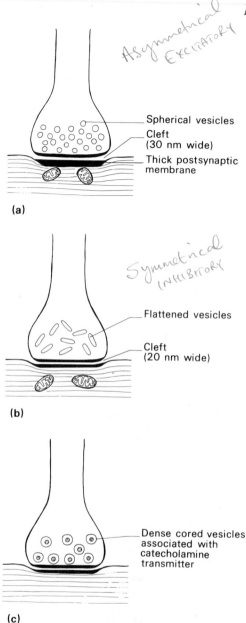

Asymmetrical EXCITATORY

Spherical vesicles
Cleft (30 nm wide)
Thick postsynaptic membrane

(a)

Symmetrical INHIBITORY

Flattened vesicles

Cleft (20 nm wide)

(b)

Dense cored vesicles associated with catecholamine transmitter

(c)

Fig. 5.4. Types of synapse in the CNS revealed by the electron microscope when glutaraldehyde fixation is used. Symmetrical synapses (b) are considered to be inhibitory and asymmetrical, (a) to be excitatory, (c) are excitatory or inhibitory.

that is unique to the nervous system, and that poses special problems as far as the distribution of intracellular materials is concerned. Since the turn of the century the concept that the soma is a trophic centre supporting its periphery has been basic to interpretations of the axonal degeneration that occurs distal to axonal interruption. It can be shown experimentally that axoplasm will dam up in fibres proximal to a chronic constriction and subsequently redistribute along the emaciated distal portion of these fibres on release of the constriction. This is taken as evidence, albeit indirect, of a slow but continuous somatofugal movement of most, if not all, of the axoplasmic constituents, at a rate of 1–2 mm/day. During the last 20 years, many workers using radioactively labelled molecules, e.g., ^{3}H-leucine, have recorded intra-axonal transport rates at least a hundred times faster than this bulk axonal displacement. The subdivision of the fast system into different phases is controversial. However, it is thought that most of the soluble protein is carried by the slow component of flow (at least 80% of the protein transported down the axon is carried in a soluble form). Particulate matter, including some of the axoplasmic and somal organelles, neurotransmitters (or their precursors) and metabolites, is carried more rapidly; fast axonal transport appears necessary for synaptic transmission and, in part, for the maintenance of postsynaptic cells. The renewal of more than 98% of the proteins and glycoproteins at the synapse is effected by components which have been synthesized in the soma and have subsequently migrated in the fast phase of axonal transport, many of them apparently within the smooth endoplasmic reticulum. The various rates of intra-axonal flow are probably caused by more than one mechanism.

The idea that the soma somehow regulates the energetic state and metabolic requirements of its periphery implies a feedback of information from the periphery to the soma. There is some evidence to support the existence of a retrograde flow of material within normal nerve fibres, based largely upon time-lapse cinemicrographic recordings.

Axonal transport

In many neurons the nucleus and cytoplasm of the cell body are separated from the peripheral ramifications of the cell by relatively vast distances (up to one metre): a spatial separation

Peripheral nerve fibres

In the PNS, axons are associated along their length with chains of Schwann cells in functional units called peripheral nerve fibres, which may be myelinated or unmyelinated.

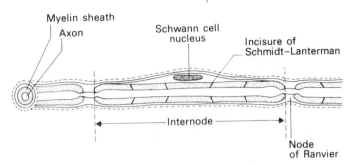

Myelin sheath
Axon
Schwann cell nucleus
Incisure of Schmidt–Lanterman
Internode
Node of Ranvier

Fig. 5.5. Diagram of a myelinated nerve fibre.

MYELINATED NERVE FIBRES

In a myelinated nerve fibre adjacent Schwann cells are separated at nodes of Ranvier: the length of axon associated with each Schwann cell territory is an internode (Fig. 5.5). The part of the internode next to the node is termed the paranode. In both immature and mature myelinated fibres there is only one Schwann cell per internode. Internodal length, which in mammalian fibres ranges from 300 to 1500 μm, increases in thicker fibres.

In conventionally prepared material, the internodal axon is a smooth-walled cylinder 2–15 μm in diameter; it becomes reciprocally indented throughout the paranodal region where the myelin sheath is crenated. At the node of Ranvier, in all but the thinnest fibres, the axon regains its smooth contour but becomes dramatically thinner.

Myelin sheath; Schmidt–Lanterman incisures; nodes of Ranvier

The myelin sheath, elaborated by the Schwann cell in the peripheral nervous system and by the oligodendrocyte in the central nervous system, is formed of apposed and subsequently compacted layers of satellite cell plasma membrane, and contains cholesterol, phospholipids, glycolipids, acidic and basic proteins and bound water.

At intervals along the peripheral internodal sheath the myelin is interrupted by inclusions of Schwann cytoplasm which constitute the Schmidt–Lanterman incisures, the length of internode between adjacent incisures being known as a cylindricoconical segment. The junction between two myelinating satellite cells is called the node of Ranvier. In the peripheral nervous system this region is more structurally complex than its central counterpart. In peripheral nerve fibres the paranodal myelin expands into a characteristic paranodal bulb which exhibits a proximodistal asymmetry

thought to be related to growth of the region in which the nerve lies. The space between two apposed paranodal bulbs is the node proper. It contains an amorphous gap substance bounded externally by a continuous Schwann cell basal lamina. Histochemical studies have shown that the gap substance contains sulphated glycosaminoglycans; it has been described as forming a polyanionic matrix around the nodal axon.

Myelination

Bundles of axons, 0.1–1.5 μm in diameter, grow into the periphery in cell-to-cell contact. During development the bundles are invaded by similarly migrating Schwann cells. These cells dissect the axonal population into smaller bundles, each bundle lying within an invagination of Schwann cell plasma membrane. As a result of repeated Schwann cell division and continued active segregation of the axons, a situation is rapidly reached in which the majority of Schwann cells contain only one promyelin axon, i.e. the 1:1 relationship between axon and satellite cell of the mature myelinated fibre has been established.

The initiation of myelinogenesis is associated with both a cessation of Schwann cell division and a period of Schwann cell hypertrophy. The axons lie at first in shallow surface depressions of Schwann cell plasma membrane which become progressively deeper. The lips of Schwann cell cytoplasm, bounding what is now a deep invagination, become apposed, thereby forming a short 'mesaxon' by which the axon appears suspended within the Schwann cell (Fig. 5.6). One explanation of myelinogenesis which has been widely accepted but is now thought to be too simple is that the mesaxon becomes elongated and spiralled around the axon; compact myelin formed as a result of the 'zippering' together of double leaflets of Schwann cell plasma membrane, with concomitant extrusion of Schwann cell cytoplasm.

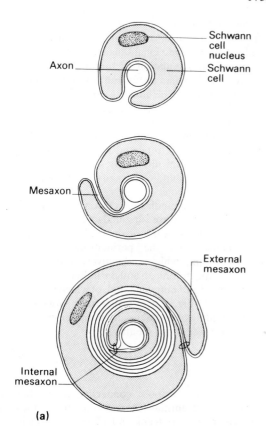

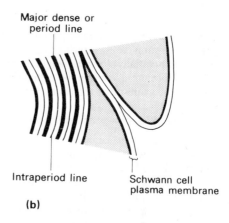

(b)

Fig. 5.6. (a) Diagram of the hypothetical mechanism of myelinogenesis in the PNS. (b) Diagram to show how major dense and intraperiod lines of myelin are produced.

UNMYELINATED AXONS

These axons are of a significantly smaller calibre than their myelinated counterparts: it is rare to find an unmyelinated axon that exceeds 1–1.5 μm in diameter, except in the large spinal roots of primates and humans. Unmyelinated axons are characteristically found in groups of 3–20, lying within individual invaginations of Schwann cell cytoplasm (Fig. 5.7). The amount of axonal surface covered by Schwann cell cytoplasm is variable. Thus each axon is bathed by extracellular fluid, and the peri-axonal space is not compartmentalized as it is in the case of the myelinated fibre by paranodal loops abutting onto the axolemma. Conduction of the nervous impulse along unmyelinated fibres, while considerably slower than along myelinated axons, is therefore continuous, the spread of current being referred to as electrotonic.

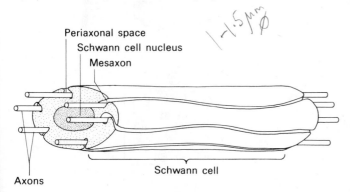

Fig. 5.7. Diagram of unmyelinated nerve fibre.

Although unmyelinated axons may branch as they near their terminations, there is no evidence to support their more proximal branching.

The Schwann cells interdigitate with one another sequentially along the length of the axon bundles, forming a continuous cellular investment for the axons other than at their terminals.

The organization of a peripheral nerve trunk

In vertebrates, a major nerve trunk, e.g., the sciatic nerve, is composed of many thousand myelinated and unmyelinated fibres which characteristically have a plurisegmental derivation from the spinal cord. In the most proximal part of their course, the individual fibres intermingle in a plexus (e.g., cervical, brachial), a formation which allows fibres from several consecutive spinal segments to be sorted out into nerve bundles destined for the supply of particular muscle groups or receptors in the limbs. The basis for this segregation, as might be expected, is embryological. The pattern of limb development, in particular the assumption of pre- and post-axial borders and the medial and lateral rotation of the limb bud, is reflected in the orderly craniocaudal sequence of dermatome innervation, and in the innervation of flexor and extensor muscle compartments. Although inevitably modified during growth, much of this

plan is retained in the adult, and can be verified by clinical testing. As the nerves are traced distally, there is a functional separation of the initial very mixed population of motor and sensory fibres into bundles or funiculi within which the majority of fibres are either motor (e.g., nerve to thyrohyoid) or sensory (e.g., lesser occipital nerve). Postganglionic sympathetic fibres are also included in these bundles. As the nerves near their destinations, repeated fasciculation (subdivision of the funiculi) occurs, so that ultimately the nerve fibre bundle may consist of fewer than one hundred axons.

As the fibre bundles pass through the tissues of the body, they are surrounded by a system of three morphologically distinct cellular sheaths, the epineurium, the perineurium and the endoneurium, which respectively surround a nerve trunk, its funiculi and the individual fibres, myelinated and unmyelinated, of which they are composed (Fig. 5.8.). Structurally organized nerve endings are essentially peripheral extensions of these three sheaths.

EPINEURIUM

Epineurium is a loose connective tissue that forms an adventitial layer around the various funiculi of a nerve trunk and, after each fascicle

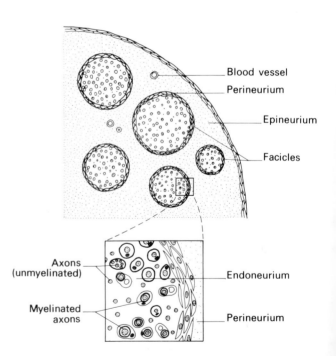

Fig. 5.8. The organization of a peripheral nerve trunk, inset showing a section at a higher magnification.

has separated from its parent trunk, is continued on as the outermost covering of the fascicles. It blends with the connective tissue sheaths of the structures through which the nerve passes. Epineurium contains fibroblasts, mast cells, macrophages, elastic fibres and irregularly disposed bundles of collagen fibrils. Blood vessels derived from regional arteries ramify throughout the epineurium before gaining access to the nerve. It is usual to find a substantial quantity of fat cells in the epineurium.

Centrally, the epineurium becomes continuous with the dura mater at the sites where the dorsal and ventral roots of a peripheral nerve enter the subarachnoid space, while at the periphery, epineurial and endoneurial spaces may communicate freely, e.g., at the motor end plate.

PERINEURIUM

Each fascicle is surrounded by a highly organized cellular sheath called the perineurium. Centrally and peripherally the perineurium terminates as an open-ended sleeve.

The perineurium is composed of several layers (up to 12) of flattened cells, whose identity is controversial. Although some authors consider them to be connective tissue, a more recent and authoritative review claims that they are modified Schwann cells. The cells are surrounded by a basement membrane, and between each layer lies a variable amount of connective tissue space containing bundles of collagen fibrils (40–80 nm diameter) running predominantly in a direction parallel with the longitudinal axis of the fibre. The cells usually display considerable pinocytotic activity. During the repair that follows degenerating or demyelinating episodes in nerve, small quantities of lipid debris are transported across the perineurium by a process of macropinocytosis.

The innermost or basal layer of perineurial cells forms a continuous sleeve around the endoneurium, the individual cells being joined by tight junctions. The perineurium is generally considered to constitute an effective diffusion barrier between epineurium and endoneurium, operational at the level of this basal layer. This barrier activity develops during the first days of neonatal life. Not only is there a barrier between epineurium and endoneurium, but also between endoneurial space and endoneurial endothelium, i.e., a blood-nerve barrier somewhat analogous to the blood-brain barrier. Thus, by these two cellular mechanisms the ionic environment of the individual nerve fibres within a peripheral nerve fibre bundle may be rigorously controlled.

ENDONEURIUM

This is the space within the basal layer of the perineurium and contains the nerve fibres and blood vessels (mostly capillaries), fibroblasts, mast cells and bundles of collagen fibrils running predominantly parallel with the long axis of the nerve. Centrally, the endoneurium continues along the nerve roots to terminate against the boundary membrane of the brain or spinal cord, while peripherally the endoneurium may become continuous with the epineurium e.g., at the motor end plate, or become greatly reduced and incorporated into the cellular investment of a receptor terminal.

Origin of the neuron

Factors involved in neuronal and glial ontogeny have been the subject of intensive and often controversial examination for well over a century. Conclusions drawn from morphological studies have always been highly inferential because of the difficulties inherent in the identification of immature tissues.

Neurons and most of the other cell types within the neuropil are derived from pluripotential cells contained in two areas of embryonic tissue, the neural tube and the neural crest. The neural tube gives rise to central nervous system neurons, ependymal cells, astrocytes and oligodendrocytes. Neurons whose somata are contained within parts of the trigeminal ganglion, and in the facial, glossopharyngeal and vagal ganglia, the ciliary ganglion, spinal sensory and autonomic ganglia, and Schwann cells and chromaffin cells of the adrenal medulla, are derived from the neural crest.

The early neural tube consists of a monolayer of functionally homogenous columnar neuroepithelial cells, bounded by internal and external limiting membranes and constituting the *ventricular germinal, primitive ependymal* or *matrix* layer. Cumulative labelling with ^{3}H-thymidine at this stage results in a linear increase in labelled cells which eventually reaches 100%, i.e., considerable proliferation is occurring (called by some workers Stage 1). The matrix layer has been subdivided accordingly into three stratae, which are, from within outwards, M (mitotic), I (intermediate) and S (synthetic). In the course of a cell cycle the matrix cell nucleus undergoes characteristic alterations in position relative to the internal limiting membrane. Thus, throughout DNA replication it lies in the S region, passes through the I region during a short pre-mitotic resting phase, lies beneath the internal limiting membrane in the M region prior to mitosis, after which the daughter cell nuclei move back through the I region to the S region. The 'elevator' movement of the nucleus has been correlated with the contraction and subsequent rounding up of the initially elongated matrix cell as it prepares to divide. If it is remembered that mitoses in the matrix layer are asynchronous it is not difficult to understand why the early neural tube has a pseudostratified appearance.

Exposure of the cells to radioisotope at a later stage yields a number of unlabelled, i.e., post-mitotic, cells which are considered to be young neurons or neuroblasts. These migrate out of the ventricular germinal zone to accumulate in a *mantle layer* of differentiating cells (Stage II). Tracts of axonal processes from these cells extend through the outer *marginal layer* into the surrounding tissue blocks. Other daughter cells of the matrix layer continue to divide, forming a *subventricular* or *subependymal* zone between ventricular germinal and mantle zones. While some post-mitotic subependymal cells differentiate into small neurons, others produce further generations of neuroblasts and, when neuroblast production has ceased, differentiate into glioblasts or macroglial precursors (Stage III). In regions such as the cerebellar cortex, numbers of subependymal cells move to a subpial position and establish new proliferative foci from which their progeny migrate to their final destinations in the developing brain where they differentiate into neurons or glia.

Although there are no morphological differences between germinal neuroepithelial cells, the old idea that neurons and glia develop from an uncommitted cell is now discredited. The possible source of these cell types is still undecided. It has been suggested (a) that a population of germ cells in the early neural tube is committed to produce neurons and another to produce glia; or (b) that neurons and glia arise consecutively from a shared cell line.

Certain facts are undisputed. Thus it is recognized that almost all neurogenesis occurs before birth, and that gliogenesis is continued after birth. Furthermore, Class I neurons arise and differentiate before Class II neurons.

Macroneurons and many microneurons are exclusively prenatal in origin; there are several sites where microneurons develop postnatally, e.g., granule cells of the cerebellum and hippocampus.

It has been suggested that whereas Class I neurons adopt a specific structure and function under strict genetic control, Class II neurons are not subject to such limitations and remain modifiable by the effects of experience (whether mediated hormonally or neuronally) until late in ontogeny.

The derivatives of the neural crest have been determined in a number of ways:
1   By examining the consequences of ablating all or part of the neural crest or of grafting parts of the crest into abnormal sites.
2   By following the fate of neural crest cells labelled autoradiographically and grafted into an unlabelled host, or after staining with vital dyes.

The mechanisms involved in the release of cells from the neural crest are unknown. During maturation of the neuroblast, neurites are extended from the soma into the surrounding tissue; one becomes differentiated as the axon, the others establish the basis of the future dendritic tree, The tips of both axons and dendrites are expanded into distinctive growth cones, from which fine filopodia are put out. The formation of synapses upon the filopodia is thought to determine the final spatial distribution of the dendrites. The degree of filopodial synaptogenesis has been shown to determine the segmental length and amount of branching of the dendrites; the expansion of the dendritic field occurs by interaction between growth cones and the axon fields through which the dendrites pass. Subsequent synaptogenesis occurs on the shaft and spines of the dendrites.

Axonal outgrowth appears to be influenced by mechanical and chemical factors. The mechanisms whereby specific connections between axon terminals and target cells are made are not known.

NEUROCHEMISTRY

The brain

UTILIZATION OF OXYGEN AND GLUCOSE

Oxygen and glucose are the most important substances required by the brain and as the brain possesses little metabolic reserve it needs a constant supply of these from the blood. It requires about 20% of the cardiac output although it represents only 2.5% of the body weight. The adult brain also consumes 20–25% of the oxygen uptake. During hard physical work the body's oxygen consumption increases by five times whilst the proportion used by the brain falls to about 5% so that the absolute amount remains the same. If the circulation to the brain is cut off for about 10 seconds the subject becomes unconscious and if the interruption is prolonged for 3 minutes irreversible damage results. Oxygen consumption does not appear to change significantly during strenuous mental effort.

Energy requirements of the brain are almost entirely provided by blood glucose, the basic substrate of cerebral metabolism. Abnormal EEG patterns are seen if blood glucose falls from the normal 80–100 mg/100 cm³ to 60 mg/100 cm³ and at a level below 40 mg/100 cm³ symptoms of hypoglycaemia become apparent. If the fall to this level or below is rapid, the symptoms can be severe and immediate effective treatment is essential if irreversible damage to the brain is to be avoided. Substances such as glutamic and succinic acids have produced arousal from hypoglycaemic coma but their action is thought to be secondary to an increase in blood adrenalin and the associated rise in blood glucose. In the hypoglycaemic state there is a decrease in cerebral energy-rich phosphates and an increase in inorganic phosphates. On the other hand, when anaesthetics are used to induce unconciousness at normal blood glucose levels, energy-rich phosphates accumulate as a consequence of less cerebral utilization of glucose.

The products of glucose catabolism in the brain are almost entirely carbon dioxide, lactic and pyruvic acids. The brain is never at rest and therefore the availability of oxygen and glucose must be maintained by a constant blood flow since the demand is the same whether thinking, resting, sleeping or day-dreaming, for which the brain utilizes about 400 calories per day!

In the brain, metabolism of glucose can be directed along any one of three pathways once it has been phosphorylated to glucose-6-phosphate. These are glycogen synthesis, glycolysis and the pentose phosphate pathway.

A small amount of glycogen is synthesized and is used as a reserve for glucose. It has a high rate of both breakdown and synthesis. Pathways of glycogenesis and glycogenolysis in brain appear to be similar to those in liver and muscle. In the brain, oxidative phosphorylation yields 33 equivalents of phosphate bonds per mole of glucose indicating a high rate of synthesis and utilization of ATP for energy requirements. In the process

glucose is finally converted to carbon dioxide and water.

The pentose phosphate pathway is more active in developing than in mature brain since it is used in lipid synthesis for production of myelin. The pathway is used for production of NADPH for reduction in synthetic reactions and synthesis of pentose for nucleotides.

The phosphorylation of glucose to glucose-6-phosphate is mediated by the enzyme hexokinase. Judging from the rate of phosphorylation of glucose only a small fraction of the potential catalytic capacity of the enzyme hexokinase is used, most of the activity of this enzyme being inhibited by its reaction product. This inhibition performs a self-limiting process in the conversion of glucose to glucose-6-phosphate and probably acts to regulate the availability of glucose-6-phosphate for utilization in any one of the three metabolic pathways.

MYELINATED NERVES

The average adult human brain weighs about 1400 grams of which about 78% is water; the dry weight composition of white matter is 55% lipid and 39% protein; in grey matter it is 32% and 55% respectively. A significant component of white matter is myelin (which confers the colour) and this is mainly responsible for the differences in chemical composition seen between white and grey matter.

During development myelin is laid down at different rates in different areas of the brain. Nerve fibres usually become fully functional after myelination is complete. The process of myelination in the human brain is almost complete by the end of the second year but may continue in some areas for at least a decade. Vitamins are essential in the normal metabolic activity of nervous tissue and a severe vitamin deficiency can interfere with normal development, growth and function of the nervous system. Vitamin deficiencies can bring about visible alterations in nervous tissue but little is known of the mechanisms involved. Vitamin B_{12} deficiency causes demyelination in the central nervous system.   Vit B₁₂

Chemical composition of myelin
Electron microscopic and X-ray diffraction techniques show that myelin is a radially repeating 'double' unit membrane having a protein–lipid–protein–lipid–protein structure 12–16 nm in thickness (Fig. 5.9).

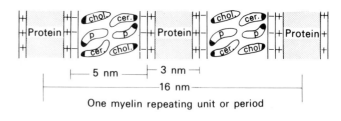

Fig. 5.9. Schematic representation of the ultrastructure of CNS myelin. The bimolecular lipid layers composed of cholesterol (chol.), phospholipid (p) and cerebroside (cer.) are shown with the polar portions of these molecules (shaded) facing the protein layers.

One myelin repeating unit or period

The lipids constitute about 75% of myelin and are mainly cholesterol, phospholipid and glycolipid (cerebroside) in the approximate molar ratio of 4:3:2; the remaining 25% is mostly protein. Studies on animal myelin have shown that its composition can vary at different periods of formation during growth. There is also some evidence of regional differences in the composition of human adult myelin, for example, the ratio of lipid to protein appears to be higher in the spinal cord than in brain. Differences in the glycolipid component also exist between peripheral and central myelin.

Proteins in central myelin generally exist as proteolipid protein and basic protein in about equal amounts, totalling approximately 70% of the total protein content, the remainder being high molecular weight proteins. Most of these proteins are found in other cells of the body but one called S-100 appears to be specific to the nervous system, as are some enzyme proteins involved in specialized functions, such as acetylcholinesterase which serves to break down acetylcholine at a nerve ending.

Chemical transmitters
(see also receptors, p. 301 and nerve conduction, p. 296)

In higher organisms it is thought that transmission between one neuron and another or between a neuron and muscle or other organ is mediated entirely by release of a chemical substance into the junction between them. Some chemical transmitters have an inhibitory effect on neurons. Recent studies indicate that gamma aminobutyric acid and glycine may be inhibitory transmitter substances in the CNS. Glutamic and aspartic acids may be excitatory transmitters.

Central and peripheral 'cholinergic' neurons, i.e. those releasing acetylcholine as a chemical transmitter, must have a readily available source of acetylcholine for release from the nerve ending. Both the enzyme choline acetyl transferase and the basic substances required for the local syntheses of acetylcholine are present at the nerve ending. The acetyl group comes from acetyl-CoA in the nerve terminal mitochondria but choline is mainly derived from elsewhere. It may be synthesized in the liver and taken up in the brain from the bloodstream by a carrier-mediated mechanism, or it may come from acetylcholine which has been hydrolysed at the nerve ending by acetylcholinesterase. The simplified reaction for the synthesis of acetylcholine is:

$$\text{acetate} + \text{choline} + \text{ATP} \longrightarrow \text{ACh} + \text{AMP} + \text{pyrophosphate}$$

Acetylcholine is currently regarded as the principal chemical transmitter in the central and peripheral nervous systems but in some neural pathways, mainly those with their cell bodies in the brainstem, there is evidence that the two catecholamines, noradrenaline and dopamine and an indolamine called serotonin, are probable chemical transmitters. The synthesis of the catecholamines is as in Fig. 5.10 and the synthesis of serotonin from tryptophan is according to the reactions in Fig. 5.11.

In adrenergic neurons, i.e. those releasing noradrenaline at the nerve ending, noradrenaline is probably derived from tyrosine in the blood then stored in granules synthesized in the nerve ending, and subsequently released into the junction when the signal arrives at the nerve ending. Noradrenaline interacts with the receptor site and subsequently is inactivated by a re-uptake mechanism into the nerve terminal. This mechanism is different from that for acetylcholine which is hydrolysed by acetylcholinesterase. An enzyme, catechol–O–methyl transferase (COMT), is present outside the adrenergic nerve ending to remove any noradrenaline not inactivated by the re-uptake process and another regulating enzyme, monoamine oxidase (MAO), is also present inside the adrenergic nerve ending and deaminates excess catecholamine which may escape from the synaptic vesicles within the nerve ending (Fig. 5.12).

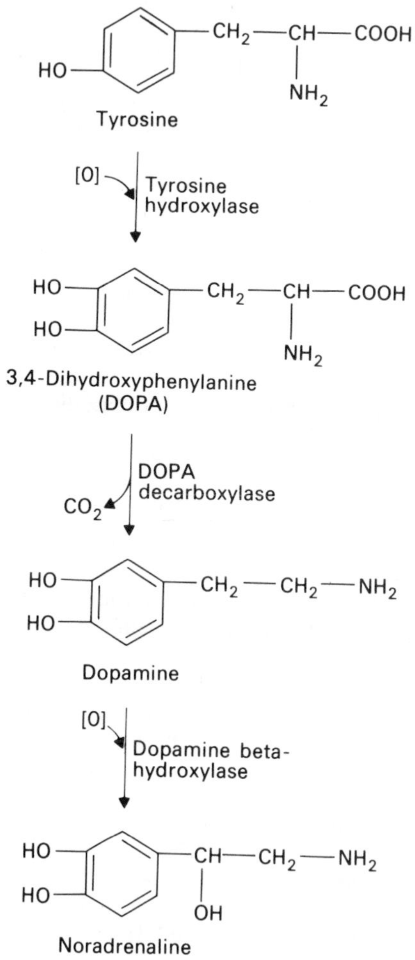

Fig. 5.10. Pathway for synthesis of catecholamine neurotransmitter noradrenaline.

Information on the putative amino acid transmitters is less well documented and evidence fulfilling the accepted criteria for their functional identification remains sparse. Gamma aminobutyric acid appears to be important as a chemical transmitter in the cerebellum, retina, hippocampus and cerebral cortex where it is released by inhibitory neurons and acts by increasing the permeability of the post-synaptic membrane to chloride ions. When it has performed its function, the transmitter substance is inactivated by a re-uptake process whereby it is transported across the pre-synaptic membrane by a carrier transfer mechanism. Glycine acts as an inhibitory transmitter by hyperpolarizing the post-synaptic membrane whilst glutamic and aspartic acids act as excitatory transmitters by depolarizing the post-synaptic membrane. These latter amino acid transmitters act predominantly in the different functional types of synapses within the spinal cord where incoming sensory information is processed by the interneurons. After release from the nerve-ending the amino acid transmitter substances may be inactivated by a re-uptake mechanism similar to that for gamma aminobutyric acid.

PHYSIOLOGY OF NERVE FIBRES

General principles

The fundamental purpose of any nerve fibre is to transfer 'information' from one point in the nervous system to another in the form of a code—namely by means of electrical impulses. Preferably it should be able to do so as faithfully, quickly and often as possible, with the minimum use of energy resources. As will become apparent, axons have evolved general properties to fulfil the above conditions in the most economical way.

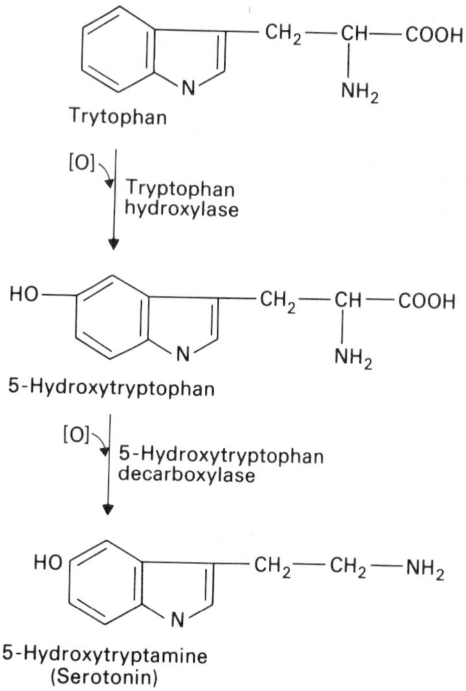

Fig. 5.11. Pathway for the synthesis of the neurotransmitter serotonin.

[handwritten: Speed { 0.1 m/sec / 120 m/sec]

The primary property of all nervous tissue is its 'excitability', or ability to respond to particular forms of energy by the production of an impulse or action potential which is simply a brief electrical pulse, usually lasting 1–2 msec, conducted along the axon. Action potentials are only produced in what are commonly called 'excitable tissues', like muscle and neural tissues.

A property of excitable tissues, although by no means exclusive to them, is the existence of large concentration differences of certain ions on the two sides of the cell membrane. A metabolically driven pump maintains a low intracellular sodium concentration. The cation concentration inside the cells is made up of a high concentration of potassium ions.

[handwritten margin note: low intracellular sodium / high intracellular potassium]

A major feature of neural transmission is the concept of threshold. An impulse will arise in a nerve fibre or nerve cell only when a certain critical level of membrane potential change occurs, corresponding to a change in the resting membrane potential of some 20 mV in a direction towards zero membrane potential. Movement in this direction is known as depolarization, (hypopolarization), whereas changes in the opposite direction, which decrease excitability, are known as hyperpolarization.

The 'all or none' law states that providing a stimulus is above threshold, an action potential of uniform, predictable amplitude is propagated without decrement from the point stimulated along the nerve fibre.

If a nerve fibre is stimulated electrically half way along its length, then the action potential will be propagated in both directions. Under normal *in vivo* circumstances nerve fibres are activated either at their origin at the cell body directly or by synaptic action, or at the peripheral receptor in sensory nerves; hence conduction is usually one way from one end of the nerve fibre to the other.

The speed at which action potentials can be propagated along an axon varies from 0.1 m/sec in the thinnest unmyelinated fibres, to about 120 m/sec in the thickest myelinated fibres. The frequency of 'firing' impulses also varies; large fibres producing a maximum of about 1000 per second whereas the smallest fibres are often incapable of firing at rates exceeding 10 per second. The upper limit to the frequency of firing is dependent on a general property of nerve fibres called the refractory period. This is the period following an action potential when a nerve fibre exhibits diminished or nil excitability.

The resting membrane potential

In close association with the membranes of nerve and muscle fibres are mitochondria and the usual cellular machinery for mobilization of large energy reserves. The membrane itself has several important properties:

1 It has high electrical resistance.

2 It maintains large differences in the concentration of ions between one side and the other.

3 It governs the size of the resting membrane potential.

If a microelectrode is inserted in a living nerve cell or axon, it can be shown that at rest the membrane is negatively charged inside, with respect to external positivity. In most nerve cells and axons the resting potential is about -75 mV. This difference in polarity arises from the unequal distribution of ions on either side of the membrane. These differences in concentration are shown in Fig. 5.13 for the most studied of all

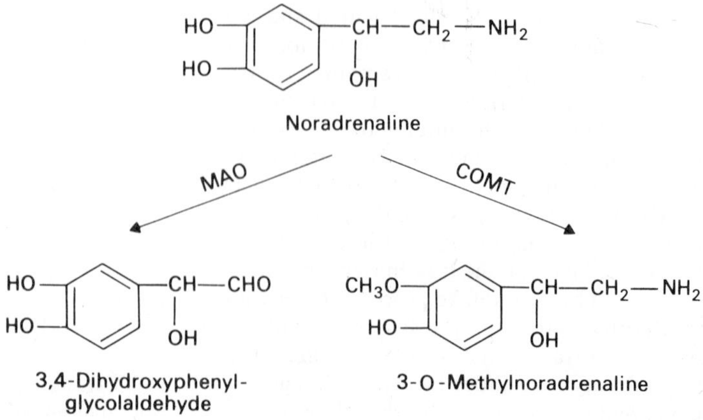

Fig. 5.12. Inactivation of noradrenaline.

Noradrenaline

MAO → 3,4-Dihydroxyphenyl-glycolaldehyde

COMT → 3-O-Methylnoradrenaline

nerve fibres, the giant axon of the squid. The major external ions are sodium and chloride whereas the major internal ions are potassium, large organic anions (Pr⁻) and some chloride.

The ionic basis of the resting membrane potential

Where one has a membrane separating two electrolyte solutions of different composition, clearly there is a tendency for the ions of higher concentration on one side to move to the other side. However, all ions do not move easily across lipid membranes, some move faster than others. If positive ions move faster than slower negative ions clearly the solution into which they are moving becomes more positive and a potential difference results which repels further movement until a situation of equilibrium occurs—the equilibrium potential for that ion.

Let us assume the membrane contains pores which allow the free passage of K^+ ions. The development of an electrical potential difference, essentially a membrane potential, can be visualized from the following reasoning. If the small K^+ ions are able to pass through the pores they will become separated from the larger negative ions (A^-) which cannot enter the pores from the inside and which have a restraining influence on the movement of the K^+ ions in their attempt to maintain electrical neutrality. Clearly diffusion forces moving K^+ outside the cell membrane are balanced by electrostatic forces tending to keep the K^+ on the inside (Fig. 5.14). Since voltage is defined as a separation of net charge, a potential difference, or membrane potential, will develop. In many living cells, and in particular in nerve cells, it is K^+ which is largely responsible for this diffusion potential. Only minute quantities of ions are needed; for example only 1/100,000th of the K^+ must move outwards to give a membrane potential of 100 mV positive on the outside.

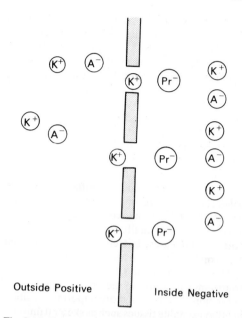

Outside Positive   Inside Negative

Fig. 5.14. Situation giving rise to a potassium diffusion potential across a membrane. A few K^+ ions diffuse through the membrane to the outside, since they pass through easily. A^- does not. This produces an excess of positive charge on the outside of membrane. As the resulting potential prevents further K^+ ions diffusing out, equilibrium ensues.

In all living cells there are differences in the ionic concentrations inside and outside the cell, and hence a diffusion potential exists which contributes to the resting membrane potential. The diffusion potential is, of course, a passive phenomenon, but it is known that very considerable active transport of ions also occurs across living membranes. Clearly, energy is required to maintain a difference in ionic constituents between the inside and outside of the cell, otherwise the ions would gradually run down their concentration gradients, as implied above. For any ion (x), the membrane potential that just stops diffusion of that ion across the membrane is called the equilibrium potential, E_x. If the measured membrane potential is the same as the equilibrium potential for a particular ion then no net movement of those ions occurs. However, as several different ions are involved, each with a different mobility, it follows that any particular membrane potential is unlikely to be the same as the equilibrium potential of any ion although it can often be very close.

The major ions involved in the resting membrane potential are Na^+, K^+ and Cl^-. In nerve and muscle cells the equilibrium potentials of the

Inside		Outside
K^+ 400 mM		K^+ 10 mM
Na^+ 50 mM	Cell membrane	Na^+ 450 mM
Cl^- 40–150 mM		Cl^- 460 mM
Pr^- 300–410 mM		–

Fig. 5.13. Concentrations of ions in intra and extracellular locations of squid giant axon. Pr⁻, large impermeable organic anions. (After Hodgkin, A.L., *Conduction of the nervous impulse*, Liverpool University Press, 1967).

Cl^- and K^+ are about -90 mV which is similar to the membrane potential (-70 mV inside). On the other hand the Na^+ equilibrium potential is nowhere near the observed resting membrane potential in these tissues. Since this is the case, Na^+ would be moving inwards across the cell membrane were it not for the sodium pump which is preventing this by actively transporting sodium against its concentration gradient. Furthermore, the membrane at rest is 75 times less permeable to Na^+ than to K^+. Thus its diffusion potential is minimal and has a negligible effect on the resting membrane potential. The principal ion causing the resting membrane potential is K^+. When the external concentration of K^+ is lowered experimentally then the membrane potential increases, but changing the external Na^+ concentration causes little change.

The position of the Cl^- seems to be that it contributes little to the membrane potential in nerve fibres but holds a more important position in other excitable tissues such as skeletal muscle.

The sodium pump

The distribution of K^+ and Cl^- across the cell membrane seems to be reciprocal. Both muscle cells and axons have a high content of K^+ and low content of Cl^-. The other anions in the cell are largely organic and cannot pass across the membrane. The small sodium ion is a particular case. The accumulation of Na^+ inside the cell is actively prevented by the presence of the sodium pump. Thus, if the pump was switched off suddenly, sodium ions would enter the cell and the membrane potential would decline towards zero. In practice the 'rundown' of the membrane potential is very slow due to the very low permeability of the resting membrane to Na^+ ions. It can be shown by the use of metabolic inhibitors (e.g. cyanide) that ATP is required for maintaining the sodium pump. This pumping mechanism is responsible for long term maintenance of the large differences in ionic composition of extra and intracellular fluids.

The action potential

THE IONIC BASIS OF THE ACTION POTENTIAL

In 1939, Hodgkin and Huxley showed that during excitation the membrane potential changed from a negative to a positive value; that is to say that at the peak of the action potential (AP) the inside of the cell became positive with respect to the outside (Fig. 5.15a). The total potential

change is from about -75 mV (RMP) to about $+50$ mV, i.e. about 125 mV overall. All the available evidence now suggests that the peak of the action potential very closely approximates the equilibrium potential for the Na ion, E_{Na}. The upstroke of the action potential is largely due to a massive sudden influx of sodium ions alone. It is still not known how the low Na^+ conductance of the resting potential is so dramatically increased on depolarization.

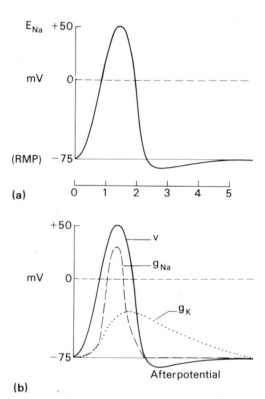

Fig. 5.15. (a) Action potential in squid giant axon, recorded by an electrode inside the cell. (b) Sodium conductance (gNa), and potassium conductance (gK) changes during the action potential (v), as theoretically evaluated. (RMP) resting membrane potential. (Redrawn from Hodgkin, 1967).

There are two reasons why this massive and sudden increase in Na^+ conductance is very brief. First, the sodium pores in the membrane stay open for a very short time and sodium conductance falls very quickly; second, potassium conductance increases shortly after the initiation of the action potential; K^+ moving in the opposite direction to Na^+ (Fig. 5.15b). This of course, will tend to restore the membrane potential to its original level. The potassium effect occurs largely as a result of the upstroke of the action potential (caused by Na^+ movement into the cell) changing the equilibrium potential for the K^+ ion. The action potential ceases when both Na^+ and K^+ conductances are restored to their original levels at the resting membrane potential. The whole process lasts about 0.5–2 msec, depending upon the type of excitable tissue involved. The total quantity of Na^+ entering and K^+ leaving the cell is minute compared to the intra and extracellular concentrations of these ions. It has been calculated that only about 3 picomoles of Na^+ pass across the membrane during the action potential.

The explosive nature of the action potential is considered to be due to 'regenerative entry' of Na^+. This means that entry of a small quantity of Na^+ powerfully facilitates the further entry of more Na^+ and so on. The energy for the process is supplied by sodium ions running down their electrochemical and concentration gradients. As the action potential rises, the sodium gates open more and consequently less energy is required. In contrast to the sodium pores, the potassium gates open more slowly and since they also close more slowly a 'positive after potential' following the action potential, can usually be recorded. This is really a temporary increase in the resting membrane potential (Fig. 5.15b).

Calcium is a divalent cation, and is therefore strongly charged positively. As such it tends to occupy sites on the nerve membrane and effectively contributes to the resting membrane potential by preventing the entry of Na^+ ions. Reducing the extracellular concentration of Ca^{2+} by any means makes the membrane unstable and the entry of Na^+ easier. From time to time enough Na^+ enters to reach the threshold, at which point an action potential is generated. When such a situation occurs on motor nerve fibres, spontaneous contraction of muscles ensues giving rise to the condition of tetany (p. 765).

CONDUCTION OF ACTION POTENTIALS

It will be recalled that action potentials are conducted along nerve fibres at speeds generally in the range of 0.1–120 m/sec, and that the process is 'non-decremental', i.e. the action potential recorded at the end of the nerve fibre has the same amplitude as that recorded at the point of initiation. Now the nerve fibre is, on superficial examination, similar to any conduction cable with an insulating sheath around it, in this case the membrane. However, its cable properties are very poor. The axoplasm and extracellular fluid are relatively poor conductors, if compared, for example, with a copper cable. The whole system is very 'leaky' electrically, and as a consequence the action potential should decrease passively or electrotonically by a considerable amount over short distances. Since it does not appear to do so, an explanation must be sought.

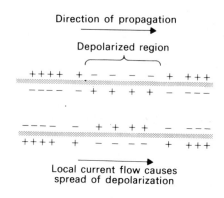

Fig. 5.16. Conduction of the nerve impulse in an unmyelinated fibre.

The action potential continually regenerates itself along the membrane of the nerve fibre. At the initial point of depolarization, caused for example by an applied electrical stimulus, sodium enters the cell and causes the upstroke of the action potential. At this instant this part of the cell is strongly positive inside with respect to adjacent portions of the resting cell, which are negatively charged inside (Fig. 5.16). Current then flows from positive to negative regions and back to the positive regions again, i.e. a local circuit is established. Negative charge is taken from adjacent regions of the membrane so that these become somewhat depolarized. This depolarization is adequate to allow Na^+ entry to become regenerative and another full-sized action potential is produced across the adjacent membrane. Evidently this process is then repeated on the next portion of membrane and so on; propagation of the nerve impulse is thus achieved. There is no theoretical limit on the distances over which such a process can be conveyed.

Chapter 5

REFRACTORY PERIOD—THE RECOVERY AFTER A NERVE IMPULSE

After a nerve impulse has been generated in an axon it is impossible to initiate another impulse until a definite period of time has elapsed. This period is known as the absolute refractory period. Following this, there is a period of time when a stronger-than-threshold stimulus is needed to produce a second impulse, this is known as the 'relative refractory period'. For mammalian nerve fibres the absolute refractory period is of the order of 0.5 msec, and relative refractory period about 3 msec. The refractory period is associated with closure of the sodium gates but its cause is largely unknown. Potassium permeability remains increased above normal levels for a time after the action potential. Both factors militate against the production of a new action potential.

The functional significance of the refractory period is that it puts an upper limit on the frequency at which action potentials can be generated in any nerve fibre.

Conduction velocity

It can be shown, both theoretically and experimentally, that conduction velocity is proportional to the square root of the diameter of the nerve fibre. Quadrupling the diameter would therefore give rise to a doubling in the conduction velocity. The speed with which the squid reacts to adverse environments is achieved by having 'giant axons' of up to 500μm in diameter. Clearly in a large vertebrate which requires some millions of fast conduction fibres for rapid relay of information there is a problem of bulk. In the vertebrate a more sophisticated means of increasing conduction velocity was achieved by the process of myelination of nerve fibres. The myelin sheath (Fig. 5.5) is essentially an insulator broken up at intervals of about 0.3–1.5 mm by the nodes of Ranvier (Fig. 5.17). The design is such that the nerve impulse literally hops from node to node rather than smoothly running along the unmyelinated nerve fibre. Normally, current flows back from the inactive node of the fibre to the active portion where the action potential is present. As in the unmyelinated fibre sufficient charge is displaced to generate an action potential at the inactive node. Such a process is sometimes referred to as 'saltatory conduction'. It is possible for action potentials to be conducted either way from a depolarized region in the experimental situation.

In part the myelin sheath acts as an insulator to prevent activation of the internode region but it also effectively reduces the electrical capacity of the fibre so that little current is lost. There appear to be very few Na^+ and K^+ gates in the membrane of the fibres at the internode region; They are all heavily concentrated at the node region. Myelination clearly increases the conduction velocity of nerve fibres enormously, usually about five-fold; the range of conduction

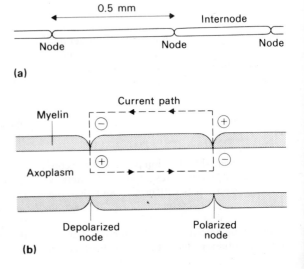

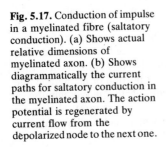

Fig. 5.17. Conduction of impulse in a myelinated fibre (saltatory conduction). (a) Shows actual relative dimensions of myelinated axon. (b) Shows diagrammatically the current paths for saltatory conduction in the myelinated axon. The action potential is regenerated by current flow from the depolarized node to the next one.

velocities for unmyelinated fibres of $0.1–1.0\,\mu m$ in diameter is about $0.1–2$ m/sec. Myelinated fibres have diameters from about $2–20\ \mu m$ in vertebrates and their conduction velocities range from $12–120$ m/sec. Large diameter fibres are normally reserved for processes requiring fast and accurate transfer of information necessitating immediate action; they are particularly important in movement control. Small fibres, on the other hand, are often, but not always, reserved for less exacting tasks; such as are carried out by the autonomic nervous system and these fibres are virtually all unmyelinated.

Action of local anaesthetics on nerve fibres
(see also Sensation)

Although the first local anaesthetics were discovered as long ago as 1860 surprisingly little is known about their mode of action. Many substances can act as local anaesthetics, but those with the most potent action, which are also most commonly used, are related to cocaine.

The primary action of cocaine-like local anaesthetics, such as procaine, lignocaine and xylocaine, is to reversibly block the conduction of the nerve impulse. These drugs do not depolarize the membrane but in some way they stabilize it by preventing or inhibiting ionic interchange. Procaine and related local anaesthetics have been shown to decrease sodium conductance. They also increase the threshold for production of an action potential, slow the propagation of an impulse and decrease the rate of rise and height of the action potential. In sufficient concentrations the propagated action potential is prevented.

Some of the actions of local anaesthetics in small doses have been compared with the effects of raised extracellular Ca^{2+} levels. Both are strongly bound by phospholipids, and procaine has been shown to compete with Ca^{2+} for uptake by phospholipids; additionally they both have the effect of increasing membrane stability. However, in contrast to local anaesthetics, increased Ca^{2+} increases the rate of rise of the action potential as well as the height. The binding sites for local anaesthetics and calcium are probably not, therefore, identical.

PROPERTIES OF SYNAPSES AND REFLEXES

Synaptic transmission

Over a hundred years ago Claude Bernard had shown that paralysis caused by curare did not prevent muscle contracting in response to direct stimulation. He concluded that a chemical substance mediated between the nerve and the muscle and caused contraction. The first definitive proof of this did not come until 1921, when Loewi showed that the vagus nerve inhibited the heart by production of the transmitter acetylcholine. Later it was shown that acetylcholine was also the agent for effecting excitatory transmission across autonomic ganglia as well as at the neuromuscular junction of vertebrates.

STRUCTURE OF THE SYNAPSE

Electron microscopy confirmed that a gap existed between the apposing membranes of nerve and muscle, and between apposing nerve cell processes. Because of this, the term synapse has been applied to both of these sites. However, as there are differences in their properties, there has been a trend towards restricting the term synapse to the gap between neurons and their processes.

In the neuromuscular junction the gap is about 50 nm (500 Ångstrom units) and about half of this in central synapses. The use of differential staining techniques established that acetylcholine esterase is present in the postsynaptic area. This is the enzyme responsible for the destruction of acetylcholine, and it is now known that it accumulates in the electron dense opacity of the postsynaptic area. Acetylcholine is stored in the axon terminal within vesicles, and its release causes changes in ionic permeability of the muscle or postsynaptic membrane. These ionic changes, if great enough, cause the generation of an action potential in the muscle cell. The synaptic cleft in the neuromuscular synapse is sufficiently wide to prevent the action potential in the axon from 'invading' the muscle cell (Fig. 5.22).

[handwritten margin note: NEURO MUSCULAR JUNCTION 50 nm]

SYNAPTIC DELAY

Sophisticated electrophysiological methods, employing microelectrodes, have shown that there is a delay, of the order of 0.2 msec, between the arrival of the action potential in the axon terminal and the generation of the action potential in the muscle. The delay is about 0.5 msec, in central synapses.

ENDPLATE POTENTIAL (THE EPP)

Similar techniques of intracellular recording have shown that the action potential in the muscle is preceded by another potential of lower amplitude. This is a depolarizing, non-propagated potential called an endplate potential, or EPP (Fig. 5.18). If the endplate potential is large enough, and it nearly always is under normal *in vivo* conditions, then an action potential is produced in the muscle. The EPP can be perfectly mimicked by the action of acetylcholine applied through a micropipette in the region of the endplate. It is possible to quantify the amount of transmitter required to produce a given number of millivolts of depolarization of the postsynaptic membrane. In each case, with the natural EPP or applied acetylcholine, the action is quite brief because acetylcholine esterase rapidly destroys the remaining transmitter once it has affected the postsynaptic membrane. The EPP therefore normally only lasts a few milliseconds.

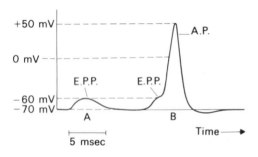

Fig. 5.18. A diagram of an action potential in muscle produced by stimulation of motoraxon and recorded intracellularly. In A the EPP amplitude is too low to evoke an action potential, whereas in B it rises above the required critical amplitude.

QUANTAL THEORY OF SYNAPTIC TRANSMISSION

It has never been conclusively proven that the transmitter resides in the vesicles, although there is plenty of circumstantial evidence that this is the case. The best view we have is that the normal EPP is composed of a large number of miniature EPPs (MEPPs) summating at the same time. Each MEPP is considered to be produced by the release of one vesicle of acetylcholine. Under resting conditions, packets of transmitter are released at a very low frequency and the MEPPs occur randomly. The EPP is the result of a massive, brief acceleration in this frequency.

CALCIUM AND NEUROMUSCULAR TRANSMISSION

Synaptic transmission needs calcium, in fact the amplitude of the endplate potential is approximately proportional to the external $[Ca^{2+}]$. This implies that calcium is essential for the release of acetylcholine from the axon terminal, but its precise role is unknown. It has been suggested that calcium changes the consistency of the axoplasm from a gel to a sol, with a resultant enormous increase in random bombardment of the presynaptic membrane by the vesicles. These fuse with the membrane and empty their contents into the cleft. This package theory of synaptic transmission is now widely known as the quantal theory of transmitter release.

Interestingly with regard to excitability of the axon, calcium has a converse action. A decrease in extracellular $[Ca^{2+}]$ leads to increased excitability of the axon itself, such that axons can spontaneously produce action potentials. Such a situation occurs in parathyroid deficiency, and may lead to many axons exhibiting spontaneous activity, causing involuntary muscular spasm, i.e. tetany.

SUMMARY

When an action potential reaches the presynaptic terminal, ionic changes occur which are similar to those in a nerve fibre that is depolarized. There is initially a rapid entry of some sodium and calcium ions. It is the calcium entry that is responsible for causing the instantaneous release of a large number of vesicles of acetylcholine into the synaptic cleft. Much of the acetylcholine then floats across to the postsynaptic membrane where it latches on to specific receptor zones. Once this occurs it is now known that an absolutely non-specific change in permeability of the postsynaptic membrane occurs with respect to all anions and cations. This causes the membrane potential to move rapidly towards zero from the resting membrane potential level of about -75 mV inside, that is to say depolarization occurs and the EPP is produced. When the EPP causes the membrane potential to fall to about -55 mV, an action potential ensues.

DRUGS AFFECTING NEUROMUSCULAR TRANSMISSION

Many substances have been discovered which affect neuromuscular transmission and some are used clinically to very good purpose. Their actions are shown in Fig. 5.19. These fall into several categories. First, there are those drugs which interfere with the enzymic destruction of acetylcholine; anticholinesterase drugs. A good example of this group is physostigmine. When a muscle is treated with this drug, a single impulse in the nerve supplying it causes a series of tetanic contractions of the muscle. The reason for this is that the impulse produces an endplate potential of quite abnormal duration, but of normal amplitude. This is due to the acetylcholine remaining in the synaptic cleft for a longer than usual time.

ter by the axon terminal. The best known of these agents is botulism toxin. This has a similar effect at all other cholinergic synapses, for example at the autonomic ganglia. Such drugs effectively give the same end result as curare, but as their mode of action is quite different, and considerably less reversible, they should not be used clinically.

A final class of drug that has been found of considerable value clinically are the depolarizing drugs such as succinyl or decamethonium choline that mimic the action of acetylcholine at the endplate. Like acetylcholine, these drugs

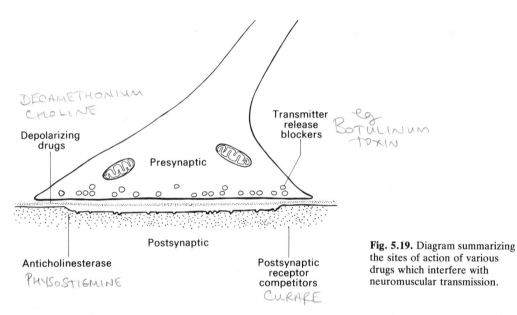

Fig. 5.19. Diagram summarizing the sites of action of various drugs which interfere with neuromuscular transmission.

A second class of drugs competes with acetylcholine for the receptor sites on the postsynaptic membrane, decreasing or preventing the depolarizing action of the transmitter. These are sometimes called curariform drugs. The active principle in curare is d-tubocurarine. An adequate intravenous dose will effectively cause muscle paralysis. They do not significantly affect the CNS because they do not readily penetrate the blood-brain barrier. This property has been utilized clinically with remarkable success in delicate operations where muscle contractions could cause problems for the operating procedure. The use of curare does, of course, cause a cessation of breathing due to its action on the intercostal neuromuscular junctions; artificial ventilation is therefore necessary.

A third class of pharmacological agent interferes with the production or release of transmit-

cause depolarization, but also raise the threshold at which the muscle membrane becomes excited by the endplate potential. For this reason depolarizing drugs are used as muscle relaxants in general anaesthesia.

TRANSMISSION IN AUTONOMIC GANGLIA SYNAPSES

The autonomic nervous system differs from the somatic nervous system in having synaptic relay stations outside the spinal cord within the efferent part of the system, but interestingly the transmitter in all autonomic ganglia, sympathetic and parasympathetic, is acetylcholine.

Neural activity arising in the spinal cord passes down preganglionic fibres to the synapses at the autonomic ganglion cells where the transmitter is rapidly released and causes a transient depolarization of the postsynaptic membrane of the autonomic ganglion cell. This depolarization is called an excitatory postsynaptic potential (EPSP) and is entirely analogous with the EPP in muscle. The EPSP, if big enough, will give rise to an action potential in the postsynaptic cell. Normally a number of EPSPs simultaneously summate to give sufficient depolarization to reach the threshold for production of a post-synaptic action potential. We shall return to this point later. This EPSP can be entirely mimicked by the application of the drug nicotine, and can be prevented from occurring by the use of cur-are which acts in a similar manner to that at a neuromuscular synapse. When ganglia are per-fused and the perfusate collected whilst the pre-ganglionic fibres are electrically stimulated, it has been shown that the amount of acetyl choline released during a few minutes of stimula-tion far exceeds the quantity of transmitter stored within the ganglion. This observation led to the widely accepted hypothesis that activation of nerve fibres not only releases transmitter from the stores, but also induces an acceleration in transmitter synthesis. Finally, in many different types of synapses some of the end-products are recovered by the presynaptic terminals as subs-trate for resynthesis of transmitter. This is par-ticularly the case in noradrenergic nerves, i.e. post-ganglionic sympathetic nerve fibres.

TRANSMISSION IN SYNAPSES OF THE CENTRAL NERVOUS SYSTEM

General features

Central synapses differ in a number of ways, both structurally and functionally, from peripheral synapses, particularly neuromuscular junctions. There are three outstanding differ-ences. First, both excitatory and inhibitory synapses occur, and second, all central synapses are very much smaller than neuromuscular synapses. The area of apposition of membranes is normally only about $1 \mu m^2$, compared with up to $300 \mu m^2$ at a neuromuscular junction. Effec-tively this means that whereas one EPP produced at the motor endplate invariably produces an action potential in the muscle cell, many EPSPs are needed to summate, by over-lapping in time or spatially, at the same post-synaptic neuron. This spatiotemporal summa-tion is an important feature of central nervous transmission (p. 306). The final difference is that there are several different transmitters in the CNS.

Functional synaptic morphology

Three types of synapses occur in the CNS, axosomatic, axodendritic and axoaxonic synapses (Fig. 5.3). In all of these, impulses travel one way only (in vertebrates), from the axon to the dendrite, soma or another axon. This unidirectional transmission at a synapse strictly distinguishes it from an axon which, in theory, can conduct either way.

There are two types of morphologically and functionally different synapses in the CNS, now classified as 'symmetrical' and 'asymmetrical' synapses. In symmetrical synapses, the apposing membranes contain electron-dense thickenings of equal density; these synapses are exceedingly abundant on the soma (Fig. 5.4). The nature of these opacities is unknown, although an analogy with the neuromuscular junction suggests that they are the sites of accumulation of the enzyme which destroys the transmitter. In 'asymmetri-cal' synapses, which are apparently almost exc-lusively axodendritic or axoaxonic, the mem-brane opacity on the postsynaptic side is thicker than that on the presynaptic side. The important point about these differences is that a consider-able amount of evidence has accumulated to show that asymmetrical synapses are excitatory whereas symmetrical are inhibitory.

EPSPs and the generation of action potentials in neurons

The processes leading to generation of EPSPs on central neurons are similar to the generation of EPPs at the neuromuscular junction. An action potential causes the release of a transmit-ter substance which, in turn, causes the genera-tion of a local potential change, the EPSP, on the postsynaptic membrane. There is a synaptic delay of about 0.5 msec which is compounded of delays in mobilization, release, and diffusion of transmitter to the postsynaptic membrane. The EPSP, like the EPP arises because of a non-specific increase in membrane permeability to all small ions, in particular Na^+, K^+ and Cl^-. Thus the membrane potential tends to move towards zero and depolarization occurs. Such a change, of course, tends to cause the produc-tion of an action potential in the postsynaptic cell. However, most EPSPs simply are not large enough to cause action potentials by themselves.

Like the EPP, the EPSP does not last more than a few milliseconds; it reaches its peak in about 0.5 msec, and then decays (Fig. 5.20b). This is mainly due to the destruction of transmit-ter by an enzyme specific for the transmitter involved. Furthermore, in common with the EPP,

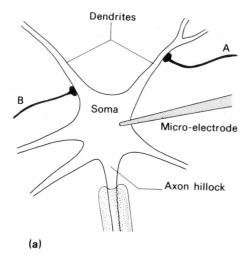

(a)

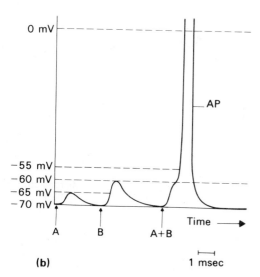

(b)

1 msec

Fig. 5.20. (a) Arrangement of axons synapsing on neuron. Recordings from inside a cell soma.
(b) Diagram showing possible events in a neuron in the generation of an action potential on stimulation of two separate axons A and B. Stimulation of nerve A produces an EPSP of 5 mV—inadequate to produce an action potential in the cell. Stimulation of nerve B produces an EPSP of 10 mV—inadequate to produce an action potential in the cell. Simultaneous stimulation of A and B produces and EPSP of sufficient amplitude to evoke an action potential.

tance away from the site at which the EPSP is generated the less its recorded size will be. This decrement with distance is known as electrotonic decrement or decay.

Convincing evidence is now available to show that action potentials in most nerve cells are generated from the axon hillock or initial segment of the axon (Fig. 5.3, 5.20a). The EPSPs in the dendrites do not cause action potentials to start in the dendrites themselves, but they depolarize the initial segment of the axon by drawing current from it, and if sufficient, cause the action potential to start there. The closer the EPSP is to the initial segment, the more effective it is. The action potential is then propagated down the axon in the normal manner, as well as being retrogradely propagated into the soma and dendrites.

As is the case in most nerve fibres, it is necessary to cause about 20 mV of depolarization, from a resting membrane potential of say −75 mV in the initial segment, to reach the threshold for producing an action potential. Most EPSPs have an amplitude of less than 10 mV at their site of production and with electrotonic decay their value could be less than 1 mV at the initial segment. EPSPs further out on the dendrites are considerably less effective than those on the soma. One EPSP is, therefore, inadequate to produce an action potential in a neuron; summation of EPSPs must occur occur if the cell is going to 'fire' an action potential. Summation occurs in a simple manner, as shown in Fig. 5.20. Activation of many converging inputs must occur more or less simultaneously in order for numerous EPSPs to 'overlap' and cause the neuron to fire. This type of summation, spatial summation, is an important principle in neurophysiology. A further related type of summation, so called temporal summation, occurs when a single presynaptic fibre is firing at a high frequency and impulses succeed each other so rapidly as to cause sequential EPSPs to build up enough depolarization to activate the cell.

Since most EPSPs only last for about 10 msec, a presynaptic fibre would have to be able to fire at more than 100 times per second (albeit for brief periods) to give temporal summation. This situation is quite common in large sensory afferents.

Inhibition in the CNS
Whilst some inputs into cells cause the generation of EPSPs with or without consequential neuronal firing, other inputs cause inhibition. Two types of

the EPSP is a local potential change, and this is most important inasmuch as it is not propagated down the postsynaptic element, be it axon, soma or dendrite. Consequently the greater the disinhibition occur; postsynaptic inhibition, which acts by causing hyperpolarization of the cell, and presynaptic inhibition, which is more complex and works by reducing the value of action potentials. In addition to the significant morphological features in inhibitory synapses, it seems that virtually all inhibition, pre or postsynaptic, in the CNS, is executed by short axon interneurons. Inhibition is, therefore, a local phenomenon occurring in various regions of the cord and between nuclei of the brain. It follows that all long tracts, sensory fibres and somatic motor fibres are probably excitatory.

Postsynaptic inhibition. Functionally, postsynaptic inhibition is the reverse of excitation. The membrane potential of a 'resting' neuron will change transiently from −75 to −80 mV on activation of a particular presynaptic axon. The hyperpolarization is called an inhibitory postsynaptic potential (IPSP) and is thought to arise because of an increase in the permeability of the membrane, mainly to chloride ions.

Inhibition in the form of IPSPs summates in a simple algebraic manner with EPSPs on the same cell. So, if we have production of an EPSP and IPSP simultaneously on the same neuron, and they both have the same value and time course, then their effects should, theoretically, cancel. The probability of the cell firing off action potentials depends on the relative amounts of inhibition and excitation influencing the initial segment of the cell at any one time.

Normally, inhibition of a neuron tends to be more profound than excitation. The reason for this is two fold, First, IPSPs tend to last longer than EPSPs; some IPSPs can last 200–300 msec. Second, inhibitory synapses are usually located closer to the initial segment of the axon and are therefore more effective. Their topographic arrangement is to stop the cell firing for variable periods of time.

Presynaptic inhibition. Presynaptic inhibition is thought to involve axoaxonic synapses only. The phenomenon is considered to operate by one afferent, A, synapsing on another afferent, B, in such a way as to reduce the amount of transmitter released by B on to a neuron, C (Fig. 5.21).

Effectively, activity in A causes prolonged depolarization of B by a mechanism which is still unknown. Action potentials in B, therefore, have a reduced amplitude overall and consequently cause the release of less transmitter on to the neuron, producing a smaller EPSP. To follow the argument it must be appreciated that it is the size of the action potential itself and not the absolute membrane potential that determines the amount of transmitter released.

Presynaptic inhibition may be important in the inhibition of sensory input into the spinal cord and seems to be mediated by short axon interneurons (p. 305). It seems to have no significance beyond primary relay cell stations. Postsynaptic inhibition is the only established means of inhibition in the brain.

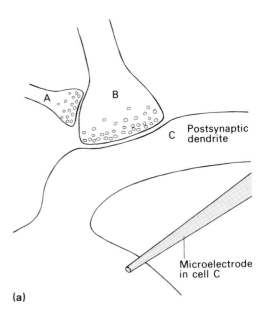

(a)

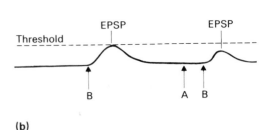

(b)

Fig. 5.21. (a) Arrangement of axoaxonic–dendrite synapses. Axoaxonic synapse of A ⟶ B causes a reduction in transmitter released by depolarizing B and thereby reduces the action potential size in B. (b) Response from microelectrode in cell C. An action potential in B causes a large EPSP on cell C. However prior activation of A reduces the size of the EPSP evoked by an action potential in B.

CHEMICAL RECEPTORS

Chemical agents such as neurotransmitters and hormones (and drugs administered during medical or dental treatment) affect cells by combining with a cellular component called a receptor. Many substances exert their effects in very low concentrations, for example, one part in 1,000 million or less. In several instances it has been calculated that the amount of the chemical in the tissue is so small that it would cover less than 1% of the cell surface. This suggests that substances bind to only a small part of a cell.

Receptors may be on the surface or inside a cell. It is thought that appropriate radicals in molecules interact with chemical groups on receptors. This combination excites the receptor, initiating a sequence of events leading to a response which might, for example, be contraction or relaxation of smooth muscle or secretion from a gland cell. Substances which excite receptors are called agonists.

A chemical can combine with a receptor by forming one or more kinds of bonds—ionic, hydrogen, van der Waals or covalent. The type and strength of bond is dictated by the chemical structures of the drug and receptor.

Receptors for transmitters in the peripheral nervous system

Before considering the types of receptor in the peripheral nervous system it is essential to review the sites where acetylcholine and noradrenaline act as transmitters.

Nerves which release acetylcholine at their terminals are called cholinergic nerves. They are:
1 All parasympathetic and sympathetic preganglionic fibres (including the sympathetic preganglionic fibres to the adrenal medulla).
2 All parasympathetic postganglionic nerves.
3 The sympathetic postganglionic nerves to some sweat glands and blood vessels.
4 The somatic nerves to skeletal muscle.

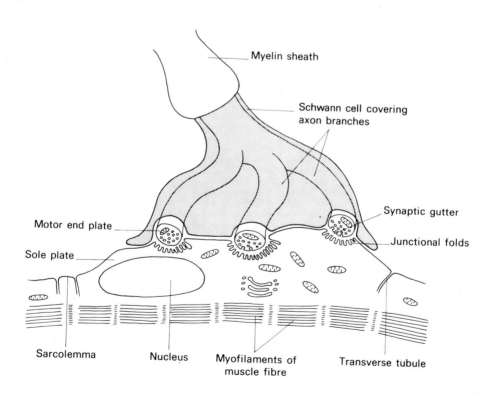

Fig. 5.22. A diagrammatic representation of a neuromuscular junction.

Nerves releasing noradrenaline at their terminals are termed adrenergic nerves and constitute all the postganglionic sympathetic nerves except a minority which, as mentioned above, supply sweat glands and some blood vessels such as in skeletal muscle and are cholinergic.

Cholinergic receptors

Acetylcholine released by postganglionic autonomic nerves interacts with receptors on target cells causing contraction of intestinal smooth muscle, increased salivary secretion and a decrease in the heart rate, to mention only a few of its effects. Such effects are also produced in food poisoning by a substance called muscarine which is present in some non-edible fungi.

Acetylcholine is also released by preganglionic autonomic nerves and excites receptors on both parasympathetic and sympathetic postganglionic neurons. Excitation of parasympathetic ganglia causes the effects listed above. Stimulation of sympathetic ganglia results in constriction of arteriolar smooth muscle causing a rise in blood pressure, and an increase in heart rate (both effects being caused by the release of noradrenaline from the postganglionic nerve terminal); adrenaline is also released from the adrenal medulla. These effects of ganglion stimulation can also be produced by nicotine which excites the cholinergic receptors in ganglia. In order to distinguish between these two groups of actions of acetylcholine mimicked by muscarine and nicotine, they are referred to as muscarinic and nicotinic actions. The associated cholinergic receptors are called muscarinic and nicotinic receptors.

Acetylcholine is also released by somatic nerves and impinges on receptors on the endplates in skeletal muscle (Fig. 5.22). Although nicotine can excite these receptors, they are different from the nicotinic receptors in the autonomic nervous system.

So far we have distinguished between different cholinergic receptors by referring to the drugs which mimic acetylcholine at the site in question, i.e. muscarine or nicotine. However, it is also possible to distinguish them by observing the effects of drugs which competitively antagonize the actions of acetylcholine at these sites. Thus it is well known that atropine antagonizes contractions of intestinal smooth muscle induced by acetylcholine, reduces salivary secretion, blocks the effect of acetylcholine on cardiac muscle, and prevents sweating. Atropine does this by combining with mus-

carinic receptors and so prevents acetylcholine from interacting with them. Similar amounts of atropine do not antagonize acetylcholine in ganglia or at endplates. The actions of acetylcholine in ganglia are antagonized by a different type of agent, e.g. hexamethonium. By preventing acetylcholine from combining with nicotinic receptors in ganglia, hexamethonium prevents the stimulation of postganglionic nerves. Hexamethonium does not affect muscarinic receptors or the nicotinic receptors on endplates. The latter are effectively blocked by tubocurarine, resulting in paralysis of skeletal muscle. Tubocurarine is the active principle of curare, a poisonous substance used by S. American Indians on their arrow heads to kill their prey. Thus, there are two types of nicotinic receptors—those in ganglia and those on endplates.

Adrenoceptors

After release, noradrenaline crosses the synaptic gap and impinges on receptors called adrenoceptors. These are found particularly in cardiac and smooth muscle cells. There are mainly two types of adrenoceptors, termed α and β for simplicity; the β-adrenoceptors can be further subdivided into β_1 and β_2. The evidence supporting the idea of two kinds of adrenoceptor was obtained by determining the relative potencies of a variety of sympathomimetic amines (amines whose actions mimic sympathetic stimulation) on tissues and organs innervated by the sympathetic nervous system. Those amines which were particularly effective in causing smooth muscle to contract had little effect on cardiac muscle. In contrast, many amines which caused smooth muscle to relax were very effective in causing an increase in the rate and force of contraction of cardiac muscle. So the idea originated that receptor α was responsible for contraction of smooth muscle, β_2 subserved relaxation of smooth muscle and β_1 increased force and rate of contraction of cardiac muscle.

This classification stems from the use of agonists. It can also be substantiated by the actions of antagonists. Thus phentolamine (an α–adrenoceptor antagonist) blocks the contractile effect of those amines which relax smooth muscle or excite the heart. Propranolol (a β–adrenoceptor antagonist) prevents the effects of sympathomimetic amines both on the heart (excitation) and on smooth muscle (relaxation). A summary of the responses of various organs and tissues to autonomic nerve stimulation and the receptors involved is given in Table 5.2. A summary of the transmitters, receptors and antagonists of autonomic and motor nerves is given in Fig. 5.23.

REFLEXES

Reflex activity in man can be described as being organized in a hierarchical manner since specific reflexes can be ascribed to different levels of organization within the nervous system. The spinal cord has certain reflexes associated with it and represents the most basic level of integration. Levels of neural organization superior to the spinal cord, such as the brain stem, medulla, midbrain and cerebral cortex are also associated with specific reflex reactions. Some examples of

Table 5.2. Responses of organs and tissues to autonomic nerve stimulation

Organs and tissues	Receptors	Autonomic nerve stimulation: sympathetic (S), Parasympathetic (P)	
		Adrenergic (S)	Cholinergic
Heart-rate and force of contraction	β Muscarinic	Increase	Decrease (P)
Lung-bronchial muscle	β Muscarinic	Relaxation	Contraction (P)
Intestine-motility and tone	α and β Muscarinic	Decrease	Increase (P)
Skin arterioles	α Muscarinic	Constriction	Dilatation (P and S)
Adrenal medulla	Nicotinic		Secretion of adrenaline and noradrenaline (S)

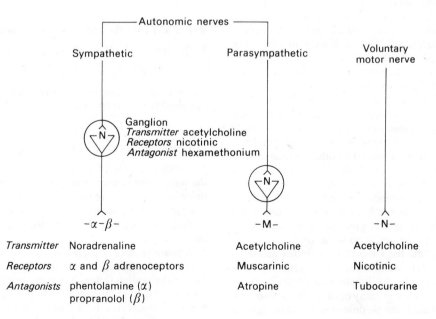

	Sympathetic	Parasympathetic	Voluntary motor nerve
Transmitter	Noradrenaline	Acetylcholine	Acetylcholine
Receptors	α and β adrenoceptors	Muscarinic	Nicotinic
Antagonists	phentolamine (α) propranolol (β)	Atropine	Tubocurarine

Fig. 5.23. A summary of the transmitters, receptors and antagonists found in autonomic and voluntary nerves. (Some postganglionic sympathetic fibres to sweat glands and some blood vessels, such as in skeletal muscle, are cholinergic.)

postural reflexes and the levels of neural organization where they are integrated are shown below. This list illustrates the concept of the hierarchical arrangement.

Level of integration	Type of reflex
Spinal cord	Stretch reflexes; supporting reactions
Medulla	Labrynthine and neck reflexes, responding to changes in the position of the head.
Midbrain	Righting reflexes.
Cerebral cortex	Optical righting reflexes.

In man and other primates the evolutionary development of the nervous system has resulted in the 'higher' centres, such as the cerebral cortex, having an increased degree of control over reflex reactions. It is now apparent that even the reflexes that are most simply organized, such as the stretch reflex, are modulated to some degree by descending influences from higher, that is, suprasegmental, areas of the brain. This is clearly illustrated when such influences are removed, as after spinal cord transection. Immediately following such an injury there is a period when reflex activity is absent, known as spinal shock. Spinal reflexes do return after a period of time, which may be as long as months in man. In contrast, spinal shock in lower animals, such as frogs, may only last a few minutes, showing the considerably greater importance of suprasegmental areas in influencing spinal reflexes in man compared to other animals. After recovery from spinal shock there remains a profound disturbance of the mechanisms involved in postural control; stretch reflexes such as the knee jerk are exaggerated due to the removal of suprasegmental inhibitory influences, but the ability to stand is lost.

However, the concept of a 'reflex action' is still a valid one and can be of great value in understanding the functioning of the nervous system. Although many of the reflex actions that will subsequently be described do have significant suprasegmental functional components, they can still be described as being 'unlearned' and 'involuntary'.

The reflex arc

The reflex arc is the basic unit of integrated neural activity and the nature and properties of the arc are fundamental in understanding the highly complex functioning of the central nervous system.

Essentially, the reflex arc consists of a sense organ, an afferent neuron, one or more synapses in a central integrating station, an efferent neuron and an effector. The number of action potentials in the afferent nerve is proportional to the strength of the applied stimulus. There is less correlation between the strength of stimulus and the frequency of action potentials in the efferent neuron, as the facility for modification of activity in the reflex arc is exerted on the connection between the afferent and efferent neurons in the central nervous system. Multiple inputs may converge on the efferent neurons.

The simplest reflex arc, where there is just one synapse between the afferent and efferent neuron is the exception rather than the rule in mammalian physiology. This type of reflex arc is monosynaptic and so reflexes occurring through them are known as monosynaptic reflexes. Reflex arcs where one or more interneurons are interposed between the afferent and efferent neurons are known as polysynaptic reflex arcs and necessarily have greater scope for modification of their activity.

Reflex action in the central nervous system

Reflex activity in the CNS is present over the whole range of physiological function. Reflexes are present in both the somatic and autonomic systems. In addition, there are the more nebulous conditioned reflexes (p. 934).

THE MONOSYNAPTIC REFLEX

The only example of a monosynaptic reflex in the body is the stretch reflex; this is described in more detail elsewhere (p. 468) but a brief discussion can serve as a guide to the understanding of more complex polysynaptic reflexes discussed later.

When a skeletal muscle with an intact nerve supply is stretched, it automatically contracts. This is the stretch reflex. The sense organ is the primary ending in the muscle spindle (Fig. 6.9), which is innervated by a single afferent fibre of large diameter (12–20 μm), called a 1a fibre. This fibre synapses directly with an α–motoneuron in the ventral horn of the spinal cord, the motoneuron thus constituting the efferent limb of the reflex arc (Fig. 5.24).

It is possible to measure the time between the application of the stimulus and the reflex response. Values for the reaction time for the knee jerk reflex in man vary between 19–24 msec. Knowing the conduction velocity for the afferent and efferent fibres and the distance from the muscle to the spinal cord, it is possible to calculate how much of the reaction time was taken up by conduction to and from the spinal cord and to subtract this from the total reaction time. The remainder corresponds to the time for transmission within the spinal cord. In man this is between 0.5–0.9 msec. As the minimal time for synaptic delay has been found to be 0.5 msec, this means that this reflex is being mediated via only a single synapse and therefore is a true example of a monosynaptic reflex.

RECIPROCAL INNERVATION AND THE INVERSE STRETCH REFLEX

Stretching a muscle, however, does not merely invoke the simple monosynaptic stretch reflex. The situation is, in reality, considerably more complex.

On entering the spinal cord the 1a afferents give off collaterals which synapse via inhibitory interneurons with the α–motoneurons innervating the antagonistic flexor muscles. The resultant activation of these inhibitory synapses causes a release of inhibitory transmitter onto the antagonistic motoneurons and so reduces the frequency of discharge in them, thus causing the flexor muscles to relax and in effect facilitating the contraction of the muscle originally stretched. This example of reciprocal innervation is clearly not monosynaptic and is thought to be essentially a disynaptic process (Fig. 5.24).

Another facet of the stretch reflex is the ability to 'switch off' the reflexly evoked contraction when the tension in the muscle reaches a certain magnitude. This is due to the inverse stretch reflex, the receptor for which is the Golgi tendon organ (Fig. 6.9). The afferents from the Golgi tendon organ synapse in the spinal cord via inhibitory interneurons with the motoneurons innervating the muscle (Fig. 10.45b). The level of discharge in these α–motoneurons is thus reduced and this effectively curtails the contraction of the muscle. The reflex arcs activated by stretching a muscle are therefore fairly complex and are certainly not restricted to those of a monosynaptic nature. There is therefore potential for modification of these reflexes by interaction with interneurons at the level of the spinal cord.

Reflexes of cutaneous origin

The reflexes described so far can all be said to be of muscular origin. There is, however, another group of reflexes also involved in the control of

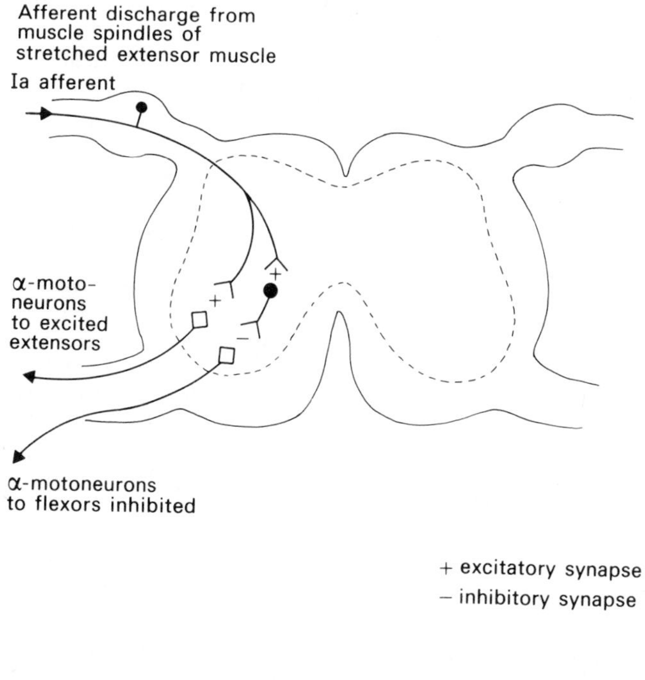

Afferent discharge from
muscle spindles of
stretched extensor muscle

Ia afferent

α-moto-
neurons
to excited
extensors

α-motoneurons
to flexors inhibited

+ excitatory synapse
− inhibitory synapse

Fig. 5.24. Reciprocal inhibition.

movement at a spinal level. These are reflexes which are basically of cutaneous origin. The sensory receptors in skin and subcutaneous tissue respond to touch, pressure, heat, cold and tissue damage. The signals from all of these receptors exert effects on spinal motoneurons via interneurons. The dominant pattern of response to cutaneous stimulation of a limb is ipsilateral flexion and, if the stimulus is sufficiently powerful, contralateral extension. This suggests that cutaneous activity of all kinds, not only that arising in response to injury, may elicit aversive responses that tend to withdraw the limb. However, it will be seen that the reflexes of cutaneous origin are not always wholly flexor. wholly flexor.

FLEXOR REFLEX

The flexor reflex comprises contraction of the flexor muscles with concomitant relaxation of the extensor muscles. Such reflexes may be initiated by inocuous stimulation of the skin as well as potentially painful and injurious stimuli. The first type consists of a contraction of one or more flexor muscles with little actual withdrawal of the limb, whereas the second type consists of a widespread contraction of flexor muscles throughout the limb that results in the abrupt withdrawal of the limb from the source of the noxious stimulus.

The flexor reflex is a good example of a polysynaptic reflex in which transmission of the impulse from the afferent to efferent limbs of the reflex arc involves one, two or possibly even more interneurons. This arrangement permits considerable modulation of the reflex in response to different stimuli and accounts for the observation that the reflex tension developed in a particular flexor muscle varies widely with the sensory nerve that is being stimulated and the distribution of afferent impulses to the motorneurons. The variety of response which is possible in a reflex can be explained by the properties of the synapses. Spatial summation at a synapse occurs when the effect of the depolarization caused by an impulse in one afferent fibre (A in Fig. 5.25) is facilitated by that due to activity in another (B) or vice versa. That is, the EPSP generated in X is larger when both A and B are activated together (or within a very short time interval) than when A or B is activated alone. If it is necessary to activate two synapses in order to reach the firing level of the neurons X, Y or Z, then in the situation where A and B are activated, X will fire but Y, although

depolarized, has not reached its firing level. However, its excitability has been increased and there is therefore subthreshold excitation in Y following activity in B. Y can therefore be said to be in the subliminal fringe of X.

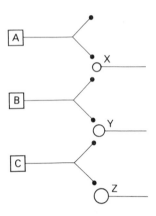

Fig. 5.25. A 'nerve net' showing arrangement of nerves that can facilitate either spatial or temporal summation.

Another phenomenon which can occur in these nerve nets is that of occlusion. In our diagram (Fig. 5.25) if neuron B is stimulated repetitively, temporal summation of the EPSPs in X and Y occurs and their magnitude is such that these neurons discharge. Similarly, repetitive stimulation of C would induce firing in Y and Z. However, repetitive stimulation of B and C simultaneously would only induce firing in X, Y and Z—this response is thus not as great as the sum of the responses to repetitive stimulation of B and C separately, because B and C share neuron Y and occlusion has occurred.

Inhibitory impulses also show spatial and temporal facilitation, subliminal fringe effects and occlusion. These properties of polysynaptic pathways have a profound influence on synaptic transmission in any pathway and it is clear that reflex activity can be modified as a result of these mechanisms. The post-synaptic membrane is continuously acting as an integrating centre for the influences impinging on it. These are algebraically summed and thus determine the level of excitability of the cell.

Because propagation of impulses across a synapse is not a foregone conclusion, the particular route taken by afferent impulses from the many anatomical pathways potentially available, is determined by the nature of this afferent activity and the level of excitability in the CNS at any one instant.

There are ample opportunities in the polysynaptic flexor reflex pathway for spatial and temporal facilitation to occur so that, as the strength of a noxious stimulus is increased, there is a spread of excitation to more and more synapses and effector flexor motoneurons. The summation of EPSPs to their firing levels occurs more readily and a shortening of the reaction time is seen. Under these circumstances a prolonged, repeated firing of the motoneurons can be observed, called an after discharge. This is the result of the continued bombardment of the motoneurons by afferent impulses continuing to arrive by complex and circuitous polysynaptic paths.

CROSSED EXTENSION

If the initial stimulus is of sufficient magnitude in the flexor reflex, not only is the ipsilateral limb reflexly activated to produce its flexion and withdrawal, but the contralateral limb is extended, thus providing support as one limb is removed. This is achieved by collaterals or interneurons which excite the extensor motoneurons of the contralateral limb (Fig. 5.26). This response is most clearly seen in experimental animals where the influence of the brain on spinal reflexes has been removed by transection of the spinal cord.

Other reflexes concerned with posture, such as joint reflexes and tonic neck reflexes (p. 472) are all polysynaptic and in man are quite complex as they involve not only the spinal cord but also suprasegmental areas.

Autonomic reflexes

The reflexes described so far have all been components of the somatic system but the autonomic system also exhibits reflex activity. Reflex activity in the autonomic system is always polysynaptic, there is no equivalent of the monosynaptic stretch reflex seen in the somatic system. It is also interesting to note that there is often an autonomic involvement in reflexes that are normally thought of as being somatic. For example, a painful stimulus that causes a flexion response as described above, can also produce a rise in blood pressure and modulation of the cardiac rate.

In some autonomic reflexes, particularly those involving the heart, there is a reciprocal action occurring centrally which adjusts the balance of activity in the two divisions of the autonomic nervous system. Because of integration of autonomic reflexes at a higher level, they are considerably more complicated than the somatic reflexes already described. Frequently, they are greatly influenced by other parts of the nervous system which are not actually integral parts of the reflex arcs. That is, autonomic reflexes rarely occur in isolation and as such do not have the

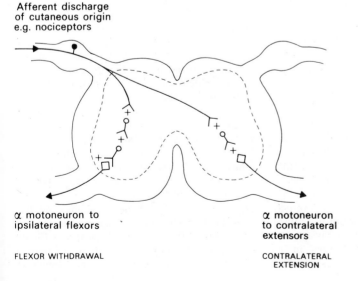

Afferent discharge
of cutaneous origin
e.g. nociceptors

α motoneuron to
ipsilateral flexors

α motoneuron
to contralateral
extensors

FLEXOR WITHDRAWAL

CONTRALATERAL
EXTENSION

Fig. 5.26. Crossed extension.

same clear-cut characteristics that may be established for spinal reflexes in the somatic system.

Reflex activity in the autonomic system is organized in ascending degrees of complexity. Simple reflexes such as bladder emptying, defaecation and sexual reflexes are integrated at the level of the spinal cord. The more complex reflexes regulating blood pressure and respiration are integrated at the level of the medulla oblongata. There is, however, considerable influence from other areas of the brain, such as the hypothalamus and cerebral cortex, upon these autonomic reflexes. The medulla oblongata is the site where integration takes place in such reflexes as swallowing, vomiting, sneezing and coughing; the neuronal mechanisms involved in these phenomena are highly complex and their precise arrangement in terms of the functional components of the reflex arcs involved has not yet been fully determined.

SENSATION

When a stimulus is applied to the body it can produce a reflex movement, a generalized alerting effect and a conscious sensation. The simplest reflex responses operate through neural circuits in the region of the central nervous system close to the point of entry of the sensory signals, whereas the alerting effect is due to the operation of diffuse neural circuits largely in the area of the mid brain and brain stem. Conscious sensation, i.e. the awareness or perception of the precise nature of a stimulus, is a function of the sensory area of the cerebral cortex.

The common route to all these neural circuits is the primary afferent (sensory) neuron. The ends of these sensory fibres are functionally specialized receptors, i.e. stimulus detectors, whereas the central processes are specialized to transmit information to other nerve cells, i.e. they synapse with cell bodies of 'second order' neurons. On appropriate stimulation the peripheral nerve endings generate signals which pass up the processes of the sensory neurons to the central nervous system. In the case of conscious perception the 'second order' sensory neurons relay the incoming signals to the thalamus where the cell bodies of 'third order' neurons are located (Fig. 5.27). The axons of the third order neurons subsequently project direct to the sensory cortex. It is important to realise that the synapses involved in these pathways are not a series of inconvenient breaks in a telephone cable; the transfer of impulses to the next neuron in the chain can be modified. Although it is common experience that our conscious perception reflects the nature of applied stimuli quite accurately, the input to the sensory cortex may be 'second hand'.

Receptors

Since both the special senses and the receptor systems involved in the reflex control of muscle length are dealt with in separate chapters, the description here will be confined to the mechanisms subserving the common sensations of touch, pressure, position, temperature and pain.

The first step in the production of sensation is stimulation of the receptor terminals of sensory neurons. Receptors having a specific sensitivity to mechanical stimulation and a very low or negligible sensitivity to other forms of energy are known as mechanoreceptors; those with a corresponding specific sensitivity to thermal stimuli are known as thermoreceptors, etc. The term 'chemoreceptor' is usually reserved for those receptors in the carotid or aortic bodies and in the brain stem, that detect and signal the local tensions of oxygen and carbon dioxide or the hydrogen ion concentration. The chemical sensitivity of nerve endings on the skin is different in that it is related to the detection of stimuli that damage tissues and release chemical substances from the damaged cells. Receptors responding only to damaging (noxious) stimuli are called nociceptors. The functional specialization of receptors, i.e. the fact that they are individually 'tuned' to particular forms of energy, is referred to as 'modality specificity'.

Histological examination of non-hairy skin shows a variety of receptor types, from nerve endings enclosed in complex laminated capsules, through forms with moderate degrees of structural complexity, down to bare nerve endings lying free in the tissue (Fig. 5.28a). Although considerable effort has been made to relate the different histological forms to specific modalities of sensation there has been only limited success. The Pacinian corpuscle, with its capsule made up of a series of layers like an onion (Fig. 5.28b), is known to be highly sensitive to mechanical stimulation, but so too are free unmyelinated nerve endings. If one looks at hairy skin one finds that it contains no encapsulated nerve endings; there are only free nerve endings and 'baskets' of unmyelinated endings around the hair roots (Fig. 5.28c), yet this is sufficient for the touch, pressure, hot, cold and pain sensitivity of the tissue. Since a very large number of

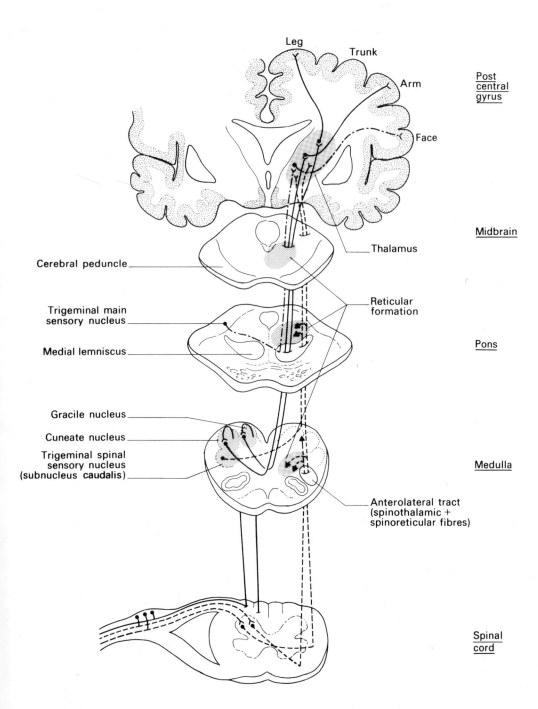

Fig. 5.27. A simplified diagram showing the main features in the somatosensory pathways. Note that the anterolateral tract contains both spinothalamic and spinoreticular fibres.

mechanoreceptors, thermoreceptors and nociceptors have the microscopic appearance of free
nerve endings, the structures determining functional specialization must lie at a submicroscopic
level. The exceptions to this generalization are
Pacinian corpuscles, muscle spindles (Fig. 6.10)
and Golgi tendon organs (Fig. 6.9).

Each afferent fibre serves many receptor endings distributed over an area of skin (Fig. 5.28d).
Such splitting of an axon to produce multiple
sensory terminals gives rise to a 'sensory unit'
analogous to the motor unit. Signals can,
however, be transmitted by the axon to the central nervous system from only one receptor at a

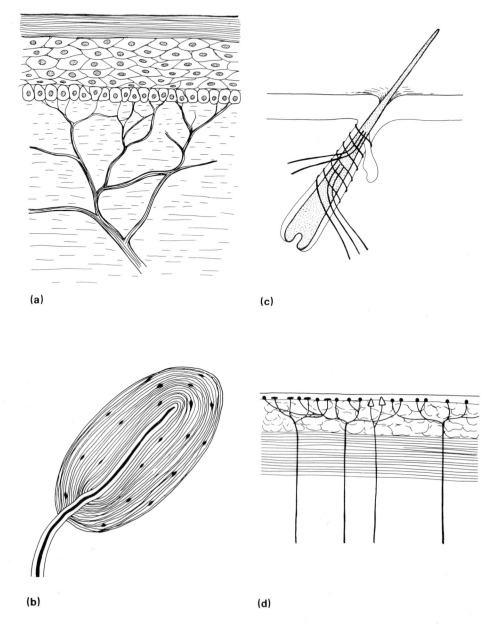

(a)

(c)

(b)

(d)

Fig. 5.28. (a) Free unmyelinated nerve endings in the
skin. (b) Pacinian corpuscle. (c) Innervation of hair
follicle. (d) Diagram showing how an area of skin may
be innervated by several sensory neurons with
overlapping receptive fields.

time. The action potentials generated by the receptor, besides passing up the afferent fibre to the central nervous system, will also pass back along the various branches towards the other receptors; in doing this they collide with the incoming signals they meet on the way and block them. The area of skin innervated by one axon is referred to as the 'receptive field' of that axon. It may vary in size from a few mm² to several hundred mm² but since the receptive fields of neighbouring axons all overlap, one axon does not necessarily have 'sole possession' of that area (Fig. 5.28d). Receptive fields tend to be smallest on the face and on the finger tips.

It is not fully established how receptors in general generate signals. Only in the case of the mechanoreceptor can some explanation of the mechanism be put forward. It is suggested that distortion of a receptor membrane changes its structural configuration so that ion permeable pores in the membrane are enlarged. This allows sodium and probably other ions to enter, so allowing the membrane potential to move away from -70 mV towards zero. This potential change in the receptor terminal is referred to as the generator potential and is related to the magnitude of the stimulus. It is, however, not related in a linear fashion but according to a logarithmic or power law, i.e. the sensitivity of the receptor to small increments of stimulus strength decreases with increase in the overall magnitude of the stimulus. The generator potential is not propagated but is confined to the tip of the fibre terminal, where it draws current from the neighbouring (more proximal) region of the nerve fibre, so depolarizing it and initiating action potentials. The size of the generator potential consequently governs the rate at which the nerve action potentials are produced. If the generator potential is small then it takes a relatively long time (perhaps several hundred milliseconds) to draw sufficient charge from the nerve fibre membrane to depolarize it to its threshold or firing level, with the result that a train of nerve impulses is generated with long intervals between each impulse. Conversely a large generator potential is associated with a high frequency of impulses. In this way the stimulus 'quantity' is signalled to the central nervous system in terms of impulse rate coding.

This explanation relates to the simple case of a steady stimulus and a steadily responding receptor. Receptors that respond in a steady fashion to the maintained intensity of a stimulus are referred to as 'tonic' (Fig. 5.29a). There are however receptors that do not respond to the maintained intensity of a stimulus but only to its rate of change. Such receptors are referred to as 'phasic' (Fig. 5.29a). They tend to respond only to the onset and cessation of stimulation and provide an example of an extreme form of 'adaptation' to persistent steady stimulation. 'Adaptation' is the term used for the progressive decrease in the frequency of firing during the application of a steady state stimulus. The Pacinian corpuscle is a good example of a phasic (rapidly adapting) receptor. Mainly because of its large size it has been studied in detail. Two mechanisms probably operate in the Pacinian corpuscle. First, the complex laminated 'onion skin' capsule around the nerve terminal exhibits viscoelastic slip so that whilst the capsule initially transmits the stimulus to the nerve terminal, the lamellae then slip or 'flow' so that stimulation of the terminal ceases. However, when the capsule is removed experimentally and a stimulus applied to the denuded terminal, there is still adaptation but at a much lower rate. There must, therefore, be an additional mechanism of adaptation in the receptor membrane.

Receptors do not all fall into these two distinct categories. Many receptors give a small phasic response to the onset of a stimulus and a slowly adapting response to its maintained steady level. The minimum stimulus that it is necessary to apply to a receptor in order to generate nerve impulses is referred to as its threshold. Receptors subserving the same modality of sensation can have different thresholds. As a stimulus has to be applied more rapidly than the receptor adapts, it follows that rapidly applied stimuli can be detected even when tissue is distorted only a few microns, whereas slowly applied stimuli of comparable magnitude may be undetected.

A mechanical stimulus applied to the surface of the body may be detected by a large number of receptors within a number of receptive fields. For any one small area the primary afferent neurons activated reflects the size of the stimulated area, the phasic response of receptors reflects the rate of application of the stimulus, and the tonic response reflects the intensity of the steady-state level of stimulation. Although the description so far has concentrated on cutaneous receptors, the same general principles apply to receptors elsewhere. In the capsules of joints, for example, some receptors respond to radial acceleration of the joint (equivalent to phasic receptors) and others to the angular position of the joint (equivalent to tonic receptors) (Fig. 5.29b). In addition to this general discrimination by the receptors, an individual receptor (or 'sensory unit') may also only be sensitive to movement or posi-

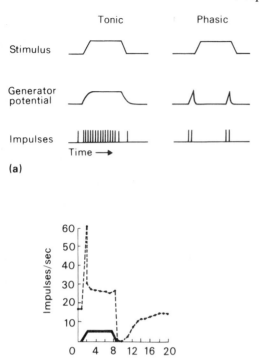

(a)

(b)

Fig. 5.29. (a) A highly diagrammatic representation of the response of a purely tonic and a purely phasic receptor. Note that the response is signalled by the rate of production of nerve impulses. (b) A plot of the impulse frequency generated by a joint receptor signalling joint position, as the joint angle is changed from one position to another and back again. The change of joint position is indicated by a solid line. Note that the receptor has an initial rate of discharge of about 17 impulses /sec reflecting the initial joint position i.e. the receptor has 'tonic' (or 'static') sensitivity. As the joint is moved there is a large discharge which falls as soon as the joint stops moving i.e. the receptor has some 'phasic' (or 'dynamic') sensitivity. The difference between the steady discharge at the new position (about 27 impulses /sec) and that at the previous position is a measure of the angle moved. In this case the movement of the joint, as it is returned to its original position, produces an 'off' effect i.e. the receptor discharge falls.

tion over a restricted range of rotation of the joint. However, the population of receptors as a whole gives information throughout joint rotation as the stimulus to the joint capsule successively activates receptors with sensitivities to different angles.

Central pathways

The ascending tracts in the spinal cord and brain are considered in detail on p. 839.

The fibres involved in sensation can be divided into two major groups on an anatomical basis, which also reflect certain physiological differences (Fig. 5.27). The first group consists of some large myelinated fibres which ascend in the dorsal columns and terminate in the cuneate and gracile nuclei.

The second group consists of both large and small diameter fibres which give off abundant collaterals that synapse with second order cells in the dorsal horn of the grey matter. The axons of these cells ascend in the anterolateral tracts.

The function of the first group is mainly in localization and discrimination of mechanical stimuli, whilst the other group is concerned with generalized responses to stimulation such as alerting and causing behavioural changes following noxious stimulation. Some information used in sensory discrimination also passes via this anterolateral route.

DORSAL COLUMNS

Activity in the ascending dorsal column is interpreted at a cortical level as a sensation of touch, deep pressure, vibration or joint position; it is also particularly important for general sensory discrimination.

Considerable processing of information can occur in the dorsal column nuclei (Fig. 5.30a). There is, first, lateral or spatial inhibition, where information coming in from one receptive field inhibits the transfer of information from neighbouring primary afferents to their second order cell. This may be by both pre- and post-synaptic mechanisms. Some idea of the utility of this mechanism can be gained by considering the case of a pressure applied to only a very small area of skin but causing distortion of the skin for several inches around, so that a large number of receptive fields are activated. In this case the rate coding of impulses might indicate bodily contact over a large area if the most stimulated receptive field was not able to inhibit transfer of information from the less stimulated fields to the higher centres.

The second form of information processing that can occur in the dorsal column nuclei is inhibition by fibres from the cortex (corticofugal system); both pre- and post-synaptic inhibitory mechanisms operate (p. 300) and will therefore control the flow of information to the next relay

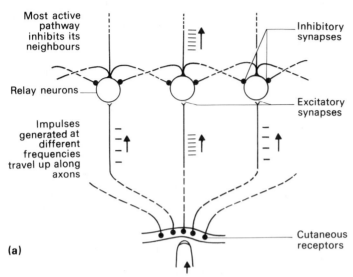

To higher centres

Most active
pathway
inhibits its
neighbours

Inhibitory
synapses

Relay neurons

Excitatory
synapses

Impulses
generated at
different
frequencies
travel up along
axons

Cutaneous
receptors

(a)

Stimulus applied causing distortion of tissue

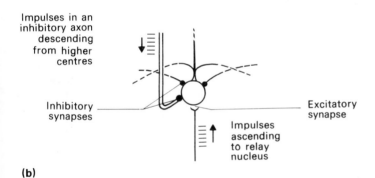

Impulses in an
inhibitory axon
descending
from higher
centres

Inhibitory
synapses

Excitatory
synapse

Impulses
ascending
to relay
nucleus

(b)

Fig. 5.30. (a) A diagram to show how mutual lateral inhibition of relay neurons on the sensory pathway can 'sharpen' the pattern of impulses arising from a group of receptors or sensory units. The collaterals from the relay neurons, shown as dotted lines, probably inhibit neigbouring relay cells via inhibitory neurons, but these have been omitted for clarity. (b) A diagram to show how impulses in a descending inhibitory pathway can block (or just reduce) the transmission of impulses at a sensory relay.

in the thalamus (Fig. 5.30b). The corticofugal system may form the basis for the direction of attention to one out of a number of simultaneously applied stimuli.

The third form of information processing is the opposite to inhibition, namely facilitation, and this also can be effected by the corticofugal fibres; it is a process akin to 'amplification' of information.

The possibility of further processing of incoming information also occurs at the thalamic relay sites. Lateral inhibition operates as it does in the dorsal column nuclei and corticofugal fibres can exert inhibitory influences at the thalamic level. The third order cells of the thalamus then project to the cortex immediately behind the

Rolandic fissure. In both thalamus and sensory cortex (Fig. 5.31) there is a representation of the body surface projected point by point. This sensory 'homunculus' is in fact distorted, the parts of the body surface that are densely innervated being disproportionately enlarged (see Fig. 19.94). The homunculus consequently has a large mouth and large hands. This somatotopic representation of the body by fibres reaching the thalamus and cortex from the medial lemniscus is the somatic area 1. Experimentally one can stimulate peripherally and record electrical activity from the corresponding area of the somatic area 1. However, additional activity can be recorded from a small area of the cortical surface below somatic area 1; this is somatic area 2. Not very much is known about this area but it seems to have connections similar to those of the primary sensory area. The system just described, involving dorsal columns, dorsal column nuclei, medial lemniscus, thalamus, thalamic radiation and somatosensory area 1, is called the lemniscal system or the specific projection system.

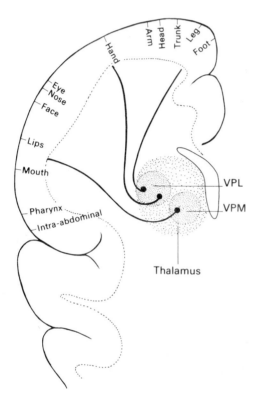

Fig. 5.31. Diagram showing the somatotopic pattern in the projection from the ventral posterolateral and posteromedial nuclei of the thalamus (VPL and VPM). The relative size of the parts of the central cortex from which sensations localized to different parts of the body can be elicited are also shown.

ANTEROLATERAL TRACTS

Fibres in the anterolateral tract carry the coding for the stimuli detected by thermoreceptors and nociceptors. Information is also transmitted through this pathway for touch, i.e. mechanoreceptor stimulation, but how this information is used is uncertain. Fibres in the anterolateral tract terminate either in the thalamus (spinothalamic) or in the ascending reticular system in

the brain stem (spinoreticular). When the spinothalamic fibres reach the thalamus their projection takes two courses. The first is to the thalamic relay nuclei, ventralis posterior lateralis and ventralis posterior medialis, where the somatotopic representation of the body is formed by the lemniscal system. This projection conveys specific sensory data for touch and temperature, which is then relayed to somatosensory area 1. The second projection is to the other areas of the thalamus and is associated with a subsequent diffuse or non-specific projection to the cortex.

Many of the fibres in the anterolateral tract are, however, not spinothalamic, but spinoreticular (Fig. 5.27). There is a close functional relationship between those parts of the thalamus associated with the diffuse or non-specific projection and the ascending reticular system to the extent that some authors consider those thalamic nuclei to be simply an extension of the reticular activating system. Experimental stimulation of the non-specific projection system in anaesthetized animals brings about changes in cortical activity that correspond to signs of alertness in the conscious animal.

When a sensory nerve is stimulated in the anaesthetized animal, electrical activity can be recorded from the contralateral sensory cortex in the area corresponding to the somatotopic (lemniscal) projection of that part of the body. This localized activity is the primary evoked response. Some 30–80 msec later there appears a secondary discharge throughout both cerebral hemispheres for which the non-specific projection is thought to be responsible.

Sensory cortex

During neurosurgical operations on man, carried out under local anaesthesia, some investigators have taken the opportunity to stimulate the primary projection area of the sensory cortex with weak electric currents. The subjects usually report only vague feelings in the somatotopically related part of the body on the opposite side. It is very significant that the spinothalamic sensations of pain, warmth or cold are virtually never reported. In the converse situation where tissue is removed from the sensory cortex, there is an initial anaesthesia of the corresponding part of the body on the opposite side. The anaesthesia has however two characteristics: first, it can have an odd distribution which may not correspond to segmental innervation by the spinal nerves, and second, it is temporary. Sensitivity to pain returns very rapidly and completely. Somewhat later some sensitivity to temperature and, to a lesser extent, touch, is restored, but the ability to discriminate the sensation of touch is permanently and severely impaired; kinaesthesia (sense of joint position) is also impaired. Consequently the ability to recognize an object solely by holding it in the hand, i.e. stereognosis, is lost. In this situation, changing mechanical stimulation of the skin and changing position of the fingers whilst handling an object normally supply information for elaboration into recognition at a cortical level. The rate and extent of restitution of any discriminative and analytical ability does, however, vary depending upon the somatotopic area of sensory cortex affected. If the cortical area lost is associated with a peripheral structure which has a bilateral projection to the sensory cortex, e.g. the mouth, then there is rapid and extensive restoration of sensory discriminative function. One must presume that this is because the discriminative function can be elaborated by the remaining projection on the opposite cortex. In contrast, if the area lost receives only a unilateral (crossed) projection, e.g. hand area, then there is a very severe permanent impairment of manual sensory discrimination.

Trigeminal (Vth cranial nerve) complex

The description of the organization of the trigeminal sensory system has not been included earlier as it is less well understood than the spinal tract systems. As in the spinal nerves, the primary afferent fibres enter the central nervous system and divide into two branches. Since one of these goes to the principal sensory nucleus of V and the other to the spinal nucleus of V, the two nuclei have in the past been considered as somewhat separate structures. However, histological examination of the spinal nucleus indicates that it is composed of three subnuclei, which in rostrocaudal order are: subnucleus oralis, subnucleus interpolaris and subnucleus caudalis (Fig. 19.75). Subnucleus caudalis is histologically similar to part of the dorsal horn and it is likely that the ascending projection, from this area only, is the equivalent of the spinothalamic system. It is also suggested that the principal sensory nucleus, together with the other two spinal V subnuclei (oralis and interpolaris) constitute the equivalent of the lemniscal projection. Despite this division into 'lemniscal' and 'spinothalamic' sections, there is a somatotopic projection of the face on to the trigeminal complex, such that the face is rep-

resented throughout the length of the nuclear complex, the ophthalmic division of V being ventral (or caudal), the maxillary division central and the mandibular division dorsal (or cranial). Second order cells in the principal sensory nucleus and the rostral subnuclei of the spinal nucleus then give rise not only to a lemniscal projection to the contralateral thalamus (specific projection system) but also to an uncrossed pathway. This carries information from the mouth and relays in the thalamus. Although it has been assumed that this uncrossed pathway gives rise to a specific projection in the cortex, there is now some dispute on this point.

The fibres arising from the nucleus caudalis terminate mainly in the non-specific projection system of the thalamus.

Pain

Pain serves as a warning that damage has occurred to the body. There seems little doubt that, in simple situations, the sensation of pain is mediated by naked endings of small diameter nerve fibres which may be myelinated (Aδ or Group III), or unmyelinated (C or Group IV) (Fig. 5.32). In the experimental situation, using controlled flash heating of the skin, it has been established that the threshold for pain is the level at which cell damage occurs. It has been suggested that, when cells are damaged, the onset of pain is due to the release, by those cells, of a variety of substances, e.g. a histamine like 'P' (pain) substance, bradykinin, K^+, etc. In the case of ischaemic muscle (muscle with a blood flow not adequate for its requirements), the pain produced is related to the accumulation of metabolites. The local presence of high levels of extracellular K^+ in the muscle has been suggested as a cause of pain; this would imply some form of 'damage' to the muscle cells.

In whatever way the nerve impulses are generated, they pass into the spinal cord and are relayed into the anterolateral tract which projects to higher centres (as described in the preceding section) where pain is perceived at a conscious level. Although this traditional view treats pain as having a simple pathway like any other sensation, it does not explain many things, for instance, why pain is unpleasant, whereas other sensations such as touch may have characteristics that are unpleasant, indifferent or very pleasant indeed! It also leaves the function of pain unclear since, when one places a hand on a hot stove, pain is not experienced until a fraction of a second after the reflex withdrawal of the hand; on functional grounds the reflex withdrawal alone would be sufficient without the pain. Admittedly pain gives rise to general aversive behaviour and in this perhaps lies a clue. Pain is a powerful stimulus in forming conditioned reflexes. It is not by chance that over the centuries certain animal trainers and penal systems have used painful stimuli in their programmes of 'education'. Pain is an excellent, if unpopular, tutor! More important, from the clinical point of view, is that if one has an inflamed area, on the back of the neck for example, which is painful when the head is moved, then the subject is conditioned into that posture in which there is minimum disturbance of the inflamed part. This, incidentally, is the best thing for the healing process. Inflammation of the peridontal membrane may similarly produce an altered jaw posture or 'bite'.

The question of which part of the brain actually perceives pain is unresolved. The removal of the somatosensory cortex results in only a transient change in pain perception. Lesions of the thalamus confined to the specific projection nuclei are ineffective in abolishing pain whereas lesions in the areas giving rise to the diffuse (non-specific) projection system are effective. As might be predicted from this, lesions of the anterolateral tracts (spinothalamic and spinoreticulothalamic pathways) abolish pain. In the case of the trigeminal nerve, fibres in the tract of the spinal nucleus can be interrupted at the level of the the subnucleus caudalis so that the trigeminal equivalent of the spinothalamic system is isolated.

The afferent fibres from the viscera that give rise to conscious sensation lie in the dorsal roots, but their peripheral processes travel with the sympathetic nerves from most of the thoracic and abdominal structures. The exceptions are, (a) some of the oesophageal and tracheal afferents travel in the vagus and (b) the afferents from pelvic structures travel in the sacral parasympathetic nerves.

All the foregoing supports the idea of a straight-line transmission system, i.e. as though one 'damage unit' in the periphery gives rise to one 'pain perception unit' centrally. A large number of examples show this not to be so. There are reports of battle casualties with extensive wounds completely denying that they are in pain and on the other hand there are syndromes where, in the absence of any tissue damage, the slightest touch causes excruciating pain. Clearly then there can be considerable modulation in the pathway: it has already been pointed out that at

each synapse on the pathway the transmission of impulses can be either inhibited or facilitated. Such influences, which can act at thalamic, dorsal column nuclei or dorsal horn relays, can arise from a number of sources, the best known of which is the cerebral cortex. There is, however, an important additional interaction in the dorsal horn between large and small diameter nerve fibres. As a generalization one can say that, with respect to the skin, the large diameter ($A\alpha$) fibres come from mechanoreceptors, many of which have moderate thresholds and exhibit moderately rapid adaptation. The small diameter ($A\delta$ and C) fibres come from thermoreceptors and nociceptors and from some mechanoreceptors which, although of widely varying characteristics, tend to be more slowly adapting than the $A\alpha$ group. Consequently the afferent impulses describing a peripheral stimulus will be partitioned differently between large and small fibres, depending upon the characteristics of the stimulus. It has been known for some time that stimulation of the large diameter nerve fibres inhibits transmission from small diameter fibres to the second order sensory cells. Thus, pain can sometimes be alleviated by lightly stroking or touching a painful area; such stimuli preferentially increase activity in large diameter fibres. Conversely, when there is loss of large diameter fibres, as in some disease, e.g. following herpes zoster virus infections, there is an associated tendency to suffer pain; the inhibitory influence is lost, leaving small fibre activity unopposed. It is also known that activity in small diameter fibres facilitates transmission of information from other small diameter primary afferents to 'second order' cells, so that any information can be amplified.

It therefore looks as though pain is not simply a question of stimulating certain small diameter fibres but of the balance between activity in small and large diameter nerves. The balance between the two has profound effects on the impulse traffic generated by the second order sensory neuron; as preponderance of small nerve activity greatly increases the activity of the second order cell.

The foregoing account is an attempt to simplify a very complex system. In Wall's 'gate control theory of pain' the large/small fibre interaction operates as a gate in the path of the sensory input, whilst descending influences also alter the ease with which the 'gate' is opened or 'shut'. The question of whether pain is perceived or not is then dependent upon whether the output of the 'second order' cell rises above some critical level and for how long it sustains that kind of activity (Fig. 5.32).

Referred pain

This is the term which describes pain felt at a site distant from the site of stimulation. The pain is usually referred to a site innervated by the same segment of the spinal cord as the site of stimulation. Pain is not usually referred across the midline, although this is not invariable. Inflammation of the pulp of a tooth may appear as pain in the other jaw, in the ear, in the temporomandibular joint or in the sinuses. It seems possible that the activity of the second order sensory cells relating to the referred site depends on two main factors. First, these cells are activated by the 'non-painful' stimuli from the referred site and second, they are also depolarized by a few, small diameter afferent fibres that come from the damaged area. Consequently when a sufficient number of small diameter fibres are activated, the second order cell is driven to discharge above the critical level (referred to in the previous section) so that pain is perceived.

Analgesia and anaesthesia

Analgesia is the loss of pain sensation whereas anaesthesia implies the loss of all modalities of sensation. The question of loss of sensation due to severance of a nerve and its sequelae are dealt with elsewhere (p. 321); the immediate effects are the same whether nerve conduction is interrupted by cutting, crushing, disease process or the injection of local anaesthetic. In the peripheral nerve, the fibres carrying the various modalities of sensation are all intermingled so that a complete chemical or mechanical lesion is liable to affect all sensations equally.

However, the susceptibility of individual nerve fibres to dilute local anaesthetics or to

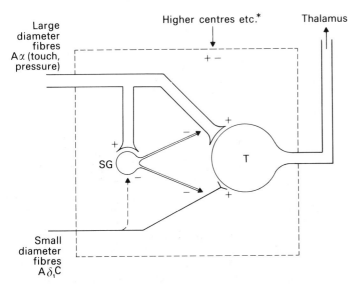

Fig. 5.32. Diagram of the postulated 'gate' control mechanism. The primary large diameter afferent fibres may divide several times on entry to the spinal cord; some branches (shown here) synapse *a* with cells in the substantia gelatinosa (SG) and *b* with the second order afferent or 'transmission' (T) cells. The SG cells presynaptically inhibit the terminals of both large and small afferent fibres. Consequently, when the SG cells are activated they reduce or stop the afferent impulses arriving at the synaptic junction with the T cell. Trains of afferent impulses in large diameter fibres will therefore only activate the T cell briefly. Conversely, afferent impulses in the small diameter fibres inhibit the SG cells so that the T cell will be activated as long as impulses arrive. Pain is coded as a continuing high level of discharge from T. Descending influences from higher centres can have an effect on the way the 'gate' operates. The precise mechanism and site of termination of descending fibres is not yet known so that the descending influences are shown as having a general effect on the complex as a whole. Excitatory synapses are shown as ' + ' and inhibitory synapses as ' − '.

asphyxia differs, depending upon their diameter, so that one can induce selective loss of sensation in some circumstances. Infiltration of nerves with dilute procaine solution in human volunteers results in blockade of C fibres first and then the A fibres, in ascending order of size. The sensation of pain is blocked first followed by those of cold and warmth which disappear at almost the same time. The sensations of touch–pressure and joint position survive until the largest myelinated A fibres fail to conduct. In contrast, pressure applied to a nerve, as by an occlusive cuff around the arm, blocks first the A fibres, followed later by the C fibres. In this case touch–pressure sensation is lost first, followed later by some loss of pain and temperature sensation. It is only when C fibres are completely blocked that all pain and temperature sensation is lost.

In order to relieve intractable pain, an operation in which the anterolateral tract is sectioned is sometimes performed. This procedure results in loss of both pain and temperature sensation on the opposite side of the body in those areas represented by spinal segments caudal to the lesion. Recently a quite different method of pain control has been tried. This depends upon increasing the activity in other pathways by electrically stimulating the large diameter afferent fibres in peripheral nerves, so that the transfer of information from the small diameter fibres at the first synapse is inhibited (Fig. 5.32).

The converse of analgesia, hyperalgesia, is experienced in or around damaged or inflamed tissue. Anyone who has been sunburnt will know that trivial stimuli can then give rise to pain. Small diameter fibres (stimulated by the products of damaged cells) probably produce just sufficient EPSP at the 'second order' cells for the additional excitation due to trivial stimulation of the tissue to drive the second order cells over the critical level so that pain is then experienced. The fact that this can condition the subject into a particular posture (or immobility) so protecting him from further injury has already been mentioned (p. 316). Hyperalgesia and spontaneous pain can also be produced by disorders of the thalamic nuclei themselves.

Whereas local anaesthetics produce their effect by disabling the mechanism of the propagated action potential (p. 295), general anaesthetics produce their effects largely by inactivating synaptic mechanisms. Signals from the periphery that would normally produce a powerful alerting response are unable to drive the multisynaptic reticular activating system into

sufficient activity. General anaesthesia does not prevent impulses reaching the sensory cortex. In fact the easiest way to demonstrate a somatotopic projection of the body on to the sensory cortex is to use a deeply anaesthetized animal. This allows impulse traffic traversing a pathway with only a few synapses, e.g. lemniscal system, to reach the cortex and produce electrical signals, which may be detected after suitable amplification, against an electrically quiet background. Under anaesthesia, the processing of information and the behavioural responses to lemniscal signals reaching the cortex do not arise, since those cortical processes are dependent upon coexisting activity in multisynaptic systems, in particular those involving the reticular system and non-specific thalamic nuclei.

HYPNOSIS, AUDIOANALGESIA, ACUPUNCTURE

Although both hypnosis and acupuncture have been practised for at least two thousand years, there is, as yet, no completely satisfactory explanation for these methods of raising pain thresholds.

Hypnosis is a state of heightened suggestion which can probably be attained by most people with practice. During this state, the subject may be directed to states of analgesia, anaesthesia, drowsiness or deep sleep. The bodily area of analgesia or anaesthesia that is suggested to the subject does not have to correspond to any segmental innervation but may be represented by the area covered by, say, a sock, i.e. parts of each of L3–5, S1 and S2. It seems possible that such analgesic or anaesthetic areas might be produced by descending inhibitory mechanisms acting on synapses within the spinal cord (see Fig. 5.30b) since the reflex responses to noxious stimuli (flexion withdrawal) are also abolished. How particular descending inhibitory pathways are activated is, however, unknown.

Audioanalgesia, the production of a 'pain free' state by playing muffled music or 'white noise' to a subject, probably functions more by reducing anxiety or distracting a subject rather than by any direct effect upon a pain appreciation system. Recent work even disputes that any analgesic effect is produced at all.

Of the three phenomena, acupuncture is perhaps the least explicable on neurophysiological grounds, and is frankly disconcerting on anatomical grounds. For example, in traditional Chinese medicine a needle would be inserted in the 'kuangming' point in the lower part of the leg in order to obtain anaesthesia of the eye! Since acupuncture offers a direct challenge to established concepts and also derives from an unfamiliar culture, there is almost as much dispute as to whether it works as to how it works. One suggestion is that acupuncture is essentially hypnosis, the subjects being conditioned by their culture or belief to respond to the insertion of needles by appropriate loss of sensation. Another suggestion is that acupuncture operates by some, as yet undiscovered, ramification of the gate control system (p. 317).

Enkephalins and endorphins

Endorphins are polypeptides with morphine-like activity, that have been isolated from the brain; enkephalins are small endorphins with a specific amino acid sequence. A polypeptide produced by the pituitary, β–lipotropin, can be split to produce endorphins and these in turn may be split to produce enkephalins. There is some uncertainty at the moment as to which of these peptides is the precursor, the metabolite and the physiologically significant molecule. The failure, so far, to detect long-chain peptides in brain tissue suggests that the enkephalins are the physiologically important peptides; they may well arise in brain tissue by ways other than by the breakdown of endorphins from β–lipotropin.

Naloxone blocks receptor sites at which morphine acts, so it is quite understandable that it might similarly block the action of naturally occurring (endogenous) morphine-like substances such as enkephalins and endorphins.

When endorphins or enkephalins are injected into the CSF or the periaqueductal grey matter of experimental animals, the reflex responses to noxious stimuli are inhibited without any motor paralysis; these 'analgesic' effects are antagonized by naloxone. Similarly in man, evidence has been advanced to suggest that these naturally occurring analgesic substances are part of a normally active 'pain control' system since the administration of naloxone can make some subjects more perceptive to pain.

THE HISTOLOGY OF THE DEGENERATION OF NERVES

There are many ways in which the nervous system can be injured. These range from the effects of mechanical trauma resulting for example, from criminal wounding, accidents or the growth of space-occupying lesions, to the effects of exposure to a variety of neurotoxic agents in the environment, both deliberately, as in glue-sniffing, or accidentally, in industrial over-exposure. The response of the nervous system however is limited to two major patterns, namely degeneration or demyelination of the neurites with concomitant chromatolysis of the relevant somata in degenerating lesions.

Chromatolysis

The classic chromatolytic reaction (seen by light microscopy) is a dissolution of the larger Nissl bodies to give either a fine powdery appearance or clear areas of cytoplasm. The nucleus usually becomes eccentric, moving away from the axon hillock and the whole cell body often swells. The severity and duration of the response vary with species, age and type and site of injury. Biochemical and histochemical analyses have revealed that following axotomy (i.e. nerve section) there is an increase in nucleolar RNA content, protein synthesis and the rate of export of proteins from the affected cell bodies to the periphery. There is a characteristic increase in neuronal acid phosphatase early in the response. This enhanced anabolism occurs even in the absence of obvious structural changes. The stimulus for chromatolysis is unknown though it is likely to involve several factors.

Degeneration

Degeneration occurs distal to a crush or cut, and involves both the axon and Schwann cells of all affected fibres, whether myelinated or unmyelinated. Because the morphological changes seen microscopically were first described by Waller, it is customary to talk of Wallerian degeneration after mechanical injury, and Wallerian-type degeneration if a similar sequence of morphological changes is produced by other means. During the first 2–3 days after injury, the myelinated internodes in the distal stump begin to break up into longitudinal chains of myelin-bound *ovoids*. This process usually starts at widened nodes of Ranvier and incisures of Schmidt–Lanterman.

Debris from degenerating myelin and axons is first sequestered in Schwann cells, which may thus be said to be autophagocytic. Considerable Schwann cell proliferation occurs during the first month after injury (as assessed autoradiographically by their uptake of ^{3}H-thymidine): it is probable that one of the stimuli for this proliferation is the presence of intra-cellular debris. The period of debris-processing (breakdown of myelin and axoplasm) lasts for about 2 weeks in the PNS: in the CNS, it can take many months. The major biochemical changes associated with Wallerian degeneration reflect the breakdown and removal of the constituents of the myelin sheath and include an early loss of basic protein, a progressive loss of phospholipids and glyco-proteins and the subsequent appearance, during the second week, of cholesterol esters and neutral lipid. Cells laden with masses of lipid droplets and whorls of myelin debris leave the basal lamina tubes that formerly contained the myelinated axons, and enter the endoneurium. Macrophages (derived from the blood stream) also enter the endoneurium: the contribution that these cells make to the removal of debris remains controversial in both the PNS and, more particularly, in the CNS. There has been much debate as to whether degeneration occurs uniformly along a nerve, or whether it progresses in a proximodistal sequence. Careful examination of teased fibres has revealed that there is a latent period (the length of which varies according to axonal calibre) prior to the onset of degeneration. Once begun, degeneration spreads very rapidly throughout the distal extent of the fibre.

Regeneration

Soon after injury the central ends of the damaged axons begin to sprout. Small (0.1–0.5 μm diameter) protrusions of axoplasm grow out across the gap into the distal stump. Many factors influence their success in penetrating the distal stump, e.g. the length of the gap to be 'bridged'; abortive growth of sprouts either back into the proximal stump or into (but not beyond) the neuroma surrounding the cut end; the mechanical barrier presented by the increased amount of endoneurial collagen that is inevitably produced after injury, and the size of the persisting Schwann cell basal lamina tubes (bands of Büngner) awaiting re-innervation in the distal stump. Axons from motor nerves can grow into Schwann cell tubes that previously housed sensory nerves and vice versa: functionally such repair is useless. Once axons become re-associated with Schwann cells in the distal stump, re-myelination can occur. Myelinated axons can grow down tubes of Schwann cells that once surrounded unmyelinated axons—it seems that the signal for (re)myelinogenesis must reside in the axon, since experiments have

shown that under these conditions, the 'host' Schwann cells will begin to make myelin. Although remyelination appears to be basically similar to myelination in the fetal and neo-natal animal, the original spectra of internodal lengths and myelin thicknesses are never regained. All re-myelinated internodes remain between 300–400 μm long, irrespective of proximal axonal calibre, and myelin sheaths remain inappropriately thin. Thus a regenerated nerve is always recognisable histologically even many years after repair. Recovery, in functional terms, obviously depends on the number of motor axons that grow back to motor end–plates and sensory axons that can re-associate with receptors, and on the success of re-myelination. Among many factors determining the extent of recovery are: the severity and causation of the lesion; the length of nerve to be regenerated (since axonal outgrowth is of the order of 1–4 mm/day, and Schwann cell tubes themselves degenerate after several months of denervation); the responsiveness of the satellite cell population, and, particularly where mixed nerves are involved, the internal architecture of the nerve bundle.

Demyelination

In demyelination, axonal continuity is maintained, while myelin is lost, either paranodally, or along complete internodes. Because loss of myelin rarely occurs along the whole extent of a nerve fibre, it is usual to talk of segmental demyelination since the intervening internodes appear to be normally myelinated. Demyelination may occur as a result of metabolic damage to the Schwann cell or oligodendrocyte (e.g. diphtheria toxin); in response to direct action of myelinolytic substances, or myelin may be 'stripped' off during an immune attack mounted by mononuclear cells sensitized against specific antigens located on or within the myelin sheath (in these cases the satellite cell is usually a passive by-stander). Once initiated, myelin breakdown is carried out either within the satellite cells or some other phagocytic cell (presumably haematogenous in origin), and demyelinated axons are subsequently re-myelinated. As in the regeneration after Wallerian degeneration, the new internodes are uniformly short (300–400 μm) and the new myelin is very thin. Loss of myelin results in a decreased internodal resistance and increased capacitance and conductance. Not surprisingly, therefore, the physiological consequences of demyelination include conduction slowing and frequently conduction block and increased refractoriness. Remyelination can restore conduction. Recent work has indicated that during the recovery period demyelinated axons can conduct continuously: there is much interest in the way in which the new Na^+ channels (necessary for electrogenesis at the new nodes) are evolved and/or redistributed along the axolemma during the repair process.

For many years it was thought that remyelination could not occur in the CNS, largely because of the intense astrocytosis and subsequent scarring that usually accompany central injury, and also because of the marked unreactivity of the oligodendrocyte population, in contrast to the Schwann cells in the PNS. It is now known that central remyelination can take place, and that both oligodendrocytes and Schwann cells can remyelinate central axons.

THE PHYSIOLOGY OF NERVE DEGENERATION AND REGENERATION

During embryogenesis neuroblasts send axonal processes out from the developing spinal cord and brain stem to innervate a variety of peripheral structures. The axons, which are destined to become sensory, motor and autonomic nerves, have some mechanism for 'seeking-out' the appropriate structures to be innervated. Innervation of the peripheral structure brings about changes in the physiology of that tissue. In the case of fetal striated muscle, which is non-innervated, the sensitivity to acetylcholine extends all over the cell surface. However, this sensitivity becomes restricted to the motor end-plate as soon as the cell becomes innervated.

To some extent the regeneration response following nerve section in the adult animal can be viewed as a repeat of the early developmental process but with some very important differences. First, since the adult neuron is a highly differentiated cell, it is incapable of mitosis. There are, therefore, no replacements for any neurons that die. Second, whereas neurons wholly within the CNS are in general incapable of re-establishing functional pathways once they are broken, those having peripheral processes can regenerate. However, they do not necessarily re-innervate the appropriate structures. Re-innervation of inappropriate structures can produce some bizarre effects.

Causes of degeneration and dysfunction

It is not necessary for a nerve to be cut for it to stop carrying propagated action potentials. Mild damage to a nerve can block the transmission of impulses without producing signs of histological damage. Pressure produces such effects either by a direct mechanical effect upon the axon or by interrupting the blood supply to the nerve. These effects can be demonstrated readily in the laboratory by inflating a pressure cuff around the upper arm to above systolic pressure. Changes in sensation occur after about 15 minutes of stasis and eventually all sensation is lost after 25–30 min. Normal sensation returns rapidly upon release of the cuff. However, the student should be aware that prolonged pressure on a nerve, or prolonged hypoxia, can produce histological signs of damage with a much delayed recovery or even a permanent loss of sensation. Intense local pressure will, of course, crush the nerve. Damage to nerves can be produced by a wide variety of conditions apart from mechanical injury. Dysfunction can also result from vitamin deficiencies (e.g. B_1), from infections (e.g. the herpes zoster virus), from poisons (e.g. lead) and from immunological responses. The big difference between, on the one hand, cutting or tearing a nerve and, on the other hand, interfering with its metabolism in some way, is that in the former case the anatomical structure of the nerve can be grossly disarranged; in the latter case it is probable that the endoneural tubes or Schwann cell sheaths are intact so that the regenerating axon has a clear path to the periphery.

Effects of degeneration and dysfunction

SENSORY NERVES

The obvious result of failure of conduction along a pure sensory nerve is loss of sensation in the area supplied by that nerve. The area of skin supplied by one sensory axon is, however, of limited size; it overlaps the territory of a number of other axons and is in turn overlapped by them. Consequently, loss of conduction in a single axon produces a loss of sensation which is therefore not likely to be particularly noticed by the subject. Loss of conduction in a large number of axons at the same time, however, leads to a large anaesthetic area which is unlikely to be overlooked. It is perhaps not so obvious that, whilst the patient is acutely aware of such a loss of sensation if it is of sudden onset, he can be less aware of the anaesthetic area if the nerve lesion has progressed very gradually, i.e. if axons have died off one at a time over a long period. In such cases, the area of anaesthesia may only come to light upon neurological examination.

Interrupted conduction in primary afferent neurons not only results in loss of conscious perception but also in the loss of reflexes that could previously be elicited by stimulating that site. This means that damaging stimuli applied to tissue will not give rise to the usual protective responses which remove the part from the stimulus. For example, in severe damage to the sensory root of the trigeminal nerve there will be a loss of the jaw opening reflex. Normal oral activity under these conditions can be hazardous as there are risks of unrecognized thermal damage to tissue, e.g. by taking drinks which are too hot or smoking cigarettes to the very end; there are also risks of involuntarily chewing lumps out of the tongue when eating! The use of local anaesthetics to block the inferior dental nerve (which in practice often means that the lingual nerve is blocked as well) gives rise to a comparable although temporary sensory deficit.

MOTOR NERVES

The effect of total failure in conduction of impulses along a motor nerve will be the immediate paralysis of the muscle supplied. Since action potentials do not reach the motor end-plates, no acetylcholine is released from them. Consequently the muscle will be flaccid, i.e. soft and flabby, and there can be neither voluntary nor reflex control over that muscle. With degeneration of the distal part of the nerve, the motor end-plates disappear.

If the muscle remains functionless for any length of time it undergoes 'disuse atrophy' i.e. the muscle cells get smaller and smaller and eventually the muscle can virtually disappear. This can be halted by artificially exercising the muscle using direct electrical stimulation.

AUTONOMIC NERVES

Lesions in autonomic nerves obviously have a variety of effects, depending upon whether sympathetic or parasympathetic pathways are affected. The effects can be worked out readily by referring to the section on the autonomic nervous system (p. 925). One condition of particular interest to the dental student is Horner's syndrome which is produced when there is failure of conduction in the cervical sympathetic chain of one side. This condition can be the result of trauma or disease processes interrupting the sympathetic chain but it has also been produced as a temporary effect by a rather poorly aimed dental injection. The subject suffers, amongst other things, from a unilateral pupillary constriction and a unilateral hot dry face. These symptoms are due to unopposed parasympathetic activity on the constrictor pupillae, absence of both cutaneous vasoconstrictor tone and sympathetic (cholinergic) innervation of the sweat glands.

DENERVATION HYPERSENSITIVITY

When a peripheral nerve fibre to a structure is divided and the synaptic junction with that structure degenerates, the postsynaptic cell membrane becomes unduly sensitive to transmitter substance. This is known as denervation hypersensitivity. Such hypersensitivity also develops following division of postganglionic sympathetic nerves. For example, the initial dilatation of arterioles due to absence of vasoconstrictor tone, is succeeded by increased vasoconstriction due to the action of circulating catecholamines on the hypersensitive tissues.

MIXED NERVES

There are few nerves in the body that are purely motor or sensory. 'Motor' nerves to muscles have in them the afferent fibres from receptors in those muscles and also from joints. 'Sensory' nerves, innervating the skin of the limbs contain sympathetic axons, i.e. efferent fibres going to sweat glands, blood vessels etc. The consequence of this is that interruption of a given nerve will be associated with mixed effects. Lesion of a 'motor' nerve may involve, in addition to paralysis, deficits in sense of joint position. Lesion of a cutaneous nerve may result not only in loss of sensation but also, in the long term, in 'trophic' changes in the skin itself, i.e. the skin becomes dry, shiny and thin. This can be explained by loss of sympathetic supply to the sweat glands and denervation hypersensitivity of the blood vessels so that local cutaneous blood flow is reduced. The additional problem is that since there is a loss of protective reflexes, the skin is frequently damaged. Moreover, because the blood supply is reduced, it only heals slowly and is likely to be chronically ulcerated.

Nerve lesions destroying proprioceptive input result in some loss of reflex control of movement and posture.

Regeneration

Nerves will not regenerate if the cause of the original degeneration is still present. In the case of a simple cut or crush injury to a skin nerve, the regeneration starts about 2 days later in the largest diameter axons, i.e. the A fibres, and is followed about 14 days later by regeneeration in the C fibres. Myelination of A fibres starts 15–30 days later and spreads peripherally. Whilst regeneration is occurring from the central cut end of a cutaneous nerve, other fibres grow into the denervated zone from neighbouring areas of skin, so decreasing the size of the anaesthetic area. During the recovery period the sensations from the area can be abnormal (paraesthesias) and may occasionally assume the character of severe burning pain (causalgia).

Regeneration of a motor nerve is not different in principle but the eventual degree of motor recovery depends upon the duration of the motor loss i.e. upon how long atrophy of the muscle fibres has been progressing before re-innervation.

If there is any interruption in the Schwann cell sheath, as could well occur in traumatic injury, then axons will regenerate as previously described, but there is no guarantee that they will enter the right sheath. Consequently one can get inappropriate innervation of structures, i.e. one can get sensory fibres destined for one area going to another or motor fibres for one muscle going to another. One may then get 'perversion of sensation' and motor disorders. If a sensory axon proceeds down what was formerly a motor sheath in a mixed nerve then the striated muscle fibres will not receive the correct innervation and will atrophy. In other cases autonomic fibres can end up innervating the incorrect structure. This can occur with injury inflicted to the parotid region, when cross innervation between autonomic fibres going to the salivary glands and to the sweat glands can arise. This can result in 'gustatory sweating', i.e. facial sweating when salivation should really occur.

FURTHER READING

Melzack R. & Wall P.D. (1965) Pain Mechanisms: a new theory. *Science* **150**, 971–979.

Wall P.D. (1978) The gate control theory of pain mechanisms: a re-examination and re-statement. *Brain* **101**, 1–18.

CHAPTER 6

Muscles

Muscle is tissue specialized for contraction, a process involving the shortening of contractile muscle cells or fibres. During contraction, chemically-bound energy in the form of ATP is transduced into molecular movements which cause protein filaments to slide over each other. These filaments are aligned parallel to the long axis of the elongated cell.

Myofilaments, the proteinaceous microfilaments of muscle cells, are composed mainly of actin and myosin (Fig. 6.3, 6.6). Microfilaments containing similar proteins are found in virtually all eukaryotic cells where they participate in phagocytosis, pinocytosis, exocytosis, and cytokinesis (p. 172). Related materials are involved in the movement of cilia and flagella, but here the proteins are arranged as microtubules (p. 172). In all these processes chemically-bound energy enables fibrous proteins to slide over each other. The difference between muscle cells and the rest lies in the quantity and arrangement of these proteins.

Muscle cells are invariably elongated in the direction in which they shorten; their cooperative action is ensured either by fusion into multinucleate units of considerable length, as in skeletal muscle, or by functional linkage through intercellular junctions, such as intercalated discs in cardiac muscle and nexuses in smooth muscle. Since each contractile unit is elongated, it is called a muscle fibre.

Muscle can be classified into three types: skeletal, cardiac and smooth. All three are derived from mesenchyme cells, but they differentiate along different routes.

Skeletal and cardiac muscle can be classified together as striated or striped muscle because their myofilaments are arranged in a pattern of alternating thin and thick bands which makes them appear transversely striped. Cardiac muscle is aptly named, since it is found only in the wall of the heart, and skeletal muscle is thus any striated muscle not found in the wall of the heart. Although most skeletal muscle is attached to the hard skeleton (hence its name) some is attached instead to connective tissue sheets or aponeuroses. Skeletal muscle is also known as voluntary muscle, implying that it is under the direct control of the will.

The third type of muscle is smooth, plain or non-striated muscle. As its name implies, its myofilaments are not arranged in a pattern producing transverse stripes. It is often called involuntary muscle because it is generally not under the control of the will, although some experts in yoga apparently can control its contraction deliberately. It is normally controlled by the autonomic part of the nervous system (as is cardiac muscle). It acts more slowly than striated muscle. Smooth muscle is found in the walls of many of the tubular structures of the body. Its fibres are arranged in encircling sheets which, by their slow and maintained contraction (tone), regulate the diameter of these tubes. Smooth muscle can undergo rhythmic contraction, with the result that waves of peristalsis pass along tubes such as the gut, pushing the contents of the tubes ahead of them. Smooth muscle fibres are always much shorter than those of striated muscle and are invariably uninucleate.

The three types of muscle are shown diagrammatically in Figure 6.1.

Although contractile fibres form the major component of any muscle, non-contractile elements are also present, and have a vital part to play in allowing and maintaining contraction. Each muscle fibre, regardless of its type, is surrounded by a delicate framework of loose connective tissue, while groups of fibres may be surrounded by denser connective tissue. Fibroblasts in the connective tissue produce inelastic collagen fibres of high tensile stregth. These tough fibres mesh with the more fragile muscle cells and transmit the forces of contraction which cause movement; that is, the fibrous framework acts as a harness. The connective tissue network also provides routes along which blood vessels, lymphatics and nerves can travel to supply fibres

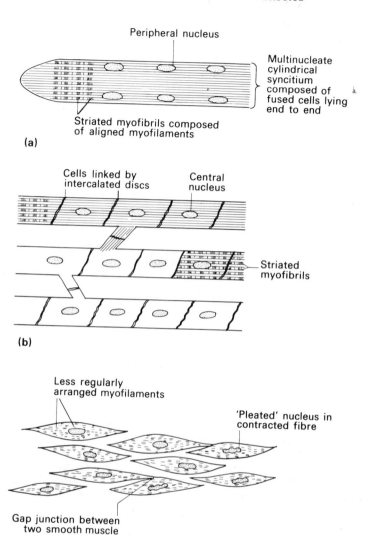

Peripheral nucleus

Multinucleate cylindrical syncitium composed of fused cells lying end to end

Striated myofibrils composed of aligned myofilaments

(a)

Cells linked by intercalated discs

Central nucleus

Striated myofibrils

(b)

Less regularly arranged myofilaments

'Pleated' nucleus in contracted fibre

Gap junction between two smooth muscle fibres

(c)

Fig. 6.1. Comparison of (a) skeletal muscle, (b) cardiac muscle and (c) smooth muscle.

deep within the muscle. The efficiency of the muscle relies on the integrity of these supply routes, as well as on the muscle fibres themselves.

SKELETAL MUSCLE

This consists of cylindrical, multinucleate muscle fibres, each about 10–40 μm in diameter and up to 30 cm long, surrounded by connective tissue. Each contractile fibre is encased in a delicate envelope of loose connective tissue, termed the endomysium, continuous with a stronger envelope, the perimysium, which surrounds the bundle or fasciculus of which the fibre is a part. The whole muscle consists of a number of fasciculi of different sizes united by a stout sheath of fibrous connective tissue termed the epimysium (Fig. 6.2).

All the connective tissue sheaths are continuous with each other and with the connective tissue of the structures lying next to the muscle and to which it is attached. A muscle may be

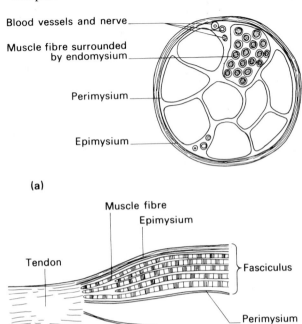

Blood vessels and nerve

Muscle fibre surrounded
by endomysium

Perimysium

Epimysium

(a)

Muscle fibre

Epimysium

Tendon

Fasciculus

Perimysium

(b)

Fig. 6.2. Diagram of (a) a transverse section and (b) a longitudinal section of a skeletal muscle, showing its connective tissue sheaths.

attached through the fibrous proteins of its epimysium to an aponeurosis, the dermis of the skin, the periosteum covering a bone, a raphe or a tendon (p. 380). In situations where the muscle is linked to bone either directly or via a tendon, collagen fibres often pass from it into the substance of the bone. As the bone grows they become firmly embedded in it, the embedded parts being known as Sharpey's fibres. Such a union is extremely strong and enables forces generated in the muscle to be transmitted to the bone with little power loss or chance of tearing.

Skeletal muscle is metabolically very active and needs a rich blood supply. Arteries enter through the epimysium, branch within the perimysium to supply the individual fasciculi, and then divide into arterioles and capillaries. The latter generally run parallel to the muscle fibres in the endomysium surrounding them. The capillaries drain into venules, which unite into veins and leave the muscle by way of the epimysium. The lymphatics of skeletal muscle are confined to the perimysium and epimysium, and thus differ from those of cardiac muscle, which are also found in the endomysium.

Nerves enter the muscle through its connective tissue sheaths, often accompanying the

arteries in neurovascular bundles. There is great variation in the number of muscle fibres supplied by a single nerve fibre. Where great delicacy of movement is required, for example in the extrinsic muscles of the eye, the ratio may be one to one. In muscle responsible for carrying out gross movements and where fine control is not required, the ratio may be a thousand to one or even higher. The muscle fibres supplied by a single nerve axon, comprise, together with that nerve cell, a motor unit. The muscle fibres of such a unit do not form a localized group but are scattered throughout the muscle. This is important since if only a weak contraction of the whole muscle is required then only a few motor units are activated and it is obviously desirable that they should be scattered through the muscle rather than grouped together. The stronger the contraction required, the more motor units are recruited.

If a nerve is examined close to the point at which it enters the muscle, that is, at the neuromuscular hilum, it will be found to contain both motor and sensory fibres. The motor fibres are the large, myelinated, efferents of the anterior horn neurons, which supply the extrafusal muscle fibres; and smaller myelinated

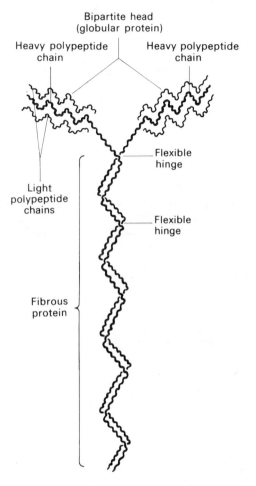

Bipartite head
(globular protein)

Heavy polypeptide chain

Heavy polypeptide chain

Flexible hinge

Light polypeptide chains

Flexible hinge

Fibrous protein

Fig. 6.3. Diagrammatic representation of a myosin molecule.

efferents which supply intrafusal muscle fibres. Intrafusal fibres lie inside muscle spindles; sense organs which monitor the extent of muscle stretch (p. 330). Delicate nonmyelinated autonomic efferents also enter skeletal muscle to supply the smooth muscle of its blood vessels. The sensory fibres are of two types: myelinated fibres which communicate with the muscle spindles and with sense organs in the tendons, and nonmyelinated pain afferents.

Structure of skeletal muscle fibres

Each skeletal muscle fibre is a single, elongated, cylindrical cell containing hundreds of peripherally arranged nuclei lying just deep to the plasma membrane or sarcolemma. The sarcoplasm (cytoplasm) contains groups of longitudinally

running myofilaments, which collectively form myofibrils about 1 μm in diameter. The myofilaments are of two types, thin and thick, the former being about 6 nm and the latter about 12 nm in diameter. They are arranged in a characteristic pattern which gives rise to transverse striations in each myofibril. The striations of adjacent myofibrils coincide, and in consequence bands or stripes appear to run across the whole width of the muscle fibre when it is examined by light microscopy (Fig. 6.1).

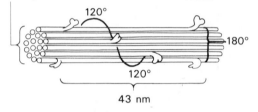

18 myosin molecules in transverse section

120°

180°

120°

43 nm

Fig. 6.4. Diagram showing the arrangement of myosin molecules in a thick myofilament.

The myofilaments and striations

Thick myofilaments are composed of the fibrous protein, myosin. A myosin molecule is an asymmetrical protein with a fibrous tail and a globular head (Fig. 6.3). A thick myofilament is a regularly arranged rope of these molecules, the globular heads projecting from the edge of the rope and forming a spiral pattern on its surface (Fig. 6.4). Across their midlines a few hundred of these ropes are tied together into fascicles by a protein, M-line protein (Fig. 6.5).

The thin myofilaments contain globular molecules of actin (G-actin) polymerized into fibres (F-actin); also the fibrous protein, tropomyosin, and the globular protein, troponin. The short (40 nm long) tropomyosin molecules are attached end-to-end, at a region containing troponin, to form a double helix about 1 μm long (Fig. 6.6). The polymerized fibres of actin are themselves arranged as a double helix which twists with the tropomyosin molecules. Thin myofilaments are attached to a midline Z-band, the directions of the actin helices being reversed on each side of the Z-band. Each Z-band also connects thin myofilaments into fascicles (Fig. 6.5).

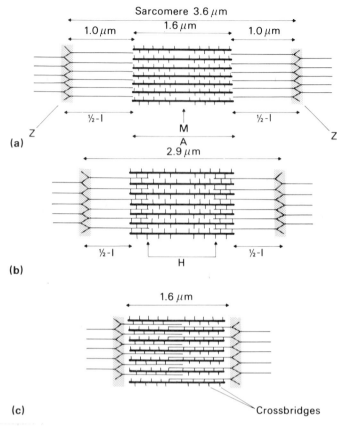

(a)

(b)

(c)

Fig. 6.5. Arrangement of myofilaments in a
sarcomere when it is (a) fully extended, (b) at rest, and
(c) fully contracted.

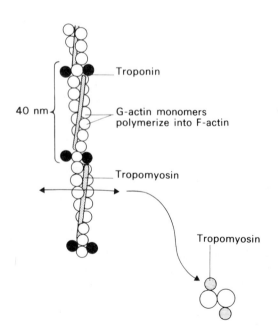

Fig. 6.6. Structure of a thin myofilament. (After
Huxley H. E. (1972) *Cold Spring Harbor Symp.
Quant. Biol.* **37**, 361.)

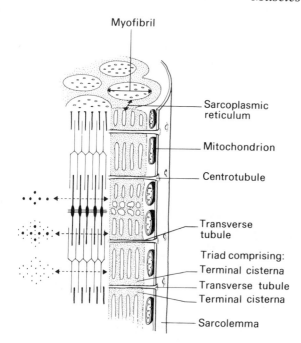

Myofibril

Sarcoplasmic reticulum

Mitochondrion

Centrotubule

Transverse tubule

Triad comprising:
Terminal cisterna
Transverse tubule
Terminal cisterna

Sarcolemma

Fig. 6.7. The ultrastructure of a skeletal muscle fibre.

Transverse to the long axis of a myofibril the thin and thick myofilaments are arranged with geometrical precision (Fig. 6.7).

In the uncontracted state, fascicles of thin filaments alternate along the length of a muscle fibre with fascicles of thick filaments (Fig. 6.5). Because the thick filaments are birefringent under polarized light and the thin filaments are not, a skeletal muscle fibre appears striated in polarized light. The resultant bands are called A-bands (aniostropic = birefringent: thick filaments) and I-bands (isotropic: thin filaments). Each band contains a thin midline striation, the M-line in the A-band, the Z-line in the I-band. When muscle contracts the thin and thick myofilaments slide over each other to produce a region where the A and I bands overlap (Fig. 6.5).

Muscle contraction

The length of a sarcomere (the smallest repeating structural unit) varies according to the amount a muscle fibre contracts: from a fully extended 3.6 μm a sarcomere can contract to about 1.6 μm. Where the thin and thick myofilaments overlap crossbridges develop between them. These crossbridges, which are the globular heads of the myosin molecules, are the only structural link between the thin and thick myofilaments. During muscle contraction the crossbridges alternately make and break contact with the thin myofilaments, so pulling them towards the centre of the sarcomere (Figs. 6.5 & 6.8).

Fine structure of the sarcoplasm of skeletal muscle fibres

Sarcoplasm is the term used for the cytoplasm of a muscle fibre. It is limited externally by the sarcolemma which has a similar structure to that of other plasma membranes. On its outer surface is a glycocalyx to which adhere the collagen fibres of the endomysium.

At regular intervals, tubular invaginations called centrotubules extend inwards from the sarcolemma. Once within the cell they are termed transverse or T-tubules because they lie in a plane transverse to the long axis of the muscle fibre, at the level of the junction between the A and I-bands (Fig. 6.7). They branch and anastomose so that each myofibril is surrounded by a T-tubule. If a muscle fibre is sectioned transversely at the level of a set of interconnected T-tubules, its cut surface resembles a sieve, with myofibrils (bundles of myofilaments) passing through the holes in the sieve. The transverse tubules, linked circumferentially to the sarcolemma via the centrotubules, are thus a con-

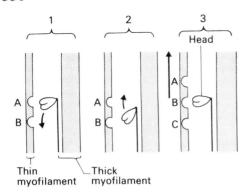

Fig. 6.8.

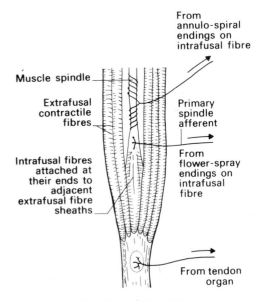

neurons enclosed within their own connective tissue capsule. The muscle fibres within this capsule are said to be intrafusal to distinguish them from those outside the spindle fibres.

The 6–14 intrafusal fibres of each spindle are of two types, termed nuclear bag and nuclear chain fibres. The nuclear bag fibres are distended centrally, forming a 'bag' within which many nuclei are clustered (Fig. 6.10). They are longer than the capsule and extend from either end of it. In contrast, the nuclear chain fibres are completely enclosed within the capsule and have their nuclei arranged in single-file. Each has a sensory and motor innervation independent of the other. Nuclear bag and nuclear chain fibres respond differently to stretching: the nuclear bag fibres have a lower viscosity than the chain fibres and are more easily deformed (p. 468).

The intrafusal muscle fibres of the spindle are supplied by two types of sensory nerve endings. Primary or annulospiral endings coil around the central regions of both bag and chain fibres, while secondary or flower-spray endings are

Fig. 6.8. One of the theories of crossbridge movement during muscle contraction. The heads of the myosin molecules swing to and fro, linking with reactive sites (A, B and C) on the adjacent thin filament, causing it to slide. 1, 2 and 3 show sequential stages in the process.

tinuation of the plasma membrane deep within the cell.

The transverse tubules are linked to intracellular membranes, collectively known as the sarcoplasmic reticulum, by tight junctions. The sarcoplasmic reticulum is the smooth endoplasmic reticulum of the muscle fibre. It is a system of branching and anastomosing tubules and cisternae which form a series of lace-like sleeves surrounding each myofibril between adjacent T-tubules. On either side of each transverse tubule, that is, at the level of the junctions between the A and I bands, the sarcoplasmic reticulum distends to form a transversely running terminal cisterna. The triple complex of terminal cisterna–T-tubule–terminal cisterna is called a muscle triad.

Muscle receptors

The amount and rate of muscle contraction are each under central neural control which is influenced by information from receptors in the muscle and tendon. The receptors are termed muscle spindles and tendon organs. The spindles lie in the substance of the muscle, in parallel with its contractile, extrafusal fibres (Fig. 6.9). The tendon organs however lie in the connective tissue harness at the end of the muscle, in series with the contractile muscle fibres.

MUSCLE SPINDLES

A muscle spindle is a group of modified striated muscle fibres supplied by sensory and motor

Fig. 6.9. Position of muscle receptors.

found on either side of the annulospiral endings. The intrafusal fibres also have a motor supply which causes contraction of those parts of the fibres which lie on either side of the non-contractile central regions. Activity in these nerves sets the sensitivity level of the spindle independent of the extrafusal fibres. These motor fibres are the γ-efferents.

TENDON ORGANS

These consist of small bundles of collagenous tendon fibres enclosed in a capsule and supplied with sensory endings of the spray type. Like muscle spindles they respond to stretching.

NEUROMUSCULAR JUNCTIONS

Skeletal muscles contract when stimulated to do so by somatic efferent (motor) nerve fibres which end upon their surfaces as *motor end plates* (Fig. 5.22). The nerve fibres enter the epimysium and generally divide, giving rise to several branches which supply different muscle fibres. Each motor neuron and the muscle fibres it supplies collectively form a *motor unit* (p. 326). When the terminal branch of a motor nerve fibre reaches its target muscle fibre, it loses its myelin sheath and its axon branches, forming the motor end plates. At these end plates the axon terminations lie in synaptic gutters, grooves in a raised zone of sarcoplasm termed the sole plate of the muscle fibre. Each gutter is covered by a thin Schwann cell process. The sarcolemma lining each gutter is thrown into a series of folds termed junctional folds. The axon terminal lying in each gutter

contains many vesicles within which is the neurotransmitter acetyl choline; when this is released into the gutter it causes permeability changes in the sarcolemma of the junctional folds. The resulting depolarization triggers a chain of events which results in the contraction of the muscle fibre.

Development of skeletal muscle

Skeletal muscle cells develop from mesenchyme cells of the embryo in specific, genetically determined areas such as myotomes and lateral plate mesoderm (Book 2). The mesenchyme cells, which are at first pluripotent, stellate cells, differentiate into myoblasts, becoming elongated and packed with myofilaments as their 'potency', in terms of developmental versatility, is reduced. The myofilaments, the intracellular fibrous proteins contained within the cells which manufacture them, become arranged in parallel bundles or myofibrils in a precisely controlled pattern which results in the production of sarcomeres (p. 328). The myoblasts next line up in columns and fuse end-to-end, forming multinucleate cylinders or myotubes. These increase in length as more myoblasts arrive at, and fuse with, their ends.

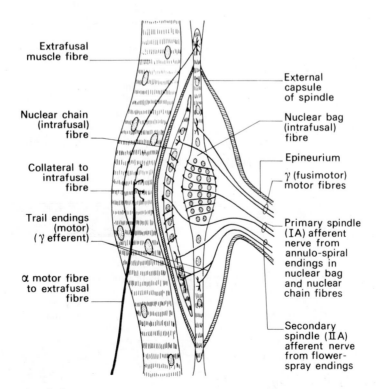

Extrafusal muscle fibre

External capsule of spindle

Nuclear chain (intrafusal) fibre

Nuclear bag (intrafusal) fibre

Collateral to intrafusal fibre

Epineurium

γ (fusimotor) motor fibres

Trail endings (motor) (γ efferent)

Primary spindle (I A) afferent nerve from annulo-spiral endings in nuclear bag and nuclear chain fibres

α motor fibre to extrafusal fibre

Secondary spindle (II A) afferent nerve from flower-spray endings

Fig. 6.10. A muscle spindle.

The fusion of myoblasts with the ends of the myotubes continues, so that they lengthen, and meanwhile their fusion becomes complete so that the cross walls are absorbed and the multicellular myotube becomes a multinucleate, syncitial muscle fibre. This process is shown diagrammatically in Fig. 6.11.

A few immature myoblasts remain associated with the skeletal muscle fibres of the adult. They are called satellite cells and lie between the sarcolemma and the glycocalyx (Fig. 6.11). They probably help to repair damaged fibres, fusing with them and adding new myofibril manufac-

turing capacity to the unit. There is no evidence for the replacement of whole muscle fibres after gross loss of muscle substance, only for the repair of individual muscle fibres.

CARDIAC MUSCLE

This consists of a system of branching and anastomosing fibres each composed of cells joined end-to-end. Instead of being resorbed, as happens in skeletal muscle fibres, the touching plasma membranes remain intact, forming inter-

1. Mesenchyme cells divide...

2. and differentiate into myoblasts...

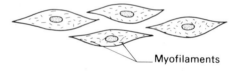

Myofilaments

3. which line up...

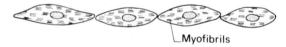

Myofibrils

4. and fuse end to end...

Myofibrils showing sarcomeres

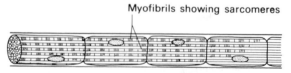

5. to form a multinucleate syncitium, the skeletal muscle fibre

Glycocalyx
Sarcolemma
Satellite cell

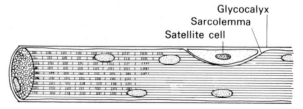

Fig. 6.11. Development of a skeletal muscle fibre.

calated discs (Fig. 6.12). Each cell generally contains a single, central, nucleus. The spaces in the network formed by the anastomosing fibres are filled with loose fibrous connective tissue.

The fibres are striated, and their myofilaments are arranged in the same pattern as in skeletal muscle fibres (p. 328). Groups of myofilaments are surrounded by sarcoplasmic reticulum, but this is sparser than in skeletal muscle and the myofibrils so formed are thus less clearly defined. T-tubules penetrate the cardiac muscle fibres at the level of the Z-bands, rather than at the junctions between the A and I bands as in skeletal muscle.

The most striking feature of cardiac muscle fibres is their intercalated discs. These represent the touching plasma membranes of adjacent cells. The membranes cross the fibres in a series

of steps (Fig. 6.12). Specialized cell junctions, desmosomes (p. 174) and gap junctions or nexuses, ensure firm mechanical linkage and free electrical conductivity respectively.

Cardiac muscle cells contain considerable quantities of glycogen and myoglobin, and numerous mitochondria, while the muscle fibres have a rich blood supply. As this suggests, cardiac muscle demands a large supply of energy and oxygen. It begins to contract in the fourth week of embryonic existence and, on average, contracts and relaxes once a second for the next 70 years. Even in maturity, cardiac muscle fibres can still grow (but not divide) in response to an increased work load; this is called compensatory hypertrophy, and involves the manufacture of more myofilaments as and where required.

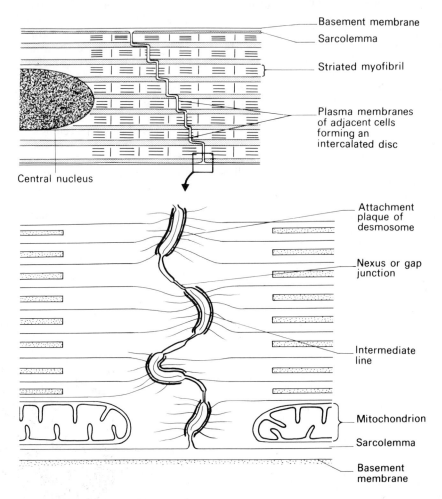

Fig. 6.12. Part of a cardiac muscle fibre showing an intercalated disc.

SMOOTH MUSCLE

Smooth muscle consists of separate, elongated, uninucleate cells, each termed a smooth muscle fibre. They range in length from 15 μm in small blood vessels to up to 500 μm in the wall of the uterus during pregnancy. The average smooth muscle fibre is about 200 μm long and about 7 μm at its widest part. The single nucleus is generally found to one side of the widest part of the cell; in relaxed muscle it has a smooth, oval outline, but in contracted fibres it often appears pleated (Fig. 6.1c). The cytoplasm contains closely packed, fine, myofilaments usually lying parallel to the long axis of the cell. Each is about 5–8 nm in diameter, and resembles the thin filaments of striated muscle. Curiously, although biochemical investigations have clearly demonstrated the presence of roughly equal quantities of actin and myosin, thick filaments are rarely found in electron micrographs of smooth muscle. As with microtubules, special conditions of fixation are necessary if they are to be preserved.

Each muscle fibre is surrounded by a glycocalyx which in turn is ensheathed by a loose endomysium of fibrous connective tissue. Individual fibres are grouped into small bundles or fasciculi by the connective tissue of the perimysium. As with striated muscle, these connective tissue infiltrations provide support for blood vessels, lymphatics and nerves, as well as for the individual muscle cells.

Development of smooth muscle

As with the other types of muscle, mesenchyme cells differentiate into myoblasts, which become elongated and synthesize myofilaments. The myoblasts remain separate, and the myofilaments never line up in a regular fashion to produce striations. Unlike most differentiated cells, mature smooth muscle fibres are able to divide.

ARRANGEMENT OF MUSCLES

Skeletal muscle

FORM OF MUSCLES

All skeletal muscles have a connective tissue framework by means of which they are attached to the connective tissue of other structures of the body, for example, the periosteum of bones or the fascia of the skin in the case of the facial muscles. Sometimes the muscle is not very obviously attached by connective tissue and the term muscular attachment is used. This however is misleading although this type of attachment is associated with a smooth area on a bone. More frequently a muscle begins and/or ends as a distinct structure called a tendon which consists of closely packed parallel bundles of collagen fibres and is usually round or oval in cross-section. Tendinous attachments are indicated by a rough area on a bone.

Tendons or tendinous areas of muscles are not necessarily found at their ends. A part of a muscle which is liable to be subjected to pressure is usually replaced by tendon and it is said that a muscle which consists of fused segments, for example the rectus abdominis muscle, has horizontal tendinous intersections along its length. Tendon is found where a muscle changes its direction, either by passing round a bony projection which acts like a pulley, for example, the superior oblique muscle in the orbit, or through a sling of fibrous tissue.

A muscle may end in an aponeurosis, a term which is used to describe a flat sheet of dense connective tissue, similar in structure to a tendon (tendons and peripheral nerves

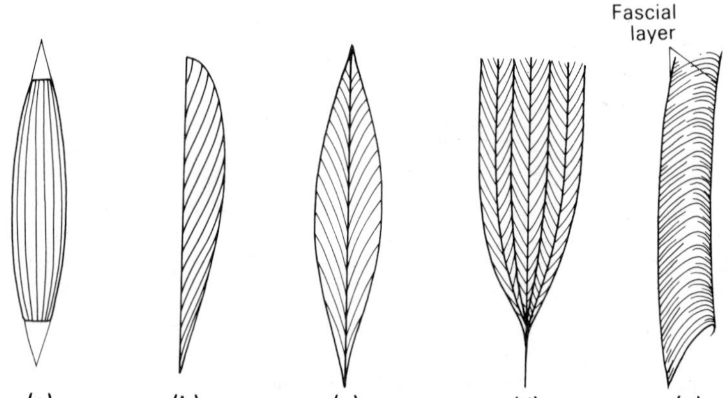

Fig. 6.13. The arrangement of the fibres in different types of muscle. (a) Strap, (b) unipennate, (c) bipennate, (d) multipennate, (e) fibres passing between two layers of fascia.

(a)   (b)   (c)   (d)   (e)

Fascial layer

were confused by early anatomists: hence the odd terminology.) Aponeuroses are best seen in the anterior abdominal wall in which the large flat muscles end in aponeurotic sheets on either side of the midline.

The arrangement of the fibres in a striated muscle varies. If the bundles of muscle fibres run parallel to one another, a strap muscle results (Fig. 6.13a). It is thought that single muscle fibres run the whole length of this type of muscle which is associated with maximum range of movement.

More frequently the muscle fibres are in bundles which run obliquely. This arrangement is reminiscent of a feather and these muscles are called pennate. If all muscle fibres run obliquely in one direction into a longitudinally running tendon it is called unipennate (Fig. 6.13b). If they converge on to the tendon from both sides the term bipennate (Fig. 6.13c) is used and if there are numerous bundles of bipennate fibres the muscle is called multipennate (Fig. 6.13d).

Since the force exerted by a muscle is directly proportional to the number of muscle fibres in it, pennate muscles tend to produce considerable power but have a limited range of movement because the individual fibres are short as compared with the fibres in a strap muscle of the same length.

The fibres in a muscle can also be arranged in a fan-shaped manner, for example, the temporalis muscle on the side of the skull. Its posterior horizontal fibres pull the lower jaw backwards and its anterior vertical fibres pull it upwards. When both sets of fibres act together they produce an oblique force. The term raphe, which means a seam, is used to describe an arrangement of muscle fibres which is best described in terms of a dictionary definition–'The seamlike union of the two lateral halves of a part or organ' (Webster's International Dictionary). This is seen in the floor of the mouth where the mylohyoid muscle on each side meets in a midline raphe.

The concept of the group action of muscles was introduced by C. E. Beevor (1854–1908). Prime movers are the muscles which produce the movement (there may be only one prime mover). Antagonists are the muscles which must lengthen in order to permit the movement produced by the prime movers (again there may be only one antagonist). It was thought that the antagonists actively relaxed; that is, they controlled the action of the prime movers by contracting and then lengthening as required. There is considerable evidence that in slow deliberate movements the antagonists lengthen passively. They may momentarily contract at the beginning of a movement and they certainly contract at the end of a rapid movement especially if the rapidly moving part has to end in a final accurate position. The antagonists then prevent overshooting.

Since a prime mover may produce an additional, unwanted movement, the name synergist has been given to a muscle which contracts to prevent this unwanted movement. The biceps brachii muscle of the upper arm both flexes and supinates the forearm. If this muscle is used to supinate the forearm the triceps brachii muscle (the extensor of the forearm) contracts in order to prevent the unwanted flexion. The term fixators is used to describe muscles which prevent movement at joints which are not acted on by the prime movers. In certain situations skilled accurate movements of the fingers are carried out and the muscles acting at the wrist and elbow joints, both the prime movers and antagonists, contract in order to fix joints in a stable position.

Gravity frequently plays an important role in movements and the movement of a part of the body may be due to gravity controlled by muscles which would normally be regarded as antagonists. For example, in the upright position, bending forwards of the trunk, a movement of flexion, is controlled by the lengthening of the long extensor muscles of the back (sometimes referred to as eccentric contraction as opposed to concentric contraction in which the muscles shorten in order to produce a movement).

RANGE OF MOVEMENT AND FORCE OF CONTRACTION

It has already been stated that strap muscles, because of their parallel fibres, produce the greatest range of movement and that this is influenced by the proportion of tendon to muscle between the attachments of the muscle. Short oblique fibres, because there are usually proportionately more per unit volume, increase the power of the muscle but decrease the range of movement. The range of movement depends on other factors and the muscle itself cannot be considered in isolation. Factors limiting the range of movement include the apposition of one part of the body against another, the shape of joint surfaces and the tension of any tissues which resist the movement. Closing and opening the jaw illustrates all of these factors.

The range of active movement can usually be increased by an external force. This movement is usually referred to as passive. It is easily demons-

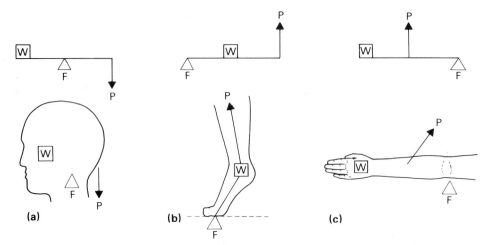

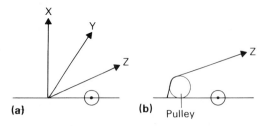

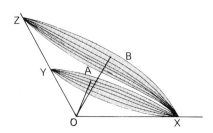

Fig. 6.14. (a) A lever of the first order; P is the pull of the muscles, F is the fulcrum (the atlanto–occipital joint), W is the weight of the head. (b) A lever of the second order; P is the pull of the calf muscles, F is the fulcrum (the metatarso- phalangeal joints), W is the weight of the body. (c) A lever of the third order; P is the pull of the flexor muscles of the forearm, F is the fulcrum (the elbow joint), W is the weight of the forearm and hand.

trated in the outstretched fingers which can be bent further backwards at the knuckles by pressure on the fingers. It may be added that the whole range of active movement can be carried out passively by an external force and this is often done during a clinical examination.

In addition to the arrangement of the fibres themselves within the muscle, the force exerted by a muscle is influenced by mechanical laws. All three types of lever are seen in the body. A lever of the first order is seen in the arrangement of the head on the vertebral column (Fig. 6.14a). A lever of the second order is seen operating when standing on one's toes (Fig. 6.14b), and a lever of the third order when holding a weight in one's hand (Fig. 6.14c).

Many muscles, because they do not pull at right angles to the part to be moved, are at a mechanical disadvantage (Fig. 6.15a).

The oblique pull, however, may be converted into a more vertical pull by means of a pulley (Fig. 6.15b). Another factor, influencing the efficiency of a muscle in terms of the force it exerts, is the distance of its attachment from the axis of movement. In Fig. 6.16 the muscle XZ will produce a greater moment at O than XY because the vertical to XZ (OB) is longer than the vertical to XY (OA).

Fig. 6.16. The muscle XZ produces a greater moment at O than the muscle XY because BO, the vertical to XZ, is greater than OA, the vertical to XY.

Fig. 6.15. (a) X exerts a greater vertical pull than Y which exerts a greater vertical pull than Z. (b) The oblique pull of Z is converted into a vertical pull by a pulley.

Smooth muscle

Smooth muscle is usually arranged in sheets in the walls of hollow organs and consists of small bundles of fibres with their long axis parallel to one another.

Smooth muscle is often described as longitudinal and circular, for example in the alimentary tract, but it has been shown that both are really helical, the former being an open spiral and the latter a tight spiral.

A distinct thickening of circular muscle is called a sphincter although it should be pointed out that skeletal muscle can also form sphincters, for example, round the opening of the mouth. Sphincters when they contract produce a narrowing or closure of an opening or the lumen of a tube.

THE CHARACTERISTICS OF CONTRACTION

The muscles of the body contribute some 40–50% of the total body weight. Their main function is the generation of force, although the skeletal muscles also serve as a major source of heat production for thermoregulation in homeotherms. The structure of the three main types of muscle (skeletal, smooth and cardiac) is described on p 325).

In smooth muscle the cells are in electrical contact with each other which means that waves of electrical excitation can pass from cell to cell, unlike the situation in skeletal muscle where any muscle fibre is in electrical isolation and will only contract when signalled to do so by the motor nerves which end on it. Smooth muscle has a different ionic basis of regulation of contraction to that of striated muscle. Cardiac muscle can be viewed as a transitional form between striated and smooth muscle. It has a similar appearance to skeletal muscle but the cells are in electrical contact.

Skeletal muscle contraction

Muscle develops a force either isotonically, when the muscle shortens under constant load, or isometrically, when it produces force without changing in length. Each of these ways of assessing the force of muscular contraction is used in the classical experiments on the isolated frog gastrocnemius muscle.

A muscle pulling a lever which writes on a drum or is attached to a pen recorder is contracting isotonically; the muscle is shortening under the constant weight of the lever. On the other hand when a 'strain-gauge' type of transducer (which generates an electrical signal or changes in electrical resistance when deformed) is used, the muscle produces force at a constant length or isometrically (i.e. without overall shortening). Analogies in everyday activities are lifting a weight (isotonic) or pushing against an immovable object (isometric). Although overall muscle length does not shorten in an isometric contraction, there is, nevertheless, internal shortening of the contractile elements. The mechanism of contraction is exactly the same in isometric and isotonic contractions.

TIME COURSE OF CONTRACTION

A single electrical stimulus applied directly through electrodes placed upon an isolated skeletal muscle depolarizes a number of indi-

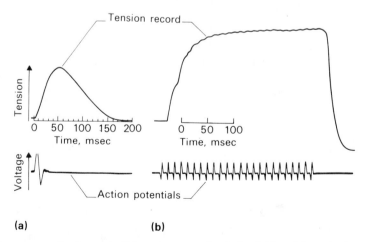

(a)　　　　　　　　**(b)**

Fig. 6.17. The time course of action potentials and tension in mammalian muscles. (a) Action potential (below) and isometric tension (above) recorded in tibialis muscle of a cat. (b) Recordings of electrical and mechanical activities of the cat extensor digitorum longus, showing development of tetanus. (After Creed *et al* (1932), *Reflex activity of the spinal cord*, Clarendon Press, Oxford.)

vidual fibres. Depending on the strength of the current used the contraction increases from the threshold of the few fibres nearest the electrodes to a maximum at large currents which depolarize fibres furthest from the electrodes.

Following depolarization to threshold, an action potential is propagated over the surface of the muscle fibre (Fig. 6.17a). After a delay of a few milliseconds contraction commences and there is a rapid rise in tension caused by the shortening of the contractile elements, followed by a somewhat slower relaxation phase. This is termed a twitch. A similar result is obtained if the nerve to the muscle is stimulated maximally to excite all the motor nerves to the muscle—except that the delay or latency is longer on account of the time for conduction of the action potential down the nerve from the stimulating electrodes and for transmission across the neuromuscular junction, in addition to the delay whilst the contractile elements are being activated. If the muscle is stimulated repeatedly, at frequencies of about 70/sec in this instance, a maximum maintained tension is reached. This is called tetanus and the tension generated is greater than that from a single twitch (cf Fig. 6.17a and b). Despite the fact that the contractions of the fibres have summated and fused together at tetanus, the action potentials in the nerve and in the muscle remain as discrete entities (Fig. 6.17b, lower trace). The ratio between the tension developed by a twitch and a tetanus is called the twitch:tetanus ratio and is characteristic for different muscle types.

SUMMATION

Why is the tetanic tension higher than the twitch tension? If a more detailed examination of the relation between tension and rate of stimulation is made (Fig. 6.18) it can be seen how the process of summation develops.

A second stimulus, given shortly after the first, causes a second twitch—but the tension developed is higher than the first because the second response starts off at a higher base line level. In the initial twitch the contractile elements have been switched on and then off again at the peak of the twitch. Before the passive elastic and connective tissue elements in the muscle have had time to relax the contractile elements are activated for the next contraction. Thus the passive elements do not have to be shortened so much before producing tension with the result that a larger overall second twitch is obtained. At progressively higher rates of stimulation, near maximal tension is maintained but still with the individual contractions superimposed (unfused tetanus). At tetanus there is a smooth maintenance of maximum tension for that muscle length.

With a single twitch the contractile process is 'switched on' for a short period during which the tension rises. If there were no components in muscle other than its contactile elements then a twitch would probably develop the same maximum tension that developed in tetanus. However, muscle contains both connective tissue and elastic elements in series and parallel to the contractile elements (Fig. 6.19). These effectively reduce the tension of a single twitch by damping or retarding shortening of the muscle because they absorb energy produced by the contractile process. It is not until these passive components have been fully shortened by the preceding contraction that a maximum tension can be generated. In a mechanical model (Fig. 6.19) the connective tissue can be viewed as a passive elastic component in parallel (PEC) with the active contractile component (CC): the elasticity of the sarcomeres themselves and elements in the tendons can be regarded as being in series (SEC) with the contractile component.

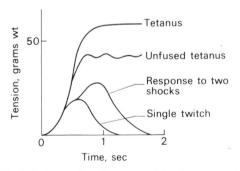

Fig. 6.18. Summation of responses following repeated stimulation of frog muscle at 0°C. After Wilkie D. R. (1968) *Muscle*, Institute of Biology. Edward Arnold, London.

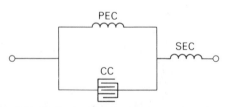

Fig. 6.19. Equivalent mechanical components in muscle, CC =contractile component; PEC = parallel elastic component; SEC =series elastic component. (After Wilkie D. R. (1968) *Muscle*, Institute of Biology, Edward Arnold, London.)

SLIDING FILAMENT THEORY OF CONTRACTION

The structure of the myofilaments in striated muscle was described above (p. 327). The basis of the sliding filament theory of contraction (developed independently in the 1950s by H. E. Huxley and A. F. Huxley) is that tension is generated by the formation of crossbridges between the actin molecules (thin filaments) and myosin molecules (thick filaments), so shortening the sarcomere.

The relationship between thick and thin myofilaments at various sarcomere lengths is illustrated in Figs. 6.5 and 6.20. At maximum extension of the muscles (Fig. 6.5a) there is no overlap between thick and thin filaments. Decreasing sarcomere length to 2.2 μm increases overlap to a position where there is maximum overlap between areas of crossbridges between the actin and myosin molecules.

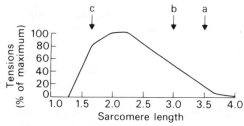

Fig. 6.20. Tension-length curve from part of a single muscle fibre (schematic summary of results). (a) fully extended, (b) at rest, and (c) fully contracted. (After Gordon A. M., Huxley A. F. & Julian F. J. (1966) *Journal of Physiology* **184**, 170.)

Tension rises linearly from zero at no overlap to a maximum tension at maximum overlap. Thus the tension developed is proportional to the number of crossbridges formed as the muscle shortens from its maximal extension.

However, if under experimental conditions the sarcomere is further shortened to less than its normal operating range, it produces no more or even less tension. The reasons are seen diagrammatically in Fig. 6.5.

TENSION-LENGTH CURVE IN WHOLE MUSCLES

In a whole muscle, the sharp inflections of the tension–length curve of the individual sarcomere become progressively more rounded because of differences in sarcomere length in different parts of the muscle and because of the presence of connective tissue. The tension–length curves obtained for some whole muscles are shown in Fig. 6.21.

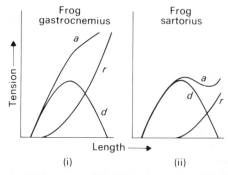

Fig. 6.21. Tension-length curves in different types of muscle. In both cases (r) shows the passive tension developed on stretching a resting muscle. This does not increase linearly with extension. On stimulation, this passive tension is superimposed on the active tension generated by contractile elements to produce the total observed tension (*a*). The actual tension developed (*d*) by the contractile elements (*a–r*) is the same for the two muscles. (After Wilkie D. R (1968) *Muscle*, Institute of Biology, Edward Arnold, London.)

A muscle generates its maximum force at or near its resting length. As it is shortened below this length so tension decreases, as it is lengthened the active tension it can generate again decreases but passive tension increases, resisting overstretching of the muscle. The connective tissue and elastic elements (mainly in the tendons) modify the response of the contractile component by absorbing energy which would otherwise have contributed to the tension produced by the muscle. The amount and distribution of these tissues vary with different muscle types, consequently observed tension–length curves vary.

FORCE AND VELOCITY OF CONTRACTION

We can now examine the relation between the force generated by a muscle and the velocity with which it shortens.

It is a well known observation that a small weight can be lifted rapidly whilst a heavy weight can be lifted only slowly. Measurement of force and speed of shortening can be made on an isolated muscle or single muscle fibre, or *in vivo* on human limb muscles. In every case, the force velocity relation obtained is part of a rectangular hyperbola which shows that maximum velocity occurs when the muscle is unloaded (i.e. no external force is produced) and maximum force is generated when the muscle is isometric and cannot shorten (Fig. 6.22).

Isometric tension is proportional to filament overlap and hence to the number of crossbridges formed. The distance over which a crossbridge can act is only a few nanometres, so during shortening crossbridges must attach, pull and detach in repeated cycles in order that filaments slide past one another. In fact, crossbridges seem to be quite rigid structures and if detachment does not occur instantaneously when the 'pull' is completed, the continued sliding motion carries the crossbridge into a region where it exerts 'push' which resists shortening.

Three important ideas follow from these considerations. First, because maximum velocity is limited by the pushing forces, a reduction in pushing force (for example, by making the crossbridges detach very quickly) will lead to an increase in maximum velocity. Put the other way around as a general statement, the maximum velocity of shortening is limited by the rate at which crossbridges detach. Second, the maximum velocity of shortening is independent of the number of crossbridges and hence, independent of filament overlap. Finally, the shape of the force–velocity relation (Fig. 6.22) is explained. As the filaments slide past each other rapidly only a few crossbridges can form. As more crossbridges are formed the tension is greater for any given speed of shortening.

MOLECULAR MECHANISM OF CONTRACTION

The mechanism by which the actin molecules of the thin filaments and the myosin molecules of the thick filaments interact to generate force involves both the formation of crossbridges between the filaments and the hydrolysis of ATP to provide the energy for contraction.

Calcium ions play an important role in this process. In isolated protein preparations of actin and myosin both calcium and ATP are necessary for the interaction of the two proteins—seen as an aggregation and a precipitation under these conditions with the simultaneous hydrolysis of ATP to ADP and inorganic phosphate. Under physiological conditions in resting muscle the free intracellular calcium is at a very low level. An action potential passing across the sarcolemma to the transverse tubules releases stores of calcium from the sarcoplasmic reticulum near the Z line. The free calcium reacts with troponin which in conjunction with tropomyosin is associated with the thin filaments (Fig. 6.6). Calcium, binding to the troponin

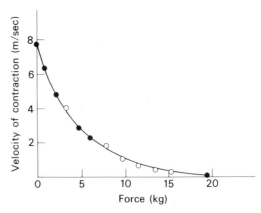

Fig. 6.22. Velocity of contraction of an arm muscle as a function of the force exerted. The abscissa values correspond to the loading of the muscle during isotonic contraction; the ordinate values give the maximum velocity of shortening of the muscle. (After Wilkie D. R. (1949) *J. Physiol.* **110**, 249.)

alters the configuration of tropomyosin in such a way that it allows the actin and myosin molecules to form crossbridges, to split ATP and to produce force. In the absence of calcium (resting muscle) troponin inhibits interaction between actin and myosin: calcium released on stimulation removes this inhibition.

ATP not only provides the energy for muscular contraction, but is necessary to keep a relaxed muscle in its physiological conformation; that is, ATP exerts a 'plasticizer' effect in keeping muscle flexible. When ATP concentration falls to a low level, as in a dying muscle for example, the muscle becomes rigid (rigor mortis).

Molecules of ATP are split to ADP and inorganic phosphate (Pi) during the formation of crossbridges between actin and myosin. Part of the myosin molecule is an ATP-ase.

$$ATP \xrightarrow{Ca^{2+}} ADP + Pi$$

However, ATP is resynthesized rapidly by exchange with a high energy phosphate donor, creatine phosphate, in a reaction catalyzed by creatine phosphotransferase.

$$ADP + creatine \sim P \rightleftharpoons ATP + creatine$$

This reaction keeps the ATP level constant during and after contraction, for example at about 3 μmol/g in an intact frog muscle. The ATP alone would only be sufficient for some 8 contractions, but the energy stored by creatine phosphate (at about 20 μmol/g) can extend this to some

80–100 contractions. However, frog muscles *in vitro* will contract for many more twitches than this. Creatine phosphate (and thence ATP) must be regenerated by energy from elsewhere. Two biochemical processes are used, one operating aerobically and the other anaerobically. First, energy is normally provided from the breakdown of glucose or glycogen to CO_2 and water through the Krebs cycle and subsequent oxidative phosphorylation. An excised frog muscle contains enough glycogen to provide energy for some 10 000–20 000 contractions under aerobic conditions. Second, the glycogen can be broken down to lactic acid under anaerobic conditions. In this case the energy provided would only be sufficient for about 600 contractions.

During sustained heavy exercise the body goes into oxygen debt with the result that energy for muscle contraction begins to be provided by the anaerobic pathway leading to a build-up of lactic acid in the muscles.

HEAT PRODUCTION OF MUSCLE

Not all the energy released by splitting ATP is turned into mechanical work, much being lost as heat. The efficiency of contraction is defined as:

$$\frac{\text{work obtained}}{\text{free energy available}}$$

Efficiency is only about 20–25% for the whole of the contraction cycle, that is contraction plus recovery (discussed above). Part of the energy absorbed in overcoming friction and viscous drag is given out as heat which, in homeotherms, is important in thermoregulation.

EXCITATION–CONTRACTION COUPLING

Skeletal muscle remains quiescent *in vivo* unless stimulated to contract by an action potential passing from the motor nerve supplying the muscle. Thus there is no active basal 'tone' unlike the situation for smooth muscle, discussed below.

Acetylcholine released at the neuromuscular junction depolarizes the muscle membrane and initiates an action potential which passes across the surface of the muscle fibre. The action potential now penetrates the interior of the fibre via the transverse tubules (p. 329) and releases calcium from stores in the cisternae of the sarcoplasmic reticulum, which diffuses into the region of the contractile proteins. Crossbridges form as previously discussed, causing the filaments to slide together and the muscle to produce tension.

After the passage of the action potential the contractile elements relax because calcium is pumped from the area of the myofilaments back into the sarcoplasmic reticulum by a calcium pump located in the membranes of the sarcoplasmic reticulum. The hydrolysis of ATP provides energy for the pump. In this way calcium ions are moved against a concentration gradient from very low calcium in the region of the myofilaments to a high concentration in the sarcoplasmic reticulum.

CONTROL OF MUSCULAR CONTRACTION

A single action potential in a motor nerve fibre to a muscle causes a single twitch. The tension developed by this twitch depends on the number of muscle fibres in the motor unit (p. 326). All the fibres in the unit contract. Since increasing the strength of the stimulus does not increase the force of contraction the motor unit is said to behave in an 'all or none' manner. In muscles where a fine gradation of movement is required, in those of the eye for example, there are on average some 7 fibres innervated by each motor nerve axon, though the ratio may even drop to 1:1. One action potential therefore produces only a very fine movement in these muscles, compared to a coarse one in the leg muscles in which the muscle:nerve ratio can be 1700:1.

If the sciatic nerve to a frog gastrocnemius muscle is stimulated electrically, then increasing the strength of single stimuli from a threshold value causes a greater twitch tension until a maximum is reached. This does not mean that the all-or-none relationship does not hold—merely that motor nerves of higher threshold are being recruited and more motor units are contributing to tension as the stimulating current is increased. Tension in a muscle may, therefore, be increased by increasing the number of motor units firing. Tension can also be increased by raising the rate at which any individual motor unit fires. As discussed earlier, the mechanical responses to two or more stimuli in rapid succession can summate so as to increase the total tension developed. Mammalian muscles develop their maximum or tetanic tension at frequencies greater than about 40 impulses/sec. The total force applied in any one direction to a bone may also be increased by bringing into play motor units in different muscles which act in the same direction, e.g. masseter and medial pterygoid.

HISTOLOGICAL DISTINCTION BETWEEN SLOW AND FAST MUSCLE FIBRES

As their names suggest, these are muscle fibres which contract at different speeds. The slow or Type I fibres produce muscle twitches lasting for about 75 msec and typify the fibres of postural muscles, where a slow, repetitive contraction is required. They are narrower than fast fibres, contain many mitochondria and oxidative enzymes, but are poor in phosphorylases. The myofibrils are ill-defined, though the Z-bands can usually be seen clearly.

Fast or Type II fibres have a twitch duration of only about 25 msec and typify muscles which have to generate forces rapidly and produce movement.

These muscle types were formerly classified as red (slow) and white (fast) respectively because of the amounts of myoglobin in them, and possibly because the red muscles receive a greater blood flow than the white muscles even at rest. These distinctions cannot be rigidly applied particularly as it has been shown that the character of muscles is not entirely inherent, but is influenced by the trophic effect of the motor nerves which supply them.

ELECTROMYOGRAPHY

In vivo, the activity of motor units can be recorded from electrodes placed on the skin overlying a muscle or from electrodes inserted directly into the extracellular space surrounding the muscle fibres (via modified hypodermic needles for example). The recording is called an electromyogram (EMG). A typical trace is shown in Fig. 6.23. The EMG is used clinically for diagnosing muscular diseases. It can indicate damage or disease in the motor nervous system, malfunction of neuromuscular transmission or degenerative changes in the muscle fibres themselves. It has also been used extensively in physiological research, for example in determining the sequences in which different muscles act during mastication or swallowing (p. 580).

NON-STRIATED OR SMOOTH MUSCLE

Unlike skeletal muscle, smooth muscle has inherent rhythmical activity (p. 617). Action potentials can pass from cell to cell by low resistance pathways provided by gap junctions (nexuses) between cells. Intracellular recordings of the membrane potential from smooth muscle

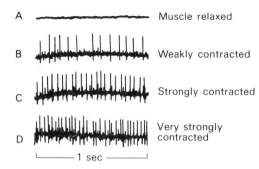

Fig. 6.23. Electromyogram of an eyelid muscle. When it is fully relaxed no electrical (or mechanical) activity can be recorded from the muscle. As the strength of contraction rises, so the frequency at which the motor unit is firing increases–to a maximum of about 30/sec in D. In addition to the motor unit being monitored, potentials from neighbouring motor units can also be seen intruding on the record as they are recruited with stronger contractions. They appear smaller on the record because they are further away from the recording electrodes–action potentials in all muscle fibres are exactly the same size. (After Bell, Davidson & Scarborough (1968) *Textbook of Physiology and Biochemistry*, Livingston, Edinburgh.)

(Fig. 6.24) contrast markedly with those from skeletal muscle (Fig. 6.17). The potential is generally less negative, some -50 mV with respect to the outside of the cell (compared to -70 to -80 mV in skeletal muscle) and is unstable. It gradually and spontaneously rises with time, reaches threshold (about -30 mV) and produces an action potential followed by a contraction, but not on a one twitch per pulse basis–rather a form of slow summation occurs (Figs. 6.24 & 6.25).

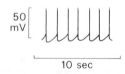

Fig. 6.24. Transmembrane potentials in isolated guinea pig's taenia coli. (After Bülbring, Burnstock & Holman (1958) *Journal of Physiology* **142**, 420.)

The instability of the membrane is thought to arise from its basic leakiness to sodium ions, which continuously diffuse into the cell from the extracellular fluid and in consequence depolarize the membrane. Once the threshold is reached, an action potential is propagated. The increase in potassium permeability during the latter phase of the action potential restores the membrane potential to a value somewhat less than that of the potassium equilibrium potential (p. 291), from which point sodium leaking into the cells again causes a decline in the membrane potential towards threshold. This pattern gives the characteristic spontaneous electrical activity of smooth muscles.

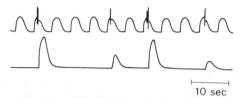

10 sec

Fig. 6.25. Electrical and mechanical activity in intestinal smooth muscle. Monophasic electrical activity (top) and mechanical activity (bottom) recorded from an isolated segment of cat jejunum with a pressure electrode attached to a force transducer. (After Bortoff A. (1976) *Physiological Review*, **56**, 418.)

Contraction, however, initiated by the action potential, is much slower than in striated muscle and is in the region of seconds or tens of seconds compared to less than 100 msec for a twitch in skeletal muscle. This means that smooth muscle has not fully relaxed before the next action potential and subsequent contraction. Thus smooth muscle remains in a permanent state of 'tone' whose tension depends on the frequency of the spontaneous action potentials.

Stretching smooth muscle causes depolarization and subsequent contraction. In most smooth muscles the overall activity seems to be guided by pacemaker regions, generating impulses which spread radially for a short dis-tance, producing waves of contraction in the tissue (Fig. 6.25). Unlike heart muscle these pacemaker regions are not definable histologically and they may move from site to site in the muscle. Conduction is not as complete as in the heart—the waves of depolarization may be propagated or blocked according to local conditions, such as the state of stretch or the release of acetylcholine or noradrenaline. As an example of smooth muscle activity, intestinal motility is described on p. 617. The physiology of cardiac muscle is considered on p. 703.

The molecular mechanism of contraction is thought to be essentially similar in skeletal and smooth muscle. Both contain actin and myosin but in smooth muscle the myofilaments are not as regularly packed as in striated muscle. Calcium is also involved in the contractile process, but it is not stored intracellularly in the same way as in skeletal muscle and diffusion of calcium into cells from the extracellular fluid is probably sufficient to activate the contractile mechanism. Such a diffusion mechanism for calcium could operate satisfactorily because smooth muscle cells have a smaller diameter than skeletal muscle fibres and a slower contractile process.

FURTHER READING

EBASHI S. (1974) Regulatory mechanism of muscle contraction with special reference to the calcium–troponin–tropomyosm system. In: P. N. Campbell & F. Dickens (eds.) *Essays in Biochemistry*, **10**, Academic Press, London.

SIMMONS R. M. & JEWELL B. R. (1964) Mechanics and models of muscular contraction, 87. In: R. J. Linden (ed.) *Recent advances in physiology*, Churchill-Livingstone, Edinburgh.

WILKIE D. R. (1976) *Muscle*, 2nd edn., Institute of Biology Series 11, Edward Arnold, London.

CHAPTER 7

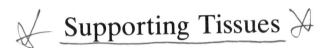

Supporting Tissues

CHEMISTRY OF CONNECTIVE TISSUES

The connective tissues comprise the calcified tissues (bone, cartilage, dentine, cementum) and the fibrous tissues (tendon, ligaments, dermis, elastic tissues, aortic walls, basement membrane, etc.).

Virtually all are constructed on the same principle. The tissues-forming cells concerned—fibroblasts, osteoblasts, chondroblasts, odontoblasts and cementoblasts each produce fibrous proteins (collagen, elastin, reticulin) which are embedded in an interfibrillar ground substance (GS), the latter comprised of large heteropolysaccharide molecules (the glycosaminoglycans, GAGs) linked with protein components, the two together constituting the proteoglycans (PGs).

The ground substance also includes small quantities of glycoproteins, each characteristic of the tissue concerned. The ground substance varies in consistency from a jelly-like fluid to the rigid structure characteristic of cartilage.

Although the ground substance plays an important role in connective tissue structure, it is the fibrous proteins which constitute the greater component and provide the molecular basis for most of the mechanical properties which the connective tissues are designed and fitted to perform.

The fibrous protein components of connective tissue

COLLAGEN

The most dominant fibrous protein in connective tissue is collagen, described on p. 66 and p. 357. It would be advisable to study these accounts before proceeding further.

In summary the connective tissue-forming cells manufacture the triple helical collagen macromolecules (tropocollagen), which aggregate into 3-dimensional, quarter-stagger arrays to form the primary collagen microfibrils. These further organize into the characteristic tissue collagen fibres (Fig. 3.29) which impart to the tissues its high mechanical strength.

The enzymic dismantling of perfectly formed collagen structures by clostridial exotoxin collagenases is a feature of gas gangrene—a potentially lethal disease which takes its heaviest toll in war-time conditions when antibiotic and chemotherapy is not readily available, as in World War I. The symptoms characteristic of chronic rheumatoid arthritis may be due to the excessive levels of collagenase claimed to be associated with the synovial fluid of sufferers from this condition. Likewise periodontal disease and caries of the dentine ultimately involve an irreversible enzymic dissolution of the collagen in gingival tissue and dentine respectively.

ELASTIN

Elastin is found to some extent in most of the soft connective tissues, though with the exception of the ligamentum nuchae connecting vertebrae, never in vastly greater amounts than collagen. As the name implies it brings the quality of elasticity to a tissue as well as high mechanical strength. It is more in abundance in tissues where extensibility and flexibility are required —as in larger arteries, skin, lungs and neck ligaments. These contrast with the pliant but non-extensible framework structures characteristic of the collagen fibres in the organic matrices of dentine, ligaments, tendons etc.

Elastin differs markedly from collagen in composition, the most notable difference being the relatively low content of the polar side-chains from basic and acidic amino acids. It resembles collagen in a high glycine (27%) and proline (13.5%) level, but there is only about 1% hydroxyproline, and no hydroxylysine. There are high levels of non-polar amino acid side-chains—valine and alanine together constitute more than a third of the total residues. It is a highly crosslinked protein involving unique structures (desmosines and isodesmosines) formed from modified side-chains of lysine residues by mechanisms similar to crosslink formation in collagen (p. 69).

Elastin fibres have an amorphous core of polymerized tropo-elastin surrounded by glycoprotein. Tropo-elastin is a globular protein which tends to form into plates. Fibres only form when plate formation is restrained by the presence of glycoproteins.

RETICULIN

Less is known about the third fibrous protein component of connective tissue, reticulin. Its composition is very like collagen and the electron micrographs show that it has a characteristic 64–68 nm repeat structure. However, it is strongly associated with lipid and carbohydrate molecules; indeed it is often shrouded by the latter, which suggests that it has some special properties that distinguish it from the true collagens.

The ground substance components: (GAGs, PGs and GPs)

GLYCOSAMINOGLYCANS (GAGs) (p. 141)

The major group of carbohydrate containing components in the ground substance consist of the glycosaminoglycans (earlier called the mucopolysaccharides), which are heteropolysaccharides, almost uniquely characterized by repeating disaccharide units comprised of a sulphated hexosamine and a uronic acid (or sulphated galactose) residue. GAGs include the two chondroitin sulphates (4- and 6-) dermatan sulphate, hyaluronic acid and heparin. Keratan sulphate is distinguished from the other GAGs by galactose in place of the uronic acid component in its disaccharide repeat unit (Table 3.16).

PROTEOGLYCANS (PG) (p. 143)

An important feature of the connective tissue GAGs is their association with protein molecules to form large polysaccharide–protein complexes known as the proteoglycans (originally called mucoproteins). The exact structure of these aggregated complexes is still debated but Fig. 3.96 shows a currently proposed structure. Thus, in the chondroitin sulphates the GAG units combine with a single protein core to form massive structures whose molecular weights are between 3–6 million. The GAGs are joined to the protein core by covalent links formed between the hydroxyl groups of serine side-chains on the polypeptide with terminal xylose residues on the GAG units. The GAG carbohydrate components form 90% of the PG molecules.

The most important property deriving from the PGs is their ability, in combination with collagen, to hold within their 3-dimensional molecular mesh-work, large quantities of water. This open polyanionic network of negatively charged groups, is able to bind relatively enormous volumes of water within its interstices accounting for the 60–70% water content found in the non-calcified connective tissue structures (Fig. 3.97). This is important, for example, in maintaining the turgidity of skin and other soft collagenous tissue.

The proteoglycan components of connective tissues are the molecular basis for their ability to resist compression whereas the fibrous protein components provide their mechanical strength.

The hyaluronic acid-containing proteoglycans are important constituents of the vitreous humour of the eye and the umbilical cord. They are also responsible for the efficient lubricating property of synovial fluid.

GLYCOPROTEINS (GP)

Glycoproteins superficially resemble proteoglycans in that they consist of polypeptide chains linked covalently along their length with numerous carbohydrate side-chains. The GP molecules are much smaller than the PG complexes, and usually contain 5–10% carbohydrate components. Exceptions are salivary GPs with 50% or more carbohydrate present.

The hexosamine units in the carbohydrate side-chains of glycoproteins form the covalent links to the protein core, usually via serine or asparagine residues. The carbohydrate chains comprise—in varying amounts according to tissue—N-acetyl glucosamine, N-acetylgalactosamine, mannose, galatose, glucose, fucose and sialic acid (n-acetyl neuraminic acid). The latter often terminate the carbohydrate side-chains, endowing them with a strongly negative (anionic) character (Fig. 7.1). These carbohydrate chains may be short, with 2 or 3 residues only, or, as in certain parotid secretion glycoproteins, all 7 may constitute the chain (Fig. 7.1).

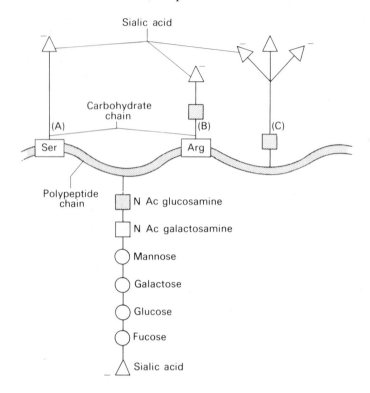

Fig. 7.1. Three different types of carbohydrate side-chain may be present in different glycoproteins: longer chains are found in glycoproteins from parotid saliva (A); short chains, with 2 or 3 residues (B); branched chains in bone sialoproteins (C).

A glycoprotein is therefore a long molecule consisting of a protein core to which is attached a host of oligosaccharide side-chains, each terminated by a group bearing a strong negative charge. This outer surface 'shroud' of negative charges repels neighbouring molecules, accounting for the slippery quality of the 'mucus' fluids in connective tissues, and saliva (Fig. 7.2).

Biochemistry of bone

The major fibrous protein is collagen, constituting 18% of the total tissue weight and 90% by weight of the total organic matter. There are subtle compositional differences distinguishing the α-chains of bone collagen and the soft tissue collagens in skin and tendon, from those in cartilage and other tissues. Some, as yet uncertainly identified, structural features must account for both the calcifiability of the bone matrix and also for its relatively greater insolubility. The latter may be due to crosslinks involving hydroxylysine (p. 69) as this amino acid is

present in greater abundance in bone than tendon collagen.

A recent hypothesis proposed to explain bone's mineralizing potential is based on the observation that the intrafibrillar space between adjacent collagen macromolecules (tropocollagen) is twice as great in bone as in soft tissues. It is postulated that this larger gap between the parallel tropocollagen molecules (0.6 nm compared with 0.3 nm) in hard tissue collagen allows phosphate ions (diameter 0.4 nm) passage within the fibril units, so facilitating intramolecular mineralization. The overall larger 'internal volume' of the fibrils could accommodate more than 50% of the inorganic components in bone (see also p. 392).

The glycosaminoglycan components in bone comprise some 1% of the total tissue, half of it chondroitin sulphate, the rest mainly keratan sulphate.

Bone matrix also contains 0.4% sialic acid, 60% of which is accounted for in a unique bone sialoprotein. This glycoprotein (Fig. 7.3) has a molecular weight of 23 000 and it constitutes 1% of the bone matrix. Its biological significance is not established, though it is thought that it may play some role in calcification.

The inorganic component of the bone tissue —and indeed of all human calcified tissues— is calcium hydroxypatite, described in the following section.

Inorganic components of hard tissues

CHEMICAL NATURE OF HYDROXYAPATITE (HA)

All the hard tissues of the animal body contain calcium phosphate salts as the predominant components of their inorganic mineral phase. Referred to generally as 'bone salt,' this same mineral phase occurs in enamel, dentine, cementum and cartilage. Chemically, bone salt is decribed as a basic calcium phosphate, i.e.

$$3Ca_3(PO_4)_2 . Ca(OH)_2$$

This represents it as a mixed crystal containing three calcium phosphate units in association with one unit of calcium hydroxide. However bone salt has been shown to belong to a family of crystal lattice structures known as the apatites, and it is more usual, and correct, to refer to it as calcium hydroxyapatite, written as follows:

$$Ca_{10}(PO_4)_6(OH)_2$$

The unit cell of a crystal lattice structure is a conceptual representation (rather than a real entity) of the minimal crystal structure that includes and describes the ionic components in the total lattice structure, and their spatial relationships. Unit cells are described in terms of three axes, a, b & c, in three dimensions of space. In the unit cell for hydroxyapatite (Fig. 7.4a) these axes are 0.944 nm, 0.944 nm and 0.688 nm respectively, with an overall rhomboid shape. Fig. 7.4b shows how six unit cells (4 whole and 4 'half' cells) can form an hexagonal apatite crystal, as found in enamel.

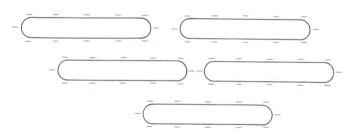

Fig. 7.2. Long negatively-charged glycoproteins.

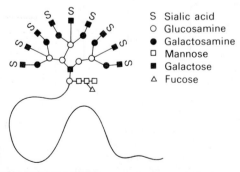

S	Sialic acid
O	Glucosamine
●	Galactosamine
□	Mannose
■	Galactose
△	Fucose

Fig. 7.3. Possible structure for the carbohydrate moiety of bone sialoprotein. (After Herring.)

In a perfect hydroxyapatite crystal the Ca/P ratio, therefore, will be $10/6 = 1.67$, but in the calcified tissues a range of values varying from 1.3 to 2.0 have been reported for the mineral phase. This departure from the theoretical 1.67 ratio is due to a variety of causes. One is a presence of mineral components such as calcium carbonate, which accounts for about 5% of the ash value. Its presence, therefore, will raise the Ca/P ratio. Conversely a removal and replacement of Ca^{2+} ions by other ions such as Na^+, Sr^{2+} and Mg^{2+} leads to lower than theoretical Ca/P ratios. Also the hydroxonium ion, H_3O^+ may

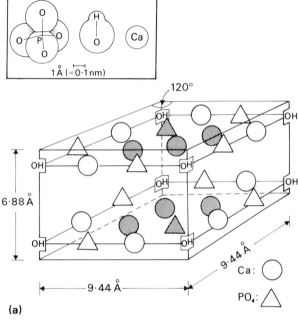

Fig.7.4 (a) The unit cell of hydroxyapatite. The two planes represent the rhomboid shaped upper and lower surfaces. The three Ca²⁺ ions (hatched circles) in the centre of each plane belong only to the unit cell, whilst the eight Ca²⁺ ions on the periphery (open circles) are shared with neighbour units, so that four only belong exclusively to the unit cell. The two phosphate ion groups in the centre (hatched triangles) belong only to the unit cell, with the eight PO_4^{3-} ions at the periphery (open triangles) shared with four adjacent unit cells: thus only four belong exclusively to this unit cell. The eight OH^- ions at the four vertical edges of the cell are shared by a total of eight unit cells, i.e. four unit cells share two OH^- ions at each vertical edge. Each unit cell has four vertical edges therefore there are only two OH^- ions to each unit cell. Fluoride ion exchange occurs at the OH group sites. The ratio of atoms maintained in the continuous crystal lattice structure gives the formula $Ca_{10}(PO_4)_6(OH)_2$. In the diagram the actual ionic sizes (see inset) are not represented: in the unit cell proper they pack close together. (b) Hexagonal lattice: The shaded part shows how six unit cells (4 whole and 4 half cells) can form a hexagonal crystal. (c) Diagrammatic representation of hydroxyapatite hydration shell.

(a)

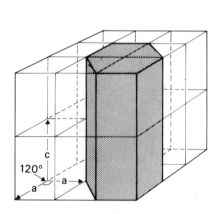

(b)

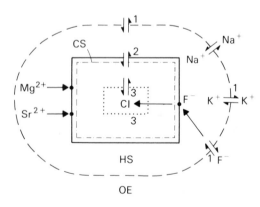

CI: Crystal interior
CS: Crystal surface
HS: Hydration shell
OE: Outer environment

(c)

substitute for Ca^{2+} in the hydroxyapatite lattice.

Bone mineral contains between 1–2% Na^+, 0.5–1% Mg^{2+} and 0.2% of K^+ and Cl^- ions. Trace amounts of Fe, Cu, Pb, Zn, Mn, Mo, Al, Sr, Sb and B are present.

AMORPHOUS CALCIUM PHOSPHATE (ACP)

The major source of the observed variations in bone mineral composition is the presence of a non-crystalline form of calcium phosphate known as amorphous calcium phosphate (ACP). The precise arrangement of the constituent ions is not clear but X-ray diffraction data and compositional studies show that it is not a hydroxyapatite structure. The molar Ca/P ratios reported for ACP are much lower than 1.67 and vary from 1.44 to 1.55, depending on the method of preparation.

Clearly the presence of significant amounts of ACP in a mineralized tissue will contribute to an overall lowering of the Ca/P ratio for the total mineral phase compared with pure hydroxyapatite. Investigations have shown that in fetal animal bones the ACP constitutes 60–70% of the mineral phase, falling to between 35–40% in the adult bone. Even in the latter the ACP therefore accounts for much of the lowered Ca/P ratio observed in most bone salt analyses.

Such observations also infer that maturation of the calcified tissues from fetal to adult form is probably associated with a conversion of ACP to hydroxyapatite form (p. 390). The rate of this conversion is determined, at any particular point in time, by the level of hydroxyapatite already formed rather than by the ACP content. The detailed mechanism of the change of form has not been determined.

SHAPE AND FORM OF HYDROXYAPATITE CRYSTALS

As viewed under the electron microscope hydroxyapatite crystals in bone, dentine and cementum are needle like structures about 10–20 nm length and 5 nm width. For reasons not yet clear hydroxyapatite crystals in enamel are much larger—up to 140 nm long by 80 nm in width. X-ray diffraction data indicate a rectangular plate-like form for hydroxyapatite, and it is possible that this may be the true form, with the plates shattering into needle-like crystals when microtome sections are cut.

Each hydroxyapatite crystal is enshrouded by a fairly substantial hydration shell of surrounding water (Fig. 7.4c).

Many changes in hydroxyapatite composition are caused by ion-exchange reactions, when calcium, phosphate and hydroxyl ions are removed and replaced in the lattice by other ions of similar shape and charge (iso-ionic exchange). Such exchanges are governed by equilibria set up in relation to the hydration shell. Firstly monovalent ions such as Na^+, K^+ and F^- are in dynamic equilibrium (1) between the shell (HS) and the outer environment (OE) but do not become concentrated within the shell. Secondly ions such as Mg^{2+} and Sr^{2+}, and the anion citrate, can concentrate within the HS and so form a loosely bound layer at the crystal surface, CS, by surface ion exchange (2). Thirdly certain ions within the HS, such as the fluoride ion, F^-, can enter into similar ion exhange reaction (2) with the OH on the crystal surface, but can also penetrate further within the lattice (3) to the crystal interior (CI). The important dental and biological consequences of this fluoride ion exchange reaction are discussed elsewhere (p. 400).

The presence of significant levels (1%) of citrate in bone salt still awaits an unequivocal explanation. One view is that it merely reflects a passive ion-exchange with PO_4^{3-} ions in the lattice; another that it accumulates from a specific metabolic process wherein citrate is thought to play a key role as a complexing agent in Ca^{2+} mobilization during bone resorption.

STRUCTURE AND FUNCTION OF CONNECTIVE TISSUES

Histology, development and growth

Three of the basic tissue classes, epithelial (covering and glandular), nervous and muscular, are discrete and clearly defined. The rest of the tissues are the connective tissues. They form a motley group, consisting of:

1 Soft connective tissue
   Loose
      areolar
      adipose
      reticular
   Dense
      regular (collagenous or elastic)
      irregular
2 Skeletal tissue
   Notochord
   Cartilage
      hyaline
      elastic
      fibrous

Connective tissues develop from the mesenchymal component of the embryonic mesoderm, and consist of widely-spaced cells separated by a matrix for the most part secreted by them. Exceptions to this definition are adipose tissue, where the cells are tightly packed together; and blood and lymph, where the material between the cells is not secreted by them.

Connective tissues account for over half the weight of the average man or woman. As their name suggests, they connect the other tissues together, allowing them to act as a highly efficient whole, but they are far from being simply inert linking agents. Healthy connective tissues can adapt by remodelling if the stresses to which they are subjected change: a familiar example of this is the alteration in the structure of the mandible following the removal of a tooth and the subsequent change in the pattern of stresses induced during mastication. If connective tissues become damaged or diseased, and are incapable of making the appropriate responses, the result can be crippling or even fatal.

Connective tissues consist of cells and intercellular materials (matrix) comprising, generally, ground substance and fibres (collagen and elastin).

The matrix forms the bulk (except in the case of adipose tissue) and determines the mechanical properties of each tissue type. In bone the matrix contains calcium salts making it rigid and somewhat brittle.

Running through the ground substance are fibres of collagen and/or elastin. Collagen resists stretching, and increases the tensile strength of the tissues, while elastin can stretch and recoil, allowing the tissues containing it to return to their original shape after deformation. The arrangement of collagen fibres in a tissue can also confer a certain resilience upon it. The elasticity of normal young skin is due mainly to the arrangement of its collagen fibres in a three dimensional lattice. If the lattice is pulled it lengthens so that the fibres become more parallel, although the fibres themselves have little extensibility. Once the force is removed the lattice returns to its normal shape. It is unfortunate that when skin is damaged the scar tissue which repairs the injury contains randomly arranged collagen rather than a lattice, often making it cripplingly inextensible. The proportions of collagen and elastin vary from one connective tissue to another. Tendons, which transmit the pull of a muscle to a bone, and which therefore must not stretch, consist mainly of parallel bundles of collagen, whereas the ligamenta flava, which connect the laminae of adjacent vertebrae and must be able to stretch gradually and recoil as the vertebral column is flexed and extended, consist mainly of elastic fibres.

Apart from structural considerations, the other properties of connective tissues depend mainly on the types of cells they contain. The insulation conferred by adipose tissue, for example, depends on fat storage in specialized cells, while the ability of most connective tissues to replace damaged regions by scar tissue is due to the activity of the fibroblasts they contain.

SOFT CONNECTIVE TISSUE

This consists of several cell types surrounded by a variety of proteinaceous fibres embedded in extensive ground substance containing sufficient proteoglycans to give it the consistency of a soft jelly. It is described as loose if the fibres form a loose network and dense if they are tightly packed.

Loose areolar (Fig. 7.5)
This is the commonest and least specialized of the ordinary connective tissues and can be considered as the prototype. It has been said that when all the other tissues of an embryo have differentiated, whatever remains of the mesenchyme becomes areolar tissue. Its distribution certainly suggests this, for it fills up the spaces between the more specialized tissues. It is found, for example, surrounding and separating individual muscle fibres, around nerves and blood vessels, beneath the epithelia of the skin (the papillary layer of the dermis) forming the nonfatty regions of superficial fascia, supporting and binding together the lobules and lobes of compound glands such as the parotid and pancreas, and attaching the parietal peritoneum to the body wall. Wherever there is a crevice, a loose connective tissue fills it, and more often than not that tissue is of the areolar type.

Areolar tissue is delicate, slippery material, which can stretch slightly but is weak and easily torn. Its ground substance contains many potential spaces in which tissue fluid can lodge: when filled, these areolae (small spaces) are often con-

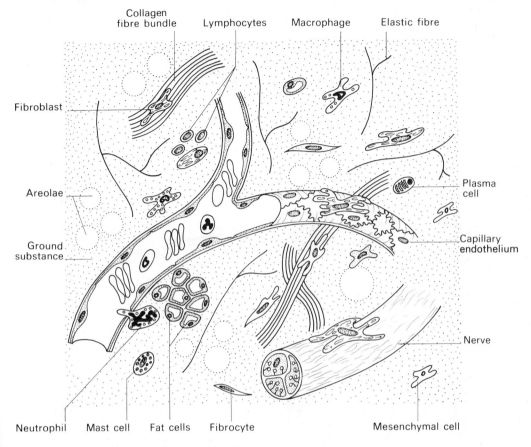

Collagen fibre bundle · **Lymphocytes** · **Macrophage** · **Elastic fibre**

Fibroblast · Areolae · Ground substance

Plasma cell · Capillary endothelium · Nerve

Neutrophil · Mast cell · Fat cells · Fibrocyte · Mesenchymal cell

Fig. 7.5. Diagram of loose areolar connective tissue.

spicuous and their presence led to areolar tissue being so named.

Areolar tissue contains two distinct populations of cells: sessile and wandering. The sessile group consists of fibroblasts, mesenchymal cells, fat cells and fixed macrophages or histiocytes, collectively concerned with the formation, turnover and maintenance of the tissue. The wandering group consists of mast cells, plasma cells and leucocytes, and is mainly concerned with the response of the tissue to infection. The proportion of each cell type depends on the position and activity of the tissue.

Fibroblasts. These are the cells which, in areolar and many other connective tissues, manufacture the organic components of the extracellular matrix.

The term 'fibroblast' was originally used to describe a cell which manufactured connective tissue fibres, i.e. a fibre generating cell (blast

=germ). It is only in recent years that it has become recognized that these cells also have other functions. Each function alters the cell morphology so much so that they can be classified into three different types; actively synthesizing young fibroblasts, less active mature fibroblasts (sometimes called fibrocytes), and contractile myofibroblasts. (Fig. 7.6).

Young fibroblasts: These are cells which, although sessile, are potentially motile, and able to secrete components of the ground substance (p. 356), and the precusors of collagen (p. 357) and elastin (p. 359). If lying on collagen or elastin fibres they are generally fusiform, while if on the ground substance they tend to be stellate. The ultrastructure of the fibroblast resembles that of any other cell actively engaged in the synthesis and secretion of proteins.

If the cell is particularly active in protein synthesis it may contain so much rough endoplasmic reticulum that its cytoplasm is basophilic,

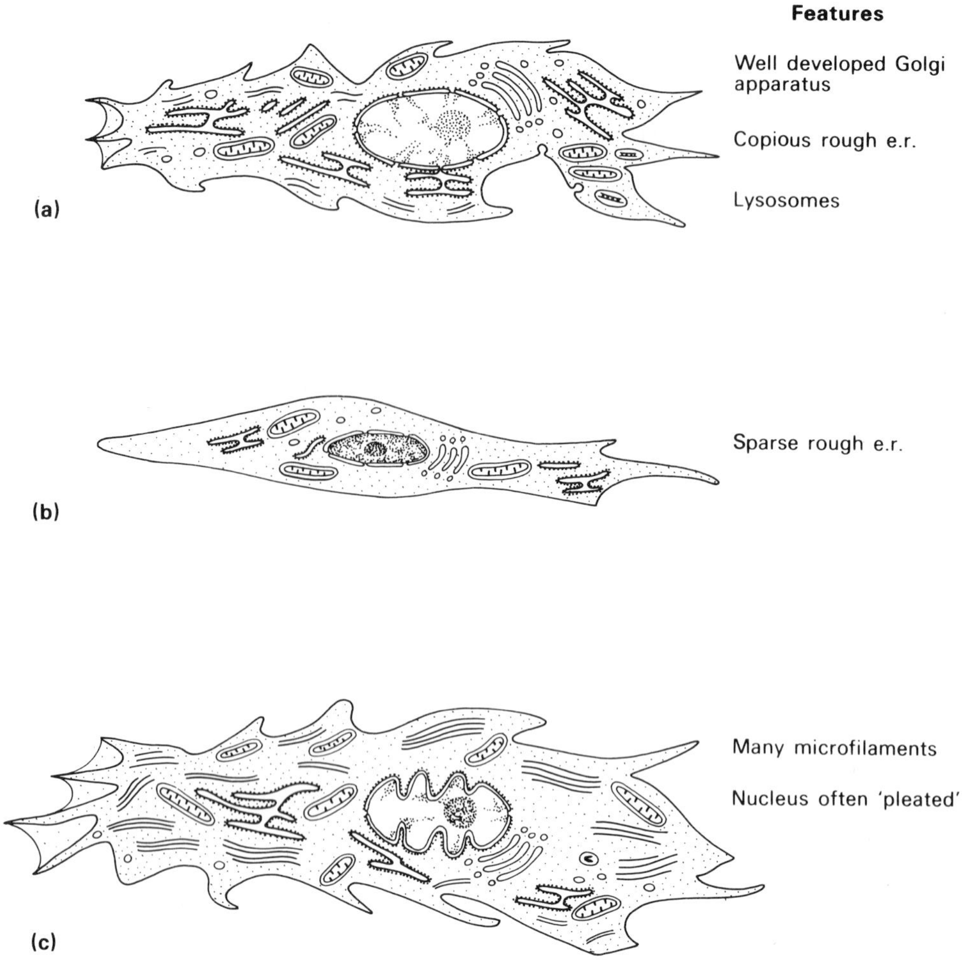

Features

Well developed Golgi
apparatus

Copious rough e.r.

Lysosomes

(a)

Sparse rough e.r.

(b)

Many microfilaments

Nucleus often 'pleated'

(c)

Fig. 7.6. (a) A young fibroblast, (b) mature fibroblast
(fibrocyte) and (c) a myofibroblast.

but more usually it remains slightly acidophilic
so that in sections stained with haematoxylin and
eosin it is often quite difficult to distinguish from
the surrounding matrix which stains in a similar
manner. As well as synthesizing collagen, fibroblasts can also phagocytose and degrade it with
their lysosomal enzymes. Recent studies have
shown that the fibroblast is the cell responsible
for both these processes in the periodontal
ligament, a connective tissue with a high rate of
remodelling.

The actual uptake of material involves the
activity of the enzyme alkaline phosphatase. The
next step is the fusion of acid phosphatase-
containing lysosomes with the collagen-
containing phagosomes to give secondary lyso-

somes (or phagolysosomes) in which the collagen
is digested. The released amino acids may be used
by the same cell to form new collagen.

Mature fibroblasts (fibrocytes): As fibroblasts
mature their ability to synthesize exportable
protein decreases; they lose much of their rough
endoplasmic reticulum, and their cytoplasm
becomes increasingly acidophilic. They are smaller than their younger, more active, relatives,
and have effectively gone into a retirement from
which they can be recalled if there is a need for
the synthesis of more matrix materials.

Myofibroblasts: These are a contractile type
of fibroblast, thought to develop from young
fibroblasts, but which become specialized for
contraction and resemble smooth muscle cells

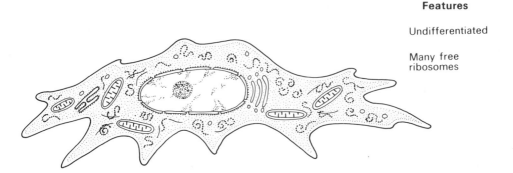

Fig. 7.7. A mesenchymal cell.

morphologically, chemically, antigenically and functionally. They contain bundles of micro-filaments with actomyosin-like properties and are linked to neighbouring myofibroblasts by desmosomes and 'gap' junctions. They are commonly found in connective tissue after injury, when their contraction is thought to help pull the edges of the wound together.

It is often stated that fibroblasts are differenti-ated cells which do not develop into other con-nective tissue types. This is now known to be incorrect. Fibroblasts can, for example, accumu-late lipid to such an extent that they may even-tually become indistinguishable from fat cells (Fig. 7.8), while the myofibroblast is virtually identical to a smooth muscle cell.

As to their origin, it seems most likely that they arise either as a result of the differentiation from mesenchymal cells or by the division of pre-existing fibroblasts, although the latter is unlikely in adults except in response to tissue damage. The once popular idea that the leuco-cytes which gather at the sites of injury could transform into fibroblasts has now been abandoned.

Mesenchymal cells. These stellate, multipotent cells are characteristic of the embryonic mesen-chyme from which all connective tissues develop. Although most mesenchymal cells dif-ferentiate into other connective tissue cells, some remain undifferentiated even in the adult. These probably retain the ability to differentiate into any kind of connective tissue cell, or even into the smooth muscle fibres of blood vessels, and may do so in response to changed environ-mental conditions.

Mesenchymal cells (Fig. 7.7) are generally smaller than fibroblasts, and can be disting-

uished from them by their ultrastructure, having abundant free ribosomes, and sparse rough endoplasmic reticulum and Golgi apparatus. They are most frequent along the outer surfaces of blood vessels, especially capillaries.

Fat cells (adipose cells or adipocytes). These cells specialize in the synthesis and storage of lipid, mainly in the form of triglycerides (Fig. 3.99). They develop by the differentiation of mesenchymal cells, and possibly also from fibro-blasts. Their appearance changes with the amount of lipid that they contain (Fig. 7.8). Unless special precautions are taken, the lipids dissolve out of the fat cells during processing, with the result that in sectioned tissue they look like rings, with the nucleus representing a solit-ary gem. Where a number of fat cells are packed closely together they become polyhedral in shape.

Fat cells begin to differentiate during the 30th week of gestation, and are added to by the dif-ferentiation of mesenchymal cells throughout the rest of gestation and during early childhood. The final number formed may depend on nutritional and hormonal influences during this period. From then onward their number can only decrease as cells die, for like neurons they cannot be replaced. Each cell can, however, vary the amount of lipid it stores thereby varying the load of fat carried by an individual, the limit being determined by the number of fat cells available. Fat babies transformed by over-indulgent parents into chubby children may have more difficulty than their leaner brethren in avoiding becoming overweight, simply because they developed more fat cells when young.

The number of fat cells present in loose areo-lar tissue is very variable, as is their distribution which is, in part, sexually dimorphic. They are

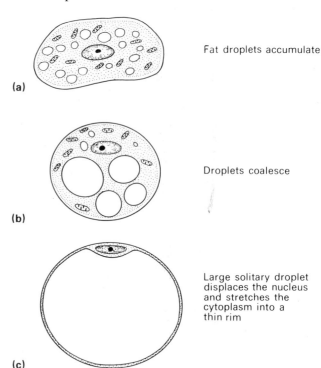

(a)   Fat droplets accumulate

(b)   Droplets coalesce

(c)   Large solitary droplet displaces the nucleus and stretches the cytoplasm into a thin rim

Fig. 7.8. Fat cells in progressive stages of development.

generally grouped around blood vessels, and if in any region they are the commonest cell type, then the tissue there is termed 'adipose' rather than 'areolar.'

Fixed macrophages (histiocytes, clasmatocytes or phagiocrine cells). These cells specialize in phagocytosis or pinocytosis, and are therefore part of the reticuloendothelial system (p 663). Although normally sessile, they can become motile if stimulated. They act as scavengers, taking up and digesting invading organisms and tissue debris. They may also be able to increase the effectiveness of antigens before passing them on to the B lymphocytes (p. 679).

There are about as many fixed macrophages in normal loose areolar tissue as there are fibroblasts. They can be distinguished from the latter by the following features: they contain less rough endoplasmic reticulum; they contain more primary and secondary lysosomes; their nuclei are smaller and more heterochromatic, and are indented on one side; they generally cluster around the blood capillaries and venules, while the fibroblasts appear to be randomly arranged; and unlike fibroblasts, they can ingest

injected vital dyes, such as trypan blue, India ink and lithium carmine.

The phagocytic abilities of macrophages can be exploited to separate them from other cell types in cultures. One ingeniuous method is to encourage them to ingest iron carbamyl, and then to remove them from the non-phagocytic cells with a magnet!

Macrophages are capable of collaborative effort. If they are individually too small to engulf a large foreign body, they can fuse to form a (syncitial) giant cell which can do so.

The origin of the fixed macrophages of loose areolar tissue is uncertain. They may differentiate *in situ* from mesenchymal cells or fibroblasts. Another possibility is that they are simply temporarily resting 'wandering' macrophages which originated elsewhere in the body.

Mast cells. These are cells which synthesize and store large numbers of basophilic granules rich in heparin and histamine. Heparin is a glycosaminoglycan which, if present in sufficient concentration, makes the granules metachromatic. Toluidine blue, for example, stains them purple rather than blue. Heparin (p. 693) is an

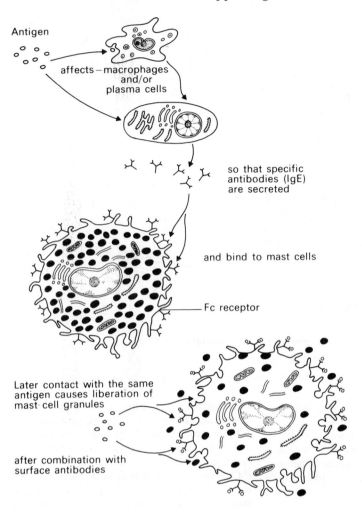

Antigen

affects — macrophages and/or plasma cells

so that specific antibodies (IgE) are secreted

and bind to mast cells

Fc receptor

Later contact with the same antigen causes liberation of mast-cell granules

after combination with surface antibodies

Fig. 7.9. The release of mast cell granules.

anticoagulant, and may prevent the clotting of plasma after it has leaked out of the blood vessels and entered the fluid-filled spaces of the ground substance. Histamine is a potent vasodilator and a stimulator of wound healing. It also increases the permeability of blood capillaries and venules, and causes contraction of some types of smooth muscle, in particular that around the bronchioles. Mast cell granules can be extruded in response to trauma or the action of antibodies (Fig. 7.9). Extrusion is an energy-consuming process and seems to involve the activity of microfilaments, for if mast cells are treated with cytochalasin, a substance which depolymerizes the microfilaments, degranulation is inhibited. Massive degranulation may be followed by anaphylaxis; this is a rare but severe allergic response involving sudden collapse and

sometimes death. It is caused by contact with an antigen to which the body has been sensitized (p. 680).

Mast cells are most common near the blood vessels. They are generally spherical or ovoid, with many filopodia. The nucleus is small and centrally placed.

Plasma cells (plasmacytes). These develop from B lymphocytes (p. 680) and specialize in antibody production. Their presence in loose areolar tissue is generally associated with infection.

Plasma cells (Fig. 7.10) are large, ovoid structures, ranging from about 6–20 μm in diameter. Russell bodies are seen in a few plasma cells. These have been variously described as temporary storage sites for antibodies synthesized in the

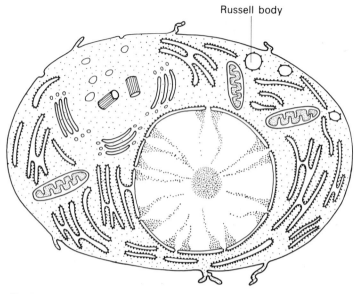

Russell body

Features
Copious rough e.r.

Well developed Golgi apparatus

'Clockface' nucleus

Fig. 7.10. Diagram of a plasma cell.

Russell bodies formed from dilated cisternae of rough e.r.

rough endoplasmic reticulum, and as symptoms of cellular ageing.

The antibodies made by the plasma cells may be produced in response to molecular information passed on by macrophages, which enhances the antigenicity of certain proteins. Other antibodies can be made without macrophage involvement.

Leucocytes (p. 676). These enter loose areolar tissue by migrating through the walls of the blood capillaries and venules.

Lymphocytes are especially common in areolar tissue prone to infection, such as the lamina propria of the alimentary tract (including gingiva) and respiratory channels, as are the phagocytic neutrophils (polymorphonuclear leucocytes) and monocytes.

Like the rest of the ordinary connective tissues, areolar tissue has a matrix composed of ground substance and fibrous proteins.

Ground substance. This is an amorphous material in which the other components of the tissue (that is the cells and fibres) are embedded. Its physical properties are those of a viscous solution or a thin gel. In fresh tissue it is colourless and transparent. It consists of the following: proteoglycans, glycoproteins, soluble proteins (such as blood proteins and the precursors of collagen and elastin), nutrients, waste products, dissolved blood-gases and water.

Often several proteoglycans aggregate, forming macromolecules of high viscosity which interact with each other and with any nearby collagen fibres, linking to form a three-dimensional network. It is this which is largely responsible for the consistency of the ground substance. Water-binding sites on the glycosaminoglycans of the proteoglycans attract and hold fluid which leaks out of capillaries. The proteoglycans then act as a sponge, retaining the tissue fluid in which they themselves become suspended and permitting the diffusion of metabolites between cells and capillaries (see pp. 140–145).

The 'areolae', after which loose areolar tissue is named, are minute droplets of tissue fluid, each limited by a retaining wall of compressed matrix protein. When extra fluid, such as a local anaesthetic, is injected into the ground substance, it remains at the site of injection for a while, being also walled off by matrix protein. The 'wall' is, however, permeable, and the fluid gradually diffuses away. The enzyme hyaluronidase hydrolyses hyaluronic acid, the commonest 'brick' in the 'wall', and can be combined with the anaesthetic to speed diffusion around the injection site. It is interesting that some of the most invasive bacteria secrete hyaluronidase which presumably acts in a similar way by removing some of the barriers to their progress through the connective tissues.

Collagen. This forms the collagenous and reticular fibres of loose areolar connective tissue. Both consist of the same molecular units but differ in size and in staining characteristics. Reticular fibres are argyrophilic and thinner than collagen fibres which are acidophilic.

Collagen is the most abundant of all body proteins. It plays a passive but vital role as the supporting framework for every organ of the body, spacing and suspending the tissues so that they can function effectively. Collagen literally holds us together, defining the shape and size of our tissues and organs, keeping them in the right place.

Collagen fibres have the following unique combination of mechanical properties: high tensile strength, inextensibility (to all intents and purposes), and structural stability.

The collagen fibres of loose areolar tissue form an irregular lattice whose structure and units are more readily appreciated in tissue spreads viewed with a stereo-microscope than in sections: mesentery is ideal for the purpose. Individual fibres vary in thickness from 1–20 μm. Each is a bundle of fibrils, about 0.2–0.5 μm wide, arranged in parallel array. The number of fibrils determines the width of the collagen fibre. To explore their structure further, electron microscopy has to be used (Fig. 7.11).

Each fibril is a bundle of microfibrils. These have regular cross-striations with a repeating pattern having a 64–70 nm periodicity.

Normally the tropocollagen molecules, which have a definite polarity, are arranged in head to tail fashion along the length of the microfibrils. Each line of tropocollagens lies parallel to its neighbours but in a staggered fashion such that adjacent molecules are overlapped by about a quarter of their length. This overlapping results in the 64 nm periodicity of the microfibrils.

The bands are caused by the alignment of similar regions within each parallel molecule of tropocollagen which forms the microfibrils.

Tropocollagen is a rod-like molecule about 280 nm long and 1.5 nm wide. It consists of 3 helically-coiled polypeptide chains called α-units which are twisted round each other in a right-handed spiral.

It has been suggested that the lines of molecules are arranged in groups of five, each group forming a hollow cylinder (Fig. 7.11). This arrangement would be compatible with the periodicity of native collagen fibres and would be very stable under bending stresses, since in cross section the ratio of molecules to lumen would be very high. The structure of tropocollagen is described on p. 68.

Collagen biosynthesis (p. 246). In most connective tissues, collagen precursors are secreted by the fibroblasts in soluble form, converted to the precipitable molecule tropocollagen at the cell surface, and then aligned extracellularly to form collagen fibres, the final structure being stabilized by intermolecular crosslinks. The stages in the process are outlined below and shown diagrammatically in Fig. 7.12, which should be referred to while the following is read.

1   The first step is the assembly of the α-units by polyribosomes, using the coded information in specific mRNA molecules.

2   The polyribosomes attach themselves to the outer surface of a rough endoplasmic cisterna and the polypeptide chain penetrates the membrane so that it hangs down into the cisterna. It continues lengthening as more amino acid residues are added forming units called protocollagen.

3   Lysine and proline residues of protocollagen are hydroxylated by enzymes (PPH) which are apparently bound to the membranes of the cisternae. Fully formed, hydroxylated, polypeptide chains are called procollagen α-units. Hydroxylation is essential for the secretion of the collagen precursors. If it is inhibited, for example by vitamin C deficiency, then they remain within the cells. The structural importance of hydroxylation is that it allows the nascent α-units to assume stable H-bonded structures intracellularly and so take up a triple-helical form, and to provide sites for glycosylation which adds further to molecular stability.

4   Some of the amino acid residues at the NH_2–terminal of the α-units become linked by disulphide bonds. Once three units are linked in this way the rest of the chains can coil into a triple helix. Positioning and coiling takes place within the cisternae of the rough endoplasmic reticulum after the release of the procollagen α-units from the ribosomes.

5   The next step is glycosylation of selected

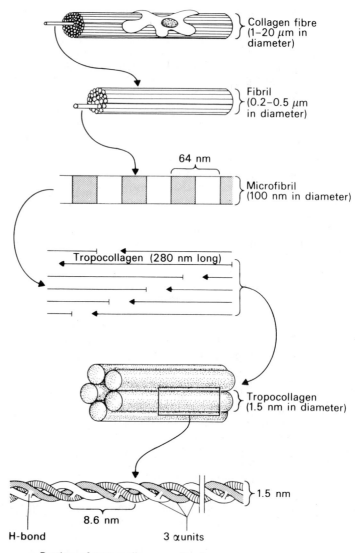

Fig. 7.11. The structure of collagen fibres.

hydroxylysine residues. This completes the synthesis of the procollagen molecule.

6 Procollagen is now carried to the Golgi apparatus in transport vesicles. These fuse together to form Golgi saccules. While progressing through the Golgi stack, the procollagen molecules become arranged in anti-parallel fashion, and it is in this form that they leave the Golgi apparatus in secretory vesicles.

7 Microtubules now act as transport conduits along which the secretory vesicles move towards the plasma membrane with which they fuse, liberating their contents. If the microtubular sys-

tem is damaged, for example by treatment with colchicine or vinblastine, secretion of procollagen is blocked.

8 Located at the surface of the fibroblast are groups of procollagen peptidase enzymes. These proceed to split peptides from the non-helical terminals of the α-units, converting each procollagen molecule into a tropocollagen. The process occurs in stages, with different enzymes acting sequentially to produce first heavy collagen (H-collagen) then tropocollagen.

Although in loose areolar connective tissue the pattern of collagen fibres appears irregular,

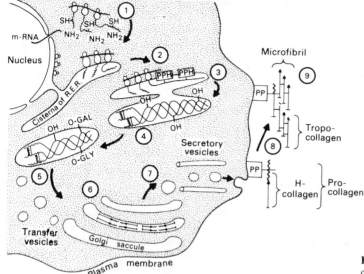

Fig. 7.12. Biosynthesis of collagen.

in many tissues the fibres are arranged in a geometrically precise and predictable way. They are laid down along lines of stress; that is, they develop where they are most required. This is particularly noticeable in bone and tendon. If the forces acting on the tissues change, then the pattern of the fibres alters. Exactly how this is achieved is uncertain. One suggestion is that some of the molecules of the matrix, possibly collagen itself, react piezo-electrically to deformation; that is, deformation produces minute electric currents which affect the movements of the fibroblasts, causing them to aggregate along the lines of maximum stress and lay down fibres along these lines.

Elastin. Loose areolar connective tissue contains thin elastic fibres. These are branching structures (unlike collagen fibrils which are not branched), yellow in fresh tissue, but staining black with Weigert's and Verhoef's elastin stains.

Elastic fibres can stretch to 1.5 times the original length without breaking, and show almost perfect recoil once the stretching force is removed. At maximum stretch they are much weaker than collagen. The resilience of elastin decreases with advancing age, when elastic fibres may gradually become calcified and brittle.

In some sites, for example, the human periodontium and the adventitia of blood vessels, oxytalan fibres can be found. Since these stain in the same way as immature elastic fibres

and resemble them ultrastructurally, it is very likely that this is what they are.

Adipose tissue

This is a loose connective tissue in which fat cells or adipocytes (p. 354 and Fig. 7.8) are the commonest cell type present. In men, it accounts for about 10–20% of the body weight and in women for about 15–25%. The 10% figure represents enough stored energy for about 40 days existence; very obese people may store enough fat to provide their energy requirements for over a year.

The fat stored in most adipocytes is constantly being used and replaced. This is necessary for although we use up energy continuously, we eat only intermittently.

The other functions of adipose tissue are: to cushion against shock (the fat pads in the palms of the hands and the soles of the feet perform this function particularly well); to give thermal insulation (the subcutaneous fat is especially important in this respect); to act as a packing and spacing tissue between the various organs and between the tissues within organs; and to provide a source of heat which can rapidly raise the body temperature (this function can be vital in new-born babies and in animals awakening from hibernation).

Adipose tissue is of two types: ordinary, yellow or unilocular; and brown or multilocular.

Ordinary adipose tissue. Here each adipocyte typically contains a single, large lipid droplet, the colour of which depends on the diet; the typical pale-yellow coloration is caused by dissolved carotenoids. The tissue is separated into lobes and lobules by septa of loose areolar, reticular or dense irregular connective tissue, in which run blood vessels and nerves. Delicate connective tissue strands extend out from the septa, framing each adipocyte in supporting reticular fibres, and carrying with them capillaries and unmyelinated nerve fibres.

Triglycerides in adipocytes are formed in any of the following ways: from glucose within the adipocyte; from lipoproteins transported from the liver to adipocytes in the blood plasma; and from chylomicrons (p. 612) in the blood plasma.

Blood-borne triglycerides are hydrolysed in the capillaries by lipoprotein lipase, giving fatty acids and glycerol which are transported through the endothelial cell cytoplasm in pinocytic vesicles. They are released into the ground substance surrounding the capillary and then enter the nearby adipocytes through more pinocytic vesicles. After recombining into triglycerides (neutral fats) they accumulate and form lipid droplets within the cell.

Adipose tissue begins to accumulate in the 30th week of gestation, and by birth the subcutaneous unilocular variety is of uniform thickness throughout the body, forming the panniculus adiposus. At puberty the sex hormones influence various parts of this fatty layer differentially, and the contours typical of the male and female body develop. Unilocular fat is also found in both sexes in the omenta, mesenteries, and in specific retroperitoneal regions (for example, around the kidneys). The fat in all the zones noted above can be drawn on as a supply of energy during periods of fasting or starvation.

Unilocular fat is also present within the orbit (following starvation the eyes sink deep into their sockets), in the palms of the hands and the soles of the feet, and within the capsules of many joints; in these sites its prime functions are to support and protect, and it is only depleted as a last resort in cases of severe starvation.

Brown adipose tissue. Here the adipocytes contain a large number of small lipid droplets, hence the alternative term 'multilocular.' They also have more cytoplasm than the adipocytes of ordinary adipose tissue. Brown adipose tissue is extremely vascular, the blood vessels being arranged in the type of pattern seen in a compound gland.

The brown coloration is caused by the large amount of cytochrome contained in the mitochondria of the adipocytes. Curiously, the mitochondria of the adipocytes are spherical; in most cells they are elongated and sausage-shaped.

Brown adipose tissue mainly acts as a source of heat, especially in the newborn infant. As in ordinary adipose tissue, noradrenaline stimulates the conversion of the stored triglycerides into fatty acid and glycerol by lipases. This is followed by oxidation and the liberation of heat rather than by the formation of ATP which is the result in most other tissues. Adipocytes can liberate heat preferentially because their mitochondria can uncouple oxidative phosphorylation from the rest of the respiratory process when heat is required. By warming the blood circulating through the adipose tissue this heat is distributed throughout the rest of the body. Oxidative phosphorylation can be recoupled when the heating emergency is over and then ATP is produced in the usual way (p. 177).

Brown adipose tissue develops at specific sites before birth, particularly in the axillae and in the posterior triangles and nape of the neck. Small collections of brown adipocytes are also found near the thyroid, along the carotid sheath, and at the hilum of each kidney. The tissue comprises about 2–5% of the body weight at birth, when it is vitally important in helping to maintain body temperature. In well-fed adults some of the brown adipocytes may become unilocular and the tissue morphologically indistinguishable from ordinary adipose tissue. Emaciation, however, is accompanied by its reversion to the fetal form.

Reticular tissue
This consists of reticular cells and reticular fibres produced by them, embedded in ground substance similar to that of loose areolar tissue but penetrated by linking, fluid-filled channels (Fig. 7.13). The reticular fibres are argyrophilic and are arranged in three-dimensional networks; they consist of delicate bundles of fine collagen fibres. The reticular cells are stellate and develop from mesenchymal cells; they were originally called reticular cells because they collectively form a reticulum or network. Reticular tissue forms the framework of the haemopoeitic and lymphopoeitic regions, for example in bone marrow and spleen, and its reticular cells were once thought to be the progenitors of blood and lymph cells. It is now generally accepted that reticular cells may become either fibroblasts or fixed macrophages, and that the precursor cells

of the blood and lymph lie between them (p. 672, 677).

Dense connective tissues

This differs from loose connective tissues in containing more fibres and less ground substance, and in being stronger and less flexible. It is termed 'regular' if the fibres are arranged in a predictable pattern, for example in parallel bundles, and 'irregular' if they seem to be arranged at random.

Regular dense connective tissue

This can be further subdivided into collagenous and elastic types.

Collagenous. Here the main fibres are collagen fibres, and these are arranged in a clearly defined pattern according to the mechanical requirements of the region. The orientation of the bundles is determined by the direction of the stresses to which the tissue is exposed. Since collagen is virtually inextensible, the laying down, for example, of parallel bundles of fibres in line with the direction in which a traction force is operating, enables that force to be transmitted with little loss to some other tissue which can thus be moved.

Tendons (Fig. 7.14): these consist of collagenous regular dense connective tissue in which the fibres are arranged in parallel bundles, and which can therefore efficiently convey the traction forces generated by muscle to bone. The collagen fibre bundles merge with the epimysium at one end of the tendon and with the periosteum at the opposite end. The strength of the attachment to the bone is enhanced by the incorporation of some of the fibres into the calcified bony matrix. Such fibres are termed Sharpey's fibres.

Macroscopically, tendons are white, fibrous and glistening. In sections observed with the microscope it can be seen that each 'fibre' is actually a fibre bundle surrounded by a little ground substance. Columns of mature fibroblasts (fibrocytes) ensheath each bundle; they are elongated in the same direction as the collagen fibres. These primary bundles are grouped into secondary bundles, separated from each other by loose areolar connective tissue in which run a few blood vessels and nerves. The whole tendon is ensheathed in a layer of dense connective tissue continuous with, and analogous to, the epimysium and fibrous periosteum. In some tendons this ensheathing layer is split into two and lined by squamous cells of mesenchymal origin.

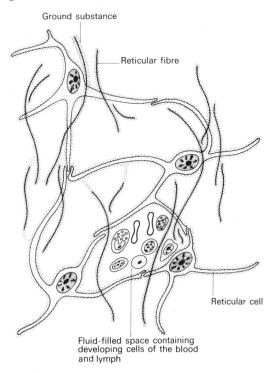

Fig. 7.13. Diagram of reticular tissue.

The two layers of the sheath are separated by a film of viscous fluid containing proteoglycans which allow the tendon to slide freely within its sheath.

Ligaments: With a very few exceptions ligaments, like tendons, are also collagenous, non-elastic structures. They are usually associated with joints which allow movement, helping to maintain the stability of the joint by connecting one bone to another. Ligaments are similar to tendons in structure, although their collagen fibre bundles are often somewhat less regularly arranged. It should be remembered that the stability of joints largely depends on the activity of the muscles which move its associated bones.

Fibrous sheets: As well as discrete cords, such as tendons and ligaments, regular dense connective tissue of the collagneous type can also form sheets. These consist of a flat layer of parallel bundles of collagen fibres, interspersed with traces of ground substance and the fibroblasts which have secreted both. Generally several sheets are superimposed, and in each the fibres run in a different direction; a few fibre bundles run from one sheet to another, joining them together. Examples of this type of tissue

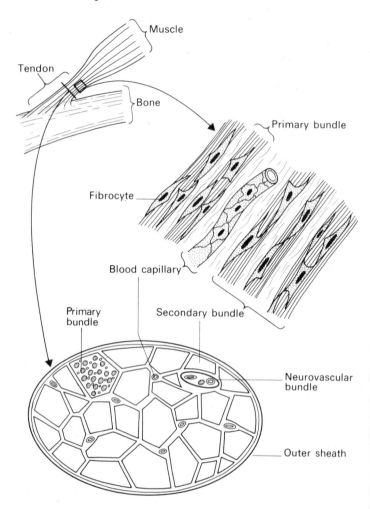

Fig. 7.14. Tendon.

are aponeuroses, fasciae, periostea, perichondria, sclera and the corneal stroma. The last of these, the corneal stroma, is interesting in that it is extremely regular, the collagen fibres of adjacent sheets running at 90° to each other and being very evenly spaced; it has been suggested that the proteoglycans of the ground substance control this spacing, and that the regularity is partly responsible for the transparency of the cornea, ensuring that any scattered light rays cancel each other by destructive interference.

Elastic. Here the majority of fibres are elastic. When fresh, such tissue is yellow (hence the term 'yellow elastic tissue'), but when prepared for light microscopy it is frequently stained black by one of the elastin stains.

The fibres are either arranged in bundles or in sheets. The bundle arrangement is found in, for example, the ligamenta flava (p. 426) and the conus elasticus. Here the bundles are loosely ensheathed by stellate fibroblasts and separated by traces of ground substance. In the sheet arrangement fenestrated lamellae of elastin are connected in superimposed layers by networks of fine, irregular, elastic fibres; fibroblasts and ground substance lie between the elastic lamellae. The sheet arrangement is typically found in the walls of hollow vessels subjected to fluctuating pressure from within; for example, the aorta and the trachea.

Irregular dense connective tissue
This contains mixtures of both collagenous and elastic fibres arranged in an irregular three-dimensional network. It differs from loose areolar tissue in that the fibre bundles are thicker and closer together; it is also less cellular and con-

tains less ground substance. The fibres are arranged in such a way that the tissue can be stretched in any direction, and can recoil once the deforming force is removed. Examples of this type of tissue are the reticular layer of the dermis (Fig. 8.4) and the capsules of many glands.

SKELETAL TISSUES

These are the hard supporting tissues of the body. Unlike the ordinary connective tissues, which differ from each other only in the arrangement and relative proportions of their various components, the skeletal tissues show more profound differences: each can give mechanical support but the methods by which they do so depend on their architecture and on their chemical composition, and these are highly variable.

Notochord

This is the axial rod which contributes to the support of the embryo and the fetus. It lies just below and in line with the neural tube, and consists of a group of radially arranged, vacuolated, turgid cells packed closely together within a collagenous sheath (Fig. 7.15). The pressure of the (incompressible) fluid in the vacuoles of these cells against each other and against the firm sheath stiffens the whole structure which thus acts as a hydrostatic skeleton, and in this respect differs from all other skeletal tissues where the matrix, that is the intercellular material, is responsible for support.

During the development of the vertebral column the notochord is eroded and replaced. Vestiges of it remain throughout life, though in modified form, in the nucleus pulposus of each intervertebral disc.

Cartilage

This is a tough, gristly tissue found wherever strength combined with resilience are required. Like bone, it has an extensive matrix which is sufficiently firm for it to be able to give mechanical support. However, unlike bone, cartilage is rarely calcified except as a preliminary to the replacement of cartilage by bone or in certain pathological conditions. This lack of calcium salts makes cartilage less resistant to pressure than bone but also less brittle.

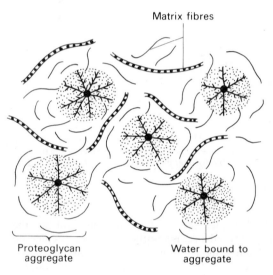

Fig. 7.16. Distribution of proteoglycans in the matrix of cartilage.

The mechanical properties of cartilage are related to the composition of its matrix. This is characterized by a large amount of glycosaminoglycan (GAG) which attracts and traps water, so that water makes up about 75% of the weight of cartilage. The GAGs also have a preponderance of negatively charged groups and it is possible that enough of these may remain free (from Na^+ and Ca^{2+} binding) for them to repel each other, causing the GAGs to stay uncoiled and stiffly extended in the matrix (Fig. 7.16). The combination of hydration and molecular extension gives the matrix, and hence the tissue, a firm consistency. It also increases its resilience. When subjected to pressure, for

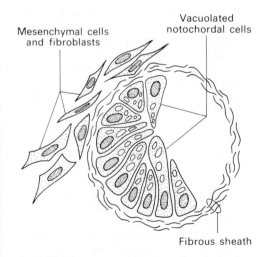

Fig. 7.15. Transverse section through notochord.

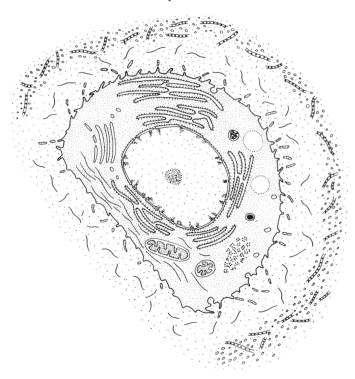

Fig. 7.17. Ultrastructure of a chondrocyte; showing numerous extensions of the surface increasing the area available for metabolite exchange, stored fat and glycogen, copious rough endoplasmic reticulum and Golgi apparatus, lysosomes, secretory vesicles and surrounding matrix.

example, the GAGs probably coil as the imposed force is absorbed and water is squeezed out as though from a sponge; when the stress is removed the GAGs extend again and water is reabsorbed. In synovial joints the production of water by articular cartilage under pressure augments the synovial fluid and is called weeping lubrication (p. 386).

Another feature of cartilage is its smoothness. Although most cartilaginous surfaces are covered by a layer of ordinary dense fibrous connective tissue (the perichondrium), those exposed to pressure are not, for example the articular surfaces of the cartilages in joints. These surfaces are extremely smooth and slippery, and provide a sliding contact for the levers of the joint, thus facilitating movement. The coefficient of friction of articular cartilage is about 0.013, making it almost three times as slippery as ice. This smoothness is a property of the cartilaginous matrix.

The view adopted in this section is that synovial fluid does not lubricate joints; indeed, it actually impedes sliding movements and its function is primarily nutritive.

The matrix is secreted and maintained by cartilage cells known as chondrocytes (Fig. 7.17). Each cell is completely surrounded by matrix through which all vital metabolities must diffuse. Cartilage has no blood supply but the diffusion is generally adequate to supply its low metabolic needs. If diffusion is impaired, for example by calcification, then the chondrocytes die. The source of the metabolites is either a capillary outside the cartilage or synovial fluid.

The tensile strength and elasticity of cartilage is related to the type and distribution of the protein fibres of its matrix. The most common type of cartilage is hyaline: its matrix contains fine collagen fibres which enable it to withstand moderate pressures and tensions. In regions subjected to heavy loads and strong tensile forces the matrix contains thicker, more numerous collagen fibres; this type of cartilage is called fibrocartilage. In other positions, where greater elasticity is required, the cartilage contains fibres of elastin as well as collagen; this third type is called elastic cartilage. The ground substance and cells are similar in all three types.

Cartilage has: a low metabolic rate; a low antigenicity; no blood vessels or lymphatics; a dense matrix which can impede the passage of cells; and no nerve supply. Considered together, these features probably explain why cartilage can generally survive transplantation and so is useful in reconstructive surgery. The absence of a nerve supply means that cartilage can be damaged without an immediate awareness of pain and since it has a poor capacity for repair the damage may be permanent. This is serious particularly where the sliding surfaces of joints are involved.

Hyaline cartilage. This type of cartilage forms most of the skeleton of the embryo. Though much of it is gradually replaced by bone, some remains as the epiphysial discs between the diaphysis and epiphyses of developing long bones.

In the adult, it is found at the anterior ends of the ribs; in the larynx, trachea and bronchi; and forming the articular cartilage within many joints.

Fresh hyaline cartilage is translucent and bluish-white in colour. It has a 'glassy' appearance and the consistency of firm rubber. Like all other connective tissues, it consists of cells and a matrix composed of ground substance and fibres.

The cells in hyaline cartilage are called chondrocytes. Those close to the surface of the cartilage are elliptical and lie with their long axes parallel to the surface, while those deeper within the matrix tend to be isodiametric (Fig. 7.18). They are often arranged in small isogenous groups or cell nests of up to eight cells, each group being the result of successive divisions of a chondroblast. In the hyaline cartilage of the epiphysial discs and in articular cartilage the cells are arranged in columns roughly at right angles to the surface. Chondrocytes capable of dividing (i.e. chondroblasts) are found within these columns (Fig. 7.24).

Cells dividing deep within the expansible matrix cause the cartilage to grow from within; this is called interstitial growth. Cells dividing at the surface cause it to grow by accretion; this is called appositional growth. Both methods of growth can take place simultaneously.

When cartilage is prepared for light microscopy, the chondrocytes shrink more than the matrix. This produces the appearance of lacunae, which are artefacts.

Chondrocytes (Fig. 7.17) manufacture all the proteins of the matrix; these include the proteoglycan chondroitin sulphate and type II collagen.

The matrix in hyaline cartilage consists of ground substance and fine collagen fibres. In fresh cartilage both have a similar refractive index which, together with the fineness of the fibres, means that the collagen cannot be distinguished by light microscopy. The commonest proteoglycan is chondromucoprotein, a copolymer of chondroitin-4-sulphate (chondroitin sulphate A) and chondroitin-6-sulphate (chrondroitin sulphate C). Keratan sulphate is also present in quantities which seem to be related to the hardness of the hyaline cartilage and age.

The collagen of the cartilage matrix accounts for about 30–40% of the dry weight. The fibrils are unbanded except in articular cartilage, where they have the 64nm periodicity typical of collagen. There are fewer fibrils in the immediate vicinity of the chondrocytes than elsewhere (Fig. 7.18).

Fibrocartilage. This is rarer than hyaline cartilage. It is found in regions subjected to considerable pressure and tensile stresses: for example, in intervertebral discs; in the secondary cartilaginous joints (e.g. the sternomanubrial joint); at the sites where some tendons are attached to bones; and covering the articular surfaces of the temporomandibular (see below) and sternoclavicular joints, where its presence may be related to the dermal origin of at least one of the bones involved in each joint. It is intermediate in structure between hyaline cartilage and dense fibrous connective tissue. It usually has most of the features of the former except that coarse bundles of collagen fibres replace the delicate collagen fibrils. At sites subjected to high tensile stresses, such as the insertion of a tendon into a bone, the fibre bundles are aligned parallel to the direction in which the stresses act, and the chondrocytes lie between them (Fig. 7.18).

In the temporomandibular joint the 'cartilage' is almost entirely dense fibrous connective tissue but contains a few chondrocytes, which can be recognised by their narrow surrounding rim of chondroitin sulphate. The number of chondrocytes increases with age.

Elastic cartilage. This is the rarest of the three types of cartilage. It is found in regions where

Hyaline cartilage
fibres:
   Fine collagen
   Reticulin

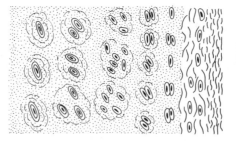

Moderate elastic recoil
Moderate tensile strength

Elastic cartilage
fibres:
   Fine collagen
   Reticulin
   Elastin

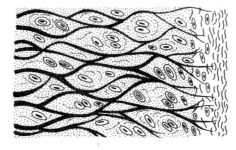

High elastic recoil
Moderate tensile strength

Fibrocartilage
fibres:
   Coarse collagen

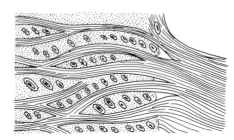

Moderate elastic recoil
High tensile strength

Fig. 7.18. Comparison of three types of cartilage.

there is a need for a great degree of flexibility as well as support: the pinna of the ear; the lateral wall of the external auditory meatus; the auditory tube; the epiglottis and parts of the larnyx.

Its cells and matrix resemble those of hyaline cartilage except that it contains large numbers of elastic fibres as well as fine collagen fibrils. The elastic fibres form a three-dimensional network in the interstitial matrix and extend into the perichondrium: their presence gives the cartilage a yellowish colour when fresh.

Hyaline cartilage, fibrocartilage and elastic cartilage are compared in Fig. 7.18.

Development, growth and repair. In the embryo, cartilage develops from mesenchymal cells which round up and crowd together forming protochordal tissue at genetically determined centres of chondrification. They divide rapidly and repeatedly and differentiate into chondroblasts, cells which are defined by their ability to synthesize chondroitin sulphate and the other components of the matrix and to divide.

The products of the division of a single chondroblast at first form isogenous groups or cell nests but eventually become separated by matrix.

Fibroblasts gathering around the developing cartilage form a fibrous perichondrium which merges with the surrounding ordinary connective tissue at its outer surface and with the cartilage at its inner surface. Within the fibrous perichondrium is an inner chondrogenic layer. The cells in this zone are generally considered to be undifferentiated mesenchymal cells which by their division and differentiation are responsible for appositional growth of cartilage. This layer generally remains latent in the adult. Although the cartilage proper has no blood vessels, lymphatics or nerves, the perichondrium is well supplied with them.

The presence of cell nests deep in a tissue sample is an indication that it is growing interstitially. Such growth is limited by the capacity of the matrix to expand. As this capacity becomes less, due, for example, to the deposition of keratan sulphate, interstitial growth is proportionately reduced. The chondroblasts stop dividing and settle down to a life devoted to the slow turnover of the cartilage matrix: they become mature chondrocytes. Old matrix is degraded by matrix dense bodies; these are fragments of cytoplasm, surrounded by a membrane and containing lysosomes, which have separated from the chondrocytes. As old matrix is removed it is replaced by new matrix materials secreted by the cells.

As the cartilage grows it often develops cartilage canals. These are formed when some of the cells of the perichondrium develop the capacity to erode the existing cartilage and excavate canals into which the perichondrium and its associated blood vessels grow. Such cells are termed chondroclasts. The blood vessels are continuous with those of the superficial perichondrium and help to nourish the deeper parts of the cartilage.

Hyaline cartilage may become calcified, that is, impregnated with crystalline hydroxyapatite (Fig. 7.4). This is a normal step in the replacement of cartilage by bone and may also occur during ageing. The chondrocytes become walled in by a material that impedes the diffusion of nutrients to the cells which in consequence degenerate and die (the cells are their own executioners). They are then autolysed (digested by their own lysosomes) leaving spaces in the matrix called primary areolae. The details of the calcification mechanism are uncertain but it appears that in cartilage the matrix dense bodies (often incorrectly described as matrix vesicles) are the primary site of hydroxyapatite deposition (p. 393).

The poor capacity for repair is probably related to the avascularity of mature cartilage. The way in which articular cartilage responds to injury is of particular importance because injury affects joint action. The response varies with the depth of the defect. If it is superficial there is no inflammatory component to the repair response; the cells next to the defect divide and increase their rate of matrix production but these changes are rarely sufficient to produce enough replacement cartilage to make good the defect. If the injury is deeper and extends through the cartilage into the underlying vascular bone, then inflammation followed by the production of granulation tissue and scarring are involved, with the final transformation of the scar into fibrocartilage. Since this differs from articular cartilage in its mechanical properties, it may eventually affect the action of the joint.

Bone
All mineralized tissues consist of an organic matrix in which inorganic crystals have grown. With the exception of enamel, the matrix consists of collagen and ground substance. The ground substance largely consists of water, proteoglycans, protein and lipids. Again with the exception of enamel, the mineralized tissue contains cells and/or cell processes. The present section is concerned only with bone.

Bone is a skeletal tissue with a calcified matrix which makes it rigid and well suited to providing mechanical support and protection. These and other functions of bone are described on p. 381.

Bone is less resilient than cartilage, incapable of interstitial growth, and its surfaces are less smooth. In many respects bone and cartilage are complementary and as such are associated together in the skeleton.

Bone has the following properties: high tensile strength; high resistance to pressure; slight elasticity; great strength for its weight; and a capacity for constant remodelling and adaptation to changing stresses. Its structure and properties are supremely adapted for its functions. As with many strong structures such as reinforced concrete and fibreglass, bone consists of two phases (p. 368).

Macroscopical features. If a long bone is sectioned longitudinally (Fig. 7.19) and the cut surface examined, two distinct arrangements of bone tissue can be distinguished. Forming an outer covering is an apparently solid yellowish-white material, termed compact bone. Lying within this cortex is the medulla which consists of a labyrinth of interlacing, interconnecting, bony beams or trabeculae separated by communicating spaces: this is spongy or cancellous bone. Both compact and cancellous bone can be distinguished towards the ends of a long bone, but the shaft often seems to consist solely of a hollow cylinder of compact bone. The cavity in the shaft is called the marrow cavity: in life it contains extremely delicate spicules of bone interspersed with reticular tissue (Fig. 7.13) and variable amounts of haemopoietic and adipose tissue giving it the colours and hence the names red marrow and yellow marrow respectively.

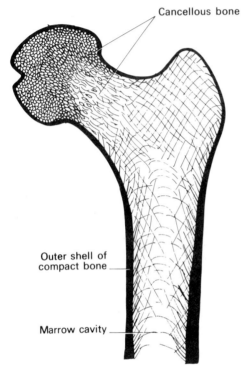

Fig. 7.19. Longitudinally sectioned femur (proximal end).

The shaft of a long bone is called the diaphysis and the ends are the epiphyses. Each of these regions develops from a separate centre of ossification. While the bone is still growing a plate of hyaline cartilage, the epiphysial plate, separates each epiphysis from the diaphysis. On the diaphysial side of this plate are trabeculae of newly formed cancellous bone whose growth and remodelling add to the length of the bone: this region is termed the metaphysis. Those surfaces of the epiphyses which contribute to the joints are covered by a layer of articular cartilage. The epiphysial plate is concerned with growth and ossification of the diaphysis; the deep surface of the articular cartilage is con-

cerned with growth and ossification of the epiphysis.

Most of the outer surface of the bone is covered by the two layers of a special connective tissue called the periosteum. Its inner layer consists of osteogenic or bone-forming cells and is well vascularized. Its outer layer is a dense fibrous connective tissue which merges with loose connective tissue peripherally. The periosteum is bound to the bone by collagen fibres which are partly embedded in the bone: these are called Sharpey's fibres.

Those regions of a bone which are capped by articular cartilage, or which are sites for the attachment of muscles, tendons or ligaments, are not covered by periosteum, with the result that no osteogenic cells cover these surfaces. The absence of osteogenic cells from these regions means that here damaged bone cannot be repaired with new bone; scar tissue forms instead.

All surfaces inside a bone are covered by a thin layer of cells called the endosteum. This consists of various kinds of cells, some with the capacity to form bone (osteoblasts) and others able to erode bone (osteoclasts).

In the flat bones of the cranium the term pericranium is used for the periosteum covering the outer cortical layer, and endocranium for the periosteum covering the cortical layer facing the brain. Except in the regions of the venous sinuses the endocranium is fused with the dura mater, the outermost of the cranial meninges (p. 886). It should be noted that although the pericranium is a type of periosteum, the endocranium is not a type of endosteum.

Composition of bone tissue

Cells. Bone contains three types of cells; osteoblasts, actively secreting the organic part of the matrix and controlling its mineralization; osteocytes, surrounded by fully-formed bone; and osteoclasts, which erode the bone.

All bone cells develop from osteogenic (osteoprogenitor) cells found in the loose connective tissue adjacent to growing bone and in the periosteum and endosteum of all bones. These are of two distinct types; preosteoblasts, which give rise to osteoblasts that later become osteocytes; and preosteoclasts which give rise to osteoclasts. These cells collectively form a single, though discontinuous, layer (Fig. 7.40) on the surfaces of bony tissue (Fig. 7.20). Their secretion is highly proteinaceous and is specific to bone. It is called osteoid.

They have all the structural characteristics

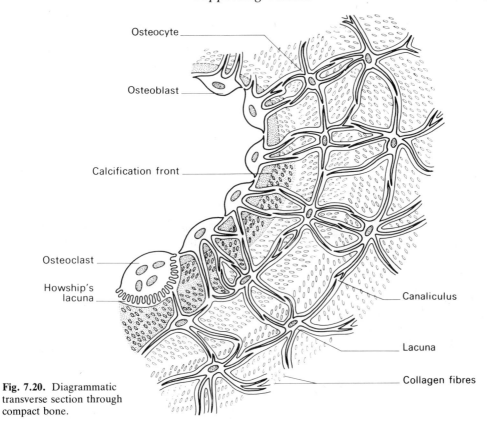

Osteocyte

Osteoblast

Calcification front

Osteoclast

Howship's lacuna

Canaliculus

Lacuna

Collagen fibres

Fig. 7.20. Diagrammatic transverse section through compact bone.

normally associated with cells involved in protein secretion. When secreting osteoid they contain histochemically detectable levels of alkaline phosphatase. Adjacent cells are linked together by spidery extensions of cytoplasm. Osteoblasts range in form from squamous to columnar, their height being directly related to the level of their activity.

Osteocytes form the majority of the cells in mature bone. They are squamous with an elliptical body from which numerous fine cytoplasmic processes extend towards similar processes of adjacent cells (Fig. 7.20). When the osteoblasts stop secreting osteoid and become surrounded by mineralized tissue they become osteocytes. They shrink, leaving spaces in the bone through which tissue fluid can percolate and conduct metabolites between the cells and the blood capillaries. Thus their cell bodies lie in lacunae and the processes in canaliculi. Since the processes of osteoblasts are contiguous, adjacent canaliculi form a continuous linking network of patent tubes extending through the substance of the bone. The presence in bone of a rich blood

supply and an interconnecting system of canaliculi enables the osteocytes and other bone cells to remain alive even after the matrix has been calcified.

Chondrocytes are entombed by calcification, but osteocytes are merely imprisoned and can be released by the action of the third type of bone cell, the osteoclast which resorbs the surrounding bone. Bone is constantly being remodelled in response to changing mechanical stresses and to the requirements of the body for calcium and phosphate. This remodelling involves the erosion of formed bone as well as the synthesis of new tissue (Fig. 7.20). The cells which erode bone are the osteoclasts. They vary in form from small uninucleate to giant multinucleate cells. The latter may contain up to 50 nuclei and be up to about 100 μm in diameter; they are most probably formed by the fusion of uninucleate osteoclasts or preosteoclasts. Recent evidence suggests that the preosteoclasts are derived from blood cells, probably monocytes.

Osteoclasts generally lie in concavities, Howship's lacunae, eroded in the bone. The part of the plasma membrane in contact with the osteoid is deeply infolded forming a constantly moving ruffled border which increases the area for reaction between the cell and the matrix. Several conflicting explanations for the resorption mechanism have been proposed. There is experimental evidence for both acid dissolution and chelation of mineral (chelation means the removal of ions by 'clawing' them from their surroundings even at a neutral pH), and destruction of ground substance by lysosomal acid hydrolases. The argument is really about which of the processes initiates resorption. It has been suggested that mineral is first removed thereby exposing the matrix which is then ingested by the brush border of the osteoclast and digested intracellularly. Collagenase has been identified in various bone preparations and this enzyme can degrade undenatured collagen at physiological pH. Osteoclasts are very sensitive to parathyroid hormone. This stimulates the release of lysosomal enzymes and increases the production of citrate and lactate ions which chelate and dissolve calcium salts respectively.

Matrix. The chemical constituents of bone are described on p. 346. Bone matrix is acidophilic due to its high content of collagen whereas cartilage, in which ground substance predominates, is basophilic.

Microscopical features. There are two common and microscopically distinct types of bone: embryonic, immature, primary, coarse-fibred or *woven*; and adult, mature, secondary, fine-fibred or *lamellar*. The basic difference between them lies in their collagen fibres: in woven bone they are coarse and irregularly arranged, while in lamellated bone they are slender and regularly arranged (Fig. 7.21).

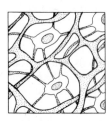 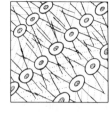

Woven bone   Lamellated

Fig. 7.21. Woven bone contains large, irregularly arranged cells and coarse irregular fibres. Lamellated bone, both compact and trabeculated, contains small cells arranged parallel to the plates of bone. The fibres are fine and regularly arranged.

Woven bone. This develops during intrauterine life and during fracture repair. It is generally a temporary structure which is replaced by lamellar bone although traces of it remain even in adults, for example near the sutures of the flat bones in the skull. Immature bone has the following features:

1 The collagen fibres are irregularly arranged.
2 Osteocytes, although regularly spaced, are irregularly orientated and the lacunae are larger than those in lamellar bone.
3 It is more cellular than lamellar bone.
4 The blood vessels occupy larger, more twisted canals than do those of lamellar bone.

Lamellar bone. This has the following features.

First, the collagen fibres are regularly arranged. Typically they are grouped in lamellae about 30–70 μm thick, some of which either lie parallel to each other while others are arranged concentrically around a Haversian canal containing blood vessels, nerves and loose connective tissue. There is still some disagreement about the detailed arrangement of the collagen fibres, but most histologists are of the opinion that the fibres in each lamella lie parallel to each other and at an angle to those in adjacent lamellae. Where the lamellae are concentrically arranged around a canal, the fibres are helically coiled with respect to the longitudinal axis of the canal, and the pitch of the helix varies from lamella to lamella (Fig. 7.22).

Second, the osteocytes are regularly spaced and regularly orientated, lying between adjacent lamellae with their longitudinal axes in line with the surface of the lamellae. Their bodies lie within lacunae in the matrix and their spidery cytoplasmic processes in linking canaliculi (Fig. 7.22). It is also less cellular than immature bone and its blood vessels lie in narrower, straighter canals than do those of immature bone.

Most mature cortical bone consists of mainly Haversian systems (osteons), a concentric series of bony lamellae surrounding a central canal. This type is sometimes called Haversian bone. Up to 20 concentric lamellae may surround each Haversian canal which is linked with its neighbours, with the bone marrow and with the periosteum by transversely or obliquely running Volkmann's canals.

Interlinking blood vessels run through the network of canals which is formed when bone is laid down around them. Most Haversian bone shows evidence of episodes of remodelling in the form of the remains of old Haversian systems which have been partly eroded by osteoclasts

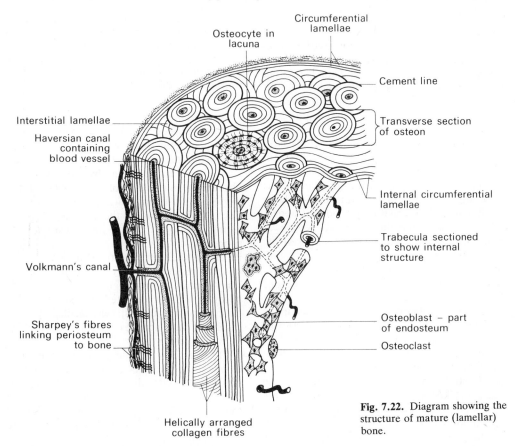

Interstitial lamellae

Haversian canal
containing
blood vessel

Volkmann's canal

Sharpey's fibres
linking periosteum
to bone

Osteocyte in
lacuna

Circumferential
lamellae

Cement line

Transverse section
of osteon

Internal circumferential
lamellae

Trabecula sectioned
to show internal
structure

Osteoblast – part
of endosteum

Osteoclast

Helically arranged
collagen fibres

Fig. 7.22. Diagram showing the structure of mature (lamellar) bone.

and replaced by new systems. These remains are called interstitial systems since they occupy the spaces between intact Haversian systems.

Haversian bone is generally coated by a few sheets of lamellated non-Haversian bone (Fig. 7.22).

The alveolar bone consists in part of bundle bone, an unusual type of mature bone (Book 2, p. 218). Collagen fibres from the periodontal ligament are embedded in the bone—Sharpey's fibres. The concentration of these fibres is far higher than in other types of mature bone and their arrangement in bundles has led to it being termed 'bundle bone'.

Development, growth and remodelling of bone
Bone normally develops within one or other of two types of connective tissue, gradually replacing it. Although the basic mechanism of bone formation is the same in both they are generally defined separately.

Dermal bones develop and grow by spreading through a 'dermis' underlying an epithelium. Endochondral bones develop and grow by replacing the cartilage in a growing cartilaginous model. Most of the flat bones of the skull such as the frontal, parietal and occipital, and the clavicle are dermal bones. Sometimes the term membrane bone is used because they develop in the membrane-like dermis. All the remaining bones are endochondral bones; for example the long bones and the vertebrae, but in these the part immediately beneath the periosteum is developed from cells differentiating from the inner layer of the periosteum (intramembranous ossification). Such bones begin to form and increase in length by endochondral ossification, but increase in thickness by subperiostial deposition.

Dermal Bones. Intramembranous ossification is most readily studied in bones such as the frontal and parietal. They develop as follows:
1 Early in gestation, the mesenchyme in the zone destined to become a dermal bone con-

denses into a richly-vascularized part of the dermis.

2 Within this layer primary centres of ossification form. The cells in these regions begin to differentiate into osteoblasts. They form thin strands of osteoid at positions roughly equidistant from the blood vessels. Since the vessels form a branching network, so do the strands or trabeculae of osteoid.

3 More cells differentiate into osteoblasts to form sheets on the surfaces of the trabeculae. Their basophilia increases as they become equipped with rough endoplasmic reticulum; they enlarge and begin to secrete another layer of osteoid within which they become trapped. The osteoblasts remain in contact with each other through their cytoplasmic extensions (Fig. 7.20).

4 The unmineralized osteoid is rapidly mineralized (p. 392) and becomes the matrix of bone.

5 As the osteoblasts become imprisoned in the calcified matrix they develop into osteocytes which retain their connection with the surface via the canaliculi and lacunae surrounding their processes and bodies.

6 The trabeculae continue to increase in length and in thickness as more mesenchymal cells are recruited to the ranks of the osteoblasts. Division of more peripheral mesenchymal cells adds to the pool of available cells of this type. The osteoblasts themselves probably never divide.

7 The spreading bones grow until they meet at sutures so that a shell of dermal bone develops around the cranium, face and mouth.

8 In the regions destined to form cortical plates of compact bone the gaps between the trabeculae become filled by Haversian systems (primary osteons), each developing around a central blood vessel. The outermost lamella of bone is the first to form, and as successive lamellae are laid down the Haversian canals become narrower.

9 Between its inner and outer cortical plate each bone remains cancellous but is constantly being remodelled as development proceeds. As well as trabeculae, this region contains cells which develop into reticular and haemopoietic tissue (red bone marrow).

10 Those parts of the connective tissue membrane which remain at the periphery of the bones adjacent to the cranial cavity eventually develop in to the (outer) pericranium and (inner) endocranium. At the sutures between adjacent cranial bones these two layers are continuous, and ossification continues at these joints until the final size of the cranium is attained. At birth large areas of the membranes are still unossified, forming the fontanelles of the skull.

Endochondral Bones. Endochondral ossification is best studied in the diaphysis of a long bone (Fig. 7.23).

1 Mesenchymal cells aggregate and divide, forming a blastemal skeleton, a compact cellular mass roughly the shape of the future limb bones. Within this mass chondroblasts differentiate and lay down cartilage thereby converting the blastemata into a set of miniature cartilage models representing each presumptive bone. Each model grows in the manner typical of young cartilage, that is both interstitially and appositionally.

2 In the middle of a cartilage model the chondrocytes begin to hypertrophy (increase in size). They accumulate glycogen and their cytoplasm becomes highly vacuolated. The swelling chondrocytes absorb the adjacent cartilage with the result that their lacunae enlarge and the cartilage between them is reduced to thin septa.

3 The cartilage remaining around the hypertrophied chondrocytes calcifies and the swollen entombed cells die. Lysosomal enzymes released from the dying chondrocytes enlarge the lacunae further, forming primary areolae, and autolyse any protoplasmic fragments they contain (Fig. 7.23c).

4 Meanwhile the first bone of the diaphysis is formed by subperichondrial deposition (intramembranous ossification). Mesenchymal cells in the perichondrium of the presumptive diaphysis differentiate into osteoprogenitor cells, some of which divide and become osteoblasts. These cells produce a narrow cylinder of immature bone called the periosteal collar, what was perichondrium is now termed periosteum, and further bone deposition is said to be subperiosteal.

5 A second type of osteoprogenitor cell, the preosteoclast, invades the periosteum, probably from the local blood vessels. Such cells develop into osteoclasts which erode the immature bone. Blood vessels penetrate through these holes in the bone to become a focus for the initiation of osteogenesis, the primary centre of ossification. The capillary loops are accompanied by mesenchymal cells which differentiate into either bone cells or haemopoeitic stem cells (Fig. 7.23d).

6 Erosion of the calcified matrix of the cartilage is continued by the lysosomal enzymes of the dying chondrocytes and of living osteoclasts. It has also been suggested that the endothelial cells

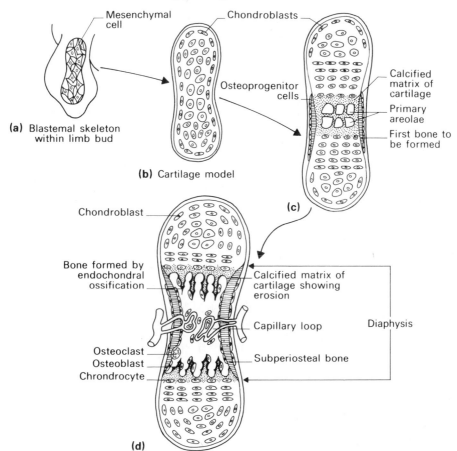

Mesenchymal cell

Chondroblasts

Osteoprogenitor cells

Calcified matrix of cartilage

Primary areolae

First bone to be formed

(a) Blastemal skeleton within limb bud

(b) Cartilage model

(c)

Chondroblast

Bone formed by endochondral ossification

Calcified matrix of cartilage showing erosion

Capillary loop

Diaphysis

Osteoclast

Osteoblast

Chrondrocyte

Subperiosteal bone

(d)

Fig. 7.23. Development of the diaphysis of a long bone.

of the capillaries may have chondrolytic activity. The net result is that adjacent primary areolae become confluent as the septa between them are broken down and secondary areolae are formed.

7   Many of the mesenchymal cells which move into the primary centre of ossification with the blood vessels become preosteoblasts. Vascularization of the centre increases its oxygen supply and the fact that osteoblasts, rather than chondroblasts, now differentiate may be related to this. Bone is laid down by the osteoblasts, whose numbers are augmented by the division of the preosteoblasts, on the surface of the disintegrating septa of the calcified cartilaginous matrix. Since this first formed woven bone is acidophilic it is readily distinguishable from the basophilic matrix of the cartilage.

8   Osteoclasts hollow out the middle of the developing diaphysis forming a marrow cavity in which blood cells can develop.

Increase in length of a long bone (Fig. 7.24) This is accomplished by division of chondrogenic cells at the edge of the cartilage, division of chondroblasts within the cartilage, and production of more cartilage. Bone tissue is increased by replacing this cartilage.

1   When the chondrogenic cells (precursors of chondroblasts) at each pole of the primary centre of ossification undergo division, they do so at right angles to the longitudinal axis of the developing bone. Those daughter cells nearer the primary centre become chondroblasts while others remain chondrogenic. The chondroblasts lay down cartilage and then become (inactive) chondrocytes. In this way columns of chondroblasts and chondrocytes are formed. Chondrocyte hypertrophy, matrix calcification, cell death and matrix erosion, follow each other sequentially, and in such a way that the pool of chondrogenic cells is nearest to the ends of the diaphysis,

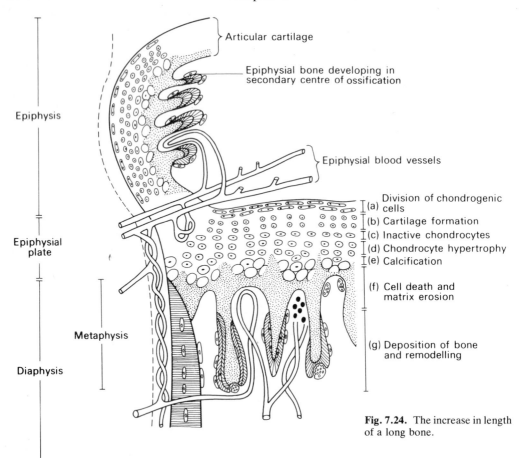

Articular cartilage

Epiphysial bone developing in
secondary centre of ossification

Epiphysis

Epiphysial blood vessels

(a) Division of chondrogenic
     cells
(b) Cartilage formation
(c) Inactive chondrocytes
(d) Chondrocyte hypertrophy
(e) Calcification

Epiphysial
plate

(f) Cell death and
     matrix erosion

Metaphysis

(g) Deposition of bone
     and remodelling

Diaphysis

Fig. 7.24. The increase in length
of a long bone.

while the tips of the columns, the sites of erosion,
are nearest to the centre of the diaphysis. Bone is
deposited on these columns.

2   The periosteal collar of bone increases in
length at the same rate as the rest of the
diaphysis, but does so by subperiosteal deposition.

3   The next stage is the formation of secondary
centres of ossification, usually one at each end of
the developing long bone. These give rise to the
bone of the epiphyses. They differ from the
primary centre in that their growth is radial
rather than longitudinal. Also their cartilage is
never wholly replaced by bone, unlike the
diaphyseal cartilage, for a cap of articular
(hyaline) cartilage remains at the free surface.
The same sequence of stages occurs as in the
endochondral ossification of the diaphysis, the
only difference being that there is no associated
subperiosteal deposition.

4   The epiphysis and diaphysis remain separated by a plate of growth cartilage, the
epiphysial plate, until the bone has attained its
final length. The only way that the bone can
increase in length is through the activity of this
plate of cartilage. A similar sequence of changes
to that described for the primary centre of ossification takes place but in a more orderly manner.

(a)   Chondrogenic cells divide on the side of the
plate nearest to the epiphysis, and mainly in a
plane at right angles to the longitudinal.
(b)   Chondroblasts differentiate and lay down
cartilage.
(c)   The chondroblasts stop manufacturing
matrix and become chondrocytes.
(d)   The chondrocytes hypertrophy and erode
much of the cartilage they earlier secreted.
(e)   The remaining cartilage becomes mineralized.

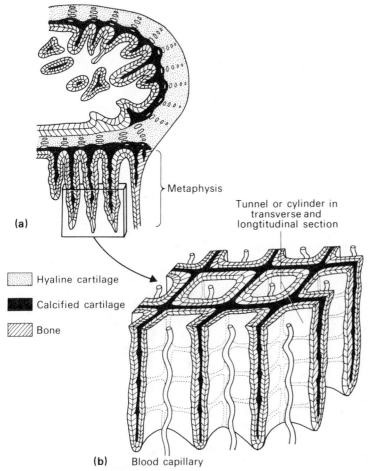

(a)

Metaphysis

Tunnel or cylinder in
transverse and
longtitudinal section

[ ] Hyaline cartilage

[■] Calcified cartilage

[▨] Bone

(b)   Blood capillary

Fig. 7.25. (a) Longitudinal
section through the end of a
growing long bone.
(b) Three-dimensional diagram
to show the arrangement of the
bone and cartilage in the
metaphyseal region. (After Ham
A.W., *Histology*, 6th Edition.
Lippincott, Philadelphia.

(f)   The chondrocytes die and most of the calcified cartilage is removed.

(g)   Woven bone is deposited on the few remaining spicules of calcified cartilage.

5   When the calcified cartilaginous matrix is eroded, the transverse septa separating adjacent chondrocytes within the same column of cells break down before the longitudinal septa between the columns. This results in the formation of a series of hollow cylinders or tunnels which run from the diaphysis into the cartilaginous plate, and inside whose walls the osteoblasts lay down bone. This transitional region between bone and cartilage, where the diaphysis widens and meets the epiphysis, is termed the metaphysis (Fig. 7.25).

6   The first bone deposited is of the woven type, but is later replaced by lamellated bone. The calcification front extends rapidly into the newly formed seam of osteoid and in health is rarely more than $1\mu m$ behind it.

7   As the diaphysis lengthens the cylinders of new bone in the metaphysis remain the same length because erosion at the diaphyseal end keeps pace with growth at the epiphyseal end. Growth of a long bone ceases when the cartilage of the epiphyseal plate is completely replaced by bone. This event is under hormonal control, particularly that of the gonadal hormones.

Increase in width of long bones. Unlike increase in length, which is ultimately due to cartilage growth, increase in width of the shaft of a long bone is entirely due to subperiosteal deposition of bone. Layer after layer of lamellated bone is laid down by osteoblasts differentiated from the osteogenic cells of the periosteum surrounding the diaphysis. At the same time the shaft is

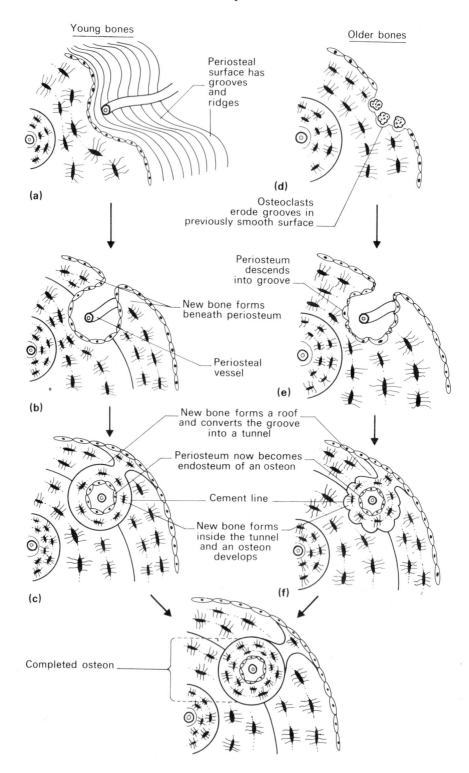

Fig. 7.26. Increase in the width of bones.

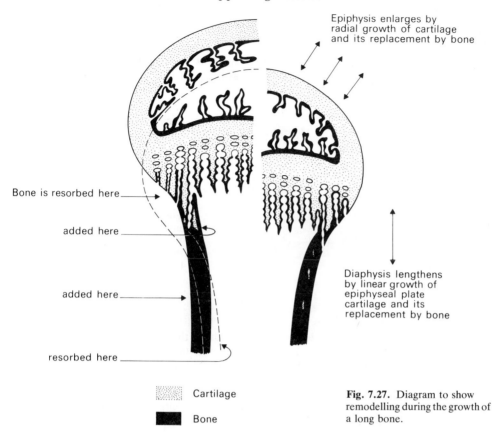

Epiphysis enlarges by radial growth of cartilage and its replacement by bone

Bone is resorbed here

added here

added here

resorbed here

Diaphysis lengthens by linear growth of epiphyseal plate cartilage and its replacement by bone

Cartilage

Bone

Fig. 7.27. Diagram to show remodelling during the growth of a long bone.

resorbed from within, thereby enlarging the medullary cavity. Much of the new bone is laid down in Haversian systems around longitudinally running blood vessels linked to those of the periosteum (Fig. 7.26).

Remodelling of bone. Although bones greatly enlarge during development, their proportions generally remain approximately the same. The original shape of a long bone is maintained by constant remodelling particularly in the region of the metaphysis. Here the situation described above for the widening of a bone is reversed: there is a progressive erosion of bone from the outside of the shaft and deposition of bone on the inside (Fig. 7.27).

The first bone to be laid down is always of the woven type, although since it is deposited in cylinders around blood vessels it may appear similar to the Haversian systems of lamellated bone. The production of the true Haversian systems of lamellated bone involves the internal remodelling of the woven bone. This takes place as follows.

1　Osteoclasts erode absorption cavities in the immature bone.

2　These cavities enlarge and coalesce, forming long cylinders through which run blood vessels.

3　Osteoclast activity ceases and osteoblasts move into the cylinders where they produce concentric lamellae of fine fibred bone. The site of the change-over from erosion to deposition is marked by a reversal line.

4　Osteoblast activity stops once the osteons (Haversian systems) have been completed.

The remodelling process begins prenatally and continues until death; old bone is constantly being replaced by new generations of Haversian systems. It takes about 4 weeks to complete such a system, bone being deposited at a rate of about 1 μm per day.

Bone turnover is very important for it allows the bone to be remodelled in accordance with the mechanical stesses placed upon it; if these change then the architecture of the bone

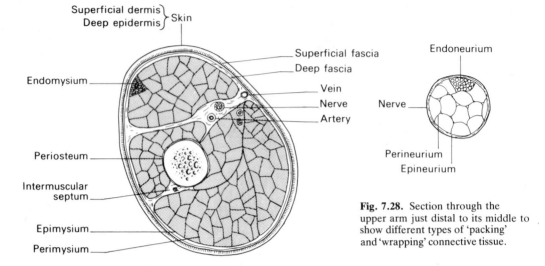

Fig. 7.28. Section through the upper arm just distal to its middle to show different types of 'packing' and 'wrapping' connective tissue.

changes. The trabeculae in the cancellous part of a bone such as the femur, for example, develop in such a way that they are ideally placed to resist the forces to which they are subjected (Fig. 7.19). If the forces change, then so do the positions of the trabeculae. This of course implies the existence of a detection system and the response of the bone cells to its signals (p. 399).

The repair of bone. If a bone is injured the damaged fragments are removed by macrophages and the wound is filled by granulation tissue (as in other connective tissues). The cells of this tissue are recruited from the periosteum and endosteum. However instead of forming fibrous scar tissue at the site of the defect, the granulation tissue acts as a skeletal blastema and replacement bone is regenerated. First chondroblasts differentiate within the granulation tissue and produce a fibrocartilaginous callus which bridges the defect. Woven bone is formed by endochondral ossification within this callus and by subperiosteal deposition at its periphery. Bony trabeculae grow out and eventually unite with the undamaged bone beyond the callus. As ossification proceeds the fibrocartilaginous callus is gradually replaced by a callus of woven bone but this is soon replaced by osteons of mature bone. The remodelling process ensures that the new bone tissue is arranged in the most efficient way to resist the stresses placed upon it.

Replacement is most rapid when the damaged surfaces of a fractured bone are correctly aligned and when there has been little loss of bone sub-stance. This limits the need for callus formation and reduces the need for remodelling.

The importance of all the connective tissues in maintaining the integrity and well-being of the body cannot be over emphasized. They are literally vital materials and without their maintenance in a healthy state, disorganization and death are inevitable.

Gross anatomy

LOOSE CONNECTIVE TISSUE

A brief description of the location and histology of the various types of connective tissue has already been given (p. 349). In this section the gross anatomy and function of connective tissues in specific sites will be considered.

The areolar tissue found deep to the skin is called superficial fascia (Fig. 7.28) and is of variable thickness in different parts of the body. Since the skin consists of an outer epidermis and inner dermis which consists of connective tissue, it may be difficult to determine at what level the dermis can be separated from the superficial fascia. This is frequently complicated by the presence of fibres connecting the skin with the underlying fascia. In some parts of the body, for example the palm of the hand and the sole of the foot, the skin is firmly bound down to the underlying tissue and is almost immobile. In most parts of the body it is impossible to pick up the skin without the superficial fascia. For example, on the back of the hand the 'skin' feels thin, on the back of the forearm it feels thicker (that is, there is more superficial fascia) and on the anterior abdominal wall it is obvious that the skin and superficial fascia are being picked up together. It appears then that the mobility of the 'skin' is very variable in different parts of the body. This attachment of the skin to the underlying tissue is of considerable importance in the healing of skin defects and only relatively small defects are repaired by movement of the skin (really the pulling in of the skin). Frequently skin grafting is necessary.

Fat is found in superficial fascia and the amount varies considerably in different parts of the body. Where it tends to accumulate, the term adipose tissue is used. There are some places, for example, the eyelid, where fat is never found in the superficial fascia. The distribution of fat varies with age, sex, race and climate. In an infant there is a pad of fat in the cheek. This is probably important in suckling. After the age of about 40 years, there is a tendency for fat to be deposited in the trunk, particularly in the anterior abdominal wall, and in those parts of the limbs adjacent to the trunk. This may be due to changed eating habits or lack of exercise, or may be hormonal. In women as compared with men, the subcutaneous fat is distributed throughout the body and this is one factor in producing the different female shape as compared with that of men.

DENSE CONNECTIVE TISSUE

The deep fascia of the body refers to a layer of dense connective tissue lying deep to the superficial fascia (Fig. 7.28). However, although it can be easily demonstrated in the neck and the limbs, particularly the lower, it is not apparently present in all parts of the trunk. Because it is inelastic and strong, deep fascia often provides attachment for muscles, and specially thick parts form slings and partitions (septa) in many parts of the body. Fibro-osseous tunnels (Fig. 7.29) may be formed by the attachment of the deep fascia to the edges or prominences of bones. In the region of the ankle and wrist, thickened, deep fascia forms bands called retinacula which hold down the tendons and prevent their bowing when the muscles contract. The deep fascia of the lower limb may have a circulatory function in that it acts as an inelastic stocking and thus assists the venous return which occurs when the muscles contract. Definite layers of deep fascia may determine the direction in which fluids track from one part of the body to another. For example, fluid in the lower part of the neck may have tracked from the vertebrae in the upper part of the neck due to the presence of a layer of deep fascia in front of the vertebrae and the muscles anterior to them.

Deep fascia may be regarded as a wrapping tissue of the whole body. In the same way dense connective tissue forms a wrapping tissue around a whole skeletal muscle (epimysium), the bundles of muscle fibres within a muscle (perimysium), and the individual muscle fibre in a bundle (endomysium). Similarly a typical peripheral somatic nerve has a wrapping of dense connective tissue (epineurium) within which are bundles of nerve fibres enclosed in a perineurium and each nerve fibre has a covering called the endoneurium (Fig. 7.28). The connective tissue framework of a skeletal muscle has an important function in relation to its contraction (p. 338). The amount of these connective tissues in a nerve of about two to three millimeters in diameter makes it difficult to tear a nerve during dissection, (the student must not try too hard to test the truth of this statement), and the endoneurium may have an important function in

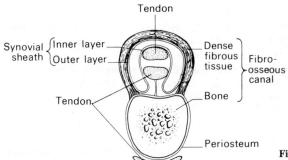

Fig. 7.29. Section through the proximal phalanx of the middle finger.

the regeneration of a peripheral nerve fibre following degeneration due to trauma. This connective tissue endoneurium is not found in the brain and spinal cord.

The outer coat of arteries, veins, and large lymph vessels (tunica adventitia) consists of connective tissue which, on the whole, is better described as loose rather than dense (Fig. 7.28). It varies, however, in different types of vessels being thin in elastic arteries and relatively thicker in muscular arteries. In large veins, the tunica adventitia is thicker than the tunica media and may contain longitudinally oriented smooth muscle fibres.

A much more dense layer of connective tissue is found around bones (periosteum) and hyaline cartilage (perichondrium). There is no perichondrium over an articular surface covered by cartilage. Both periosteum and perichondrium have a thick outer layer consisting mainly of collagen and a thin inner layer containing elastic fibres.

SPECIAL TYPES OF CONNECTIVE TISSUE

The tendons and aponeuroses of muscles (p. 334) and the ligaments of joints are specialized forms of dense connective tissue. Tendons and ligaments are relatively avascular but they have a comparatively rich sensory nerve supply which conducts impulses interpreted as either painful or indicating changes in tension. The latter are often called mechanoreceptors. The ligaments of joints are often present as rounded cords of varied thickness or as flat bands or sheets consisting of collagen fibres in layers which run in different directions. They are important in maintaining the stability of joints and determining the direction and limit of movements at joints. The tensile strength of tendons and ligaments is considerable.

The term ligament is not confined to dense collagenous structures found in the region of a joint. It is also used to describe different types of structures both with regard to their origin embryologically, their composition and their function. For example, a double fold of pleura below the hilus of the lung is called the pulmonary ligament and there are many similar double folds of peritoneum, especially in relation to the liver, which are called ligaments. These consist of connective tissue, but of the loose type, and have little tensile strength. The ligamentum arteriosum, between the left pulmonary artery and the aorta, was the ductus arteriosus in the fetus and its lumen became obliterated after birth. Structurally, it could be described as consisting of relatively dense connective tissue.

Synovial membrane is the name given to connective tissue with the property of secreting synovial fluid, a nutrient and a lubricant. This will be discussed more fully in the section on joints (p. 384). Synovial membrane, where it lines the fibrous capsular ligament, consists of an outer layer of loose connective tissue and an inner layer of cells which are either polyhedral or flattened. The commonest type of cell is probably both secretory and absorptive.

Synovial membrane also occurs in relation to tendons where they are enclosed in tunnels usually consisting partly of bone and partly of dense connective tissue. It is then known as a tendon synovial sheath (Fig. 7.29). This consists of a double fold of loose connective tissue. These folds are continuous with each other at their ends and where the inner fold is reflected back on to the outer. In other words, the tendon is invaginated into its synovial sheath. It should be added that frequently along part of its length the site of reflexion breaks down so that the two layers of the synovial sheath form two cylinders, separated by a small amount of synovial fluid secreted by the contiguous surfaces of the two layers. The presence of these synovial sheaths enables the tendons to glide easily in the compressed space within which they lie and have to move. If a tendon is enclosed within the capsular ligament of a joint, it lies outside the synovial membrane into which it is invaginated and an extension of the synovial membrane accompanies the tendon for a short distance after it has emerged from the capsular ligament.

Another structure with similar functions is called a bursa. These structures are hollow and consist of an outer layer of connective tissue of varying thickness and density of fibres, lined by synovial membrane. Inside there is a small amount of synovial fluid. Bursae are found between skin and underlying bone and may act as a water (saline) cushion to relieve pressure on the underlying skin. They also enable the skin to move more easily over the bone. Bursae are also found between a tendon and a ligament in the vicinity of joints. These bursae can become inflamed and enlarged. This type of pathological change is commonly seen in the bursa in front of the knee-cap or in the bursa between the skin and bone on the back of the elbow. The former is called housemaid's knee and the latter student's elbow.

The coelomic cavity of the embryo becomes subdivided into three cavities each of which is

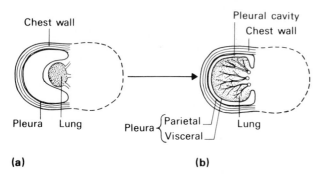

Chest wall

Pleural cavity
Chest wall

Pleura   Lung

Pleura { Parietal
        { Visceral   Lung

(a)   **(b)**

Fig. 7.30. Transverse section of thorax to show invagination of pleural sac by lung.

lined by a serous membrane (Fig. 7.30). The pleural cavity surrounds the lungs and its serous membrane is called the pleura, the pericardial cavity surrounds the heart and its serous membrane is called the pericardium and the abdominal cavity is lined by the peritoneum.

The word serous is a little misleading. It refers to fluid which is derived from the serum of blood, but its composition differs considerably from that of serum in that the secretion from serous glands and serous membranes consists almost entirely of water. There is also a serous membrane around the testis. Because organs invaginate into serous membranes, these membranes are present in the form of double layers, an outer layer called parietal and an inner called visceral (Fig. 7.30). Each layer consists of loose connective tissue and their opposing surfaces are covered by flattened (squamous) cells forming a mesothelium. A small amount of serous fluid is found in the cavity or potential cavity between the two layers. The two layers can therefore glide easily over one another and it can be seen that serous membranes are found around organs which expand and contract (the heart and the lungs) or show rhythmic movements as in the case of the intestinal tract. The two layers of any of the serous membranes may become adherent to each other as a result of disease, and the consequent limitation of function can be severe. The peritoneum may have additional functions. It is absorptive and protective. The latter function is especially found in relation to the large, free-hanging apron of peritoneum called the greater omentum.

The functions of the skeleton
1 That the skeleton gives shape and rigidity to the body is obvious, since without the skeleton, the body would be a shapeless, amorphous mass.
2 The many pieces of the skeleton together

with the joints and muscles provide the body with a system of jointed levers which enable movement to take place. The bones must, therefore, be able to withstand the forces to which they are subjected by muscular contractions and the transference of the weight of the body, not only in standing and walking, but also in running and jumping. As will be seen later, the bones are so constructed that they can perform these functions efficiently.
3 Parts of the skeleton are protective, most notably, the skull in relation to the brain, the ribs in relation to the heart and lungs and the vertebral column in relation to the spinal cord.
4 The bones are also a storehouse for calcium which is removed if the circulating calcium falls below a certain level.
5 Finally, many of the bones contain red bone marrow which is haemopoietic.

The form of an adult bone
The adult form of a bone is determined by a number of factors; fundamentally it is genetically determined. However, nutritional, hormonal and physical (mechanical) factors play a part in determining the way in which a bone grows and what its final shape will be.

Among the mechanical factors are the pull of muscles and tendons, the pressure of overlying structures, the pressure of nerves and vessels, the stresses and strains due to the transmission of weight and the normal alignment of one part of the skeleton in relation to another. Examples of each of these will illustrate their significance.
1 The mastoid process of the temporal bone is said to be produced by the pull of the muscles attached to this region of the bone.
2 There are many depressions and ridges on the inside of the skull and these correspond with the gyri and sulci of the cerebral hemispheres.
3 Grooves on the inner surface of the ramus of

the mandible correspond with nerves which lie in close relation to the bone.

4   The left side of the bodies of the fifth and sixth thoracic vertebrae is flattened due to the pressure of the thoracic aorta.

Of more importance is the internal pattern of the lamellae of bone. These are laid down so that the bone can withstand compression and tension forces. Classically this is best seen in the beautiful architecture of the head and neck and the upper part of the body of the femur. It is also seen as the thickened strut of bone anteriorly between the ramus and body of the mandible. Examples of the effect of changed alignment are most obvious in pathological situations where gross changes produce marked effects on the shape of bones.

Mechanical properties of bone
Because of its structure, bone can resist considerable compression and tension stresses. This is possible because of the combination of inorganic and organic material. Bone has a breaking strain similar to that of cast iron (about 2500 kg/cm^2) and yet is about three times lighter and more flexible. Bone also has to resist torsion, shearing and bending stresses and is capable of resisting forces considerably greater than that of the body weight. It is estimated that in normal walking, at one stage of a step, the upper end of the femur is subjected to a force which is five or six times the body weight: in running and jumping the force is much greater. It is not surprising that in older people, who often show a reduction in the mass of bones (osteoporosis), fracture of the neck of the femur is not uncommon following a comparatively minor torsional stress applied to the femur near the hip joint.

The blood and nerve supply of bone
Long bones have a complex blood supply especially during their development and growth as compared with that of other types of bone. The three main sources of blood are the nutrient artery to the body (shaft), a circle of arteries at the metaphysis (the region between the body and the bone end) and the periosteal vessels. In the growing bone, the metaphyseal arteries are separate from the epiphyseal arteries, which come from a periarticular plexus. There is usually one nutrient artery which enters by a distinct foramen in the body of the bone. The arteries entering the region of the bone ends do so by a large number of foramina. The nutrient artery supplies the medullary cavity and also the bone

almost as far outwards as the periosteum. That this is the main source of blood to the bone is a recent observation as it was believed, and still is by some authorities, that the main blood supply to the body of a long bone comes from the vessels of the periosteum. The branches of the nutrient artery to the bone anastomose with periosteal arteries, and at the ends of the bone, with the metaphyseal arteries. The growth cartilage on both its surfaces is nourished by blood from both the epiphyseal and metaphyseal arteries. When growth ceases and the growth cartilage is ossified, the epiphyseal and metaphyseal arteries anastomose to some extent. It should be added that the periosteal arterial plexus communicates with the arterial plexus of muscles attached to the bone. The metaphyseal arteries arise from main vessels in the region and the epiphyseal arteries form a circle of vessels in the capsule of the joint, the circulus articularis vasculosus.

The venous drainage of a long bone does not follow the arterial supply. A large amount of the blood to the bone itself, although reaching the bone from the nutrient artery, joins the periosteal veins as does the metaphyseal blood. There are, however, metaphyseal veins and usually a nutrient vein.

Short bones, flat bones and irregular bones receive arterial blood from their periosteal vessels and large irregular bones, for example the hip bone, have nutrient arteries. The large basivertebral vein emerging from the posterior surface of the body of each vertebrae deserves special mention. It is said to be related to the haemopoiesis which takes place in the cancellous bone of the vertebral body.

There are small myelinated and non-myelinated nerve fibres in the periosteum, and their branches pass into the underlying bone. They may be related only to the blood vessels, but there in some evidence that they may end in relation to the bone itself. Both the periosteum and bone are very sensitive to stimuli any of which are interpreted as painful.

Terms used in describing bones
The names given to individual bones are often Latin or Greek names which have persisted, but these names frequently have some descriptive basis.

The main part of a bone is usually called the body. Somewhat elongated projections from the body are called processes and these have qualifying terms such as the transverse, spinous and articular processes of vertebrae. A rounded pro-

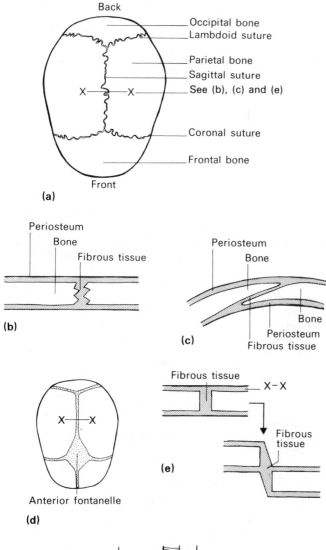

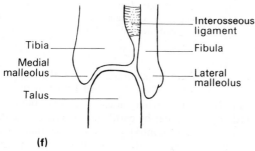

Fig. 7.31. Fibrous joints (a) superior view of the vault of the skull showing the main sutures (b) section through a serrated suture (X–X) (c) section through a squamous suture (d) sutures in a new born infant (e) section of suture in a new born infant to show the possibility of movement (f) fibrous joint between the tibia and fibula just above the ankle joint.

jection is called a tubercle (a variation is tuberosity) and a linear projection a line or ridge. A linear depression is called a groove (sulcus) and a rounded depression a fossa (ditch). A round hole is called a foramen and if it has any length it is called a canal. An opening with width but no depth is called a fissure. The end of the body of a bone is often called the head and a constricted part between the head and body is referred to as the neck. The term condyle refers to a prominence like a knuckle. A thin flat area of bone is called a plate.

It should be remembered that where tendons and ligaments are attached to bone, it is usual for the bone to present a roughened surface. Sometimes the area projects sufficiently for it to receive a specific name such as ridge or tubercle. This is said to be due to the spread of ossification into the tendon or ligament due to the pull exerted by that structure, but it has to be admitted that the area of attachment of a tendon may be represented by a depression and not a projection.

JOINTS

Joints are included in this section because all the tissues comprising a joint are different forms of connective tissue. A joint may be defined as the union between two or more bones. The best classification of joints is based on the way in which the bones are held together. A functional grouping into movable and immovable joints, is not very satisfactory because there is movement at joints of very different structure, and movement may be present, for example, in an infant and not in an older child. On a structural basis there are three types of joints–fibrous, cartilaginous and synovial.

In fibrous joints the bones are held together by fibrous tissue. The fibrous tissue is continuous with the periosteum on the surfaces and edges of the bone. The result is a rigid joint, as a rule. These joints are found between the bones of the skull and are called sutures (Fig. 7.31a & b). If the edges are irregular and interlocked they are called serrated sutures and if they overlap with reciprocal bevelled surfaces, they are called squamous (Fig. 7.31c). With increasing age, after the age of 30 years, the fibrous tissue in some of the suture is replaced by bone (synostosis), but many of the sutures remain indefinitely. It is obvious that if there is sufficient fibrous tissue, movement between the bones is possible, and this may be seen in the newborn child. During labour the size of the infant's head is frequently reduced by the bones of the vault of the skull overlapping each other (Fig. 7.31d & e). After birth the bones move back to their former position. It may be added that the edges of these sutures are not serrated in the infant.

There are other regions which might not be thought of as joints. These are where bones are joined together by fibrous tissue, for example, the tibia and fibula just above the ankle joint (Fig. 7.31f) and the radius and ulna. It would

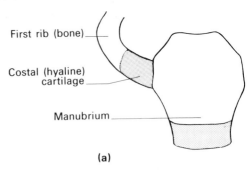

(a)

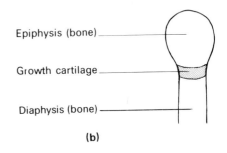

(b)

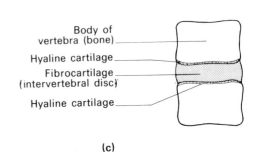

(c)

Fig. 7.32. Cartilaginous joints. (a) A primary cartilaginous joint between the first rib and the sternum and a secondary cartilaginous joint between the manubrium and body of the sternum. (b) A primary cartilaginous joint between an epiphysis and diaphysis. (c) The secondary cartilaginous joint between the bodies of two adjacent vertebrae.

seem appropriate to call the costotransverse joints of the 11th and 12th ribs fibrous joints.

In cartilaginous joints the bones are held together by cartilage. This type of union is subdivided into primary and secondary. At primary cartilaginous joints, the bones are united by hyaline cartilage (Fig. 7.32a). This arrangement is common in the growing child in whom a bony epiphysis is joined to a bony diaphysis by a plate of cartilage (Fig. 7.32b). This is also found in the base of the skull between the basilar part of the occipital bone and the body of the sphenoid bone. It should be emphasized that the periosteum of the bones and the perichondrium of the cartilage are continuous with each other. By the age of 25 years, all of these joints have usually disappeared because the cartilage has been replaced by bone. The first rib remains united to the manubrium sterni by hyaline cartilage.

Secondary cartilaginous joints have a more complex structure and all lie in the midline of the body. The articulating surfaces are covered by hyaline cartilage and a disc of fibrocartilage unites the hyaline cartilage (Fig. 7.32c). Since the fibrocartilage is relatively thick, some movement can be expected at these joints which are found:

1 Between the manubrium and body of the sternum.
2 Between the bodies of the vertebrae (Fig. 7.32c).
3 Between the pubic bones of the pelvis anteriorly in the front line (the symphysis pubis).

The union of the two halves of the mandible anteriorly in the midline is called a symphysis (symphysis menti) but bony union takes place by the end of one year and nothing resembling a secondary cartilaginous joint exists after that time. All the parts of this type of joint are united by the continuity of the outer layers of tissue, the periosteum and perichondrium. The symphysis pubis is completely immobile except during pregnancy during which some softening of the fibrous elements of the connective tissue may occur and bone absorption may take place. This can result in an enlargement of the cavity of the bony pelvis thus assisting the passage of the fetal head during labour. The tissues return to their normal state after pregnancy and immobility is restored.

The manubriosternal joint allows some increase in angulation between the manubrium and body on inspiration. After 40 years of age these two parts of the sternum become joined by bony tissue and the joint disappears.

The intervertebral discs between the bodies of the vertebrae are important in movements of the vertebral column and have a special structure. This will be considered more fully with the vertebral column as a whole (p. 423).

All synovial joints have four basic features; the bones forming the joints are separate; they are held together by a capsular ligament (the capsule); the capsule is lined by synovial membrane; and the bone ends are covered by articular cartilage (Fig. 7.33a). Not unexpectedly, there are exceptions, but only minor ones. The

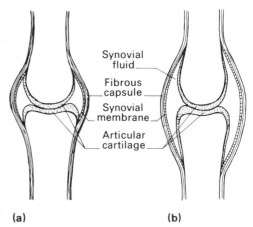

Fig. 7.33. Vertical section through a typical synovial joint to show its structure. (a) The capsule is attached at the edge of the articular cartilage, (b) The capsule is attached beyond the edge of the cartilage.

cartilage on the bone ends in the sternoclavicular and acromioclavicular joints is fibrocartilage and the articulating surfaces of the temporomandibular joint are covered by fibrous tissue. That the bones are separate makes movement more likely but the amount of movement depends, among other things, on the shape of the joint surfaces. To take the two extremes, two flat surfaces firmly bound together by a capsular ligament permit only very little movement in any direction. A ball and socket joint on the other hand permits considerable movement in all directions although limitation may be imposed by structures such as ligaments and tendons of muscles.

The capsular ligament is usually attached to the bone at the edge of the articular cartilage, but not infrequently, it is attached beyond the edge (Fig. 7.33b). The capsule is on the whole very strong and together with the muscles around the joint is able to hold the bone ends together and can resist the normal forces which would tend to separate the bones. The capsule is frequently thickened in one or more places and forms intrinsic ligaments. Sometimes these ligaments are completely separate from the capsule (extrinsic ligaments). The ligaments strengthen the capsule, but they also limit or prevent movements. Similarly different parts of the capsule are loose or tight allowing or preventing movement.

The ligaments and capsule have a rich sensory nerve supply. Large diameter fibres with encapsulated nerve endings are involved in perceiving

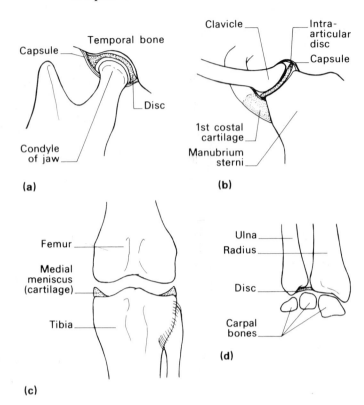

Fig. 7.34. Vertical sections through several joints to show the intra-articular fibrocartilage. (a) Temporomandibular joint. (b) Sternoclavicular joint. (c) Knee joint. (d) Wrist joint.

movements so that the individual is aware of changes in position. The spiral arrangement of the collagen bundles assists this function of the capsule. These nerve endings also subserve complex reflex activities such as walking. Smaller diameter fibres are associated with pain. They are free nerve endings and pain is experienced as a result of excessive twisting and stretching.

The synovial membrane lines the capsule as far as the articular cartilage. If the capsule is attached beyond the cartilage, the synovial membrane is reflected on to the bone as far as the cartilage (Fig. 7.33b). The part of the synovial membrane next to the capsule consists of loose connective tissue and contains sensory nerve fibres associated with pain, but the synovial membrane adjacent to the joint cavity has no sensory innervation. There is a well marked capillary network of blood vessels in the deeper parts of the synovial membrane and also some lymphatic vessels.

Synovial fluid (synovia) is produced by the synovial membrane and acts as a lubricant. It can be regarded as a dialysate of blood plasma.

Hyaluronic acid is synthesized by the lining cells of the synovial membrane and the viscosity of synovial fluid varies directly with the amount of hyaluronic acid present. The binding of the hyaluronic acid to protein is important in the lubrication of joints.

Besides producing synovial fluid, the synovial membrane has other functions. It helps to nourish the articular cartilage adjacent to it (synovial fluid also does this) and it is absorptive. The structure and function of articular cartilage has been discussed previously.

The relation of the synovial membrane to the capsule and articular cartilage has also been mentioned. In some joints, there are ligaments and tendons inside the capsule. These always lie outside the synovial membrane into which these structures are invaginated. In addition, in the case of tendons, a sleeve of synovial membrane surrounds the tendon for a variable distance beyond the capsule. There may be pads of fat between the capsule and membrane, and these assist in lubrication by spreading the synovial fluid within the joint during movements. They also fill spaces which are formed in some joints

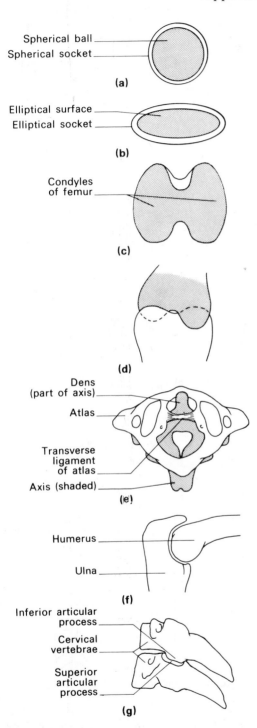

Spherical ball
Spherical socket

(a)

Elliptical surface
Elliptical socket

(b)

Condyles
of femur

(c)

(d)

Dens
(part of axis)
Atlas
Transverse
ligament
of atlas
Axis (shaded)

(e)

Humerus
Ulna

(f)

Inferior articular
process
Cervical
vertebrae
Superior
articular
process

(g)

Fig. 7.35. Types of synovial joint. (a) Ball and socket, (b) ellipsoid, (c) condyloid, (d) saddle-shaped, (e) pivot, (f) hinge, (g) plane (gliding).

as a result of movements. All these structures are better described as intracapsular rather than intra-articular.

Some joints have intra-articular structures called discs or menisci. These are not covered by synovial membrane and consist mainly of dense fibrous tissue with some islands of cartilage. In the temporomandibular and sternoclavicular joints (Fig. 7.34a & b) the discs completely separate the joint cavity into two, although in the former the disc may be perforated. In the acromioclavicular joint, the disc extends only partly across the cavity and in the knee joint there are two crescentic menisci at the periphery of the joint attached to the upper end of the tibia (Fig. 7.34c). There is also a triangular disc separating the radiocarpal (wrist) joint from the inferior radio-ulnar joint (Fig. 7.34d). Attempts have been made to assign one function or origin to all of these discs or menisci. It would appear that their presence absorbs some of the effects of pressure and thus protects the articular cartilage and it has been reported that after removal of the menisci in the knee, pathological changes in the articular cartilage are more likely to occur. Another suggested function is to spread the synovial fluid during movement, so that there is always some lubricant between the joint surfaces. Another theory emphasizes that these structures are present in joints where two types of movement take place at the same time, for example, the temporomandibular and knee joints (rolling and gliding). Whatever their theoretical functions may be, at both these joints the discs or menisci make incongruent surfaces more congruent.

Synovial joints are classified according to either the shape of the joint surfaces or the type of movement which occurs (Fig. 7.35). Their names are: ball and socket, for example, the shoulder joint; ellipsoid, for example, the wrist joint; condyloid, for example, the knee joint in which the condyles (projections) of the femur are parallel, or both the temporomandibular joints in which the condyles are in series; saddle, for example, the carpometacarpal joint of the thumb in which the joint surfaces are reciprocally concavoconvex; pivot, for example, the joint between the dens of the axis, and the anterior arch of the atlas and its transverse ligament; hinge, for example, the elbow joint; plane or gliding, for example, the joints between the articular processes of cervical or thoracic vertebrae.

Movements at joints are usually described as taking place about different axes, and these are

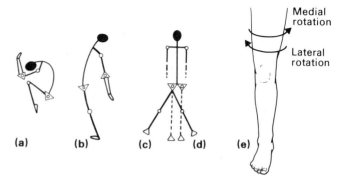

Fig. 7.36. Movements at joints.
(a) Flexion, (b) extension, (c)
abduction, (d) adduction, (e)
lateral and medial rotation.

(a) **(b)** **(c)** **(d)** **(e)**

either transverse, anteroposterior, or vertical relative to the body. At a ball and socket joint movements can take place about all three axes and at an ellipsoid joint about the first two and not about a vertical. At condyloid and hinge joints movements take place about a transverse axis, but some rotation about a vertical axis is possible at a condyloid joint. At a pivot joint, movement about a vertical axis occurs. There is little movement at a plane joint, but a limited amount of gliding, rotation and tilting is possible. Movements about all three axes are possible at a saddle joint but rotation about a vertical axis is limited.

Movements about a transverse axis are called flexion (forwards) and extension (backwards) (Fig. 7.36a & b); about an anteroposterior axis abduction (away from the midline of the body) and adduction (towards the midline) (Fig. 7.36c, d); and about a vertical axis rotation (lateral, so that the anterior surface faces laterally, medial, so that the anterior surface faces medially) (Fig. 7.36e). There are, however, many special terms used to describe movements at different joints, for example, at the temporomandibular joint the terms used are lowering and elevating, and protrusion and retraction of the mandible.

More recently, emphasis has been placed on the type of movement which occurs at the joint surfaces. Given two flat surfaces, sliding and tilting are possible (Fig. 7.37a). If one surface is concave in all directions (female) and one convex in all directions (male), rotating (spin), sliding and rolling movements are possible (Fig. 7.37b). If one surface is concave in only one direction and the other convex in only one direction, spin is impossible. Usually, in either type of joint sliding and rolling occur together (Fig. 7.37c). It can be seen that the shape of the joint surfaces is paramount in determining the type

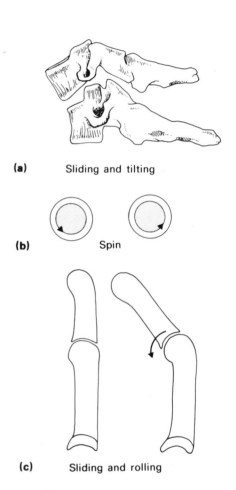

(a)   Sliding and tilting

(b)   Spin

(c)   Sliding and rolling

Fig. 7.37. Types of movement. (a) Sliding and tilting (two flat surfaces), (b) spin, sliding and rolling (one surface concave in all directions, the other surface convex in all directions), (c) sliding and rolling (one surface concave in one direction, the other surface convex in one direction).

and also the range of movements possible. Other factors enter into this, however, and these include the capsule and ligaments and the muscles attached near the joint. Opposition of one part of the body against another, as in the meeting of the teeth, obviously can limit movement. The range of active movement, that is the limits of movement reached by an individual at a particular joint, can often be increased by an external force. This additional movement is called passive movement, although this term is used to describe any movement produced by an external force. Noting the range of active and passive movements is part of the routine investigation of any joint.

MECHANISMS OF CALCIFICATION

The term mineralization refers to the deposition of any mineral. Calcification is the deposition of calcium salts in an extracellular organic matrix. The term ossification refers to the calcification of bone. The relatively insoluble inorganic calcium salt is a mixture of two phases, non-crystalline amorphous calcium phosphate, $CaHPO_4$, and crystalline hydroxyapatite in which the basic unit consists of 18 ions with the formula $Ca_{10}(PO_4)_6(OH)_2$. The crystals of hydroxyapatite can be seen in electron micrographs and are distributed throughout the organic matrix of the calcified tissue. Each crystal in bone is seen as an electron-dense needle approximately 5 nm thick by 30 nm long.

Calcification mechanisms operate not only during the embryonic development and growth of bones but throughout life because bone is continually being deposited within (and removed from) the skeleton (remodelling p. 371). Cementum and dentine are calcified connective tissues which also continue to form throughout life. Initial deposition of calcium salts at primary sites (fetal bone) probably involves a different mechanism from that at sites where calcium salts are continuing to form at an existing calcification front (adult bone).

Complex physiological and physicochemical mechanisms are involved in calcification and these interact in the initiation, spread and subsequently the limitation (perhaps the most important of all) of calcification at very specific sites within selected connective tissues. Reactions between ions and components of the extracellular matrix and the activity of the cells result in the controlled deposition of calcium salts followed by crystal growth.

General mechanisms

Hydroxyapatite (HAP) is the final product of calcification, but before reaching this stage the (Ca^{2+}) and (HPO_4^{2-}) concentrations must increase sufficiently in order to combine and form calcium phosphate. The ions then become arranged into a unit cell of the HAP nucleus. As each side is only about 0.8 nm the unit cell is not resolvable by the electron microscope. A nucleus is defined as the smallest grouping of ions which, given an adequate supply of new ions, will spontaneously grow into the macroscopic form of the crystal. The nucleus is the seed for the next stage during which crystals grow and are orientated into a pattern typical of calcified bone or dentine. Biological calcification, therefore, occurs in three sequential stages, or three levels of organization: first the localized accumulation of Ca^{2+} and HPO_4^{2-} ions: second, the formation of insoluble calcium salts and HAP nuclei: and third, crystal growth and orientation.

Three different experimental approaches have contributed to our understanding of the mechanism of calcification. First, the behaviour of calcium and phosphate ions in the rigidly controlled environment in *in vitro* physicochemical experiments; second, the influence of macromolecules on these inorganic reactions; third, the ultrastructure of the cells and the environment in which the biochemical processes are taking place.

CONTROL BY INORGANIC COMPONENTS

The formation of HAP is represented as:

$$10\ Ca^{2+} + 6\ HPO_4^{2-} \rightarrow Ca_{10}(PO_4)_6(OH)_2 + 2\ H_2O + 8\ H^+$$

For precipitation to occur the product of the concentrations of ions in solution must exceed a 'constant' for the given set of conditions: this constant is the solubility product. Differences in temperature or pH alter the value of this product; also the solubility product is raised if many different ions are present, because the number of effective ionic collisions is reduced.

Provided that the product (Ca^{2+}) and (HPO_4^{2-}), each measured in mmols, is greater than 4.3 mmol², nuclei of HAP spontaneously develop in a solution *in vitro*. Following the appearance of nuclei, crystals of HAP can grow in solutions even if the product is as low as 0.83 mmol². As the $(Ca^{2+}) \times (HPO_4^{2-})$ product in tissue fluid is around 1.67 mmol², HAP cannot precipitate from normal extracellular fluids

$(Ca^{2+}) \times (HPO_4^{2-})$ product is 1.67mmol², HAP cannot ppt without a local ionic booster, catalyst or concentrating mechanism, but once nucleation of HAP has been achieved, crystals can rapidly grow in the ionic concentrations found in body fluids. Two problems arise: how is the ionic product locally raised to 4.3 mmol² to initiate crystal nucleation and how is the rate of crystal growth kept in check?

In newly formed bone where nucleation and crystal growth are rapid, as much as 70% of the mineral is in the form of amorphous calcium phosphate, (ACP), whereas in older bone only 36% is ACP. ACP prepared *in vitro* by precipitation from buffered solutions changes into crystalline HAP. Electron micrographs of samples taken at intervals from the start of the reaction demonstrate that HAP crystals form in close association with ACP spheres and gradually completely replace the ACP. In electron micrographs of newly formed bone, similar ACP spheres are seen around the edges of calcifying regions and between the forming crystals. ACP is short lived, either dissolving or changing into HAP crystals. Nevertheless, its role as an intermediate in calcification cannot be ignored. There is *in vitro* evidence that bone calvaria contain a soluble calcium phosphate, $CaHPO_4 2H_2O$, a highly hydrated aggregate of $CaHPO_4$ which could be the progenitor of ACP.

Although the $(Ca^{2+}) \times (HPO_4^{2-})$ product required to form ACP *in vitro* is lower (2.5 mmol²) than that required to initiate HAP crystals (4.3 mmol²), it is still above the ion product of the body fluid (1.67 mmol²). In fact, in studies with calvaria in physiological solutions, the Ca × Pi product (i means inorganic) is stable up to 3 mmol² (Fig. 7.38). Mineral is not precipitated because of the continuous metabolic production of lactate by the osteoblasts which lowers the pH of the medium to below 6.2. If lactate production is prevented *in vitro*, pH rises and the ionic product falls. Such a cellular control of pH in the bone matrix *in vivo* could provide a mechanism for regulating crystal growth and maintaining Ca^{2+} ion levels in the body fluids. Although the pH of bone matrix is probably kept about 6.8, it seems that there is a mechanism which allows ACP to form even at the ionic product present in plasma. A local increase in pH would then encourage the ACP to change to HAP. Even so, calcium salts do not readily precipitate and grow into macroscopic crystals in the absence of any pre-existing crystals; one reason being that aggregations of ions are highly unstable. These minute crystals very easily redissolve because the surface area available for the escape of ions is large compared with the small number of ions inside the crystal tending to hold them in place. This effect could account for the existence of what appear to be sharp mineralizing fronts, as for example at the predentine–dentine border. Within the predentine, crystals are so small as to be undetected or lost due to their high solubility, but when they reach a certain size their solubility decreases and their growth accelerates tremendously with the result that a sharply delineated mineralizing front appears.

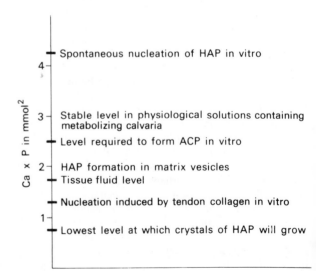

Fig. 7.38. Products of Ca and P (in mmol²) required for nucleating and growing crystals.

CONTROL BY ORGANIC MATRIX COMPONENTS

With the exception of enamel, the matrix into which calcium salts are deposited contains water, collagen, proteoglycans, citrate, lipids, and plasma constituents. The cells concerned with the development of the hard tissues all contain unusually large quantities of the enzyme, alkaline phosphatase. Not unnaturally each of these components has been, and still is being, investigated to find out whether or not it has a role in calcification. Could they, in some way, raise the calcium and/or phosphate concentrations locally, and so cause HAP nuclei to form, and could they then support the growth of the nuclei into crystals?

Two principal calcification theories have evolved over the past 50 years;

1 Ionic concentrations are boosted locally above the levels present in plasma to bring about precipitation of an insoluble calcium phosphate salt;

2 There is a molecular template that captures ions available in tissue fluid in the correct spatial arrangement required for them to grow into a HAP crystal.

Alkaline phosphatase (booster) theory

Robison (1923) noted in his studies on alkaline phosphatase activity that in the presence of Ca^{2+} and Ba^{2+} buffer systems their insoluble phosphates formed. He also observed that calcifying cartilage contained much higher levels of alkaline phosphatase than non-calcifying cartilage. He therefore proposed the theory that this enzyme hydrolysed organic phosphate substrates present in plasma and calcifying tissue fluids, so locally raising the inorganic phosphate concentration. This boosting effect caused the solubility product of calcium phosphate to be exceeded which, therefore, precipitated as $Ca_3(PO_4)_2$ at the site of the enzyme (bone salt was not known to be HAP at the time), e.g.

Glucose-1-phosphate $\xrightarrow[\text{\textit{phosphatase}}]{\textit{Alkaline}}$ Glucose $+ P_i$

$$\text{Plasma} \begin{cases} Ca^{2+} \\ P_i \end{cases}$$

$$Ca_3(PO_4)_3 \text{ ppt} \\ \text{(bone salt)}$$

His theory was criticized for various reasons: first his observations had been based on *in vitro* work on an abnormal tissue namely, rachitic cartilage. Also it did not explain why other tissues showing alkaline phosphatase activity did not normally calcify. Furthermore, subsequent investigations showed that although *in vitro* calcification was inhibited by fluoride, iodoacetate and phloridzin, these substances showed no direct inhibitory effect on alkaline phosphatase.

ATP was found to stimulate *in vitro* calcification and glycogen was shown to be abundant in cells at the onset of calcification but disappeared with its progression. These facts, coupled with the knowledge that the inhibitors of calcification acted on enzymes in glycolysis, led to Robison's 2nd mechanism. This envisaged glycogenolysis (p. 189) as the source of a series of phosphorylated intermediates. These acted as substrates for the alkaline phosphatase-catalysed release of inorganic phosphate, as originally postulated. However, the 'booster' theory was still subjected to stringent criticisms. Apart from those stated, it was calculated that insufficient organic phosphate substrates were present in bone tissue fluid to provide the necessary 3-fold increase in P_i concentration required to cause $Ca_3(PO_4)_2$ precipitation. There was also further *in vitro* evidence that tissue slices from normal healthy animals were calcifiable in solutions containing Ca^{2+} and PO_4^{3-} concentrations below the $Ca_3(PO_4)_2$ solubility product level. Such observations and criticisms stimulated the search for other explanations of tissue calcification.

Neuman proposed a very different role for alkaline phosphatase. In his view it did not supply excess phosphate ions but removed an inhibitor in the matrix which prevented calcification. Subsequently Fleisch and coworkers clearly demonstrated *in vitro* that pyrophosphate in plasma prevents deposition of calcium salts and that alkaline phosphatase added to plasma before incubation destroys this inhibitor and allows calcification to proceed. Fleisch therefore proposed that pyrophosphate acts as a crystal poison, effectively preventing crystal growth by blocking a site in the crystal. This role of alkaline phosphatase, namely to remove inhibitors of crystal growth may be particularly important in calcifying cartilage which is in close contact with plasma in the zone of erosion.

Recently alkaline phosphatase has again been linked with the provision of HPO_4^{2-} ions from organic phosphates. However, it is now thought that the reactants are enclosed within a matrix electron-dense body, the matrix vesicle (p. 393). This allows sufficient excess of ions, even from small amounts of organic phosphate, to accumulate within the vesicle, exceed the solubility product and precipitate. The mechanism is particularly evident in calcifying cartilage and it is interesting to see how Robison's original ideas now fit the new experimental evidence from matrix vesicles.

The collagen template-nucleation theory

During investigations on the ability of blood and extracellular fluids to precipitate bone mineral, the effect of adding collagen preparations to the solutions was tested. In early experiments, it was found that when calf skin collagen was added, calcium salts were not precipitated, whereas with tendon collagen they were. Furthermore, tendon collagen initiated calcification at ionic products of 1.3 mmol² which is lower than blood levels. It was therefore proposed that the collagen fibres had some directing influence on calcification. It was suggested that certain amino acid residues, with charged side chains, provided a specific spatial arrangement that constituted a template matching that of an HAP nucleus. The requisite ions were attracted to these sites, the HAP nucleus formed, and subsequently the crystals grew at the expense of the Ca^{2+} and HPO_4^{2-} in the tissue fluid. The nucleation phenomenon is known as epitaxy. The protein template normally occurs only at calcifying sites, and crystals are nucleated at the calcium/phosphate ionic product values normally present in plasma and tissue fluids. A necessary corollary of this seeding theory is that connective tissues which do not calcify may, therefore, have spatial arrangements of charges in their collagens which do not constitute a template for HAP nuclei formation. Alternatively, certain key charged sites on the template may be protected by chemical groupings (e.g. ground-substance components), with calcifying tissues having some mechanism for exposing them and creating the active template. This latter hypothesis provides a possible explanation for pathological calcification in soft tissues.

Considerable attention has been directed towards characterizing those features of collagen molecules which might act as the epitactic surface for HAP nuclei. It has been demonstrated *in vitro* that alone amongst the various artificially reconstituted collagens (Fig. 3.28) only those having the 64 nm periodicity calcify. This suggests that it is the 3-dimensional organization of the collagen macromolecule rather than the tropocollagen molecule that creates the nucleating template. The 64 nm bands of collagen can be accounted for in terms of particular amino-acid residues, and early in the development of the hypothesis it was suggested that certain lysine and hydroxylysine groups might be important as specific ion-binding sites in crystal nucleation. Phosphate ions were considered to be the first to bind at these sites and so initiate calcification. Recent work has focused attention on Ca^{2+} ion binding sites, and has shown that a reasonable proportion of the carboxyl sites (COO^-), associated with the aspartic and glutamic acid residues, are free and probably involved in nucleation.

Support for the template concept comes from early electron microscope studies which demonstrated that in many calcified tissues, the HAP crystals are regularly arranged with their long axes parallel to that of the collagen fibres; also that the smallest detectable crystals, around 5 nm, are associated with the light bands of the 64 nm repeating unit of collagen.

Another interesting alternative explanation of why certain collagens calcify and others do not has been put forward. The HPO_4^{2-} and Ca^{2+} ions must diffuse through intrafibrillar pores and spaces in order to reach the nucleating sites which are postulated as *inside* the collagen fibril. Whereas the gaps between adjacent tropocollagen molecules in the fibrils in bone are considered large enough (diameter 0.6 nm) to allow the HPO_4^{2-} ions (0.4 nm) through, the corresponding gaps in soft tissue collagens (0.3 nm) are too small. Therefore, bone collagen calcifies within the fibrils whereas soft tissue collagen cannot; some 60% of the inorganic phase of bone in fact is found inside the collagen fibrils. This concept is advanced in support of the theory that bone collagen is an *in vivo* catalyst for HAP deposition, but it does not explain how the extrafibrillar matrix calcifies and in particular how cartilage calcifies.

Lipids

There is abundant evidence which links the distribution of lipid with calcification centres in bone, dentine and cartilage, but there is no clear direct experimental proof that lipids are necessary for calcification. Decalcified bone or dentine cannot be made to recalcify if all the lipid is extracted, but will calcify if part of the lipid remains within the matrix. The method of extracting the lipid is important. Neutral chloroform-methanol extracts a lipid which will not calcify, yet the remaining matrix will recalcify *in vitro*; conversely acidified chloroform-methanol extracts a lipid which will calcify, leaving a matrix which cannot calcify. The lipid fraction associated with the mineral is a phospholipid containing phosphatidyl serine and phosphatidyl inositol. A calcium–phospholipid–phosphate complex has been isolated from young bone and found to induce apatite formation *in vitro* from metastable calcium phosphate solutions. (These are solutions in which the product of the Ca^{2+} and HPO_4^{2-} ions exceeds the solubility product of apatite). Acidic phospholipids extracted from dentine have also been shown to precipitate apatite *in vitro*. Similar phospholipids are also associated with the matrix vesicles in calcifying cartilage (Fig. 7.25), and these cell-derived bodies are the earliest foci of calcification.

Glycosaminoglycans (GAGs) and proteoglycans (PGs)

The precise role of these matrix components in calcification is still uncertain, but many observations suggest that they have a controlling influence. PGs and GAGs isolated from calcifying tissues bind Ca^{2+} ions whereas those from non-calcified tissue do not. Furthermore they inhibit *in vitro* nucleation and growth of apatite, probably by sequestrating Ca^{2+} ions; partial degradation of PGs *in vitro* allows formation of apatite to proceed. Similar degradation occurs in the cartilage matrix within the calcifying zone and this is an important factor in controlling growth of the calcified phase. It seems most likely that these components of the matrix do not initiate calcification, but first inhibit, then later regulate, the rate of calcium precipitation. Secretion of PGs and GAGs and their subsequent depolymerization is controlled by the cells within the matrix.

CONTROL BY CELLS

The cell plays a dominant role in the control of calcification. It controls secretion of the organic matrix, enzymes and metabolic products, and in addition may control the supply of calcium and phosphate.

Ion-storage and release

Studies with (radioactive) ^{45}Ca have shown that calcium passes into the cells through the plasma membrane and then into the matrix. Osteocytes in mouse calvaria go through a 15 day cycle of loading and unloading calcium and phosphate complexes within the cytoplasm. The cells unload at the same time as new calcium deposits can be detected in the adjacent extracellular matrix. A calcium pump at the plasma membrane probably transports Ca^{2+} and HPO_4^{2-} ions. A possible unloading mechanism is described below.

Mitochondria

Mitochondria are known to accumulate Ca^{2+} and HPO_4^{2-} ions and to form ACP deposits which are seen in electron micrographs as very dense granules 30–50 nm in diameter. These always remain as ACP, probably due to the stabilising influence of Mg^{2+} ions. The mitochondria in calcifying tissues contain more of these granules than those in non-calcifying tissues, which suggests that they may have a special role in calcium metabolism. In this context it is perhaps significant that mitochondria *in vitro* rapidly release Ca^{2+} ions if their ATP is converted into ADP and that this release is accelerated by vitamin D and parathyroid hormone. Even so, it has not been proven that mitochondria are concerned in forming 'packages' of Ca^{2+} and HPO_4^{2-} ions for subsequent export into the matrix.

Matrix vesicles

The recent identification of cell-derived matrix vesicles at early calcification sites suggests yet another role for the cell. These membrane-bound vesicles, 100–200 nm in diameter, are found within the organic matrix, destined to become membranous bone; within predentine matrix prior to any calcification; and within the precalcifying zone of growth cartilage. The investing membrane of the vesicle is similar to the plasma membrane and the contents of the vesicle are rich in phospholipids with a strong affinity for calcium. At the onset of calcification the first HAP crystals appear inside the matrix vesicles. Subsequently, calcification spreads from these foci forming calcospheretic masses of HAP crystals. Matrix vesicles, isolated from calcifying tissues by tissue fractionation procedures, induce precipitation of HAP *in vitro* from solutions containing Ca^{2+} and HPO_4^{2-} ions. The minimum solubility product ($Ca \times P_i$) for crystal formation in the presence of vesicles was found to be 2 mmol^2 contrasting with 5–6 mmol^2 in the absence of vesicles. This suggests that matrix vesicles have a nucleating potential and in some way concentrate Ca^{2+} and HPO_4^{2-} ions sufficiently to allow formation of HAP nuclei. Calcium ions may bind to phospholipid to form a nucleation site within the vesicle. As matrix vesicles also contain much of the alkaline phosphat-

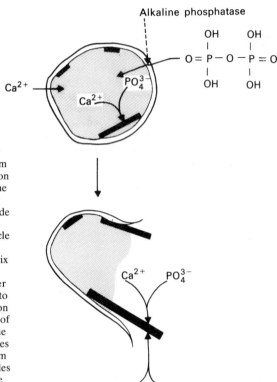

Fig. 7.39. Diagram to show how calcification may start from matrix vesicles. During Phase 1. Calcium ions are sequestered within the vesicle by association with the phospholipid matrix. This either occurs as the vesicle is formed by the cell or by active transport across the vesicle membrane. Phosphate ions are made available through enzymic hydrolysis of inorganic pyrophosphate by alkaline phosphatase at the vesicle membrane. The intra-vesicular ionic product is thereby raised above that of the surrounding matrix resulting in formation of nuclei of hydroxyapatite. Nuclei of HAP form inside the vesicle where the inner membrane provides nucleation sites. These grow into crystals of sufficient size to demonstrate by electron microscopy (thick bars in figure). Continued growth of the crystals is from the ions available in normal tissue fluid. Nucleation of crystals spreads from these sites throughout the surrounding matrix. (Modified from Anderson H.C. (1973) Calcium accumulating vesicles in the intercellular matrix of bone, in 'Hard Tissue Growth, Repair and Remineralization'. Ciba Foundation Symposium II. Elsevier, Amsterdam.

ase present in calcifying cartilage, inorganic pyrophosphate can be hydrolyzed thereby raising the ion concentrations above the $Ca \times P_i$ solubility product so that HAP precipitates. The removal of pyrophosphate also withdraws its influence as a crystal poison. The membrane of the vesicle then ruptures or breaks down. Crystal growth continues at the ionic levels of the tissue fluid and nucleation of crystals spreads throughout the surrounding matrix (Fig. 7.39).

In rickets the low levels of Ca^{2+} and HPO_4^{2-} ions in the body fluids are not sufficient for crystal growth although HAP crystals do form within the matrix vesicles.

In summary, it seems probable that there may be two mechanisms of calcification in most hard tissues. The first, extrafibrillar calcification, results directly from cellular activity via the matrix vesicles; the second, intrafibrillar calcification, depends upon provision of epitactic sites on the collagen fibrils and control of the supply of ions by cells and matrix macromolecules.

CONTROL BY A BONE-MEMBRANE

It has been established in the foregoing sections that crystals grow when supplied by an adequate concentration of calcium and phosphate ions in their fluid environment. This premise poses two problems: how is accretion of new bone mineral halted, and how can the mobilization of calcium ions from the skeletal reservoir into plasma be effected under certain circumstances (p. 762)?

The fluid bathing bone tissue must have a Ca^{2+} ion concentration which is in equilibrium with bone mineral such that crystals neither grow nor dissolve. In contrast, tissue fluid away from the bone surface has a higher Ca^{2+} ion concentration, in equilibrium with the plasma (Fig. 7.40). It has been proposed that the 'bone-fluid' and tissue-fluid compartments are separated by a layer of cells known as the bone-membrane. Since there is a concentration gradient across the bone-membrane, calcium is continuously diffusing in but it is also continuously

Bone mineral   Bone fluid   Interstitial fluid   Plasma

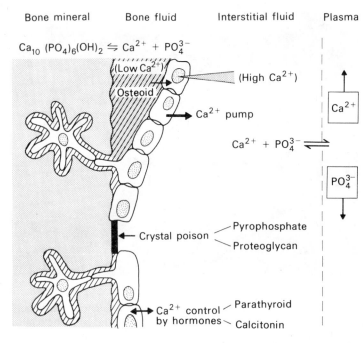

$$Ca_{10}(PO_4)_6(OH)_2 \leftrightharpoons Ca^{2+} + PO_4^{3-}$$

(Low Ca^{2+})

Osteoid

(High Ca^{2+})

Ca^{2+} pump

$$Ca^{2+} + PO_4^{3-} \rightleftharpoons$$

Ca^{2+}

PO_4^{3-}

Crystal poison ← Pyrophosphate

Proteoglycan

Ca^{2+} control ⟨ Parathyroid
by hormones ⟨ Calcitonin

Fig. 7.40. Diagram to show how a bone membrane may act as a biological control system. Bone fluid is in equilibrium with the bone mineral but not with plasma or interstital fluid. The gradient of Ca^{2+} between opposite sides of the cell layer is maintained by a calcium pump. Where cells do not cover the surface of bone, crystal growth is stablized by an inhibitor. Hormones are able to influence the level of Ca^{2+} in the plasma by altering the ability of these cells to move Ca^{2+} ions in and out of the bone fluid, probably by acting on the Ca^{2+} pump. As far as an understanding of this concept is concerned it does not matter whether phosphate is expressed as PO_4^{3-} or HPO_4^{2-}. The amount of the PO_4^{3-} moiety is infinitesimally small at the pH of biological fluids. (After Simkiss K. (1975) *Bone and Biomineralization.* Studies in Biology No. 53. Inst. of Biol. Edward Arnold, London.)

being pumped out by some active cellular process.

A morphologically distinct cellular membrane covers the periosteal and endosteal surfaces of forming bone. In regions not covered by a complete layer of cells it is suggested that ionic exchange is prevented by a crystal poison or inhibitor of crystal growth, either a pyrophosphate or proteoglycan. If the bone-membrane is able to regulate the level of Ca^{2+} and HPO_4^{2-} ions in the bone fluid, then it can participate not only in the formation but also in the dissolution of the HAP. These cellular activities may be modulated by the parathyroid hormone, calcitonin, and 1,25-dihydroxycholecalciferol (p. 763).

Another function of the bone-membrane might be removal of protons, since biocalcification involves not only the precipitation of cations (Ca^{2+}) and anions (HPO_4^{2-}) but also the displacement of protons (H^+), i.e.

$$10\,Ca^{2+} + 6\,HPO_4^{2-} \rightarrow Ca_{10}(PO_4)_6(OH)_2 + 2\,H_2O + 8\,H^+$$

These protons must be removed from sites of calcification, which would otherwise become acidic, and this is probably brought about by a pump in the cell membrane. In contrast, a local accumulation of protons might be one mechanism promoting bone resorption.

Finally there are different rates of formation and degrees of calcification in the calcified tissues throughout the body. These differences are shown as incremental growth lines and are a result of changing patterns of cell activity. Frequently these increments are very regular and can be shown to be due to daily patterns of cell activity, coordinated by physiological mechanisms acting through the cell membranes lining the forming calcified tissues.

PHYSIOLOGY OF BONE

Skeletal homeostasis (maintenance of skeletal integrity)

A constant bone mass is maintained after bone growth has ceased and before the ageing process sets in, despite the fact that some 3–5% of the total skeleton is continually being remodelled. Within any small histological specimen of normal bone it is usual to detect small areas of resorption separated by only a few microns from areas showing deposition of new bone (Fig. 7.41). Although no one knows how these activities are planned at the cellular level, overall remodelling seems to be required in order for adult bones to adapt to various

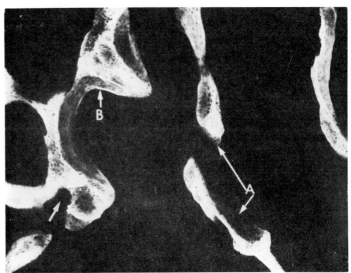

Fig. 7.41. A microradiograph of trabecular bone in which new bone tissue is taking place at A and has just ceased at B. Arrow indicates possible site of active resorption. The site of bone deposition which has recently ceased at (B) is lined by a characteristic thin, high density border × 60. (After Jowsey *et al* (1965) *Journal of Bone and Joint Surgery* **47**A, 785–806.)

mechanical stresses; to provide cavities for haemopoiesis, and to contribute to plasma calcium homeostasis. The small size of the bone crystals gives them an enormous surface area relative to their mass and they can thus act rather like a mixed ion exchange resin for certain ions in plasma. It has been calculated that nearly five grams of calcium is immediately available in the young adult skeleton for exchange and of this about 200 mg is exchanged daily. Appreciable quantities of phosphate, sodium and magnesium are also present in the skeleton and some of this is exchangeable.

The skeleton is affected by mechanical stress and by genetic, metabolic, and hormonal influ-

ences (Fig. 7.42). These influences exert their most profound effects in the growing child. Particular regions of a growing bone are sensitive to particular influences (Fig. 7.43). In a young adult the remodelling is controlled in such a way that the amount of bone resorbed from the skeleton is balanced by the deposition of new bone. As age increases there is no change in the chemical composition of the bone but the balance is disturbed in favour of increased resorption. In non-weight-bearing bones, the endosteal surfaces are resorbed without sufficient compensation by new periosteal bone (Fig. 7.44a), whereas in weight bearing bones it is the trabeculae which are resorbed. Between the

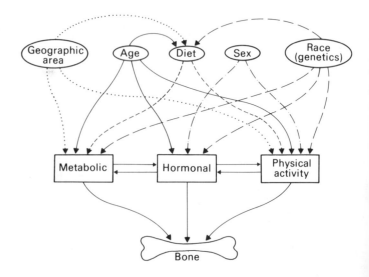

Fig. 7.42. Schematic representation of the factors which influence bone. (After Smith (1967) *Federation Proceedings* **26**, 1737–1747.)

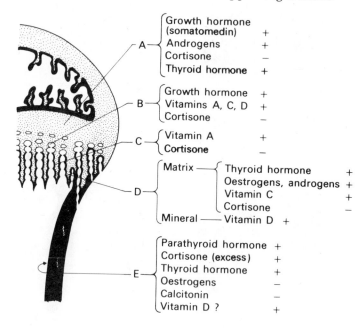

Growth hormone
(somatomedin) +
A { Androgens +
Cortisone −
Thyroid hormone +

Growth hormone +
B { Vitamins A, C, D +
Cortisone −

C { Vitamin A +
Cortisone −

D {
Matrix {
Thyroid hormone +
Oestrogens, androgens +
Vitamin C +
Cortisone −
}
Mineral —— Vitamin D +

E {
Parathyroid hormone +
Cortisone (excess) +
Thyroid hormone +
Oestrogens −
Calcitonin −
Vitamin D ? +
}

Fig. 7.43. Diagrammatic representation of the key stages in bone development at which nutritional and hormonal factors can exert their influence. A, division and proliferation of cartilage cells; B, hypertrophic cartilage cells within tunnels of calcifying cartilage; C, destruction of calcified cartilage; D, osteoblast activity in bone matrix formation and mineralization; E, resorption of bone. Closure of the epiphysis by connective tissue is influenced by oestrogens and testosterone. Stimulatory and inhibitory effects are shown as + or − respectively.

ages of 40 and 80 years men lose about 15% of their bone tissue and women up to 40% (Fig. 7.44b). It is not known whether this generalized rarefaction (osteoporosis), so marked in women, is merely a manifestation of normal ageing or should be regarded as pathological.

DISTURBANCES OF SKELETAL HOMEOSTASIS AND GROWTH

The quantity of bone tissue in any region or in the whole body can be changed by disturbing the normal remodelling processes in four different ways; either by increasing or decreasing the rate of bone resorption, or by increasing or decreasing the rate of bone formation. As is so often the case many of the physiological factors normally controlling these processes were discovered following observations of patients in whom this normal control had been disturbed.

Increased bone loss

Parathyroid hormone (PTH) is directly concerned with maintaining normal plasma levels of calcium (p. 763). The skeleton is called on by PTH to supply calcium in times of need and can act as a reservoir in times of plenty although excess calcium is largely excreted. Any condition which lowers plasma calcium stimulates the secretion of PTH and, if the level is high enough, the mobilization of calcium from the skeleton. For example, both excess thyroid hormone and cortisone decrease intestinal absorption of calcium; the resulting fall in plasma calcium is corrected by mobilization of skeletal calcium.

Many and varied conditions are associated with increased bone loss. One of the most common is the lack of oestrogens in post-menopausal women. Another is renal disease and kidney failure in which there is:

1 Retention of excess hydrogen ions in the plasma which increases bone dissolution,
2 Too much circulating PTH because of a failure to destroy the hormone by healthy kidney tissue at normal rates and
3 Impaired formation of the active vitamin D_3 metabolite in the kidney (p. 766) with a consequent reduction in intestinal calcium absorption.

Immobilization and prolonged bed-rest are associated with an increased excretion of calcium in urine as well as a measurable decrease in bone density. In a recent study this fall in bone density reached 29% in the femoral head after six months immobilization of the legs. Other bones showed smaller changes, but the urinary and faecal calcium figures suggested an overall loss of about 25g of skeletal calcium. As one author cogently expresses it, 'the skeleton passes out through the urethra'.

Decreased bone formation

Normal growth depends on adequate levels of growth hormone (p. 773) and thyroxine (p. 757). Growth hormone affects chondrogenesis but works through an intermediary produced in

(a)

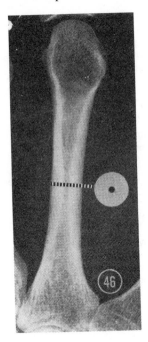
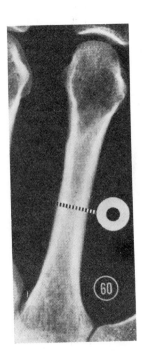

(b)

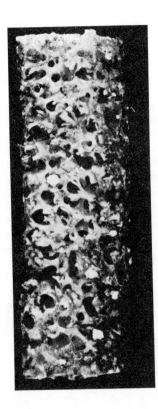
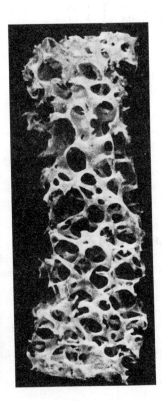

Fig. 7.44. (a) Age changes in the radiographic appearances of second metacarpals of a woman in her 46th year (left) and in her 60th year (right). The medullary cavity enlargement and decrease in cortical area are shown diagrammatically at the sites of measurement. (After Garn *et al* (1967) *Federation Proceedings* **26**, 1729–1736). (b) Fat-free dry bone cylinders from the iliac crest of a twenty-year old (left) and sixty-year old person (right). The enormous reduction in true bone tissue is obvious in the older bone.

the liver called somatomedin; a deficiency in infancy causes dwarfism. Thyroxine is thought to affect osteogenesis; a deficiency in infancy causes cretinism.

A deficiency of vitamin D during childhood results in rickets, in which there is a failure of cartilage and osteoid to calcify with a subsequent overgrowth and weakness of the epiphyses (p. 820). The corresponding condition in adults is osteomalacia, in which many bone surfaces are replaced by poorly mineralized osteoid. These effects cannot be entirely explained by a lowering of plasma calcium resulting from reduced intestinal absorption. It has been proposed that osteoblasts are a target for vitamin D since in its absence they produce a less calcifiable matrix.

Vitamin C is necessary for collagen synthesis. In cases of severe deficiency, the number of osteoblasts is reduced, less osteoid is formed and a thin brittle network of calcified cartilage replaces the normal epiphyses.

The anti-anabolic effects of steroids such as hydrocortisone and cortisone are manifested by a reduction in the rates at which collagen and chondroitin sulphate are synthesized.

Increased bone formation

Excess production of growth hormone (p. 773) in children produces gigantism and in adults produces acromegaly. It acts via somatomedin on cartilage and areas of potential chondrogenesis.

The spurt in skeletal growth which is observed at puberty is usually attributed to the output of adrenal androgens in both boys and girls. Sexual maturation in fact initiates the ossification of epiphyses and the termination of body growth, but this seems to be controlled by the gonads rather than by the adrenal glands since in eunuchs or cases of hypo-gonadism the epiphyses of the long bones remain open, leading to an exaggerated length of the limbs.

Oestrogens, like androgens, are anabolic steroids; they influence the formation of osteoid. Administration of oestrogens to young animals produces complex effects; limb bone growth is stopped prematurely with the result that the bones are short despite the fact that bone deposition in the endosteum may have been encouraged.

Reduced bone resorption

The action of PTH in mobilizing bone calcium is opposed by that of calcitonin which slows the rate of resorption (p. 765).

Deficiency of vitamin A hinders the remodelling of calcified cartilage and leads to stunted bone development. It is thought that the vitamin is required for the synthesis and subsequent release from lysosomes of acid hydrolases. Osteoclast activity is also suppressed so that the remodelling of bone is impaired. When too much bone is formed around foramina the nerves become gradually compressed and there is paralysis. It was due to this observation on puppies suffering from hypovitaminosis A that it was originally, incorrectly, thought that vitamin A was necessary for nerve function.

Oestrogens have been administered in an attempt to reverse the bone loss which is triggered by endocrinal changes at the menopause. A transient improvement both in the appearance of bone and in calcium balance has been reported in many but not all studies. Oestrogens may 'protect' bones from the effects of parathyroid hormone.

STRESSES AND STRAINS ON BONE

Both the apatite crystals and collagen fibres in bone are regularly arranged, but because the arrangement is not perfectly regular it is said that they have a preferred orientation. For this reason the mechanical strength of bone differs according to the plane in which forces are applied. The matrix deforms under load and distributes the stress to the crystals. With progressively increasing loads, bone is first elastic (elastic range), then becomes plastic (plastic range), and finally breaks. If tensile stresses within the plastic range are continuously applied to bone via the collagenous tendons, new bone is laid down in the direction of tension. If the stresses exceed the plastic limit, the connective tissues disrupt with the result that the stress is removed from the bone and bone growth ceases.

If a horizontal force is applied to a tooth for 2 or 3 days, the tooth tilts in its socket and osteoclasts differentiate on the surfaces of alveolar bone in the compression zones and, a little later, osteoblasts differentiate in the tension zones (Fig. 7.45). It might be said that pressure causes resorption and tension causes deposition.

It is not known how pressure leads to the differentiation of osteoclasts. When pressure has been applied to a tooth it moves and the periodontal ligament is compressed. However, this does not prove that the adjacent bone is subjected to an increase in pressure. Fluid might just be displaced to the other side of the tooth, the tension region. One suggested mechanism is that the microcirculation is altered differently on the compression and tension sides with the result

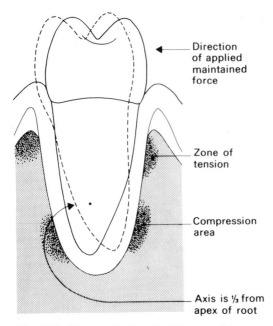

Direction
of applied
maintained
force

Zone of
tension

Compression
area

Axis is ⅓ from
apex of root

Fig. 7.45. Diagram showing the effects upon the alveolar bone of a maintained horizontal force applied to the crown of a premolar. The compression or pressure areas show resorption of bone, whereas at the tension zones new bone will be deposited.

that the metabolism of the cells is altered in such a way that they respond by resorbing and depositing bone respectively.

Another system proposed is that the mechanical energy of deformation is converted into potential chemical energy. Tension applied to bone is thought to decrease the bond energy between molecules of the solid, thus raising the solubility so that calcium enters the bone cell enviroment and stimulates osteoblasts or inhibits osteoclasts. Compression presumably has the opposite effect. The response of the bone cells thereby alters the structure of bone in such a way as to release it from the mechanical stress.

Finally a piezo-electric effect could be involved. It has been shown that when a rod of bone is bent, the side under tension becomes negatively charged and that under compression becomes positively charged (Fig. 7.46). The effect, which is due to the properties of collagen and apatite and their arrangement, is similar to the piezo-electric effect produced when crystals such as quartz are deformed. It is possible that the charges developed on the surfaces of deformed bone provide the stimulus for the differentiation of the appropriate cell type.

The chemical reactions involved in bone

resorption by osteoclasts and osteocytes are still uncertain. Some of the views are discussed elsewhere (p. 370).

SUMMARY

The underlying theme in this section is that bone is a dynamic, living tissue which is subject to a variety of influences; genetic, physical, nutritional and hormonal. Though the means by which these affect bone are beginning to be understood in biochemical terms the processes concerned in the remodelling of bone at a cellular level are still largely unknown.

DEPOSITION OF FLUORIDE

Mechanism of incorporation
Fluoride ions are incorporated into calcified tissues by exchange with hydroxyl ions within the lattice and on the surface of hydroxyapatite crystals both during and after their formation and growth according to the equation:

$$Ca_{10}(PO_4)_6(OH)_2 + 2 F^- \rightarrow Ca_{10}(PO_4)_6F_2 + 2 OH^-$$

Fluoride is also held in the hydration shell around the apatite crystals.

As the crystals are extremely small they present an enormous surface area to their fluid environment so that there are considerable opportunities for surface exchange. The partial conversion of hydroxyapatite to fluorapatite is easily effected because the OH^- and F^- ions are approximately the same size.

Fluoride in bone
The deposition of fluoride in the skeleton is related to the fluoride intake in food and water

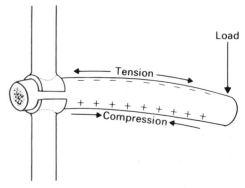

Load

Tension

Compression

Fig. 7.46. The piezo-electric effect on a rod of bone which is being bent.

and to the age of an individual. Fluoride is more readily incorporated in the bones of children because of their greater rates of growth and formation, but it continues to accumulate slowly and steadily over the whole life span.

In individuals over 70 years of age there is a slight deviation from the almost linear relationship between fluoride in bone and age (Fig. 18.7). This may be the result of a preferential removal of endosteal bone (having a lower fluoride concentration than periosteal bone), which gives rise to an apparently higher fluoride content of the whole bone. Deposition of fluoride in the skeleton is not an irreversible process however. Individuals moving from an area with a high concentration of fluoride in the drinking water to one with a lower level mobilize and excrete a small fraction of their skeletal fluoride. After several years of ingestion of fluoride at a particular level there is a situation approaching but not quite reaching an equilibrium between the fluoride concentration in extracellular fluid and that in the hydration shells and exposed crystal surfaces (Fig. 7.4c). Consequently plasma fluoride increases as the skeletal fluoride levels rise with age.

Skeletal fluorosis
Prolonged ingestion of fluoride in amounts many times greater than those either advocated as a dental public health measure or found naturally in many water supplies can cause skeletal fluorosis. This condition has been reported in grazing cattle exposed to industrial dust containing fluoride and in farm workers in hot countries like India who drink large quantities of water containing high concentrations of fluoride to relieve their thirst. Mild skeletal fluorosis is characterised by an increase in bone density (osteosclerosis) which may be symptomless but may progress to the crippling form of the condition in which there is thickening of vertebrae, compression of the spinal cord, calcification of ligaments, and exostoses. It seems probable that some of the changes in skeletal fluorosis are due to the action of fluoride on sensitive enzyme systems in osteoblasts.

FURTHER READING

MELCHER A.H. & EASTOE J.E. (1969) In *Biology of the Periodontium*. Editors A. H. Melcher and W. Bowen, pp. 167–343. Academic Press, London.

ISRAEL H. (1967). Loss of bone and remodelling-redistribution in the craniofacial skeleton with age. *Federation Proceedings*, **26**, 1723.

SMITH R.W. (1967). Dietary and hormonal factors in bone loss. *Federation Proceedings*, **26**, 1737.

VAUGHAN JANET M. (1970) *The Physiology of Bone*. Clarendon Press, Oxford.

CHAPTER 8

Lining Tissues

EPITHELIUM

Epithelia are tissues which cover surfaces with continuous sheets of cells: the surfaces may be large, as in the case of the skin, or small, as in the case of the lining of ducts in salivary glands. Epithelial cells are usually in close contact with each other over a substantial part of their surfaces, there being very little intercellular material. The category of epithelial cells can be extended to include the parenchymal cells of solid organs and glands developed from epithelial surfaces.

Epithelia generally originate from ectoderm or endoderm. Surface layers derived from mesoderm, known as mesothelia, cover extensive areas in the body such as the opposing surfaces of the pleural and peritoneal cavities. It is difficult to avoid including mesothelia in any morphological classification of epithelia but it must be remembered that the component cells differ from epithelial cells not only in their origin but also in their behaviour and, most importantly, in their pathology.

Epithelial cells are usually distinctly polarized; that is to say one end of the cell (basal) differs in structure and function from the other (apical) end. Where the epithelium consists of a single layer of cells the basal end of each cell (facing towards mesoderm) is in contact with a basal lamina. In stratified epithelia (Fig. 8.2d) only the basal cells have such contact; cf. junctional epithelium of the tooth (Book 2).

Basement membrane and basal lamina

A basal lamina is found beneath all normal epithelia (Fig. 8.1). As it is less than 100 nm thick it can only be seen in the electron microscope. It consists of two layers, a lamina lucida which appears clear, and a lamina densa which appears stippled. The amount of material in each of these layers is very small but it is believed that the glycoproteins present include type IV collagen (p. 66). The components of the basal lamina are produced by the epithelial cells. A basal lamina is always present between the junctional epithelium and the surface of a tooth (Book 2).

Beneath the basal lamina is a thicker layer of reticulin and fine collagen fibres. This layer is readily stained (by some silver solutions, and the PAS reaction for example) and seen in sections studied by light microscopy. Under the light microscope only a single stained membrance, presumably consisting of the basal lamina and the reticular layer, can be seen. It is called the basement membrane.

Classification of epithelia

1 By the number of cell layers:

(a) Simple—a single cell layer with all cells in contact with the basal lamina.

(b) Stratified—several layers of cells but only basal cells in contact with the basal lamina.

(c) Pseudostratified—all cells in contact with the basal lamina but with nuclei at different

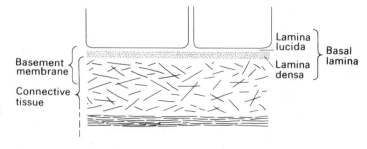

Fig. 8.1. The position of basal lamina in epithelium.

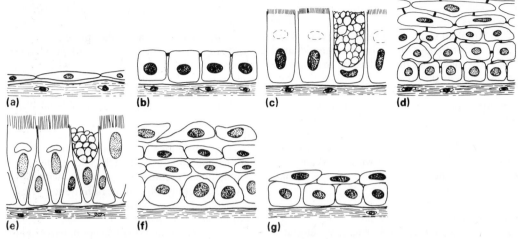

Fig. 8.2. Epithelia. a) Simple squamous, b) simple cuboidal, c) simple columnar (with mucous cell), d) stratified squamous (non-keratinized), e) pseudostratified columnar ciliated (mucous cell), f) transitional (organ contracted), g) transitional (organ dilated).

levels. Some cells do not reach the surface giving a false appearance of stratification.

2 By the shape of the cells:
  (a) cuboidal
  (b) columnar
  (c) squamous (flattened)

3 By the presence or absence of cilia (where relevant).

4 By the presence or absence of keratin (where relevant).

SIMPLE EPITHELIA

Simple squamous epithelium (Fig. 8.2a)
A single layer of flattened, often more or less hexagonal cells in surface view, simple squamous epithelia are uncommon but line the smaller ducts of some glands. Simple squamous epithelium lines Bowman's capsules, the descending limbs of the loops of Henlé in the kidney and the air spaces of the lungs. The category is sometimes broadened to include mesothelia, lining serous cavities (e.g. pleura and peritoneum) and endothelia lining blood vessels.

Simple cuboidal epithelium (Fig. 8.2b)
The cells appear square in vertical section although they fit together as polyhedrons to cover the surface. This epithelium is seen in glands such as the thyroid, in many ducts from different glands, on the surface of the ovary and in the choroid plexuses.

Simple columnar epithelium (Fig. 8.2c)
In a vertical section columnar epithelial cells are much taller than cuboidal cells. In a typical example the nuclei are oval and all at the same level, usually slightly nearer the basal pole of the cell. The Golgi apparatus is commonly found at the apical pole of the nucleus and may show as a paler-staining area in the light microscope.

Simple columnar epithelium lines most of the alimentary canal from the cardiac sphincter of the stomach to the anal canal and the cells are divisible into different functional types such as mucous and absorptive cells. It also lines the larger ducts of glands, for example the salivary glands.

The apical surfaces of columnar cells can have various modifications, indeed a simple flat surface is most unusual. In the gut many of the cell surfaces are specialized to form elaborate series of microvilli producing what, for obvious reasons, are known as brush borders.

A special modification is the possession of apical cilia. Ciliated simple columnar epithelium lines the bronchioles of the respiratory tract and the uterus and Fallopian tubes.

STRATIFIED EPITHELIA

In truly stratified epithelia, the cells are arranged in layers. Only the basal layer is in contact with the basal lamina: the basal cells do not extend upwards into the other layers.

The cells of the basal layer are capable of

mitosis and provide a constant supply of new cells which pass upwards into the more superficial layers.

In stratified squamous epithelium (Fig. 8.2d) the cells become progressively flattened until they are shed from the surface as squames. In many sites, as they differentiate, the cells progressively synthesize more of the fibrous protein keratin so that ultimately the squames shed from the surface are dead and completely cornified. This form, which is known as keratinized stratified squamous epithelium, covers the external surface of the body where it is called the epidermis of the skin. It also lines part of the oral cavity (p. 530).

Stratified columnar epithelium
This is found in very few places, usually at a junction between one tissue lined or covered with columnar epithelium and another lined with stratified squamous epithelium. It forms part of the conjunctiva, and lines part of the urethra, the anal mucous membrane, pharynx, epiglottis and the ducts of some glands.

Pseudostratified columnar epithelium (Fig. 8.2e)
This is a much more common type of epithelium whose ciliated variety lines the greater part of the respiratory tract. It differs from a truly stratified epithelium in that all the component cells have contact with the basal lamina. However, only the tall superficial cells, reach the surface; the remainder are basal or supporting cells. This arrangement leads to an appearance of stratification because in a vertical section the nuclei of the cells are at different levels and unless the section is quite vertically orientated many of the superficial cells are not seen to reach the basal lamina. In its non-ciliated form this epithelium is only rarely seen; for example in the main ducts of salivary glands and in the male urethra.

Ciliated pseudostratified columnar epithelium
This is one of the commonest epithelia of the body, lining as it does most of the respiratory mucosa. In this situation some of the 'superficial' cells are mucous goblet cells; the intervening cilia beat to create a gentle flow in the film of mucus secreted on to the surface.

Transitional epithelium (Figs. 8.2f and g)
This special type of epithelium is not easily related to the forms already described. Despite its name it is not transitional between stratified squamous and simple columnar epithelia. Trans-

itional epithelium lines organs which are capable of distension and contraction—the most characteristic being the urinary bladder. Thus when such organs are contracted the epithelium covers a much smaller surface area and possesses a basal cuboidal or columnar layer with several more superficial layers of irregularly shaped cells. There is no flattening of the cells towards the surface—indeed the surface cells have elevations projecting into the lumen of the organ in question. When the organ (e.g. the bladder) becomes distended, the cells of the transitional epithelium slide across each other to form an epithelium of greater surface area but with fewer layers, generally two, of more flattened cells.

Epithelial cell structure
The components of individual epithelial cells are dealth with in Chapter 4. Particular attention should be paid to some groups of organelles. The surfaces of epithelial cells are frequently specialized and several important adaptations must be borne in mind, notably; microvilli, cilia, desmosomes and hemidesmosomes, tight junctions and terminal bars (p. 174). In addition, many epithelia contain specialized cells and reference should be made to relevant sections for details. Such cell types include:
1　Mucous cells—found in many places especially in the gastro-intestinal and respiratory tracts.
2　Cells of the pigment-forming system.
3　Myoepithelial cells in salivary glands.
4　Some endocrine cells: e.g., argentaffin cells.
5　Taste buds.

Regeneration of epithelia

The special subject of wound healing will not be dealt with in detail. Epithelia always contain cells which are capable of mitosis. These may be scattered randomly or they may be arranged in localized areas or special regions. Examples of the latter arrangement are found in the epidermis where all the dividing cells are situated in the basal layer of a stratified squamous epithelium, and in the small intestine where mitosis occurs only in the depths of the crypts of Lieberkühn. In these cases the architecture of the epithelium is such that the daughter cells of mitoses are restrained to migrate in well-defined directions and while doing so they differentiate in their own specific way, ultimately to be shed or lost (Fig. 8.3). This process is regulated within close limits so that the loss of cells is exactly balanced by the number of mitoses. It is possible to measure the

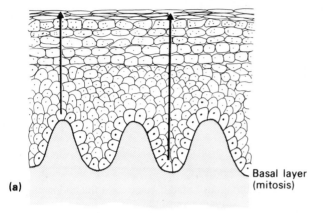

(a)

Basal layer
(mitosis)

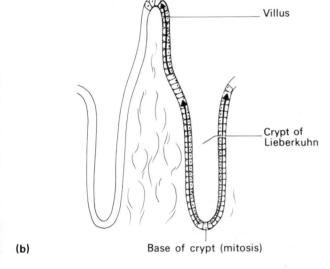

Villus

Crypt of
Lieberkuhn

(b)   Base of crypt (mitosis)

Fig. 8.3. Regeneration of epithelium. a) Pathway of migration in stratified squamous epithelium. b) Mitosis in base of crypt of Lieberkühn.

speeds at which these cells move and their rate of turnover in several different ways.

The mitotic index is defined as the number of mitoses found at any one time in 1,000 of the potentially mitotic cell population (e.g. basal cells). The higher the mitotic index, the more rapid the turnover of the tissue. Estimates may also be made of the time taken for any cell to pass through the whole process of differentiation (e.g. from basal cell to keratinized squame), or of the time taken for all the cells in a given tissue to be replaced.

The rate of turnover of a tissue can be influenced by various factors. There is usually an in-built diurnal rhythm and generally the rate of turnover declines with increasing age. The rate may also be influenced by hormone levels and injury. When tissue is lost due to injury the rate of mitosis in the surviving cells increases to make up the deficiency. The control of mitosis may be

due to the release of a chemical substance (chalone) by non-dividing cells.

In the healing of epithelial wounds cells may migrate to cover the underlying connective tissue before the mitotic rate increases. In the skin and oral mucosa, 'non-mitotic' cells of the stratum spinosum migrate over the exposed (healing) mesoderm before the cells of the stratum basale increase their mitotic rate. Subsequently cells of the stratum basale insinuate themselves over the connective tissue.

After a large area of skin has been damaged, the mode of healing depends on the depth of the injury. If epidermal appendages such as hair follicles survive in the bed of the wound epidermal cells will migrate from this source. When damage extends beyond the dermis epidermal healing is possible only from the edge of the wound. During regeneration, large wounds contract with resultant scarring due to the formation

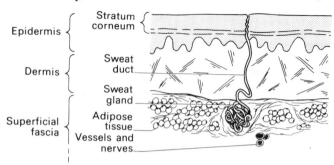

Fig. 8.4. A section of skin on sole of foot.

of fibrous tissue. To minimize the deformity and to accelerate repair, whole skin grafts are used. Alternatively the exposed tissue may be 'seeded' with mitotic epidermal cells as in split-skin grafts or pinch-grafting.

STRUCTURE AND FUNCTION OF SKIN

The skin is a compound structure and from structural, functional and clinical points of view is best regarded as a separate organ of the body.

The skin consists of two parts (Fig. 8.4), the epidermis which provides the outer epithelial covering, has a protective function and is mainly of ectodermal origin, and the dermis which is mainly supportive in function and is of mesodermal origin. In addition there are hairs and hair follicles, nails, sebaceous glands, sweat glands and apocrine glands to be considered as well as the pigment-forming system of the epidermis.

The hypodermis or superficial fascia is that tissue deep to the dermis: it is not anatomically part of the skin even though its functions may affect the properties of the skin itself.

Epidermis

The epidermis is a keratinized stratified squamous epithelium. Its thickness varies from little more than 0.1 mm over the abdomen and flexor surfaces of the arms to about 1.5 mm on the sole of the foot. Variations in the thickness of the epidermis are due to the thickness of the outermost horny layer of dead cells and are partly a response to friction and pressure and partly genetically determined. Regional variations are present at birth.

In regions such as the soles of the feet, finger tips and palms of the hands there is an elaborate system of ridges and grooves on the surface of the epidermis. The overall pattern is typical of the area of the body but the detail is unique to the individual and forms the basis of dermatoglyphics (finger printing) and palmistry. The pattern is not innate to the epidermis but depends on the dermis for its initiation and maintenance.

HISTOLOGICAL STRUCTURE

The epidermis is conventionally described as a sequence of cell layers (Fig. 8.5):
1 Stratum basale or germinativum (basal layer).
2 Stratum spinosum (spinous or prickle cell layer).
3 Stratum granulosum (granular layer).
4 Stratum corneum (cornified layer).
In some situations a stratum lucidum separates 3 and 4.

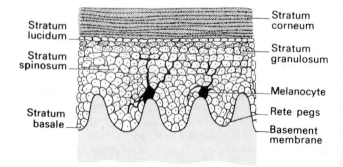

Fig. 8.5. The detailed structure of the epidermis.

The stratum basale is in contact with the basal lamina; it is a single cell thick and contains cells capable of mitosis. The stratum spinosum, the thickest layer, contains larger polyhedral cells joined by prominent 'intercellular bridges'—the 'spines' or 'prickles' of the layer. The short, spiny, cellular processes are joined by desmosomes. The stratum granulosum is characterized by basophilic keratohyalin granules. There is a clearly defined boundary between this layer and the stratum corneum beyond which all cellular detail is replaced by an acidophilic mass of keratin. However, the cell boundaries remain quite distinct in the stratum corneum.

In the sole of the foot and the palm of the hand a clear layer, the stratum lucidum, separates the stratum granulosum from the stratum corneum.

Stratum basale

The basal cells of the epithelium lie close to the basal lamina which is considered in more detail above. The cells are cuboidal or rounded with large nuclei. The cytoplasm is basophilic because of the ribonucleic acid (RNA) present in numerous free ribosomes. Endoplasmic reticulum is practically absent showing that the protein synthesis in which the RNA is involved is for growth and intracellular use and not for the synthesis of secretory products. The cells adhere to the basal lamina by means of hemidesmosomes and to each other by desmosomes (Fig. 4.12). The desmosomes are closely related to bundles of cytoplasmic fibrils (tonofilaments) in the epidermis.

Mitosis is restricted to the basal layer. The number of mitoses per thousand basal cells or 'mitotic index' is a measure of the rate of cell production. It is approximately 3 per 1000 in human epidermis and is higher at night than in the daytime. One daughter cell from each mitosis loses the ability to divide and migrates towards the surface.

Stratum spinosum

As the migrating cells differentiate, the cytoplasm increases in bulk. Free cytoplasmic ribosomes remain very numerous and the number of dense bundles of tonofilaments increases progressively. Intercellular spaces are small but many processes form where the cells are joined by desmosomes. These processes give the cells a spiny appearance. There is no cytoplasmic continuity at these sites, i.e. they are not truly intercellular bridges.

Towards the upper part of the stratum spinosum, the cells begin to flatten out and develop tiny cytoplasmic granules. These are quite unlike keratohyalin granules (see later) and cannot be seen in the light microscope. At a later stage the granules are discharged from the cells into the intercellular spaces where they add to the intercellular material and act as a barrier to permeability.

Stratum granulosum

Flattening of the cells and accretion of tonofilaments continues. A new component, keratohyalin, appears in the form of granules. These vary in size from about 0.5 μm to 5 μm, they stain basophilically and are known to contain RNA. They have a relatively high content of sulphur-containing amino acids (cysteine).

Stratum lucidum

In stained sections of epidermis from the sole of the foot and palm of the hand a narrow transparent layer is seen between the stratum granulosum and stratum corneum where the squames are filled with refractile droplets known as eleidin. The nature of the change occurring here is not known and the stratum lucidum is not always visible.

Stratum corneum

The cells of the stratum granulosum undergo two major changes. First the plasma membrane increases in thickness by the addition of material, possibly lipid, to its inner surface. Immediately after membrane thickening practically all the cell contents including the nucleus, ribosomes, mitochondria and keratohyalin granules disperse and can no longer be separately distinguished. The contents now consist of a fibrous material embedded in a homogeneous amorphous matrix. The desmosomes gradually break down and the cornified 'squames' are finally lost from the surface.

KERATINIZATION

Keratin is an extremely insoluble fibrous protein with great chemical and physical stability. Its composition varies considerably according to its origin but is most notable for the amount of sulphur which is present in the form of $-SH$ groups in the amino acid cysteine. Metabolic studies of the skin using radioactively labelled amino acids have shown that keratin synthesis begins in the basal layer and continues actively in all layers up to the stratum granulosum. Keratin accumulates in the cytoplasm and as it does so the degree of crosslinking in the keratin molecules increases with the conversion of cysteine to cystine.

The keratin of the stratum corneum contains two fractions. One is fibrous, contains little sulphur and is derived from the tonofilaments. The other is amorphous, contains much more sulphur and may be derived from the kerato-hyalin granules. The thickened plasma membrane provides a water-resistant envelope in which the keratin is enclosed. Epidermal cells take 35–80 days to pass through the full process of keratinization in human skin.

Dermal–epidermal junction

In section the junction is irregularly shaped with numerous rete pegs apparently protruding from the epithelium and interlocking with matching dermal papillae. A surface view of the dermal–epidermal junction shows either a peg (dermis) and socket (epidermis) arrangement or a system of ridges and valleys.

The pattern of the dermal–epidermal junction is not related to any surface ridges of the stratum corneum but is known to be correlated with the direction of the major shear stresses on the surface. This supports the concept that it is a device for increasing the mechanical strength of the junction. At the same time the folds increase the surface area of the basal layer and this may be of importance in relation to the blood supply and cell kinetics of the epithelium.

Dermis

The connective tissue immediately underlying the epidermis is known as the dermis (Fig. 8.4). It is analogous to the lamina propria of the alimentary canal. Its thickness varies from approximately 0.5 mm on the eyelids to more than 3 mm on the soles of the feet and palms of the hands. Its boundary with the epidermis, the basement membrane, has already been described (Fig. 8.1). The deeper boundary is indistinct because it cannot be readily separated from the underlying superficial fascia (hypodermis or subcutaneous layer).

The dermis consists of dense fibrous connective tissue in which the collagen fibres run parallel to the surface interspersed with elastic fibres especially near glands and hair follicles. It contains cells typical of connective tissues; fibroblasts, histiocytes (macrophages), capillary endothelial cells and perivascular cells, and cells from the blood such as lymphocytes. Capillary blood vessels and lymphatics, loops of small nerves and nerve endings are also found. Fat cells are seldom present. The sebaceous glands and hair follicles of the skin are situated in the dermis but sweat glands are often found deep to it.

The dermis may also contain smooth muscle fibres, for example in the perineum and scrotum. The striated muscle fibres of the muscles of facial expression are inserted into the dermis.

Superficial fascia (see also p. 378)

Without being part of the organ which is defined as skin, the superficial fascia contributes to the character of the skin, especially its mobility and flexibility. In most situations the superficial fascia is a loose fibrous tissue that allows the skin to slide over the underlying deep fascia which is a dense fibrous tissue. In some places however it may be thick and densely fibrous, holding the dermis closely to the underlying tissues as on the sole of the foot (Fig. 8.4). It may be thick but largely adipose, as over the abdomen and it may be very thin and only moderately fibrous, as on the eyelids. The tissue contains larger blood vessels, lymphatics and nerves.

Hypodermic injections for therapeutic purposes are given into the superficial fascia, which being loose, can be distended without causing pain. Intradermal injections (into the dermis) are painful because the injected fluid distends and tears the dense fibres. They are given only for special purposes such as sensitivity testing where a localized reaction visible on the surface is required.

Pigmentary system

The colour of skin is dependent on the total thickness of the epidermis including its stratum corneum. To thin skin, the blood in the vessels imparts a pink colour providing the subject is warm and well-oxygenated. True pigmentation is due entirely to the presence of melanin. The amount of melanin is influenced by genetic, racial and environmental factors, by disease processes, and by external agents.

The pigment-producing cells (melanocytes) are found in the basal layer of the epidermis. They enter the epidermis during embryonic life and are derived from cells which have migrated from the neural crest. The number of melanocytes is approximately 10% of the total number of basal cells but varies from area to area in the body. There is little or no racial variation in the number of melanocytes for a given body area. Racial differences in colour are due to the quantity of melanin produced. Melanocytes are also found in albinos but they produce no pigment.

Melanocytes do not have desmosomal connections with other epidermal cells. They have a clear cytoplasm and long thin branching processes which stretch up into the stratum spinosum. The cells contain an enzyme system which includes tyrosinase by means of which the amino acid tyrosine is converted to DOPA (dihydroxyphenylalanine) and thence to the protein-complex pigment, melanin. The pigment exists in melanocytes as small bodies or melanosomes. Some of these remain in the melanocyte but most of them are injected by this cell into the adjacent epidermal cells. The greater the degree of pigmentation the greater the number of layers of pigment-containing epidermal cells.

The normal activity of melanocytes in skin depends on their content of tyrosinase. However they can be demonstrated in skin or other tissues by incubating sections with DOPA. The cells then synthesize increased amount of the brown pigment melanin and so become visible. Epidermal cells other than melanocytes are not capable of independent melanin synthesis.

Cutaneous appendages

THE NAIL (Fig. 8.6)

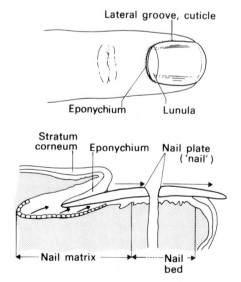

Fig. 8.6. The structure of a finger nail.

The nail proper or nail plate consists of a modified stratum corneum in which the squames contain a variant of keratin, known as hard keratin, which is comparable to that found in the cortex of hair. The nail plate is firmly adherent to the underlying epidermis or nail bed. Only the most proximal part of the nail bed or lunula contributes significantly to nail growth. Epidermal cells of the nail bed rest on the ubiquitous basal lamina beneath which a densely fibrous dermis is closely adherent to the periosteum of the distal phalanx. At the lunula basal cell proliferation is followed by a process of differentiation whose course is similar to that described for the epidermis as a whole. The major differences lie in the greatly increased quantity of tonofilaments and the absence of keratohyalin granules.

HAIR (Figs. 8.7 and 8.8)

Individual hairs vary in structure according to their location. Coarse facial and scalp hairs consist of a central medulla of soft keratin and an outer cortex of hard keratin. Surrounding the whole hair is a cuticle of minute overlapping scales. Each hair grows from a hair follicle which is a downgrowth of the epidermis into the dermis. At its deeper end, the follicle expands to form the bulb-like structure into which a small connective tissue papilla is invaginated.

The basal layer of the bulb is continuous with the hair follicle wall or outer root sheath which is in turn continuous with the epidermis. The bulb of the follicle comprises a mass of rapidly dividing cells whose daughter cells are forced to move upwards and in so doing differentiate into the various parts of the hair. The most central cells accumulate soft keratin and give rise to the thin medulla where it is present. Those more radially placed produce the hard keratin of the cortex and even further out the scales of the cuticle. The cuticle slides along the inner surface of the outer root sheath which is (soft) keratinized in its upper part where it is continuous with the epidermis.

Hair grows in cycles. In the human scalp an individual hair grows for a period of several years to be followed by a period of decline and then inactivity which may last for two or three months.

Detailed examination of hairs may be required in forensic investigations. The species from which hairs have come can be determined by examination of the surface pattern of the cuticular scales. Microscopical examination may

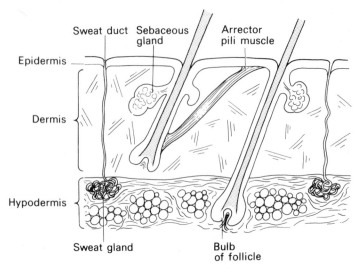

Fig. 8.7. Diagram of a section of scalp showing location of hair follicles, sweat glands, sebaceous glands, arrector pili muscles.

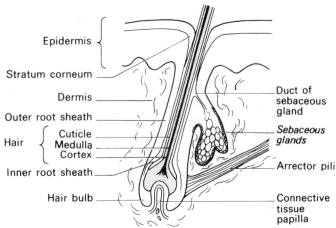

Fig. 8.8. Hair follicle.

also show the race and pigmentation of the individual

Arrector pili muscles
All hairs are associated with muscles (arrector pili) and sebaceous glands.

The arrector pili muscle is a thin band of smooth muscle running from the superficial layer of the dermis to the connective tissue sheath of the bulb of the hair follicle. When it contracts the hair is raised to the vertical position and the surrounding epidermis is slightly depressed. This response to cold, fear and excitement is the basis for several commonly used expressions such as 'goose-flesh', 'making the flesh creep' and 'hair standing on end'.

Sebaceous glands
In most parts of the body sebaceous glands are

related to, and develop from, hair follicles (Fig. 8.8). Clearly therefore it would be expected that areas lacking hair would also lack sebaceous glands. This is true over the soles of the feet and palms of the hand. However sebaceous glands are found unrelated to hair follicles in a few places. Examples of such sites are the eyelids and the corners of the mouth. Abberrant sebaceous glands sometimes occur in the oral mucosa as Fordyce spots.

Each hair follicle usually supports several sebaceous glands which develop from the 'embryonic' follicle. Each gland is a pear-shaped structure opening by a broad duct into the side of the follicle. The periphery of the gland is surrounded by a thin connective tissue capsule and a basal lamina. The epithelial cells adjacent to this basal lamina are mitotic. The daughter cells of the mitoses migrate away from the basal layer into the mass of gland cells. As they do so they swell due to a progressive accumulation of lipid while their other contents degenerate. Ultimately the necrotic cells are liquefied and pass from the gland along the side of the hair and on to the surfaces of the body. This form of secretion achieved by the shedding of whole cells, is called 'holocrine'.

Sebaceous glands produce a water repellant layer on the skin surface. They are responsible for the natural surface 'grease' of skin.

SWEAT GLANDS (Fig. 8.7)

There are two types of sweat gland in human skin. The more numerous is the ordinary (eccrine) sweat gland. The rarer is the so-called axillary, odoriferous or 'apocrine' sweat gland.

Ordinary sweat glands are very numerous but particularly so over the palms of the hands, soles of the feet and the finger tips. They are absent at the margins of the lips and over the glans penis. Sweat glands are simple, tubular glands opening from a straight or spiral duct on to the surface of the epidermis. The secretory part of the gland is found in the dermis or the superficial fascia and is coiled into a knot-like ball. The coiled tubule is surrounded by a thin connective tissue capsule and contains three types of epithelial cell. Clear cells, separated by complex intercellular canaliculi are responsible for fluid or ion transport and secrete the main components of sweat. Dark cells contain dense secretory glycoprotein granules in their cytoplasm. Between these cells and their basal lamina are myoepithelial cells similar to those in the salivary glands (p.547).

Sweating is of course stimulated by heat but also by emotions such as excitement and fear. The eccrine sweat glands are innervated by the sympathetic nervous system, but, unusually, by cholinergic endings.

'Apocrine', 'axillary', or 'odoriferous' sweat glands are much fewer in number. They are situated mainly in the axillae and perineal region. Unlike ordinary sweat glands they are frequently associated with hair follicles. Histologically they are much larger and the constituent cells are all dark cells. The large secretory granules are released by exocytosis (p. 418). The secretion is viscous and contains little salt. Development of these glands is controlled by sex hormones and is related to the onset of puberty. The names given to them are all misleading. They are not apocrine in the classic sense (p. 417), not restricted to the axilla

and the secretion is odourless until acted upon by bacteria at the skin surface.

Blood supply

In the superficial fascia (hypodermis) there is a network of small arteries derived from cutaneous branches of nearby larger arteries. From this plexus small branches pass upwards to the dermis and others pass deeper to supply the subcutaneous fat and those hair follicles which extend beyond the dermis. The branches to the skin supply the hair follicles, sweat and sebaceous glands and then form a plexus of arterioles immediately beneath the epidermis. Capillary loops extend from this plexus into the dermal papillae to supply the epidermis which is itself avascular. Arteriovenous anastomoses or shunts are found in the dermis of the fingers and toes.

Nerve supply

The skin is the largest and most important single organ of common sensation. All common sensory modalities except that of proprioception are mediated by skin. The nerve supply is therefore overwhelmingly sensory but also includes very important autonomic elements.

Cutaneous nerve trunks running in the superficial fascia give off fairly thick bundles which form a coarse plexus in the subcutaneous tissues. Smaller branches from this plexus pass up into the dermis and form a series of layers of very fine plexuses the most prominent of which is known as the dermal plexus. From these plexuses, non-myelinated autonomic nerves are distributed to the sweat glands and sebaceous glands, blood vessels and arrector pili muscles of the hair follicles. The sensory input to the dermal nerve nets is derived from a series of nerve endings. They may be non-encapsulated (free axonal) endings in the dermis or the epidermis or encapsulated endings in the dermis and deeper tissues. Many different encapsulated nerve endings have been described but only two special ones are now generally recognized. These are Pacinian corpuscles (Fig. 5.28b) and Meissner's corpuscles. Pacinian corpuscles are large and appear onion-like in section and are associated with pressure reception. They are widely distributed in deep tissues especially along fascial planes, around joints and in mesenteries. In the dermis they are most numerous in the fingers and toes. A Meissner's corpuscle consists of a coiled nerve ending in a complex fibrous capsule closely associated with the epidermis. Meissner's corpuscles are found only in the skin of the hands and feet and are believed to be associated with the sensation of touch. All other encapsulated endings are grouped together as mucocutaneous nerve endings and appear as sausage-shaped rolls or coils of fine fibres. They are most numerous in glabrous (non-hairy) skin.

Cleavage lines

If a conical object is driven into the skin and then withdrawn it leaves a linear, rather than circular, wound. This surprising result is due to the parallel arrangement of bundles of collagen fibres in the dermis: the separated fibres return to their original positions when the cone is withdrawn. The lines along which skin cleaves (Langer lines) have been mapped for the whole body. Surgical incisions made parallel to Langer lines heal with less scar tissue than those made across Langer lines.

Functions of skin

SENSATION

The skin is the largest single organ of sensation and has a very substantial sensory innervation. The histological basis for sensory function is dealt with on p. 310. The importance of the sensory innervation especially the modalities of touch, pain and hot and cold are obvious.

PROTECTION

Skin protects the body from its environment. Keratin is a mechanically strong fibrous protein and the outer horny layer is particularly well developed in areas where repeated trauma is encountered e.g. the soles of the feet. Such development is genetically determined but can be increased by increased trauma. Some thickening of the stratum corneum elsewhere can be brought about by increased trauma alone. The folds of the dermal–epidermal interface prevent the two components being readily sheared apart. Shearing forces are also dissipated by movement of the skin over the loosely woven superficial fascia. The dermis is the only really tough component of the skin. It enables folds of skin to be lifted without tearing (off the back of the hand for example) and to be sutured. Minor injuries successfully restricted to the skin are rapidly repaired by virtue of the regenerative powers of dermis and epidermis.

Skin also protects the body from invasion by micro-organisms. Intact skin is proof against practically all bacteria, fungi and viruses but a break in the epithelial surface whether due to injury or disease can lead to infection of underlying tissues or the skin itself. Many bacteria survive for long periods on the surface of the skin. Even elaborate decontamination procedures will fail to remove them probably because some persist in sweat ducts or hair follicles. It is also true that some bacteria fail to survive on the skin surface. The reasons are uncertain but the acidity of the sweat over most of the body and the bactericidal activity of unsaturated fatty acids of sebaceous secretion are probably important factors.

WATERPROOFING

Man lives in a dry environment and the skin functions as a means of preventing fluid loss. Whereas the mechanical properties of the stratum corneum are due to the mechanical strength of keratin, impermeability to water is maintained by the thickened lipid wall of the keratin squames. Passage of water between the squames is prevented by a material secreted from the cells in the stratum granulosum and carried towards the surface with the migrating cells (p. 0000). Impermeability extends to other compounds particularly if they are water-soluble. It does not extend to many synthetic organic chemicals which are often fat-soluble. Trinitrotoluene (TNT) is a famous example of a substance rapidly absorbed through skin (dating from its use in the manufacture of explosive projectiles in the First World War); but many other chemicals constitute industrial and agricultural hazards by virtue of their ability to penetrate the intact skin.

The secretions of sebaceous glands spread over the surface of the skin and repel water. In the special situation of the outer ear modified sweat glands or ceruminous glands secrete a water-repellent wax.

WATER BALANCE

Because of the activity of sweat glands the skin plays an important part in water balance. Measurement of water input and output in the body must always take account of insensible and largely unmeasurable loss from the skin (and from respiration). A figure of 500–900 cm^3/day is a rough measure of water loss from skin in a temperate climate, when no sweating is apparent. It may of course increase dramatically during exertion with high ambient temperatures, reaching as high as 2 dm^3/hour in extreme conditions. Salt loss becomes significant long before such high levels are reached so that athletes and heavy manual workers often require salt as well as watery fluids.

HEAT REGULATION

In the absence of an external covering such as clothing or hair the surface temperature of the skin regulates the rate at which heat is lost from the body.

The hair in man does not generally provide thermal insulation but reflex erection of hairs by the arrector pili muscles occurs in response to cold. Similarly the use of hair in defensive or offensive responses is not a feature of man's behaviour but the reflex persists in fear, anger and excitement.

PROTECTION AGAINST RADIATION

Skin provides protection against ultra-violet radiation, normally from sunlight, by virtue of its pigmentation. This is genetically controlled accounting for individual and racial variation: but it may also increase in response to increased exposure to radiation as in sun-tanning, especially in the 'white' races.

Vitamin D is produced in skin during ultra-violet irradiation.

SECONDARY SEXUAL CHARACTERISTICS

Skin possesses secondary sexual characteristics and displays sexual dimorphism. The apocrine glands respond to sex hormones. The more overt secretory characteristics of these glands are overlaid in many societies by the use of external agents such as deodorants and perfumes.

CHAPTER 9

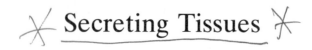

Secreting Tissues

CLASSIFICATION OF GLANDS

Rhodin has defined glands as those organs or tissues in which there are cells 'engaged in the synthesis, storage and discharge of secretory products'.

There are two major categories of gland in the body.

Endocrine glands

Endocrine glands synthesize hormones and secrete them into extracellular spaces from which they enter the blood stream or lymphatic system. These glands do not possess a duct system to transport the secretion away from its site of secretion and were once known as ductless glands. The secretion enters the blood stream rapidly and it does not leave the body tissues until it is ultimately metabolized or excreted. An endocrine gland may be closely related structurally to an exocrine gland, as for example in the case of the endocrine islets of Langerhans in the exocrine pancreas. Further details of the histology of the endocrine glands will be found in the sections devoted to individual glands.

Exocrine glands

In exocrine glands the secretion is discharged from the secretory cells on to a surface and not into the extracellular spaces. Frequently, though by no means always, the secretion first passes through a system of ducts which transports it to the surface or the site of discharge. The ducts of an exocrine gland are not necessarily a passive transport system but may themselves modify the secretion by adding to it or subtracting from it. The secretion may not of course actually leave the body but may be discharged on to an internal surface such as the lining of the alimentary canal. However this is quite a different matter to the discharge into extracellular spaces which characterizes endocrine secretions. It is with exocrine glands that most of this section is concerned.

DEVELOPMENT OF GLANDS

All multicellular glands consist of tissues derived from at least two primary germ layers. The secretory cells and the lining of the duct system are of epithelial origin, either ectoderm or endoderm, and these cells possess many of the physiological, histological and pathological properties of epithelial cells. It is to the attributes of these epithelial cells that we generally turn in describing the properties and character of each individual gland. The second element is the connective tissue or mesodermal part of the gland and this is often relegated to a secondary position. It is true that it is less important to the student of histology but it is a vital integral part of the gland, which carries the blood and nerve supply and which determines its physical character. The nature of the connective tissue is particularly important to the surgeon.

All glands, whether exocrine or endocrine, begin their development in a similar way (Fig. 9.1a). The first evidence of their presence is an invaginating proliferation of cells from an epithelial surface. For exocrine glands the site of this invagination is generally related to the point at which the duct system will ultimately discharge at the surface. The parotid gland serves as an example. In the adult the parotid duct opens into the vestibule of the mouth at a small papilla opposite the crown of the second maxillary molar tooth. The parotid gland is the first of the salivary glands to appear during development and it does so during the fifth week of embryonic life soon after the rupture of the buccopharyngeal membrane. The 'anlage' or 'primordium' of the gland is seen in the ectoderm of the stomatodaeum.

The invaginating bud of epithelial cells resulting from local proliferation pushes down into the underlying mesenchyme. In an exocrine gland such as the parotid, the epithelial bud lengthens into a more or less cylindrical mass of cells. As it increases in length so the growing tip divides and

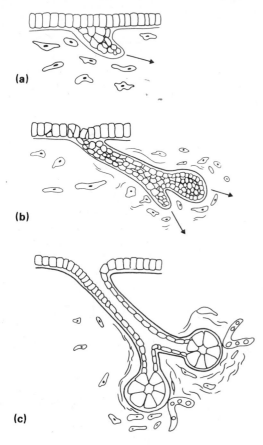

(a)

(b)

(c)

Fig. 9.1. The development of an exocrine gland.

redivides into the tree-like outline of the duct system of the mature gland (Fig. 9.1b). Ultimately the terminal branches of the system differentiate into the tubules and secretory acini of the gland. Later the solid cords of cells linking them to the surface canalize to produce a system of ducts (Fig. 9.1c).

As the proliferating glandular cells grow down from the surface they come into contact with proliferating mesenchyme cells, which develop simultaneously with the epithelium, to give rise to the connective tissue elements of the gland. Mesenchyme cells exert an important controlling influence on the development of glands.

Isolation and recombination experiments have shown that the information required for epithelial cells to differentiate into a particular gland is derived from the mesenchyme cells. If the epithelial anlage of a gland is removed at a sufficiently early stage and then grown in organ culture with the mesenchyme from a site of development of a different gland, the structure which develops resembles the gland from which the mesenchyme was taken (the pancreas is an exception to this generalization). If the epithelium or the mesenchyme are grown alone in organ culture, no recognizable glandular morphology appears. The reaction between epithelium and mesenchyme in development of a gland has some similarity to that observed in development of the tooth germ.

Endocrine glands differ in their development. The cord of epithelial cells grows down into the mesenchyme and its distal end proliferates to form a mass of secretory cells. The cord of cells connecting the gland to the surface disappears at an early stage and does not canalize. As in other situations where epithelial cells normally degenerate, anomalies can occur where the connection with the surface persists. One well known example is a persisting thyroglossal duct.

MORPHOLOGICAL CLASSIFICATION OF EXOCRINE GLANDS

The glands of the body can be classified according to the histological arrangement of the epithelial elements and the system of ducts.

Unicellular glands

The simplest gland consists of a single cell which discharges its secretory product directly on to the surface without the necessity for a duct. In man all unicellular glands are mucous glands. They may be very numerous on surfaces such as the lining of the respiratory tract. Where such secretory cells entirely cover a surface, for example in the surface epithelium of the gastric mucosa, the epithelium might be regarded either as a collection of unicellular glands or as the simplest form of multicellular gland.

Multicellular glands

SIMPLE GLANDS

Except for the above situation where an entire sheet of epithelial cells constitutes a gland, multicellular glands contain ducts. Where the duct leading from a small group of secretory cells to the surface is unbranched it is known as a simple gland. Where the duct is branched it is known as a compound gland. Simple glands may be further categorized according to the arrangement of the secretory cells discharging into the duct. They may line a secretory tubule, a secretory acinus or both. Thus there are:

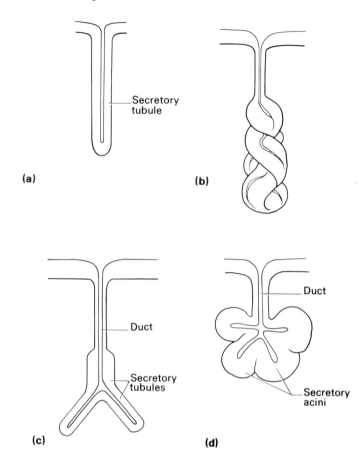

Fig. 9.2. Different types of simple glands. (a) Simple tubular gland, (b) simple coiled tubular gland, (c) simple branched tubular gland, (d) simple branched acinar gland.

Simple tubular glands (Fig. 9.2a)

In these glands the secretory cells line a tubular continuation of the unbranched duct. In the most numerous example, the crypts of Lieber-kühn in the duodenum, the whole gland is lined with secretory cells and there is no duct.

Simple coiled tubular glands (Fig. 9.2b)

The unbranched duct leads into a single elon-gated secretory tubule which is coiled upon it-self. Example—ordinary sweat glands (Fig. 8.7).

Simple branched tubular glands (Fig. 9.2c)

A single duct gives rise to a number of tubules lined by secretory cells. The secretory part of the gland is branched but the duct is simple and unbranched. Example—lingual salivary glands.

Simple branched alveolar (acinar) glands (Fig. 9.2d)

The unbranched duct leads into a short branched secretory tubule; each branch ends in a secretory alveolus. Example—sebaceous glands (Fig. 8.8).

COMPOUND GLANDS

As larger glands are examined the complexity of the duct system is seen to increase. Glands in which the duct system branches repeatedly from the main secretory duct are called compound glands: this category includes all the larger glands of the body. As with simple glands sub-categories may be devized which rely on the arrangement of the terminal secretory portions:

Compound tubular glands

The smallest peripheral ducts are continuous with tubules lined with secretory cells. This arrangement is found in mucous glands such as many of the minor salivary glands which do not possess terminal acini.

Compound alveolar glands

The majority of large exocrine glands belong to this category. They have an extensive branching duct system and each terminal duct gives rise to a group of bulb-like alveoli (or acini) containing secretory cells. Such an arrangement can produce a vast area of secretory cell surface. The secretory surface may be further increased by the presence of intercellular canaliculi allowing cells to secrete from their sides. The number of cells secreting into the lumen of an alveolus may be increased by an arrangement such as that of the serous demilunes in salivary glands where a more peripheral group of cells pass their secretions into the alveolar lumen through canaliculi which penetrates between the cells comprising the acinus.

COMPOUND TUBULOALVEOLAR GLANDS

Some glands are a mixture of tubules and alveoli.

Mode of secretion

A further classification of exocrine glands is based on the type of secretory mechanism which can be deduced from light microscope studies. However the information accumulated in the last twenty five years or more with the electron microscope has produced a clearer picture of the cellular basis of secretion which, in many cases, casts doubt on this long established classification. Nevertheless the older classification still has its uses and holds good in a number of instances. It is based on the amount of the cell cytoplasm supposed to be lost during secretion.

HOLOCRINE SECRETION

This is the extreme process in which the secretion from a gland consists of complete, usually degenerate, cells. The outstanding example is the sebaceous gland of the skin and there is no reason to doubt the existence of this secretory mechanism.

APOCRINE

In apocrine glands a variable but substantial amount of cytoplasm is supposed to be lost during secretion. In most instances, for example the mammary gland and the 'axillary' sweat glands it is now known that very little or even no cytoplasmic ground substance is lost when the secretion leaves the cell.

MEROCRINE SECRETION

Here it was believed that the secretory product diffused from the cell so that no cellular contents were lost. This, the commonest form of secretion, will be considered further in the description of ultrastructure.

Type of secretion

Many glands may be classified as serous, mucous or mixed (mucous and serous). These glands contain fairly readily identifiable cells each of which can be classified as mucous or serous secreting. The original basis for this classification was the appearance and viscosity of the secretion. A serous secretion is a clear, low-viscosity fluid containing proteins. A mucous secretion is opaque with high viscosity and a peculiarly viscid quality. It contains a high proportion of glycoproteins (p. 345). A fairly precise description of the cells responsible for these two types of secretion is possible.

Serous cells (Fig. 9.3) often have a central or basal, rounded nucleus and contain numerous large but discrete secretion droplets. Their cytoplasm is basophilic (due to a high concentration of RNA). They contain large quantities of rough endoplasmic reticulum distributed through much of the cytoplasm. The Golgi apparatus is well-developed, usually apical to the nucleus and gives rise to the secretion droplets by dilatation of its sacs with synthesized protein. The droplets are therefore contained within membranes derived from the walls of the sacs of the Golgi apparatus. The contents of the droplets usually

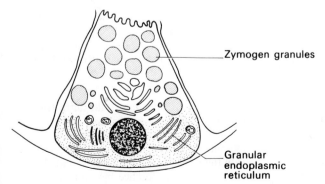

Zymogen granules

Granular endoplasmic reticulum

Fig. 9.3. A serous cell.

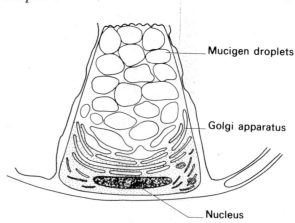

Fig. 9.4. A mucous cell.

stain intensely, often with basic dyes such as haemotoxylin, and as a result of their protein content they have a dense appearance in electron micrographs.

A mucous cell (Fig. 9.4) frequently has its nucleus flattened towards the base of the cell and its cytoplasm reduced to a comparatively narrow rim at the base and sides of the cell. It contains considerable amounts of RNA and of rough endoplasmic reticulum in the compressed cytoplasm. The Golgi apparatus is prominent and produces very large dilated secretion droplets which tend to fill the main body of the cell accounting for the paucity of intervening cytoplasm. The mucous droplets are frequently acidophilic (stain with eosin) and are translucent in electron micrographs. The droplets contain carbohydrates (deduced from their positive reaction to the periodic acid–Schiff stain) as well as protein.

In both serous and mucous cells the basic processes of synthesis and secretion are similar (Fig. 9.5). The precursors of protein synthesis are amino acids which are incorporated into polypeptide chains in the ribosomes of the granular endoplasmic reticulum. They are segregated within the membranous cisterns of the endoplasmic reticulum and are then transported to the sacs of the Golgi apparatus. Further synthetic processes, notably the incorporation of carbohydrates (glycosylation) and sulphate occur in the Golgi apparatus. Each secretion droplet is enclosed in a sac derived from the membrane of the Golgi apparatus. When the droplet is extruded, this membrane fuses with the cell surface membrane and is incorporated into it (Fig. 9.5). The contents of the droplet are now in continuity with the extracellular space and move out of the cell into the extracellular region. This process is some-

times referred to as reversed pinocytosis although it has no physiological relationship with pinocytosis. The term exocytosis is preferable. Repeated exocytosis during secretion should lead to a build-up of membrane round the cell. There is evidence that secretory cells are able to take in excess membrane by pinocytosis and then recycle the chemical components. In this way there may be continuous circulation of membrane throughout the life of a cell.

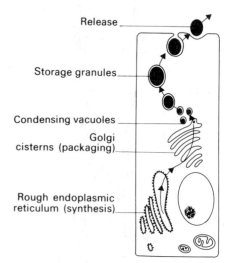

Fig. 9.5. Schematic representation of the formation, packaging and release of protein from a cell. (After Finean *et al* 1978).

The above description is the ultrastructural analysis of merocrine secretion and it is also known to describe the secretion process in most 'apocrine' glands.

On the basis of light microscopy and electron microscopy the difference between serous and mucous glands is quite clear-cut. The biochemical basis for this classification is less clear since it is now known that many if not all the cells of exocrine glands secrete glycoproteins. Serous and mucous secretions differ largely in the degree of glycosylation of the protein end product, i.e. the concentration of carbohydrate in the glycoproteins present.

Connective tissue elements of glands

All glands have a connective tissue stroma. This is a capsule which may vary from well-developed and thickened (often part of the fascia of the subcutaneous tissues) to practically non-existent. It consists of bundles of collagen and elastic fibres with fibroblasts and other connective tissue elements. Extending inwards from the capsule, septa divide the gland into lobes and then into lobules. The septa contain arteries, veins, lymphatics, nerves and ducts. The ducts are known, according to their position, as lobar and interlobular ducts. Smaller, intralobular, ducts run in the substance of the lobule and are connected to the secretory tubules and acini by intercalated ducts.

Blood and nerve supply of glands

The description of an individual gland is not complete without a description of its nerve and blood supply. Arterial blood is distributed to glandular tissue by vessels which run in the connective tissue septa. Capillaries then ramify closer to the secretory cells. The nerve supply to a gland may contain an ordinary sensory element but its most important contribution is likely to be from the autonomic part of the nervous system, either sympathetic or parasympathetic of both. Stimulated nerves may increase or reduce secretion by a direct action on the glandular tissue or ducts—the secretomotor effect, or an indirect action by reducing or increasing the blood supply—the vasomotor effect. The part played by each differs from gland to gland.

THE SECRETORY PROCESS

Secretion is often wrongly considered to be synonymous with extrusion. In fact it consists of first the transport of water and raw materials into the cell from plasma; second their movement through the cytoplasm together with synthesis and storage; and finally the extrusion of the product into a lumen, or in the case of an endocrine gland, into plasma.

Movement of water and solute through membranes

The movement of water through a cell can be the result of pressure gradients across the membranes created by hydrostatic or osmotic forces. In some glands the secreted fluid contains one or more constituents in higher concentration than in plasma; these exert an osmotic pull on fluid across the cell into the secretion. Some solute is passively transferred by hydrostatic and osmotic forces, but this is limited by water and lipid solubility and the charge, size and shape of the molecules. Several other transport mechanisms are available.

FACILITATED DIFFUSION

The passive diffusion of solutes implies transport down a concentration gradient and does not require cellular energy. Sometimes a cellular trapping mechanism effectively reduces the concentration of the free solute in a cell thereby increasing the concentration gradient and therefore the rate of diffusion.

Movement can be speeded up by the presence of carriers in the membrane which form complexes with the solute. If this carrier can move at similar rates in both directions the rate of facilitated diffusion is faster than in the absence of the carrier, but is still dependent on the concentration gradient. If, having discharged its load, the carrier cannot return for more solute because for example, it has been metabolized, a one-way ferry is produced and the availability of carrier becomes the factor which limits the rate of movement.

In some cases a carrier is not ion specific. For example, a carrier may take sodium ions in one direction and potassium ions in another.

ACTIVE TRANSPORT

This describes an energy-dependent process which transports a substance against an electrochemical gradient. As it depends on metabolic energy, transport is impaired by drugs such as 2,4-dinitrophenol (DNP) or cyanide, which interrupt metabolic pathways.

Considerable energy is used in the active 'uphill' extrusion of sodium from cells. The driving force is sometimes called the sodium pump. It is normally self-regulating, with a key enzyme, adenosine triphosphatase (ATPase), being activated by a rise in the intracellular concentration of sodium. This enzyme is probably involved in the secretion of some glands because ouabain, a drug which inhibits the enzyme, decreases the secretion of these glands.

Sometimes an ion which is being carried allows a different ion to be tagged on. Chloride can 'cadge' a lift on sodium ions in some glandular cells.

The acid-producing cells in gastric mucosa afford another example of an 'uphill' movement of ions. In parietal cells the H^+ concentration is about $1 \times 10^{-7}M$ whereas the extracellular acid which they have produced has a concentration of about $1 \times 10^{-2}M$. A recent theory suggests that energy is involved in such transport to induce transient conformational changes in membrane proteins. These changes control the passage of materials into and out of the cell.

Intracellular control and stimulus-secretion coupling

A feature common to all protein-secreting systems and many others which depend on stimulation by a neurotransmitter or hormone for their activation, is the presence of an intracellular control system which couples the stimulus received at the cell membrane to the secretion process. Cyclic AMP and calcium ions contribute separately or together in this control and are sometimes known as 'cell messengers'. The most likely sequence of events (Fig. 9.6) is that the stimulus latches on to a receptor-site and activates (or inhibits) adenyl cyclase, which in turn causes more (or less) cAMP to be formed from ATP. By the action of cAMP phosphodies-terase a kind of balance is set up between the rates at which cAMP is formed and destroyed. The overall response in the cell depends on the intracellular level of cAMP which has been established. In some way, still uncertain, the cAMP activates enzymes and possibly also changes in cell membrane structure and permeability and so effects the secretory process.

Just where calcium fits in to this sequence is not clear. It seems probable that a critical calcium level has to be established at some site within the secretory cell. If the permeability of the cell membrane to calcium is increased as a result of conformational changes in its structure on receipt of a stimulus, then there might be a straightforward flux of calcium into the cell from a high calcium ion environment in intersitial fluid. Alternatively, intracellular stores of calcium, notably in mitochondria, may be persuaded to release their calcium. Different secretory cells use different mechanisms to achieve these changes in their calcium concentration. Contradictory evidence in the literature concerning the effects of depletion of extracellular calcium upon secretion is largely due to difficulties involved in such experiments in altering the calcium bound to organelles.

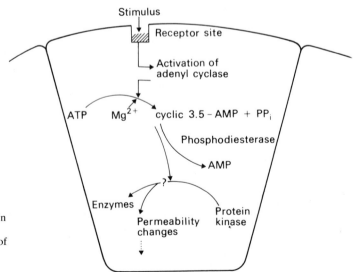

Fig. 9.6. Intracellular events in stimulus-secretion coupling. Because of the uncertain role of calcium, this ion has not been included in this diagram.

FURTHER READING

WOODBURY J.W. (1965) The cell membrane: ionic and potential gradients and active transport. In *Physiology and Biophysics*, ed. T.C. Ruch and H.D. Patton. W.B. Saunders, Philadelphia. pp. 1–25.

MATTHEWS E.K. (1970) Calcium and hormone release. In: *Calcium and Cellular Function*, ed. A.W. Cuthbert. Macmillan, London. pp. 163–182.

DOUGLAS W.W. (1968) Stimulus-secretion coupling: the concept and clues from chromaffin and other cells. *British Journal of Pharmacology*, **34**, 451–474.

FINEAN J.B., COLEMAN R. & MICHELL R.H. (1978) *Membranes and their Cellular Functions*, 2nd Edition. Blackwell Scientific Publications, Oxford.

CHAPTER 10

✳ The Locomotor System ✳

INTRODUCTION TO TOPOGRAPHICAL ANATOMY

The anatomical position is the one by which parts of the body are described and interrelated: the body is erect with the head facing forwards, the upper limbs are at the sides of the trunk with the thumb pointing outwards, and the lower limbs are together and parallel to each other with the feet pointing forwards. Three cardinal planes are used (Fig. 10.1):

1   The sagittal, a vertical plane in the midline running anteroposteriorly.
2   The coronal (frontal), a vertical plane at right angles to the sagittal.
3   The transverse or horizontal plane running at right angles to the other two.

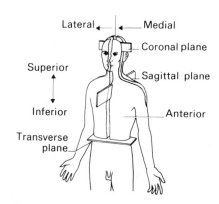

Fig. 10.1. Body planes and other terms used in anatomical terminology.

The sagittal plane is often called the median and planes parallel to the sagittal are called parasagittal. All vertical planes at right angles to the sagittal are called coronal. The front surface of the body is anterior and the back surface is posterior. The terms ventral and dorsal (used when describing all other vertebrates) are synonymous with anterior and posterior respectively.

These terms are also used to describe relative positions of parts of the body to one another. Medial and lateral refer to the midline. The former is nearer the midline; the latter is further away from the midline. For example, in the anatomical position the little finger is medial to the thumb and the thumb is lateral to the little finger. The terms superior or cranial, and inferior or caudal, are used to indicate a vertical relationship. For example, the head is superior to the neck. The terms superficial and deep refer to the surface of the body on any of its aspects.

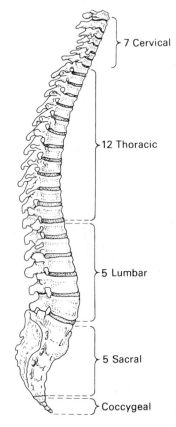

Fig. 10.2. Vertebral column.

Superficial is nearer the surface and deep nearer the inside. External and internal are used in a similar way but refer especially to cavities or hollow organs. In the limbs proximal refers to nearer the trunk and distal to nearer the fingers or toes.

TRUNK AND LIMBS

It is customary to divide the skeleton into axial (the vertebral column, ribs, sternum and skull) and appendicular (the pectoral girdle and upper limb bones, and the pelvic girdle and lower limb bones). Trunk and limbs are dealt with together and the skull (including the mandible) is dealt with separately.

Vertebral column (Fig. 10.2)

The segmented nature of the vertebral column reflects the basically segmental pattern of the human body, however much of this pattern has been lost during development. It should be added that many features of the adult human body, for example the innervation of the muscles and skin of the limbs, indicate a segmental arrangement which has become somewhat obscured. In the human body there are usually seven cervical vertebrae in the neck (cervix means a neck), twelve thoracic in the thorax (sometimes called dorsal), five lumbar in the lower part of the back (lumbus means a loin, the part between the last rib and the pelvis), five sacral wedged posteriorly as one piece between the two hip bones and three or four coccygeal.

A TYPICAL VERTEBRA
(Fig. 10.3a & b)

A vertebra has certain basic features which are best seen in a middle thoracic vertebra. It has a cylindrical part anteriorly (the body) which varies in shape in different parts of the column being more oval transversely in the cervical and lumbar regions. It increases in size from above downwards because the lower a vertebra the more weight it must transmit. Anteriorly and laterally the body is convex horizontally and slightly concave vertically. Posteriorly the body is concave from side to side. On all sides there are small foramina for arteries, but one or two large foramina on the posterior surfaces are for veins. The edges of the upper and lower surfaces are smooth. More centrally these surfaces are rough. An intervertebral disc is attached to each of these surfaces. Posterolaterally on each side of the body at its upper and lower margins are facets for the head of a rib (these are present in only the thoracic vertebrae). Behind the body is the vertebral (or neural) arch which, together with the back of the body forms the vertebral foramen in which lie the spinal cord, its meninges and blood vessels. The anterior part of the arch on each side is called the pedicle and the posterior part is called the lamina. The pedicles are short and rounded and the laminae are flattened and somewhat longer. The pedicle is attached to the upper part of the body so that there is a very shallow superior vertebral and a deep inferior vertebral notch. When two adjacent vertebrae are articulated, the pedicles and notches form part of an intervertebral foramen which is completed in front by an inter-

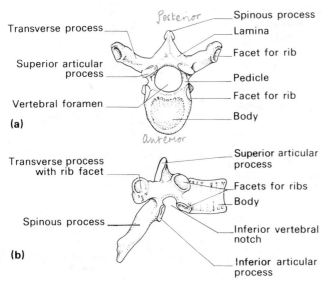

Transverse process — Posterior — Spinous process
— Lamina
Superior articular process — Facet for rib
Vertebral foramen — Pedicle
(a) — Facet for rib
— Body
Anterior

Transverse process with rib facet — Superior articular process
— Facets for ribs
— Body
Spinous process — Inferior vertebral notch
(b) — Inferior articular process

Fig. 10.3. Typical thoracic vertebra: (a) superior aspect; (b) lateral aspect.

vertebral disc and behind by the joint formed by two adjacent articular processes. A spinal nerve lies in the foramen. The two laminae are directed medially and backwards and meet in the midline. Projecting backwards in the midline from the vertebral arch is the spinous process which varies considerably in length and direction in different parts of the vertebral column. Projecting upwards and downwards from the arch at the junction of the pedicle with the lamina on each side are the superior and inferior articular processes (zygapophyses). Projecting laterally from the vertebral arch on each side between the superior and inferior articular process is the transverse process. In the cervical and lumbar region the rib (costal process) has fused with the transverse process.

CERVICAL VERTEBRAE
(Fig. 10.4a & b)

A cervical vertebra is recognized by the presence of the foramen transversarium in the transverse process. The first and second cervical vertebrae are modified in some ways and the seventh has several individual characteristics.

A typical cervical vertebra has a relatively small, oval body with its long axis from side to side. The spinous process projects backwards and somewhat downwards and is bifid except in the first and seventh vertebrae. The articular facets are on a relatively stout piece of bone not seen on any other part of the vertebral column and when the vertebrae are articulated together the articular processes form a pillar of bone which is weight-bearing.

The first cervical vertebra is called the atlas and has no body or spinous process (Fig. 10.5). It consists of a bony ring which is divided into a smaller anterior arch and a larger posterior arch by two lateral masses. The anterior arch is flattened anteroposteriorly and has a small anterior tubercle on the middle of its convex anterior

surface. On the middle of the concave posterior surface of the anterior arch is a round facet for articulation with the dens of the axis (the second cervical vertebra).

On the medial side of the lateral mass there is a tubercle to which is attached the transverse ligament which passes behind the dens of the axis. This ligament completes the ring in which the dens rotates when the atlas and head rotate to the right and left. Posterior to the transverse ligament are the spinal cord and its meninges.

The second cervical vertebra (the axis) (Fig. 10.6) has projecting upwards from its body the dens (odontoid process). There is a constriction between the dens and the body of the axis. The transverse ligament of the atlas lies in the posterior part of this constriction and anteriorly there is an oval facet for articulation with the anterior arch of the atlas. Each alar ligament is attached to a tubercle on the side of the dens above the constriction. The ligaments pass upwards and laterally into the skull. On either side of the dens, on the body and pedicle, there is a relatively flat, oval facet facing upwards and laterally, for articulation with the atlas.

The seventh cervical vertebra usually has a small foramen transversarium because only an accessory vertebral vein lies in it. The spinous process is not bifid, but it is long and can be seen projecting under the skin on the back of the neck. Although called the vertebra prominens it is not as a rule the most prominent spinous process, which is usually that of the first thoracic vertebra. The anterior part of the transverse process may form a separate bone of varied length. This is called a cervical rib.

THORACIC VERTEBRAE
(Fig. 10.3a & b)

A typical vertebra has already been described above.

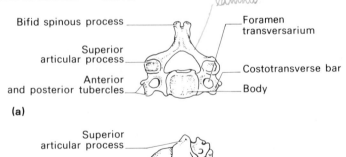

Fig. 10.4. Typical cervical vertebra: (a) superior aspect; (b) lateral aspect.

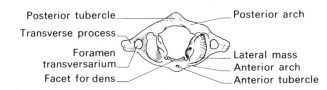

Posterior tubercle — Posterior arch
Transverse process —
Foramen — Lateral mass
transversarium — Anterior arch
Facet for dens — Anterior tubercle   **Fig. 10.5.** Atlas superior aspect.

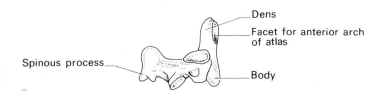

Dens
Facet for anterior arch
of atlas
Spinous process —
Body   **Fig. 10.6.** Lateral aspect of axis.

LUMBAR, SACRAL AND COCCYGEAL VERTEBRAE

The lumbar vertebrae do not have a foramen transversarium or facets on the body. The body is large relative to that of a typical thoracic or cervical vertebra, and is wider from side to side than anteroposteriorly.

The sacrum in the adult is a flattened triangular bone consisting of the five fused sacral vertebrae. The sacral canal contains the end of the subarachnoid space, the cauda equina and the filum terminale.

The coccyx is usually in two pieces and consists of four rudimentary vertebrae. It is curved forwards. It articulates above with the sacrum both in the midline and laterally. The sacrum and coccyx form the posterior wall of the lesser pelvis (meaning a basin) which is completed on each side by a hip bone. The hip bones meet anteriorly at the symphysis pubis which forms the anterior part of the pelvis in the midline. The pelvis will be considered in more detail later on (p. 436).

INTERVERTEBRAL DISCS

These are found between the bodies of the vertebrae from the second cervical to the fifth lumbar. They constitute about a fifth of the total height of the vertebral column but are thinner in the thoracic region than in the cervical and lumbar regions, in which they are wedge-shaped with the thicker part of the wedge anteriorly thus contributing to the anterior convexity of these regions.

Each disc consists of an outer anulus fibrosus and inner nucleus pulposus (Fig. 10.7c). The anulus is made up of layers of collagen fibres arranged spirally. Adjacent layers are at right angles to each other. Some cartilage is found in the inner parts of the anulus. The collagen fibres are attached to thin plates of hyaline cartilage on the adjacent surfaces of the vertebral bodies and also to the anterior and posterior longitudinal ligaments. The nucleus is much more fluid than the anulus and consists of a gelatinous mass, containing, during the first ten years of life, notochordal cells, as well as thin bundles of collagen and elastic fibres. It also contains a considerable amount of structureless material. With advancing age the nucleus becomes more fibrous and finally fibrocartilaginous and almost indistinguishable from the anulus. There is a high water content in the discs and this decreases during the day so that an individual is not as tall in the evening as in the morning. This water content decreases with age especially that of the nucleus. Only the peripheral part of the disc has nerve fibres and some blood vessels. The main part of the disc receives its nutrition by diffusion from the bodies of the vertebrae.

Functionally, as well as providing a strong union between the vertebrae, the discs are shock-absorbers. They permit a limited amount of movement due to the spiral arrangement of the collagen fibres. They can be compressed on one side and stretched on the opposite side as well as rotated. They can resist considerable increases in pressure such as occur when heavy weights are lifted.

VERTEBRAL COLUMN AS A WHOLE

Viewed from the front, the vertebral column is seen to consist of bodies and intervertebral discs increasing in size from the second cervical to the second sacral vertebra. Directly or indirectly the weight of the head, upper limbs, thorax and its contents, and abdomen and pelvis and their contents is transferred to the upper half of the sacrum and thence directly to the hip bones and the lower limbs. The pillar of bone formed by the articular processes of the cervical vertebrae referred to (p. 424), is weight-bearing. The transverse processes of the cervical vertebrae are prominent when the column is viewed from in front but those of the thoracic and lumbar regions project backwards as well as laterally and are less easily seen.

From the side the most striking features of the column are the curves and the intervertebral foramina. In the cervical and lumbar regions the curves are convex forwards (secondary curves), in the thoracic and sacral regions they are concave forwards (primary curves). The fetus with its flexed posture is assumed to have one primary curve forwards. The baby, holding its head up at between six weeks and three months after birth, develops a secondary cervical curve. At about six months the baby sits up and after nine to twelve months stands up, during which time the secondary lumbar curve develops. It is more marked in the female than in the male. The primary curves are due to the posterior parts of the vertebral bodies being higher than the anterior parts, and the secondary curves are due to similar but reverse differences in the intervertebral discs. This is particularly marked in the wedge-shaped intervertebral disc between the fifth lumbar vertebra and the first sacral, so that there is a distinct backward bend at the lumbosacral junction.

Probably the main function of the curves is to give the vertebral column resilience in its weight-bearing, comparable with that of an arched bridge. It is said that the sites of change in the direction of the curves (seventh cervical and first thoracic, twelfth thoracic and first lumbar, and fifth lumbar and first sacral) are the weakest parts of the column.

From behind, the most obvious features are the spinous processes, the laminae and the transverse processes. Attention is drawn to the gap between the spinous processes of the second and third, and third and fourth lumbar vertebrae. A hollow needle can be inserted between the spinous processes into the subarachnoid space (a procedure known as lumbar puncture). This is below the level of the spinal cord which ends at the first lumbar vertebra and above the lowest level of the subarachnoid space which ends at the second sacral vertebra. Between the spinous processes medially and the transverse processes laterally, overlying the laminae and the articular processes, is a longitudinal groove

extending the whole length of the vertebral column. The erector spinae muscle lies in this groove.

JOINTS OF VERTEBRAL COLUMN (Fig. 10.7)

There is a typical secondary cartilaginous joint (p. 385) between the adjacent bodies of the vertebrae from the second cervical to the first sacral. The adjacent surfaces of the bodies are therefore covered by hyaline cartilage between which is a disc of fibrocartilage, the intervertebral disc. These joints are very stable and they are strengthened by the anterior and posterior longitudinal ligaments.

The joints between the articular processes of adjacent vertebrae are synovial of the gliding type.

There are additional ligaments between the vertebrae, the most important of which are the ligamenta flava (meaning yellow ligaments because they contain a large amount of yellow elastic fibres). (Fig. 10.7).

The supraspinous ligaments pass between the tips of the spinous processes and the interspinous ligaments between the upper and lower borders of these processes. In the neck the supraspinous and interspinous ligaments are replaced by the ligamentum nuchae (nucha means the back of the neck) which is attached to the occipital bone above in the midline (behind the foramen magnum) and to the posterior tubercle of the atlas and the spinous processes of the cervical vertebrae (Fig. 10.8). It has some depth and muscles are attached to its surfaces on either side of the midline.

The joints between the occipital bone and atlas (atlanto-occipital) and atlas and axis (median atlanto-axial and lateral atlanto-axial, one on each side) have special features. The atlanto-occipital joints are synovial of the ellipsoid type. The articular surface of the condyle which is oval and points inwards and forwards is convex in both directions, and the articular surface on the upper aspect of the lateral mass of the atlas is reciprocally concave. The anterior and posterior atlanto-occipital membranes are additional ligaments joining the anterior arch and the posterior arch to the occipital bone in front of and behind the foramen magnum respectively. The vertebral artery and the first cervical spinal nerve lies laterally between the posterior membrane and the posterior arch.

The median atlanto-axial joint is a synovial joint of the pivot type between the dens of the axis and a ring formed by the posterior surface of

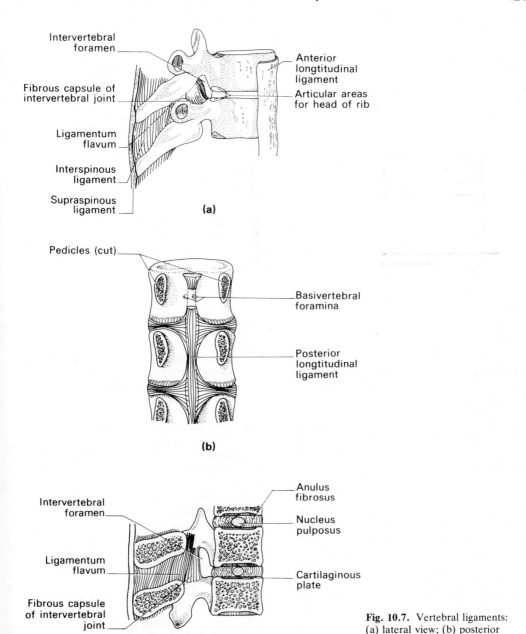

Fig. 10.7. Vertebral ligaments: (a) lateral view; (b) posterior view; (c) sagittal section.

the anterior arch of the atlas and the transverse ligament of the atlas, which is attached laterally to the medial side of its lateral mass. The facets on the anterior arch of the atlas and dens form one joint surrounded by a fibrous capsule and the posterior surface of the dens is separated from the transverse ligament by a bursa. There are also some vertical fibres in the midline passing upwards and downwards from the middle of

the transverse ligament. The upper fibres pass through the foramen magnum to the occipital bone and the lower fibres downwards to the back of the body of the axis. The vertical fibres and transverse ligament together form the cruciform ligament. The membrana tectoria is an upward continuation of the posterior longitudinal ligament and lies posterior to the cruciform ligament. The membrane is attached to the occipital

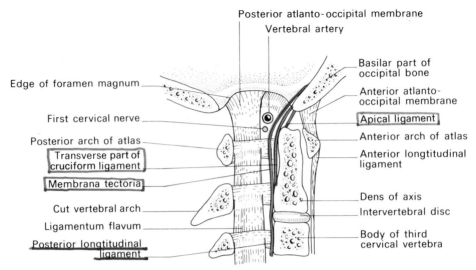

Posterior atlanto-occipital membrane
Vertebral artery

Basilar part of
occipital bone

Anterior atlanto-
occipital membrane

Edge of foramen magnum

Apical ligament

First cervical nerve

Anterior arch of atlas

Posterior arch of atlas

Anterior longtitudinal
ligament

Transverse part of
cruciform ligament

Membrana tectoria

Dens of axis

Intervertebral disc

Cut vertebral arch

Ligamentum flavum

Body of third
cervical vertebra

Posterior longtitudinal
ligament

Fig. 10.8. Sagittal section through foramen magnum showing ligaments attaching skull to vertbral column.

bone. The apical ligament is attached to the apex of the dens, passes upwards deep to the cruciform ligament and is attached to the occipital bone. The alar ligaments, one on each side, are attached to the dens, pass upwards and laterally through the foramen magnum and are attached to the occipital bone on the medial side of the condyles. The lateral atlanto-axial joints are synovial of the gliding type and have no special features.

VERTEBRAL MUSCLES AND FASCIAE

The most superficial muscles of the back of the trunk are attached to the vertebral column and the pectoral girdle or humerus. Deep to these is a longitudinally running mass of muscle from the sacrum to the occipital bone, known as the erector spinae (sacrospinalis). This muscle is divided into three, both vertically and from lateral to medial, so that there are nine named muscles. The important features of the erector spinae are that it is attached by a common tendon to the back of the sacrum; the muscle is attached to the backs of the ribs for a distance of about 5 cm from their heads as well as to the transverse and spinous processes of the vertebrae; its lateral border is marked by a groove visible on the back in the living and the direction of its fibres is mainly vertical. Deep to the erector spinae are a large number of muscles most of which are short. These muscles pass between transverse processes and spinous processes, or between adjacent transverse processes or bet-

ween adjacent spinous processes. The direction of their fibres may be oblique, usually upwards and medially, or vertical. The only two muscles named here are the longissimus capitis which is attached to the temporal bone and the semispinalis capitis which is attached to the occipital bone. Both are attached inferiorly to the transverse processes of the upper thoracic vertebrae. A third muscle not belonging to either of the large groups already mentioned is the splenius capitis which is in the back of the neck superficial to the erector spinae. It spirals upwards and laterally from the spinous processes of the upper thoracic vertebrae to the temporal bone (Fig. 10.31), superficial to the longissimus capitis and deep to the sternocleidomastoid.

The nerve supply of all these muscles comes at the appropriate levels from the dorsal rami of the spinal nerves, from the second cervical to the lower sacral.

There is a small group of muscles deep to the semispinalis capitis called the suboccipital muscles. They are attached to the axis, atlas and occipital bone and can be seen in Fig. 10.9. Three of them form the suboccipital triangle in which lie the posterior arch of the atlas, the vertebral artery and the dorsal ramus of the first cervical nerve which supplies all these muscles. Their importance lies in making fine adjustments to the position of the head on the vertebral column. These muscles contain a large number of muscle spindles.

There is a layer of fascia related to the erector

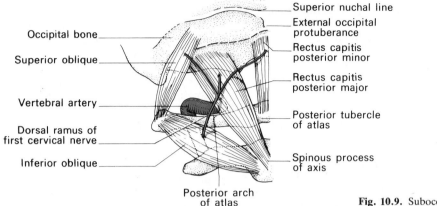

Occipital bone

Superior oblique

Vertebral artery

Dorsal ramus of
first cervical nerve

Inferior oblique

Superior nuchal line

External occipital
protuberance

Rectus capitis
posterior minor

Rectus capitis
posterior major

Posterior tubercle
of atlas

Spinous process
of axis

Posterior arch
of atlas

Fig. 10.9. Suboccipital triangle.

spinae muscles, the thoracolumbar fascia. It is most marked in the lumbar region where it consists of three layers; the posterior which is attached to the spinous processes of the lumbar vertebrae; the middle which is attached to the tips of the transverse processes and lies between the erector spinae and quadratus lumborum; and the anterior which is attached to the middle of the anterior surface of the transverse processes in front of the quadratus lumborum and behind the psoas. The three layers fuse laterally and provide attachments for some of the muscles of the anterior abdominal wall. In the thoracic region the fascia is thin, extends laterally as one layer posterior to the erector spinae and is attached to the ribs at their angles.

There are prevertebral muscles in the neck and lumbar region. The longus colli has a vertical part attached to the front of the bodies of the cervical vertebrae, a superior oblique part which passes upwards and medially from the transverse processes of the middle cervical vertebrae to the anterior tubercle of the atlas and an inferior oblique part from the front of the bodies of the upper three thoracic vertebrae upwards and laterally to the transverse processes of the middle cervical vertebrae. Its nerve supply is from the anterior primary rami of the second to the sixth cervical spinal nerves. The longus capitis is attached to the transverse processes of the lower cervical vertebrae and passes upwards and medially to the occipital bone in front of the foramen magnum. Its nerve supply is from the ventral rami of the upper cervical spinal nerves.

There are two small muscles attached to the atlas and the occipital bone similar to the small muscles of the suboccipital triangle. Rectus capitis anterior is attached below to the anterior arch of the atlas to the side of the midline and above to the occipital bone in front of the foramen magnum; rectus capitis lateralis is attached below to the front of the lateral mass of the atlas and above to the anterior aspect of the occipital condyle. Both are supplied by the ventral ramus of the first cervical nerve.

There are three scalene muscles (Figs. 10.21 & 10.22). The scalenus anterior is attached to the transverse processes of the third to the sixth (the typical) cervical vertebrae and passes downwards and slightly laterally to the scalene tubercle on the medial border of the first rib and the adjacent part of its upper surface. There are many important structures related to this muscle. The sternocleidomastoid covers it almost completely and the omohyoid runs upwards and medially between them. The subclavian vein is anterior to the muscle on the first rib and the phrenic nerve passes downwards over its anterior surface. Branches of the subclavian artery pass laterally across the muscle superficial to the phrenic nerve. Posterior to the muscle the subclavian artery passes laterally on the first rib and emerging between it and the scalenus medius are the nerves forming the brachial plexus. Medial to the muscle are the vertebral and inferior thyroid arteries and sympathetic trunk and on the left side the thoracic duct.

The previous three muscles are attached to the anterior tubercles of the transverse processes. The scalenus medius and posterior are attached to the posterior tubercles of the cervical vertebrae. The medius is attached below to the upper surface of the first rib behind the subclavian artery and the posterior to the outer border of the second rib. All the scalene muscles are supplied by the ventral rami of cervical spinal nerves. The prevertebral fascia which lies in front of all the prevertebral muscles will be described with the deep fascia of the neck.

In the lumbar region, the psoas major (the fillet steak of cattle) is attached to the bodies and intervertebral discs of the lumbar vertebrae by a series of arches which span the middle of the bodies, and to the anterior surface of the transverse processes. The muscle passes downwards lateral to the lumbar vertebrae, then round the brim of the pelvis and enters the thigh deep to the inguinal ligament. It is joined on its lateral side by the iliacus and both are attached to the lesser trochanter of the femur. The quadratus lumborum is attached above to the twelfth rib and below to the posterior part of the iliac crest. Medially it is attached to the tips of the transverse processes of the lumbar vertebrae. Both muscles are supplied by the ventral rami of the upper lumbar spinal nerves. A thick layer of fascia cover the psoas (psoas fascia). On each side its upper border forms a medial arcuate ligament which is attached medially to the body and laterally to the transverse process of the first lumbar vertebra and gives origin to some of the fibres of the diaphragm.

FUNCTIONS AND MOVEMENTS OF
VERTEBRAL COLUMN

The vertebral column protects the spinal cord from injury and during movements both the cord and the spinal nerves can slide sufficiently to prevent damage by stretching or tearing.

The column also transmits the weight of the head, neck, upper limbs and trunk to the lower limbs, via the sacrum, sacro-iliac joints and hip bones. The column is so constructed that it carries out this function very efficiently but its segmentation, which allows movement between the segments, interferes with its weight-bearing functions. This combination of weight-transmission and mobility is probably the cause of the high incidence of backache in the general population over the age of 30 years.

The bodies of the vertebrae become successively larger from the second cervical to the second sacral and then diminish rapidly in size. The sacro-iliac joint does not extend beyond the middle of the third sacral vertebrae. Weight is transmitted through the bodies but in the cervical region it also passes through the two columns of bone formed, one on each side, by the articular processes. Although in the upright position

the vertical line through the centre of gravity of the head lies in front of the transverse axis passing through the atlanto-occipital joints, there is very little activity in the muscles in the back of the neck. This somewhat unexpected finding indicates that the structure of the joints and the arrangements of the ligaments, especially the posterior ligaments, stabilize the cervical part of the vertebral column so that the head can be held in position with very little expenditure of energy.

The weight of the upper limbs is transmitted to the pectoral girdle and thence to the vertebral column mainly through muscles. The thoracic contents and walls transmit their weight through the ribs and their articulations with the thoracic vertebrae. The muscular walls of the abdomen are attached to the ribs and some of the muscles are also attached indirectly to the vertebral column. The weight of all these structures passes to the fifth lumbar vertebra which tends to slide forwards and downwards. This is resisted by strong ligaments passing from its transverse processes to the hip bones, by a very thick wedge-shaped intervertebral disc between it and the first sacral vertebra and by the almost coronal direction of the lumbosacral joints. The sacrum is prevented from being pushed downwards and forwards and rotating in these directions by very strong posterior ligaments between it and the hip bones, and by the interlocking of the articular surfaces of the sacro-iliac joints.

The curves of the vertebral column can be compared with a series of vertically arranged arches which to a limited extent can bend and return to their original form.

Movements of the vertebral column are flexion (forward bending), extension (backward bending), lateral flexion to the right or left (bending to the side) and rotation to the right or left. The first two movements take place about a transverse axis, the next about an anteroposterior axis and the last about a vertical axis. Similar movements of the head on the vertebral column also occur. Flexion of the trunk in the upright position is controlled by all the vertebral muscles of the back on both sides whether the fibres run vertically or obliquely. In the cervical region the trapezius and splenius capitis are also involved. The small muscles of the suboccipital region control the forward bending and rotation of the head. When supine the anterior muscles produce flexion of the head, neck and trunk. The longus capitis and longus colli, the rectus capitis anterior and lateralis, the scalenes, the sternocleidomastoid on both sides are active in flexing the head and neck. The anterior abdominal muscles (p. 588) (especially the rectus abdominis) and the psoas flex the trunk. In the upright position extension is controlled by the flexors just described. In the prone position the posterior vertebral muscles of both sides and the trapezius and splenius capitis and the suboccipital muscles produce extension. Lateral flexion to the right in the upright position would be expected to be controlled by the left anterior and posterior vertebral muscles. There is evidence that the stability of the vertebral column makes it necessary for the right vertebral muscles to contract so that the head, neck and trunk are pulled to the right in the coronal plane. Similarly the left vertebral muscles are involved in left lateral flexion. Rotation to the right is produced by posterior oblique muscles on the left running upwards and inwards and posterior oblique muscles on the right running upwards and outwards. The right splenius capitis turns the head and neck to the right. The left sternocleidomastoid turns the head (and neck) to the right.

The greatest range of flexion and extension takes place between the occipital bone and atlas (about 40°). Lateral flexion between the occipital bone and atlas, and atlas and axis is relatively limited, and rotary movements take place between the atlas and axis at the median and lateral atlanto–axial joints (i.e. the head and atlas rotate round the dens of the axis). These movements are controlled by the large number of small muscles passing between these three bones—the occipital, the atlas and the axis.

Thorax

BONES AND JOINTS OF THORAX

The trunk is divided into the thorax and abdomen by the diaphragm (p. 435). The bones forming the thoracic cage are the twelve thoracic vertebrae and their intervertebral discs posteriorly in the midline, the twelve ribs and their costal cartilages, which form the lateral walls and part of the posterior and anterior walls, and the sternum in the midline anteriorly (Fig. 10.10).

A typical rib (Fig. 10.11) has the following features. The main part, called the body (shaft), is flattened so that it has an upper and lower border and an external and internal surface. About 8 cm lateral to the posterior end of the rib the body bends forwards at the angle where the rib is also twisted so that the posterior part faces

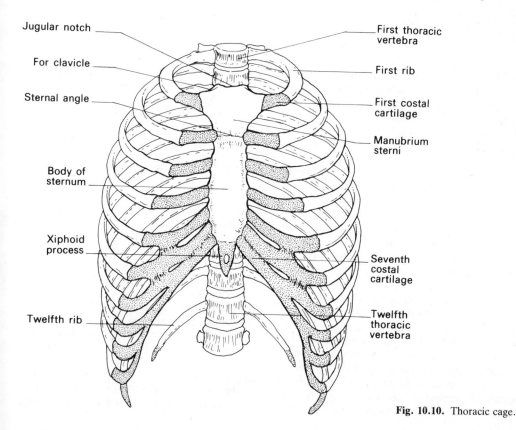

Jugular notch — First thoracic vertebra

For clavicle — First rib

Sternal angle — First costal cartilage

Manubrium sterni

Body of sternum

Xiphoid process — Seventh costal cartilage

Twelfth rib — Twelfth thoracic vertebra

Fig. 10.10. Thoracic cage.

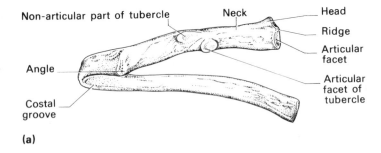

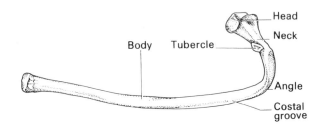

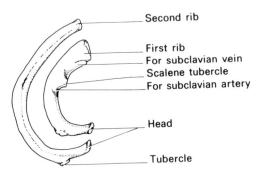

Fig. 10.11. Typical rib: (a) left rib viewed from behind; (b) right rib viewed from left.

slightly upwards and the anterior faces downwards. The anterior end of the body is considerably lower than the posterior. Medial to the angle the erector spinae is attached to the outer surface, and lateral to the angle the serratus anterior (upper eight ribs), the external oblique (lower eight ribs) and latissimus dorsi (lower four ribs) are attached. On the inner surface posteriorly there is a groove just above the inferior border, the costal groove, in which lie the intercostal nerve and posterior intercostal vessels. The intercostal muscles are attached to the upper border of the rib and also to the lower border of the rib above, the external and internal muscles lying superficial to the vessels and nerve, and the intimus deep to these structures.

The posterior end of the rib is called the head which has two facets separated by a transverse ridge. The facets articulate with facets on the bodies of two adjacent vertebrae as a rule, the rib corresponding in number with the lower vertebrae (Fig. 10.13a & b). The first, tenth, eleventh and twelfth ribs articulate with a single facet on their corresponding vertebrae. Lateral to the head is the neck, lateral to which is the tubercle. The medial part of the tubercle is smooth where it articulates with the transverse process of the vertebra and the lateral part, to which is attached a ligament, is rough. The anterior end of a rib is oval and has a concave

Fig. 10.12. Superior aspect of first and second ribs.

facet where it becomes continuous with a costal cartilage.

The above description refers to the third to the tenth ribs. The first rib (Fig. 10.12) is usually the smallest and is much more curved than the others. It has an outer and inner border and upper and lower surface. The tubercle and angle are merged. The upper surface has two grooves separated by the scalene tubercle on the inner border of its anterior part. The scalenus anterior is attached to the tubercle and the subclavian artery and upper trunk of the brachial plexus lie in the posterior groove. The subclavian vein lies in the anterior groove. The scalenus medius is attached to the upper surface behind the artery

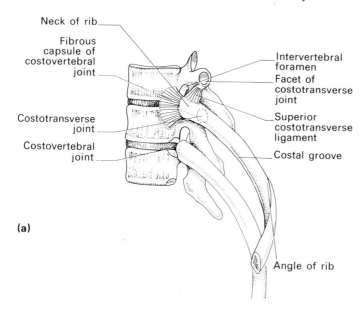

Neck of rib

Fibrous capsule of costovertebral joint

Costotransverse joint

Costovertebral joint

Intervertebral foramen

Facet of costotransverse joint

Superior costotransverse ligament

Costal groove

(a)

Angle of rib

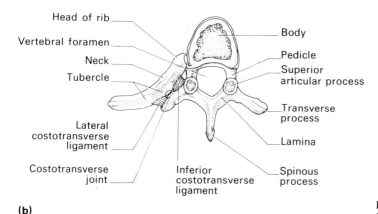

Head of rib

Vertebral foramen

Neck

Tubercle

Lateral costotransverse ligament

Costotransverse joint

Inferior costotransverse ligament

Body

Pedicle

Superior articular process

Transverse process

Lamina

Spinous process

(b)

Fig. 10.13. (a) Costovertebral joints; (b) Costotransverse joint.

and the suprapleural membrane to the inner border. The first rib has no costal groove. The second rib (Fig. 10.12) tends to have upper and lower surfaces and outer and inner borders. The scalenus posterior is attached to the outer border. The eleventh and twelfth ribs are much shorter than the typical ribs and do not have a neck, tubercle or costal groove.

The costal cartilages (Fig. 10.10) are attached to the anterior ends of the ribs. The first seven articulate with the sternum (true ribs). The eighth, ninth and tenth articulate with the costal cartilage above (false ribs) producing the costal margin. The eleventh and twelfth costal cartilages are short and end in the abdominal wall (floating ribs). The medial end of the first costal cartilage superiorly forms part of the sternoclavicular joint. The internal oblique and rectus abdominis are attached to the lower costal cartilages anteriorly and the transversus abdominis and diaphragm to the internal surface of the lower six cartilages. In old age the costal cartilages, which consist of hyaline cartilage, become partly calcified and also ossified.

The sternum (meaning the breast), a typical flat bone, consists of three parts, the manubrium, body and xiphoid process (Fig. 10.10). The manubrium is roughly quadrilateral in shape with a notch on its superior border (jugular or suprasternal notch). The upper lateral angle has two notches, a more medial for the clavicle and a lower for the first costal cartilage.

At the lower lateral angle there is a notch for the second costal cartilage. The sternocleidomastoid is attached to the superolateral angle of the anterior surface. The lower border articulates by a secondary cartilaginous joint (p. 384) with the upper border of the body. This is easily palpable and is called the sternal angle. The xiphoid process articulates with the lower border of the body by a fibrous joint and ends below in a pointed extremity in the abdominal wall. The muscles of the anterior abdominal wall are attached to it, as is the diaphragm to its deep surface. It often remains incompletely ossified in the adult.

There are synovial joints between the costal cartilages of the second to the seventh ribs and the sternum (chondrosternal joints), and also where the seventh, eighth, ninth and tenth costal cartilages articulate with one another. The eleventh and twelfth costal cartilages end in the abdominal wall. There is a primary cartilaginous joint between the first rib and the manubrium and a secondary cartilaginous joint between the manubrium and body of the sternum.

The thorax is roughly conical in shape with a relatively small inlet above and a much larger outlet below (Fig. 10.10).

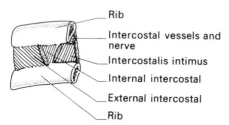

Rib
Intercostal vessels and nerve
Intercostalis intimus
Internal intercostal
External intercostal
Rib

Fig. 10.14. Intercostal muscles and neurovascular bundle.

MUSCLES AND FASCIA OF THORAX
(INCLUDING DIAPHRAGM)

The muscles attached to the thorax and acting mainly on the upper limb or the vertebral column or the abdominal walls are excluded. There are three sets of intercostal muscles, the external, internal and innermost (intimi) (Fig. 10.14). There are eleven pairs of each of these muscles between adjacent ribs. Posteriorly the fibres of the external muscles pass downwards and laterally, at the side they pass downwards and forwards, and anteriorly they pass downwards and medially. The fibres of the internal intercostals run in the opposite direction to those of the external and those of the intimi run in the same

direction as the internal intercostal fibres. Anteriorly the external intercostal muscle is replaced by the anterior intercostal membrane and posteriorly the internal intercostal is replaced by the posterior intercostal membrane. The sternocostalis muscle is attached to the inner aspect of the lower part of the sternum and its fibres radiate upwards and outwards to the upper costal cartilages. The subcostal muscles pass between the inner surfaces of adjacent ribs posteriorly. The levatores costarum are found posteriorly between the tip of a transverse process of a thoracic vertebra and the posterior surface of the rib below it. Their fibres pass downwards and laterally. There are two thin sheets of mainly tendinous muscles on the posterior surface of the thorax between the spinous processes of the upper thoracic vertebrae and the upper ribs (serratus posterior superior) and the spinous processes of the lower thoracic vertebrae and the lower ribs (serratus posterior inferior). The nerve supply of these muscles is from the intercostal nerves which are the ventral rami of the thoracic spinal nerves. The levatores costarum are supplied by the dorsal rami.

The endothoracic fascia refers to a layer of loose connective tissue between the chest wall and parietal pleura. It is thickened over the dome of the pleura in the neck and forms the suprapleural membrane, a distinct fibrous layer which is attached above to the transverse process of the seventh cervical vertebra and below to the inner border of the first rib.

The diaphragm (Fig. 10.15) is a dome-shaped musculotendinous sheet separating the thoracic from the abdominal cavity. It is muscular peripherally and tendinous in its centre. The muscle fibres are attached to:
1 The deep surface of the xiphoid process of the sternum (sternal part).
2 The inner surface of the lower six costal cartilages and ribs where they interdigitate with the fibres of the transversus abdominis (costal part).
3 The lateral arcuate ligament (the thickened upper border of the fascia over the quadratus lumborum), the medial arcuate ligament (the thickened upper border of the psoas fascia) and by two crura to the sides of the lumbar vertebral bodies, the upper three on the right and the upper two on the left (lumbar part).
The muscle fibres pass upwards and converge onto a central tendon. The medial fibres of the right crus pass to the left side so that the oesophagus passes through the right crus (the oesophageal opening). The central tendon is trefoil in shape with an anterior leaf and two

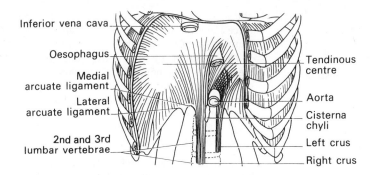

Inferior vena cava

Oesophagus

Medial arcuate ligament

Lateral arcuate ligament

2nd and 3rd lumbar vertebrae

Tendinous centre

Aorta

Cisterna chyli

Left crus

Right crus

Fig. 10.15. Diaphragm.

posterolateral leaves. The upper surface of the tendon is attached to the pericardium. Normally the diaphragm, apart from some openings, completely separates the thoracic from the abdominal cavity due to the peripheral muscular attachments.

Several structures pass through (or behind) the diaphragm. The aorta passes behind the diaphragm near the midline between the crura at the level of the twelfth thoracic vertebra, and the thoracic duct and the azygos vein pass upwards through the same opening to the right of the aorta. The oesophagus passes through the right crus, as described above, about 2 cm to the left of the midline at the level of the tenth thoracic vertebra. The gastric nerves and some branches of the gastric arteries to the oesophagus also pass through this opening. The inferior vena cava passes through the central tendon 3 cm to the right of the midline at the level of the eighth thoracic vertebra. The edges of the opening are adherent to the wall of the vena cava and the right phrenic nerve passes through this opening. The sympathetic trunk enters the abdomen behind the medial arcuate ligament and the subcostal nerve passes behind the lateral arcuate ligament. The splanchnic nerves pass through the crura.

Above the diaphragm on each side are a lung and its pleura and in the middle are the heart and pericardium. Below on the right side are the right lobe of the liver, right kidney and right suprarenal gland, and on the left are the left lobe of the liver, the fundus of the stomach, the left kidney, the left suprarenal gland and the spleen.

The right half of the diaphragm is supplied by the right, and the left half by the left phrenic nerve which comes from the third, fourth and fifth cervical spinal nerves, mainly the fourth. About one-third of the fibres are sensory. The lower six intercostal nerves also supply the peripheral parts of the diaphragm with sensory fibres.

FUNCTIONS OF THORAX AND THORACIC MUSCLES

The bony thorax protects the lungs and heart; it also provides fixed areas for the action of many muscles to the extent that respiration, the most important function of the thorax, is temporarily suspended in strong muscular effort.

In quiet inspiration the central part of the diaphragm moves down about 2 cm due to the contraction of the peripheral muscle fibres (Fig. 10.16). It has been suggested that the diaphragm lifts the lower ribs, and because this raises the sternum, the upper ribs, which are attached to it, are also raised. The way in which they move is determined by the shape of the costotransverse joints. Another suggestion is that the scalene muscles in the neck lift the first rib and the others are thus made to move. It should be appreciated that the amount of movement is small and hardly measurable. However in the upright position the movements of the ribs account for about one-third of the increase in the volume of the chest. The result is an increase in the transverse and anteroposterior diameters of its upper part. The axis of movement of the upper ribs is a line through the costovertebral and costotransverse joints (Fig. 10.17). Because the lateral and anterior parts of the upper ribs are lower than the posterior an increase in two diameters takes place. The lower ribs rotate outwards about a vertical axis through the neck so that only the transverse diameter increases (Fig. 10.17). The difference in the shape and plane of the costotransverse joints is associated with these differences in movement.

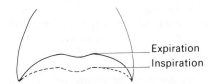

Expiration
Inspiration

Fig. 10.16. Diaphragm movement in quiet respiration.

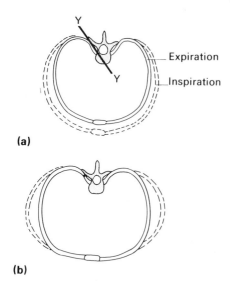

(a)

(b)

Fig. 10.17. Movement of ribs during respiration: (a) upper ribs; (b) lower ribs.

Expiration is largely a passive act due to the elastic recoil of the lungs. The diaphragm relaxes and moves upwards, the abdominal viscera move up and the abdominal muscles move in. The ribs return to their 'resting position'.

In deep breathing the total excursion of the diaphragm is about 9 cm. Associated with this, are the increased descent of the abdominal viscera and the increased pushing out of the anterior abdominal wall in inspiration. In deep expiration the upward movement of the diaphragm is produced by active contraction of the muscles of the anterior abdominal wall, especially the oblique muscles at the sides. The excursion of the ribs is also increased and both the external and intercostal muscles are active in inspiration and expiration in deep breathing. It has been suggested that their function is to prevent the intercostal spaces from being sucked in during inspiration and blown out in expiration.

In forced respiration, which by definition is respiration against an obstruction, every muscle which can increase the volume of the thorax is said to be 'active'. In inspiration the diaphragm and the intercostals are markedly contracted, the sternomastoids and scalenes contract maximally and it is said that any muscle which can act on the chest wall is brought into play.

Forced expiration is associated with marked contraction of the muscles of the anterior abdominal wall, especially the oblique muscles. The latissimus dorsi also contracts. Coughing and sneezing which are good examples of normal forced expiration, are associated with marked contraction of these muscles.

The position of the body influences the amount of movement of the diaphragm. It is greatest when lying down, least when sitting up and leaning forwards, and intermediate when standing up.

CONTENTS OF THORAX

Most of the thoracic cavity is occupied by the lungs, one in each half, with the heart lying between them. Each lung is covered with pleura (visceral) which is continuous on its medial side with a layer of pleura (parietal) lining the chest wall. The heart is covered by the pericardium. Entering and leaving the heart are the large venous and arterial vessels. Most of these lie above or behind the heart. The space between the lungs is called the mediastinum. This is divided in a superior and inferior mediastinum by an imaginary plane through the manubriosternal joint and the liver border. The inferior is further subdivided into an anterior in front of the heart, a middle containing the heart and a posterior behind the heart. The superior mediastinum contains the oesophagus and trachea posteriorly, the remains of the thymus anteriorly, and the large blood vessels in between. In the posterior mediastinum are the oesophagus, thoracic duct and vagus nerves, the thoracic aorta and the sympathetic trunks, and the azygos veins. The middle mediastinum contains the heart and the beginning or end of the large blood vessels and the phrenic nerves. There is only some areolar tissue in the anterior mediastinum.

Abdomen and pelvis

BONES, JOINTS AND MUSCLES OF ABDOMEN AND PELVIS

The abdominal cavity extends into the thorax to the level of the fifth or sixth intercostal space anteriorly. The abdominal cavity extends downwards into the pelvis which is divided into the greater (false) pelvis above the level of the superior pelvic aperture (also known as the pelvic brim or inlet), and the lesser (true) pelvis below the level of the superior aperture (Fig. 10.18). The greater pelvis can be regarded as part of the abdominal cavity, and deal separately with the lesser pelvis, although it is continuous with the abdominal cavity.

The walls of the abdomen are mainly muscular especially anteriorly but the muscular interval

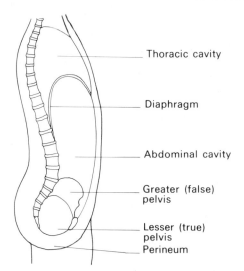

Thoracic cavity

Diaphragm

Abdominal cavity

Greater (false) pelvis

Lesser (true) pelvis

Perineum

Fig. 10.18. Sagittal section of trunk showing body cavities.

between the lowest rib and the bony pelvis (the loin) laterally and posteriorly is quite small (about 8 cm). The posterior wall in the middle is formed by the lumbar vertebrae (p. 425). More laterally it is formed by the psoas and quadratus lumborum (p. 430). The rest of the wall is formed by the anterior muscles of the abdominal wall.

The bony pelvis consists of the hip (innominate) bone on each side and anteriorly, and the sacrum posteriorly. Each hip bone (Fig. 10.19) consists of three bones, the ilium, the ischium and the pubic bone. All three bones meet and contribute to the deep hollow on the outer side of the hip bone, the acetabulum, with which the head of the femur articulates to form the hip joint. The upper boundary of the ilium is called the crest to which many muscles of the abdominal wall and the lower limb are attached.

NECK (COLLUM; CERVIX)

Although it may be considered superfluous to define the neck as that part of the body between the head and thorax, it is important to realize that the neck is much more extensive posteriorly than anteriorly. All the cervical vertebrae are considered to be in the neck and the lower border of the mandible is at the level of the third cervical vertebra. Anterior structures which are comparatively superficial in the neck lie at a much deeper level in its upper part and cannot be seen very clearly without removing the mandible and extending the head on the vertebral column. The neck develops largely from the pharyngeal arches and is not present in the early embryo, that is, at about three weeks. Functionally it may be regarded as part of a movable column which can turn the head and particularly the eyes in the desired direction, as a passageway for large vessels from and to the thorax and head, and as a communication between the beginnings of the respiratory and alimentary tracts and their continuations lower down. In the neck there are also branches of some of the

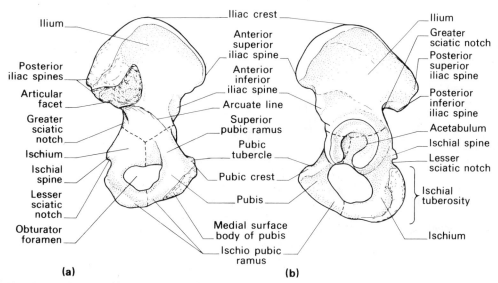

Fig. 10.19. Hip bone: (a) inner aspect; (b) outer aspect.

lower cranial nerves, particularly the vagus, and
the termination of the large lymphatic vessels.
Two of the large salivary glands and the thyroid
gland are situated in the neck.

Bones, joints and muscles of the neck

The cervical vertebrae and their joints lie posteriorly with their anterior (prevertebral) and
posterior muscles. More anteriorly there are also
skeletal elements derived from the pharyngeal
arches. The hyoid bone (Fig. 10.20) develops
from the skeleton of the second and third arches
and some of the laryngeal cartilages from arches
lower down.

Anteriorly the hyoid bone has a body which if
followed backwards becomes the greater cornu.
It is at approximately the same level as the body.
At the junction of the body and greater cornu,
the lesser cornu projects upwards and backwards. The hyoid bone does not articulate with

any other bone or cartilage but has a large
number of muscles attached to it and is kept in
place and moved by these muscles. The muscles
are divided into two groups, the suprahyoid and
infrahyoid, above and below the bone respectively (Figs. 10.20 & 10.21).

The suprahyoid muscles include the digastric,
stylohyoid, mylohyoid, middle constrictor of the
pharynx, the hyoglossus and the geniohyoid.
The digastric muscle has two bellies. The posterior belly is attached to the mastoid (digastric)
notch of the temporal bone and passes downwards to the body of the hyoid bone to which it is
attached by a tendon. From this tendon the
anterior belly passes upwards and becomes
attached to the inner surface of the mandible
lateral to the midline near the lower border. The
stylohyoid muscle is attached to the styloid process of the temporal bone and passes downwards
with the posterior belly of the digastric to the
hyoid bone. The posterior belly and the

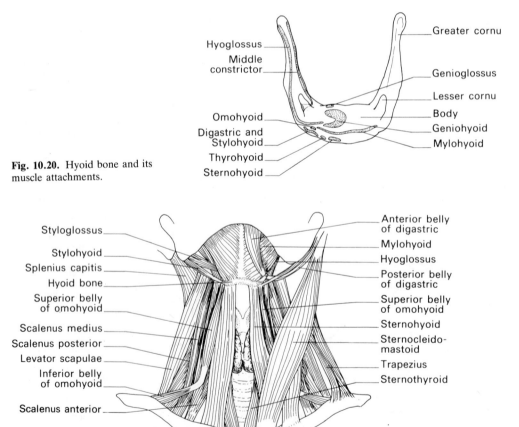

Fig. 10.20. Hyoid bone and its muscle attachments.

Fig. 10.21. Muscles of neck from in front.

stylohyoid are supplied by the facial nerve. The mylohyoid muscle is attached to the inner surface of the ramus of the mandible along the mylohyoid line and passes medially and slightly downwards. Most of its fibres form a midline raphe but some become attached to the body of the hyoid. The mylohyoid muscles form the floor of the mouth and separate neck structures below from mouth structures above. The mylohyoid and anterior belly of the digastric are supplied by the nerve to the mylohyoid muscle, a branch of the inferior alveolar nerve, a branch of the mandibular nerve. The middle constrictor is attached to the greater and lesser cornua and fans out into the wall of the pharynx and the hyoglossus is attached to the greater cornu and passes upward into the base of the tongue. The middle constrictor is innervated by the pharyngeal plexus (the motor branch is from the vagus) and the hyoglossus by the hypoglossal nerve. The geniohyoid is attached to the inner surface of the mandible near the midline and to the body of the hyoid bone. It is supplied by the first cervical nerve.

The infrahyoid muscles include the sternohyoid, thyrohyoid, and omohyoid. The sternothyroid muscle is included since it functions with this group. The sternohyoid is attached inferiorly to the upper part of the deep surface of the manubrium of the sternum and passes upwards to the body of the hyoid bone. The thyrohyoid is attached inferiorly to the lamina of the thyroid cartilage and above to the body of the hyoid. The sternothyroid is attached below to the upper part of the deep surface of the manubrium sterni and above to the lamina of the thyroid cartilage. The omohyoid muscle has two bellies, the inferior is attached to the upper border of the scapula (omo means a shoulder) and passes upwards and forwards deep to the sternocleidomastoid. The intermediate tendon has a fascial sling attaching it to the region of the sternoclavicular joint and the superior belly passes upwards to the hyoid bone. All these muscles are supplied by one or more of the ventral rami of the first three cervical nerves.

The infrahyoid group of muscles stabilize the hyoid bone so that the suprahyoid muscles can act in chewing and swallowing. They are active in phonation. With the hyoid bone fixed, the anterior belly of the digastric and the mylohyoid muscles are active in opening the mouth against resistance.

The lesser cornu of the hyoid bone is attached above to the styloid process of the temporal bone by the stylohyoid ligament. The body and greater cornua are attached below to the laminae and superior cornua of the thyroid cartilage by the thyrohyoid membrane. This membrane passes upwards deep to the body of the hyoid bone and is attached to its upper border. There is usually a bursa between the membrane and the posterior surface of the body. The epiglottis passes upwards behind the body of the hyoid and is attached to it by the hyo–epiglottic ligament.

The hyoid bone ossifies in cartilage, the upper part of the body and lesser cornua from the cartilage of the second pharyngeal arch and the lower part of the body and the greater cornua from that of the third arch. There is a centre of ossification for each cornu and each half of the body. They appear towards the end of intrauterine life except for those for the lesser cornua which appear about puberty. The lesser cornua often remain attached to the body by fibrous tissue until late in life and not infrequently ossification extends into the stylohyoid ligament.

The platysma is a muscle in the superficial fascia of the anterolateral part of the neck. It extends upwards over the mandible into the cheek and angle of the mouth and downwards over the clavicle into the chest. It is grouped with the muscles of facial expression (p. 464) and is innervated by the facial nerve.

There are two large superficial muscles in the neck, the trapezius at the back and the sternocleidomastoid in front. The trapezius arises from the superior third of the superior nuchal line of the occipital bone, the external occipital protuberance, the ligamentum nuchae and the spines of all the thoracic vertebrae. It is inserted into the lateral third of the clavicle and the upper border of the spine of the scapula. The sternocleidomastoid (Figs. 10.21 & 10.22) is attached inferiorly and anteriorly to the upper, lateral part of the manubrium sterni by a tendinous head and to the medial half of the clavicle by a muscular head. The muscle passes upwards and backwards round the side of the neck and is attached to the posterior part of the lateral side of the mastoid process of the temporal bone and the lateral third of the superior nuchal line of the occipital bone. Deep to its attachment to the temporal bone are the splenius capitis and longissimus capitis.

The sternocleidomastoid divides the neck into two regions—one in front of it called the anterior triangle and one behind it (limited by the trapezius) called the posterior triangle. These will be described later in more detail. Superficial

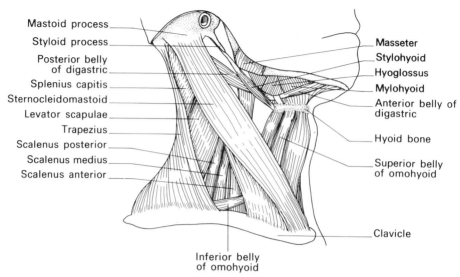

Mastoid process

Styloid process

Posterior belly
of digastric

Splenius capitis

Sternocleidomastoid

Levator scapulae

Trapezius

Scalenus posterior

Scalenus medius

Scalenus anterior

Masseter

Stylohyoid

Hyoglossus

Mylohyoid

**Anterior belly of
digastric**

Hyoid bone

Superior belly
of omohyoid

Clavicle

Inferior belly
of omohyoid

Fig. 10.22. Muscles of neck from the side.

to the sternocleidomastoid is the external jugular vein and some cutaneous branches of the cervical plexus. Just above the clavicle the muscle is superficial to some of the infrahyoid muscles and the anterior jugular vein. Above these, the large vessels (subclavian and carotid arteries and internal jugular and subclavian veins and some of their branches and tributaries) are deep to the muscle. The brachial and cervical plexuses are partly covered by the sternocleidomastoid. Its nerve supply is the spinal accessory and the ventral rami of the second and third cervical spinal nerves. The latter are sensory.

When one sternocleidomastoid contracts the head is turned to the opposite side and tilted to the same side. Both muscles contracting at the same time are flexors of the head.

TRIANGLES OF NECK

For convenience of description, the neck is divided into a number of triangles (Fig. 10.22). The anterior triangle is bounded laterally by the anterior border of the sternocleidomastoid, anteriorly by the midline of the neck and superiorly by the lower border of the mandible. This triangle is further subdivided into three triangles. The submandibular (digastric) triangle is bounded by the two bellies of the digastric muscle below and by the lower border of the mandible above. There are several structures in this triangle including the submandibular salivary gland, submandibular lymph nodes and mylohyoid muscle. Deep to the mylohyoid are

the deep part of the submandibular gland, the hyoglossus muscle and the hypoglossal and lingual nerves. The carotid triangle is bounded posteriorly by the anterior border of the sternocleidomastoid muscle, above by the posterior border of the digastric muscle and in front by the superior belly of the omohyoid. The main structures in this triangle are the internal and external carotid arteries and the branches of the latter artery, hence the name of the triangle. The muscular triangle is bounded above and laterally by the superior belly of the omohyoid, below and laterally by the anterior border of the sternocleidomastoid and medially by the midline of the neck. In this triangle are the infrahyoid or strap muscles deep to which lies the thyroid gland. The submental triangle is inferior to the mandible and is bounded by the anterior bellies of the digastric muscles and the hyoid bone.

The posterior triangle (Fig. 10.22) is bounded posteriorly by the anterior border of the trapezius, anteriorly by the posterior border of the sternocleidomastoid and inferiorly by the middle third of the clavicle. Although called posterior this triangle winds round the side of the neck. Its apex is related to the occipital bone posteriorly and its base is anterior. The posterior triangle has a muscular floor. The muscles from below upwards are the scalenus medius, levator scapulae and splenius capitis. At the apex some vertically running fibres of the semispinalis capitis can be seen. At the anterior inferior corner there is a small part of the scalenus anterior. The inferior belly of the omohyoid passes upwards and forwards across the lower part of the floor and runs deep to the sternocleido-mastoid. The posterior triangle is divided by the omohyoid into a lower supraclavicular triangle and an upper occipital in which several cutaneous branches of the cervical plexus can be seen emerging from the posterior border of the sternocleidomastoid muscle. These pass upwards or forwards or downwards. Crossing the floor of the occipital triangle and running downwards and backwards is the spinal accessory nerve which goes deep to the trapezius. In the supraclavicular triangle the third part of the subclavian artery passes laterally and becomes the axillary artery and the trunks of the brachial plexus and some of its branches lie superior to the artery.

Cervical fascia

The neck is enclosed in a well marked sheath of deep fascia, called the cervical fascia. In addition to the ensheathing layer there are several fairly distinct structures of a fascial nature and these are regarded as subdivisions of the cervical fascia (Fig. 10.23). The ensheathing layer, unfortunately named the superficial layer, is attached posteriorly to midline structures—the external occipital protuberance, the ligamentum nuchae and the spinous process of the first thoracic vertebra. When followed laterally it is seen to enclose the trapezius and meet at its lateral border. It then covers the posterior triangle and is often referred to as the roofing layer because there is another deeper layer of fascia covering the floor of the triangle. The investing layer then splits and encloses the sternocleidomastoid and continues over the anterior triangle to the midline anteriorly where it becomes attached to the hyoid bone and the laryngeal prominence. Inferiorly it is attached to the middle third of the clavicle and in the midline to the upper border of the manubrium sterni. Just above the jugular notch the deep fascia splits and encloses a space, the suprasternal space, in which are the anterior jugular veins. Superiorly the deep fascia is attached to the inferior border of the mandible. About halfway between the symphysis menti and angle of the mandible the fascia splits to enclose the submandibular salivary gland. Near the angle the fascia encloses the parotid gland and above the gland is attached to the zygomatic arch and the supramastoid crest. If followed posteriorly it is seen to enclose the sternocleidomastoid and trapezius muscles along the superior nuchal line.

The prevertebral lamina of the deep cervical fascia lies anterior to the prevertebral muscles, that is in front of the longus colli, longus capitis, scalene muscles and levator scapulae, and can be followed laterally over the posterior triangle deep to the ensheathing layer and deep to the trapezius where the fascia fades out. The subclavian artery is deep to the prevertebral fascia and carries a layer into the axilla (axillary sheath) round the axillary artery. The accessory nerve as it crosses the posterior triangle lies superficial to the prevertebral fascia, that is, between the two layers of fascia covering the muscles in the floor of the triangle. In the midline the prevertebral fascia is separated anteriorly from the posterior wall of the pharynx by the retropharyngeal space which contains loose areolar tissue and, inferior to the skull, a few lymph nodes. The prevertebral fascia superiorly fuses with the periosteum of the skull and inferiorly with the anterior longitudinal ligament of the vertebral column. As is the case elsewhere in the body the nerves of the region (the cervical and brachial plexuses) are external to the fascia.

The carotid sheath surrounds the common and internal carotid arteries, the internal jugular vein and the vagus nerve and extends from the thorax to the base of the skull. It is thicker medially next to the arteries than laterally near the vein to allow for distension of the vein.

The pretracheal lamina of the deep cervical fascia lies in front of the trachea in the lower part of the neck. If followed upwards, it forms a sheath for the thyroid gland and becomes attached to the lamina of the thyroid cartilage. Inferiorly the pretracheal fascia passes into the thorax and fuses with the fibrous pericardium.

The various parts of the deep cervical fascia determine to some extent the way in which infection spreads in the neck. Infection deep to the prevertebral fascia near the midline tends to be spread laterally into the posterior triangle. In the midline, pus anterior to the fascia bulges into the pharynx. Pus deep to the pretracheal layer can spread downwards into the mediastinum,

General arrangements of structures in neck (Fig. 10.23)

This is probably best appreciated by examining a simplified transverse section at, for example, the level of the seventh cervical vertebra. It is important to recognize that most of the section is occupied by the vertebra and the muscles attached to it. In front of the body of the vertebra lies the oesophagus. Higher up this is replaced by the pharynx which extends upwards to the base

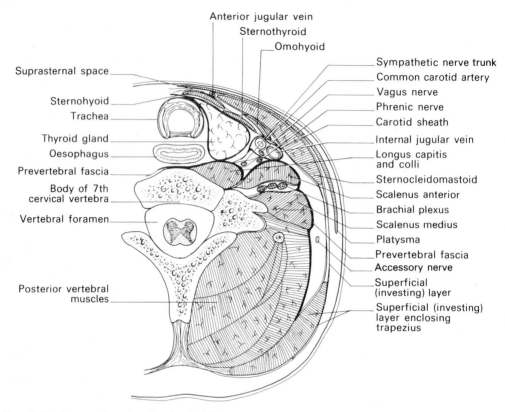

Fig. 10.23. Cross section of neck at level of 7th cervical vertebra showing fascia.

of the skull. The trachea, and its upward continuation, the larynx, are anterior to the oesophagus. The larynx begins at the level of the third or fourth cervical vertebra and can be regarded as an anterior diverticulum from the pharynx. If the front of the neck is examined in the living, laterally the greater cornua of the hyoid bone can be felt, as well as its body in the midline. This is roughly at the level of the mandible if the head and neck are not extended. About 1 cm inferior to the hyoid bone, the laryngeal prominence (Adam's apple) can be felt in the midline and the upper part of the laminae of the thyroid cartilage on either side. The lower part is more difficult to palpate because on each side the lobes of the thyroid gland extend about halfway up the laminae. Immediately inferior to the thyroid cartilage the anterior arch of the cricoid cartilage can be felt. This is a circular structure with a flattened plate posteriorly. The cricoid cartilage marks the level of the body of the sixth cervical vertebra and also where the larynx and pharynx end and the trachea and oesophagus begin. Inferior to the

cricoid cartilage the upper rings of the trachea can be felt above the jugular notch. The two lobes of the thyroid gland are joined by an isthmus which is anterior to the second, third and fourth rings of the trachea.

The main blood vessels of the neck and head lie anterior to the transverse processes of the cervical vertebrae. These are the common and internal carotid arteries and the internal jugular vein. The common carotid artery divides into the internal and external carotid arteries at the upper border of the lamina of the thyroid cartilage and the internal continues upwards in line with the common carotid artery. The external gives off a large number of branches to the structures of the neck and head (outside the skull). The vagus nerve runs downwards in the neck posterior to and between the artery and vein. The sympathetic nerve trunk runs vertically upwards embedded in the prevertebral fascia, posterior and medial to the carotid sheath. The phrenic nerve runs downwards on the scalenus anterior deep to the prevertebral fascia. The ventral rami of the cervical spinal nerves, as they pass laterally, emerge between the scalenus anterior and scalenus medius and form the cervical (upper four) and brachial plexuses (lower four together with the ventral ramus of the first thoracic nerve).

HEAD

The skeleton of the head, the skull, may be regarded as a number of bony cavities containing structures related to the nervous system and also as the beginning of the respiratory and alimentary systems. The largest of these, the cranial cavity, contains the brain and the beginning or end of the cranial nerves. The orbit contains the eyeball and the structures related to it. The nasal cavity is associated with respiration and smell and the oral cavity with sucking, chewing, swallowing, taste and respiration. The temporal bone contains organs related to hearing and equilibrium. In addition individual bones contain air spaces the function of which in man are somewhat obscure. There are two groups of muscles, one associated with mastication and the other with facial expression. The latter have retained their more primitive functions in relation to the orifices of the orbit and mouth, namely to open and close them, but this function has been lost with respect to the nasal cavity and external ear.

Instead in man the muscles are associated with the expression of emotion to an extent far exceeding that seen in any other animal, and the muscles round the orifice of the oral cavity are involved in sucking, chewing, swallowing and the production of sounds recognized as language.

Skull

The skull consists of two parts, the cranium and the mandible. The cranium consists of an upper box-like part, the calvaria, which contains the brain, and a lower anterior part which forms the facial skeleton (Fig. 10.24). Frequently the word skull is used to mean cranium. There is a large number of bones in the skull articulating with each other by fibrous joints, called sutures, at which after birth (p. 384), there is no movement. The mandible articulates with the base of the skull by means of a condyloid synovial joint. A detailed knowledge of the skull demands a study of the individual bones but it is probably better to be familiar with the situation of the main bones and follow this with a detailed examination of the skull as a whole.

From the side, the upper part of the cranium is seen to consist from in front backwards of the frontal, parietal and occipital bones (Fig. 10.24). The frontal bone articulates with the parietal at

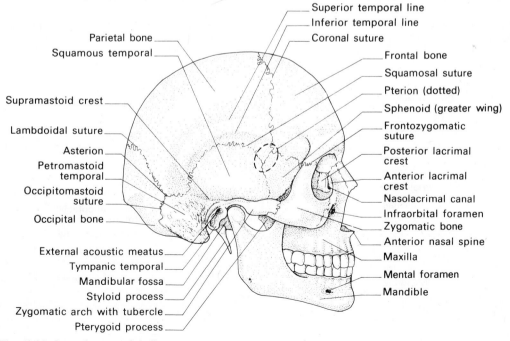

Fig. 10.24. Lateral aspect of skull.

the serrated coronal (frontal) suture and the occipital with the parietal at the lambdoidal suture, also serrated. Inferior to the parietal bone is the temporal bone and the articulation between them is the squamosal suture at which the bones overlap. The temporal bone posteriorly articulates with the occipital at the occipitomastoid suture. In front of the temporal bone a part of the sphenoid bone is seen articulating with the frontal and the parietal bones at an H-shaped suture called the pterion. Projecting forward from the temporal bone is its zygomatic process which meets the zygomatic (cheek) bone and completes the zygomatic arch. Below and in front of the zygoma, and in a deeper plane, is the maxilla with a curved lower border carrying the upper teeth.

Although the bones bounding the opening of the orbit can be seen from the side of the skull (the frontal bone above, the zygomatic bone laterally and the maxilla below and medially) they are more obvious from in front (Fig. 10.25). Between the openings of the two orbits the maxillae articulate with the frontal bone above, and medially with the nasal bones which meet in the midline. The large opening into the nasal cavity is bounded by the maxilla on each side and below, where the maxillae meet, and above by the nasal bones.

Inferiorly the occipital bone is seen to extend into the base of the skull (Fig. 10.26). In this part of the bone is the large foramen magnum on each side of which is an occipital condyle. Lateral to the condyle the occipital bone articulates with the temporal bone. In front of the foramen magnum the occipital bone is narrow and fuses with the sphenoid bone which can be followed forwards to the posterior nasal apertures and laterally to the side of the skull. The temporal bone projects medially and forwards between the sphenoid bone in front and the occipital bone behind. More laterally the temporal bone projects forwards and meets the lateral part of the sphenoid bone. The anterior part of the skull in the middle projects downwards to a lower level as compared with that of the rest of the skull. This projection is largely formed by the two maxillae which constitute most of the hard palate. The posterior part of the hard palate is formed by the palatine bones. The sphenoid bone projects downwards behind the maxillae on each side and forms the lateral boundary of the posterior nasal apertures. Between the two apertures is the vomer (ploughshare).

Inside the skull the floor of the cranial cavity posteriorly is formed by the occipital bone (Fig. 10.27). In front of the foramen magnum it fuses with the sphenoid bone which extends laterally to the side of the skull. Between the lateral parts of the occipital and the sphenoid bones is the temporal bone. Anteriorly the sphenoid bone articulates with the frontal bone except in the

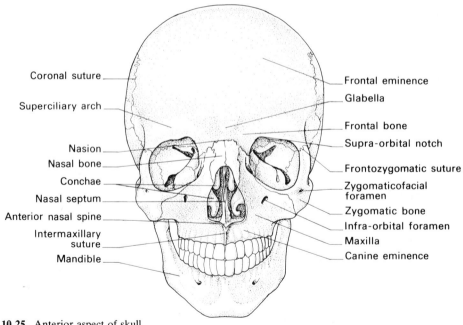

Fig. 10.25. Anterior aspect of skull.

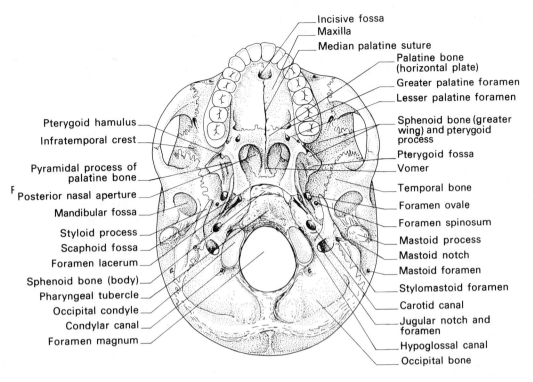

Fig. 10.26. Inferior aspect of skull.

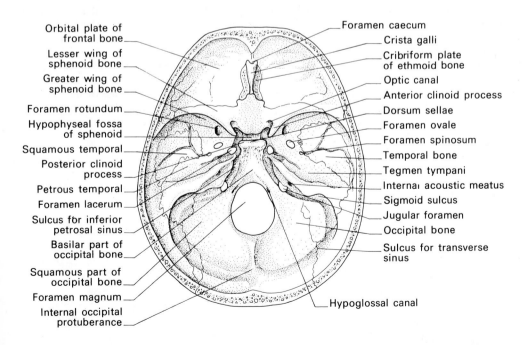

Fig. 10.27. Floor of cranial cavity.

middle where a gap between the orbital plates of the frontal bone is filled by part of the ethmoid bone.

Once the names and position of the main bones of the skull are known, it is necessary to examine the skull more closely in order to become acquainted with the position of a large number of openings (foramina and fissures) and surface projections (spines and lines, tubercles and tuberosities, plates and processes) to which reference is frequently made in describing the course of a nerve or blood vessel or the attachment of a muscle or ligament.

SUPERIOR ASPECT OF SKULL
(Fig. 10.28)

The calvaria is smooth, rounded and usually oval in shape. There is great variation in the shape of the skull from being markedly oval to almost round and the ratio of one diameter to the other is used as an index by means of which skulls are classified (Book 2). The bones seen are anteriorly the frontal bone and laterally and posteriorly the parietal bones. Between the parietal bones in the midline is the sagittal suture and between the parietal bones and the frontal bone running tranversely is the coronal suture. Posteriorly part of the lambdoid suture, between the parietal bones and the occipital bone, can be seen as well as a small part of the occipital bone. The junction between the sagittal and coronal sutures is called the bregma and the junction between the sagittal and lambdoid sutures the lambda. At the lambda small bones are often found (sutural or Wormian bones). The highest point of the skull is called the vertex. About 3 cm anterior to the lambda on each side of the sagittal suture there is a parietal foramen through which an emissary vein connects the

veins of the scalp with intracranial veins. The frontal eminences, one each side, can be seen anteriorly and occasionally the frontal (metopic) suture persists into adult life. This is a sagitally placed suture indicating the two halves from which the frontal bone develops. The parietal eminences, one on each side, can also be seen. The diameter between them is usually the widest diameter of the skull and these eminences obscure the zygomatic arches when the skull is looked at from above.

ANTERIOR ASPECT OF SKULL (Fig. 10.25)

The frontal eminences can be seen superiorly below the domelike outline of the calvaria. The frontal bone forms the sharp upper margin of the orbital opening. Laterally the frontal bone articulates with the zygomatic bone at the frontozygomatic suture which can be felt in the living as a depression on the lateral side of the opening. About 2.5 cm from the midline there is a notch in the supra-orbital margin, the supra-orbital notch, which may be a foramen, in which lie the supra-orbital nerve and vessels. Above the medial half of the upper margin of the orbit is the superciliary arch forming a prominence of varying size in different skulls. On the medial side of the orbital opening the frontal bone articulates with the frontal process of the maxilla. The only bony attachment of the orbicularis oculi muscle is to the frontal bone and maxilla on the medial side of the orbital opening. The bridge of the nose is formed by the nasal bones on each side of the midline. Each nasal bone articulates with the frontal process of the maxilla laterally and the frontal bone above. The nasion is the depression above the bridge of the nose. The glabella (glaber means smooth), used in making measurements of the skull, is the prominence just above the nasion.

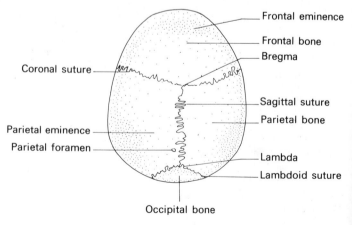

Fig. 10.28. Superior aspect of skull.

The prominence of the cheek is formed by the zygomatic bone which forms the lateral and part of the lower margin of the orbital opening. The articulation between the zygomatic bone and maxilla runs downwards and laterally from the middle of the lower border of the orbital margin. The zygomaticofacial foramen from which emerges the nerve of that name is on the facial surface of the bone.

Almost all of the upper skeleton of the face below the orbit is formed by the two maxillae which meet in the midline below at the intermaxillary suture. The piriform (pear-shaped) opening of the nasal cavity is formed below and laterally by the maxillae and above by the nasal bones. Projecting upwards in the midline, just above the suture, is the anterior nasal spine. The facial surface of the maxilla has the infraorbital foramen 1 cm below the inferior border of the orbital opening and 2.5 cm from the midline. The infra-orbital vessels and nerve emerge from this foramen. Several of the muscles of the openings of the mouth and nose are attached to the facial surface of the maxilla and zygomatic bone. The narrow part of the face below the zygomatic bones is formed by the alveolar processes of the maxillae, the lower borders of which form the alveolar arch. In the arch are the sockets of the teeth (the alveoli of the alveolar arch) corresponding to which are elevations on the surface of the maxilla. The most prominent is the canine eminence about 2 cm from the midline. Lateral to the eminence is the canine fossa and medial to it is the incisive fossa.

Within the nasal cavity the bony part of the nasal septum can be seen in or near the midline, together with the conchae or turbinate bones which project from the lateral nasal wall. The walls of the cavity will be described later. The lower part of the front of the skull is formed by the mandible which will be dealt with as a separate bone. The main features of the walls of the orbital cavities are best described here.

Each orbit has a roof, a floor and a lateral and medial wall (Fig. 10.29). The lateral wall slopes medially at it passes backwards and the medial wall is in a parasagittal plane. The back of the orbit is therefore much smaller than the front and is often referred to as the apex. At the apex is the superior orbital fissure the main communication between the orbit and the cranial cavity. The orbit contains the eyeball with its muscles, nerves and vessels as well as part of the lacrimal apparatus and some fat.

The roof is formed mainly by the orbital plate of the frontal bone with the lesser wing of the sphenoid bone behind. The frontal sinus extends backwards for a variable distance in the medial part of the roof. Lying on the roof are the meninges and frontal lobe of the brain. Anterolaterally the roof is hollowed out to some extent and forms the fossa for the lacrimal gland. Anteromedially the trochlea (pulley) for the superior oblique muscle of the eyeball lies just within the orbital margin (Fig. 10.30). Above the medial end of the superior orbital fissure the optic canal for the optic nerve and ophthalmic artery is seen in the lesser wing of the sphenoid.

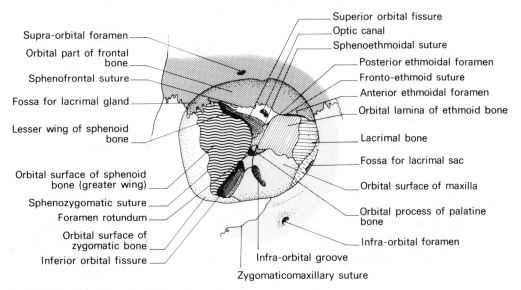

Supra-orbital foramen
Orbital part of frontal bone
Sphenofrontal suture
Fossa for lacrimal gland
Lesser wing of sphenoid bone
Orbital surface of sphenoid bone (greater wing)
Sphenozygomatic suture
Foramen rotundum
Orbital surface of zygomatic bone
Inferior orbital fissure

Superior orbital fissure
Optic canal
Sphenoethmoidal suture
Posterior ethmoidal foramen
Fronto-ethmoid suture
Anterior ethmoidal foramen
Orbital lamina of ethmoid bone
Lacrimal bone
Fossa for lacrimal sac
Orbital surface of maxilla
Orbital process of palatine bone
Infra-orbital foramen

Infra-orbital groove
Zygomaticomaxillary suture

Fig. 10.29 Anterior view of orbital cavity.

A tendinous ring is attached above, medial to and below the optic foramen.

The floor of the orbit is formed by the orbital surface of the maxilla which separates it from the maxillary sinus inferiorly. The orbital process of the palatine bone forms a small part of the floor posteriorly. The floor slopes upwards and narrows as it passes backwards. The inferior orbital fissure lies between the floor and the lateral wall posteriorly and forms a communication between the region behind the maxilla and the orbit. The maxillary nerve, infra-orbital vessels and zygomatic nerve pass through this fissure. The infra-orbital groove passes forwards from the fissure into the infra-orbital canal which lies in the anterior part of the floor. The canal leads to the infra-orbital foramen on the anterior surface of the maxilla. The inferior oblique muscle is attached to the anteromedial part of the floor. The zygomatic nerve enters the zygomatic foramen on the orbital surface of the zygomatic bone, which forms a small part of the floor anteriorly.

The lateral wall of the orbit is formed anteriorly by the zygomatic bone and posteriorly by the greater wing of the sphenoid bone. The zygomatic bone separates the orbit from the temporal fossa. Between the greater and lesser wings of the sphenoid, that is, between the lateral wall and the roof, the superior orbital fissure is seen passing downwards and medially. Its medial end is wider than its lateral and trans-

mits a number of nerves and the ophthalmic veins. The tendinous ring round the optic canal bridges the medial end of the fissure.

The medial wall of the orbit (Fig. 10.30) is formed from before backwards by part of the frontal process of the maxilla, the lacrimal bone, the orbital plate of the ethmoid bone and a part of the lateral surface of the body of the sphenoid bone. The ethmoidal air cells lie medial to the lacrimal bone and the orbital plate of the ethmoid and may extend into the roof and floor of the orbit. The body of the sphenoid contains the sphenoidal air sinus. On the anterior part of the medial wall the lacrimal groove containing the lacrimal sac is formed by the lacrimal bone and the maxilla. The groove is limited anteriorly by the lacrimal crest of the maxilla and posteriorly by the lacrimal crest of the lacrimal bone. The lacrimal sac passes downwards into a foramen formed by the fusion laterally of the lower ends of the two lacrimal crests. Between the medial wall and the roof the anterior and posterior ethmoidal foramina lead into canals of the same name. The canals open into the cranial cavity and contain vessels and nerves. The nasal cavity, separated by the ethmoidal air sinuses, lies medial to the medial wall of the orbit.

POSTERIOR ASPECT OF SKULL (Fig. 10.31)

Superiorly the parietal bones separated by the sagittal suture pass from one side to the other.

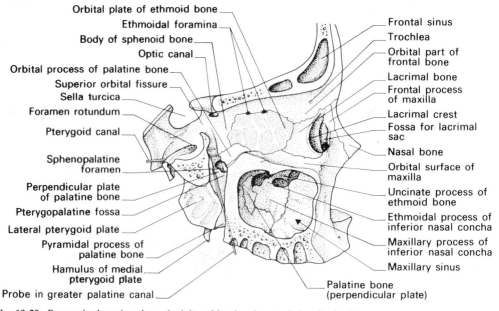

Fig. 10.30. Parasagittal section through right orbit, showing medial wall of orbit.

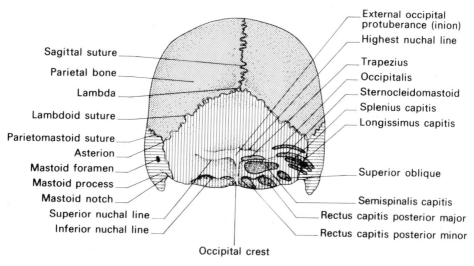

Sagittal suture

Parietal bone

Lambda

Lambdoid suture

Parietomastoid suture

Asterion

Mastoid foramen

Mastoid process

Mastoid notch

Superior nuchal line

Inferior nuchal line

Occipital crest

External occipital protuberance (inion)

Highest nuchal line

Trapezius

Occipitalis

Sternocleidomastoid

Splenius capitis

Longissimus capitis

Superior oblique

Semispinalis capitis

Rectus capitis posterior major

Rectus capitis posterior minor

Fig. 10.31. Posterior aspect of skull with muscle attachments.

Inferiorly the squamous part of the occipital bone articulates at the arched lambdoidal suture with the posterior edges of the parietal bones. Lateral to the occipital and inferior to the parietal bone is the posterior part of the temporal bone, the lateral part of which projects downwards as the mastoid process. The mastoid foramen for an emissary vein is just medial to and above the mastoid process. Medial to the process inferiorly is the mastoid notch to which the posterior belly of the digastric is attached. The occipitomastoid and parietomastoid sutures meet the lambdoid suture at the asterion.

The external occipital protuberance (the inion) is a prominence about the middle of the squamous part of the occipital bone. Passing downwards in the midline from the protuberance is the external occipital crest which reaches the posterior edge of the foramen magnum. Highest, superior and inferior nuchal lines pass laterally from the protuberance and crest. The most marked is the superior nuchal line. Several muscles are attached to the lines and the areas between them (Fig. 10.31).

LATERAL ASPECT OF THE SKULL (Fig. 10.24)

No new features of the occipital and parietal bones can be seen, but the asterion where these two bones meet the temporal bone is more easily identified. The temporal bone can be examined in more detail. Basically it consists of four parts, the squamous which forms part of the lateral wall of the cranium inferior to the parietal bone, the petromastoid postero-inferiorly which extends into the base of the skull, the tympanic which forms the bony part of the external acoustic (auditory) meatus and the styloid process which is embedded in the petrous part behind the tympanic part and projects downwards and forwards. The squamous part extends forwards as the zygomatic process, meets the zygomatic bone and completes the zygomatic arch. The squamous part also extends medially in front of the external acoustic meatus into the base of the skull and forms the mandibular (glenoid) fossa with which the mandible articulates. The zygomatic process if followed backwards divides into two, an anterior root which turns medially and passes in front of the mandibular fossa and a posterior which passes backwards above the external acoustic meatus. There is a tubercle towards the posterior end of the zygomatic process and the lateral ligament of the temporomandibular joint is attached to it.

The tympanic part of the temporal bone is in the form of a cylinder deficient postero-superiorly. The defect is filled by the squamous part of the temporal bone. The squamotympanic suture lies in front of the meatus and behind the mandibular fossa. The outer edge of the tympanic part is rough and the cartilaginous part of the external meatus is attached to it. The tympanic part extends downwards in front of the styloid process.

The mastoid process is the lateral part of the petrous part of the temporal bone. The process is continuous anteriorly with the squamous part, but forms sutures with the parietal bone above and the occipital bone behind. Above the mastoid process the supramastoid crest is continuous anteriorly with the upper border of the zygomatic process and posteriorly with the superior temporal line which arches upwards and forwards on the parietal bone. The suprameatal triangle is bounded above by the suprameatal crest, in front by the posterosuperior edge of the external meatus, and posteriorly by a vertical line running along the posterior edge of the meatus. This triangle is the surface marking of the mastoid (tympanic) antrum of the middle ear. The antrum in an adult is about 15 mm from the surface but is only 3–5 mm from the surface in a child about one year old.

The styloid process is about 2 cm medial to the lateral surface of the mastoid process and has attached to it a number of muscles and ligaments. It is attached to the lesser cornu of the hyoid bone by the stylohyoid ligament and was part of the second pharyngeal arch.

The main features of the anterior part of the lateral aspect of the skull have already been described. The zygomatic bone articulates with the frontal bone above, the maxilla inferiorly and anteriorly and the zygomatic process of the temporal bone posteriorly and laterally. Posteriorly and more medially it articulates with the greater wing of the sphenoid bone. The anterolateral (facial) surface of the maxilla is inferior to the opening of the orbit and the zygomatic bone.

Two lines on the lateral surface of the cranium can be seen. Although called the temporal lines, superior and inferior they are not entirely on the temporal bone but rather in the temporal region. At their beginning and end they form one line. Anteriorly they begin at the suture between the zygomatic and frontal bones and then arch upwards over the frontal bone and backwards over the parietal bone where two distinct lines can be seen. They then pass downwards and form one line which passes forwards over to the squamous part of the temporal bone to become continuous with the supramastoid crest. The temporal fascia is attached to the superior line and the temporalis muscle to the inferior. The Frankfort plane is a plane passing through the lower border of the orbital opening and the upper border of the external acoustic meatus. In the upright position this line is horizontal and can be used to hold the skull in the correct position when the lateral aspect is being examined.

Three fossae can be seen from the lateral side of the skull. The temporal fossa refers to the space between the zygomatic arch and the lateral wall of the cranium (Fig. 10.32). The upper limit of the fossa is regarded as the temporal lines so that its medial wall in front and superiorly is formed by parts of the frontal and parietal bones, and inferiorly by the greater wing of the sphenoid in front of the squamous part of the temporal bone. The anterior limit of the fossa is the temporal surface of the zygomatic bone. The H-shaped articulation, the pterion, between the

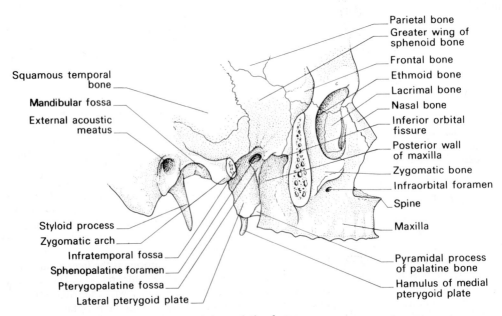

Fig. 10.32. Temporal, infratemporal and pterygopalatine fossae.

frontal, parietal, temporal and sphenoid bones is on the medial wall. The main structures in the space are the temporalis muscle and its vessels and nerves. The temporalis fascia roofs over the space because it is attached to the zygomatic arch. A foramen on the surface of the zygomatic bone facing the fossa is the point of emergence of the zygomaticotemporal nerve.

The infratemporal fossa is medial to the anterior part of the temporal fossa. The greater wing of the sphenoid bone has a vertical part on the lateral wall of the cranium and a horizontal part in the base of the skull. The junction of these two parts of the greater wing is marked by a ridge of bone, the infratemporal crest (Fig. 10.26). The anterior limit of the infratemporal fossa is the posterior wall of the maxilla and its posterior limit is the articular eminence (tubercle) in front of the mandibular fossa. Medially is the lateral surface of the lateral pterygoid plate of the sphenoid bone. Between the anterior end of the lateral pterygoid plate and posterior surface of the maxilla there is the pterygomaxillarry fissure leading medially to the pterygopalatine fossa. The details of the infratemporal fossa are best seen when the base of the skull is examined but it contains a number of important structures, the pterygoid muscles, the maxillary artery and vein and branches of the mandibular nerve.

The third fossa in this region is the pterygopalatine, a narrow space between the posterior wall of the maxilla anteriorly and the pterygoid process of the sphenoid bone posteriorly (Figs. 10.30 & 10.32). Medially it is limited by the perpendicular plate of the palatine bone. A large number of important structures traverse or lie in this fossa. The maxillary artery enters from the lateral side through the pterygomaxillary fissure and divides into its terminal branches. The maxillary nerve enters the upper part of the fossa from behind through the foramen rotundum, and leaves anteriorly to enter the orbit through the inferior orbital fissure which is in the superior and anterior part of the fossa.

Within the fossa is the sphenopalatine ganglion which receives a large branch from the maxillary nerve and gives off a number of branches which pass

1   Medially through the sphenopalatine foramen and enter the nasal cavity;
2   Downwards and go to the palate through the greater palatine canal, and
3   Backwards through the palatovaginal canal to the upper end of the pharynx.

Opening on to the posterior wall of the fossa is the pterygoid canal through which the nerve of the pterygoid canal enters the fossa.

INFERIOR ASPECT (BASE) OF SKULL (Fig. 10.26)

Posteriorly is the occipital bone with the foramen magnum in the middle. Anterolateral to the foramen magnum on each side is an oval occipital condyle which encroaches on the edge of the foramen magnum and points medially as well as forwards. The articular surface is concave transversely and anteroposteriorly. Posterior to the occipital condyles the posterior atlanto-occipital membrane is attached to the edge of the foramen magnum and anterior to the condyles the anterior atlanto–occipital membrane is attached to the anterior edge. The spinal cord, its meninges, the spinal accessory nerves and the vertebral arteries pass through the foramen magnum. Superolateral to the front part of the condyle is the opening of the hypoglossal canal through which passes the hypoglossal nerve. Behind the condyle in a depression is the opening of the condylar canal through which passes an emissary vein.

The part of the occipital bone lateral to the condyle is called the jugular process. Laterally it articulates with the petrous part of the temporal bone and anteriorly it is hollowed out and forms the jugular notch which is the posterior wall of the jugular foramen. Medial to the foramen the occipital bone forms the petro-occipital suture with the temporal bone. The sigmoid sinus passes through the lateral part of the jugular foramen and becomes the internal jugular vein. The accessory, vagus and glossopharyngeal nerves leave the cranial cavity through the middle of the foramen and the inferior petrosal sinus passes through the medial part of the foramen and joins the beginning of the internal jugular vein. Posteriorly the external occipital crest passes backwards in the midline from the foramen magnum, and anteriorly the basilar part of the occipital bone in front of the foramen fuses with the body of the sphenoid bone. The pharyngeal tubercle is in the midline of the basilar part about 1 cm anterior to the foramen magnum. The superior constrictor of the pharynx is attached to the tubercle.

The petromastoid part of the temporal bone lies anterolateral to the occipital bone. The mastoid process is directly lateral to the jugular process and the petrous part extends forwards and medially and meets the basilar part of the occiptial bone. It is separated from the body of the sphenoid by a gap called the foramen lacerum which in the living is closed in its lower part by cartilage. Above the cartilage the pterygoid canal opens on to the anterior wall of the foramen. Medial to the mastoid process is the mastoid notch to which the posterior belly of the digastric is attached. On the inferior surface of the petrous part the styloid process projects downwards about 1 cm medial to the anterior edge of the mastoid process. Immediately behind the styloid process is the stylomastoid foramen from which the facial nerve emerges. Anteromedial to the foramen is the large opening of the carotid canal for the internal carotid artery and its sympathetic plexus of nerves. Posterior to the carotid canal the temporal bone forms the anterior wall of the jugular foramen. The tympanic branch of the glossopharyngeal nerve enters the temporal bone on the small ridge between the carotid canal and the jugular foramen and goes to the medial wall of the middle ear.

Anterior and lateral to the styloid process is the anteroinferior surfaces of the tympanic part of the temporal bone. It extends down the anterior surface of the styloid process as the vaginal process. Anterior to the tympanic part is the mandibular fossa. In front of the fossa there is the articular eminence. Between the tympanic and the squamous parts is the squamotympanic fissure, which medially is divided into an anterior petrosquamous and posterior petrotympanic fissure by a downward projecting piece of the petrous temporal. The chorda tympani, a branch of the facial nerve, emerges from the petrotympanic fissures. The articular eminence if followed laterally turns forward into the zygomatic process and arch. Medially the squamous temporal articulates with the lateral part of the greater wing of the sphenoid. The petrous temporal articulates with the posterior part of the greater wing. Posteromedial to this articulation there is a groove which if followed laterally leads into the canal in the petrous temporal in which the bony part of the auditory (Eustachian) tube runs. The cartilaginous part of the tube lies in the groove.

The body of the sphenoid bone appears to pass forwards above the posterior nasal apertures. On either side of the apertures the pterygoid process of the sphenoid projects downwards. Each pterygoid process has an everted lateral and a narrower medial pterygoid plate. The posterior border of the medial is prolonged downwards and laterally as the pterygoid hamulus. In the disarticulated bone the lower ends of the plates are separated. This gap is filled by the pyramidal process of the palatine bone which separates the maxilla from the sphenoid. The hollow between the plates is called the pterygoid fossa and above and medial to the fossa is a small elongated groove called the scaphoid fossa. The lateral and medial pterygoid muscles are attached to the pterygoid plate and the superior constrictor and pterygomandibular ligament to the hamulus. The tensor veli palatini is attached to the scaphoid fossa and its tendon winds round the lateral side of the hamulus.

The inferior surface of the greater wing of the sphenoid is seen lateral to the superior part of the lateral pterygoid plate. The greater wing extends as far forwards as the inferior orbital fissure, backwards to where it articulates with the petrous temporal and laterally where it bends upwards and forms part of the lateral wall of the cranium. In the greater wing of the sphenoid lateral to the lateral pterygoid plate is the foramen ovale through which pass the mandibular division of the trigeminal nerve and the accessory meningeal artery. Behind and lateral to the foramen ovale there is the foramen spinosum through which pass the middle meningeal artery and the nervus spinosus. The foramen spinosum receives its name from the spine of the sphenoid which is posterior and lateral to the foramen. The sphenomandibular ligament is attached to the spine of the sphenoid. This region forms the main part of the infratemporal fossa.

Inferior to the body of the sphenoid are the choanae (posterior nasal apertures), one on each side of the midline. They are separated by the posterior edge of the vomer which forms the postero-inferior part of the nasal septum. Each aperture is vertical and about 2.5 cm high and 1 cm wide. The lateral boundary is formed by the medial pterygoid plate articulating anteriorly with the perpendicular plate of the palatine bone, the horizontal plate of which forms the lower boundary. The superior boundary is more complicated. When followed upwards the midline vomer divides into two alae passing laterally and meeting the vaginal process of the sphenoid which is a medial extension of the upper end of the medial pterygoid plate. The ala and vaginal process overlap inferior to the body of the sphenoid. The upper end of the vertical plate of the palatine bone divides into a lateral orbital process seen in the floor of the orbit, and a medial sphenoid process which articulates with the inferior surface of the body of the sphenoid and its vaginal process forming the palatinovaginal canal through which passes the pharyngeal branch of the sphenopalatine ganglion.

At a lower level than the rest of the base of the skull the hard palate is seen in front of the lower ends of the posterior nasal apertures. It is bounded anteriorly and laterally by the alveolar process of the maxilla. The processes form the horseshoe-shaped alveolar arch in which are the sockets for the teeth. The hard palate is concave from side to side and is formed mainly by the palatal processes of the maxillae. The posterior quarter of the hard palate is formed by the horizontal plates of the two palatine bones. The posterior border of the hard palate forms a sharp free ridge to which is attached the aponeurosis of the muscles forming the soft palate.

The median palatine suture runs anteroposteriorly between the two halves of the hard palate. Just behind its anterior end there is a depression, the incisive fossa, into which open several foramina containing branches of the nasopalatine (long sphenopalatine) vessels and nerves. Posterolaterally the greater palatine foramen opens between the maxilla and palatine bone, and behind this foramen are several lesser palatine foramina in the palatine bone.

INTERIOR OF SKULL (Fig. 10.27)

This can be examined by means of a horizontal cut so that the inside of both the skull-cap and the base can be seen, or by means of a sagittal section. The horizontal cut is usually made about 4 cm above the nasion and the external occipital protuberence. The skull-cap then consists of a small triangular piece of the occipital bone posteriorly, almost the whole of the parietal bones laterally and part of the frontal bone anteriorly. The sutures, coronal, sagittal and lambdoid, may not be very obvious or even obliterated if the skull is that of an individual more than 40 years of age at death.

The section may pass through the upper ends of the frontal sinuses next to the midline anteriorly. In the midline of the frontal bone above the sinuses there is the frontal crest to which the falx cerebri is attached. Passing backwards from the crest along the midline is a groove on the frontal, parietal and occipital bones. This is the sagittal sulcus which widens posteriorly and contains the superior sagittal sinus. Posteriorly it extends beyond the sawcut to the internal occipital protuberance. On either side of the sulcus a number of depressions can be seen. These contain the arachnoid granulations which project into the superior sagittal sinus and are the main structures involved in the return of cerebrospinal fluid to the circulation. The bone is often very thin over the granulations. Grooves passing upwards and backwards over the parietal bone are related to branches of the middle meningeal vessels. The deepest of these, which may form a tunnel, runs just behind the coronal suture and indicates the position of the anterior branch; it is not infrequently a site of tearing due to injury.

The interior of the base of the skull (Fig. 10.27) is divided for descriptive purposes into three fossae:
1   Anterior, extending as far back as the lesser wings of the sphenoid bone
2   Middle, which has a median portion, the body of the sphenoid, and a lateral part on each side, formed mainly by the greater wing of the sphenoid and extending backwards as far as the upper border of the petrous temporal bone and
3   Posterior, behind the middle fossa and limited at the sides and posteriorly by the transverse groove on the occipital bone.

Anterior cranial fossa

Parts of three bones form this fossa but the main contribution is from the orbital plates of the frontal, which have ridges corresponding with the sulci on the surface of the cerebral hemispheres. Between the orbital places, part of the ethmoid bone is seen. This is the cribriform plate of the ethmoid with the crista galli which projects upwards in the sagittal plane and has the falx cerebri attached to it. Through the holes of the cribriform plate bundles of olfactory nerve fibres pass from the roof of the nasal cavity to the olfactory bulb lying on the plate. Between the ethmoid and frontal bones the anterior and posterior ethmoidal foramina are seen. Anterior to the crista galli the foramen caecum is the site of an emissary vein between the nasal cavity and the inside of the skull. The third bone is part of the sphenoid. Immediately posterior to the cribriform plate, and articulating with it, is the part of the body of the sphenoid called the jugum sphenoidale behind which is a groove. At the lateral ends of the groove on each side is the optic canal which is anterior to the medial end of the lesser wing of the sphenoid. Lateral to the optic canal the lesser wing articulates anteriorly with the orbital plate of the frontal bone. When followed medially the posterior edge of the lesser wing curves backwards and forms a sharp projection called the anterior clinoid process to which is attached the free edge of the tentorium cerebelli. The internal carotid artery passes upwards medial to the process which may be joined to the middle of the side of the body of the sphenoid and form a foramen through which the artery passes.

Middle cranial fossa

This consists of two lateral parts and a median part formed by the upper surface of the body of the sphenoid. This surface is hollowed out and forms the sella turcica or hypophyseal fossa. The sphenoidal air sinus is immediately inferior to the fossa. The posterior boundary of the fossa is formed by a transverse ridge (dorsum sellae) with small lateral projections called the posterior clinoid processes to which are attached the anterior ends of the attached margin of the tentorium cerebelli. The hypophysis cerebri (pituitary gland) lies in the hypophyseal fossa and is covered by a part of the dura mater called the diaphragma sellae which is attached to the four clinoid processes and the anterior and posterior edges of the fossa. The internal carotid artery lies in a groove running anteroposteriorly lateral to the fossa.

Laterally part of the floor of the middle fossa is formed by the greater wing of the sphenoid, which is separated by the superior orbital fissure from the lesser wing of the sphenoid. The posterior edge of the lesser wing marks the anterior limit of the middle fossa. The fissure has been seen from its orbital aspect. When looked at from behind it is seen to pass upwards, laterally and forwards. Its medial end is much wider than its lateral end. The oculomotor, trochlear and abducent nerves and the three main branches of the ophthalmic division of the trigeminal nerve pass through the fissure with the ophthalmic veins.

Immediately behind the medial end of the fissure is the foramen rotundum which leads anteriorly into the pterygopalatine fossa and transmits the maxillary nerve. The foramen ovale is about 1 cm posterior and slightly lateral to the foramen rotundum and leads downwards into the infratemporal fossa. The mandibular nerve leaves the cranial cavity through the foramen ovale. The foramen spinosum is posterolateral to the foramen ovale and also leads downwards into the infratemporal fossa. The middle meningeal vessels enter the cranial cavity through the foramen spinosum from which a groove runs anterolaterally on to the squamous part of the temporal bone forming the lateral wall of the lateral part of the middle fossa. The groove on the squamous temporal runs forwards

and laterally towards the inner aspect of the pterion and divides into anterior and posterior branches. The anterior branch runs mainly upwards over the pterion and the posterior branch runs backwards.

The anterosuperior surface of the petrous temporal bone forms the posterior wall of the middle fossa. The foramen lacerum lies between the medial end of the petrous temporal and the sphenoid bone. The carotid canal in the temporal bone opens on to the upper surface of the cartilage in the foramen lacerum. The internal carotid artery here turns forwards and enters the cavernous venous sinus which lies lateral to the hypophyseal fossa and on the greater wing of the sphenoid bone.

There are two grooves on the anterosuperior surface of the petrous temporal. The lateral groove leads medially to the foramen ovale and contains the lesser petrosal nerve. The medial leads to the foramen lacerum and contains the greater petrosal nerve which joins the deep petrosal nerve from the carotid sympathetic plexus and forms the nerve of the pterygoid canal. This canal has an opening in the anterior wall of the foramen lacerum above the cartilage and leads to the pterygopalatine fossa.

On the upper border of the petrous temporal there is a groove in which lies the superior petrosal venous sinus running laterally and joining the transverse sinus. The medial end of the upper border is flattened and on this area deep to the sinus lie the sensory and motor roots of the trigeminal nerve. On the most medial area on the anterosuperior surface of the petrous temporal lies the trigeminal ganglion which extends over the edge of the foramen lacerum. Above and slightly lateral to the grooves for the petrosal nerves there is an elevation called the arcuate eminence indicating the position of the anterior semicircular canal of the internal ear. Lateral to the eminence is the tegmen tympani, the thin roof of the tympanic cavity and mastoid antrum.

Posterior cranial fossa

Anteriorly, in the middle, this fossa is bounded by the dorsum sellae and posterior clinoid processes of the sphenoid bone. The body of the sphenoid passes downwards and backwards from the dorsum sellae to the basilar part of the occipital bone. Anteriorly and laterally on each side is the posterosuperior surface of the petrous temporal which medially reaches the body of the sphenoid. On this surface of the temporal bone about 2 cm lateral to the sphenoid is the internal acoustic meatus into which pass the vestibulocochlear and facial nerves and the labyrinthine artery. Laterally the cranial surface of the mastoid process has a deep wide groove, the sigmoid sulcus, which passes downwards and then medially across the occipitomastoid suture on to the occipital bone.

The occipital bone forms the rest of the posterior cranial fossa. In the middle anteriorly, the basilar part is continuous with the body of the sphenoid. The foramen magnum is in the floor of the fossa and is narrowed to some extent by the encroachment of the occipital condyles. The hypoglossal canal is seen opening above the middle of the medial edge of the condyle. Lateral to the condylar canal which is on the lateral side of the condyle, the jugular process forms the posterior boundary of the jugular foramen, whose anterior boundary is formed by the petrous temporal bone. Leading to the anteromedial part of the jugular foramen is the petro–occipital suture in which lies the inferior petrosal sinus. The petrosal sinuses drain the blood from the cavernous sinus.

Laterally and posteriorly the upper limit of the posterior fossa is formed by the upper of the two transverse ridges which bound the sulcus for the transverse venous sinus. If followed backwards the sulcus leads to the internal occipital protuberance. Most commonly the superior sagittal sinus becomes the right transverse sinus. Vertically in the midline the internal occipital crest runs downwards from the protuberance to the posterior edge of the foramen magnum. The region of the protuberance is called the confluence of the sinuses.

The squamous part of the occipital bone forms the main part of the floor and posterior walls of the fossa and in it lie the cerebellar hemispheres. These are covered by the tentorium cerebelli the attached edge of which is fixed to the edges of the transverse sulcus, to the upper border of the petrous temporal and to the posterior clinoid process. The tentorium thus roofs over the posterior fossa except anteriorly in front of the free edge of the tentorium, where the midbrain lies on the body of the sphenoid. Inferior to the midbrain, the pons and medulla oblongata lie on the basilar part of the occipital bone with the basilar artery intervening.

STRUCTURE OF BONES OF SKULL

Most of the bones in the skull consist of two plates of compact bone containing a layer of cancellous bone. The bones of the vault are on the whole of a uniform thickness although the thickness of the cancellous bone as compared with that of the compact bone is somewhat variable. The cancellous bone is called diploe and contains veins (diploic veins). These veins have very thin walls, show small dilations along their course and are about 3 mm wide when seen in X-rays of the skull. They are found in the frontal, parietal, squamous temporal and occipital bones and communicate with the intracranial and extracranial veins. They begin to develop at about the age of two years.

The bones of the vault of the skull within certain limits possess elasticity. A blow on the side of the head sometimes results in a fracture

Table 10.1. Ossification of skull. Development and growth of skull are described in Book 2.

Type of Ossification	Region of skull	
Membranous	*Vault*	*Face*
	Occipital above highest nuchal line	Maxilla
		Zygomatic
	Squamous temporal	Lacrimal
	Parietal	Nasal
	Frontal	Palatine
	Greater wing of sphenoid	Vomer
Endochondral	*Base*	*In Nasal Capsule*
	Occipital below highest nuchal line	Ethmoid
		Inferior concha
	Petromastoid and styloid process of temporal	Sphenoidal concha
	Body and lesser wing of sphenoid	

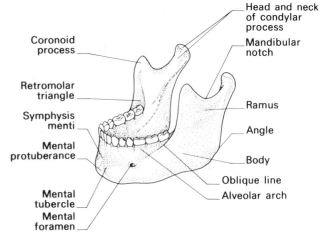

Coronoid process

Retromolar triangle

Symphysis menti

Mental protuberance

Mental tubercle

Mental foramen

Head and neck of condylar process

Mandibular notch

Ramus

Angle

Body

Oblique line

Alveolar arch

Fig. 10.33. Mandible, viewed obliquely from the left.

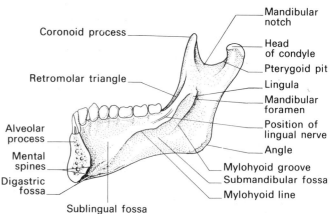

Coronoid process

Retromolar triangle

Alveolar process

Mental spines

Digastric fossa

Sublingual fossa

Mandibular notch

Head of condyle

Pterygoid pit

Lingula

Mandibular foramen

Position of lingual nerve

Angle

Mylohyoid groove

Submandibular fossa

Mylohyoid line

Fig. 10.34. Medial aspect of right half of mandible.

of the inner plate with an intact outer plate of bone. This is due to the outer plate being subjected to compression forces which are resisted more easily than the tensile forces to which the inner plate is subjected.

Some bones or part of the bones of the skull are reduced to a thin plate of bone. This is seen in the nasal and lacrimal bones and the orbital plate of the frontal bone. In other situations the amount of compact bone is increased to such an extent that there is no cancellous bone. This is seen in the zygomatic process of the frontal bone and the medial part of the petrous temporal bone. The structure of different parts of the bones reflects the pressures to which they are subjected.

Ossification of Bones of Skull
Table 10.1 is a useful generalization about the ossification of these bones.

Mandible, temporomandibular joint, muscles of mastication and maxilla

MANDIBLE

This bone has a horizontal horseshoe-shaped anterior body and on each side a vertical part called the ramus (Figs. 10.33–10.36). The body has internal and external surfaces and upper and lower borders; at birth it is in two halves. The upper alveolar part of the body has an arch in which are the sockets (alveoli) for the teeth. The posterior end of the arch is medial to the posterior end of the body.

The region where the two halves of the mandible are united in the midline anteriorly is called the symphysis menti. The mental protuberance is the name given to a triangular elevation on the lower half of the external surface of the symphysis and the mental tubercle, one on each side, is a projection at the lower lateral angle of the

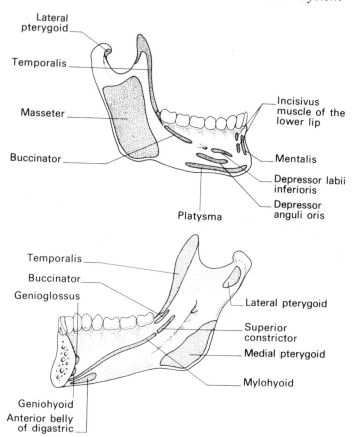

Fig. 10.35. Lateral aspect of right half of mandible showing muscle attachments.

Fig. 10.36. Medial aspect of right half of mandible showing muscle attachments.

protuberance. The lower border is thickened as compared with the rest of the body. About 2.5 cm lateral to the symphysis, midway between the upper and lower borders of the external surface, is the mental foramen which faces backwards and upwards, and from which emerge the mental nerve and vessels. The oblique line passes upwards and backwards from the mental foramen and becomes continuous with the anterior border of the ramus. Some of the muscles surrounding the opening of the mouth are attached between the symphysis and the mental foramen; the buccinator is attached to the oblique line and the platysma to the lower border of the body. The digastric muscle is attached to the digastric fossa, a small depression near the midline on the lower border.

The mylohyoid line divides the internal surface of the body into upper and lower parts. This line begins behind and below the crown of the third molar tooth and runs downwards and forwards just above the digastric fossa to the symphysis menti. The mylohyoid muscle is attached to this line.

The pterygomandibular ligament, superior constrictor of the pharynx and the buccinator are attached to the posterior end of the line. The submandibular salivary gland lies in the submandibular fossa below the line and the sublingual salivary gland lies in the sublingual fossa above the line. The lingual nerve lies just above the posterior end of the line on the bone and immediately below the crown of the third molar tooth. A groove passing downwards begins just below the posterior end of the line (the mylohyoid groove). In the groove lie the mylohyoid nerve and vessels. On the inner aspect of the symphysis above the anterior end of the line there are four tubercles, two on each side, one above the other. These are known as mental spines or genial tubercles to which the genioglossus (upper tubercles) and the geniohyoid (lower tubercles) are attached. Left and right, or upper and lower tubercles may be united. Behind the lower incisor teeth on each side lies an inferior alveolar foramen transmitting a small artery. Between the genial tubercles superiorly lies a small pit, the genial pit. Occasionally a bony prominence of varying size (torus mandibularis) lies above the mylohyoid line and projects into the floor of the mouth.

The ramus is quadrilateral in shape and its upper border has two projections, an anterior, the coronoid process and a posterior, the condyloid process. Between the two processes is the mandibular notch in which lie the masseteric vessels and nerve. The coronoid process is triangular with its apex superior and is deep to the zygomatic arch when the mouth is closed. The temporalis muscle is attached to the process, to the anterior border of the ramus and to a vertical ridge, the temporal crest, posterior to the anterior border of the ramus on its medial surface. At their lower ends, the anterior border of the coronoid process and the temporal crest diverge behind the third molar tooth to delineate a retromolar triangle. The condyloid process is enlarged superiorly to form a head which has a long axis running transversely and somewhat backwards from the lateral to the medial side. The lateral projection of the head can be palpitated just anterior to the tragus of the auricle. Below the head is a narrow neck with an anteromedial pit to which the lateral pterygoid muscle is attached. The capsular ligament of the temporomandibular joint is attached to the neck. A thickened ridge of bone is seen on the medial surface of the ramus passing downwards from the medial end of the condyle across the neck towards the mandibular foramen. This is a bony strut resisting compressive forces.

Where the posterior border of the ramus meets its inferior border the angle of the mandible is formed. The maximum curvature of the angle is called the gonion. The stylomandibular ligament is attached to the angle. The posterior border of the ramus is in contact with the parotid gland, and its anterior border is continuous inferiorly with the oblique line on the outer surface of the body.

The outer surface of the ramus has several oblique ridges to which the masseter is attached. Immediately in front of the attachment of the masseter there is frequently a notch on the lower

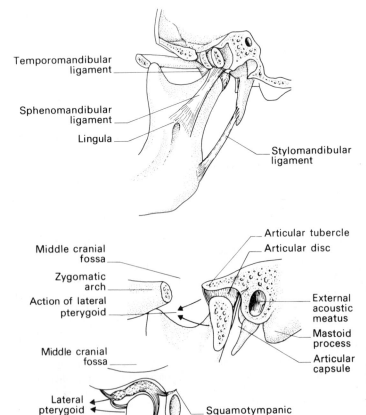

Fig. 10.37. Temporomandibular joints and ligaments.

Fig. 10.38. Temporomandibular joint showing articular disc.

border of the ramus in which lies the facial artery as it passes from the neck on to the face. The notch is about 4 cm anterior to the angle. In the middle of the inner surface of the ramus is the mandibular foramen which leads to the mandibular canal. This runs downwards and forwards in the body and contains the inferior alveolar nerve and vessels. The lingula is an upward projection of bone above and medial to the foramen. The sphenomandibular ligament is attached to the lingula and the mylohyoid groove begins below and behind it and runs downwards and forwards on to the body.

TEMPOROMANDIBULAR JOINT
(Figs. 10.37 & 10.38)

This is a condyloid synovial joint and although it is obvious that there are two joints, left and right, from a functional point of view the two joints may be regarded as one. The term condyloid refers to both joints at the same time since by definition a condyloid joint has two condyles (or elevations like knuckles). Each joint is between the head of a condylar process of the mandible and the mandibular fossa of the squamous part of the temporal bone and the articular eminence in front of the fossa. The two heads point backwards as well as medially and their articular surface is convex from front to back. If extended medially they meet at an anterior obtuse angle of about 150° just in front of the foramen magnum. The medial pole of the condyle projects much more than its lateral pole. The articular surface of the fossa and tubercle is concavoconvex from back to front. Anteriorly the slightly roughened articular surface extends forwards over the articular eminence while posteriorly it extends as far back as the squamotympanic fissure. The lateral end of the articular eminence at the posterior end of the zygomatic arch is especially prominent. The posterior edge of the fossa is prominent laterally and forms the postglenoid tubercle in front of the external acoustic meatus. Medially the fossa is closely related to the spine of the sphenoid and may form an elevation, the entoglenoid process. Superiorly the capsular ligament is attached just anterior to the squamotympanic fissure, to the edge of the fossa and to the front of the eminence. Inferiorly it is attached to the neck of the condyloid process of the mandible and the medial and lateral ends of the head of the process. The bone separating the deepest part of the articular fossa from the middle cranial fossa is particularly thin.

There are three ligaments associated with the joint. The unimportant stylomandibular, attached to the tip of the styloid process and the angle of the mandible, is regarded as a thickened part of the deep cervical fascia. The sphenomandibular ligament is attached superiorly to the spine of the sphenoid and inferiorly to the lingula on the inner surface of the ramus of the mandible. This ligament develops from the periosteum of the skeletal elements of the first pharyngeal arch and can be followed through the petrotympanic fissure to the anterior process of the malleus, an auditory ossicle which develops from the first pharyngeal arch. The ligament is related to a number of important structures. Between it and the ramus of the mandible are found the auriculotemporal nerve, the maxillary vessels and the inferior alveolar vessels and nerve. The lateral pterygoid muscle is lateral and the medial pterygoid medial to the ligament. The nerve and vessels to the mylohyoid muscle pierce it. The lateral ligament (formerly called the temporomandibular ligament) is attached to the tubercle at the posterior end of the zygomatic arch, passes downwards and backwards and is attached to the lateral and posterior aspects of the neck of the mandible. There is a deeper, more horizontal part of this ligament attached to the tubercle and disc anteriorly and to the lateral pole of the condyle and the disc posteriorly.

The synovial membrane of the joint lines the capsule and is reflected upwards on to the neck as far as the articular surfaces which are lined by fibrous tissue containing a few cartilage cells in older individuals. This mainly fibrous tissue is thick over the whole of the articular surface of the condyle but superiorly it is thin in the roof of the fossa and thick posteriorly and anteriorly.

The articular disc completely divides the joint cavity into upper and lower compartments. It consists largely of dense collagen fibres with some elastic fibres posteriorly. Occasionally it contains a few cartilage cells, recognizable because they are surrounded by glycosaminoglycans typical of cartilage.

In sagittal section the disc is concavoconvex above, moulding on to the articular eminence and fossa, and concave below where it fits around the head of the condyle. Anteriorly it is attached in front of the articular eminence and to the lateral pterygoid muscle; laterally and medially it is firmly attached to the poles of the condyle together with the capsular ligament with which it blends; posteriorly it splits into two parts, the upper being attached to the bone in front of the squamotympanic fissure and the

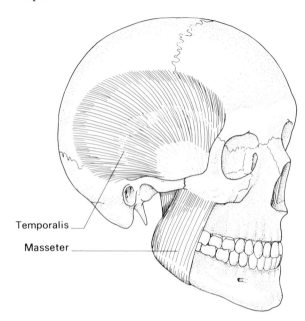

Temporalis

Masseter

Fig. 10.39. Masseter and temporalis muscles.

lower to the borders of a triangular area behind and below the head of the condyle.

The central part of the disc is the most dense and is thinnest in its middle part facing the anterior wall of the fossa whence it passes downwards medially and laterally (Fig. 10.38). This dense part of the disc is poorly supplied by vessels and nerves. The upper portion of the posterior bilaminar part consisting of loose connective tissue contains many elastic fibres and is richly supplied by nerves and vessels. The inferior portion is more fibrous. The anterior bilaminar region is looser than the central part.

The blood supply of the joint is derived from neighbouring arteries, the superficial temporal and the maxillary and the nerve supply from neighbouring nerves, the auriculotemporal and masseteric.

MUSCLES OF MASTICATION

This term is used to include the more important muscles which move the mandible rather than all the muscles involved in chewing. The masseter is attached superiorly to the lower border and deep surface of the zygomatic arch and inferiorly to the outer surface of the ramus of the mandible (Fig. 10.39). It is said to have three layers. The superficial is attached to the lower border of the zygomatic arch and possibly the zygomatic process of the maxilla and passes downwards and backwards to the ridges on the posteroinferior surface of the ramus. The middle layer is more

vertical and posterior. It is attached to the deep surface of the zygomatic arch and the posterior part of the lower border to which the superficial layer is not attached. The fibres pass to the outer surface of the ramus above the attachment of the superficial part. The third part is deep to the middle layer and superiorly is attached to the deep surface of the zygomatic arch and inferiorly to the base of the coronoid process and the adjacent area of the ramus. It is closely associated with the most superficial fibres of the temporalis muscle.

The upper part of the superficial head of the masseter is tendinous and when the jaw is tightly clenched the line joining the superior tendinous portion and the inferior muscular part is easily determined. The parotid duct passing transversely across the middle of the muscle can be palpated especially where it turns medially round the anterior border of the muscle. The parotid gland overlaps the masseter posteriorly and branches from the facial nerve pass forwards over the muscle. Anteriorly the deep surface of the muscle overlaps the temporalis and buccinator muscles and the buccal nerve. There is a considerable quantity of fat between the masseter and the buccinator.

The temporalis muscle (Fig. 10.39) is attached to the inferior of the two temporal lines, to the bones of the temporal fossa except the zygomatic and to the overlying temporal fascia. Its posterior fibres are almost horizontal and the anterior are vertical or even pass slightly backwards. The whole muscle is fanshaped and the fibres converge deep to the zygomatic arch. They are inserted on to both surfaces of the coronoid process (but largely medially), the anterior border of the ramus of the mandible and also to the adjacent temporal crest on the inner surface of the ramus. The attachments to the anterior border and the ridge are separate and if followed down are seen to diverge behind the third molar tooth and leave an area of bone (the retromolar triangle) to which no muscle fibres are attached. The temporalis fascia overlying the muscle is attached superiorly to the superior temporal line. Inferiorly it divides into two. The superficial part is attached to the outer surface of the zygomatic arch and the deeper part to its deep surface.

When the teeth are clenched, the anterior part of the temporalis can be palpated above and behind the orbital opening. Passing upwards superficial to the muscle are the superficial temporal vessels, the auriculotemporal and zygomaticotemporal nerves and branches of the facial nerve. Anteriorly the temporalis overlies the lateral and medial pterygoid muscles, the maxillary artery and the buccal nerve.

The lateral pterygoid muscle (Fig. 10.40) has two heads which are continuous with each other. The inferior head is attached to the lateral surface of the lateral pterygoid plate, and the superior to the inferior surface of the greater wing of the sphenoid bone as far laterally as the infratemporal crest. Most of the fibres of the lateral pterygoid pass horizontally backwards and laterally and are attached to a pit anterior to the neck of the mandible. Some of the upper medial fibres are attached to the capsule of the temporomandibular joint and through the capsule to the articular disc. The latter attachment pulls the disc forwards but the attachment of the disc to the poles of the condyle ensures that it will move forward if the condyle moves in this direction. The lowest fibres of the inferior head pass upwards as well as backwards.

The maxillary artery is superficial to the lateral pterygoid and then passes deep to it either between the two heads or inferiorly. The mandibular nerve is deep to it and its branches may pass laterally above it (temporal and masseteric) or through it (buccal) or inferior to it (lingual and inferior alveolar).

The medial pterygoid muscle (Fig. 10.40) has a deep head attached to the medial surface of the lateral pterygoid plate and a superficial head attached to the tuberosity of the maxilla at the posterior end of the alveolar process and the pyramidal process of the palatine bone which lies between the divergent lower ends of the lateral and medial pterygoid plates. Its fibres pass obliquely downwards, backwards and laterally and are attached to the inner surface of the angle of the mandible and to the postero–inferior part of the inner surface of the ramus. The area of attachment is indicated by ridges which extend as high as the mandibular foramen and as far backwards as the groove for the mylohyoid nerve. In the gap between the medial pterygoid and the ramus are the maxillary artery, the lingual and inferior alveolar nerves, the spheno-mandibular ligament and a small part of the parotid gland. The deep surface of the medial pterygoid is related to the upper part of the lateral wall of the pharynx formed by the superior constrictor from which it is sepa-

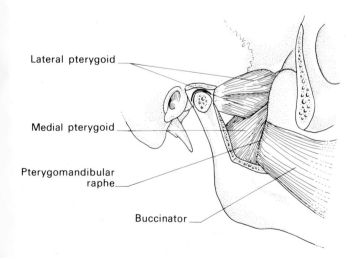

Lateral pterygoid

Medial pterygoid

Pterygomandibular raphe

Buccinator

Fig. 10.40. The lateral and medial pterygoid and buccinator muscles.

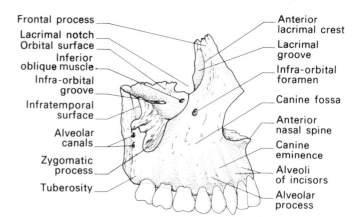

Frontal process

Lacrimal notch
Orbital surface
Inferior
oblique muscle
Infra-orbital
groove
Infratemporal
surface
Alveolar
canals
Zygomatic
process
Tuberosity

Anterior
lacrimal crest
Lacrimal
groove
Infra-orbital
foramen
Canine fossa
Anterior
nasal spine
Canine
eminence
Alveoli
of incisors
Alveolar
process

Fig. 10.41. Lateral view of right maxilla.

rated by the stylopharyngeus and the styloglossus.

It is convenient to consider that the main muscles of mastication are arranged in layers from lateral to medial. The first layer is the masseter and zygomatic arch, the second is the temporalis and the coronoid process, the third is the lateral pterygoid and the condyle of the mandible and the fourth is the upper part of the medial pterygoid. The next layer is the lateral wall of the pharynx. The mandibular nerve is deep to the lateral pterygoid but posterior to the medial pterygoid.

The action of all these muscles, except the lateral pterygoid, is to pull the jaw upwards as in closing the mouth. The deepest fibres of the masseter and the horizontal posterior fibres of the temporalis, particularly the latter, pull the upper part of the mandible backwards, an important part of the action of closing the jaws. The medial pterygoid because of its obliquity downwards and outwards may help to pull the lower jaw to the opposite side. The six muscles, the masseter, temporalis and medial pterygoids, can exert a considerable force, about 15 kg. The pain experienced by accidentally biting one's tongue or cheek while chewing is a more homely example of the force exerted by these six muscles. The lateral pterygoid pulls the condyloid process and articular disc forwards, an essential part of the movement of opening the mouth.

The mandibular division of the trigeminal nerve supplies all these muscles. This nerve leaves the skull through the foramen ovale in the greater wing of the sphenoid bone and lies deep to the lateral pterygoid muscle. The nerve is only about 1 cm long before it divides into anterior and posterior branches. Before it does so, it gives off the nerve to the medial pterygoid. The

anterior branch supplies the temporalis usually by two nerves which pass laterally above the lateral pterygoid muscle, the masseter by a nerve which also passes laterally above the lateral pterygoid and then through the mandibular notch, and the lateral pterygoid by a branch which goes directly into the muscle.

The mylohyoid muscle, the geniohyoid and the anterior belly of the digastric (p. 438) can be included in the muscles of mastication (Fig. 10.21). These muscles are attached inferiorly to the hyoid bone and superiorly to the mandible and they can pull the mandible downwards if the hyoid bone is fixed. Gravity also assists in this movement, which may be controlled to some extent by the graded relaxation of the elevators of the mandible. The nerve to the mylohyoid, a branch of the inferior alveolar nerve, supplies the mylohyoid and anterior belly of the digastric, and the geniohyoid is supplied by the first cervical nerve through the hypoglossal nerve.

The movements which take place at the temporomandibular joint during mastication are very complex and are dealt with in some detail elsewhere (p. 565).

THE MAXILLA (Figs. 10.41 & 10.42)

The two maxillae are the largest of the bones of the facial skeleton, and together form the upper jaw. The main part of the maxilla is called the body from which there are four projections. The lower medial horizontal projection is the palatine process. The frontal process projects upwards from the anteromedial part of the body. The inferior part in which the teeth are lodged is the alveolar process which forms half an arch. Superolaterally is the zygomatic process, a flattened rough area for articulation with the zygomatic bone.

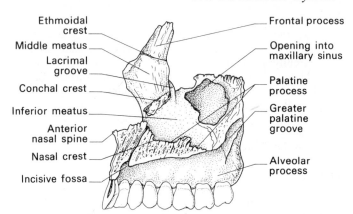

Ethmoidal crest
Middle meatus
Lacrimal groove
Conchal crest
Inferior meatus
Anterior nasal spine
Nasal crest
Incisive fossa

Frontal process
Opening into maxillary sinus
Palatine process
Greater palatine groove
Alveolar process

Fig. 10.42. Medial view of right maxilla.

The body has four surfaces and has been likened to a pyramid lying on its side with its base medially and its apex laterally. The orbital surface forms most of the floor of the orbit and a small part of the inferior margin of the orbit. On this surface, are, from behind forwards, the infra-orbital groove, canal and foramen in which lie the infra-orbital vessels and nerve. The inferior oblique muscle of the eyeball is attached to the anteromedial part of the orbital surface.

The anterior surface is actually antero–inferolateral and is better described as the facial surface. It can be palpated through the cheek below and lateral to the orbit. The infraorbital foramen opens on to this surface, 1 cm below the orbital margin, about 2.5 cm from the midline. The canine tooth produces an elevation and lateral to it is a depression called the canine fossa. Medial to the canine eminence is the incisive fossa. The medial border of the facial surface forms the major part of the edge of the piriform opening into the nasal cavity. This opening is completed superiorly by the lower edge of the nasal bone. Some of the muscles of facial expression are attached to the facial surface. (Fig. 10.43, 10.44).

The infratemporal surface is posterior and forms the anterior wall of the infratemporal fossa and more medially the anterior wall of the pterygopalatine fossa. (Fig. 10.30) In the former are some of the masticatory muscles, the mandibular nerve and its branches and part of the maxillary artery. In the latter are the maxillary nerve and some of its branches, the sphenopalatine ganglion and the terminal part of the maxillary artery. Superiorly this surface is separated from the greater wing of the sphenoid bone by the inferior orbital fissure. Inferiorly

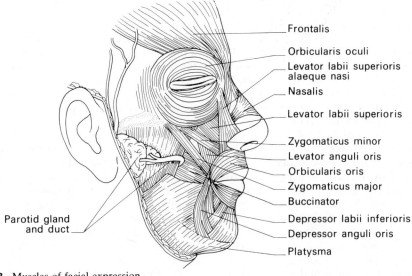

Frontalis
Orbicularis oculi
Levator labii superioris alaeque nasi
Nasalis
Levator labii superioris
Zygomaticus minor
Levator anguli oris
Orbicularis oris
Zygomaticus major
Buccinator
Depressor labii inferioris
Depressor anguli oris
Platysma

Parotid gland and duct

Fig. 10.43. Muscles of facial expression.

and laterally this surface projects behind the third molar tooth and forms the tuberosity of the maxilla to which the medial pterygoid muscle is attached. Although the maxilla apparently articulates posteriorly with the pterygoid process of the sphenoid bone, the pyramidal process of the palatine bone intervenes. Above this lies the entrance to the pterygopalatine fossa, the pterygomaxillary fissure, between the maxilla and the pterygoid process. (Fig. 10.30) In the posterior wall are openings and canals for the superior alveolar nerves. A ridge of bone passes upwards from the first molar tooth and separates the anterior from the infratemporal surface.

The nasal surface of the maxilla forms a large part of the lateral wall of the nasal cavity and in the disarticulated bone has a large almost circular opening about 2 cm in diameter. (Fig. 10.42) This leads into the cavity in the body of the maxilla, the maxillary sinus. On the nasal surface anterosuperiorly is the lacrimal groove in which lies the nasolacrimal duct. If followed upwards this groove is continuous with a groove on the lateral surface of the frontal process of the maxilla. The perpendicular plate of the palatine bone articulates with the posterior part of the nasal surface and extends over the opening of the maxillary sinus. A groove which passes downwards on this articular surface is called the greater palatine groove. A similar groove on the perpendicular plate of the palatine bone converts these grooves into the greater palatine canal in which lie the greater and lesser palatine nerves. In front of the lacrimal groove is the conchal crest for articulation with the inferior concha. Superior to the conchal crest is the ethmoidal crest for articulation with the ethmoid bone. In the living subject the opening into the maxillary sinus is very much reduced in size by the encroachment of neighbouring bones: the palatine, ethmoid, lacrimal and inferior concha.

The alveolar process forms half an arch, the alveolar arch, in which are the sockets for the teeth. The palatine process projects medially from the upper part of the alveolar process and forms the major part of the hard palate. It separates the oral from the nasal cavity. With the two maxillae together, the incisive fossa is seen to lie behind the incisive teeth. Opening into the fossa are the incisive canals, one in each maxilla, passing upwards into the two halves of the nasal cavity. In each canal are the nasopalatine nerve and sphenopalatine vessels. The medial border of the palatine process forms a ridge projecting upwards, the nasal crest. The vomer lies in the groove formed by the ridge of the two maxillae.

The anterior end of the ridge projects forwards and forms the anterior nasal spine. The posterior edge of the palatine process articulates with the anterior edge of the horizontal plate of the palatine bone. The inferior surface of the palatine process has a number of foramina for vessels and depressions for glands.

The frontal process articulates superiorly with the frontal bone, anteriorly with the nasal bone and posteriorly with the lacrimal bone. On its lateral surface there is a vertical ridge, the anterior lacrimal crest. Behind the crest there is a vertical groove which, with a similar groove on the lacrimal bone, forms a hollow for the lacrimal sac. If followed downwards the groove is seen to be continuous with the groove on the nasal surface of the maxilla. Anterior to the lacrimal crest is a smooth area to which part of the orbicularis oculi is attached. (Fig. 10.44) The medial palpebral ligament is attached to the crest itself. The medial surface of the frontal process forms part of the nasal cavity. The ethmoid crest, already referred to, is on this surface and part of the middle meatus lies between it and the conchal crest.

The maxillary sinus is described in detail on p. 479.

Muscles of facial expression (Fig. 10.43)

This term is used to distinguish a group of muscles from those of mastication, some of which are also in the face. These muscles are all derived from the mesoderm of the second branchial arch. They differ from almost all other voluntary muscles in the body in that they run from bone to skin, rather than to another bone or to a raphe. It is for this reason that they move the skin. At its simplest, the lips can be thought of as containing a ring of muscle fibres whose contraction closes the mouth, like a purse-string. From the edges of this ring, muscle fibres pass out to be attached to adjacent bone or into the buccinator. When these fibres contract they pull the ring out, up or in.

The orbicularis oris (Fig. 10.44) consists of two sets of fibres, those which enter the lips, and those which are confined to the lips. The latter fibres which form a ring within the lips either pass obliquely from the skin to the mucous membrane (most of these fibres remain on one side but some of the deeper cross the midline) or are attached to the upper and lower jaws over the lateral incisors and pass laterally towards the angle of the mouth.

The muscles entering the upper lip from above

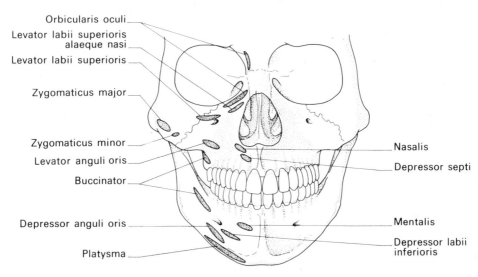

Orbicularis oculi
Levator labii superioris alaeque nasi
Levator labii superioris
Zygomaticus major
Zygomaticus minor
Levator anguli oris
Buccinator
Depressor anguli oris
Platysma

Nasalis
Depressor septi
Mentalis
Depressor labii inferioris

Fig. 10.44. Attachments of muscles of facial expression.

are attached superiorly to the frontal process of the maxilla or its canine fossa and to the zygomatic bone. From medial to lateral they are the levator labii superioris alaeque nasi (part of this muscle is attached to the alar cartilage of the external nose), levator labii superioris, levator anguli oris (from the canine fossa), zygomaticus minor and zygomaticus major. The levator anguli oris and zygomaticus major pass into the angle of the mouth and the other three into the upper lip more medially.

The muscles entering the lower lip from below are the depressor labii inferioris and the depressor anguli oris. The former is attached to the body of the mandible between the symphysis menti and the mental foramen and passes upwards into the lower lip. The latter is attached to the mandible inferior and lateral to the former and passes upwards to the angle of the mouth. The mentalis is attached to the mandible lateral to the midline above the mental protuberence. The fibres pass upwards to the skin of the lip and chin. The mentalis pulls the skin of the chin upwards and everts the lower lip.

There are three additional muscles attached to the angle of the mouth. The most superficial is the risorius which is attached laterally to the fascia over the parotid gland and medially to the skin over the angle of the mouth. The platysma (Fig. 10.23) lies in the superficial fascia of the neck. It extends inferiorly, distal to the clavicle, and passes upwards into the neck. Medially it is attached to the lower border of the mandible but more laterally it passes over the lower part

of the face and is attached to the overlying skin as well as mingling with the other muscles which pass to the angle of the mouth. The third of these muscles is the buccinator.

The buccinator forms the main part of the cheek between the maxilla and the mandible. It is attached posteriorly to the pterygomandibular raphe which is attached above to the hamulus at the inferior end of the medial pterygoid plate and below to the posterior end of the mylohyoid line. The tensor veli palatini hooks round the hamulus and the buccinator is attached to fibrous tissue which arches over the tensor between the hamulus and the adjacent area of the maxilla. The superior constrictor of the pharynx is attached to the posterior border of the raphe. The buccinator has a bony attachment to the outer surface of the alveolar process of the maxilla and mandible, opposite the molar teeth. The fibres of the buccinator pass forwards towards the mouth. At the angle, the upper part of the upper fibres and the lower part of the lower fibres pass directly into the upper and lower lips respectively but the middle fibres decussate. The deep surface of the buccinator is lined by the mucous membrane of the mouth to whose lamina propria it is firmly attached. Superficially the facial vessels pass almost vertically over it and the buccal nerve and branches of the facial nerve pass transversely across it. The parotid duct pierces it at the level of the upper second molar tooth. More posteriorly there is a pad of fat between it and the masseter and ramus of the mandible.

The modiolus is the name given to the site at the angle of the mouth where fibres from eight muscles interlace–the levator and depressor anguli oris, levator labii superioris, depressor labii inferioris, zygomaticus major, risorius, platysma and buccinator.

All the muscles are supplied by the facial nerve, its buccal branch supplying the superior muscles and its mandibular branch the lower whilst the cervical branch supplies the platysma. The actions of the muscles are suggested by their names and their attachments. Their use in facial expression can also be worked out to some extent. For example, smiling, in which the angles of the mouth are pulled laterally, involves the risorius (from risor meaning a laugh) and buccinator. Sharp intermittent pulling downwards of the angles of the mouth is the best way to demonstrate the subcutaneous platysma on both sides. The buccinator expels the air violently after blowing out the cheeks and is also used in pushing the food between the teeth from the vestibule of the mouth while chewing.

These labial muscles are necessary in chewing and swallowing; eating, drinking and especially sucking in an infant are also important functions in which these muscles are used.

The main muscle of the eyelids is a sphincter, the orbicularis oculi (Fig. 10.43) which is in three parts. The orbital part is attached medially to the nasal part of the frontal bone, the frontal process of the maxilla and the medial palpebral ligament which is attached between these bony attachments. The fibres form complete ellipses round the opening of the orbit without any bony attachment but some of the fibres are attached to the superficial fascia. The palpebral part, thinner and paler than the orbital, is attached medially to the medial palpebral ligament and the adjacent bone. The fibres pass across the eyelids and interlace at their lateral ends. The lacrimal part is the name given to a group of fibres attached to the lacrimal bone and lying behind the lacrimal sac. They pass laterally into the eyelids and some of the fibres are attached to the tarsus of each eyelid. The medial palpebral ligament lies in front of the lacrimal sac and is attached medially to the frontal process of the maxilla and laterally to the tarsal plates.

The orbicularis oculi is supplied by the temporal and zygomatic branches of the facial nerve. The palpebral part closes the eyelids gently, intermittently as in blinking and continuously as in sleep. The orbital part closes the eyelids tightly and pulls the skin on the lateral side of the orbital opening medially. The lacrimal part pulls the eyelids medially and may dilate the lacrimal sac which lies in front of it. Opposing the action of this sphincter are those muscles opening the lids, the levator palpebrae superioris, occipitofrontalis and possibly the inferior rectus of the eyeball (p. 951).

The corrugator supercilii is attached to the frontal bone at the medial end of the superciliary arch. Its fibres pass laterally into the skin overlying the lateral end of the eyebrow. On contraction it produces the vertical furrows seen over the bridge of the nose in frowning. It is supplied by the facial nerve.

The muscles related to the external nose and auricle are small and unimportant. They are supplied by the facial nerve.

The scalp consists of hairy skin, deep to which is a layer of superficial fascia firmly bound to an underlying aponeurotic layer containing muscles. The aponeurotic layer is separated from the periosteum (pericranium) of the skull by a loose connective tissue layer. The vessels and nerves of the scalp are in the superficial fascia. The layer with muscles in it is called the epicranial aponeurosis. The muscles the frontalis and occipitalis are both supplied by the facial nerve.

The aponeurosis with its associated muscles is attached anteriorly to the skin over the eyelids, laterally to the zygomatic arch and temporal fascia, and posteriorly to the highest nuchal line and external occipital protuberence. Fluid deep to the aponeurosis spreads widely—laterally as far as the zygomatic arch and anteriorly into the eyelids (a blow on the scalp can cause a black eye). Fluid (or blood) deep to the pericranium is limited in its spread by the sutures.

The frontalis muscle elevates the skin of the forehead together with the eyebrows and produces transverse creases in the forehead.

POSTURE

Posture is the attitude that the parts of the body take in relation to one another and the position of the whole body in space. In animals without a skeleton, such as the jellyfish, posture is determined mostly by gravity and the physical characteristics of the supporting environment. Man, on the other hand, can counter the effects of gravity, survive in a low density environment and move about in that environment. Movement requires adjustments in posture to control the forces predicted by Newton's third law. In order to do all these things man has a skeletal system, a muscle system and a nervous system. How the nervous system uses the other systems to produce what is known as posture is the subject of this section.

The bony endoskeleton provides a basic anti-gravity system for maintaining an upright body. In order to move, this skeleton must be provided with joints thereby sacrificing the ability a solid skeleton would have to resist gravity. This weakening is compensated by the powerful anti-gravity (extensor) muscles and by special arrangements within the nervous system which gives some priority to these muscles. The basic properties of the bony skeletal system and the muscle system have been given in other sections. Here we will be mostly concerned with the mechanisms which the nervous system uses to coordinate the effector (muscular) system.

Reflexes

Basic to an understanding of posture is the concept of the reflex (p. 304). A great number of

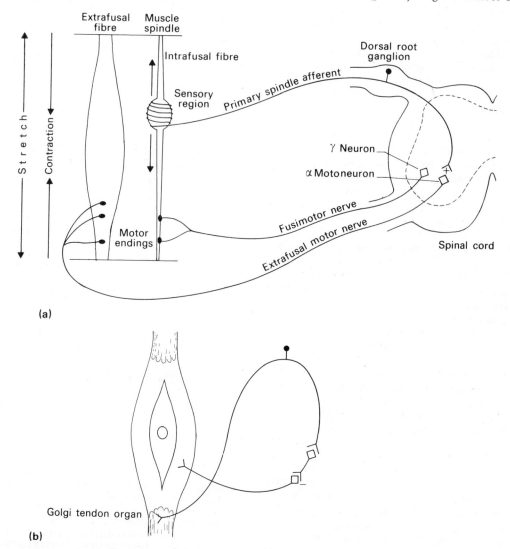

(a)

(b)

Fig. 10.45. (a) Schematic representation of nervous pathways involved in stretch reflex. Stimulation of the sensory ending in the intrafusal fibre (the muscle spindle) excites the ventral motoneuron which causes contraction of extrafusal muscle fibres. The sensitivity of the sensory region to applied stretch can be increased by stimulation of fusimotor neurons which cause contraction of the intrafusal muscle fibre in the direction shown by arrows. (b) Pathway in golgi tendon reflex. Stimulation of the high-threshold receptor in the tendon causes relaxation of the muscle by inhibition of the ventral motoneuron.

reflexes are coordinated and used for the maintenance of any particular posture, but only a few 'classic' reflexes have been selected to illustrate the general principles of integration and control.

STRETCH REFLEX

If the legs are crossed while sitting down and the patellar tendon of the freely swinging leg is tapped with a soft rubber hammer, the knee extensor muscle (quadriceps) contracts and the leg quickly extends and then relaxes. This knee jerk reflex is an example of a fundamental piece of neural machinery, a stretch reflex.

The sensory or afferent side of a stretch reflex comes from the sensory region of the muscle spindle (Figs. 6.9 & 6.10). A description of the muscle spindle and its innervation has been given (p. 330). The nerve carrying the sensory information to the spinal cord is called the primary spindle afferent or IA nerve (Fig. 10.45a) to distinguish it from another, smaller nerve (IIA) which comes from the flower spray or secondary sensory endings also in the muscle spindle. The smaller nerve is called the secondary spindle afferent and participates in other reflexes. The muscle spindle lies 'in parallel' with the extrafusal fibres (Fig. 6.9). When a muscle is stretched, for example by tapping the stretched patellar tendon, the spindle is stretched and the number of action potentials in the afferent nerve is increased (Fig. 10.46b). Like most receptors, stretch receptors vary in their thresholds and in consequence differing degrees and rates of stretch can be monitored and the reflex contraction adjusted to the stimulus. The primary spindle afferent nerve is a large nerve fibre which conducts action potentials very rapidly (70–80 m/sec in man) and synapses directly (monosynaptically) with the extrafusal (α) motoneurons supplying the muscle from which the afferent nerve originates (Fig. 10.45a). In our example the quadriceps (extensor) muscle would contract.

Another stretch reflex is the jaw jerk; when the jaw is relaxed and the chin is tapped with a soft rubber hammer the jaw closing muscles (masseters and temporalis) are stretched. Their muscle spindles are also stretched and action potentials are transmitted by the primary spindle afferent nerve. This nerve synapses directly with the motoneurons of the jaw closing muscles and if the number of action potentials in the nerve is sufficiently great, the masseter motoneurons are stimulated. This activation causes the masseter muscle to contract. The contraction is brief

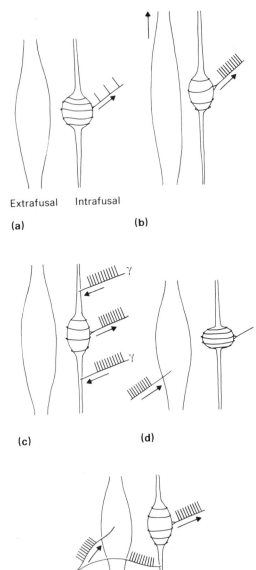

Extrafusal   Intrafusal

(a)   (b)

(c)   (d)

(e)

Fig. 10.46. Representation of activity in afferent and efferent innervation of intra- and extrafural muscle fibres. (a) When the intra and extrafusal muscle fibres are relaxed few action potentials travel in the primary afferent fibre; (b) when the spindle and extrafusal fibres are stretched the number of action potentials in the afferent nerve is increased; (c) γ-efferent discharge causes the intrafusal fibre to contract so that threshold of the muscle spindle is reached, as a result the number of action potentials in the primary afferent is increased; (d) the muscle spindle may shorten (relaxes) when the extrafusal fibres contract but usually the α and γ-efferent systems are activated together as shown in (e).

because it is self-limiting. The stretching of the muscle spindle nuclear bag is reduced by the reflex contraction because of the parallel arrangement between the muscle spindle and the contracting muscle fibres. The relaxation of the sensory region terminates the action potential sequence (Fig 10.46a)

The stretch reflex tends to keep a muscle at a constant length because an increase in length (stretching) causes the muscle to shorten (contraction). Too much shortening however, causes so much relaxation of the muscle spindle that even if the muscle is lengthened by external forces (e.g. gravity) acting upon it, action potentials are not generated in the primary afferent nerve. But at what length ought the muscle to be set and can the setting of the length be varied? The answer is that the nervous system is able to choose the optimum muscle length in order to maintain a particular posture.

A very simple neural device allows the length to be set at whatever length is required within the limits of the force that the muscle can generate. At each end of the muscle spindle sensory region are small intrafusal muscle fibres (Figs. 6.10 & 10.46c).

The intrafusal muscle fibres receive most of their motor innervation from small fusimotor neurons (γ-efferents). These, and the extrafusal (α-efferent) motor neurons, constitute two different, independent motor systems. They are usually activated together (Fig. 10.46e) but they can be activated separately under some circumstances.

In contrast to the shortening of the spindle following contraction of extrafusal muscle fibres (Fig. 10.46d), the non-contractile bag is stretched when the intrafusal muscle fibres contract. If the threshold length of the nuclear bag is reached the number of action potentials in the primary afferent nerve increases (Fig. 10.46c) and the extrafusal muscle contracts reflexly because of the monosynaptic connection between the primary muscle spindle afferent and the extrafusal motoneuron. The extrafusal muscle continues to contract until the tension imposed by intrafusal contraction upon the sensory region of the muscle spindle is relieved.

In recent years it has been found that there are two types of nuclear bag endings known as bag 1 and bag 2. Bag 1-type endings are innervated by γ-efferent, dynamic motoneurons (γ-d) rapidly adapting and specialized to transmit information about 'high frequency' changes in the length of the muscle, i.e. vibration. The bag 2-type intrafusal fibre is innervated by the static motoneurons (γ-s). These receptors are considerably less sensitive to vibration than bag 1 type; they are less quickly adapting and therefore are able to provide signals regarding the length of the

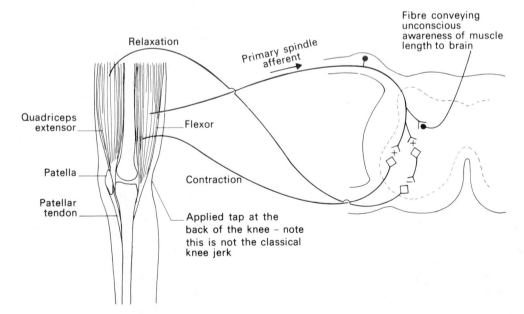

Fig. 10.47. Reciprocal inhibition — The reflex excitation of the flexor motoneurons elicited by stretching of the spindles in the flexor muscle results in inhibition of the extensor motoneurons and consequent relaxation of the extensor muscles.

muscle; γ-s afferents also innervate the nuclear chain fibres which are specialized to provide information about the static stretch of the muscle.

For a given posture the nervous system can impose the required length on the extrafusal muscle fibres by setting the tension on the muscle spindle via the γ-efferents to the spindle. If the muscle lengthens further the spindle fires and the muscle contracts. If the contraction goes too far the spindle stops firing and the muscle relaxes. This type of system is known to engineers as a 'servo' system. Mechanical servo systems are widely used in industry for automatic controls. A very common servo system in the home is thermostatically controlled central heating. Setting the temperature in the thermostat is equivalent to setting the tension of the spindle.

The nervous system uses this stretch reflex in a number of ways. An obvious example is the maintenance of a standing posture. The forces of gravity act to flex the major articulations at the knee, hip, spine and head. Once the length of the anti-gravity (extensor) muscles has been set by the fusimotor (and other) systems, any tendency for the joint to collapse (flex) is immediately resisted by the stretch reflex.

The effects of the stretch reflex are not limited to antigravity muscles or only to the motor neurons innervating the muscle from which the primary spindle afferent originates. The stretch reflex is also found in flexor muscles (Fig. 10.47). This type of innervation allows for an automatic 'servo' adjustment to any external force which would act to disturb a posture set by the nervous system. If a sharp blow is applied with the edge of the hand to the flexor tendon behind the knee one can see and feel the quadriceps (knee extensors) relax. This is an example of reciprocal inhibition (Fig. 10.47). Excitation of the flexor motoneurons elicited by stretching of the spindle in the flexor muscle is accompanied by inhibition of the extensor motoneurons.

✕ GOLGI TENDON ORGAN ✕

Another sensory receptor in the muscle system is the Golgi tendon organ which is most often found near the tendon–muscle junction. Because of their location (Fig. 6.9) most tendon organs are connected 'in series' with the extrafusal muscle fibres and are therefore activated by both excessive stretch and in isometric contraction. Tendon organs can be called tension receptors and their behaviour is often contrasted with

muscle spindles which are thought of as muscle length receptors.

The afferent nerve from the Golgi tendon organ enters the spinal cord and forms a disynaptic inhibitory connection with motor neurons which innervate the muscle from which the afferent originates. (Fig. 10.45b) Because of this inhibitory arrangement too much stretch on a contracting muscle may lead to inhibition of further contraction. This reflex has been described as a 'safety valve' to prevent excessive muscular contraction but recent investigations have shown that the role of the Golgi tendon in posture and movement is more complex than this. When during the closing phase of a chewing cycle the opposing teeth come into contact with hard food, further shortening of the jaw closing muscles is prevented, though isometric contraction (clenching) may continue. When tension reaches a critical level this can cause stimulation of Golgi tendon organs in part of the anterior temporalis muscle and inhibition of the motoneurons to this muscle in readiness for jaw opening.

CONTROL OF POSTURAL REFLEXES

All the reflexes described above (with the exception of those in chewing) are used to maintain an erect posture. There are other, equally important, postural relationships that use other reflexes. Special neck reflexes, for example, are used to maintain an approriate position of the head to the rest of the body. These reflexes are so well integrated into the nervous system that extraordinary methods must be used to study them. To study spinal cord reflexes in isolation it is necessary to 'dis-integrate' them from the rest of the nervous system by cutting between the brain and spinal cord. For animals with long necks this is a relatively easy experiment. Such an operation produces a 'spinal' animal.

A chicken with its head removed by traditional means is capable of running a short distance after the chop. This demonstrates that much of the running and walking behaviour is organized by spinal cord neural mechanisms. A similar lesion in a mammal produces a much reduced range of movement and a loss of posture; in fact, there is very little nervous activity of any sort directly after spinal cord transection. This is called the period of spinal shock. After this phase, stretch reflexes and withdrawal (flexor) reflexes become apparent but the animal cannot stand. These observations tell us something of how reflexes are organized and what part of the nervous system contains the

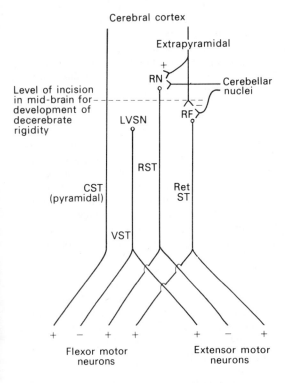

RN   Red nucleus and RST rubrospinal tract

RF   Reticular formation and Ret ST reticulospinal tract

LVSN Lateral vestibulospinal nucleus and
      VST vestibulospinal tract

CST   Corticospinal tract

Note that the descending tracts terminate on internuncial neurons and γ motorneurons; only a few corticospinal fibres synapse directly on α motorneurons

Fig. 10.48. Diagram to show main descending spinal pathways and the neural elements in the brain which are responsible for posture.

various bits of neural machinery (p. 304).

It turns out that many of the neural components used to regulate posture are in the brain stem (Fig. 10.48). The brain stem is very complex both anatomically and physiologically and a variety of techniques are used to study it.

If a careful incision is made at the upper end of the brain stem the animal is rendered unconsious and incapable of voluntary movement, but unlike the spinal animal, it can 'stand' if it is helped. This animal is called 'decerebrate' because the cerebrum has been separated from the brain stem and spinal cord. The animal can stand because all its anti-gravity muscles are contracted into spasm, it has to be helped because it cannot 'balance.' The least disturbance from any direction causes the animal to fall over and having fallen over, it is unable to get up.

The main neural elements responsible for the decerebrate posture are the lateral vestibular nucleus and the reticular formation (Fig. 10.48). These structures are located in the lower two-thirds of the brain stem and are below the incision. The lateral vestibular nucleus provides both a powerful monosynaptic excitation to extensor motor neurons which innervate intra- and extrafusal muscle fibres and inhibition to flexor motor neurons. The major excitatory drive to flexor motor neurons is provided by the red nucleus and the corticospinal (pyramidal) tract. The red nucleus normally supplies powerful inhibition to the extensor motor neurons but the surgical incision removes these influences on the motor neurons. The result is the exaggerated contraction of the extensor muscles which are not opposed by extensive flexor contraction.

If an incision is made above the midbrain but below the thalamus, the animal is able to stand unsupported. There is, of course, no voluntary movement. If this 'midbrain' animal is pushed and falls over it can recover a standing posture. If the recovery to the standing posture is carefully studied it is seen to involve a whole series of reflexes which are carried out in a pre-set, predictable order. These reflexes are called 'righting reflexes.' Some of these 'righting reflexes' require receptors in the labyrinths, others depend on receptors in the neck muscles.

Normally, when 'righting' ourselves to an erect posture we use information from more sources than are available to the 'midbrain' animal. We use additional cues from visual systems and cutaneous and joint receptors which have been processed in the thalamus. All of these cues are so well integrated that our 'righting' movements are far from stereotyped. In fact, since they are so precisely correlated with environmental events at the moment the righting is invoked, they are never likely to be exactly the same.

Many of the reflexes described above are called 'segmental reflexes' because the input and output of the reflex is contained in a very small segment of the spinal cord. Other reflexes are described as belonging to a restricted region of the nervous system, e.g. the upper brain stem. There are, however, reflexes that require the entire nervous system as their substrate. Such responses require nearly $1/20$th of a second and follow a pathway through the sensory and motor cortex of the brain. Their function is not very well understood.

Only a few of the known mechanisms by which the nervous system uses the muscular system to maintain posture have been described. What has been shown in a very limited way are the 'wiring diagrams' of a very few of the simplest reflexes. The methods that the nervous system uses to co-ordinate sensibly all these reflexes are fascinating, but are still only imperfectly known.

VOLUNTARY MOVEMENT

From the previous section it should be clear that posture and voluntary movement are closely integrated and that it is impossible to separate them. Every voluntary movement requires postural adjustments. The great majority of these adjustments are automatic and make use of the reflex systems already discussed. Complex movements, such as walking, involve complicated sequences which are controlled without conscious attention. These sequences can be voluntarily interrupted and other movements superimposed upon them. This section is concerned with the neural machinery used for making voluntary movements.

For many years it has been popular to divide the nervous system into regions such as respiratory centres, speech centres, hearing centres, voluntary movement centres and so forth whose functions have been assigned by observing the effects of destruction in or around these centres. The concept of centres has been a very productive one. In years past, before many of the modern diagnostic tools were available, it enabled physicians to locate disease in the nervous system, at times with stunning accuracy. Among the many interesting questions raised by the concept is; where is voluntary movement initiated?

Neurophysiologists have been impressed by the range of movement and the fine control demonstrated by the human hand. Experiments on monkeys and man showed that large areas of the cerebral cortex are devoted to fine movements of the hand, mouth, tongue and feet (Fig. 19.94). Further studies demonstrated a large conspicuous pathway from a part of the cerebral cortex, just anterior to the central sulcus, into the brain stem and so on to the spinal cord. Finally, lesions such as strokes (haemorrhages) or tumours in this motor area were known to result in profound disturbances of movement. The large motor pathway running from the cortex into the spinal cord was called the pyramidal tract (after the pyramid in the brain stem). All other pathways involved in movement were called extrapyramidal.

Experiments showed that most of the large pyramidal shaped (Betz) cells in the motor cortex were connected polysynaptically through chains of excitatory and inhibitory neurons to the extrafusal alpha motor neurons. In primates about 10% of the pyramidal tract fibres are connected monosynaptically to extrafusal motor neurons. This monosynaptic pathway was thought to be of special use for the rapid voluntary movements of the hand and this view agreed with theories which attached great importance to the pyramidal system in the control of movement. Other experiments, however, lead to a reappraisal of the supremacy of the pyramdial system. When very careful lesions were made in pyramidal tracts in monkeys it was found that only the finest of the finger movements were lost, especially those of the thumb and index finger. A great variety of voluntary movements remained.

The supposed supremacy of the pyramidal system quite naturally suggested the motor cortex as a likely candidate for the origin of voluntary movements. Experiments were devised which allowed recordings to be made from pyramidal tract cells in awake monkeys trained to perform certain movements. As would be expected from a motor control centre, the pyramidal tract neurons discharge action potentials 50–100 msec before a movement begins. The question which naturally follows on from this is what are the functions of other brain structures known to be involved in movement? Structures such as the cerebellum and basal ganglia (Fig. 19.34b) are known to play a subsidiary but nevertheless important role in the control of voluntary movement. Though movements are not normally elicited when these structures are stimulated electrically, profound disturbances of movement result from their damage or disease. It was believed (and still is, judging from many of the text-books) that the cerebellum might supply feedback information mainly from joint and muscle receptors to the motor cortex which would determine the corrections needed for the evolving pattern of movement. If this concept was correct then the cerebellum ought to show activity at some finite period after the motor cortex discharged its first commands to the 'lower' centres. In fact, recordings from neurons in the cerebellum and in the basal ganglia show that activity in relation to a movement begins at approximately the same time as activity from the motor cortex. From evidence such as this, it is becoming increasingly clear that movement is initiated by the entire motor nervous system. No one centre is above all others or controls the rest. A coordinated sensible voluntary movement is initiated by the concerted, integrated action of the cerebellum, motor cortex, basal ganglia and all other areas in the pyramidal and extrapyramidal systems.

Having stressed the integration of the various parts of the motor system, can anything meaningful be said about the function of the parts? It can, as long as it is remembered that no one function is the exclusive prerogative of any one part.

The cerebellum functionally consists of a midline portion and a lateral portion (p. 858). Lesions in the midline portion seriously affect balance and equilibrium. The lateral cerebellar lobes and the dentate nucleus are more involved with voluntary movement. Destructive lesions in the lateral cerebellum result in decreased muscle tone. This is because the excitatory drive to the fusimotor (γ) system is decreased and the muscle spindles are slack. Movements are also late in starting and they are not accurately terminated. If a patient with a cerebellar lobe lesion is asked to point at a target, his finger shoots past it. The 'past-pointing' is over corrected and again the target is missed. This back and forth movement is often called an intention tremor. The main function of the lateral lobes and nuclei of the cerebellum appears to be to assist in ordering the sequence of contraction in different muscles and to ensure that the contractions occur at the right moment during a voluntary movement. In other words, the cerebellum can be said to receive an 'advance report' of activity in the pyramidal tract. Proprioceptive information processed by the cerebellar cortex influences and modifies the output of the cerebellar nuclei and subsequently the motor centres and plays an important role in the co-ordination of voluntary movement.

In animals such as birds and reptiles, the basal ganglia are the major motor centres. In animals higher on the phylogenetic scale, the cortex is greatly expanded and appears to 'take over' many of the functions which in lower animals were carried out by the basal ganglia. Lesions in the basal ganglia result in purposeless unwanted movements (p. 875). There is no comprehensive hypothesis for the function of the basal ganglia in man.

The uppermost part of the motor cortex contains neural elements that project mainly to the motor neurons that supply the leg and foot muscles, the middle area to the arm motor neurons and the lower area to facial and tongue motor neurons. The motor cortex contains numerous different cell types many of which have an uncertain or unknown function. The main output from this area is from the pyramidal shaped cells. These project to both pyramidal and extrapyramidal pathways. This in part explains the profound paralysis which results from destruction of the motor cortex while pyramidal tract damage results only in loss of very fine movement. The pyramidal tract projects to both the extrafusal and intrafusal motor neurons. Studies upon the nerves of human subjects performing voluntary movements have shown that both the extrafusal and intrafusal motor systems are activated together in the production of a movement. What is the purpose of this co-activation? During a voluntary movement the extrafusal muscle is contracting and tending to relieve the stress on the muscle spindle. The intrafusal muscle system is also contracting so as to maintain the tension on the nuclear bag. If any external disturbance prevents the movement, the extrafusal shortening is halted but the intrafusal contraction continues. This places an additional stretch on the muscle spindle sensory region and elicits increased activity in the primary afferent nerve to the motor neuron pool of the contracting muscle so that a greater contraction results in order to overcome the resistance to the movement. This illustrates how the stretch reflex is used for both postural and voluntary control and how co-activation of the two motor systems (α and γ) allows for automatic compensation for any change in resistance to a movement.

It is important to appreciate that a smooth voluntary movement requires that the nervous system acts as an integrated whole. The concept of centres for this or that function is misleading both factually and because it detracts from this fundamental principle of integration.

FURTHER READING

BROOKS V.B. & SONEY S.D. (1971) Motor mechanisms: The role of the pyramidal system in motor control. *Physiological Reviews* **33**, 337.

MATTHEWS P.B.C. (1972) Mammalian muscle receptors and their central actions. *Physiological Society Monograph.* London, Arnold.

CHAPTER 11

The Respiratory Passages

ANATOMY

External nose and nasal cavity

The external nose consists of bone and cartilage with some fibrous tissue (Fig. 11.1). The bony part is superior and consists of the nasal bones which articulate with each other in the midline, with the frontal bone superiorly and the frontal process of the maxilla laterally. The root of the nose is usually depressed as compared with the lowest part of the forehead lying immediately above it. The cartilages form the major part of the external nose. The lateral nasal cartilage is triangular and is attached superiorly to the nasal bone, laterally to the maxilla and inferiorly to the major alar cartilage, which is folded so that its opening faces backwards. Inferiorly this cartilage forms the anterolateral part of the external nose and in the midline passes inferior to the septal cartilage forming the mobile part of the nasal septum. The two nasal openings are called the nares or anterior nasal apertures. The blood supply is from branches of the facial, ophthalmic and infraorbital arteries and its main sensory nerve supply is from the ophthalmic nerve (ex-

ternal nasal and infratrochlear branches). The lateral edge of the nares receives a branch from the maxillary nerve (infraorbital branch).

The nasal cavity lies above the oral cavity and below the cranial cavity, inferomedial to the orbits. It is divided into two by the vertical nasal septum which is usually to one side of the midline. The nasal cavity opens anteriorly at the nares and posteriorly by the vertical choanae or posterior nasal apertures into the nasopharynx. Each half of the nasal cavity has four sides; a lateral wall, a roof, a floor and a common medial wall, the septum (Figs. 11.2, 11.3).

The septum is partly bony, partly cartilaginous. The bony part is posterior and superiorly is formed by the perpendicular plate of the ethmoid bone. The vomer extends posteriorly inferior to the body of the sphenoid, and anteriorly beyond the perpendicular plate. The inferior border of the vomer lies in the ridge formed by the palatine processes of the maxilla and the horizontal plates of the palatine bones. The septal cartilage is roughly quadrilateral and is attached to the perpendicular plate posteriorly, the vomer inferiorly and the cartilages of

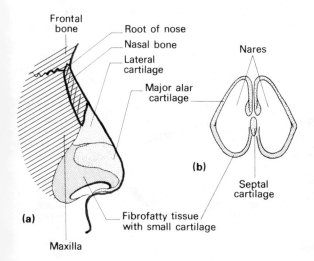

Frontal bone
Root of nose
Nasal bone
Lateral cartilage
Major alar cartilage
Nares
Septal cartilage
Fibrofatty tissue with small cartilage
Maxilla

(a)
(b)

Fig. 11.1. The external nose.
(a) Lateral view; (b) inferior view.

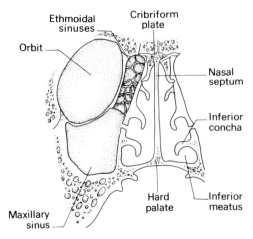

Fig. 11.2. Coronal section through the nasal cavity (diagrammatic).

sive canal on each side passes downwards and forwards to the incisive fossa on the oral surface of the hard palate.

The lateral wall (Figs. 11.2, 11.4 & 11.5) slopes upwards and medially so that the upper part of the nasal cavity is much narrower than the lower. This wall is irregular because of the presence of three conchae projecting medially and then downwards into the cavity. They are called inferior, middle and superior. The inferior is a separate bone and the other two are part of the ethmoid bone. Occasionally the ethmoid has a small supreme concha above the superior. The space between a concha and the lateral wall of the nose is called a meatus. There are three meatuses, inferior, middle and superior. The narrow space at the top of the nasal cavity between the ethmoid laterally and the sphenoid medially is called the sphenoethmoidal recess. The nasolacrimal duct opens into the anterior part of the inferior meatus. The frontal and maxillary air sinuses and the anterior and middle ethmoidal air cells open into the middle meatus. The posterior ethmoidal air cells open into the superior meatus and the sphenoidal air sinus into the posterior wall of the sphenoethmoidal recess.

In order to understand the structure of the lateral wall of the nasal cavity, the details of some of the bones involved have to be considered. The medial (nasal) surface of the maxilla has a large opening somewhat posterior and superior in position, the maxillary hiatus, leading into the maxillary sinus. The lacrimal groove lies anterior to the opening and posterior to a ridge forming the conchal crest. This ridge is the lower border of the medial surface of the frontal process of the maxilla which has a horizontal ridge (the ethmoidal crest) about its middle. Behind the opening the bone is roughened for

the external nose superiorly and anteriorly. The vomeronasal organ (of Jacobson), the remains of a structure associated with the sense of smell in animals such as reptiles, is a blind-ending recess passing backwards along the lower edge of the septal cartilage: it opens at the side of the cartilage just behind the incisive canal.

The roof of the nasal cavity has a horizontal part formed by the cribriform plate of the ethmoid, a posterior sloping part by the body of the sphenoid and an anterior sloping part by the nasal part of the frontal bone and the nasal bones.

The floor (Figs. 11.2 & 11.3) is horizontal and almost flat. The anterior three-quarters are formed by the palatine processes of the maxillae and the posterior quarter by the horizontal plates of the palatine bones. About 1 cm behind the anterior nasal spine of the maxilla the inci-

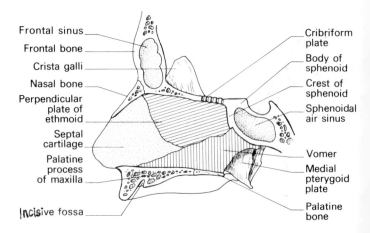

Fig. 11.3. The left side of the nasal septum.

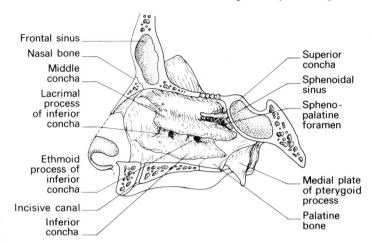

Frontal sinus
Nasal bone
Middle concha
Lacrimal process of inferior concha
Ethmoid process of inferior concha
Incisive canal
Inferior concha

Superior concha
Sphenoidal sinus
Spheno-palatine foramen
Medial plate of pterygoid process
Palatine bone

Fig. 11.4. The right lateral wall of the nasal cavity.

articulation with the palatine bone. Running downwards in the lower part of this rough area is a groove which, together with a similar groove on the palatine bone, forms the greater palatine canal. The palatine bone has a perpendicular plate the lateral surface of which articulates with the medial surface of the maxilla (Figs. 11.6 & 11.7). This plate overlaps the posterior edge of the maxillary hiatus. On the nasal surface of the perpendicular plate there are two horizontal ridges, the upper is the ethmoidal crest and the lower the conchal crest.

The ethmoid bone has a midline perpendicular plate which forms part of the septum and a horizontal cribriform plate which forms the roof of the nasal cavity. The part of the perpendicular plate projecting above the cribriform plate is called the crista galli. Suspended from the lateral edge of the cribriform plate is the ethmoidal

labyrinth most of which is occupied by the ethmoidal air cells. The medial (nasal) surface ends below as the middle concha which extends beyond the labyrinth anteriorly and posteriorly and projects medially and then downwards thus forming the middle meatus which is lateral to it. The middle ethmoidal air cells form a swelling in the middle meatus called the bulla ethmoidalis. Projecting downwards and backwards from the lower anterior part of the labyrinth is the uncinate process of the ethmoid. The hiatus semilunaris leads upwards into a canal in the labyrinth called the infundibulum which leads to the frontal air sinus. The anterior ethmoidal air cells open into the infundibulum.

The inferior concha (Figs. 11.4 & 11.5) is an elongated, thin, curved plate of bone which forms most of the medial wall of the inferior meatus. It extends forwards to articulate with

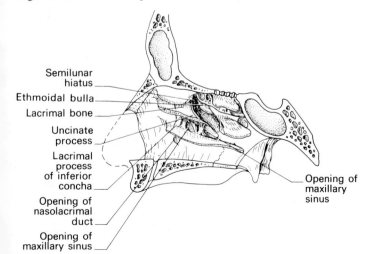

Semilunar hiatus
Ethmoidal bulla
Lacrimal bone
Uncinate process
Lacrimal process of inferior concha
Opening of nasolacrimal duct
Opening of maxillary sinus

Opening of maxillary sinus

Fig. 11.5. The right lateral wall of the nasal cavity after removal of most of the three conchae.

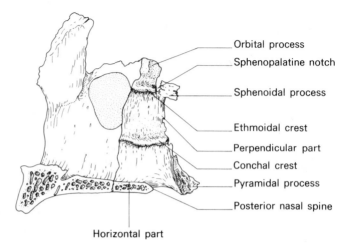

Fig. 11.6. Right palatine bone articulating with the right maxilla.

Orbital process
Sphenopalatine notch
Sphenoidal process
Ethmoidal crest
Perpendicular part
Conchal crest
Pyramidal process
Posterior nasal spine
Horizontal part

the conchal crest of the maxilla and backwards to articulate with the conchal crest on the perpendicular plate of the palatine bone. Between these articulations there is anteriorly an upwards projecting process which meets a downward projection of the lacrimal bone. These two projections lie over the anterior part of the maxillary hiatus. They also exclude the nasolacrimal duct from the middle meatus so that the duct opens into the inferior meatus. There is a projection upwards from about the middle of the inferior concha which articulates with the uncinate process. There is also a posterior projection which articulates with the part of the palatine bone covering the posterior part of the hiatus. Normally the maxillary sinus opens into the posterior part of the hiatus semilunaris and there may be a second opening inferior to the hiatus.

The choanae (posterior nasal apertures) are vertical openings on either side of the midline about 2.5 cm high and 1 cm wide (p. 444). They are separated by the posterior edge of the vomer, the ala of which, together with the vaginal process of the medial pterygoid plate, inferior to the body of the sphenoid, form the upper boundary of the choana. The lateral wall is formed by the medial surface of the medial pterygoid plate. This plate is directly continuous anteriorly with the perpendicular plate of the palatine bone. Inferiorly the posterior edge of the horizontal process of the palatine bone forms the boundary of the choana. The soft palate is attached to this edge.

The nasal cavity behind the vestibule is lined by two types of epithelium. The olfactory epithelium is found in the roof and adjacent parts of the lateral walls and septum. It is yellowish and thicker than the adjoining epithelium. The rest of the cavity is lined by columnar, ciliated, mucous epithelium, which may be pseudostratified. Besides the goblet cells there are serous and mucous glands deep to the epithelium and separated from it by a layer of fibrous tissue containing lymphocytes. The lin-

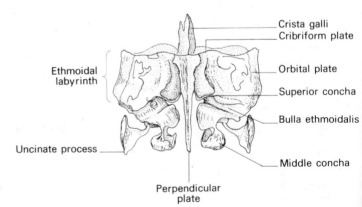

Ethmoidal labyrinth
Uncinate process
Crista galli
Cribriform plate
Orbital plate
Superior concha
Bulla ethmoidalis
Middle concha
Perpendicular plate

Fig. 11.7. Posterior view of the ethmoid bone.

ing differs in thickness in various parts of the cavity being thickest over the conchae, especially the inferior, and the septum. It is thin in the floor of the cavity and the meatuses. The amount of subepithelial cavernous tissue, that is regions of dilated thin-walled capillaries with arteriovenous communications, determines the thickness of the lining. The total area of the lining is obviously increased by the presence of the conchae on the lateral wall. Apart from the olfactory function of the nasal cavity, the serous and mucous secretions moisten the inspired air and produce a sticky surface to which particles adhere. The special cavernous tissue warms the air while the cilia beat backwards and convey the mucus towards the nasopharynx whence it passes downwards and is swallowed. It is thought that the conchae cause turbulence of the inspired air thereby giving their former name, turbinate bones, a functional as well as a structural significance.

The structural advantages of the nose may often exaggerate the effects of infection. Swelling of an already thick lining together with increased mucous secretion frequently blocks the nasal cavity and the openings into the sinuses, especially that of the maxillary sinus. It is also important to realize that the lining of the nasal cavity is continuous with that of the paranasal sinuses, the nasolacrimal duct and the nasopharynx, and indirectly with that of the auditory tube and middle ear. Thus nasal infections can readily spread to the middle ear, especially in children who, compared to adults, have a short auditory tube.

The arteries to the nasal cavity are derived from the ophthalmic (anterior and posterior ethmoidal), the maxillary (sphenopalatine and greater palatine) and the facial (labial). The vestibular area of the septum receives, in addition to the sphenopalatine and labial branches, an ascending branch from the greater palatine artery which enters the nasal cavity through the incisive canal. The veins correspond with the arteries, with the important addition of venous communications between the nasal cavity and the veins on the inferior surface of the frontal lobe of the brain through the foramen caecum and cribriform plate.

The nerves of general sensation are derived from the maxillary nerve except for a small area, anteriorly and superiorly, which is supplied by the ophthalmic (anterior ethmoidal nerve). The infraorbital nerve supplies the vestibule, the anterior superior dental nerve the anterior and inferior parts of the septum, floor and lateral wall, and branches from the pterygopalatine ganglion supply the rest of the lining. These include the nasopalatine and other branches which enter the nasal cavity from the pterygopalatine fossa through the sphenopalatine foramen situated near the posterior end of the middle concha.

There are also important sympathetic vasomotor fibres to the blood vessels and parasympathetic secretomotor fibres to the glands. These run in the sensory nerves.

Paranasal air sinuses

These are found in the frontal, maxillary, ethmoid and sphenoid bones. The frontal sinuses lie at the side of the midline above the nasion and posterior to the superciliary arches. Each sinus is pyramidal in shape and is about 2–3 cm in height, depth and width. The septum separating the sinuses is rarely in the midline and a sinus can extend laterally and backwards over most of the roof of the orbit. If the sinus is large there are often ridges of bone projecting from the walls into the cavity of the sinus. The sinus is related inferolaterally to the orbit, inferiorly to the nasal cavity and laterally to the meninges and frontal lobe of the brain. It opens into the middle meatus by the frontonasal duct (the infundibulum). The nerve supply is from the supraorbital nerve, and its arterial supply from the supraorbital and anterior ethmoidal arteries.

The maxillary sinus (Fig. 11.8) is the cavity in the body of the maxilla. It is shaped like a four-sided pyramid with its base on the lateral wall of the nose. The facial wall is anteroinferolateral and can be felt through the cheek below the zygomatic bone. In this wall are branches of the superior alveolar nerves. The medial part of the posterior wall is related to the pterygopalatine fossa in which lie part of the maxillary artery, the pterygopalatine ganglion and the maxillary nerve. More laterally is the infratemporal fossa containing part of the maxillary artery, the pterygoid muscles and branches of the mandibular nerve. In the posterior wall are branches of the posterior superior alveolar nerve. The roof of the sinus forms most of the floor of the orbit and in it run the infraorbital vessels and nerve. The floor of the sinus is usually separated by bone from the roots of the second premolar and the first and second molar teeth. A very large maxillary sinus may be close to the first premolar and third molar teeth.

The medial or nasal wall forms a large part of the lateral wall of the nose. In the disarticulated

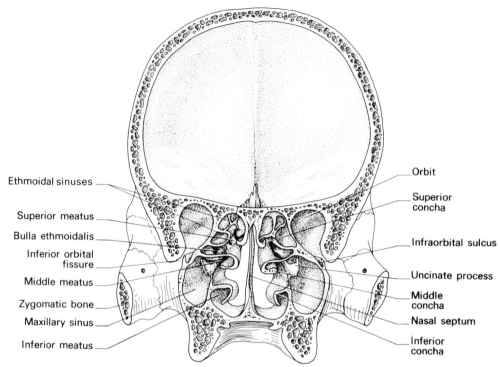

Ethmoidal sinuses

Superior meatus

Bulla ethmoidalis

Inferior orbital fissure

Middle meatus

Zygomatic bone

Maxillary sinus

Inferior meatus

Orbit

Superior concha

Infraorbital sulcus

Uncinate process

Middle concha

Nasal septum

Inferior concha

Fig. 11.8. A coronal section through the skull at the level of the second molar tooth.

bone it has a large opening. This however is reduced in size by the encroachment of neighbouring bones (p. 476), the palatine, ethmoidal and inferior concha, so that a small opening into the hiatus semilunaris of the middle meatus remains. There may be a second opening inferior to the hiatus. Anteromedial to the sinus is the nasolacrimal duct. The nerve supply of the sinus is from the nerves in its walls (the infraorbital and the superior alveolar) and its arterial supply is from the facial and maxillary arteries.

The sphenoidal sinuses are cavities in the body of the sphenoid bone and are separated by a thin septum which is seldom in the midline. The hypophysis cerebri and the optic chiasma are superior and the cavernous sinus and internal carotid artery are superolateral. The size of the sinuses varies but together form a space about 2 cm in height, depth and width. Rarely the sinuses extend backwards into the occipital bone, laterally into the lesser and greater wings of the sphenoid or downward into its pterygoid process. The sinus can then become closely related to the optic, ophthalmic or pterygoid nerves. The sinuses lie behind the superior part of the nasal cavity and open into the sphenoethmoidal

recess. The anterior wall of the sinus takes the form of a thin plate of bone in the upper half of which is the opening into the nasal cavity. Occasionally it is necessary to remove the pituitary gland. A convenient approach to this region through the sphenoidal air sinus is via the back of the nasal cavity. The nerve supply of the sinus is from the posterior ethmoidal nerve and its arterial supply from the posterior ethmoidal artery.

The ethmoidal air cells (sinuses) lie in the labyrinth of the ethmoid. Their number varies inversely to their size. There are usually between ten and fifteen, divided into anterior, middle and posterior. The anterior open into the infundibulum of the ethmoid, the middle into the bulla ethmoidalis (both open into the middle meatus) and the posterior into the superior meatus. Many of the ethmoidal cells are completed by neighbouring bones, the frontal, lacrimal, maxilla and palatine. The plate of bone separating the cells from the orbit is very thin. Their nerve supply is from the anterior and posterior ethmoidal nerves and their arterial supply from arteries of the same name.

All the sinuses are lined by ciliated mucous columnar epithelium continuous with that of the

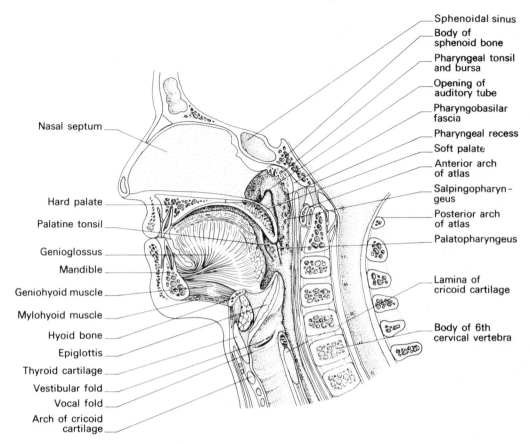

Sphenoidal sinus
Body of sphenoid bone
Pharyngeal tonsil and bursa
Opening of auditory tube
Pharyngobasilar fascia
Pharyngeal recess
Soft palate
Anterior arch of atlas
Salpingopharyn-geus
Posterior arch of atlas
Palatopharyngeus
Lamina of cricoid cartilage
Body of 6th cervical vertebra

Nasal septum
Hard palate
Palatine tonsil
Genioglossus
Mandible
Geniohyoid muscle
Mylohyoid muscle
Hyoid bone
Epiglottis
Thyroid cartilage
Vestibular fold
Vocal fold
Arch of cricoid cartilage

Fig. 11.9. Sagittal section of part of head and neck to show the three parts of the pharynx.

nasal cavity. Beneath the epithelium is a thin lamina propria which is fused with the underlying periosteum. The epithelium is, however, thin except at the openings of the sinuses. They are all supplied mainly by the ophthalmic nerve except the maxillary sinus which is supplied by the maxillary nerve. Comparative anatomy suggests that they have temperature regulating and olfactory functions in other animals. These functions have been lost in man but the sinuses have persisted with the result that they are said to make the head lighter and add resonance to the voice. There is no evidence that air enters and leaves the sinuses during respiration.

Clinically they are important because of the ease with which infection can spread to them from the nasal cavity. The commonest to be infected is the maxillary sinus and constitutes the sinusitis or antrum of the layman (the maxillary sinus was called the antrum of Highmore).

Because of the position of the opening and its small size, drainage from the maxillary sinus, in the upright position, is poor. Because many of the superior dental nerves pass along the walls of the maxillary sinus they may be irritated by a sinusitis. The resultant pain may be indistinguishable from toothache. In the past this sometimes led to the extraction of all the cheek teeth. When the pain persisted, it was then realized that the cause of the pain was sinusitis. When extracting teeth, it is not uncommon to fracture a root. During subsequent surgery for the removal of one of the roots of the upper cheek teeth, great care is necessary to avoid pushing a root into the maxillary sinus. In the event of such an accident it is usually necessary to make a hole into the sinus through the alveolar bone behind the canine tooth in order to remove the root.

In edentulous patients the alveolar bone may be resorbed so much that the maxillary sinus lies just below the oral mucosa. It will be appreciated that the maxillary sinus is extremely important to the dental surgeon.

All the sinuses are small or absent at birth. They grow slowly to the age of seven or eight years and then rapidly during the eruption of the second dentition.

Pharynx, auditory tube and palate

PHARYNX

Although this structure is usually regarded as part of the alimentary tract, the nasopharynx behind the nasal cavity is entirely respiratory, the oropharynx behind the mouth is both respiratory and alimentary and only the laryngopharynx is almost entirely alimentary (Fig. 11.9). It is also convenient to describe the pharynx with the respiratory passages.

The pharynx is a muscular tube about 12 cm long extending from the base of the skull to the level of the sixth cervical vertebra. It is wider above (about 4 cm) than below (about 1.5 cm) where it becomes continuous with the oesophagus. Its anterior wall is largely deficient and from above downwards, the pharynx opens into the nasal cavity, the oral cavity and the larynx. Posterior to the pharynx are the prevertebral fascia and muscles in front of the cervical vertebrae. The muscular wall is formed mainly by the three constrictors, superior, middle and inferior (Figs. 11.10 & 11.11). These muscles form the posterior and lateral walls. Three additional muscles pass into the pharyngeal wall from above, the stylopharyngeus, palatopharyngeus and salpingopharyngeus.

The superior constrictor has its main attachment to the posterior edge of the pterygomandibular raphe which extends from the hamulus of the medial pterygoid plate to the posterior end of the mylohyoid line on the inner surface of the mandible. The buccinator muscle is attached to the anterior edge of the raphe and the inner surface of the cheek continues onto the surface of the pharynx. The constrictor extends onto the neighbouring bone at each end of the raphe onto the medial pterygoid plate and the mucous membrane over the mandible adjacent to the mylohyoid line. Some muscle fibres of the tongue extend into the superior constrictor. The highest fibres arch backwards and upwards and are attached to the pharyngeal tubercle on the basilar part of the occipital bone. Since the hamulus is at a lower level than the tubercle there is a space between the upper border of the

muscle and the base of the skull. This is filled by the membranous pharyngobasilar fascia passing, as its name suggests, between the pharynx and the base of the skull (Fig. 11.11). The auditory tube with the levator veli palatini (levator palati) above and medial, and the tensor veli palatini (tensor palati) below and lateral lie in this space. The rest of the fibres of the superior constrictor fan out and enter the fibrous pharyngeal raphe running longitudinally in the middle of the posterior wall of the pharynx. Some of the superior fibres are joined by muscle fibres from the soft palate (palatopharyngeus), and, on contraction of the palate, form a ridge on the posterior wall of the nasopharynx, the ridge of Passavant. This ridge becomes prominent in patients with a cleft palate. It seems that the muscle becomes hypertrophied in attempts to close off the nasopharynx from the oropharynx during swallowing.

The middle constrictor is attached to the greater and lesser horns of the hyoid bone and extends upwards onto the stylohyoid ligament. The muscle fans out as it passes backwards and then medially into the posterior raphe. It is external to the superior but internal to the inferior constrictor. The inferior constrictor is attached to the thyroid and cricoid cartilages. The part of the inferior constrictor attached to the oblique line on the lamina of the thyroid cartilage and to a fibrous arch over the cricothyroid muscle is called the thyropharyngeus, and the part attached to the lateral surface of the arch of the cricoid cartilage is called the cricopharyngeus. Its lowest part is horizontal and is continuous with the circular fibres of the oesophagus and acts like a sphincter. The inferior constrictor passes backwards and is inserted into the posterior raphe.

The stylopharyngeus (Figs. 11.10 & 11.11) is attached to the medial side of the base of the styloid process and passes downwards superficial to the superior constrictor and deep to the middle constrictor, between the two muscles. It is attached to the posterior border of the thyroid cartilage and its fibres mingle with those of the middle constrictor. The salpingopharyngeus is attached to the lower border of the cartilaginous part of the auditory tube, passes downwards on the inner surface of the constrictors and mingles with the fibres of the palatopharyngeus. The palatopharyngeus (Fig. 11.12a) has two layers of muscle in the soft palate. The upper is immediately deep to the mucous membrane of the pharyngeal surface and the lower is deep to the levator veli palatini. Laterally the two layers join

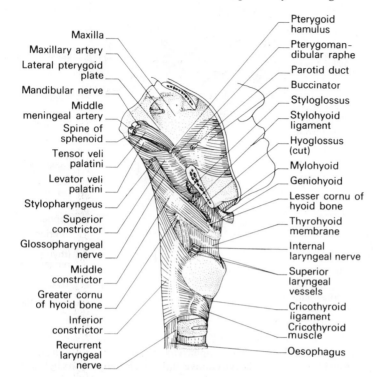

Maxilla
Maxillary artery
Lateral pterygoid plate
Mandibular nerve
Middle meningeal artery
Spine of sphenoid
Tensor veli palatini
Levator veli palatini
Stylopharyngeus
Superior constrictor
Glossopharyngeal nerve
Middle constrictor
Greater cornu of hyoid bone
Inferior constrictor
Recurrent laryngeal nerve

Pterygoid hamulus
Pterygomandibular raphe
Parotid duct
Buccinator
Styloglossus
Stylohyoid ligament
Hyoglossus (cut)
Mylohyoid
Geniohyoid
Lesser cornu of hyoid bone
Thyrohyoid membrane
Internal laryngeal nerve
Superior laryngeal vessels
Cricothyroid ligament
Cricothyroid muscle
Oesophagus

Fig. 11.10. Lateral view of the right constrictor muscles of the pharynx.

and pass downwards in the palatopharyngeal fold behind the palatine tonsil. Within the soft palate the muscle is attached to the palatal aponeurosis and the posterior edge of the hard palate. In the pharyngeal wall the fibres spread out and with the stylopharyngeus form a longitudinally running layer of muscle internal to the constrictors. Some of the fibres of the palatopharyngeus posteriorly join the pharyngeal raphe and anteriorly are attached to the thyroid cartilage.

Posterior to the pharynx are the bodies of the cervical vertebrae covered by some of the prevertebral muscles and fascia. Laterally are the carotid sheath and its contents and the ascending pharyngeal artery as they lie anterior to the transverse processes of the cervical vertebrae. Anteriorly there are the openings already referred to. Several nerves and vessels are related to the constrictors. The glossopharyngeal nerve is lateral to the superior constrictor and runs downwards along the posterior border of the stylopharyngeus before crossing superficial to that muscle and entering the tongue deep to the hyoglossus together with the lingual artery. The internal laryngeal nerve and an accompanying artery lie between the middle and inferior constrictors before entering the larynx through the

thyrohyoid membrane, and the external laryngeal nerve runs downwards on the inferior constrictor and pierces it to supply the cricothyroid muscle. The recurrent laryngeal nerve and a laryngeal artery pass upwards deep to the inferior constrictor on their way to the larynx. The lingual and facial arteries loop upwards on the middle constrictor and the facial artery may reach the lateral surface of the superior constrictor. In this position the artery lies lateral to the palatine tonsil which is medial to the superior constrictor.

The nerve supply of the stylopharyngeus is from the glossopharyngeal nerve. The remaining five muscles are supplied by the pharyngeal plexus which lies on the external surface of the middle constrictor. The pharyngeal branch of the vagus nerve is the motor nerve of the plexus and is derived from the cranial accessory nerve. The cell bodies of the fibres supplying all the muscles are in the nucleus ambiguus of the medulla oblongata. Most of the lining receives its sensory nerve supply from the glossopharyngeal nerve which also partly supplies the tonsillar region and the soft palate. The maxillary nerve supplies the region of the nasopharynx and the recurrent laryngeal nerve the lowest part of the pharynx. The arteries of the

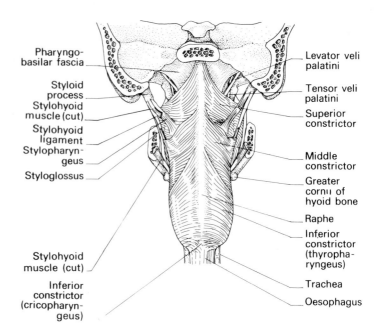

Pharyngo-basilar fascia

Styloid process

Stylohyoid muscle (cut)

Stylohyoid ligament

Stylopharyn-geus

Styloglossus

Stylohyoid muscle (cut)

Inferior constrictor (cricopharyn-geus)

Levator veli palatini

Tensor veli palatini

Superior constrictor

Middle constrictor

Greater cornu of hyoid bone

Raphe

Inferior constrictor (thyropha-ryngeus)

Trachea

Oesophagus

Fig. 11.11. Posterior view of the constrictor muscles of the pharynx.

pharynx come from the ascending pharyngeal, the facial (ascending palatine and tonsillar), the maxillary (pharyngeal, greater palatine) and the lingual. The veins go to the internal jugular and facial veins.

The pharynx is divided into three parts and the lining of each of these has features of considerable importance (Fig. 11.9). The nasopharynx, lying in front of the atlas behind the nasal cavity, is roofed over by the basilar part of the occipital bone and the body of the sphenoid. Below it is continuous with the oropharynx at the level of the soft palate. Anteriorly are the choanae and on the posterior wall there is a mass of lymphoid tissue called the pharyngeal tonsil (adenoid). It is much larger in children than in adults. It may project so far forwards that it obstructs the choanae. Passing backwards in the upper part of the tonsil there is a recess called the pharyngeal bursa. On the lateral wall of the nasopharynx there is the opening of the auditory (Eustachian, pharyngotympanic) tube. This opening is marked by the projection of the medial end of the tube superiorly and posteriorly, and lies about 1 cm behind the inferior meatus of the nasal cavity. A catheter (always called a Eustachian catheter) can be passed along the floor of the nasal cavity and inserted into the tube. There is a recess behind the tube called the pharyngeal recess. The pharyngeal tonsil may extend laterally as far as the posterior wall of the opening of the tube and superiorly onto the roof.

The oropharynx communicates with the nasopharynx above and the laryngopharynx below. It lies in front of the second and third cervical vertebrae and its anterior boundary is formed by the palatoglossal folds (anterior pillar of the fauces). The palatine tonsil, a mass of lymphoid tissue, lies behind this fold and in front of the palatopharyngeal fold (posterior pillar of the fauces) in a recess called the tonsillar sinus. The palatine tonsil, usually called the tonsil, extends upwards into the soft palate, medially into the tongue and forwards into the palatoglossal fold. It is much larger in the child than in the adult. Laterally it is separated from the superior constrictor by a fibrous capsule. Its medial surface has a number of pits, tonsillar crypts, and is covered by a small fold of mucous membrane inferiorly, the plica triangularis. The intratonsillar cleft is a deep recess in the upper medial part of the tonsil.

The tonsillar artery, a branch of the facial artery, enters the lower pole of the tonsil after piercing the superior constrictor. A large vein passes downwards from the soft palate lateral to the tonsil and then pierces the pharyngeal wall. It is at risk when the tonsils are removed. The tonsil receives a sensory nerve supply from the glossopharyngeal nerve and also the maxillary nerve (lesser palatine branch).

The laryngopharynx (Figs. 11.9 & 11.12a) lies in front of the fourth, fifth and sixth cervical vertebrae. Anteriorly it extends from the upper edge of the epiglottis to the lower border of the cricoid cartilage. The opening of the larynx is the most obvious feature in the anterior wall. The arytenoid cartilages articulate with the upper lateral angles of the posterior surface (lamina) of the cricoid cartilage. Between the lateral edge of the epiglottis and arytenoid cartilage is the aryepiglottic fold which on each side bounds the laryngeal opening. Between this fold and the lamina of the thyroid cartilage, lateral to the opening, is the piriform fossa. The internal laryngeal nerve, having pierced the thyrohyoid membrane, passes to the larynx deep to the mucous membrane lining the fossa.

The pharynx is usually described as consisting of three coats, an inner mucous membrane, a middle fibrous coat (submucosa) and an outer muscular layer. The lamina propria of the mucous membrane is covered by stratified squamous epithelium in the oro- and laryngopharynx and by ciliated mucous columnar epithelium in the nasopharynx where there are also mucous glands. The fibrous layer is thickened superiorly where it forms the pharyngobasilar fascia between the upper edge of the superior constrictor and the base of the skull. The auditory tube is superior to the fascia which is also attached to the posterior edge of the medial pterygoid plate and is continuous inferiorly with the pterygomandibular raphe.

Briefly, the functions of the pharynx are respiratory and alimentary. It conducts air from the nasal cavity and mouth to the larynx and food from the mouth to the oesophagus. The walls of the nasopharynx are relatively rigid and its cavity is always patent unlike that of the oro- and laryngopharynx. The auditory tube is opened during swallowing and allows air to enter or leave the middle ear thereby equalizing the pressure on the two sides of the tympanic membrane between the external and middle ear. The salpingo- and palatopharyngeus muscles are probably responsible for this. The stylo- and palatopharyngeus muscles due to their attachment to the thyroid cartilage lift up the larynx in swallowing. The constrictors by a descending wave of contraction propel the food downwards. The details of the act of swallowing are considered on p. 578.

AUDITORY (PHARYNGOTYMPANIC) TUBE (Figs. 11.9 & 11.12a & b)

This is a communication between the nasopharynx and the cavity of the middle ear. In the adult it is about 3.5 cm long and is directed laterally, upwards (about 30° from the horizontal) and backwards (about midway between the coronal and sagittal planes) from the nasopharynx. Its lateral third is a bony canal in the petrous part of the temporal bone. The medial two-thirds are cartilaginous and lie between the petrous temporal and greater wing of the sphenoid. The cartilage is an inverted J-shaped plate, folded over so that there is a gap inferiorly and laterally filled by fibrous tissue (Fig. 11.12b). Its lateral end is attached to the ragged medial end of the bony part. The prrojecting medial end in the nasopharynx has already been described (p. 484), and is the widest part of the tube which is narrowest at the junction of the bony and cartilaginous parts. The tube is lined by ciliated mucous columnar epithelium continuous with that of the nasopharynx and middle ear.

If one looks at the position of the tube in the skull, the foramen spinosum and foramen ovale are seen to be anterior to the tube with the foramen ovale medial to the spinosum. The middle meningeal artery and the mandibular nerve are therefore anterior to the tube. The tensor veli palatini is attached to the anterolateral surface of the tube and intervenes between the tube and the mandibular nerve. The levator veli palatini is attached to its posteromedial surface.

In babies and young children the tube is more horizontal and the bony part wider than in the adult. It is thought that upper respiratory infections in early life spread more readily to the middle ear because of these differences.

As already stated, the function of the tube is to equalize the pressure on the two sides of the tympanic membrane. If the tube is blocked for a long time, the air in the middle ear is absorbed, the auditory ossicles are dislocated and one form of conduction deafness results.

PALATE

This structure forms the floor of the nasal cavity (p. 476) and the roof of the mouth. Its nasal surface is covered by ciliated mucous columnar epithelium and its oral surface by stratified squamous epithelium. The palate is divided into an anterior hard palate and posterior soft palate.

The hard palate (Fig. 11.9) is formed anteriorly by the palatal processes of the maxillae (three-quarters) and posteriorly by the horizontal plates of the palatine bones. It is bounded laterally and anteriorly by the alveolar processes of the maxillae covered by the gingivae, and the soft palate is attached to its posterior edge. The

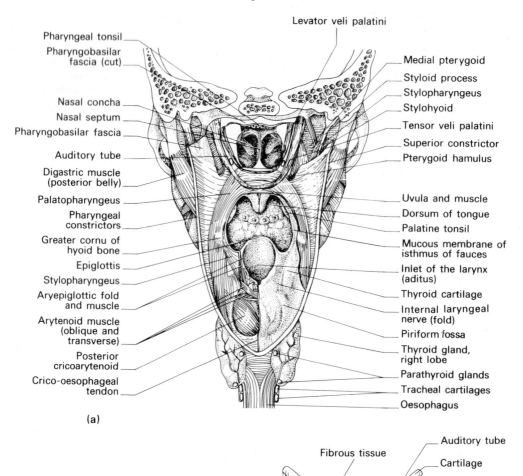

Pharyngeal tonsil
Pharyngobasilar fascia (cut)
Nasal concha
Nasal septum
Pharyngobasilar fascia
Auditory tube
Digastric muscle (posterior belly)
Palatopharyngeus
Pharyngeal constrictors
Greater cornu of hyoid bone
Epiglottis
Stylopharyngeus
Aryepiglottic fold and muscle
Arytenoid muscle (oblique and transverse)
Posterior cricoarytenoid
Crico-oesophageal tendon

Levator veli palatini
Medial pterygoid
Styloid process
Stylopharyngeus
Stylohyoid
Tensor veli palatini
Superior constrictor
Pterygoid hamulus
Uvula and muscle
Dorsum of tongue
Palatine tonsil
Mucous membrane of isthmus of fauces
Inlet of the larynx (aditus)
Thyroid cartilage
Internal laryngeal nerve (fold)
Piriform fossa
Thyroid gland, right lobe
Parathyroid glands
Tracheal cartilages
Oesophagus

(a)

Fibrous tissue
Auditory tube
Cartilage
Tensor veli palatini
Hamulus
Palatine aponeurosis

(b)

Fig. 11.12. The muscles of the soft palate and pharynx. (a) The pharyngeal raphe is divided vertically; (b) the tensor veli palatine.

mucous membrane on both its surfaces is firmly bound down to the underlying periosteum. The oral mucous membrane is separated from the periosteum by a thick submucosa which contains mucous glands posteriorly and fat anteriorly. The lamina propria of the mucous membrane is firmly bound down to the periosteum by Sharpey fibres and the holes occupied by these fibres can be seen in the dried maxilla. In the midline the submucosa is very thin and the lamina propria is united to the suture separating the two halves of the palate at the palatine raphe. The softer region which can be palpated in the angle between the alveolar process and the middle of the palate contains the greater palatine artery and nerves. Injections made into this region (for the purpose of extracting a tooth) are less painful than injections into the rest of the palate because the soft tissue can swell to accommodate the volume of fluid injected.

The anterior part of the oral surface is transversely ridged (rugae) and there is a small midline papilla overlying the incisive fossa. A midline bony swelling, the torus palatinus, is occasionally seen. Just anterior to the junction between hard and soft palate there are frequently

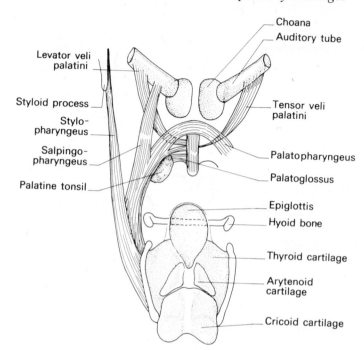

Fig. 11.13. Diagrammatic representation of the muscles of the soft palate as seen from behind.

two small hollows, the palatine foveae, one on each side of the midline. They are probably the openings of the ducts of large mucous glands.

The soft palate (Figs. 11.12 & 11.13) consists of a number of muscles attached to an aponeurosis covered by a mucous membrane on both its surfaces. It is attached to the posterior edge of the hard palate and hangs down between the mouth and oropharynx so that its surfaces can be described as anterior (inferior or oral) and posterior (superior or pharyngeal). The uvula is a conical projection of varying length, 5–15mm long, hanging downwards in the midline from the posterior free edge. This edge, if followed laterally, divides into an anterior palatoglossal arch containing the palatoglossus muscle and a posterior palatopharyngeal arch containing the palatopharyngeus muscle.

The palatine aponeurosis is attached to the posterior edge of the hard palate and is the expanded tendon of the tensor veli palatini to which the other muscles are attached. The anterior part of the aponeurosis is much thicker than its posterior part and has few muscle fibres attached to it.

Two muscles enter the soft palate from above (Figs. 11.10 & 11.12a). The tensor veli palatini is attached to the scaphoid fossa of the pterygoid

process of the sphenoid bone and the lateral surface of the cartilaginous part of the auditory tube. It is outside the pharynx and its tendon winds round the hamulus of the medial pterygoid plate, passes between the hamulus and the buccinator muscle and is attached to the palatine aponeurosis. The levator veli palatini is attached to the inferior surface of the petrous temporal anteromedial to the carotid canal and from the medial surface of the auditory tube. It is inside the pharynx, enters the soft palate between the two layers of the palatopharyngeus and becomes attached to the upper surface of the aponeurosis.

Two muscles leave the soft palate and pass downwards. The palatoglossus is attached to the inferior surface of the aponeurosis and passes laterally and downwards into the palatoglossal fold in front of the tonsil. The muscle enters the upper lateral part of the tongue. The palatopharyngeus has been described on p. 482.

The musculus uvulae consists of two slips attached anteriorly to the posterior nasal spine. The fibres pass backwards on either side of the midline within the aponeurosis and end at the mucous membrane of the uvula.

The tensor veli palatini is innervated by the mandibular nerve. The remaining muscles are

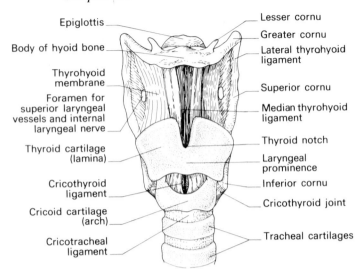

Epiglottis — Lesser cornu

Body of hyoid bone — Greater cornu

— Lateral thyrohyoid ligament

Thyrohyoid membrane — Superior cornu

Foramen for superior laryngeal vessels and internal laryngeal nerve — Median thyrohyoid ligament

Thyroid cartilage (lamina) — Thyroid notch

— Laryngeal prominence

Cricothyroid ligament — Inferior cornu

Cricoid cartilage (arch) — Cricothyroid joint

Cricotracheal ligament — Tracheal cartilages

Fig. 11.14. The 'skeleton' of the larynx, anterior view.

supplied by the pharyngeal plexus, the motor branch of which is the pharyngeal branch of the vagus. The cells of origin of the latter nerve fibres are in the nucleus ambiguus in the medulla oblongata and the fibres leave the medulla in the cranial accessory nerve which joins the vagus nerve. The sensory innervation of both surfaces of the whole palate is almost entirely from the maxillary nerve (greater and lesser palatine and nasopalatine). A small part of the soft palate receives sensory fibres from the glosso-pharyngeal nerve. Some taste fibres from the oral surface of the soft palate are branches of the facial nerve and reach the palate via the greater

petrosal nerve, pterygopalatine ganglion and lesser palatine nerve.

Branches of the facial (ascending palatine), maxillary (greater palatine and sphenopalatine), and ascending pharyngeal (palatine) arteries supply the palate. Venous drainage is mainly to the pterygoid plexus.

The soft palate, together with the ridge produced by part of the superior constrictor and the palatopharyngeus closes off the nasopharynx from the oropharynx during swallowing and phonation except in the production of nasal consonants. The actions of the soft palate are described with swallowing (p. 578).

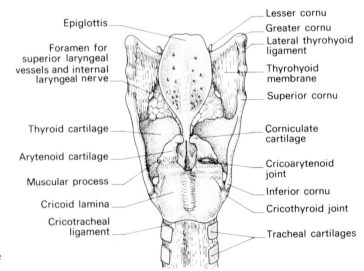

Epiglottis — Lesser cornu

— Greater cornu

— Lateral thyrohyoid ligament

Foramen for superior laryngeal vessels and internal laryngeal nerve — Thyrohyoid membrane

— Superior cornu

Thyroid cartilage — Corniculate cartilage

Arytenoid cartilage — Cricoarytenoid joint

Muscular process — Inferior cornu

Cricoid lamina — Cricothyroid joint

Cricotracheal ligament — Tracheal cartilages

Fig. 11.15. The 'skeleton' of the larynx, posterior view.

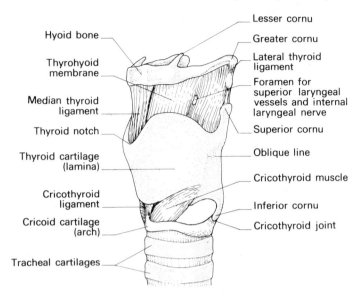

Hyoid bone

Thyrohyoid membrane

Median thyroid ligament

Thyroid notch

Thyroid cartilage (lamina)

Cricothyroid ligament

Cricoid cartilage (arch)

Tracheal cartilages

Lesser cornu

Greater cornu

Lateral thyroid ligament

Foramen for superior laryngeal vessels and internal laryngeal nerve

Superior cornu

Oblique line

Cricothyroid muscle

Inferior cornu

Cricothyroid joint

Fig. 11.16. The 'skeleton' of the larynx, left anterolateral view.

Larynx

The larynx is that part of the air passages between the oropharynx and the trachea and lies in the middle of the anterior part of the neck opposite the fourth, fifth and sixth cervical vertebrae. It is smaller in the female in all its dimensions; this difference becomes marked at puberty.

SKELETON OF LARYNX

This consists of a number of cartilages connected by membranes (Fig. 11.14, 11.15 & 11.16). The largest of the cartilages is the thyroid (thyreos means a shield) which consists of two quadrilateral laminae joined anteriorly at an angle to form a forward projection called the laryngeal prominence (Adam's apple). This is much more marked in men than in women. The two laminae meet at an angle of about 90° in men and an angle of about 120° in women. Immediately above the prominence there is the thyroid notch. The posterior borders of the laminae project upwards and downwards as the superior and inferior cornua. On the external surface of the lamina the oblique line runs downwards and forwards from the superior cornu towards the lower border (Fig. 11.16).

The cricoid cartilage is shaped like a ring with an anterior arch and a posterior lamina. The lower border of the arch and lamina is horizontal: the upper border of the arch when followed

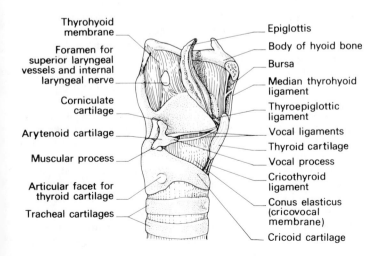

Thyrohyoid membrane

Foramen for superior laryngeal vessels and internal laryngeal nerve

Corniculate cartilage

Arytenoid cartilage

Muscular process

Articular facet for thyroid cartilage

Tracheal cartilages

Epiglottis

Body of hyoid bone

Bursa

Median thyrohyoid ligament

Thyroepiglottic ligament

Vocal ligaments

Thyroid cartilage

Vocal process

Cricothyroid ligament

Conus elasticus (cricovocal membrane)

Cricoid cartilage

Fig. 11.17. The skeleton of the larynx from the right side. The right lamina of the thyroid cartilage has been removed to show right conus elasticus (cricovocal membrane) and arytenoid cartilage.

backwards rises considerably and becomes continuous with the upper border of the lamina. Where the arch becomes the lamina there is a small facet on the middle of the surface for articulation with the inferior cornu of the thyroid cartilage at the synovial cricothyroid joint (Fig. 11.17).

There are two arytenoid cartilages each of which has four triangular surfaces. The anterolateral surface is markedly concave. The base articulates with the cricoid cartilage at the crico-arytenoid joint. The apex curves backwards and medially and on it is the corniculate cartilage which elongates the apex. The inferior border of the medial surface is prolonged forwards as the vocal process. The posterior surface of the arytenoid cartilage is flat and its inferior border is prolonged laterally as the muscular process. The remaining surface faces anterolaterally.

The epiglottis consists largely of elastic cartilage shaped like a leaf, with its narrow end below where it is attached to the posterior upper part of the angle between the laminae of the thyroid cartilage just below the thyroid notch (Fig. 11.15). The broad upper part of the epiglottis lies behind the tongue and the hyoid bone to the upper border of which it is attached by the hyo-epiglottic ligament. The lateral borders of the epiglottis are continuous through the aryepiglottic folds with the arytenoid cartilages. The cuneiform cartilage lies in the aryepiglottic fold anterior to the corniculate cartilage. The posterior surface of the epiglottis has a projection in its lower part called the tubercle, and a number of pits which contain mucous glands.

The thyroid cartilage is attached to the hyoid bone by the thyrohyoid membrane. This passes upwards to be attached behind the upper border of the arch of the cricoid cartilage and the bone. There is a bursa between the membrane and the body. Inferiorly the membrane is attached to the upper border of the laminae and the anterior surface of the superior cornua of the thyroid cartilage.

The cricothyroid ligament (Fig. 11.14) has a median thickened part between the upper border of the arch of the cricoid cartilage and the lower border of the laminae of the thyroid cartilage. More laterally it is attached to the upper border of the cricoid arch and passes upwards deep to the lamina of the thyroid cartilage (Fig. 11.17). This part is called the conus elasticus or cricovocal membrane: it has a free upper edge attached posteriorly to the vocal process of the arytenoid cartilage and anteriorly to the deep

aspect of the laryngeal prominence. This edge, which is called the vocal ligament, forms the skeleton of the vocal fold. The conus elasticus is the lower part of the fibroelastic membrane of the larynx, the upper part of which is called the quadrangular membrane. This extends from the vestibular fold to the aryepiglottic fold.

The epiglottis is attached to the thyroid cartilage by the thyroepiglottic ligament. Inferior to the free part of the epiglottis its anterior surface is connected to the back of the tongue by a median glosso-epiglottic fold and two lateral glosso-epiglottic folds, one on each side. The space on either side of the median fold is called the vallecula.

The epiglottis, the corniculate and cuneiform and the apices of the arytenoid cartilages consist of elastic cartilage and the thyro-epiglottic, hyo-epiglottic and the cricothyroid ligaments (conus elasticus) consist largely of elastic fibres. The elastic cartilages do not ossify, but the others (the thyroid, cricoid and most of the arytenoid cartilages) begin to ossify as early as 30 years and by 60 years some ossification is usually present in all of them.

MUSCLES OF LARYNX

These are often divided into extrinsic and intrinsic. The former include all the infrahyoid, some of the suprahyoid muscles (p. 438) and some of the pharyngeal muscles (for example, the stylopharyngeus).

The following are the intrinsic muscles. The cricothyroid (Fig. 11.16) is attached to the lateral surface of the arch of the cricoid cartilage. The upper fibres pass backwards to the lower border of the thyroid lamina and the lower fibres to the inferior cornu. The inferior constrictor is attached to a fibrous arch passing over the muscle and the conus elasticus is medial to it. The muscle is supplied by the external laryngeal nerve, a branch of the superior laryngeal. When the cricothyroid muscles contract the lower part of the thyroid cartilage rotates about the cricothyroid joints and moves downwards and forwards, or alternatively the upper part of cricoid cartilage moves upwards and backwards. In either case the vocal folds are tensed. They may also be lengthened.

The arytenoideus muscle, unpaired, passes between the posterior surfaces of the arytenoid cartilages, and is attached as far laterally as the muscular processes. The deep fibres are transverse and the more superficial are oblique. The latter cross in the midline passing from one mus-

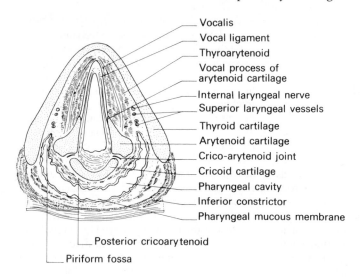

Vocalis
Vocal ligament
Thyroarytenoid
Vocal process of arytenoid cartilage
Internal laryngeal nerve
Superior laryngeal vessels
Thyroid cartilage
Arytenoid cartilage
Crico-arytenoid joint
Cricoid cartilage
Pharyngeal cavity
Inferior constrictor
Pharyngeal mucous membrane
Posterior cricoarytenoid
Piriform fossa

Fig. 11.18. A horizontal section of the larynx and pharynx through the middle of the thyroid cartilage seen from above.

cular process upwards towards the opposite apex and some of them continue into the aryepiglottic fold forming the aryepiglottic muscle. The muscle is supplied by the recurrent laryngeal nerve. When it contracts it pulls the two arytenoid cartilages together at the crico-arytenoid joints and thus approximates (adducts) the vocal folds. The part in the aryepiglottic folds pulls the folds together and closes the entrance to the larynx.

The posterior crico-arytenoid muscle is attached to the posterior surface of the lamina of the cricoid cartilage and passes upwards and laterally to the muscular vocal process. The lowest fibres are almost vertical. The muscle is supplied by the recurrent laryngeal nerve. Its action is to abduct the vocal fold by rotating the arytenoid cartilage at the crico-arytenoid joint: the vertical fibres also pull the arytenoid cartilage backwards thereby tensing the vocal fold.

The lateral crico-arytenoid muscle is attached to the upper border of the cricoid arch and passes upwards and backwards to the muscular process of the arytenoid cartilage. It is supplied by the recurrent laryngeal nerve. The muscle adducts the vocal fold by rotating the arytenoid cartilage at the crico-arytenoid joint. This muscle together with the other adductors of the vocal folds has a very important role in increasing intra-abdominal pressure for example during defaecation or childbirth. The lungs are expanded and the intrathoracic pressure is raised while attempting to exhale with the vocal folds adducted to prevent the air escaping. The raised intrathoracic pressure acts against the diaphragm.

The thyro-arytenoid muscle is attached to the inner aspect of the lamina of the thyroid cartilage near the midline and passes backwards to become attached to the anterolateral surface of the arytenoid cartilage. The most medial fibres lying lateral to the vocal ligament constitute the vocalis muscle and are attached to the ligament. The superior fibres extend into the aryepiglottic fold and form the thyro-epiglottic muscle. The muscle is supplied by the recurrent laryngeal nerve. The thyro-arytenoid muscles rotate the arytenoid cartilages at the crico-arytenoid joints so that the vocal folds are adducted. They also pull the arytenoid cartilages forwards and thus relax the vocal folds. The vocalis is said to alter the functioning length of the vocal folds since its fibres are attached to the posterior half of the vocal ligament. When they contract they cause relaxation of the posterior half and the anterior half of the fold remains tense. The thyro-epiglottic muscle may pull the aryepiglottic folds laterally and enlarge the laryngeal opening.

INTERIOR OF LARYNX

This is divided into three parts by two pairs of folds lying approximately anteroposteriorly and projecting into the cavity of the larynx. The upper are called the vestibular folds (false vocal cords) and the lower the vocal folds (true vocal cords). The part of the larynx above the vestibular folds is called the vestibule. Its upper limit is the opening of the larynx which communicates with the laryngopharynx. It is bounded anteriorly by the upper edge of the epiglottis, laterally by the aryepiglottic folds containing the aryepiglottic muscle and the cuneiform cartilages, and posteriorly by the arytenoid cartilages with the corniculate cartilages and the mucous membrane between them. The anterior wall of the vestibule is much longer than the posterior wall because of the upward projection of the epiglottis. The tubercle or lower part of this cartilage projects into the cavity of the vestibule. The lower limit of the vestibule is defined by the vestibular folds and leads into the second part of the larynx through the space between the folds (rima vestibuli). Each fold consists of fibrous tissue, the vestibular ligament, covered by mucous membrane and is attached anteriorly to the inner aspect of the lamina of the thyroid cartilage near the midline just above the attachment of the vocal fold, and posteriorly to the anterolateral surface of the arytenoid cartilage.

The middle part of the larynx is limited above by the vestibular folds and below by the vocal folds. Since these project into the cavity of the larynx there is a lateral space between them. This is called the sinus of the larynx. Anteriorly the sinus leads upwards into a small cavity called the saccule which is lateral to the vestibular folds. The thyro-arytenoid muscle is lateral to the sinus and saccule. There are also some muscle fibres medial to the saccule between it and the vestibular fold. These fibres may be responsible for closing the vestibular folds in swallowing and even in speech in certain situations. The saccule contains a large number of mucous glands and the muscle fibres on either side can press on the saccule and force the secretion on to the vocal folds which have no glands or goblet cells. The extent of the saccule varies in different animals; in many apes it extends up into the neck and even into the axilla.

The vocal folds are attached anteriorly to the inner surface of the lamina of the thyroid cartilage near the midline and posteriorly to the vocal process of the arytenoid cartilage. The space between them is called the rima glottidis (Fig. 11.18) which is described as extending backwards between the arytenoid cartilages thus forming an anterior intermembranous part and a posterior intercartilaginous part. The vocal fold is strikingly pearly white in the living because the stratified squamous epithelium which covers the fold is tightly bound to the underlying tissue which is avascular. Within the vocal fold is the vocal ligament which is the upper edge of the conus elasticus, and the vocalis muscle which is lateral to the ligament.

The vocal folds can be adducted (moved towards the midline) and abducted (moved away from the midline). They can also be made more or less tense, and to a very limited extent, lengthened or shortened. Their functioning length, however, can change considerably, as can their thickness. There is some vocal cord movement during respiration and swallowing and changes in tension, length and thickness as well as movements occur in speech.

The part of the larynx below the vocal folds has no special features. The inner surfaces of the conus elasticus and cricoid cartilage, covered by mucous membrane, form its walls. Its cavity is continuous inferiorly with that of the trachea.

Most of the larynx is covered by ciliated mucous columnar epithelium. Stratified squamous epithelium is found over the vocal folds, along the upper edge of the aryepiglottic folds and the anterior surface of the epiglottis. Reference has already been made to the mucous glands in the pits of the epiglottis and in the saccule. They are also found in the aryepiglottic folds near the arytenoid cartilages. There are some taste buds on the posterior surface of the epiglottis. Their nerve supply is from the vagus nerve. There is a considerable amount of subepithelial loose connective tissue in the aryepiglottic folds and vestibule of the larynx. Swelling due to effusion of fluid into this tissue can cause obstruction to breathing, largely because the fluid cannot drain beyond the vocal folds in which the subepithelial tissue is tightly bound to the vocal ligament.

ARTERIES AND NERVES OF LARYNX

The arteries come from the thyroid arteries, the superior laryngeal from the superior thyroid and the inferior laryngeal from the inferior thyroid. The nerve supply of the muscles is from the recurrent laryngeal nerve, except that of the cricothyroid which is supplied by the external laryngeal nerve. It is important to note that the external laryngeal nerve runs with the superior thyroid artery and the recurrent laryngeal nerve with the inferior thyroid artery. The sensory nerve supply of the lining of the larynx above the vocal folds comes from the internal laryngeal nerve which enters the larynx with the superior laryngeal artery through the thyrohyoid membrane. When this nerve is stimulated it initiates the cough reflex, one of whose functions is to prevent a foreign body passing down the larynx. Below the vocal fold the sensory innervation comes from the recurrent laryngeal nerve which reaches the larynx by passing deep to the inferior

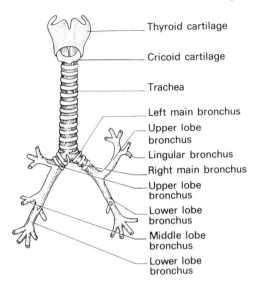

Fig. 11.19. The trachea, main bronchi and segmental bronchi.

constrictor together with the inferior laryngeal artery.

Trachea and main bronchi

The trachea (Fig. 11.19) extends from the cricoid cartilage (at the level of the sixth cervical vertebra) into the thorax where it divides slightly to the right of the midline into the right and left main bronchi (at the level of the fourth or fifth thoracic vertebra). It is about 10 cm long and about 2 cm in diameter. It is flattened posteriorly so that its lumen is D-shaped.

The trachea is superficial in the neck as compared with its position in the thorax. This is largely due to the thorax projecting anteriorly relative to the vertebral column and to the backward curve of the thoracic vertebrae. In the neck the trachea is covered by skin and fascia in which are the anterior jugular veins which anastomose in front of the trachea. The isthmus of the thyroid gland lies in front of the second, third and fourth tracheal rings, and the lobes of the gland lie laterally extending downwards to about the level of the sixth tracheal ring. On each side the common carotid artery is lateral to the trachea deep to the thyroid lobe. The oesophagus is posterior to the trachea and the recurrent laryngeal nerve lies in the groove between them. The inferior thyroid arteries are lateral to the trachea and constitute its main source of blood. In the thorax the trachea and oesophagus are in the space called the mediastinum which divides the thoracic cavity into right and left sides. The relationships of important structures in the mediastinum at the level of the third and fourth thoracic vertebrae are shown in Figs. 11.20 and 11.21 respectively.

The trachea consists of an inner mucous membrane and a fibrous tissue outer wall in which are the tracheal cartilages (Fig. 11.22). These number about fifteen to twenty and are C-shaped with the deficiency posteriorly where transverse smooth muscle fills the gap. The smooth muscle has a sympathetic and parasympathetic (vagus) nerve supply. The intervals between the cartilages are about 1 mm and the cartilages about 4 mm in height. The first cartilage is attached to the cricoid cartilage by the cricotracheal ligament. The cartilage at the bifurcation has a backward directed hook-shaped process which lies between the two main bronchi and produces a projection called the carina, a conspicuous ridge in bronchoscopy.

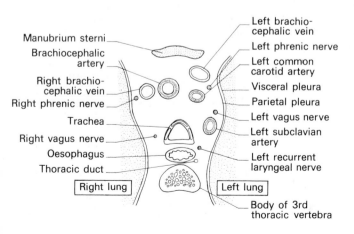

Fig. 11.20. Transverse section through the thorax at the level of the third thoracic vertebra. This is the upper surface of the section as seen from below.

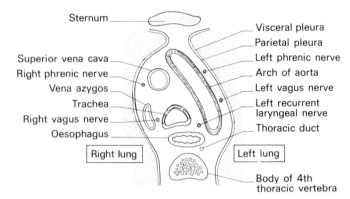

Fig. 11.21. Similar to Figure 11.20; the section is at the level of the fourth thoracic vertebra.

The mucous membrane is covered by pseudostratified ciliated mucous columnar epithelium. The cilia beat upwards towards the larynx. Besides the ciliated and mucous cells other types have been described. Some of these have microvilli and are called brush cells. These are of two kinds. One is probably a sensory receptor cell (brush) and the other an immature cell which will replace brush cells which have been shed from the surface of the epithelium. Another type of cell is thought to be effector in function and is concerned with the integration of secretory processes since it contains neuro-secreting granules (small granule cell). Finally a very immature cell (basal or short) has also been described. In the submucous tissue there are numerous lymphocytes and also longitudinal elastic fibres. The sensory nerve supply of the lining comes directly from the trunk of the vagus and from its recurrent laryngeal branches.

The cartilages have the very important function of ensuring that the lumen remains patent. Their posterior deficiency allows the oesophagus to expand when food passes down its lumen. The elastic fibres allow the trachea to elongate and return to its original length and the transverse smooth muscle can within narrow limits alter the size of the lumen although it is difficult to visualize the advantage of narrowing the trachea. The parasympathetic nerves cause the muscle to contract and the sympathetic cause it to relax. The epithelium continues the process

of cleansing the air on its way to the lungs.

The right main bronchus (Fig. 11.19) is about 2.5 cm long and passes to the right from the division of the trachea to the hilum of the right lung. It is more vertical, wider and shorter than the left main bronchus, which is 5 cm long. The pulmonary artery lies in front of it and the vena azygos arches forwards above it. The bronchus and the pulmonary artery and veins form the root of the lung. The veins are, on the whole, inferior to the bronchus and artery. The vagus nerve passes posterior and the phrenic nerve anterior to these structures, and there are anterior and posterior plexuses of autonomic nerves related to the root of the lung, together with a number of lymph nodes.

The left main bronchus (Fig. 11.19) passes to the left lung and forms part of its root. It is anterior to the oesophagus and thoracic aorta. The root of the left lung has similar relations to that of the right—autonomic nerve plexuses, lymph nodes, vagus and phrenic nerves.

The structure of the main bronchi resembles that of the trachea. The cartilage, however, is not in the form of C-shaped pieces but varies considerably in its shape. It is never circular but is often spiral in its arrangement.

The arterial blood supply of the trachea comes from the bronchial arteries, branches of the thoracic aorta or posterior intercostal arteries at the level of the fifth and sixth thoracic vertebrae. The sensory nerve supply is from the vagus. The

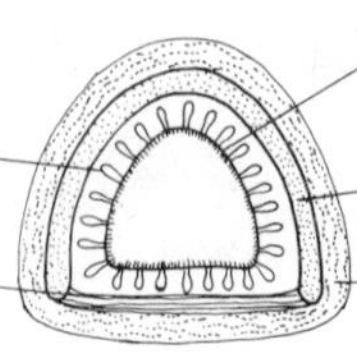

Fig. 11.22. Diagram of the structure of the trachea.

smooth muscle is supplied by sympathetic nerves (bronchodilator) and parasympathetic nerves (bronchoconstrictor). The functions of the main bronchi are similar to those of the trachea. Due to the right main bronchus being more vertical than the left, foreign bodies are more likely to enter the right than the left bronchus.

Pleurae

There are two pleural sacs, one for each lung. Each sac is a double layer of serous membrane, one covering the lung (pulmonary or visceral) and the other lining the thoracic cavity (parietal). The two layers join at the hilum of the lung. The pulmonary pleura extends into the fissures of the lungs and is firmly adherent to the underlying lung tissue.

The costal pleura is that part of the parietal pleura which lines the ribs, sternum and vertebrae from which it is separated by the endothoracic fascia. The diaphragmatic pleura covers the upper surface of the diaphragm and the mediastinal pleura is on the lateral wall of the mediastinum (p. 436). The part of the parietal pleura covering the apex of the lung, which extends into the neck above the first costal cartilage and the anterior part of the first rib, is called the dome of the pleura or cervical pleura. Posteriorly the cervical pleura reaches the neck of the first rib. It is covered by the suprapleural membrane, a fairly dense layer of connective tissue attached superiorly to the transverse process of the seventh cervical vertebra and inferiorly to the medial border of the first rib.

The costal pleura is continuous with the diaphragmatic pleura along the outer margin of the diaphragm and this marks the lowest limit of the parietal pleura. The corresponding border of the lung (between its costal and diaphragmatic surfaces), does not extend as far downwards as the parietal pleura. This leaves a potential space between the costal and diaphragmatic parietal pleura, the costodiaphragmatic recess. The lung in quiet respiration does not fill this recess and is about 4 cm above it. In deep inspiration the lower border of the lung moves down much more and enters the recess. There is a similar recess between the costal and mediastinal parietal pleurae anteriorly behind the costal cartilages and sternum. This is the costomediastinal recess.

The pleura consists of a loose connective tissue whose collagen fibres give it strength. There is a single layer of flattened cells called a mesothelium on the contiguous surfaces of the pulmonary and parietal pleurae. The loose connective tissue of the pleura contains blood, lymphatic vessels and nerves.

Normally during respiration the adjacent surfaces of the pleura, including those in the lung fissures, slide smoothly on each other but due to their being slightly moist they do not separate.

Lungs

The two lungs are the organs within which gaseous exchange takes place between the air-containing respiratory passages and the blood. The lungs occupy most of the space in the thoracic cavity and are separated by the structures in the mediastinum, mainly the heart and large blood vessels. Each lung lies within its own pleural sac within which it can expand and contract. Its only attachments are the reflexion of the pleura on its medial surface and the structures which enter and leave the hilum forming the root of the lung.

The mottled surface is seen to be due to the surface delineation of small polyhedral areas by lines which are made obvious by the deposition of fine particles of carbon which have been inhaled and deposited in the areolar tissue near the surface of the lung. In a newly born child this mottling is not seen and the lung is pink. In people who have lived in industrial areas the mottling is much more marked than in those who have lived in the country.

Each lung is cone-shaped with its apex superior. Inferiorly the surface in contact with the diaphragm is called the base and is hollowed out. The convex surface in contact with the ribs and costal cartilages is called the costal surface. The medial surface is mainly flat and is related anteriorly to the mediastinum and posteriorly to the vertebral column. The edges between the base and costal surface, between the base and medial surface and anteriorly between the costal and medial surfaces, are sharp. This is in contrast with the rounded edge posteriorly between the costal and medial surface where a large mass of the lung lies in a deep hollow formed by the sides of the vertebrae and the posterior ends of the ribs.

The apex projects into the neck due to the obliquity of the inlet of the thorax (Fig. 11.23). It is covered by the dome of the pleura which fits closely over it and which is related to the important structures shown in Fig. 11.24.

The diaphragm separates the base of the right lung from the right lobe of the liver and the base of the left lung from the left lobe of the liver, the

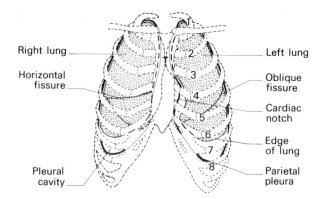

Right lung

Horizontal
fissure

Pleural
cavity

Left lung

Oblique
fissure

Cardiac
notch

Edge
of lung

Parietal
pleura

Fig. 11.23. Surface projection of
the lungs and pleurae as seen
from the front.

fundus of the stomach, the spleen and the left
kidney. The main features of the mediastinal
surfaces of the right and left lungs are shown in
Figs. 11.25 and 11.26.

The hilum of the lung has already been
described. It is a term used to indicate the site of
entry and exit of vessels (and other structures)
into and out of the lung. Broadly speaking the
arrangement of the largest structures is the same

for both lungs—the main bronchus is posterior,
the pulmonary artery is anterior to the bronchus
and one pulmonary vein is in front of the artery
and the other inferior to the bronchus and artery
(Figs. 11.25 & 11.26).

One further feature the two lungs have in
common; each lung is divided by an oblique
fissure (Fig. 11.23). This begins at the upper,
posterior part of the hilum and passes upwards

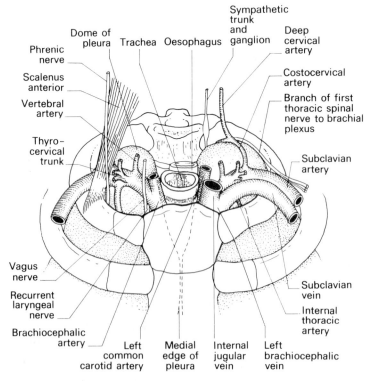

Phrenic
nerve

Scalenus
anterior

Vertebral
artery

Thyro-
cervical
trunk

Dome of
pleura   Trachea Oesophagus

Sympathetic
trunk
and
ganglion

Deep
cervical
artery

Costocervical
artery

Branch of first
thoracic spinal
nerve to brachial
plexus

Subclavian
artery

Vagus
nerve

Recurrent
laryngeal
nerve

Brachiocephalic
artery   Left
          common
        carotid artery

Medial
edge of
pleura

Internal
jugular
vein

Left
brachiocephalic
vein

Subclavian
vein

Internal
thoracic
artery

Fig. 11.24. Drawing of the structures at the inlet of the
thorax (the thoracic duct which is on the left side has
been omitted).

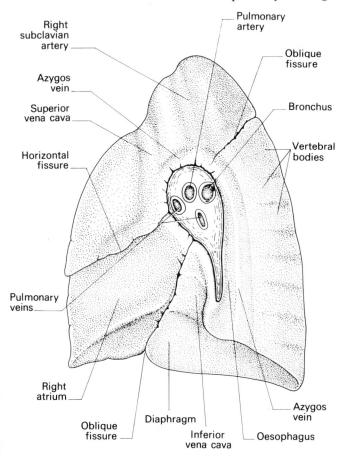

Right
subclavian
artery

Azygos
vein

Superior
vena cava

Horizontal
fissure

Pulmonary
veins

Right
atrium

Oblique
fissure

Diaphragm

Inferior
vena cava

Pulmonary
artery

Oblique
fissure

Bronchus

Vertebral
bodies

Azygos
vein

Oesophagus

Fig. 11.25. Medial surface of the
right lung.

and backwards to the posterior border at a point about 6 cm below the apex. It then extends round the costal surface downwards and forwards to the lower border near its anterior junction with the medial surface and finally passes upwards and backwards on the medial surface to the lower border of the hilum. The left lung consists of two lobes divided by the oblique fissure. The upper (superior) lobe includes the apex and parts of the costal and medial surfaces; the lower (inferior) lobe includes the remainder of the costal and medial surfaces, most of the base and a large part of the rounded posterior border which lies at the side of the vertebrae.

In the right lung there is, in addition to the oblique fissure, a horizontal fissure which passes forwards from the anterior edge of the hilum to the anterior border and across the costal surface to meet the oblique fissure in the midaxillary line. The superior lobe is thus divided into a middle lobe and an upper lobe. The middle lobe is wedge-shaped.

There is another difference between the right and left lungs. The anterior border of the left lung deviates to the left for about 4 cm at what corresponds with the fourth left costal cartilage, and then turns downwards to the lower border which it meets at the level of the sixth costal cartilage. This is called the cardiac notch. The pleura does not deviate to the left to the same extent so that the heart and its pericardium at this site are covered by only two layers of pleura.

STRUCTURE OF THE LUNG

The lung is divided into lobes and each lobe into segments called the bronchopulmonary segments which may be defined as subdivisions of a lobe each supplied by a segmental bronchus and all its branches. The segments can be regarded as independently functioning units. Each has an almost independent blood supply from a branch of the pulmonary artery but the pulmonary veins

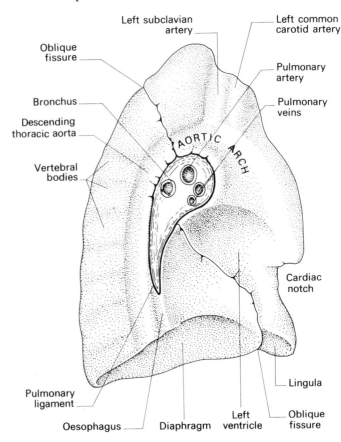

Fig. 11.26. Medial surface of the left lung.

of adjacent segments are not so markedly separate nor are the lymphatics which form connections between segments. After their bifurcation from the trachea each main (primary) bronchus is thus divided into lobar (secondary) bronchi and each lobar bronchus is divided into segmental (tertiary) bronchi.

A segmental bronchus divides and subdivides within its own segment becoming smaller in diameter with each subdivision. The histological structure of the segmental bronchus and its subdivisions is similar to that of the main bronchi. They are lined by a mucosa of pseudostratified, ciliated, mucous, columnar epithelium with its underlying lamina propria containing some muscle fibres (muscularis mucosae): outside this the submucosa contains a framework of cartilage bars, smooth muscle, glands and elastic fibres. The term bronchus may be applied to about ten generations of subdivisions; when the diameter of a subdivision is about 1 mm, the air passage is called a bronchiole. As the bronchi become smaller the arrangement of the cartilage becomes less regular and the smooth muscle instead of

lying in bundles between the ends of cartilage plates forms circles or spirals internal to the cartilage. The wall decreases in thickness due to a reduction in the height of the epithelial cells and in the thickness of the lamina propria and submucosa. The elastic fibres form a skeleton of elastic tissue, those in the lamina propria being longitudinal and those in the submucosa being more circular. In the wall of the bronchus there are glands, with both mucous and serous cells, and in the lining epithelium there are mucous cells. The glands decrease in number and the mucous cells increase to some extent as the bronchi become smaller. Neither are found in the bronchioles. The mucous cells produce four kinds of acid glycoproteins but there is doubt as to whether each is produced by a different cell type.

The bronchioles can be distinguished by their histological structure as well as their size. They have neither cartilage nor glands and the smooth muscle, although no longer a continuous sheet, is proportionally thicker in relation to the thickness of the wall. There are no mucous cells but in

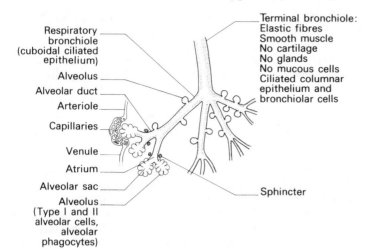

Respiratory bronchiole (cuboidal ciliated epithelium)
Alveolus
Alveolar duct
Arteriole
Capillaries
Venule
Atrium
Alveolar sac
Alveolus (Type I and II alveolar cells, alveolar phagocytes)

Terminal bronchiole:
Elastic fibres
Smooth muscle
No cartilage
No glands
No mucous cells
Ciliated columnar epithelium and bronchiolar cells

Sphincter

Fig. 11.27. Histological structure of the respiratory unit of the lung.

addition to the ciliated columnar cells there are tall nonciliated cells called bronchiolar (Clava) cells. They project beyond the ciliated cells and give the epithelial lining a wavy appearance. These cells vary in structure in different species but in man they have large mitochondria and their apical cytoplasm is densely packed with agranular reticulum. The function of their secretion is not known. The adjacent walls of all the epithelial cells interdigitate and the capillaries next to the bronchial wall have fenestrations. This structural arrangement is related to water transport across the epithelium.

The last or terminal bronchiole divides into respiratory bronchioles (Fig. 11.27). The term lobule is sometimes used when referring to a terminal bronchiole and all its subdivisions together with the associated blood vessels, lymphatics and nerves. These lobules are separated from each other by connective tissue. On the surface of the lung they are about 1 cm² in area and can be seen with the naked eye. Within the lung the lobules are smaller and their separation by connective tissue is less well defined. The term respiratory bronchiole is justified because their walls have outpouchings, called alveoli, which have a respiratory function, but the rest of the wall has the same structure as that of a bronchiole. Respiratory bronchioles divide and form alveolar ducts. Each alveolar duct forms dilations called atria which lead into spaces called alveolar sacs on the walls of which are outpocketings called alveoli. There are also alveoli on the walls of the alveolar ducts.

Smooth muscle is found in the walls of the the respiratory bronchioles, alveolar ducts and atria. The alveoli are the functioning parts for

the atria. The respiratory bronchiole is lined with low columnar ciliated cells and bronchiolar cells. Where there are no alveoli the wall of the alveolar duct is similar to that of the respiratory bronchiole. Elastic fibres form a network round the respiratory bronchioles, alveolar ducts and atria. The alveoli are the functioning parts for respiratory exchange. In man there are estimated to be in one lung about 300 million alveoli, each with a diameter of about 200 μm and a total surface area of about 75 m².

Some of the alveolar cells secrete a lipoprotein called surfactant which lowers the surface tension of the film of liquid coating the alveoli, thereby preventing the collapse of smaller alveoli and facilitating their expansion.

The capillary wall adjacent to the alveolar wall consists of flattened endothelial cells similar in thickness to the squamous cells of the alveolus. The two cell layers are separated by a basement lamina about 0.1 μm thick. These three structures constitute such a thin barrier that gases can be rapidly exchanged. Where the capillaries and alveoli are not in close contact a network of elastic and collagen fibres supports the capillaries.

Another cell associated with the alveoli is the alveolar phagocyte (alveolar macrophage, duct cell) which lies on the outer surface of the alveolar epithelium. They are part of the defence mechanism of the respiratory system and are very active in ingesting particles which reach the alveolar lumen.

The pulmonary artery enters the hilum of the lung and divides into lobar branches and then segmental branches. Further subdivisions correspond with those of the bronchi and finally a capillary network is formed in relation to the alveoli. The capillary plexus drains into venules which form pulmonary veins. These do not run with the branches of the pulmonary artery and bronchi until they become quite large; finally two pulmonary veins emerge from the hilum of each lung and go the left atrium.

The bronchial arteries come from the thoracic aorta or the upper posterior intercostal arteries. They enter the lung at the hilum and accompany the bronchi and their subdivisions to the level of the respiratory bronchioles. They supply oxygenated blood to the walls of the air passages and the structures contained therein, as well as the walls of the large branches of the pulmonary artery and veins (vasa vasorum). Some of the blood in the bronchial arteries returns by way of the pulmonary veins. The rest of the blood, mainly from the main bronchi, drains into bronchial veins which enter a plexus deep to the pulmonary pleura and the hilar lymph nodes. The veins end in the azygos system of veins.

There are anastomotic channels between the bronchial and pulmonary arteries near the smaller bronchi. These may in turn form arteriovenous connections with the pulmonary veins. Arteriovenous shunts between pulmonary arteries and veins have been demonstrated at the level of the terminal bronchioles.

The lungs are innervated by both parasympathetic nerves from the vagus and sympathetic nerves from the ganglionated trunk in the thorax. There is a large posterior pulmonary plexus and a smaller anterior pulmonary plexus each receiving both types of autonomic nerve fibres. The nerves enter the lung at the hilum and run in the walls of bronchi and round the blood vessels. The fibres supply the smooth muscle, glands and epithelium of the bronchi and the walls of the vessels. The vagus causes contraction of the muscle of the bronchi down to the alveolar ducts and the sympathetic causes relaxation. The vagus is secretomotor to the glands and the sympathetic causes vasoconstriction. There are sensory fibres to the visceral pleura, the connective tissue of the septa and the epithelium of the air passages. These are almost entirely vagal.

RESPIRATION

Respiration involves the delivery of oxygen to all the cells of the body according to their requirement, the utilization of the oxygen and the removal of carbon dioxide. The subject can be broken down into three main subheadings:

1 The movement of air in and out of the lungs, to provide oxygen and remove carbon dioxide—sometimes termed external respiration.
2 The loading of the blood with oxygen and the removal of carbon dioxide, and the transport of these gases around the body.
3 The utilization of oxygen and production of carbon dioxide by the cells (internal respiration).

Different tissues require different amounts of oxygen; the kidney uses oxygen at a rate of 5 cm³/100g/minute while skin uses only 0.2cm³/100g/minute. The overall requirement of the body at rest is about 250 cm³/minute, but this can be greatly increased to a maximum of about 4 dm³/minute during exercise. The flexibility required to accommodate this degree of variation is achieved by altering the blood supply and thus the rate of supply of oxygen to the tissues. These alterations are brought about by increasing the cardiac output and by locally changing vascular resistance. However, in order to satisfy an increased demand for oxygen, more must be available in the lungs to load the blood during its rapid transit through the pulmonary capillaries.

The account that follows will only deal with external respiration and the way in which gases are carried in the blood. The blood supply to tissues is considered on p. 715 and the utilization of oxygen by the tissues (internal respiration) is dealt with on p. 199.

The first consideration is the mechanism for moving air in and out (ventilation or breathing).

The mechanism of respiration

THE PLEURAE AND INTRAPLEURAL PRESSURES

In order to understand this subject, the significance of the structure of the thoracic cavity must be considered (Fig. 11.23), in particular the roles of the parietal and the visceral pleurae and the elasticity of the lungs. The pressure in the pleural cavity is below atmospheric pressure due to the fact that the lungs exert an elastic recoil which tends to collapse them whereas the thoracic wall exerts a recoil in an outward direction. The lungs can collapse only when air or fluid (blood, pus or serum) enters the pleural cavity and the pressures are allowed to equilibrate. This is known as pneumothorax.

The intrapleural or intrathoracic pressure can be measured fairly easily by recording the pressure in a small partially inflated balloon which has been swallowed and held in the lower part of the oesophagus. At the end of a normal expiration the pressure is about −3 mmHg.

The size of the thoracic cavity increases on inspiration but the two layers of pleura remain in contact, with the result that the inward pull of the lungs (the elastic recoil) increases and the intrapleural pressure becomes more negative; thus during normal inspiration the pressure is about −7 mmHg. In deep inspiration the pressure may reach −30 mmHg. When a forced expiratory effort is made against a closed glottis (Valsalva's manoeuvre) as occurs in coughing and defaecation, the pressure becomes positive and may reach 100 mmHg and be so maintained for a few seconds.

As the size of the thorax is increased during inspiration, the lungs are drawn outwards and increase in size. Since the lumen of the lungs is in open contact with the atmosphere, air passes into the lungs. On expiration, the size of the thoracic cavity is reduced, the lungs recoil as a result of their elasticity, and the air is expelled. During normal breathing the pressure within the lungs (intrapulmonary or intra-alveolar pressure) hovers around atmospheric becoming lower during inspiraion (−2mmHg) and slightly higher as expiration begins (+2mmHg). Larger pressure changes are seen when sucking, coughing or playing a wind instrument.

RESPIRATORY MUSCLES

From the above account, it is clear that the movement of air in and out of the lungs is dependent on changes in intrathoracic volume. These changes are brought about by the activity of the diaphragm, the external and internal intercostal muscles and a number of accessory muscles of respiration (p. 435).

Estimates of the contribution of the various muscles to respiration vary considerably from person to person. Without doubt, the diaphragm is the most important and in quiet breathing accounts for at least 75% of the increase in thoracic volume. As breathing becomes deeper, the contribution decreases to about 60%.

The only active process in quiet breathing is the muscular contraction which results in inspiration. Expiration is the result of a relaxation of the inspiratory muscles which allows the elastic recoil of the lungs. Only in deep breathing do the expiratory muscles become active and decrease the volume of the thoracic cavity beyond the normal expiratory volume. Thus air which in normal quiet breathing would stay in the lungs is forced out.

WORK OF BREATHING

If the lungs were perfectly elastic and no other factors needed to be taken into consideration, their expansion would be proportional to the change in intrapleural pressure which in turn would be proportional to the work done by the inspiratory muscles. Due to a number of complicating factors the situation is not so simple. Work is done during inspiration in overcoming frictional resistance and surface tension in lung tissue and resistance to airflow in the branched airways.

As respiration deepens these resistances become more significant and a greater proportion of the work done by the respiratory muscles is spent in overcoming them. These sources of resistance become important in certain diseases, for example, in emphysema where much of the lungs' elasticity is lost, and in asthma where the resistance to airflow is increased.

Compliance is a term frequently used in studies of the work of breathing, and is simply a measure of the ability of the lungs and chest wall to stretch. When the rigidity of the lungs or chest wall increases, the value drops. Elasticity is the reciprocal of compliance and is a measure of the ability of the lungs to recoil.

LUNG VOLUMES

A person at rest breathes about 16 times a minute and each breath has a volume of about 400 cm³ (tidal volume). Therefore the volume of air moved in and out of the lungs in one minute is about 6 dm³: this is known as the respiratory minute volume (RMV). There is a wide variation in these and all other so called 'normal' respiratory values. Tidal volume measurements may be between 350 and 600 cm³ and respiratory rate between 12 and 18 per minute, giving a range of 6–8 dm³ for RMV. This large variation from person to person is not surprising when the size of different people's thoracic cavities is considered.

If at the end of normal inspiration a maximal inspiratory effort is made, the extra volume of air taken into the lungs is called the inspiratory reserve volume and is normally about 2.5 dm³. Similarly, if at the end of normal expiration a maximal expiratory effort is made, the extra air expired is called the expiratory reserve volume and is about 1.5 dm³. The amount of air moved

TIDAL VOL   400ml
INSPIR. RES. VOL.   2·5 L
ExP. RES. VOL.   1·5 L
VITAL CAPACITY   4·4 L.
RESIDUAL VOL   1·5 L

RESP. MIN. VOL = 400 × 16
                = 6·4 L/min

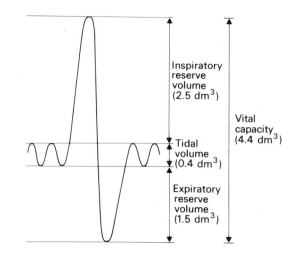

Fig. 11.28. A diagram showing different lung volumes as measured on a spirometer.

from maximal inspiration to maximal expiration is known as the vital capacity and is the sum of the other three volumes (4.4 dm³) (Fig. 11.28). Even at the end of maximal expiration the lungs are not totally collapsed, they still contain about 1.5 dm³ of air and this volume is known as the residual volume; it can be expelled if the lungs are collapsed by a pneumothorax. The residual volume and expiratory reserve volume together form the functional residual capacity.

In Fig. 11.28, the various volumes have been measured with a spirometer (p. 806). They can also be represented diagrammatically in a way which relates the size of the lungs to the various respiratory volumes (Fig. 11.29). It can be seen that with a maximal inspiration the lungs are fully expanded but with a maximal expiration they still contain the residual volume. A normal quiet inspiration causes only a small increase in the volume of air already in the lungs.

The values for the various volumes given in the above account can only be considered as an example: the 'normal' variation is enormous. A group of healthy men have vital capacities ranging from 3 to 7 dm³ and yet all may be considered 'normal'. In general terms the vital capacity of the young is larger than that of the old, the fit larger than the unfit; and of course a person with a large thoracic cavity is likely to have a larger vital capacity than a person with a small thoracic cavity.

It must also be realized that a normal individual's vital capacity may vary under different circumstances. For example, differences in posture result in the abdominal contents exerting different degrees of resistance to the movement of the diaphragm. Vital capacity is greater when standing upright than when lying down. The

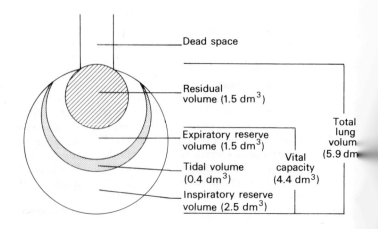

Fig. 11.29. A diagrammatic representation of the lung volumes showing their relationship to the degree of expansion of the lungs.

same explanation accounts for the observation that vital capacity progressively declines during pregnancy.

This extensive variation makes vital capacity a poor indicator of pulmonary function, although it is true that in progressive lung disease, vital capacity decreases. However, vital capacity measured when the subject expires as rapidly as possible can serve as an important pulmonary function test. This is called the forced expiratory volume (FEV) and is recorded on fast moving calibrated paper as shown in Fig. 11.30. The healthy subject had a forced vital capacity of 5.85 dm³ and of this, 4.80 dm³ were expired in the first second. The forced vital capacity in health is the same as the vital capacity measured slowly, but in some lung diseases it is much less. The $FEV_{1.0}$ is expressed either in dm³ or as a percentage of the vital capacity. In our example, the $FEV_{1.0}$ is 82% of the forced vital capacity and is within the range of values expected in a healthy subject.

The importance of this test is that in a condition such as asthma, the vital capacity, particularly when measured slowly, may appear normal but the $FEV_{1.0}$ values are greatly reduced. The asthmatic subject in Fig. 11.30 had the same vital capacity as the normal subject but took 6 seconds to expel it, the $FEV_{1.0}$ value being 42%. In conditions such as asthma the resistance encountered in breathing through constricted airways prevents rapid expiration.

During vigorous exercise, RMV increases from about 6 dm³ to a maximum of over 100 dm³ due to an increase in both the rate and depth of respiration. The tidal volume increases from its normal value of about 400 cm³ to possibly 3 dm³ by encroaching on the inspiratory and expiratory reserve volumes. The vital capacity is obviously unchanged. Thus it is important to define the conditions under which different lung volumes are measured.

The ability to increase RMV is the basis of a test of lung function known as the maximum ventilatory volume (MVV). This test involves breathing as rapidly and deeply as possible for a period of 15 seconds and collecting the expired air. The volume of expired air is measured and expressed as dm³/minute; in normal subjects the range of values is 120–170. This value decreases dramatically in people who suffer from conditions which prevent rapid expiration, such as asthma, and is also reduced in many different types of impaired lung function.

DEAD SPACE

About 400 cm³ of air passes into the respiratory tract in each breath. Not all of this reaches the regions where gas can be exchanged. That which only reaches the trachea and bronchi is expired unchanged. This part of the respiratory tract is known as the dead space. Unfortunately two different types of dead space must be considered, anatomical and functional. The anatomical dead space is that part of the respiratory tract which is not lined with the respiratory epithelium through which gases are exchanged. The functional or physiological dead space on the other hand, is that part of the respiratory tract in which air does not equilibrate with blood. In a healthy subject the two are normally the same, but in some diseases the functional dead space may be much larger than the anatomical. The difference arises from the fact that gas is not exchanged in some alveoli because, for

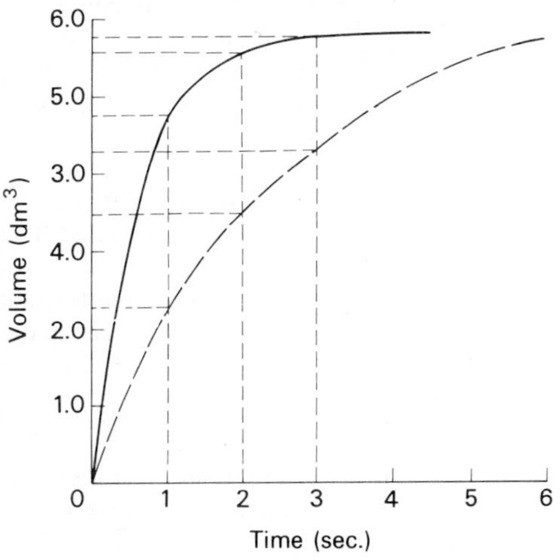

Fig. 11.30. Trace obtained by recording the rapid expiration of the vital capacity on a fast moving paper, with a normal subject (continuous line curve) and an asthmatic subject (broken line curve). The dotted lines are drawn to indicate the volumes expired at 1, 2, and 3 seconds. For explanation see text.

example the ventilated alveoli receive no pulmonary blood supply or because some alveoli are not ventilated adequately.

Dead space can be measured indirectly from measurements of tidal volume and the composition of alveolar and expired airs. The formula for this is:

$$V_D = V_T \frac{(C_A - C_E)}{C_A}$$

where V_D = dead space
where V_T = tidal volume
$\quad\quad C_A$ = %CO_2 in alveolar air
$\quad\quad C_E$ = %CO_2 in expired air.

The 'normal' value for dead space varies considerably; 150 cm³ is the most commonly quoted figure.

ALVEOLAR VENTILATION

As has already been discussed the RMV is the amount of air moving in and out of the respiratory tract in 1 minute. RMV is calculated by multiplying the tidal volume by the number of breaths per minute:

$$\begin{array}{ccc} 400 \text{ cm}^3 & \times \quad 16 & = 6.4 \text{ dm}^3 \\ \text{(tidal volume)} & \text{(rate)} & \text{(RMV)} \end{array}$$

As about 150 cm³ of each breath is dead space air and never reaches the part of the lungs where gas exchange occurs, only 250 cm³ actually gets into the alveoli. Thus the effective ventilation of the alveoli is not 6.4 dm³ but is:

$$\begin{array}{cccc} (400 & - & 150) & \times \quad 16 & = 4.0 \text{ dm}^3 \\ \text{(tidal} & & \text{(dead} & \text{(rate)} \\ \text{volume)} & & \text{space)} \end{array}$$

This is known as the alveolar ventilation.

The importance of alveolar ventilation can be seen by considering the effects of increasing the depth and rate of respiration. Suppose the tidal volume is doubled to 800 cm³ and the rate halved to 8 per minute, the RMV is unchanged:

$$\text{RMV} \quad = \quad 800 \quad \times 8 = 6.4 \text{ dm}^3$$

But alveolar ventilation = $(800-150) \times 8 = 5.2$ dm³. Thus, although the RMV is unaltered, the alveolar ventilation is increased by 30%.

In another example, if the tidal volume is halved to 200 cm³ and the rate is doubled to 32 per minute, the RMV is again unchanged:

$$\text{RMV} = 200 \times 32 = 6.4 \text{ dm}^3$$

But alveolar ventilation = $(200-150) \times 32 = 1.6$ dm³. In this case there is a 60% reduction in

alveolar ventilation without any change in RMV.

These examples demonstrate clearly that in respect of alveolar ventilation, it is more efficient to increase the depth of breathing than the rate. This is important in clinical conditions in which there is rapid, shallow breathing, because respiration becomes inefficient in terms of alveolar ventilation. On the other hand, it must be remembered that as respiration becomes deeper an increasingly large proportion of the work done by the respiratory muscles is spent in overcoming the resistance to breathing (see p. 501). In practice, as will be seen later, both rate and depth are generally increased when respiration is stimulated.

VENTILATION: PERFUSION RATIO

This is a term which is commonly used in respiratory physiology and its meaning should be understood. It is simply the ratio:

$$\frac{\text{alveolar ventilation}}{\text{pulmonary blood flow}}$$

A normal value for alveolar ventilation ($\dot{V}_A$) is 4.0 dm³/minute and for the quantity of blood flowing through the lungs ($\dot{Q}$) is 5.0 dm³/minute. Thus the ventilation: perfusion ratio is:

$$\frac{4.0}{5.0} = 0.8$$

It must be remembered however, that this is for the lungs as a whole. If the ratio is worked out for different regions of the lungs there may be considerable differences due to local variations in ventilation or blood flow, even in a healthy subject. For example, at rest in the supine position alveolar ventilation is reasonably uniform, but when the body is upright the alveoli at the base of the lungs have both a higher blood flow and greater ventilation than those at the apex. The increase in perfusion at the base is relatively greater than that of ventilation so the $\dot{V}_A/\dot{Q}$ is decreased. The ratio at the base is about 0.6 whereas at the apex it is about 3.0. In disease, the lungs may become very unevenly ventilated. The $\dot{V}_A/\dot{Q}$ for a particular region may deviate considerably from the normal expected value for that region, but this may have a minimal effect on the ratio for the lung as a whole.

Blood gases

From an evolutionary standpoint, respiration is an aquatic process and this is still true in the mammalian lung. Oxygen must dissolve on the

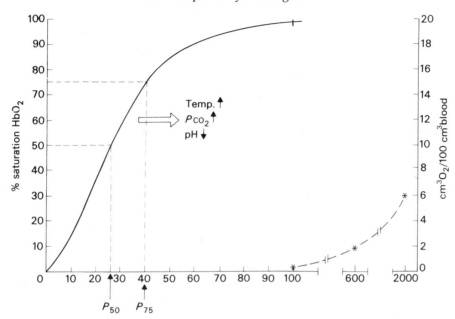

Fig. 11.31. Sigmoid relationship between % O_2 saturation of haemoglobin and O_2 partial pressure—the oxygen dissociation (association) curve.

The broken line on the right indicates the volume of oxygen dissolved in plasma at pressures above those found normally in alveolar air.

wet surface of the alveolus before it can pass, by diffusion, across the alveolar walls into the plasma and thence into the red blood corpuscle. Similarly, CO_2 passes from the aqueous phase in the reverse direction to the gaseous phase.

OXYGEN

A normal man requires about 240 cm³ of O_2 per minute while he is at rest and this requirement increases more than ten-fold in exercise. Suppose that man had no haemoglobin. Any gas dissolves in blood in proportion to its partial pressure (Henry's Law) and its solubility. Oxygen has a low solubility and at a partial pressure of 100 mmHg in the alveolus only 0.003 cm³ of O_2 could be carried away from the lungs in each cm³ of blood. If all the oxygen had been given up from the blood to the tissues in one passage and the venous blood returning to the heart contained no oxygen, then the volume of blood to be pumped per minute would be:

$$\frac{240}{0.003 - 0} = 80\ 000 \text{ cm}^3 \text{ or } 80 \text{ dm}^3.$$

This represents an impossible task for the heart, even when the body is at rest. The problem is overcome by the presence of haemoglobin which in normal amounts (about 15g per 100

cm³) allows about a seventy-fold increase in the carriage of oxygen since one gram of haemoglobin can carry up to 1.36 cm³ of O_2.

Oxygen dissociation curve and transport of oxygen
To understand the function of haemoglobin in oxygen transport we have to become familiar with the oxygen dissociation curve (Fig. 11.31) or, as it could equally well be termed, the oxygen association curve. This curve relates the partial pressure of oxygen (PO_2) either to the amount of oxygen carried in the blood or to the percentage haemoglobin which is saturated with oxygen. The curve is constructed from measurements obtained using whole blood equilibrated *in vitro* with gases of known composition. These measurements are made at a fixed PCO_2 and pH and at body temperature. The relationship obtained is a sigmoid curve (Fig. 11.31), a shape which has many implications.

Association
Let us consider, first of all the chemical nature of the association between blood and oxygen.

Each molecule of haemoglobin contains four distinct binding sites for oxygen, one associated with each haem ring. The ease with which oxygen is bound by the ferrous atom in a haem ring (to form oxyhaemoglobin) varies with the degree of oxygenation and this partly accounts for the S shaped or sigmoidal dissociation curve. After the first ring has taken up its oxygen (at a PO_2 of 17 mmHg) a disturbance is induced in the quaternary protein structure (p. 73) which is transmitted to the site of the second haem ring. The disturbance enables this ring to bind oxygen more easily when exposed to an increased oxygen tension and it becomes saturated by a smaller rise in PO_2 than does the first ring. The same applies to the third haem ring. The behaviour of the second and third haem rings is responsible for the steep part of the oxygenation curve. The fourth haem, like the first, requires a larger rise in PO_2 to saturate it.

Although we have considered the reaction between haemoglobin and oxygen from the point of view of O_2 uptake, the same principles apply to unloading oxygen as the PO_2 falls. For example, the oxygen tension must fall to about 40 mmHg before the fourth haem ring releases all its oxygen.

Haemoglobin is almost fully saturated (97%) at a partial pressure of only 100 mmHg; the partial pressure which is provided in the alveoli of man breathing normally. It is because haemoglobin is comfortably close to full saturation at this alveolar O_2 tension that the maintenance of alveolar PO_2 is not normally a critical factor in driving ventilation in mammals. The fine control of ventilation is set to maintain a constant PCO_2 (p. 511); moderate variations in alveolar PO_2 have little influence on oxygen uptake.

Between a PO_2 of 70 to 100 mmHg there is an increase of only 0.56 cm³ of oxygen combined with haemoglobin in every 100 cm³ blood. This relatively flat plateau of the curve is important in two main circumstances. If a man is at an altitude of only a few thousand metres, although the blood and the alveolar PO_2 fall to about 70 mmHg the haemoglobin is still 94% saturated. Likewise with reductions in respiratory efficiency, such as occur for instance with increasing age and in some respiratory diseases, the blood can still be reasonably saturated.

Dissociation

The main cause of the dissociation of oxygen from oxyhaemoglobin is ultimately a low PO_2 in the tissues through which the blood is passing. Metabolically active cells rapidly consume oxygen from the tissue fluid; oxygen diffuses from the plasma into the tissue fluid; the reduced PO_2 in the plasma then causes the dissociation of oxygen from oxyhaemoglobin.

Consider the effect on oxyhaemoglobin of passing from 100 mmHg PO_2 down to 70 mmHg and then to 40 mmHg, a partial pressure which corresponds to that in mixed venous blood. From Fig. 11.31 it seems that during the first step the blood would unload 0.56 cm³ of oxygen per 100 cm³ but in the second step in the steep part of the curve, the figure would rise to 3.9 cm³. But this is only true *in vitro*; the situation is more complex *in vivo*.

In an active tissue, such as exercising muscle, the temperature and the PCO_2 rise, and glycolysis produces lactic and pyruvic acids. Each one of these factors moves the oxygen dissociation curve to the right: that is to say, for a particular PO_2 the oxyhaemoglobin releases more oxygen (Fig. 11.31). In addition to this increase in the extraction of oxygen there is also a more plentiful supply of oxygen due to the greater flow of blood to active tissues.

Changes in pH have a large effect on dissociation. At a PO_2 of 30 mmHg and a pH of 7.4 haemoglobin retains 57% of its oxygen but this falls to 45% if the pH is 7.2

The effect of PCO_2 on dissociation, which is known as the Bohr effect, is too complex to analyse here. The CO_2 becomes hydrated and the H^+ so formed lowers the affinity between haemoglobin and O_2. A conformational change in the globin molecules could be responsible for this physiologically important effect. It is sufficient to note that an increase in PCO_2 enhances the supply of oxygen to tissues. In addition, as will be seen later, CO_2 uptake by the blood is enhanced by greater amounts of deoxygenated haemoglobin. However, it must be stressed that the release of oxygen from oxyhaemoglobin is not dependent on a reciprocal uptake of carbon dioxide.

High temperatures (i.e. above 37°C) can markedly increase the dissociation of oxyhaemoglobin but the effect is small when the partial pressure of oxygen is high. It is worth noting at this point that low temperatures move the curve far to the left. The effect of this is seen, for example, in the bright red colour of the blood in the ears of very cold subjects. Because oxygen cannot dissociate from the haemoglobin under these circumstances the red colour of oxyhaemoglobin persists.

The effects of increased temperature, decreased pH and increased PCO_2 are very important at the oxygen tensions found in active tissues but have little influence on the uptake of oxygen at normal alveolar oxygen tensions. The opposite effects of low P_{CO_2} and high pH move the curve to the left and this is valuable in oxygenating haemoglobin at high altitudes where alveolar P_{O_2} is reduced.

It has become a practice in recent years to compare the blood from different species or from individuals of different ages by noting the P_{50} (Fig. 11.31). This is the P_{O_2} at which the blood is 50% saturated *in vitro*. For normal human adult blood the figure is 26 mmHg, whereas it falls to 20 mmHg for fetal blood. This, of course, acts in favour of the transfer of oxygen from the maternal to the fetal blood across the placental wall, for it means that fetal blood binds oxygen more readily than does maternal blood. Also marked in Fig. 11.31 is the 75% saturation point, which normally corresponds to a P_{O_2} of about 40 mmHg. This is the percentage saturation and the P_{O_2} which are commonly found in mixed venous blood (blood in the pulmonary artery) of resting man. The condition of a resting man, with a normal amount of haemoglobin, is vastly different from the hypothetical character with no haemoglobin who was considered earlier. His cardiac output is not 80 litres per minute but only

$$\frac{240}{20-15} \times 100 \text{ cm}^3/\text{minute} = 4.8 \text{ dm}^3$$

Further, he has a large reserve of O_2 in his blood which can be imparted to active muscles if he decides to exercise himself.

In recent years, great interest has been generated in a substance called 2, 3-diphosphoglycerate (2,3-DPG) which interacts powerfully with the haemoglobin molecule as it becomes deoxygenated and promotes dissociation. The higher the cellular 2,3-DPG the more readily haemoglobin gives up its oxygen. Fetal red cells have lower levels of 2,3-DPG and consequently have a higher affinity for oxygen; this allows them to take up oxygen from maternal blood. Red cells contain a specific enzyme, 2,3-DPG mutase, which converts 1, 3-diphosphoglycerate (an intermediate in the normal glycolytic pathway) into 2,3-DPG. The activity of 2,3-DPG mutase is inhibited by increasing concentration of 2,3-DPG. The stimulus within the cell for increasing the activity of the enzyme is not known.

So far, we have been considering the normal condition. However, suppose the subject has only half the normal quantity of haemoglobin. Although the shape of the curve in Fig. 11.31 would be the same (for example, the haemoglo-

bin, although less in amount, would still be 97% saturated at 100 mmHg) the total amount of oxygen carried as oxyhaemoglobin would be only 9.3 cm³/100 cm³ blood and our earlier calculations would be incorrect. Thus, anaemia of any sort is of extreme importance in the carriage of oxygen. We can, if we wish, regard poisoning with carbon monoxide as a particular form of anaemia because carbon monoxide binds very tightly with the haemoglobin molecule and, even if breathing only 0.1% for over an hour, 50% of the haemoglobin would be in the HbCO form and thus unavailable for oxygen carriage.

TRANSPORT OF CARBON DIOXIDE

Because CO_2 is about 20 times as soluble as O_2, more CO_2 than O_2 can be carried in the plasma in simple solution. The amount in this form is linearly related to the P_{CO_2} (Henry's Law). At 37°C blood can dissolve 0.03 mmol CO_2 per mmHg pressure of CO_2. Mixed venous P_{CO_2} is about 6 mmHg higher than arterial P_{CO_2} so that it dissolves $6 \times 0.03 = 0.18$ mmol/dm³ more CO_2.

CO_2 can also be carried in the red cell in the carbamino form where CO_2 substitutes for H^+ on amino groups projecting from the sides of the protein chain. This reaction may be written:

$$\text{Hb} - \text{N} \Big\langle {}^{H}_{H} + CO_2 \quad \rightarrow$$

$$\text{Hb} - \text{N} \Big\langle {}^{H}_{COO^-} + H^+$$

Finally, CO_2 is transported in blood as bicarbonate in both the red cell and, more importantly, in the plasma.

CO_2 diffuses from areas of high concentration in the tissues into the tissue fluids and thence to the plasma. We can now consider some of the changes which take place when the CO_2 dissolved in the plasma passes into the red blood cells (Fig. 11.32).

Within the red blood cell, carbonic anhydrase plays a vital role in accelerating the forward reaction:

$$CO_2 + H_2O \rightleftharpoons H_2CO_3 \rightleftharpoons H^+ + HCO_3^-.$$

The red cell membrane is relatively impermeable to cations but permeable to small anions, so that, as the concentration of HCO_3^- rises in the cell, it passes into the plasma and is replaced by another anion, chloride thus preserving electrical neutrality. It has been found that as the concentration of HCO_3^- rises in venous blood there is a net increase of Cl^- ions within the red cell.

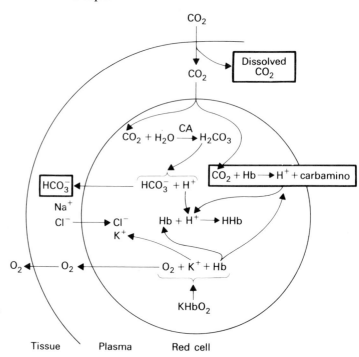

Fig. 11.32. Sequence of reactions taking place between a red blood cell and tissue. CA=carbonic anhydrase; Hb=haemoglobin.

The reciprocal movement of Cl^- and HCO_3^- is known as the chloride shift.

Now consider the H^+ ions. The carriage of CO_2 molecules as bicarbonate and carbamino haemoglobin involves the release of an equivalent number of protons (H^+) which must be rapidly and effectively buffered (p. 748). Deoxygenated haemoglobin (Hb) is less acid than oxygenated haemoglobin (HbO_2): the pK of Hb is 7.9 and of HbO_2 is 6.7, because during the oxygenation of haemoglobin there is a change in the ionization of the $-NH^+$ group in the histidine residues. When O_2 is released to the tissues the β-protein chains in the globin molecule move apart and H^+ ions are taken up at the histidine sites. The straightforward buffering by the free carboxyl and free amino groups in the globin molecule is of minor importance.

CO_2 which is not converted into HCO_3^- can form a carbamino compound with Hb. Deoxygenated haemoglobin binds more CO_2 as carbamino compound than HbO_2. Note that in both the above cases the discharge of O_2 enhances the capacity of the red blood cell to take up CO_2.

There is a net increase in the number of molecules within the red cell when it is carrying more CO_2, hence its osmotic pressure tends to rise and water is taken in. Thus the haematocrit of venous blood is slightly greater than that of

arterial, and similarly, venous blood is slightly more easily haemolysed in hypotonic saline solutions.

The relative amounts of O_2 and CO_2 in arterial and venous blood are shown in Table 11.1.

It should be noted from Table 11.1 that considerable quantities of bicarbonate are present in both arterial and venous blood. This is important because the bicarbonate : CO_2 ratio in plasma provides a vital system for controlling the pH of the blood (p. 748). Carbon dioxide is transported in various forms from the tissues to the lungs. Bicarbonate accounts for most of the carriage, but the carbamino haemoglobin has a particular importance because its formation and breakdown are so rapid and are so intimately linked to the degree of oxygenation of haemoglobin. The amounts of carbonic acid and protein-bound CO_2 in plasma are insignificant.

When CO_2 content of blood is plotted against P_{CO_2}, dissociation curves of the types shown in Fig. 11.33 are produced. It is clear that the oxygen saturation of haemoglobin markedly affects the amount of CO_2 carried. Blood with no oxygen can take up more CO_2 than fully oxygenated blood (the Haldane effect) for two reasons. First, as already mentioned, deoxygenated Hb can combine with more CO_2 to form carbamino compound and second, it is a better

Table 11.1. Mean values for blood O_2, CO_2 and pH.

	Arterial	Mixed venous
O_2 pressure (mmHg)	100	40
O_2 content (cm³O_2/100 cm³ blood)	20.3	15.5
Dissolved	0.3	0.1
Combined with Hb	20.0	15.4
% saturation of Hb with O_2	97	75
CO_2 pressure (mmHg)	40	46
Total CO_2 (cm³CO_2/100 cm³ blood)	48	52
Dissolved in plasma	3	3.5
Bound as HCO_3^- in plasma	42	44.5
Bound as carbaminohaemoglobin	3	4
pH	7.40	7.36

acceptor of H^+ ions. The formation of carb-amino haemoglobin is also aided by this removal of H^+ ions as accumulation of H^+ would cause the $-NH_2$ groups to form $-NH_3^+$ rather than $-NHCOOH$. The physiological CO_2 dissociation curve is really a vector or line drawn between two curves, one for 75% HbO_2 and the other for arterial blood (97.5% HbO_2) over the PCO_2 range between alveolar air (40 mmHg) and mixed venous blood (46 mmHg).

The elimination of CO_2 from the lungs reverses the processes which were considered in the tissues (Fig. 11.32). The mixed venous blood in the pulmonary artery, at a PCO_2 of 46 mmHg, is in intimate contact with the alveolar air at a PCO_2 of 40 mmHg. Because of this partial pressure gradient, CO_2 leaves the blood. As the haemoglobin takes up oxygen it becomes a stronger acid and so drives CO_2 from the bicarbonate in the red blood cell. Bicarbonate enters the cell once more from the plasma, combines with H^+ released from haemoglobin during its oxygenation, and under the influence of carbonic anhydrase, the H_2CO_3 is rapidly converted into CO_2 and water. The haemoglobin also releases much of its CO_2, not because of the lowered PCO_2, but largely because of the oxygenation. It is remarkable that these reactions are able to proceed nearly to equilibrium in less than 0.75 seconds—the time spent by the red cells in the pulmonary capillaries.

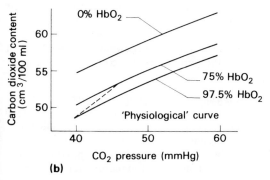

(a)

(b)

Fig. 11.33(a). Carbon dioxide dissociation curves for completely deoxygenated blood (upper), mixed venous blood (middle) and normal arterial blood (lower). (b) Representation of the physiologically important part of the curves. As arterial blood releases oxygen to the tissues there is an upward shift towards the curve for 75% HbO_2—this is shown by the broken line. More CO_2 is carried for a given change in PCO_2.

The control of respiration

The first consideration is the origin of the normal pattern of respiration at rest; and second the many factors which can interrupt it either for a transient period, such as in speaking, coughing or swallowing, or for a prolonged period, such as at high altitude.

THE ORIGIN OF NORMAL QUIET
RESPIRATION

In normal, quiet respiration, the inspiratory muscles are intermittently active, each contraction being followed by relaxation. This pattern is due to a repeating pattern of activity in the motor nerves supplying the muscles. These are the phrenic nerves to the diaphragm, which leave the spinal cord at the level C3–5 and the intercostal nerves at levels T1–T12. If the spinal cord is sectioned above C3 respiration ceases, even though the motor innervation of the inspiratory muscles is intact, indicating that the stimulus is initiated at a higher level. This has been recognised ever since it was observed that head injuries often affect respiration.

In 1812 Legallois demonstrated that an area in the medulla was associated with respiration and in 1923 Lumsden found another area in the pons. The importance of these regions of the brain stem in maintaining the normal pattern of quiet breathing has been investigated in three main ways;
1   By observing the effect on respiration of sectioning the brain stem at different levels.
2   Electrically stimulating various areas.
3   Recording electrical activity of groups of neurons by microelectrodes.
These experiments have led to many conflicting views about the functional organization of the different regions which exert an influence over respiration. We shall exclude consideration of much of the experimental evidence in presenting the following summarised scheme (Fig. 11.34). It must be emphasized that several alternative schemes are possible.

An area in the upper (rostral) part of the pons, the pneumotaxic centre, seems to control an intrinsic pattern generated in the medulla. This generator consists of neurons which directly control medullary cells, which in turn drive the inspiratory and, under some circumstances, expiratory muscle motoneurons. There is some kind of reciprocal activity between these two closely located groups of medullary inspiratory and expiratory cells. The rhythm exhibited by the generator is influenced principally by the P_{CO_2} in arterial blood perfusing the brain but there are also feedback loops through the pneumotaxic 'centre' and through afferent impulses reaching the medulla through the vagus nerves from receptors in the lung and possibly chest wall which are stimulated on lung inflation. The evidence for the pneumotaxic centre comes from rather crude experiments in anaesthetised animals in which the vagal afferent fibres were first cut and the brain then sectioned at different levels. When the level was in the mid pons, the slow deep breathing characteristic of the animal after vagal sectioning changed to one with much longer phases of inspiration—apneustic breathing. This suggests that a mechanism for terminating inspiration had been removed by the section. The level of sectioning implied that another group of neurons in the lower pons, the apneustic centre, might mediate in this mechanism. The so-called 'respiratory centre' is not an anatomical structure, but rather the diffuse, loosely defined groups of neurons and associated circuitry which together control rhythmical breathing.

Pulmonary stretch receptors
Two observations implicate vagal afferents in normal quiet breathing. First, if both vagus nerves are cut in an anaesthetized animal, respiration becomes slower and deeper. Second, if afferent impulses travelling up a vagus nerve are recorded, bursts of activity are seen on inflation of the lungs and these decline on expiration. The level of this activity in the vagus has been shown to be proportional to the degree of inflation.

The receptors responsible for this vagal activity are found in the walls of the bronchi and bronchioles and are sensitive to stretch. The action of these receptors was first investigated by Hering and Breuer, by whose names the reflex is now known.

Thus inflation of the lungs in normal quiet breathing appears to be one of the sources for inhibiting active inspiration. The role of the Hering–Breuer reflex has been clearly demonstrated in animals and newborn babies but it is of doubtful importance in a conscious, adult man.

Respiratory muscle proprioceptors
The muscles of respiration, like other skeletal muscles, contain muscle spindles and Golgi tendon organs. The intercostal muscles have large numbers of both but the diaphragm has few muscle spindles and numerous tendon organs.

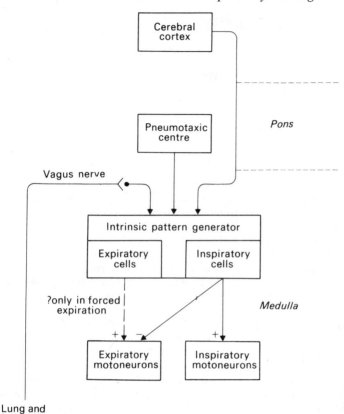

Fig. 11.34. A scheme to illustrate functional organization of different areas of the brain which influence respiration.

Afferent impulses from these receptors enter the spinal cord by way of the dorsal root and are relayed to the respiratory centre. During the past 20 years, the role of these receptors has been the subject of much investigation. They are phasically active during normal quiet breathing and although their exact role has still to be elucidated it seems likely that in man they may perform a similar function to the lung stretch receptors (Hering–Breuer reflex) in lower animals.

Role of chemical control in quiet breathing
Normal quiet breathing undoubtedly depends on the tensions of CO_2 and O_2 in arterial blood; their role is described below.

FACTORS AFFECTING RESPIRATION

Any variation in the pattern of respiration must be mediated by a change in the activity of the motor nerves supplying the respiratory muscles. As with the control of skeletal muscle, there are two variables; the frequency of discharge of the motoneurons and the number of active motoneurons. Thus an increase in the respiratory rate is brought about by an increase in the frequency of the bursts of activity, whereas an increase in the depth of inspiration mainly involves the recruitment of more motoneurons.

Chemical stimuli
In order to understand the chemical control of respiration, the two gases, CO_2 and O_2, which are actively involved in respiration will be considered separately, but it is important to realize that the physiological situation often involves a change in both together.

Carbon dioxide. The normal arterial blood tension or partial pressure of carbon dioxide is 40 mmHg and any tendency for this to increase (hypercapnia) results in stimulation of respiration and an increase in RMV (hyperpnoea). This can be demonstrated very simply: a subject inspiring from a bag containing, for example, 5%

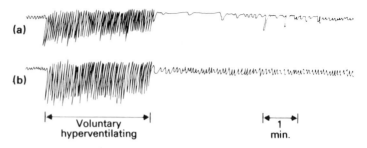

Fig. 11.35. Recording made using a stethograph to measure chest movements during and following voluntary overbreathing. (a) With inspired room air; (b) with inspired air containing 5% CO_2.

CO_2 in air, may reach an RMV around 30 dm^3/minute instead of the normal 6–8 dm^3/minute. In the opposite situation, if there is a reduction in the arterial P_{CO_2} there is a reduction in the ventilation. This is seen after a subject voluntarily hyperventilates for two or three minutes and then stops: there is a period during which ventilation ceases (apnoea) followed by intermittent short bursts of respiration until the normal pattern is resumed. This pattern is known as Cheyne–Stokes respiration and is illustrated in Fig. 11.35a. Apnoea does not occur in all subjects following a period of hyperventilation, but is replaced by a period of reduced ventilation. Cheyne–Stokes respiration is sometimes seen in young children when they are asleep and also in adults sleeping at high altitude.

Cheyne–Stokes breathing is explained in the following way. During voluntary hyperventilation the P_{CO_2} in alveolar air is reduced and this causes less carbon dioxide to be carried in the arterial blood, with the result that the P_{CO_2} is reduced from the normal 40 to possibly 15 mmHg. Thus the drive to respire promoted by the normal P_{CO_2} in arterial blood is removed and respiration only starts again when the P_{CO_2} builds up to the normal level. The truth of this explanation can be demonstrated by asking the subject to repeat the hyperventilation with inspired air containing 4–5% CO_2. There is no apnoea in this case because the hyperventilation has not reduced the P_{CO_2} (Fig. 11.35b). This experiment also eliminates an alternative explanation—that the apnoea is induced by the raised P_{O_2} in arterial blood in hyperventilation.

The arterial P_{CO_2} exerts a control over respiration by affecting a region in the medulla. It was at first thought that this sensitive region corresponded with the medullary respiratory centres but it now seems that they are anatomically separate. It is usual to refer to the CO_2 sensitive regions as the central chemoreceptors. Most evidence suggests that carbon dioxide acts indirectly by altering the hydrogen ion concentra-

tion of the cerebrospinal fluid (CSF). This latter explanation depends on the fact that CO_2 readily penetrates the blood–brain barrier and enters the CSF. It is rapidly converted into bicarbonate and hydrogen ions and since the CSF is without buffer substances, the local concentration of hydrogen ions in the CSF rises in proportion to the P_{CO_2} of the arterial blood. It is probable that a direct action of CO_2 also plays some part.

Oxygen. The overall effects of oxygen lack (hypoxia) are considered in detail in the next section, but the effect of hypoxia on respiration is briefly considered here. In general, hypoxia stimulates respiration, although the magnitude of the effect depends on the cause of hypoxia. Chemoreceptors situated in the carotid bodies (at the bifurcation of the common carotid arteries) and the aortic bodies (in the region of the arch of the aorta) are supplied by branches of the glossopharyngeal and vagus nerves respectively (Fig. 15.64). In order to avoid confusion with the central chemoreceptors discussed above, they are often referred to as the peripheral chemoreceptors. They are stimulated in two main ways; first, by a reduction in the P_{O_2} of the arterial blood and second, by a reduction in their blood supply. It must be stressed that an increase in the P_{CO_2} of arterial blood is only a very weak stimulus to the peripheral chemoreceptors.

Hypoxia, besides stimulating the peripheral chemoreceptors, directly depresses neuronal activity and therefore the respiratory centres. Thus the net effect of hypoxia on respiration is governed by the extent of its direct and indirect effects.

If pure oxygen is breathed at sea level the P_{O_2} of arterial blood is increased to well above the normal 100 mm Hg. The resulting slight reduction in pulmonary ventilation suggests that normal quiet respiration is to a small extent driven by the peripheral chemoreceptors (Fig. 11.36). H^+ *concentration.* An increase in $[H^+]$ stimu-

$CO_2 \rightarrow H^+$ ions in CSF

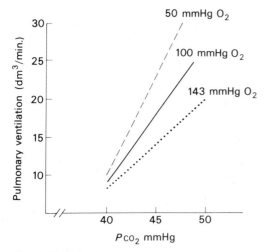

Fig. 11.36. Effect of variations in alveolar air P_{CO_2} at three P_{O_2} levels on pulmonary ventilation. The reduced response when P_{O_2} is above normal suggests that arterial P_{O_2} normally exerts a small drive on respiration.

lates the peripheral chemoreceptors and causes a small increase in pulmonary ventilation. A fall in [H$^+$] brings about a reduction in RMV.

Evaluation of the control of respiration by oxygen and carbon dioxide
When hypercapnia and hypoxia are combined (asphyxia) they cause a large increase in pulmonary ventilation (Fig. 11.36). It is possible to sort out the relative contributions of each by the following simple experiment. A subject is connected to a spirometer filled first with room air which is rebreathed for a few minutes. His respiration gradually becomes faster and deeper until he is 'fighting for breath' (dyspnoea) and the test has to be terminated. After recovery the test is repeated but this time the spirometer is filled with pure oxygen. It is found that the trace on the spirometer is virtually identical with that of the first test, both in the degree of the increase and its rate of onset. This result indicates that the stimulus must be the accumulation of carbon dioxide rather than deficiency of oxygen since at the end of the second experiment there is still a high percentage of oxygen left in the spirometer. Finally, in a dangerous experiment, which must only be performed under qualified supervision, the spirometer is filled with room air and a soda-lime canister is put in to absorb the carbon dioxide. As the percentage of oxygen in the spirometer gradually falls, there is some stimula-

tion of respiration, but its onset is slower and its magnitude much less than in the previous tests. In addition, the subject who in the previous test has been struggling for breath and has begged for the termination of the experiment, goes on breathing happily, quite unaware of any impairment of mental function and impending loss of consciousness due to lack of oxygen!

It is quite clear that hypercapnia is a much stronger stimulus to respiration than hypoxia. This conclusion from experiments in which the two conditions are separately induced however gives a false impression about the importance of hypoxia. There is now evidence that a degree of hypoxia, which alone is a weak stimulus to respiration, has a much greater effect if it is coupled with some hypercapnia. This conclusion can even be drawn from the results illustrated in Fig. 11.36.

Other factors affecting respiration
In addition to the control of respiration by the mechanisms already described, e.g. chemical control and the Hering–Breuer reflex, there are a number of factors which affect respiration, usually in a transient way. These different effects will now be considered separately.

Higher centres. There is a degree of voluntary control over breathing. Most people can hold their breath for about a minute before reaching a breaking point which is caused by the accumulation of carbon dioxide. If the P_{CO_2} is reduced by voluntary hyperventilation, the breath can be subsequently held for much longer. Conversely, if carbon dioxide accumulates faster, as after exercise, the breath can only be held for a few seconds.

Consider the voluntary control of respiration in speaking and singing. Both are essentially long controlled periods of expiration followed by short inspiratory gasps (p. 521). This voluntary control is obviously cortical in origin. Other centres can modify respiration in response to such stimuli as pain and emotion.

Protective mechanisms. There are three reflex mechanisms which protect the respiratory tract. These are: the inhibition of respiration during swallowing; the expulsion of irritant material from the respiratory tract by coughing and sneezing; and the inhibition of respiration following irritation of the mucous membranes of the upper respiratory tract.

With regard to swallowing (p. 578) it is sufficient to say here that just before swallowing, impulses pass along the glossopharyngeal nerve from the pharynx to the respiratory centre and cause the temporary inhibition of respiration. In a dental context it is important to remember that during general anaesthesia, this protective reflex along with all other reflexes, is depressed and there is a risk that tooth fragments, or even whole teeth can be inhaled.

There are several reflex responses to irritation of the mucous membranes in various parts of the respiratory tract. Coughing results from irritation of the trachea and bronchi and starts with a deep inspiration. An expiratory effort is then made against a closed glottis: the glottis is suddenly opened and there is an explosive outflow of air at high velocity. Sneezing, caused by irritation of the mucous membranes of the nasal passage, is a similar expiratory act, but intrathoracic pressure is not increased because the glottis remains open. Both of these reflexes tend to expel irritant particles and help to keep the airways clear.

In addition to their role in sneezing, the mucous membranes of the upper respiratory tract, particularly the nasal passages, are the source of powerful reflexes which cause the inhibition of respiration. Irritant gases such as ammonia or smoke drawn through the nasal passages in an anaesthetized animal cause reflex apnoea due to afferent activity in the trigeminal nerve. This defence mechanism prevents the entry of irritant gases into the respiratory tract. Water in the nasal passages has the same effect and also has marked cardiovascular effects. It is likely that this latter reflex could be of importance in diving mammals.

Cutaneous sensation. Anyone who has stepped into a cold shower will know the effect that an unpleasant cutaneous stimulation has on respiration. It is a deep inspiration or 'gasp'. It is difficult to attribute any specific function to this reflex in man. In the newborn baby it may be one of the mechanisms involved in causing the baby to take its first breath after leaving its more comfortable uterine environment. Although this is unlikely to be the full explanation, it may well play a part, because if a baby is reluctant to take its first breath at birth, cutaneous stimulation is the first form of encouragement tried.

Joint receptors. It has been shown in both experimental animals and man, that ventilation is increased in passive exercise, and as this still occurs when the veins from the limbs are occluded, the stimulus is likely to be nervous

rather than humoral in origin. It is presumably due to some form of receptor around the joints, but little is known about the mechanism. The effect is very small: the passive movement of a human leg at 100 times per minute causes less than a 50% increase in RMV. Nevertheless it may contribute to the hyperpnoea that develops during exercise, which will be discussed later.

Baroreceptors and cardiovascular changes. It has been shown that large increases in blood pressure which stimulate the baroreceptors in the carotid sinus and aortic arch to inhibit the vasomotor centre, also inhibit respiration. This reflex, however, is very much a secondary effect and is probably of little or no importance in the nervous control of breathing. Although it does not concern the baroreceptors, it is important to realize that any cardiovascular change, whether elicited reflexly or by drugs, which alters the blood flow in the carotid arteries, may affect respiration by the alteration of blood flow to, and therefore oxygen supply of, the carotid body chemoreceptors.

Hiccups and yawning. These are two modifications of the respiratory pattern, the physiological significance of which remains a mystery.

ALTITUDE AND EXERCISE

Most of the foregoing influences on respiration cause only transient effects. There are two physiological situations which, in the normal healthy individual, result in respiration being driven at a greatly increased level, possibly for prolonged periods. However, the cause of the hyperventilation is different in altitude and exercise.

Altitude
This subject is considered in more detail in the section on hypoxia (p. 516).

Exercise
At rest, oxygen consumption is about 250 cm^3/minute and this is provided by a RMV of 6–8 dm^3/minute. In severe exercise, the oxygen consumption can increase to 4 dm^3/minute or more and to provide this the RMV goes up to over 100 dm^3/minute. In the preceding account of the various factors which control respiration, there are several which might contribute to this massive increase.

1 Cortical control. Ventilation often increases before exercise actually starts. This is an anticipation effect and obviously involves the cerebral cortex. In addition, it is probable that the further rapid increase in ventilation at the start of exercise is also initiated by the cortex, as it occurs before any of the other possible factors could come into operation. However, once started, the hyperventilation cannot be voluntarily stopped which suggests that it is then driven by other mechanisms. Immediately exercise stops there is a rapid substantial reduction in the ventilation, followed by a slow return to normal. It is likely that the rapid reduction is partly due to removal of the cortical stimulus.

2 Joint receptors. As mentioned earlier, movement of the limbs can cause a small increase in RMV (about 50%). Nevertheless, it may be an important factor.

3 PO_2 and PCO_2. It is often thought that because of the increased level of muscular activity, the level of CO_2 in the arterial blood must rise and that of O_2 fall and that these cause the hyperventilation of exercise. Studies of arterial blood gas tensions during exercise show little deviation from normal. The increase in ventilation checks any appreciable rise in PCO_2. It is uncertain therefore, to what extent gas tensions in arterial blood stimulate respiration during exercise. It has been suggested that there are chemoreceptors in veins, which would obviously be much more effective than those in arteries, but much more evidence is needed before this mechanism can be substantiated.

4 Lactic acid. During exercise lactic acid is produced and passes into the blood stream where it increases the hydrogen ion concentration in arterial blood despite the buffering effect of plasma bicarbonate. This stimulates peripheral chemoreceptors and certainly contributes to the hyperventilation that occurs during exercise. The lactic acid has a more specific role when exercise has ceased and after the initial rapid reduction in respiration. It causes the ventilation to be maintained at an increased level for maybe as long as 90 minutes. During this time the O_2 debt that the body has incurred during exercise is gradually paid off.

5 Sympathetic nerve activity and adrenaline. During exercise the sympathetic nervous system is active and adrenaline is released into the blood stream from the adrenal medulla. It is possible that these contribute a stimulus for hyperventilation by constricting the blood vessels supplying peripheral chemoreceptors which are then stimulated by the resulting inadequate oxygen supply.

6 Temperature. It has been shown that pulmonary ventilation is increased by an increase in body temperature. The rise in body temperature during exercise could well promote hyperventilation.

It is clear from the consideration of these six factors that no single one provides a full explanation of the hyperventilation that occurs as a result of exercise. It is doubtful that even if the effects of all six are added they would be sufficient. There is, however, evidence of an additional mechanism which co-ordinates some of the above factors and which may provide an integrating synergistic effect. During exercise there appears to be an increase in the sensitivity of the central chemoreceptors to PCO_2. Thus although the level of CO_2 in arterial blood may not be elevated as discussed in (3) above, it may now provide an increased drive to respiration. The increased sensitivity could be caused by the higher temperature and the action of adrenaline.

EMERGENCY ARTIFICIAL RESPIRATION

The object of artificial respiration must be to:
1 Achieve adequate ventilation of the lungs as soon as possible after spontaneous respiration has stopped, and
2 Encourage spontaneous respiration to start again.
If the heart has stopped beating it is necessary to apply external cardiac massage since there is no point in artificial respiration in the absence of a pulmonary circulation.
Respiration can fail as a result of such things as drowning, electric shock, carbon monoxide poisoning, inhalation of a foreign body, food or vomit, and asphyxia from smoke. In all methods it is essential to ensure that the airway is clear and that the tongue does not drop back to cause a blockage.

1 Mouth to mouth method
In this method the operator applies his mouth to the patient's mouth (or nose) and blows his expired air into the patient's lungs at about the normal respiratory rate of 15 times a minute.

The degree of inflation is adjusted to give normal chest movement. The obvious advantage of this method is that the operator can immediately see that his efforts are ventilating the lungs. The common criticism, that 'second-hand air' is being used, is invalid because expired air still contains plenty of oxygen, at least 16% and probably more, as the operator will be hyperventilating (the 4–5% carbon dioxide acts as a respiratory stimulant). A more important criticism is that the positive pressure applied to the lungs causes the intrapleural pressure to become positive (above atmospheric). This tends to prevent venous return, in contrast to the normal negative pressure which assists venous return. Pulmonary capillary blood flow is also impaired by this positive pressure. It is therefore essential to maintain the normal respiratory rate, which ensures long periods of normal intrapleural pressures between inflations, and to refrain from exerting too much pressure when expiring into the patient.

2 Holger–Nielsen and Sylvester methods

These two methods both involve the application of external pressure to the thoracic cavity which forces air out of the lungs, followed by movement of the arms and shoulders which brings about expansion of the thorax and draws air into the lungs. An advantage of these methods is that expansion of the thorax reduces intrapleural pressure and this aids return of blood to the heart. This contrasts with the effects of the mouth to mouth method.

HYPOXIA AND HYPERCAPNIA

Definitions

Hypoxia refers to conditions in which there is an inadequate supply of oxygen to tissues or in which the cells are unable to utilize the oxygen brought to them. This second type is called histotoxic hypoxia and is common in tissues in which there is an accumulation of fluid (oedema) hindering the passage of oxygen from blood to tissues.

Hypercapnia is the accumulation of carbon dioxide in tissues. Hypercapnia often accompanies hypoxia though it is a common error to think that this is inevitable. There are several reasons why it is not obligatory for hypercapnia to be associated with hypoxia. Carbon dioxide is much more soluble than oxygen so that in conditions where fluid accumulates in alveoli, CO_2

readily passes out of the blood into the alveoli whereas the opposite movement of O_2 is restricted. Although cellular production of CO_2 obviously depends on the supply of O_2, confusion stems from the observation that skeletal muscles working under hypoxic conditions seem to produce large quantities of CO_2. This, however, is misleading, as the carbon dioxide originates from plasma bicarbonate during the buffering of lactic acid and not from the metabolism of hypoxic muscle.

The combined effects of hypoxia and hypercapnia are more profound than either alone. These two conditions occur together in hypoventilation and also when there is circulatory impairment as in shock or haemorrhage.

All tissues require a particular amount of oxygen per minute in order to satisfy their particular needs. Nervous tissue has a high oxygen consumption and is consequently very quickly affected by hypoxia. In discussing the response of the body to any stress, both the severity and duration must be considered. As we shall see later, the response to a few minutes of severe oxygen depletion differs from that to several hours of mild hypoxia and this in turn differs from exposure to more prolonged hypoxia—say over several days or weeks.

Hypoxia affects all the tissues of the body when the underlying cause is defective oxygenation of blood in the lungs (hypoxic hypoxia) or when there is a decrease in the O_2-carrying capacity (anaemic hypoxia). This generalized hypoxia can also result from reduced cardiac ouput and deficient blood flow to tissues (stagnant hypoxia). Sometimes hypoxia is localized to only one part of the body as when the blood flow to the hands and feet is restricted on a cold day.

Hypoxic hypoxia

The characteristic defect here is reduced oxygenation of blood in the lungs, thus the P_{O_2} and percentage saturation of haemoglobin both fall, so that insufficient oxygen is delivered per minute to the tissues. The decrease in the P_{O_2} of blood in the capillaries puts at risk all those cells which are farthest away from the vessels because of the reduced diffusion gradient.

Causes of this form of hypoxia include:

1   Exposure to reduced P_{O_2} in the atmosphere, as at high altitude.
2   Insufficient supply of oxygen, during general anaesthesia for example.
3   Hypoventilation or shallow breathing due to

airway obstruction as when a foreign body is inhaled; when airway resistance is increased, as in asthma, and when lung movement is impaired.

4 Congenital heart abnormalities which shunt blood away from the lungs so that blood entering the left side of the heart is only partially oxygenated.

RESPONSES TO REDUCED ALVEOLAR PO_2

Acute hypoxia

The responses to acute hypoxia at high altitude can be studied experimentally in a decompression chamber.

As the total barometric pressure falls, the PO_2 in alveolar air falls relatively more than the PO_2 in the inspired air. This is because water vapour and carbon dioxide are continually being produced in the lungs and they exert a relatively constant pressure in alveolar air which is independent of altitude.

Because of the shape of the oxygen dissociation curve (Fig. 11.31) haemoglobin is still surprisingly well oxygenated even when the alveolar PO_2 has fallen to 60 mmHg.

The first signs of hypoxia in the resting subject occur when the alveolar PO_2 reaches about 60 mmHg (corresponding to about 12 000 feet above sea level). There is a slight increase in pulmonary ventilation, which may be hardly noticeable until light exercise is begun. The ventilation increases to a maximum 2–3 fold when the alveolar PO_2 falls to about 35 mmHg, but below this respiration is depressed in an unacclimatized person. Experiments have shown that the stimulating effect is relatively mild because the co-incident 'blowing off' of CO_2 (hypocapnia) and the decreased H^+ concentration remove the normal stimuli to respiration and oppose the effects of oxygen lack. Cheyne–Stokes or periodic breathing (p. 512 and Fig. 11.35) can develop at reduced atmospheric pressures.

In addition to hyperventilation, there is tachycardia, a redistribution of blood away from the constricted cutaneous vessels and a raised blood pressure.

Increased amounts of 2,3-DPG (p. 507) have been found in red blood cells on exposure to a low atmospheric PO_2 and in patients with chronic obstructive lung disease. This serves to shift the dissociation curve to the right and aids the release of oxygen to the tissues. However, as a result of a lowering of PCO_2 due to hyperventilation, and an increase in pH, the dissociation curve shifts upwards and to the left, so that the effect of DPG is really just offsetting this.

As the hypoxia becomes more severe, dilatation of the pupils, cold sweating and tachycardia indicate that the sympathetic nervous system is stimulated. Mental aberration, lassitude, decreased visual acuity and sometimes a feeling of euphoria indicate that the central nervous system is also disturbed. Frontal headache and vomiting are common. The symptoms have been likened to drunkenness.

Sudden exposure to conditions corresponding to an altitude of 21 000 ft. (i.e. an alveolar PO_2 of about 40 mmHg) causes loss of consciousness within 10 minutes and death in a few hours. The critical arterial oxygen saturation is about 40%.

Chronic hypoxia

Various forms of adaptation take place following more prolonged exposure to hypoxic hypoxia. It was previously thought that the inability to tolerate hypoxia was in part due to the severe effects of the accompanying hypocapnia, such as cerebral vasoconstriction and respiratory depression, but it now seems that the body can adapt to low alveolar PCO_2 levels. The respiratory system becomes less depressed by hypocapnia, partly because the pH shift has been corrected by renal excretion of excess alkali. Pulmonary ventilation is therefore raised further. Slowly acclimatized subjects can remain fully conscious with arterial partial pressures as low as 30 mmHg (O_2) and 10 mmHg (CO_2). Tachycardia also tends to disappear.

One of the most useful adaptations is an increase in the rate at which red blood cells are formed. Because of the increased number of red blood cells it is not uncommon for the arterial blood to be carrying normal quantities of oxygen at quite low alveolar PO_2 levels. When the kidneys are rendered hypoxic by either hypoxic or stagnant hypoxia they release erythropoietin. This hormone is responsible for the bone marrow response.

Anaemic hypoxia

In conditions such as anaemia and carbon monoxide poisoning the oxygen carrying capacity is low but the arterial PO_2 is almost normal (Fig. 11.37). If produced suddenly, as after a severe haemorrhage, the effects of anaemic hypoxia are complicated by the accompanying fall in blood pressure and cardiac output. In chronic anaemia

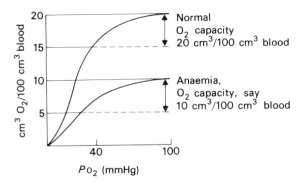

Fig. 11.37. O₂ dissociation curves of normal and anaemic subjects. Note in the case of anaemia that the oxygen requirements of the tissues can only be met by having a lower P_{O_2} (about 28 mmHg) in mixed venous blood. At a tissue P_{O_2} of 40 mmHg only about 3 cm³ O₂ would be released by 100 cm³ blood.

there is a marked decrease in circulation time which usually allows an adequate supply of oxygen to tissues so long as the subject is at rest but he is unable to meet the demands of exercise. There is little or no stimulation of peripheral chemoreceptors since the arterial P_{O_2} is only very slightly reduced.

Stagnant hypoxia

The reader is referred to the section on haemorrhage and shock (p. 727).

COMBINED HYPOXIA AND HYPERCAPNIA

As the respiratory response to an elevated P_{CO_2} is enhanced by a fall in P_{O_2}, their combined effect upon pulmonary ventilation is very marked (Fig. 11.36). The increased depth of breathing causes a reflex tachycardia which, together with stimulation of the vasomotor centre, raises the blood pressure. Cutaneous vessels tend to dilate because of a local action of CO_2.

If the situation is not alleviated by these measures, the subject will experience dyspnoea. As the condition worsens, the force of contraction of heart muscle becomes reduced, cardiac output falls, and a crisis develops when the brain cannot be adequately perfused despite cerebral vasodilatation.

Cyanosis

A feature of persons suffering from hypoxic hypoxia is the bluish colouration of the skin, particularly the lips, nail beds and mucous membranes of the mouth. This is due to the colour of deoxygenated haemoglobin, the absolute concentration of which has increased in the arterial blood entering the capillaries. When more than 5g is present per 100 cm³, the blue colour of

cyanosis appears. The actual shade of colour varies according to the state of the superficial cutaneous blood vessels. If these are dilated, as when hypercapnia accompanies hypoxia, the colour is more intense and more mauve, but if they are constricted there is an ashen blue-grey colour. Cyanosis is also commonly seen in stagnant hypoxia because the slow blood flow allows the tissues to extract more oxygen from a given volume of blood than at normal faster rates. Cyanosis is not found in anaemic hypoxia as the total haemoglobin concentration is then lower than normal so that there is insufficient deoxygenated haemoglobin to exceed the critical concentration.

SPEECH

General functions of the larynx

The larynx is primarily protective both in swallowing and (less commonly) when food regurgitated from the stomach is vomited. In these processes the vocal cords are drawn together, respiration is stopped, and the larynx is raised so that its inlet lies protected under the base of the tongue. Should this mechanism fail, foreign particles entering the larynx are prevented from descending further by a sensory mucosa whose stimulation results in the cough reflex.

Introduction

Speech is the most sophisticated of the many forms of communication between animals. Lack of speech in monkeys and apes, at least as we recognise it, can be attributed to a deficiency in either the development of their central nervous system or the anatomy of their vocal apparatus.

The very complex mechanism of speech basically involves the decision to put a thought into

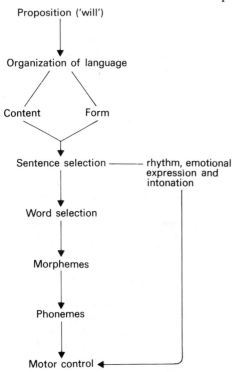

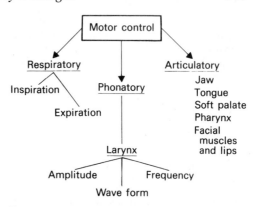

Fig. 11.39. Summary of motor activity in speech.

Fig. 11.38. Suggested 'mental' sequence in the generation of speech.

words, and the organization of these words into a particular sequence and grammatical context (Fig. 11.38). The production of sounds follows and requires highly coordinated movements of the abdominal, thoracic and laryngeal muscles, and of the soft palate, jaws, tongue and lips for the modification of the sound to form consonants and vowels (Fig. 11.39). Although these movements are obviously under voluntary control they are executed without conscious direction so that the highly automated process has been described as an example of 'involuntary motor activity'.

Because of the technical difficulties in carrying out studies on the human larynx, our knowledge of the speech mechanism is rather limited. This deficiency is partly compensated by a substantial amount of information on the neurophysiology of animal larynges, development and disorders of speech; linguistics; and sound physics and communication technology.

Development and generation of speech

Many factors are necessary for the normal development of speech. An adequate hearing mechanism is an essential, not only in young children who are attempting to mimic the spoken words made by others, but also in adults, since aural monitoring is perhaps the most important feedback mechanism in controlling our own speech. The frequent lack of variation and emotional quality in the voices of congenitally deaf persons who have been taught to speak is attributed to their inability to monitor their speech and to introduce inflections and changes in pitch.

The young child also requires adequate stimulation from the environment. This comprises audible, tactile and visual stimuli. Associations are formed in the cerebral cortex between the motor areas for speech and the various areas connected with the recognition of these stimuli.

Maturation and correct structure and function of many intricate systems are essential for normal speech. These systems, cerebral, respiratory, phonatory and articulatory are both executive (motor) and perceptual or proprioceptive.

Last, but not least, there is a required level of intelligence and emotional stability, the most important feature of which seems to be the desire to communicate.

The sequence of events in the generation of speech is summarized in Fig. 11.38. Any suggestion of timing is of course rather ridiculous when one thinks of the rapidity of these processes.

The basis of spoken language is the building up of language sounds (phonemes) into syllables (morphemes). In the English language there are 40 phonemes of which nearly half are vowels. The syllables are put together to form words, then these are arranged to form sentences. The whole operation has to be thought out and planned, probably in the reverse order, ahead of the actual speech utterance. (Hence the order shown in Fig. 11.38.) The cerebral motor area controls the motor neurons whose activity ultimately determines the production of voice and recognizable speech. If we reflect on the stages of speech development in infants we can isolate some phases of this so-called sequence (Fig. 11.38).

SPEECH AREAS (See also p. 939)

The anatomical location of cortical and subcortical speech areas remains a hoary problem because of the relatively crude methods available for locating precisely those brain lesions which are associated with speech defects. However, there is considerable evidence that an area in the temporoparietal region of the left cerebral hemisphere (the dominant hemisphere in right-handed people) is one of the principal speech areas, though coordination between many areas of the brain is necessary (Figs. 11.40 & 11.41).

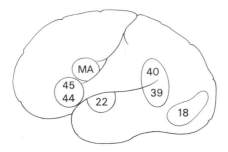

Fig. 11.40. Areas of the left cerebral hemisphere concerned with speech. The primary motor area (MA) is in the pre-central area of the left hemisphere in most individuals. It is necessary for initiating vocalization and articulation. Areas 39 and 40 are for formation of thoughts. The role of areas 44 and 45 is to 'put thoughts into words'. Area 18 is concerned with interpretation of visual recognition associated with language. Area 22 is an auditory area and is intimately concerned with the speech process.

Motor aphasia is a general term which describes the inability to express thoughts in spoken words when there is no abnormality in the effector speech organs or their innervation.

Many areas mediate in the feedback system while others are concerned with the maintenance of muscle tone. Failure of any one of these will cause forms of speech disturbance (Fig. 11.41). Lesions in the cerebellum for example, cause loss of tone, incoordination and loss of synergism in laryngeal muscles (dysarthria).

Feedback systems

Although hearing is the most dominant monitoring system in controlling speech there is experimental evidence that laryngeal structures signal position, movement and tension. Receptor end-organs of various types have been located in the laryngeal mucous membrane, muscles, tendons, perichondrium and joint capsules (Fig. 11.41). These constitute an efficient input. There is still disagreement about the presence of stretch receptors and a fusimotor γ-system in the intrinsic laryngeal muscles. The equivalent role of spindles in the muscles of limbs and digits has probably been taken over in the larynx by joint mechanoreceptors, which, in the cat at least, have been shown to influence the intrinsic muscles reflexly.

Motor systems (Fig. 11.39)

The physiological processes through which speech is effected are respiration, phonation and articulation, and although these are highly integrated and interdependent we must, for simplicity only, consider each in isolation.

RESPIRATION

In producing a sound, a subglottic pressure is built up so that expired air is forced through the constricted glottis past the vocal folds. This provides the necessary force against which the vocal folds vibrate in the production of sound waves. The air escapes as a series of puffs or waves and complex air motion is set up adjacent to the larynx. The magnitude of the subglottic pressure determines the loudness of the sound (amplitude of the waves) as well as the stress and length of speech utterances. During normal speaking the pattern of breathing is significantly altered; the tidal volume is increased from about 500 to 1500—2000 cm^3 and the respiratory rate is reduced, with inspiration occurring rapidly at the end of sentences. Expiration is prolonged and carefully controlled. The output of speech per expiration is roughly constant for an individual but is markedly altered by emotion. Many of us have experienced difficulty in talking associated with breathlessness caused by nervousness or by taking vigorous exercise. Some forms of stuttering are due to incoordination in the speech-breathing apparatus.

During speech the elastic recoil of the lungs is augmented by the increased inspiratory volume. The rapidity and force of expiration is minim-

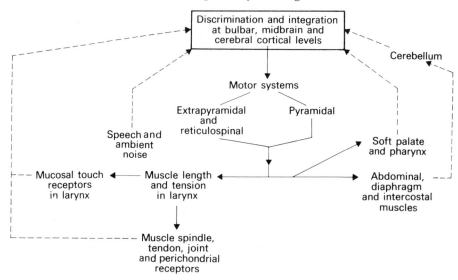

Fig. 11.41. Summary of principal sensory and motor mechanisms in speech.

ized by contraction of the opposing (external) intercostal muscles. Towards the end of a long speech utterance and particularly at the end of a long phrase in singing (Fig. 11.42) the internal intercostal and abdominal muscles are often required to produce an active expiratory effort.

PHONATION

Phonation is the mechanism of voice production. At rest the vocal cords are separated in the 'phonation neutral position'. At the beginning of a sound they are set in motion by the expired air pressure which drives them apart. From this position they recoil; first, due to their composition of elastic and muscle elements and second, due to the Bernouilli force, which is a negative pressure created by the rapid flow of air through the constricted glottis. The expired air pressure now drives them apart again and so the process goes on. The vocal cords traverse an elliptical path, the movement being mainly horizontal but also slightly vertical. Changes in pitch (frequency of sound waves) and quality (wave form or overtones) are produced by rapid changes in the shape, length and tension of the vocal cords, and by variations in their points of contact. This description is sometimes known as the 'myoelastic aerodynamic' theory.

From direct observation one can see that the rima glottidis changes its shape in the production of different sounds; the point of contact can extend along the whole length or be confined to only one portion. These differences are made possible by the different directions of the thyroarytenoid muscle fibres. At high frequencies only the edges of the cords vibrate and these hardly make contact, whereas at low frequencies the motion is very complex with considerable apposition of the cords, particularly when the sound is loud.

Records of the electromyographic activity in the larynx have shown that muscle length and tension are pre-set 1/3–1/2 second before any isolated sound is emitted. Some adjustment could conceivably take place by reflex activity from receptors in the larynx during this interval. The fact that a trained singer with perfect pitch can produce a particular note without any apparent 'search' also suggests that the larynx

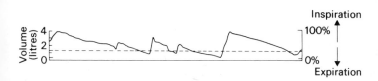

Fig. 11.42. Lung volume changes during singing by an experienced amateur singer. The broken line shows normal expiration. At two points the subject inspired almost maximally.

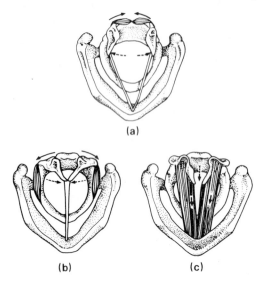

(a)

(b)   (c)

Fig. 11.43. (a) Contraction of posterior crico-arytenoid causes abduction of cords. (b) Adduction of cords caused by contraction of the lateral crico-arytenoid muscles. (c) Adduction and shortening of cords caused by contraction of vocalis (medial) and thyroarytenoid muscles (lateral to vocalis). (After *Diseases of the ear, nose and throat*, Vol. 1, 4th edn. (1979). Editors, J. Ballantyne & J. Groves. London, Butterworth.)

may be accurately set before the sound is made. Such a system might involve a 'template' in the cerebral cortex which sets the tensions of all the relevant muscles and monitors the response. It is known that in normal speech the musculature of the larynx and oropharynx is 'fluid' and is always being adjusted in anticipation of the sound about to be made even while a sound is still being made. Positions are maintained for as little as 300 msec. We are probably dealing in this case with control from an 'engram' or program compiled through experience and stored in the cortex. All the instructions for the various combinations of sounds are, as it were, coded rather like shorthand symbols and these are emitted in correct sequence by the motor speech area. Any mistake cannot be corrected immediately, but is brought to the attention of the program, which is altered accordingly so that no errors are made in the future.

The control of the movements of the larynx is precise and rapid due to the high nerve:muscle ratio of less than 1:200 (compared with 1:1000 in limb muscles) and to the rapid contraction time of the muscles (about 15 msec has been recorded in the thyroarytenoid muscle). Variations in the frequency of the stimulation to some

of the adductors has a large effect on the tension developed since these muscles have tetanus-twitch ratios (p. 338) as high as 10:1.

A subtle balance between subglottal pressure and the tension and length of the laryngeal muscles has to be created for normal phonation. This is achieved by the simultaneous action of various muscles, particularly those which can rotate the arytenoid cartilages (Fig. 11.43). An example will serve to show this complex synergism. To raise pitch while retaining the same sound quality, the air flow is increased and the vocalis muscles are further contracted to stiffen the anterior vocal cords. Since an increased air-flow would necessarily force the cords apart there must be simultaneous activity of adductor muscles to prevent this. Also, contraction of the vocalis muscle would shorten the cords and draw the arytenoid cartilages forward unless this was resisted by contraction of the lateral cricoary-tenoid muscles and the cricothyroid muscles.

Normally, when the vocal cords have thick margins, low tension and increased length, a low pitch (100 Hz) is produced, whereas thin margins with short cords under high tension produce a high pitch (1000 Hz). In normal speaking, changes in the tension and shape of the cords are sufficient to achieve variations in the quality of sound. For the very high notes of a soprano (about 1200 Hz) there is actually an increase in length of the cords caused by contraction of the cricothyroid muscle, but this is more than offset by the simultaneous large increase in tension.

This aerodynamic theory of the laryngeal mechanism is the more generally accepted of two theories. In it the active force in sound production is the exhaled air pressure. In the alternative 'neurogenic' or 'neurochronaxic' theory, the air current is thought to be secondary to the laryngeal muscles and nerves. It is claimed that the vibration of the vocal cords is initiated not by the expired air but by a particular frequency of stimulation in the motor nerves supplying the transverse fibres of the thyroarytenoid muscle. EMG activity recorded from the cords has suggested that they contract and relax at a frequency which is proportional to the frequency of discharge in the nerve. More experimental work is required to resolve these conflicting views.

ARTICULATION

Articulation is the term used to describe the modification of laryngeal sound by the oral and

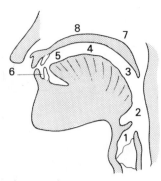

Fig. 11.44. Resonating chambers in which air-waves emanating from the glottis can be modified. Small variations in the shapes of these chambers further modify the sounds.

nasal cavities. Vowel sounds are modified by resonance and voiced consonants are modified by resonance and air flow obstruction. Resonance is created by several chambers (Fig. 11.44) whose shapes are variable. Obstruction to the air flow is offered by the lips, teeth and tongue.

The different vowel sounds are created by high amplitude waves of characteristic frequency which become modified in the mouth and pharynx to give two main harmonics plus several overtones. The air-flow is uninterrupted but is channelled or restricted by the position of the lips and tongue (Fig. 11.45).

In experimental studies both air-flow and pressures from the mouth and nose have been recorded, but unfortunately, in many of these, single consonant or vowel sounds have been used rather than a sequence of sounds as in normal speaking: the results have obscured the important concept that 'in normal speech there are no positions, only continuous movement'. For example, it has been found that the vocal cords move apart 100 msecs or more before a vowel sound ends in preparation for a succeeding voiceless consonant. The position of the soft palate is not constant for the *m* sound; it differs in duration and form in producing the *m* sounds in 'mat', 'amen' and 'camp'. The *p* in 'spin' is produced in a slightly different way from the *p* in 'pin'. The speaker organizes his instructions for the articulation of a given phoneme according to the environment in which that phoneme resides.

The consonants are sounds of low amplitude and are customarily classified by the point or area of articulation and the method of their pro-duction. Thus the *b* and *p* sounds in 'big' and 'pan' are bilabial plosives. The air-flow is obstructed by apposing the lips and followed by their sudden relaxation, whereas *t* and *d* as in 'Tom' and 'dad' are linguodental ('alveolar') plosives because the sounds are made by placing the tongue just behind the upper incisors. Some sounds are made by forcing air through constricted regions and these are called 'fricatives': *f* in 'fun' is a breathed labiodental fricative in which the upper incisors form an incomplete seal with the lower lip, and *v* as in 'van' is similar, but is voiced. Dental fricatives refer to sound made by placing the tip of the tongue between the upper and lower incisors; for example the *th* in 'thick'. When the tongue approaches but does not touch the palate firmly, we produce *s, z* which is voiced, or the unique *r* sound as in 'run'.

The above sounds are typical of most in that the nasal cavity is closed by the soft palate, but for a few, such as *m, n* and *ng,* resonance is produced in the nasal cavity and nasopharynx due to depression of the soft palate and closure of the mouth. The *m* sound is a voiced bilabial and *n* a voiced linguodental.

Articulation defects

The characteristic speech disturbance associated with cleft palate is caused by an excessive escape of air from the nose due to an incompetent soft palate. This not only leads to additional nasal resonance but leads to insufficient intraoral pressure being built up for the production of certain consonants. The *m, n* and *ng* sounds are least affected.

Dental malocclusion frequently leads to speech defects and this commonly affects the *s* and *z* sounds. In some cases of open bite, with a low tongue position, there may be too much air escaping between the top of the tongue and anterior part of the hard palate and this can produce a form of lisping. An inability to extend the lips and tongue causes difficulty in making the *f*, *v*, *p*, *m* and the *th* sounds. A recessive mandible is another cause of such defects. Class I and II malocclusions likewise affect the bilabials. In prognathism there is difficulty in pronouncing *f* and *v* but a 'muddling' of speech sounds can sometimes result because of interference with tongue movements.

The loss of upper incisors due to normal exfoliation in the young child or to extraction or injury of the permanent incisors in later life affects the *f*, *v* and *th* sounds in particular. Some children experience much unhappiness at school because of such speech difficulties.

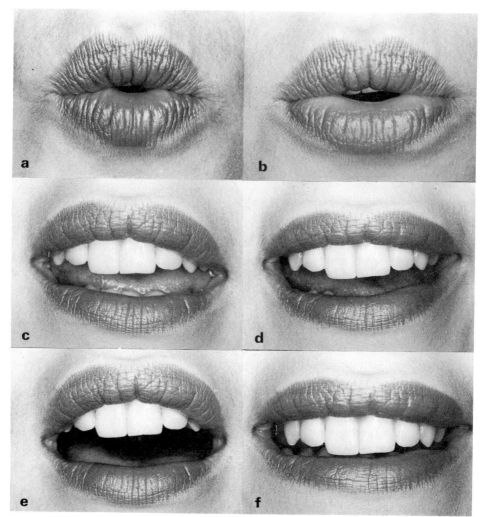

Fig. 11.45. Position of the lips in the production of various vowel sounds. It is necessary that the shape of the resonating chambers in the mouth is also altered by the position adopted by the tongue. (a) oo, (b) o, (c) eh, (d) a, (e) ah, (f) ee.

Defects in the *s, z, ch, j* and *l* sounds are quite common following the fitting of upper dentures and some orthodontic appliances, but in general the subject rapidly adapts to the new situation.

FURTHER READING

COMROE, JULIUS H. (1972) *Physiology of Respiration.* Year Book Medical Publishers, Chicago.

FRY D.B. (1971) Mechanism of normal speech. *Scott-Brown's Diseases of the ear, nose and throat,* Vol. 1, 3rd Edition pp 379–397 Edited by J. Ballantayne and J. Groves. Butterworth, London.

KESSLER H.E. (1945) The relationship of dentistry to speech. *Journal American Dental Association* **48**, 44–49.

PRESSMAN J.J. & KELEMAN G. (1955) Physiology of the larynx. *Physiological Reviews* **35**, 506.

Various contributions in Sound production in Man (1968) *Annals of the New York Academy of Sciences* **755**, 1–381.

CHAPTER 12

$\times$ The Upper Alimentary Tract $\times$

ANATOMY

ORAL CAVITY

The oral cavity (mouth) is the space bounded anteriorly by the lips and laterally by the cheeks. It is roofed over by the palate and has a muscular floor. If the lips are separated the mouth communicates with the exterior. Posteriorly it opens into the oropharynx through the isthmus of the fauces or oropharyngeal isthmus which is bounded laterally by the palatoglossal folds (Fig. 12.1). The oral cavity is divided into the oral vestibule, an outer part (between the lips and cheeks externally and the teeth and alveolar processes of the mandible and maxillae internally) and, internal to the teeth and processes, the oral cavity or mouth proper in the floor of which lies the tongue. With the teeth together the vestibule communicates with the mouth proper behind the last molar tooth. This communication is used for the passage of food when the upper and lower jaw are splinted together in the treatment of fractured jaws.

Lips

These are two fleshy folds surrounding the opening of the mouth. They consist of muscles and glands covered by skin on the outside and mucous membrane on the inside, with both coverings firmly bound to the underlying tissue. The skin and mucous membrane meet at the red margin of the lip (vermilion border). Where the upper and lower lips meet laterally at the angle of the mouth they are connected by a thin fold which is most obvious when the mouth is opened widely. This is called the labial commissure (Fig 12.16). The philtrum is a vertical, midline, shallow groove between the nose and the edge of the upper lip. The tubercle of the upper lip is a projection of the red area just below the philtrum. The nasolabial groove runs downwards and laterally from the ala of the nose where it meets the cheek, towards the angle of the mouth,

and ends about 1 cm lateral to it. It deepens with age. The labiomarginal groove makes its appearance only with advancing age and runs from the angle of the mouth downwards and slightly inwards towards the lower border of the mandible. The labiomental groove is the transverse groove between the lower lip and the prominence of the chin.

The skin of the lips is covered by keratinized stratified squamous epithelium and contains hairs, hair follicles and sebaceous and sweat glands. At the vermilion border between the skin and the mucous membrane, the epithelium is not keratinized. This, together with the vascularity of the underlying dermis, produces the red appearance. Normally when the lips are together, the line along which the lips meet lies just above the lower edge of the upper incisors so that the lower lip is in contact with the upper incisors. The vertical height of the upper lip also shows considerable variation.

The mucous membrane of the lips is covered by non-keratinized stratified squamous epithelium and contains salivary glands in considerable number (labial glands). These are sometimes large enough to be palpable. Both lips have a frenulum, a midline vertical fold of mucous membrane between their deep surface and the gingiva. The upper, which sometimes extends posteriorly onto the alveolar process between the upper incisors thereby maintaining a midline space between them, is much larger than the lower, which may be only vestigial. The main substance of the lips consists of the orbicularis oris muscle (p. 464).

Cheeks

They are similar in structure to that of the lips and consist of an outer skin, an inner mucous membrane and a layer of muscle, the buccinator, together with some of the muscles of the orbicularis oris. The cheek is much more extensive externally than internally; posteriorly the

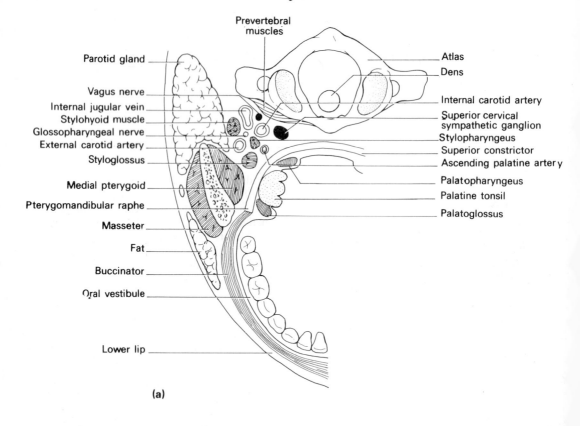

Prevertebral muscles

Parotid gland

Vagus nerve
Internal jugular vein
Stylohyoid muscle
Glossopharyngeal nerve
External carotid artery
Styloglossus

Medial pterygoid

Pterygomandibular raphe

Masseter

Fat

Buccinator

Oral vestibule

Lower lip

Atlas
Dens

Internal carotid artery
Superior cervical sympathetic ganglion
Stylopharyngeus
Superior constrictor
Ascending palatine artery

Palatopharyngeus
Palatine tonsil
Palatoglossus

(a)

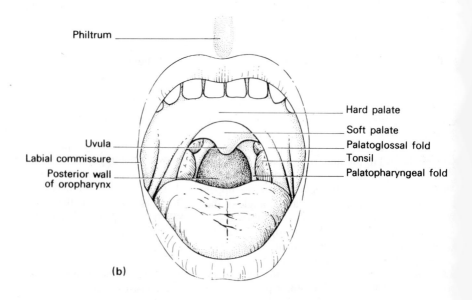

Philtrum

Hard palate

Soft palate
Uvula
Labial commissure
Palatoglossal fold
Tonsil
Posterior wall of oropharynx
Palatopharyngeal fold

(b)

Fig. 12.1. (a) Horizontal section through the head at the level of the atlas. (b) Structures seen in the open mouth.

masseter and a small part of the parotid gland lie deep to the skin. Internally the cheek is bounded above and below by the reflection of the mucous membrane from the cheek to the jaws, regions known as the upper and lower fornices of the vestibule. It is limited posteriorly by a fold of tissue between the maxillary and mandibular alveolar processes in which lies the pterygomandibular raphe. The superior constrictor of the pharynx is attached to the back of the raphe.

The cheek contains the parotid duct which pierces the buccinator and opens into the vestibule of the mouth opposite the upper second molar tooth. The opening is marked by a small elevation, the parotid papilla. There are numerous mixed glands deep to the mucous membrane, the buccal glands. Some may lie external to the buccinator muscle and open opposite the last molar tooth (the molar glands).

There is a pad of fat lateral to the posterior part of the buccinator. This extends backwards between the buccinator and masseter muscles and is continuous with the fat between the rest of the muscles of mastication. It is relatively much larger in the newborn and infants and has been called the suckling pad although there is some doubt as to whether it has a specific function in relation to suckling.

Tongue

The tongue is a muscular organ lying partly in the mouth and partly in the pharynx. For reasons based on anatomical and clinical considerations, the mylohyoid muscle is considered to separate the neck from the mouth (Fig. 12.6). Muscles above the mylohyoid muscle are in the mouth; those below the mylohyoid are in the neck.

Anteriorly the tongue has a free mobile part which at rest is relatively horizontal, and a more fixed posterior part (the base or root) which is almost vertical. The tip of the tongue is called the apex (Fig. 12.2). The upper surface of the anterior part and posterior surface of the fixed part are called the dorsum of the tongue which is divided into an anterior two-thirds and a posterior third by a V-shaped groove, the sulcus terminalis, which has its apex pointing backwards. Immediately behind the apex of the sulcus terminalis is a small pit called the foramen caecum which is the site of origin of the thyroid diverticulum. The sulcus terminalis divides the tongue into two parts which differ in development, innervation and structure.

The part of the tongue which lies in the floor of the mouth has an inferior surface which is covered by a much thinner mucous membrane than that found on the dorsum. As a result the deep lingual vein passing towards the apex can be seen (Fig. 12.3). Lateral to this vein is the fimbriated fold (of connective tissue) running in the same direction. The frenulum of the tongue is a vertical median fold passing between the inferior surface of the tongue and the floor of the mouth. Where the inferior surface becomes continuous with the floor of the mouth there is a transverse fold, the sublingual fold, which indicates the position of the sublingual salivary gland(s). At the medial end of this fold, at the side of the frenulum, there is a small papilla on to which opens the duct of the submandibular salivary gland.

The dorsal surface of the anterior part of the tongue has a longitudinally running median sulcus and different types of papillae which are described below. Posterior to the sulcus terminalis the dorsal surface is studded by small irregular elevations which are due to underlying lymph follicles (lingual follicles) and are collectively called the lingual tonsil, part of Waldeyer's ring (p. 662). Laterally this surface of the tongue is continuous with the lateral wall of the pharynx. Posteriorly there is a space between the tongue and the anterior surface of the epiglottis. A sagittal midline fold, the median glossoepiglottic fold and a fold on each side, the lateral

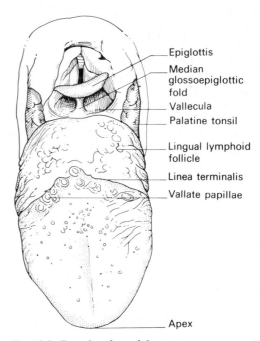

Epiglottis

Median glossoepiglottic fold

Vallecula

Palatine tonsil

Lingual lymphoid follicle

Linea terminalis

Vallate papillae

Apex

Fig. 12.2. Dorsal surface of the tongue.

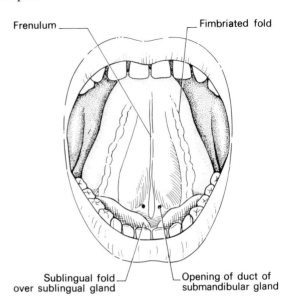

Frenulum ___   ___ Fimbriated fold

Sublingual fold ___   ___ Opening of duct of
over sublingual gland   submandibular gland

Fig. 12.3. Inferior surface of the tongue.

glossoepiglottic fold, bound two small hollows called the valleculae.

The muscles of the tongue are divided into intrinsic and extrinsic. There are three groups of intrinsic fibres, which are (by definition) those confined to the tongue itself (Fig. 12.4). These are vertical, transverse and longitudinal. The vertical fibres pass from the dorsal to the inferior surface at the sides of the anterior part of the tongue. The transverse are attached to a sagittal fibrous partition in the tongue (septum linguae) and pass laterally to the sides of the tongue. The longitudinal fibres form superior and inferior muscles running superficially along the whole length of the tongue. The vertical fibres flatten and broaden the tongue. The transverse fibres produce elongation and narrowing, and the longitudinal shortening. The superior longitudinal turn the tip upwards and the inferior longi-

tudinal turn the tip downwards. The tip of the tongue is protruded by contracting the vertical and transverse fibres while relaxing the longitudinal fibres.

The extrinsic muscles are attached to structures outside the tongue (Figs. 12.5 & 12.6). The hyoglossus is attached to the greater cornu and adjacent part of the body of the hyoid bone and passes vertically upwards forming the most lateral part of the tongue except superiorly where the fibres of the styloglossus mingle with those of the hyoglossus. The hyoglossus has a number of important relations. The stylohyoid muscle and tendon of the digastric are superficial to it and it is overlapped anteriorly by the mylohyoid muscle. The lingual and hypoglossal nerves pass downwards and forwards on its superficial surface, the lingual superior to the hypoglossal, and the submandibular ganglion is between the

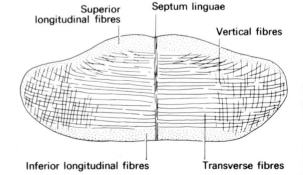

Superior   Septum linguae
longitudinal fibres

Vertical fibres

Fig. 12.4. Transverse section through the anterior free part of the tongue.

Inferior longitudinal fibres   Transverse fibres

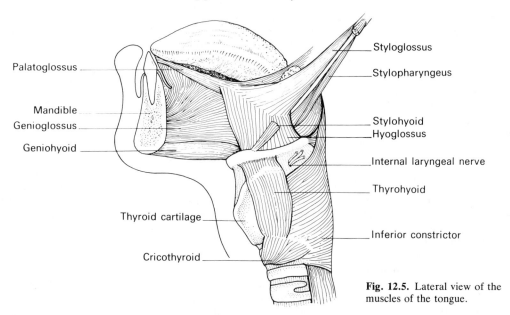

Palatoglossus

Mandible
Genioglossus

Geniohyoid

Thyroid cartilage

Cricothyroid

Styloglossus

Stylopharyngeus

Stylohyoid
Hyoglossus

Internal laryngeal nerve

Thyrohyoid

Inferior constrictor

Fig. 12.5. Lateral view of the muscles of the tongue.

nerves and suspended from the lingual nerve. The deep part of submandibular gland, its duct and a part of the sublingual gland are on the superficial surface of the muscle (in the mouth). The lingual artery and the glossopharyngeal nerve pass forwards deep to the hyoglossus. The action of the hyoglossus is to pull the tongue downwards. To do this most efficiently the hyoid bone is held down by the infrahyoid muscles.

The styloglossus (Fig. 12.5) is attached above to the anterior surface of the styloid process. It passes downwards and forwards into the tongue where its fibres mingle with those of the hyoglossus and more anteriorly with the fibres of the

longitudinal intrinsic muscle. The styloglossus pulls the tongue upwards and backwards.

The genioglossus (Fig. 12.5) is attached to the upper part of the mental spine (formerly the upper genial tubercle) of the mandible. It is a fan shaped muscle lying in the sagittal plane near the midline. Its superior fibres pass upwards and forwards into the tip of the tongue and the rest of the fibres are found throughout the whole of the tongue on either side of the midline. The lowest fibres are attached to the body of the hyoid bone near the midline. The majority of the fibres pass backwards and their main effect is to pull the back of the tongue downwards and forwards: the

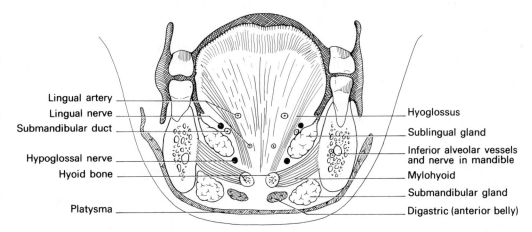

Lingual artery
Lingual nerve
Submandibular duct

Hypoglossal nerve
Hyoid bone

Platysma

Hyoglossus

Sublingual gland

Inferior alveolar vessels and nerve in mandible

Mylohyoid

Submandibular gland

Digastric (anterior belly)

Fig. 12.6. Coronal section through the mouth at the level of the second molar tooth.

more vertical, anterior fibres pull the apex of the tongue down. Acting together the two genioglossi can produce a longitudinal midline furrow in the tongue.

The palatoglossus muscle has already been described (p. 487). It is the most inferior muscle of the soft palate and runs in the palatoglossal fold in front of the palatine tonsil. In the tongue it mingles with the fibres of the styloglossus and the transverse intrinsic muscle. The palatoglossus pulls the side of the tongue upwards and/ or the soft palate downwards. It has an important role in swallowing, first helping to close the entrance from the mouth to the oropharynx before the food passes through and subsequently helping to close the entrance again when the food is in the oropharynx.

The artery of the tongue is the lingual, a branch of the external carotid. Some arterial blood reaches the tongue through the ascending pharyngeal artery and the tonsillar branch of the facial artery.

All the intrinsic muscles and the extrinsic muscles are supplied by the hypoglossal nerve except the palatoglossus which is supplied by the pharyngeal plexus. The motor nerve of this plexus is the pharyngeal branch of the vagus. The sensory innervation is general and special (taste) and differs between the anterior two-thirds and the posterior third. The lingual nerve from the mandibular nerve is the nerve of general sensation to the anterior two-thirds. The taste fibres from this part of the tongue are in a branch of the facial nerve, the chorda tympani, which joins the lingual nerve near the base of the skull. The glossopharyngeal nerve supplies the posterior third of the tongue with both general and special fibres. The taste buds of the vallate papillae, although anterior to the sulcus terminalis, are supplied by the glossopharyngeal nerve. The sympathetic nerves to the arterioles pass with the lingual artery from the superior cervical sympathetic ganglion. The parasympathetic secretomotor fibres to the serous glands, the ducts of which enter the troughs surrounding the vallate papillae, are in the glossopharyngeal nerve.

Innervation of tongue

1 *Motor.* Hypoglossal, except palatoglossus supplied by pharyngeal plexus (motor nerve is branch of vagus).
2 *Sensory.* (a) Anterior two-thirds; general —lingual nerve (mandibular); special (taste)— chorda tympani (facial).

(b) Posterior one-third; general and special— glossopharyngeal. Taste buds of vallate papillae —glossopharyngeal.
3 *Autonomic.* (a) Sympathetic, from superior cervical sympathetic ganglion.
(b) Parasympathetic to anterior two-thirds of tongue—chorda tympani; to posterior one-third—glossopharyngeal.

ORAL MUCOUS MEMBRANE

The oral mucous membrane is the tissue lining the mouth. It is analogous with the skin and has many structural features in common with skin. Its two major layers, the oral epithelium and (mesodermal) lamina propria are equivalent to the epidermis and dermis of the skin. The surface is kept permanently moist by the secretion of the major and minor salivary glands. Reduction or absence of such secretion can be a serious disability.

Underlying much of the oral mucous membrane or oral mucosa, there is a layer of connective tissue called the submucosa. Obviously the submucosa is not part of the oral mucosa but it plays an important part in its function and will therefore be included in this description.

General

SUBMUCOSA

The submucosa is the connective tissue which intervenes between the lamina propria (p. 379) and the tissue on which the oral mucosa lies (e.g. muscle, periosteum). Histologically, it can be distinguished because of its loose texture in comparison with that of the very dense lamina propria. As well as the basic elements of connective tissues it may contain fat, salivary glands and ducts, the larger blood vessels, lymphatics and nerves. A submucosa may be absent, as in the gingiva, over the midline raphe and at the periphery of the hard palate, the dorsal surface of the tongue and intermittently over the cheeks. In such areas the lamina propria is firmly bound to the fibrous investment of underlying tissue (perimysium or periosteum): when bound to a periosteum the combination of tissues is referred to as a mucoperiosteum.

The degree of mobility of the oral mucosa on underlying tissues is dictated by the submucosa. Where the submucosa is absent (gingiva) or is densely fibrous (hard palate) the oral mucosa is fixed in position. Where the submucosa is a loose areolar tissue (e.g. vestibular fornix) the mucosa is freely mobile. Both in structure and in function the submucosa is to the mucosa as the superficial fascia is to the skin.

The lamina propria comprises the dense connective tissue intimately related to the epithelium. Just as the dermis imparts strength to the skin, so lamina propria imparts strength to the mucosa. The dermal papillae project between rete pegs or folds in the basal layer of epithelium. The lamina propria contains collagen and reticulin fibres and sometimes elastic fibres together with fibroblasts and other connective tissue cells. Capillary loops and lymphatics, nerves and nerve endings enter from the submucosa or underlying tissue and ducts of salivary glands pass through the lamina propria to open on to the surface of the epithelium. There are no salivary glands in the lamina propria.

EPITHELIUM

The ectodermal component of the oral mucosa is a stratified squamous epithelium which may be keratinized or non-keratinized. It consists of a number of layers of cells which from the basal layer to the surface represent stages in a continuous differentiation of individual cells (Fig. 12.7).

Keratinized epithelium
The structure of the keratinized epithelium is virtually the same as that of the epidermis of the skin to which reference should be made (p. 406). Differences are mainly quantitative.

There are none of the epidermal appendages described for skin except for occasional sebaceous glands in the lips and cheeks. The layers of the oral epithelium are the same as those of the epidermis, i.e. stratum basale, spinosum, granulosum and corneum (a stratum lucidum is never present) (Fig. 12.7).

The characteristics of the individual layers are similar to those of skin but some degree of variation is seen in the stratum corneum. Particularly in the gingiva (p. 532) the conversion of the epithelial cells to horny squames may not necessarily be accompanied by loss of the nuclei. Where the nuclei are lost the process is referred to as orthokeratosis and where they persist it is called parakeratosis. Further consideration of this phenomenon is found in the section on gingiva (p. 532).

In man, cells of keratinized oral epithelium take about 10 days to mature and desquamate. There is regional variation in the rate of turnover which is much more rapid in oral mucosa than in skin.

Keratinized oral epithelium is impermeable. In the case of the cells this property is probably due to a thickened plasma membrane (p. 166). In the intercellular spaces it is due to a barrier of glycolipid secreted by the cells of the stratum spinosum and stratum granulosum.

Non-keratinized epithelium
In general, non-keratinized oral epithelium is thicker than keratinized oral epithelium. The stratum basale and stratum spinosum resemble those of the keratinized form but the epithelial cells flatten out towards the surface of the stratum spinosum. The remaining layers of a keratinized epithelium are not present. The cells

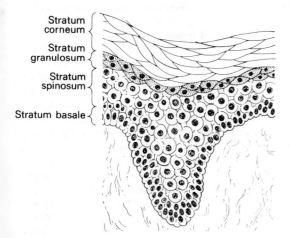

Stratum corneum
Stratum granulosum
Stratum spinosum
Stratum basale

Fig. 12.7. The layers of the oral epithelium.

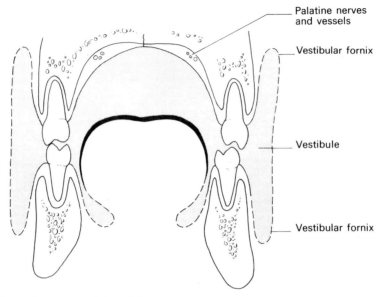

Fig. 12.8. The oral mucosa consisting of the masticatory mucosa (line), the lining mucosa (broken line) and the gustatory mucosa (heavy line).

remain nucleated until they are shed. In the superficial layers the cell membranes become thickened like those in a keratinized mucosa. Non-keratinized epithelium appears to be more permeable than keratinized epithelium and skin but only to low molecular weight organic compounds such as the drug glyceryl trinitrate.

Regional variation

The oral mucosa may be divided into three functionally and structurally different types. There are masticatory mucosa, lining mucosa and gustatory mucosa (Fig. 12.8). The vermilion border of the lip which is intermediate between skin and oral mucosa has special features of its own.

Masticatory mucosa

This lines the hard palate and most of the gingiva.

GINGIVA

The mucosa of the gingiva has two distinct parts. The part visible in the mouth is covered with keratinized epithelium but the gingival sulcus (crevice) related to the surfaces of the teeth and continuous with the junctional epithelium is non-keratinized. The keratinized and non-

keratinized epithelia are continuous with each other at the gingival margin. Figure 12.9 shows the arrangement of the gingiva. A short distance (0–0.5 mm) below the gingival margin is a shallow free gingival groove which marks externally the apical limit of the gingival sulcus. Between the groove and the gingival margin is the free gingiva whose extent depends on the depth of the gingival sulcus. Apical to the gingival groove is the attached gingiva. On the palatal aspect of the maxillary teeth the attached gingiva merges almost imperceptibly with the mucosa of the hard palate. Elsewhere there is a more or less distinct mucogingival junction between the keratinized gingival epithelium and the non-keratinized lining epithelium of the vestibular mucosa and the floor of the mouth. This junction is most distinct in the vestibule where it is seen as a scalloped line between the more opaque and hence pale pink gingival mucosa and the translucent and hence reddish or pigmented shiny alveolar mucosa. The attached gingiva has a finely pitted surface, easily seen in reflected light and is sometimes called stippled gingiva. This effect is due to. the insertion of bundles of collagen fibres into the lamina propria from the periosteum and periodontal ligament.

There is no submucosa deep to the oral mucosa of the gingiva. The epithelium with its lamina propria, and the periosteum of the alveo-

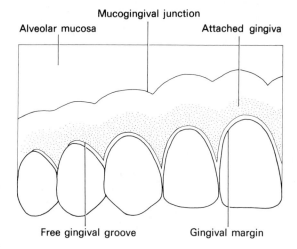

Alveolar mucosa   Mucogingival junction   Attached gingiva

Free gingival groove   Gingival margin

Fig. 12.9. The arrangement of the gingiva.

lar bone, together constitute a mucoperiosteum. The collagen fibres of the lamina propria merge with those of the fibrous layer of the periosteum and with the gingival fibres of the periodontal ligament. The attached gingiva is therefore immovable over its underlying structures.

When seen in sections the gingival epithelium has long rete pegs (Fig. 12.10): these represent sections through tall ridges which may extend far down into the lamina propria. In a random sample of human gingivae a high proportion are parakeratinized and a few may even lack keratin. It is most likely that these variations are the result of the inflammation of the gingiva found at some time in most of the population. The more rigorously and effectively the teeth and gingivae are cleaned, the greater the proportion which show orthokeratinization.

Tissue similar to gingival mucosa is also found immediately distal to the lower third molar, where there is a pad of tissue known as the retro-molar pad. The retro-molar pad has a submucosa which sometimes contains minor salivary glands. In the upper jaw this gingiva is continuous with the lining mucosa over the hook of the pterygoid hamulus.

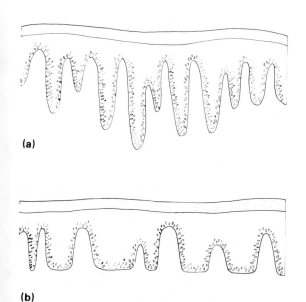

(a)

(b)

Fig. 12.10. (a) Gingival epithelium, showing long rete pegs.
(b) Epithelium of the hard palate.

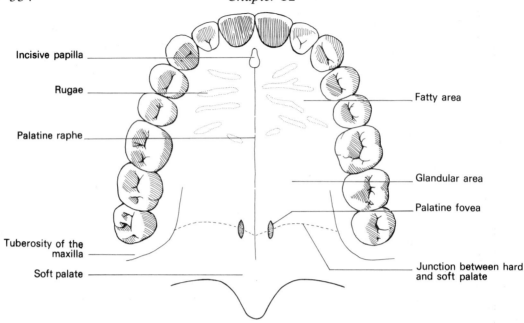

Fig. 12.11. The appearance of the hard palate.

HARD PALATE

The oral mucosa of the hard palate is continuous with that of the gingiva. It has an opaque whitish appearance anteriorly but posteriorly appears more shiny and red. There are more or less prominent ridges or rugae in the mucosa on either side of a midline raphe which ends anteriorly as a papilla (the incisive papilla) over the incisive foramen (Fig. 12.11).

In the hard palate, a submucosa is not found peripherally at the junction with the gingival mucosa or along the midline raphe. In these areas, as in the gingiva, the palatal mucosa is part of a mucoperiosteum, firmly-bound to the underlying bone. Elsewhere in the hard palate there is a submucosa between the lamina propria and the periosteum covering the palatine processes of the maxillae and the horizontal plates of the palatine bones (Fig. 12.12). Anteriorly this submucosa contains fat and posteriorly it contains palatine mucous glands. It also contains the palatine arteries, veins and nerves along the sides in a softish region which can be palpated with the forefinger. The peculiarly tough character of the submucosa is due to dense bundles of collagen fibres which run vertically from the lamina propria to the periosteum so that the palatal mucosa is virtually immovable.

In the normal hard palate the epithelium is always orthokeratinized. The basal layer is thrown into wide ridges or rete pegs but these are relatively shallow and square-cut so that, in contrast to those of the gingiva, they end at a line roughly parallel to the surface (Fig. 12.12).

GINGIVAL SULCUS

The gingival sulcus is limited coronally by the gingival margin and apically by the junctional epithelium.

Lining mucosa

The non-keratinized lining mucosa lies over the cheeks, vestibular fornices, alveolar processes, inner surfaces of the lips, soft palate, floor of the mouth and under surface of the tongue.

Much of the lining mucosa lies over muscle and here there is only a little, patchily distributed, loose submucosa. The lamina propria is close to the perimysium and the mucosa is barely mobile: in surgical procedures the lamina propria cannot be cleanly separated from the muscle. Over limited areas a more extensive submucosa is present. It accommodates the minor salivary glands and the ducts of the major salivary glands, vessels and nerves. In the vestibular fornices and alveolar vestibular mucosa, over bone and periosteum and the attachments of the buc-

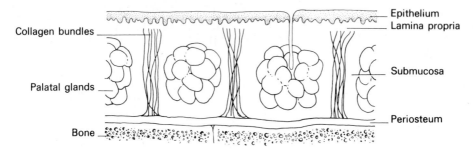

Epithelium
Lamina propria
Collagen bundles
Submucosa
Palatal glands
Periosteum
Bone

Fig. 12.12. The structure of the oral mucosa and submucosa of the hard palate.

cinator muscle (rather than the buccinator muscle itself) the submucosa is an extensive loose connective tissue which is readily split to allow the preparation of a surgical flap of mucosa. The mucosa of the soft palate is separated from the palatine aponeurosis by mucous glands and lymphoid tissue.

In the cheeks and lips isolated sebaceous glands may be present. They are visible as small white spots known as Fordyce spots. Their number increases with age.

Gustatory mucosa

The dorsal surface of the tongue is specialized to undertake mechanical and gustatory (taste) functions. Taste buds lie over the sides and dorsum of the tongue and also on the soft palate and epiglottis. The dorsal surface of the tongue is divided by a V-shaped groove, the sulcus terminalis, into two parts, an anterior two thirds and a posterior one third or pharyngeal portion (Fig. 12.2). At the posteriorly pointing apex of the V is the foramen caecum which represents the termination of the embryological thyroglossal duct derived from the thyroid diver-

ticulum. The specialized papillae of the tongue all lie anterior to this line.

On the dorsum of the tongue a keratinized epithelium covers a series of papillae overlying a dense lamina propria which is tightly bound to the perimysium of the intrinsic muscles of the tongue. There is little submucosa and the mucous and serous lingual glands are accommodated between the bundles of muscle fibres.

The papillae of the tongue are classified according to their shapes.

FILIFORM PAPILLAE

These are arranged in lines approximately parallel to the sulcus terminalis. They have a dermal core, with smaller secondary papillae. The stratum corneum over the surface is extended into several short spiky processes. During illness, when little food is eaten, the keratin is not worn away and the tongue appears furry.

FUNGIFORM PAPILLAE (Fig. 12.13)

These are scattered singly over the surface with a concentration near the tip of the tongue. They

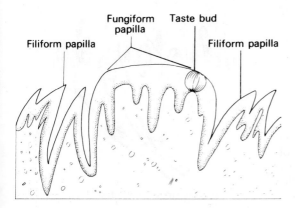

Fungiform papilla   Taste bud
Filiform papilla   Filiform papilla

Fig. 12.13. The papillae of the tongue.

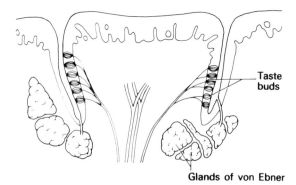

Fig. 12.14. Vallate papilla of the tongue.

Glands of von Ebner

appear red because of the vascularity of the dermal core. The epithelium is flat over the surface of the projecting rounded papillae but the core extends into secondary papillae by pushing into the basal layer of the epithelium. The epithelium of fungiform papillae contains taste buds.

VALLATE PAPILLAE (Fig. 12.14)

These are the most easily recognized papillae and are up to 12 in number. They are found just anterior to the sulcus terminalis. Unlike the filiform and fungiform papillae the vallate papillae do not project above the surface. The large, flat, upper surface is surrounded by a trough or furrow, lined by keratinized epithelium containing numerous taste buds. A number of ducts from the posterior lingual glands (or serous glands of von Ebner) open into the base of this furrow. The connective tissue core spreads out in the body of each papilla giving rise to numerous secondary papillae projecting into the epithelium.

FOLIATE PAPILLAE

These are large, red, leaf-like projections found at the sides of the tongue sometimes referred to as folia linguae. They are homologous with the papillae found in this region in other mammals (e.g. rabbits) but are of doubtful significance in man although they contain taste buds.

TASTE BUDS (Fig. 12.15)

Taste buds are ovoid bodies wholly contained within the gustatory epithelium. The long axis of a taste bud extends from the basal lamina to a small opening between the superficial epithelial cells called the gustatory pore. Each taste bud

consists of spindle-shaped supporting cells whose distal ends surround the base of a small pit beneath the gustatory pore. Interspersed between the supporting cells are the sensory (taste) cells from whose ends microvilli project into the pit.

Vermilion border of the lip

At the mucocutaneous junction of the lips there is a red border which is intermediate between the skin and the labial mucosa. No epidermal appendages are present in the vermilion border and it is not moistened by saliva except by licking the lips. The epithelium is thick with large, vacuolated, keratinized cells at the surface. The basal lamina has long irregular, tubular, invaginations which accommodate capillary loops from the lamina propria. Many of these reach to within a few cells of the surface resulting in the characteristic red colour of the lips and in their

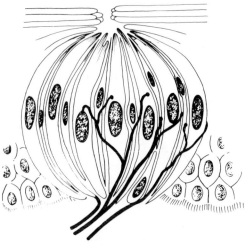

Fig. 12.15. The structure of a taste bud.

peculiar fragility and susceptibility to drying. The proximity of the capillary loops to the surface also explains the ease with which cyanosis can be detected in the lips (by their blue colour).

Pigmentation

The oral mucosa may be pigmented. In general terms the degree of pigmentation in the mouth is related to the level of pigmentation in the skin. As in the skin, pigmentation depends on the presence of melanocytes (p. 408). The number of melanocytes varies from place to place in the mouth but varies little from person to person. The amount of pigment produced is related to the activity of the cells and not to the number of cells.

SALIVARY GLANDS

The salivary glands are those glands which secrete saliva and are generally classified as major and minor.

Major salivary glands

The major salivary glands comprise three pairs of large glands: the parotid glands; the submandibular glands; and the sublingual glands.

THE PAROTID GLAND
(Fig. 12.16a, b, c & d)

The parotid gland is the largest salivary gland. In the transverse plane it is wedge-shaped with the broad base of the wedge lying superficially, covered by skin, superficial fascia and the parotid capsule (Fig. 12.16c). The apex of the wedge is the deepest part of the gland, and is separated from the internal jugular vein and lateral wall of the pharynx by the styloid process and its attached muscles and ligament. Thus the main bulk of the gland is wedged between the ramus of the mandible, masseter and medial pterygoid muscles anteriorly and the mastoid process, sternocleidomastoid and posterior belly of digastric muscles posteriorly. Anteriorly, parts of the parotid gland are packed deep to the medial pterygoid muscle and into the space between it and the mandible. In some individuals a separate, accessory, lobe of the parotid lies on the surface of the masseter muscle (Fig. 12.16b). Posteriorly, part of the gland may extend into the space between the mandibular condyle and the posterior end of the articular fossa.

The capsule of the parotid gland is formed by the deep cervical fascia, which extends upwards from the neck as the parotid fascia, to be attached above to the bone of the zygomatic arch. The poorly defined fascia deep to the gland is attached to the sheaths of nearby muscles, the styloid process and the angle of the mandible. It is thickened to produce the stylomandibular ligament which lies between the parotid gland and the submandibular gland (Fig. 12.16a).

The facial nerve enters the deep posterior aspect of the gland and divides within its substance. Its branches emerge along the anterior border of the gland (Fig. 12.16d). If the gland has to be partially or completely removed for any reason the facial nerve is at risk. If a branch of the nerve is cut the relevant muscles of facial expression are paralysed. The external carotid artery enters the gland at the deep surface of the lower pole. It supplies the gland by means of minor twigs and divides into its terminal branches, the superficial temporal artery and the maxillary artery, in the gland substance. The superficial temporal artery leaves the gland at the upper pole and the maxillary artery pierces the anterior medial surface of the gland.

The retromandibular vein is formed within the capsule by the superficial temporal vein and the maxillary vein. It runs through the gland and leaves it near the lower pole having already divided into its anterior and posterior divisions.

The gland receives a parasympathetic supply from the auriculotemporal nerve which passes through the upper pole. This parasympathetic supply is derived from the glossopharyngeal nerve (p. 538, 902). The gland also receives a sympathetic nerve supply from the superior cervical ganglion via the plexus surrounding the external carotid artery.

The parotid gland receives arterial blood from the external carotid and its branches within the gland. Blood drains into tributaries of the external jugular vein. The lymphatic drainage is to the superficial and deep cervical lymph nodes. There are a number of parotid lymph nodes within the gland and on its surface.

THE SUBMANDIBULAR GLAND
(Fig. 12.17a, b & c)

The submandibular gland is somewhat variable in size but is much smaller than the parotid. It lies partly under cover of the mandible (Fig. 12.17b) where it rests on a smooth oval depression in the bone below the mylohyoid line (Fig. 12.17a).

The mylohyoid muscle is the muscular floor of the mouth and by definition separates the mouth above from the neck below. The submandibular gland hooks round the sharply defined posterior border of the mylohyoid muscle so that a larger, superficial part of the gland is in the neck below mylohyoid and a smaller deep part is in the mouth, above mylohyoid (Fig. 12.17a & c). The superficial part is covered by skin, the platysma muscle and the investing layer of deep cervical fascia which is attached to the lower border of the mandible. The facial artery lies in a groove in the gland deep to the mandible before curving round the lower border of the mandible at the anterior edge of masseter muscle (Fig. 12.17b).

The deep part of the gland, the part in the mouth, lies between the mylohyoid and hyoglossus muscles (Fig. 12.17c). It extends forwards as far as the posterior pole of the sublingual gland.

The duct of the submandibular gland, much of it contained within the gland substance, hooks round the sharp posterior edge of mylohoid muscle and runs forward in the mouth between the mylohyoid and hyoglossus muscles. It continues forward between the sublingual gland and the genioglossus muscle to open into the floor of the oral cavity at the sublingual papilla lateral to the frenulum of the tongue. The duct is crossed by the lingual nerve (Fig. 12.17a).

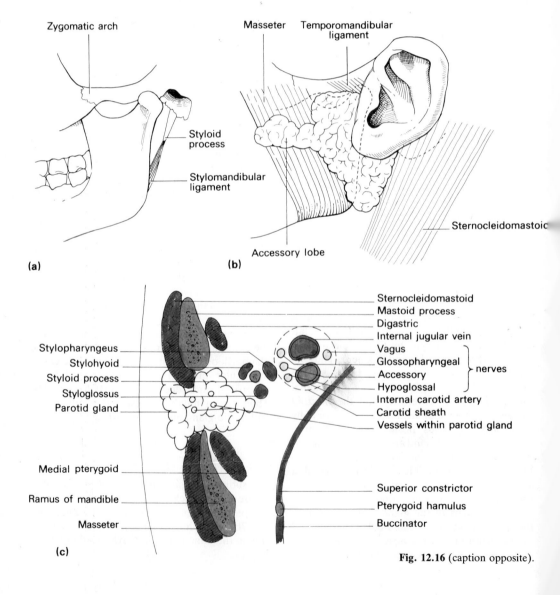

(a)

(b)

(c)

Fig. 12.16 (caption opposite).

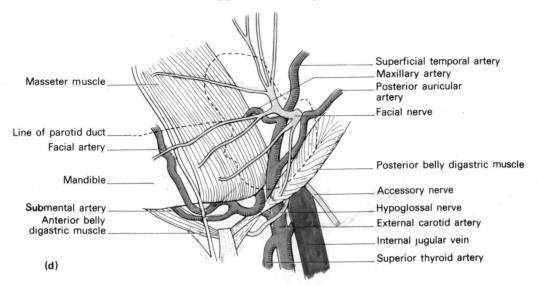

Masseter muscle

Line of parotid duct
Facial artery

Mandible

Submental artery
Anterior belly
digastric muscle

(d)

Superficial temporal artery
Maxillary artery
Posterior auricular artery
Facial nerve

Posterior belly digastric muscle

Accessory nerve
Hypoglossal nerve
External carotid artery
Internal jugular vein
Superior thyroid artery

Fig. 12.16. The parotid gland. (a) Structures deep to the gland. (b) The position of the gland relative to the ear. (c) The position shown in the transverse plane. (d) The position of the gland relative to vasculature and innervation.

The blood supply of the submandibular gland comes from branches of the facial and lingual arteries, the nerve supply from the lingual branch of the mandibular division of the trigeminal nerve. Post-ganglionic parasympathetic fibres come from the submandibular ganglion which is suspended just below the lingual nerve. The preganglionic fibres travel in the chorda tympani nerve. The sympathetic supply is derived from the cervical sympathetic trunk via the plexus round the external carotid artery.

THE SUBLINGUAL GLAND

The sublingual glands are the smallest of the major salivary glands. They lie beneath the sublingual folds of oral mucous membrane in the sublingual fossae of the mandible each side of the symphysis menti. Each gland lies on the mylohyoid muscle and extends back to the anterior pole of the deep part of the submandibular gland (Fig. 12.17a). It is related medially to genioglossus muscle, lingual nerve and submandibular duct.

The sublingual gland is drained by multiple ducts which empty into the mouth along the summit of the sublingual fold of oral mucous membrane. There is often a larger duct opening at the summit of the sublingual papilla or even into the submandibular duct.

The sublingual gland is supplied by the submental artery which pierces the mylohyoid muscle and by the lingual artery. Its nerve supply is similar to that of the submandibular gland.

Minor salivary glands

The submucosa of the oral cavity contains numerous small aggregations of glandular tissue known as the minor salivary glands. They may be classified according to their positions.

BUCCAL AND LABIAL GLANDS

Small, easily palpable nodules of poorly encapsulated glands are distributed in the submucosa of the lips and cheeks. The ducts open on the surface of the oral mucosa.

PALATINE GLANDS

In the densely fibrous submucosa of the posterior part of the hard palate lie the palatine glands. Posteriorly they increase in size and merge with aggregations of glands in the soft palate which form a thick glandular layer between the oral mucosa and the muscle of the soft palate. Inferiorly they join a group of glands lying in the palatoglossal folds (anterior pillars of the fauces).

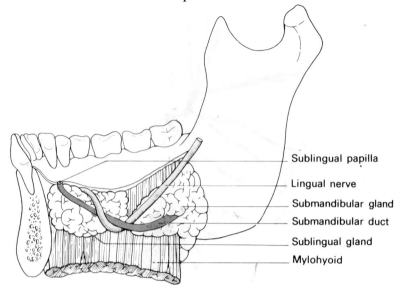

(a)

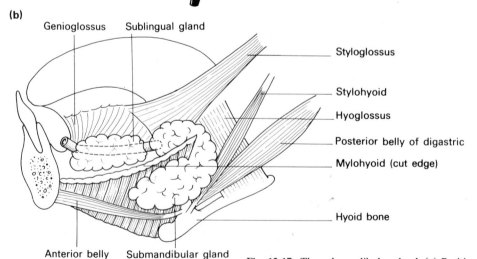

(b)

(c)

Fig. 12.17. The submandibular gland. (a) Position relative to the mandible, (b) to the facial artery, (c) and to the mylohyoid and hyoglossus muscles.

LINGUAL GLANDS

Anterior lingual glands are situated either side of the midline near the tip of the tongue with ducts opening on the undersurface of the tongue near the frenulum.

There are two distinct groups of posterior lingual glands: mucous glands which open into lingual crypts; serous glands with ducts which open into the troughs of the vallate papillae. The latter are known as the glands of the vallate papillae or glands of von Ebner.

PHYSIOLOGY OF THE MOUTH

Functions of the tongue

CLEANSING

The role of the tongue in cleansing is intimately linked with its highly developed sensory function. The ability of the tip of the tongue to explore, locate and retrieve food particles from the vestibule and buccal cavity and from between the teeth provides a good example of not only its sensitivity but also its precision of movement. Experimental evidence suggests that position sense is augmented by a proprioceptive system from the muscles of the tongue; thus the control of tongue movements and position sense are retained even after inferior alveolar and lingual nerve blocks. Despite what standard textbooks of anatomy say about the purely motor function of the hypoglossal nerve, there may be some proprioceptive fibres in this nerve.

ARTICULATION (See also p. 422)

In recent years attention has been drawn to disorders of speech and mastication in people with impaired lingual sensation. The sense of position of the tongue for articulation probably depends on both the lingual tactile receptors and on receptors in deep muscles which are deformed by the pressure of the tongue against the hard palate or teeth. The direction and velocity of movement are monitored by the proprioceptive muscle spindle system (p. 468).

PERCEPTION

The oral perception of shape, size and texture is highly developed in normal healthy people, but is less accurate than manual perception. When subjects use their hands and eyes to select test objects of similar size to those placed in their mouths, they usually select bigger objects. Appreciation of size is distorted in the oral cavity. It is important that patients should be reassured of this when they detect a cavity in a tooth or an ulcer on their tongue.

PROTECTION

The tongue and lips act as an important sensory system guarding the oral cavity and upper alimentary tract from extremes of temperature and the ingestion of noxious materials. Highly specialized nerve endings for taste perception are distributed over the dorsum of the tongue. Stimulation of these allows us to appreciate an immense range of flavours (p. 543). The saliva which covers the tongue helps to dissolve substances and distributes the solutions to a wider area.

SWALLOWING (See also p. 578)

The decision to swallow a mouthful of food is taken when information received in part from tactile endings on the dorsum of the tongue, is interpreted as indicating that the consistency is acceptable. The mass of chewed food is then separated into smaller portions by the tongue and swallowed. The bolus which has been lubricated by saliva during the movement of food around the mouth during chewing is propelled backwards by the tongue.

TOOTH POSITION AND JAW SHAPE

In a quite different role the tongue influences the position of the teeth and perhaps the shape of the dental arch. During infancy, the tongue is in continuous contact with the walls of the oral cavity proper. It has been proposed that it helps to mould the shape of the jaws and the positions of the erupting incisors, but the extent and duration of this influence is still a matter for debate. Some authorities hold the opposite view; that the tongue form is moulded by the arch enclosing it. They suggest that as the jaws increase in size and the teeth erupt, the tongue no longer 'overflows the gum pads' and being easily accommodated within the jaws it now produces less force on the surrounding structures. The subject is discussed in Vol. 1, Book 2, p. 31.

Taste

Before it can be tasted a substance must be dissolved; an important function of saliva is to provide the solvent. A stone, for example, is tasteless because it cannot be dissolved. The dissolved substances stimulate taste cells in the oral cavity and these initiate action potentials in the nerves which supply them (Figs. 12.18 & 12.21). The sensation of taste stimulates further salivation which aids in swallowing, in buffering acids, and in diluting harmful substances introduced into the mouth. It also stimulates gastric secretion. As an indicator of the edibility of substances, taste is notoriously unreliable: many poisons, particularly those in plants, have a pleasant taste.

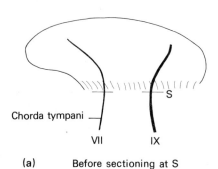

(a)   Before sectioning at S

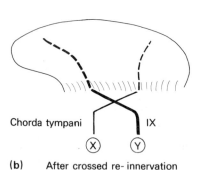

(b)   After crossed re-innervation

Fig. 12.18. Diagram of innervation of the taste cells of the tongue in cross-regeneration experiment. The cut end of the chorda tympani is anastomosed with the distal empty stump of the glossopharyngeal, and the cut end of the IXth nerve joined to the distal part of the chorda tympani. The summated electrical responses recorded at X and Y after re-innervation of peripheral cells had been achieved were different from those obtained prior to the sectioning. The response to chemicals applied to the tongue were typical of the area of the tongue which was stimulated and not the fibre which innervated it. (a) Before suturing at S. (b) After crossed re-innervation. (After Oakley & Benjamin (1966) *Physiological Reviews* **46**, 173–211.)

RECEPTORS AND NERVE PATHWAYS

The gustatory or taste cell is a modified epithelial cell which resides in a taste bud and together with its nerve supply can be regarded as a functional taste unit. When the sensory nerve is cut, the taste cell degenerates. If the nerve regenerates and reaches the epithelium the cells are renewed and function is restored. Materials are probably synthesized in the nerve cell body and carried forward by axoplasmic flow to maintain the integrity and differentiation of the gustatory cells. It is the taste cell receptor and not the nerve which determines which chemicals activate the sensory nerve (Fig. 12.18).

Taste buds are distributed over areas of the tongue which vary in taste sensitivity. The mapping of the tongue into regions of differing sensitivity (Fig. 12.19) is less precise than many textbooks would have us think. Taste buds are also found in the pillars of the fauces, hard and soft palate, epiglottis and pharynx.

Olfactory receptors contribute to the detection of some tastes. Tactile and thermal-sensitive endings may contribute to the perception of certain flavours such as mint, pepper, alcohol and curry. Upper dentures, by covering receptors in the palate, may diminish the appreciation of certain tastes.

The nature of the coupling between taste cell excitation and nerve activity is still largely unexplored. Taste-cells contain aggregates of vesicles resembling those found at synapses and nerve endings. This suggests that taste may be mediated by a chemical transmitter and the histochemical demonstration of cholinesterase in the adjacent nerve fibres lends support to this view.

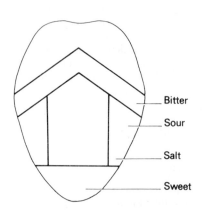

Fig. 12.19. A map of the areas of the tongue which are particularly sensitive to the four differently tasting substances.

Presumably the cholinesterase breaks down acetylcholine released by stimulated taste cells.

Many nerve fibres of the small, unmyelinated variety, innervate each taste bud and even a single taste cell can be served by many fibres, some of which enter invaginations of the cell membrane. In the rat at least, the same fibre can supply different papillae on the tongue. A plexus-like arrangement of fibres, both myelinated and unmyelinated, borders the epithelium containing the taste-buds.

When chemicals are applied to the tongues of rats and cats or when papillae are stimulated electrically, activity can be recorded at various levels up to the cerebral cortex (Fig. 12.20). These include the tractus solitarius and the cephalic part of its nucleus, the medial lemniscus and the ventromedial part of the thalamus. From here fibres project to both the motor area for mastication in the precentral gyrus and the sensory area for face and tongue in the postcentral gyrus. The cortical area for taste as such is still ill-defined.

Diverse lines of evidence, such as the finding that an injection of alcohol into the trigeminal

ganglion impairs taste sensation in some subjects (hypogeusia), suggest that there is more variability in the routes taken by taste afferents than is classically described.

MODALITIES OF TASTE

It is a common experience that we can distinguish four primary modalities of taste; sour (acid), sweet, salt and bitter, though others such as alkaline and metallic have been added by some writers. Indirect evidence for four groups of sapid substances (substances that can be tasted) comes from experiments showing that single papillae or single nerve fibres can be stimulated by members of only one of the groups. Local anaesthetics like xylocaine, when sprayed over the dorsum of the tongue abolish tastes in the order; bitter first, then sweet, salt and sour. Flavours and other complex tastes are explained by the simultaneous combination of smell and taste and simultaneous stimulation of several types of taste receptor. Tastes can change because of successive contrast; that is, the influence of a preceding stimulus on the one

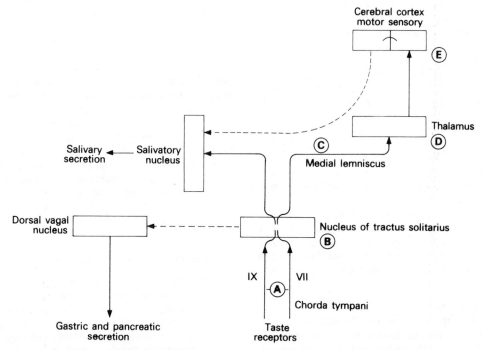

Fig. 12.20. Schematic representation of pathways taken by taste stimuli. Electrical responses have been recorded at the points labelled A–E. There is evidence for convergence of taste messages carried by different peripheral nerves (glossopharyngeal and chorda tympani) in thalamic and cortical neurons. (Based on descriptions by Oakley and Benjamin (1966), Halpern (1967). In *Chemical Senses and Nutrition*, Editors M. R. Kare & O. Maller. Hopkins Press, Baltimore.)

which follows. An example of this is the transient change in the appreciation of taste which follows the use of medicaments, dentifrices and mouth-washes containing, for example, menthol, thymol or chlorhexidine.

As might be expected, different substances which have similar tastes often have some common structural feature, though there are notable exceptions. This finding is compatible with a theory on the mechanism of taste, namely that there is adsorption of molecules onto receptor sites in the cell membrane or on to enzymes. A 'key and lock' arrangement has been suggested.

Sweet-tasting substances are commonly polyalcohols, such as the sugars and glycerol, but the synthetic sweetener, saccharine, some notorious lead and beryllium salts and chloroform are exceptions. The importance of the spatial arrangement of atoms and groups is illustrated by the progressive reduction in sweetness of equimolar solutions of sucrose, fructose, maltose, glucose and lactose.

Salt-tasting substances are, as the name suggests, caused by salts, particularly the anion, though an interaction with the cation occurs. The sodium halides afford an interesting comparison since the taste of equimolar solutions decreases in the order, chloride, bromide, iodide and finally the almost tasteless fluoride.

Bitter substances, to which the vallate papillae are particularly responsive, are mostly organic molecules such as quinine, morphine, nicotine, caffeine and bile salts, to mention a few. Some chemical groups associated with this taste are $-CN$, SCN, $-N=$, $-SH$ and $-S-S-$.

Much interest has centred around phenylthiourea (phenylcarbamide). The inability of about 30% of the population to taste this substance is an inherited characteristic. This taste 'blindness' does not extend to other bitter substances.

Sourness is associated with acidity, but since organic acids such as tartaric, citric and ascorbic are more sour than equimolar hydrochloric acid it is obvious that factors other than the hydrogen ion concentration are involved.

Taste thresholds

A taste threshold is usually defined as the minimum concentration at which the particular taste is correctly appreciated. Taste thresholds are affected by many factors such as the temperature of the solution, the presence of a conditioning stimulus, the age, health and nutritional status of the subject.

The threshold for sucrose in young adults is less than in the elderly. This reduction in sensitivity with age is paralleled by a decrease in the number of taste buds. Tests show that the salt threshold, and to a smaller extent sugar threshold, of heavy smokers are significantly higher than non-smokers of the same age. Changes in taste thresholds have been reported in certain endocrinal disturbances such as adrenal cortical insufficiency and may be due to the sensitivity of taste receptors being altered by the chemical composition of saliva flowing over them.

RECEPTOR MECHANISMS

Very little is known about the initial events which lead to the change in nerve membrane potential when certain chemicals are applied to taste cells. It is commonly suggested that specific protein receptors in taste buds bind to sapid substances. 'Sweet and bitter receptors' have been isolated biochemically. Membrane potentials have been recorded in taste cells. In response to the application of solutions with different tastes, hyperpolarization or depolarization may be seen, even in the same taste cell. These non-propagated receptor potentials then in some way cause excitation of the sensory nerves.

A second theory is based on the demonstration of high concentrations of enzymes in the region of taste buds. It has been shown histochemically that these enzymes are activated or inhibited by certain sapid substances which are not themselves the substrates for the enzymes. However, if such enzymes were involved in taste, pH changes and the presence of certain cell poisons would probably alter taste perception much more than they do. It is also difficult to explain how variations in the rate of substrate breakdown can alter a generator potential.

NEURAL CODING FOR TASTE

In common with other sensory systems, an increase in the strength of stimulus (a sapid solution) leads to an increase in the frequency of electrical activity in the sensory nerve and possibly also the recruitment of receptors with higher activity thresholds. Studies in both man and animals have related the subjective appreciation of taste to the electrical responses in taste nerves. These are an important landmark in sensory physiology.

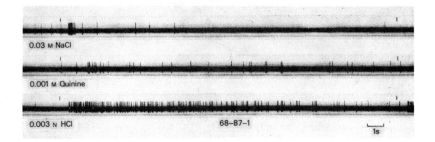

Fig. 12.21. Electrical activity recorded in a single fibre of the cat chorda tympani nerve in response to the application to the tongue of three different chemical solutions, 0.03 M NaCl, 0.001 M quinine and 0.003 NHCl. Adaptation is seen in the response to each.

Though there is a lack of specificity, the different temporal pattern of responses to different chemicals is obvious. The solutions were applied between points on and off. (From Wang M. B. & Bernard R. A. (1969) *Brain Research* **15**, 567–570, with permission.)

Taste has been investigated in animals by aversion or preference behaviour studies: an animal is taught to avoid a particular solution in one of several different drinking vessels. Obviously it can only become conditioned to one solution in preference to another if it can discriminate between their tastes. Attempts are made to relate the behaviour to measurements of the electrical activity in taste nerve fibres.

How is neural coding interpreted and recognized by the brain as a taste modality? The doctrine of specific nerve energies implies that separate modalities must have separate receptors and pathways. This view is still held for most sensory systems. However, a single fibre of the chorda tympani may respond to stimulation of the tongue by chemicals normally associated with different taste qualities (Fig. 12.21). This finding, which has been amply confirmed in many species, can be explained if one fibre innervates several different papillae, taste buds or taste cells. Each fibre and possibly even each receptor responds to a range of stimuli. As the width of this spectrum varies, both receptors and their nerve fibres are either fairly specific or 'broadly tuned'. But this still leaves the problem of how activity in a fibre is interpreted by the brain. The probable answer is that it is the frequency of firing in many fibres at the same time which provides a code for taste quality. This 'composite input pattern' or 'across-fibre profile' is analysed centrally. It has been found that the more similar are those patterned responses to different chemical stimuli the more difficult it is to discriminate between their tastes (Fig. 12.22).

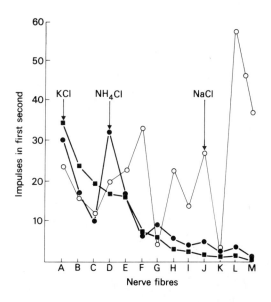

Fig. 12.22. 'Across-fibre' profiles for 13 single fibres from the rat chorda tympani nerve. These fibres are lettered A–M. The electrical activity in the first second (before significant adaptation) is recorded in response to the application of three different salt solutions to the tongue. The similarity in across-fibre profile between 0.1 M NH₄Cl and 0.3 M KCl matches the inability of animals to discriminate between these solutions in behavioural tests whereas the distinct pattern obtained with 0.1 M NaCl explains the ability to distinguish this salt from the others. (After Marshall (1968) *Physiology and Behaviour* **3**, 1–15.)

Salivation

HISTOLOGY OF SALIVARY GLANDS

A salivary gland consists of secretory cells arranged in acini, leading into tubules connected with a duct system terminating in a main excretory duct. The whole is enclosed by a fibrous tissue framework supported by septa which join an outer capsule. The connective tissue septa divide the gland into lobes and the lobes in turn into lobules (Fig. 12.23).

Human salivary glands can be classified according to the type of secretory cell they contain, serous or mucous or mixed.

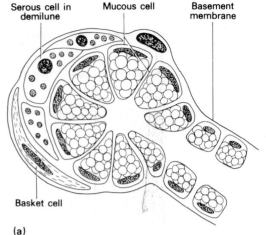

(a)

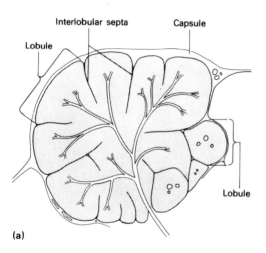

(a)

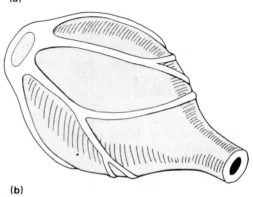

Fig. 12.24. A mucous acinus, and secretory tubule (a) and (b) basket cell clasping an acinus.

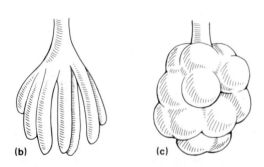

(b)   (c)

Fig. 12.23. (a) A single lobe of the submandibular gland which is divided into lobules by septa running inwards from the connective tissue capsule. Only one vessel is shown for the sake of simplicity but this could equally represent an artery, a vein or even the system of interlobular ducts. In any case it would be more complex than is shown. (b) and (c) microscopic clusters of tubular and grape-like acini.

Major salivary glands
Parotid—almost entirely serous secretory cells, possibly some mucous cells at birth declining rapidly in number with age.
Submandibular—mixed, predominantly serous.
Sublingual—mixed, predominantly mucous.

Minor salivary glands
Buccal and labial—mixed, predominantly mucous.
Palatine—mucous.
Anterior lingual—mixed.
Posterior lingual—mucous except for the glands of the vallate papillae which are purely serous.

Secretory tissue
The secretory epithelial cells are arranged in clusters of grapelike or tubular acini (Fig. 12.23). Each acinus surrounds a central lumen which may not be visible in light microscopy

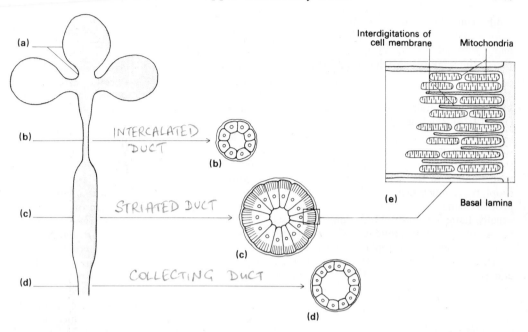

Fig. 12.25. (a) An acinus and its duct sectioned at the level of (b) an intercalated duct, (c) striated duct, (d) collecting duct. (e) Shows the nature of the striations in (c).

(Fig. 12.24). The whole acinus is surrounded by a basement membrane. The lumens of the acini are continuous with those of the other acini of the cluster and in turn with that of the secretory tubule, also lined with secretory cells. The tubule is continuous with a narrow non-secretory intercalated duct lined with cuboidal epithelium (Fig. 12.25). From the intercalated duct, the secretions enter a striated duct. This is much larger and is lined with a columnar epithelium with characteristic basal striations. It leads into the smallest collecting ducts.

The intercalated ducts, striated ducts and smallest collecting ducts are known as intralobular ducts. They run in the interstitial connective tissue between acini and not in the well-defined connective tissue septa. The smallest collecting ducts unite to form progressively larger ducts which are situated in the connective tissue septa and are known as interlobular ducts. Ultimately they join together to form tributaries to the main duct of the whole gland (Fig. 12.23).

An acinus of a salivary gland is composed of either serous or mucous cells but not both. In a mixed gland the mucous cells are concentrated locally in mucous acini while the serous cells are arranged in demilunes which sit like caps on these mucous acini (Fig. 12.24). A basement membrane surrounds the whole complex. The serous cells of the demilune do not appear to abut on to a permanent lumen. Their secretion is discharged into temporary intercellular canaliculi between the serous cells and between the acinar mucous cells.

Most salivary acini are associated with a further type of cell—the myoepithelial or basket cell (Fig. 12.24). These cells have extended cytoplasmic processes which clasp the entire acinus. Myoepithelial cells are enclosed, together with the acinar cells in a basement membrane.

CYTOLOGY

Serous cells
Secretory products within zymogen granules dominate the cytoplasm of serous cells (Fig. 12.24). They contain protein and glycoprotein including the enzyme ptyalin (amylase) or its intracellular precursor. The (acidic) granules stain intensely with basic dyes and obscure much of the detail of the cells in the light microscope. The nucleus of the cell is large and round and may lie towards the base but is not flattened against the basal plasma membrane. Ultrastructurally the serous cell is a typical protein-

synthesizing and secretory cell so that there is a large amount of granular endoplasmic reticulum and a substantial Golgi apparatus which gives rise to the secretory droplets (p. 170).

Mucous cells

Mucous cells contain large pale-staining droplets (Fig. 12.24) which are closely packed with little or no intervening cytoplasm. The structure of the droplets is more difficult to preserve in a stained preparation so that they often resemble soap bubbles in the cell. The contents of the droplets are much richer in highly glycosylated proteins than those of serous cells. The nucleus is usually flattened and curved along the basal border of the cell. In a mucous cell packed with secretory droplets the cytoplasm is a mere rim at the base and sides of the cell. It contains granular endoplasmic reticulum and a large Golgi apparatus.

Myoepithelial cells

The extraordinary myoepithelial cells have cytoplasmic extensions which clasp an acinus in octopus-like fashion. The cytoplasm contains numerous fibrils resembling those of smooth muscle cells. This cell appears to be contractile and is believed to help expel secretory products from the acini.

Ducts

Not all the ducts are passive transporters of fluid. The cells in striated ducts possess the structure characteristically observed in cells which indulge in active ion transport. The basal striations, when seen by electron microscopy, consist of mitochondria orientated in rows parallel to the long axis of the cell (Fig. 12.25). The adjacent plasma membrane of the cell is folded into the cytoplasm to form a doubled membrane which lies between the columns of mitochondria. This arrangement brings a large volume of mitochondrial material—producing energy in the form of ATP—into the immediate vicinity of a relatively huge area of plasma membrane. Plasma membranes in situations such as this often contain ATPases so that the energy is utilized very close to its source. It is known that the ionic composition of saliva is substantially changed as it passes down the ducts, a process consuming energy.

The histology of the connective tissue elements of salivary glands is not significantly different from that of similar tissues elsewhere in the body.

SALIVARY SECRETION

Because of the accessibility of the acini, ducts, nerves and blood supply, the salivary glands have been subjected to considerable study. Until recently more of this has been directed towards understanding the nature and control of secretory mechanisms than the functional significance of the secretion.

Secretion, in its broadest sense, implies the transport of raw materials into the cell, the manufacture and sometimes the storage of the constituent to be secreted and, lastly, extrusion. Salivary glands, in common with other exocrine glands, have a complex system of ducts which modify the primary (acinar) secretion so that the ducts cannot be regarded as mere conduits. The control of the secretion and its modification are each intimately linked to the control of the blood supply to the gland.

These topics, together with an overall view of reflex salivation and salivary composition will be considered. One of the factors which bedevils the literature on salivary secretion is the enormous variation between species and even between glands within one species. The discussion will be confined, as far as possible, to human secretion.

Nature of the secretory process

Acinar secretion. Since the pioneering studies of Ludwig and Heidenhain 100 years ago, it has been generally accepted that saliva is not formed by mere filtration through the blood capillaries and acinar cells, but that it is an active, metabolically dependent process which continues when ductal pressure is raised well above capillary pressure.

Salivary secretions consist of water, electrolytes, proteins, traces of lipid, and small organic molecules including amino acids, urea and glucose. By micropuncturing ducts close to the acini it is possible to collect and analyse what is effectively the acinar secretion (Fig. 12.25b). It proves to be isotonic and to contain electrolytes which in composition and concentration resemble those of plasma. The electrolyte composition does not change with alterations in the rate of secretion suggesting that in acini the secretion of electrolytes is linked to that of water.

The following changes take place during secretion. A sodium pump maintains a low intracellular level of sodium and high level of potassium in the resting cell (Fig. 12.26). When stimulated by acetylcholine liberated from parasympathetic nerve terminals close to the basal plasmalemma, the cell membrane becomes more permeable; K^+ leak out of the cell and fewer Na^+ leak in along with Cl^-, with the result that the cell becomes hyperpolarized (the inside of the cell becomes more negative). By a process of active transport Na^+ are now pumped out of the cell into the acinar lumen or intercellular spaces and these are accompanied by Cl^-. In these regions the osmotic pressure is raised and water is pulled out of the cell so contributing to the primary secretion.

Proteins such as amylase are manufactured by the rough endoplasmic reticulum, transferred in vesicles to the Golgi region and become membrane-bound, presecretory granules before maturing into zymogen granules. On receipt of the appropriate stimulus their membrane fuses with the luminal membrane and the contents are discharged (Fig. 12.27). The rate at which such proteins are synthesized is related to their rate of secretion but the nature of the feedback control is uncertain. Some salivary proteins originate from the ductal cells.

Duct function. Several different techniques have confirmed that sodium and chloride are progressively reabsorbed along the ducts, particularly in the striated ducts, and that potassium and bicarbonate are secreted; all at rates which to some extent are related to the rate of salivary flow (Figs. 12.28 & 12.29). Even at the highest flow rates, when the contact time between luminal fluid and reabsorptive surfaces is negligible,

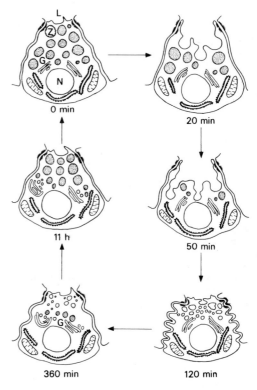

Fig. 12.27. Schematic representation of the ultrastructural changes during the secretory cycle in the rat parotid gland *in vitro*. At 0 min. the resting cell is full of zymogen granules (Z). The gland is then stimulated with isoprenaline (a β-adrenergic stimulant) and after 20 min. the apical granules have been expelled into the lumen (L); the contours of the lumen suggest that fusion of granule membrane and apical cell membrane has occurred. The process continues and the lumen appears much enlarged. By 120 min. there appear small vacuoles formed by condensation of the 'new' apical membrane. Secretory vesicles and zymogen granules appear around the Gogli apparatus (G) at 360 min. and accumulate during the remaining period up to 11 hr. (After Amsterdam, Ohad and Schramm (1969) *Journal of Cellular Biology* **41**, 753–773.)

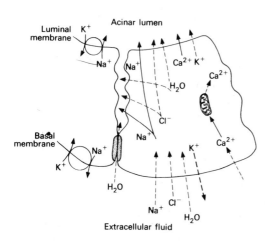

Fig. 12.26. A model for the transport process in the acinus during the formation of primary saliva. Two adjacent cells are represented; on the left is a resting cell and on the right is a cell stimulated with acetylcholine (ACh). Broken arrows indicate passive fluxes occurring along existing electrochemical gradients and fully drawn arrows represent active processes. The stimulus alters the permeability of the basal membrane to K^+ and in some way causes active Na^+ extrusion into the lumen. Modified from several papers by Petersen *et al.*

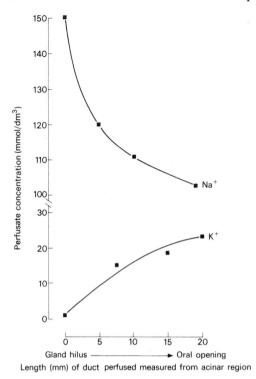

Gland hilus ⟶ Oral opening

Length (mm) of duct perfused measured from acinar region

Fig. 12.28. Final concentrations of sodium and potassium in perfusate as a function of the length of duct perfused. Isotonic saline containing ^{22}Na or ^{42}K was perfused at a slow constant rate through the main excretory duct from the rat submaxillary gland. The total length of this duct from its origin (hilus) to opening in the mouth is about 27 mm. (Modified from Schneyer (1972) *Oral Physiology* pp. 61–73. Pergammon Press, Oxford.)

the final sodium concentrations rarely reach that of the primary secretion (about 143 mmol Na/dm³). This suggests that some sodium is actively reabsorbed by a mechanism which is not affected by rate of flow.

Ductal activity (in the rat submaxillary gland) is influenced by parasympathetic and probably by sympathetic stimulation but the effects are too complex to discuss here.

In some respects duct cells have similar properties to those of the nephron. First, they are relatively impermeable to water as is the loop of Henlé. Second, some reabsorption and secretion

is selective: this leads to wide variations in the saliva/plasma ratios of different substances (Table 12.2 and Fig. 12.30). Third, hormones such as aldosterone alter the ductal reabsorption of sodium.

Nervous control of secretion

In most species including man, parasympathetic nerve activity causes a profuse flow of watery saliva. The sympathetic nerves are responsible for a sparse flow of viscous fluid. In the parotid gland, simultaneous stimulation of both autonomic nerves results in saliva with a lower flow rate and with a higher content of protein than that resulting from parasympathetic stimulation alone. Other observations also suggest that serous cells receive a dual motor supply, parasympathetic and sympathetic. For example, the electrical potential of single cells responds differently to parasympathetic and sympathetic stimulation. In addition, electron micrographs have shown cholinergic and adrenergic axons alongside a single cell (Fig. 12.31). It seems probable that myoepithelial and mucous cells also receive a dual nerve supply but the position of duct cells is less certain.

Both physiological and histological evidence suggests that several parasympathetic fibres can converge on one cell and that a change in membrane permeability is not an 'all or none' phenomenon (Fig. 12.32a). The rate at which saliva flows is proportional to the frequency of stimulation of the parasympathetic nerves over a particular range (Fig. 12.32b). Myoepithelial or 'basket' cells probably take part in the expulsion of saliva, but their precise role is not clear. It has been suggested that the onset of secretion is preceded by their contraction and that this reduces the volume of the acinar and proximal duct system and prevents any distension during secretion.

Extensive EM studies have shown that the neuroeffector 'contact' is often of the 'en passant' type, with one axon in a bundle of axons, bared of its Schwann cell investment, leaving a gap of about 100 nm between it and the effector cell. More intimate contact is also seen, in which the free axon penetrates the basement membrane to reside within some 20 nm of the cell. Along its length one axon may influence many cells.

Control of blood supply. For over a century it has been known that the blood vessels receive sympathetic vasoconstrictor nerves and that

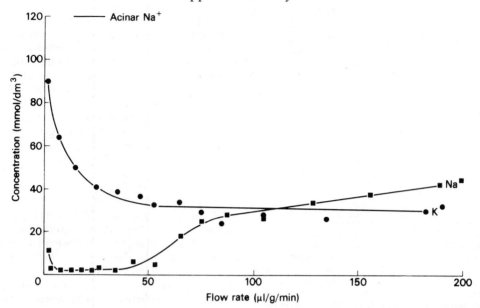

Fig. 12.29. Effect of stimulation with carbachol, a parasympathomimetic drug, upon the sodium and potassium concentrations in saliva from the rat submaxillary gland. The concentrations of potassium at the highest flow-rates is still greatly in excess of that in plasma (4.5 mmols/dm³) and in the primary secretion. Similarly sodium concentrations at these high flow-rates are much less than that in plasma (147 mmols/dm³). These findings suggest that active mechanisms independent of the flow-rate can proceed in the duct cells. In many other glands the final levels of sodium and potassium are closer to those in plasma and primary (acinar) secretion. (Young & Martin (1972) *Oral Physiology* pp. 99–113. Pergammon Press, Oxford.)

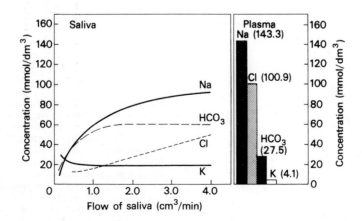

Fig. 12.30. Schematic representation of some electrolyte concentrations in human parotid saliva at different flow-rates. This is modified from the now classic graph obtained by Thaysen *et al* in 1954. *American Journal of Physiology* **178**, 155–159.

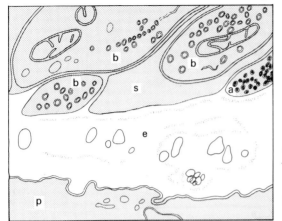

Fig. 12.31. Diagram of electron micrograph of human submandibular gland. A bundle of axons (a and b) surrounded by a Schwann cell (s) are separated from the parenchymal cell (p) by a large space (e). An axon (a) containing small granular vesicles is free of its Schwann cell envelope on one side (nearest p) and is probably an adrenergic axon; the other axons (b) have larger granular vesicles and are probably cholinergic axons. (X 35 000). (After Eneroth, Hokfelt & Norberg (1969) *Acta otolaryngologica* **68**, 369–375.)

stimulation of parasympathetic nerves increases the flow of both saliva and blood. Unlike the increased flow of saliva the functional vaso-dilation is remarkably resistant to the action of atropine (p. 522). This resistance to atropine has suggested to some that the vasodilator fibres cannot be cholinergic and that the mechanism responsible for the functional vasodilation must be sought elsewhere. It has been claimed that parasympathetic stimulation of salivary glands brings about the release of peptides which cause a local increase in blood flow.

Stimulation of secretion
The sheep parotid and rabbit submandibular glands have a resting secretion which continues in the absence of any stimulus. In man there is a small salivary flow during sleep which ensures that the mouth and throat are kept moist. It is not known whether this is a resting secretion or whether it is reflexly evoked by stimuli such as a dry mouth, swallowing or mouth movements. The mouth is bathed by the 'resting' flow of saliva for 90% of the time. A mean value for

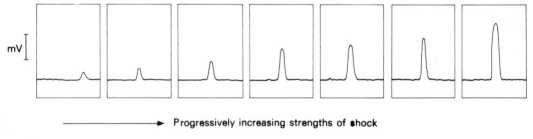

mV

⟶ Progressively increasing strengths of shock

(a)

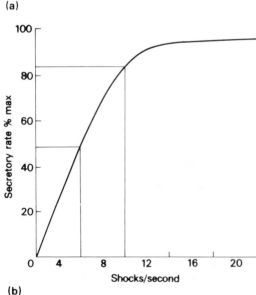

Secretory rate % max

Shocks/second

(b)

Fig. 12.32. (a) Electrical responses obtained with intracellular electrode in an acinar cell of the submandibular gland of a cat under anaesthesia. Single shocks of increasing strength applied to the chorda tympani nerve excite an increasing number of nerve fibres to the gland. (After Lundberg (1955) *Acta Physiologica Scandinavica* **35**, 1–25.) (b) Flow-rate as a percentage of maximal rate produced in response to electrical stimulation of the chorda tympani nerve to the submandibular gland in the anaesthetized dog. Between the vertical lines are the frequencies which represent the probable physiological range in that they produce flow-rates similar to the normal reflex flow-rates. (Modified from Emmelin & Holmberg (1967) *Journal of Physiology* **191**, 205–214.)

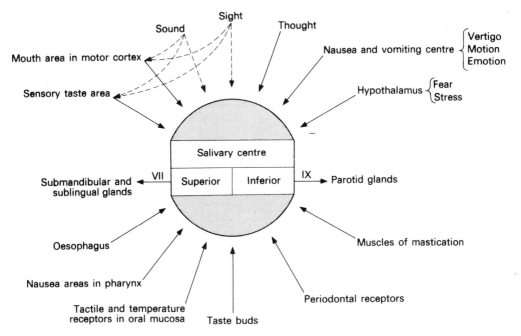

Fig. 12.33. Schematic representation of the nervous control of salivary secretion. The sympathetic innervation has been omitted since its role is still uncertain. It is probably concerned in secretion of enzymes and protein during eating. The broken lines represent the association pathways which are probably created during conditioning.

salivary flow of 20 cm³/hr has been proposed during waking hours.

Unlike other exocrine glands of the alimentary tract, there is no hormonal drive to salivary gland secretion. Some hormones may modulate the response of glands to nervous stimuli and account for the hypersalivation occasionally seen during pregnancy.

The superior and inferior salivary nuclei in the pons, receive information from many sources (Fig. 12.33).

Taste. Taste is the most potent salivary stimulant, but different modalities vary in their effectiveness, decreasing in order from sour, salt, sweet to bitter.

Mastication. When a bite (p. 570) is held lightly between the teeth a little saliva flows from the ipsilateral glands. As more pressure is exerted, receptors in the peroidontal fibres send more impulses to the brain and the rate of flow is increased. During chewing, this 'static reflex secretion' is augmented by another originating from the muscles of mastication whose effect is also mainly ipsilateral. An increase in the force or frequency of chewing is followed by an increased flow, but over the normal physiological frequency range there is little change. At very high frequencies, in experimental situations, there is a reduction in salivation; this has been attributed to inhibition of the salivary nucleus from the cortex or hypothalamus due to stress or pain.

Touch. Stimulation of trigeminal endings in the oral mucosa, particularly by irritant materials, produces a small flow of saliva. Ingestion of cold water (< 15°C) or hot water (> 55°C) has a stimulating effect. Stimulation of certain areas in the oropharynx, sometimes designated as the 'nausea' areas, because touching them with a cotton wool wisp or contact with dry powder can cause retching or a feeling of nausea, evokes secretion and is obviously a protective mechanism. Excessive distension of the upper part of the oesophagus also stimulates salivary flow.

Thought, sight, olfaction and conditioned reflexes. Pavlov demonstrated that dogs could be induced to salivate by a conditioned reflex (p. 934). In one of his famous studies the dogs

Table 12.1. Mean and range of mixed salivary flow-rates (cm³/min) in 23 students thinking about and observing a lemon being sucked.

	Control	Thought preceded sight.	
Mean	0.48	0.59*	0.73†
Range	0.12–1.17	0.10–1.57	0.14–1.93
Significance	P <0.01		P <0.01
		P <0.001	

* Five of these subjects showed no increased flow relative to control.
† Four subjects failed to show an increased flow relative to control.
The nose was clipped to eliminate olfactory effects.

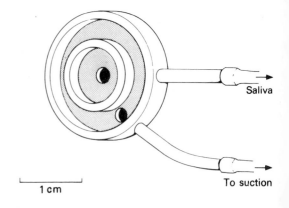

Saliva

To suction

| 1 cm |

(a)

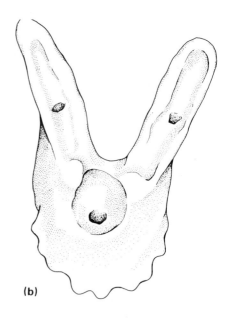

(b)

associated the chimes of a near-by church clock with feeding time in the animal-house, but after a while it was found that the clock chime, by itself, could evoke some salivation. Do we salivate in a parallel situation on hearing the sizzling of bacon in the frying pan? A recent carefully controlled study has demonstrated that some subjects can be conditioned to salivate in response to a sound or a flash of light, but opinion is still divided as to the effect of thought and sight of food on salivation, even though most people claim to have had 'mouth watering' experiences. Thought and sight of food or of lemons being sliced or sucked, generally promote an increase in salivation (Table 12.1) but some subjects do not respond. There is no dispute about the existence of an olfactory-salivary reflex.

Emotion. The legendary medieval practice of determining guilt by the dry appearance of a stone sucked by the accused is based on the physiological principle that fear inhibits salivary secretion. The response is mediated via the hypothalamus and the salivary centre but is also effected by circulating adrenaline.

Secretion is increased by nausea, in motion sickness or just prior to vomiting. This provides protection for the soft tissues of the mouth against the gastric acids which are about to be regurgitated. This reflex must surely be one of the best examples of purposeful planning in physiology.

Fig. 12.34. (a) Modified Lashley cannula. These cups can be made from perspex, aluminium or other materials. Two concentric wells are cut out from a small cylinder on a lathe and these are drained by separate small side tubes. Polythene tubing leads the saliva from the central trough out of the mouth to a collecting tube. The cup is held against the cheek by applying suction to the outer well through a small syringe which can be conveniently placed in a top pocket or attached by adhesive tape to a collar. (b) A Schneyer apparatus (viewed from below) for separate collection of submandibular and sublingual saliva. This can be constructed in acrylic resin from an impression taken of the floor of the mouth. The central depression is over the submandibular ducts and the lateral ones collect saliva from the numerous openings of the sublingual ducts.

COMPOSITION OF SALIVA (Table 12.2)

The main constituent of saliva is, of course, water; solids amount to about 1%. The fluidity of saliva makes it an excellent cleansing agent for the oral vestibule and the teeth and provides lubrication for speech and swallowing. It also promotes the dissolution of foods and thus aids in taste sensation. In man salivation does not play a role in electrolyte and water balance since the saliva is swallowed and later absorbed in the intestine, nor does it participate in evaporative cooling during heat-stress (e.g. panting in dogs).

Collection for analysis

Numerous devices have been constructed for obtaining saliva directly from salivary ducts in humans. Two types in common use are based on the Lashley cannula (Fig. 12.34a) or Curby cup for parotid saliva, and the Schneyer apparatus (Fig. 12.34b) for submandibular and sublingual secretions. The disadvantage of the latter is that it has to be tailor-made for each subject and that, because of its position, tongue movement is restricted. In experimental animals the ducts are usually surgically exposed and cannulated under an anaesthetic; and in dogs, rabbits and sheep, chronic, long-term cannulation of the ducts has been achieved.

GENERAL CONCEPTS APART FROM THOSE RELATING TO ORAL HEALTH

It is not easy to produce a meaningful table which lists the concentrations of each constituent in saliva because its composition is affected by so many factors, both within one subject and between different subjects. The percentage contribution made by each of the major gland, but 'resting' flows (spontaneous, unstimu-12.35); mechanical stimuli with little or no taste markedly raise the contribution of the parotid gland but 'resting' flows (spontaneous, unstimulated) contain a high contribution from the submandibular gland. The composition of mixed saliva must therefore vary. Variations in flowrate and in duration of stimulation of a gland have a profound influence on the composition of saliva from any one gland (Figs. 12.30 & 12.36).

Table 12.2. Salivary composition in normal adults (from Mandel (1974) *Journal of Dental Research*, **53**, 246–266)

	Parotid		Submaxillary	
	Unstimulated (0.04 cm³/min)	Stimulated (0.7 cm³/min)	(0.6 cm³/min)	Plasma
	[mmol/dm³]			
Potassium	36.7	20.0	17.0	4
Sodium	2.6	23.0	21.0	140
Chloride	24.8	23.0	20.0	105
Bicarbonate	1.0	20.0	18.0	27
Calcium	1.5	1.0	1.8	2.5
Magnesium	0.15	0.1	0.15	1.0
Phosphate (inorg)	10.0	4.0	3.0	1.2
	[mg/100 cm³]			
Urea	19.6	15.0	7.0	25
Ammonia	–	0.3	0.2	–
Uric acid	9.5	3.0	2.0	4
Glucose	<1.0	<1.0	<1.0	80
Total lipid	–	2.8	2.0	500
Cholesterol	–	<1.0	–	160
Fatty acid	–	1.0	–	300
Amino acids	–	1.5	–	50
Proteins	–	250.0	150.0	6,000
pH	–	6.8–7.2	6.8–7.2	7.35

The – sign indicates that no figures are available in these analyses and not that these substances are absent from the saliva.

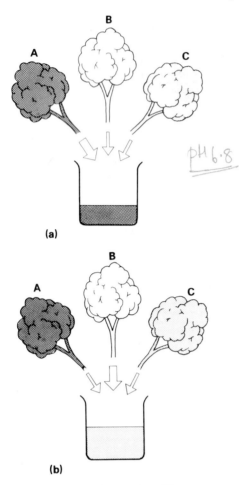

pH 6.8

(a)

(b)

Fig. 12.35. Diagram to illustrate how different types of stimulation of salivary secretion can alter the volume and composition of mixed saliva in the mouth. The three glands A, B and C differ in structure and in the nature of their secretions. (a) Mixed saliva produced on stimulation with X; (b) After Y stimulus.

The flow-rates recorded in response to the same stimulus in different people vary enormously, partly because the sizes of their glands vary.

Both the composition and the flow-rate of 'resting' and stimulated human saliva also vary throughout the day: there is a circadian rhythm (Fig. 12.37).

For convenience, the composition will be considered first in general terms and in relation to digestion and second as it affects oral health.

Organic constituents

Over twenty protein fractions have been separated from pure glandular secretions by electro-

phoresis. From the histology of the various glands it is perhaps surprising that the submandibular gland contributes less protein than the parotid gland. Glycoproteins comprise about 35% of the total protein in parotid saliva. The glycoproteins in serous glands are, however, chemically different from those in mucous glands.

Alpha-amylase. The amylase activity of human parotid saliva is more than four times that of submandibular saliva and many more times that of serum amylase, from which it is quite distinguishable. The enzyme is stable at pH 5.0–8.5 with an optimum pH of 6.8 and requires chloride ions in low concentrations for full activity. Amylase hydrolyses particular 1,4-α-glycosidic linkages in the polyglycan amylose chains in starch and glycogen. However the 1,6 linkages in amylopectin (which constitutes 70–80% of the total starch) and in glycogen are resistant to amylase. Thus these branched polymers (starch and glycogen) are in part broken down by α-amylase to maltose, maltotriose and glucose, but in addition, a mixture of branched residual cores—the α-dextrins or limit dextrins are formed. These contain the unattacked α(1–6) branches, and their size is about six glucose residues per molecule. The mode of attack of α-amylase is shown in Fig. 12.38.

In uncooked starch, which is not a very common item in human nutrition, even the amylose chains are not accessible to amylase, as the starch granule is protected by a thin protein layer. The digestive value of salivary amylase (formerly called ptyalin) is limited by the short time that food stays in the mouth, but the enzyme continues to work in the centre of a bolus in the stomach until hydrochloric acid penetrates and inactivates it.

Salivary glycoproteins (p. 345). Some of the glycoproteins act as excellent lubricants and prevent food from sticking to mucosal surfaces, reduce friction of moving parts and aid in articulation during speech and in the forming and swallowing of a bolus. They are a complex group of compounds distinguished by their high content of carbohydrate (often >50%). The relative amounts of carbohydrate and protein and the nature of the carbohydrate moieties vary. In the rather watery parotid saliva, the major glycoprotein migrates on electrophoretic strips towards the cathode whereas the principal glycoprotein in submandibular glands, which

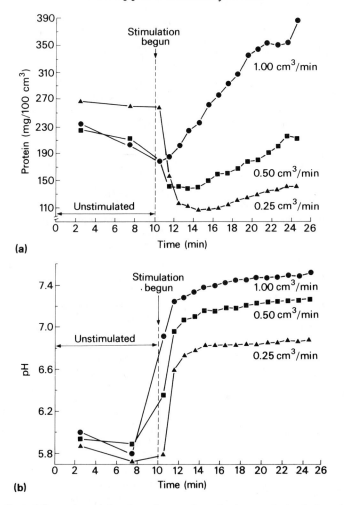

Fig. 12.36. The effect of flow-rate and duration of stimulation on the pH and protein concentration in human parotid saliva from: A, ten; B, fifteen subjects. For the first 10 minutes the salivary flow was unstimulated, but during the final 15 minutes three constant flow-rates were achieved by sucking sour candies. The pH reached almost steady values within about 5 minutes of stimulation whereas the protein levels are still rising after 15 minutes. It is obvious that an analysis taken within a few minutes of stimulation would produce very different results from those made say after 15 minutes. (After Dawes (1969) *Archives of Oral Biology* **14**, 277–294.)

gives saliva its viscosity, behaves as an anion. One glycoprotein which has been isolated from parotid secretions has a molecular weight of about 36 000, the protein core contributing 20 000 and the four carbohydrate side chains over 3000 each. These side units are made up of N-acetyl glucosamine, galactose, mannose, fucose and sialic acid. On the other hand one of the principal glycoproteins in the submandibular gland has a molecular weight approaching 2 million; the carbohydrate side chains contain galactose, glucosamine, galactosamine, fucose, sialic acid and N-acetyl galactosamine which forms a glycosidic link with the hydroxyl groups of serine and threonine in the polypeptide core. These sidechains also contain sulphate which may be responsible for part of the negative charge of these molecules. Since parotid and submandibular glycoproteins contain similar quantities of sialic acid their different viscoelastic properties cannot be entirely attributed to this charged group as was formerly supposed. Other factors such as the degree of hydrogen-bonding between side chains and the presence of sulphate

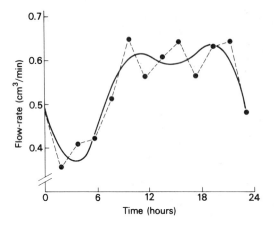

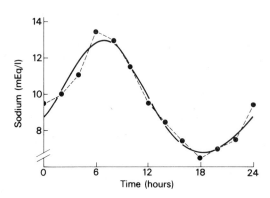

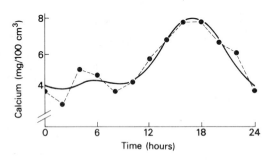

Fig. 12.37. Flow-rate and sodium and calcium concentrations in human submandibular saliva plotted against time of day for one subject. No stimulation was used to produce salivation. The solid line is a plot of the best-fitting sine curve derived mathematically from the actual data shown by the dotted line. Considerable variation has been reported in the actual patterns obtained in different subjects and in stimulated saliva from submandibular and parotid glands. (After Ferguson & Fort (1974) *Archives of Oral Biology* **19**, 47–55.)

must also be involved in dictating the shape and viscoelastic properties of these molecules in submandibular and sublingual saliva.

Other organic constituents. Many other glycoproteins are secreted, some of which are identified as the blood-clotting factors (p. 692).

About 75% of the population have a genetically determined ability to form and secrete certain fucomucins—the blood group substances. These correspond to the A and B agglutinogens and to the H agglutinogen in persons of blood group O (p. 683). Their presence is of importance in forensic science.

The immunoglobulins in saliva are discussed later.

Numerous enzymes are present in glandular secretions, for example, hexokinase, lactic dehydrogenase, esterases and lipases, acid phosphatase, peroxidase, lysozyme, carbonic anhydrase, beta glucuronidase, ribonuclease and kallikrein. Almost nothing is known of their functional significance. Many more enzymes are present in mixed saliva since these are contributed by bacteria, cells and tissue exudates. Some, such as hyaluronidase, neuraminidase and proteolytic enzymes may have clinical significance.

Traces of uric, citric and lactic acids, amino acids, creatinine, cholesterol and phospholipids are present in saliva. The substantial quantity of urea which is secreted appears to be related to the blood urea level and to protein intake.

Hormones are also present in trace amounts. Use has been made of this as a method of determining the sex of an unborn child during pregnancy, but the reliability of such tests is very low. Water soluble vitamins have been detected, but again their significance is unknown. Very low concentrations of glucose are found in saliva (<30 mg/dm^3) relative to those in blood (800–1000 mg/dm^3). Under experimental conditions it has been found that certain non-electrolytes enter saliva in amounts related to their molecular weights and their solubility in water and lipids. Thus saliva:serum concentration ratios range from 1:50 for mannitol to 1:10 for glycerol and 1:2.5 for urea.

Inorganic constituents
The concentrations of inorganic constituents show such enormous variation within and between normal individuals that mean values can be misleading. However, most readers feel cheated if they are not given some idea of the

(a) Amylose is hydrolysed to yield maltose and maltotriose. The latter is hydrolysed slowly, yielding maltose and free glucose.

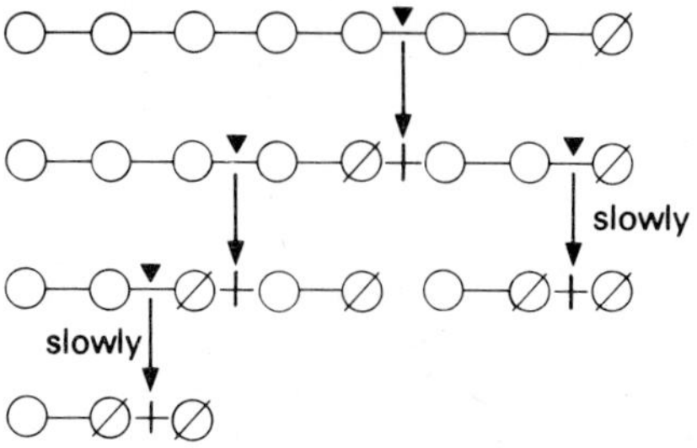

slowly

slowly

(b) In amylopectin and glycogen, α 1–6 glycosidic bonds and also adjacent α 1–4 glycosidic bonds are resistant to hydrolysis by α–amylase.

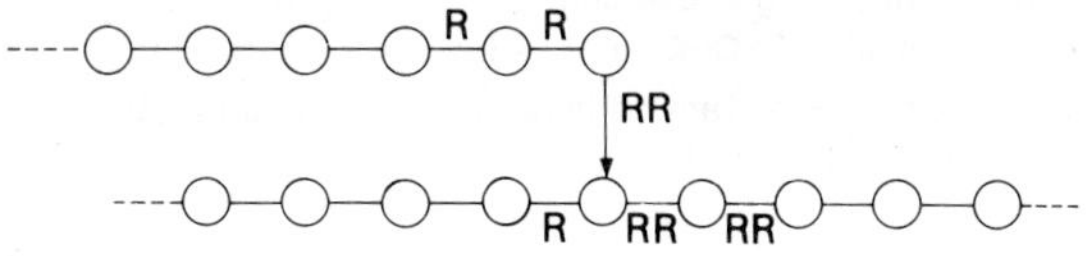

R   R

RR

R   RR   RR

(c) The major products of the action of α–amylase on starch and glycogen are maltose and limit dextrins made up of 4–7 glucose residues. The α 1–6 bond in these is subsequently hydrolysed in the small intestine by the brush border enzyme: limit dextrinase (also called isomaltose).

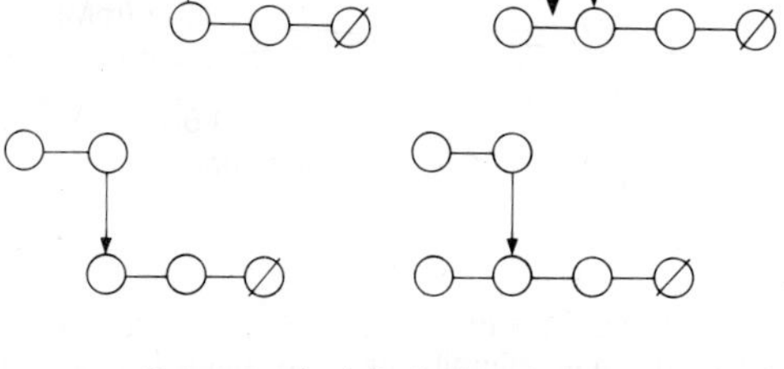

very / slowly   extremely / slowly

Some typical limit dextrins

Fig. 12.38. (continued overleaf).

(d) Structures of some typical limit dextrin molecules which result
from exhaustive hydrolysis of highly branched molecules by
α–amylase

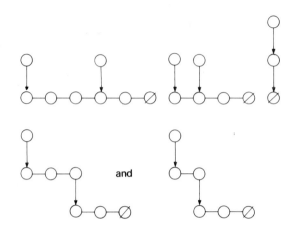

Key

O, non-reducing glucose unit; Ø, reducing glucose unit;
▼, point of attack; O—O, α, 1–4 link; α, 1–6 link;
RR, extremely resistant to hydrolysis; R, moderately
resistant to hydrolysis

Fig. 12.38. Mode of attack of α-amylase on starch and
glycogen in food.

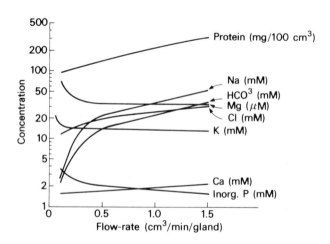

Fig. 12.39. Summary diagram of the effect of
flow-rate on the composition of human submandibular
saliva. The points from which the lines were
constructed represent the mean values for collections
made over 2–13 minutes of stimulation at particular
flow-rates in eight subjects. As the scale on the
ordinate is logarithmic one should be careful in making
comparisons with the graph for parotid saliva shown in
Fig. 12.30.

approximate composition. This is shown in Table 12.1.

pH and buffering. The pH varies from about 5.4 for parotid and 6.4 for submandibular saliva at minimal rates of flow, to about 7.5 at very fast rates. The buffering capacity increases with increased flowrate because of the increase in the concentration of sodium bicarbonate (Fig. 12.39), which, with CO_2 in solution, is the principal buffer system. This is obviously an important function of saliva. Phosphates assist in buffering and proteins too under very acid conditions. The buffering capacity is increased by a high vegetable diet, is raised shortly after meals and shows a diurnal variation.

Inorganic ions. The principal ions are Na^+, Ca^{2+}, Mg^{2+}, K^+, Cl^-, HPO_4^{2-} and $H_2PO_4^-$, but many others such as Br^- and SCN^- are present in trace amounts. Iodide is unusual because it is trapped and concentrated in salivary glands so that high salivary:plasma ratios are obtained. Fluoride levels are very low in saliva even in persons ingesting fluoridated water or fluoride tablets (p. 825).

Calcium and phosphate. Only about 50% of the total calcium concentration in duct saliva (about 1.4 mmols/dm³) is ionized. The rest is com-

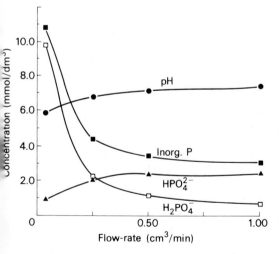

Fig. 12.40. The effect of flow-rate on pH and the concentrations of different phosphate ion species. Although the total orthophosphate concentration falls with increase in flow-rate the concentrations of HPO_4^{2-} (and minute quantities of PO_4^{3-}) are raised because of the pH shift. As pH rises, $H_2PO_4^- \longrightarrow HPO_4^{2-} \longrightarrow PO_4^{3-}$. (After Dawes (1969) *Archives of Oral Biology* **14**, 277–294.)

plexed with bicarbonate, phosphate, and citrate, and bound to proteins and to sialic acid and sulphate in some glycoproteins. Within subjects, there is a positive correlation between the flow-rate of parotid saliva and total calcium concentration but more of the calcium is bound to proteins at higher flowrates because they become more negatively charged as pH increases. Most of the inorganic phosphate (about 5 mmols/dm³) is ionized orthophosphate, the actual ionic species depending on the pH, but about 10% is pyrophosphate. Phosphate concentration falls with increased flow-rates but stabilizes at high flow-rates (Fig. 12.40).

COMPOSITION OF SALIVA IN RELATION TO ORAL HEALTH

Much effort has been expended in trying to discover if there is an association between the composition of saliva and the incidence of dental caries and periodontal disease or the rates at which calculus (tartar) is formed. Such studies are fraught with difficulties and unresolved questions. Should whole-mouth (mixed) saliva be studied, with its inherent difficulties of collection and its inevitable contamination by bacteria, epithelial cells, leucocytes and food debris, or can we use parotid saliva which is obtained more easily? Should 'resting' saliva be collected or should some well-controlled form of stimulation be used? Does diet influence salivary composition? The analysis of salivary constituents also presents problems. For example, after collection the pH tends to rise due to loss of CO_2. This leads to a change in ionic calcium and phosphate due to the precipitation of insoluble calcium phosphate salts. The viscosity is lowered due to the breakdown of salivary 'mucin' by bacteria.

Because of these difficulties and the large variations in the composition of saliva between individuals it is still questionable if there is any association between salivary composition and oral disease. About ten years ago it was concluded that 'we are still rather ignorant, but our ignorance is becoming more sophisticated all the time'. The situation has changed little since then.

Precipitation of salivary proteins and the formation of the acquired pellicle
It has been demonstrated by analyses of amino acid composition that the acquired acellular pellicle, which forms on a tooth surface a few minutes after a thorough prophylaxis, originates mainly from salivary proteins. Subsequently it

incorporates the products or residues of bacterial degradation. This pellicle, which is about 1 μm thick perhaps assists the adherence of bacterial plaque.

What causes the deposition of the pellicle? One suggested mechanism is that bacterial neuraminidase in the mouth removes sialic acid groups from salivary glycoproteins causing a change in the conformation of the molecule. The glycoprotein residues subsequently aggregate and may then be deposited on the enamel surfaces.

An alternative theory is based on the observation that several high molecular weight glycoproteins in parotid saliva are preferentially adsorbed *in vitro* by powdered enamel; the free carboxyl groups on the dicarboxylic amino acids seem to play an important role. In addition a tyrosine-rich acidic peptide of low molecular weight—statherin—has been isolated; this has a high affinity for calcium and mineral surfaces. Calcium ions in saliva or in fluid from the gingival crevice cause certain salivary proteins to aggregate and precipitate.

Calculus formation

The deposition of calcium phosphate on teeth has been attributed to spontaneous precipitation or to epitactic nucleation (p. 392).

Three possible mechanisms for spontaneous precipitation have been suggested. First, it could be related to a local rise in pH due to either the loss of CO_2 from saliva by the action of carbonic anhydrase or the production of ammonia by the action of bacterial urease. Second, the concentration of phosphate might be locally increased by the action of phosphatases in saliva, bacteria and epithelial cells on organic phosphate esters. Third, the concentration of calcium might be increased locally by its release from salivary protein at an acid pH.

Alternatively, plaque matrix or protein adsorbed to the tooth surface might act as a template for nucleation. This concept naturally leads one to consider the existence of inhibitors of nucleation or crystal growth in persons who are poor calculus formers.

However, attempts to relate the composition of saliva to the calculus-forming status of individuals have been contradictory. The source of calcium is not restricted to saliva; inflammatory exudates and crevicular fluid also influence the formation of calculus, particularly the subgingival variety whose composition resembles that of whitlockite ($Ca_{3-x} Mg_x (PO_4)_2$). Supragingival calculus is mostly brushite ($CaHPO_4 2H_2O$).

Because submandibular saliva has a higher resting pH, higher calcium concentration and lower ionic strength it is probably more saturated in respect to brushite, octacalcium phosphate and hydroxyapatite than parotid saliva. Increased flow-rates increase this degree of saturation. These findings explain the observation that calculus forms most readily on the lingual surfaces of the mandibular anterior teeth nearest to the openings of the submandibular ducts.

Saliva and dental caries

Saliva influences the caries process in a number of ways:
1 By its cleansing action,
2 By maintaining a degree of saturation of calcium and phosphate ions,
3 By buffering acids produced locally by cariogenic organisms in dental plaque and
4 By influencing bacterial metabolism.

Some salivary factors increase and some decrease the cariogenic potential of the bacterial plaque.

Flow-rate. Xerostomia (drying of the mouth), due to impaired salivation, is always accompanied by rampant caries if it persists for some time. Caries is then found on tooth surfaces which are normally little affected. In the absence of a pathological condition which severely reduces flow, it is probably correct to say that the association between flow-rate and caries incidence is poor.

Calcium and phosphate. Results relating caries incidence to the calcium and/or phosphate levels in either whole saliva or parotid and submandibular saliva are contradictory and unconvincing. One might have expected a better correlation, since an equilibrium exists between the tooth mineral and calcium and phosphate ions in saliva. *In vitro*, at pH values above about 6.0, saliva is sufficiently saturated to prevent dissolution of enamel or hydroxyapatite, but under more acidic conditions the phosphate in saliva (mainly HPO_4^{2-}) is converted to H_2PO^{4-} and the activity product in saliva of Ca^{2+} and HPO_4^{2-} will not maintain the stability of hydroxyapatite (Fig. 12.41) so it dissolves. A similar situation theoretically exists *in vivo* under an acid-producing plaque at the tooth surface; but as plaque contains higher levels of calcium and phosphate than saliva, and as it releases these ions under acid conditions, so the critical pH for dissolution would be reduced.

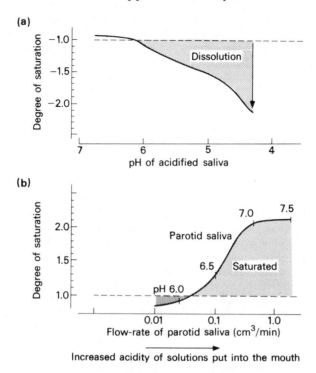

Increased acidity of solutions put into the mouth

Fig. 12.41. Schematic representation of relationship between pH of saliva and dissolution of enamel. On the ordinate is the degree of saturation of saliva; below 1.0 saliva is unsaturated with respect to enamel mineral and more dissolves than precipitates (hatched area). The results in (a) are obtained by subjecting saliva-enamel suspensions in a test-tube to increasing concentrations of acid. Mineral dissolves when the pH falls to below about 6.0. The curve in (b) was calculated from results of experiments in which acids of increasing concentration were put in the mouth. (Other suitable salivary stimulants can be used.) The parotid saliva produced in response shows an increase in flow-rate and a concomitant increase in pH. As a result, the degree of saturation also increases so that enamel is better able to resist dissolution.

When an acid beverage is drunk, or when tasty food is chewed, there is an increase in salivary flow; the pH of saliva rises so that the concentrations of HPO_4^{2-} (and PO_4^{3-}) rise at the expense of the $H_2PO_4^-$ (Fig. 12.40). This is simply the result of the dissociation characteristics of phosphoric acid. Although there is a decrease in the total concentration of inorganic phosphate and a small decrease in the ionic calcium concentration as more of the calcium becomes bound to protein at the higher pH, the overall effect is to increase the degree of supersaturation. With the increase in the buffering capacity of saliva this tends to protect the teeth from acid erosion (Fig. 12.40). As the labial surfaces of the upper anterior teeth are not well bathed by saliva they escape much of this protection. The damaging effects of drinking concentrated sweetened fruit juice (in some infants) or compulsive lemon-eating in some adults are seen on these surfaces.

pH and buffering. A significant association between salivary pH and caries has not been demonstrated but there is a statistical relationship between higher buffering capacities (mainly bicarbonate) in whole saliva and low caries rates.

Some pH-raising factors are also present. Sialin is a small peptide which can be metabolized by oral bacteria under certain conditions to produce amines which raise the pH.

Traces of ammonia are present in duct saliva, but it is also produced by the action of bacterial urease on salivary urea and by deamination of amino acids produced by some microorganisms which utilize urea as a substrate. No significant differences in the salivary levels of ammonia or urea have been found between persons of different caries status.

Antibacterial factors. Saliva has a collection of powerful antibacterial factors. One of the first proteins to be found in saliva was lysozyme, initially described by Alexander Fleming, better known for his discovery of penicillin. It is present at concentrations of 150–200 mg/dm³ in parotid saliva and is even higher in submandibular saliva. This enzyme splits the bond linking N-acetyl muramic acid to N-acetyl glucosamine in the peptidoglycan of certain bacterial cell walls particularly those of Gram positive micro-organisms, and there is some evidence to suggest that it can be adsorbed by phosphate groups in enamel and plaque. Despite its theoretical potential as an anti-caries factor, any specific role for lysozyme in caries still remains to be established and attempts to relate lysozyme levels to caries activity have been negative. The normal flora is not very susceptible to its actions which are primarily directed against pathogenic bacteria that occasionally enter the mouth.

Another factor in saliva is lactoperoxidase, an enzyme which is active against lactobacilli and some streptococci during their growth phase. It requires thiocyanate ions as a cofactor. Once again, no association has been found between the peroxidase activity in saliva and the caries status of individuals. This conclusion also applies to amylase, which, if its activity was high, might theoretically provide a more cariogenic subs-

trate by rapidly degrading starch into maltose. No differences have been found in the availability of chloride (required for optimum amylase activity) in different caries groups.

Immunoglobulins. Secretory antibodies have been detected in saliva. These take the form of immunoglobulins and constitute about a third of the total protein secreted by parotid and submandibular glands at resting flows. Both acinar and plasma cells in the salivary glands are involved in the synthesis of these antibodies. In whole-mouth saliva their concentration is related to the severity of gingival inflammation which means that the gingival exudate is a source of immunoglobulins. Crevicular fluid from healthy gums has also been shown to contain these antibodies (mainly IgG). Quantitatively, the predominant type of immunoglobin in saliva is that known as IgA. Although it seems that this secretory antibody can affect both experimental caries and the organisms causing caries in certain model systems, it is still premature to define the significance of the salivary immune system in human caries and periodontal disease.

It is appropriate to conclude by summarizing what is known about the relationship between composition and function (Table 12.3).

Table 12.3. The relationship between composition and function in saliva.

Constituent	Function in saliva
Water	Lubrication, cleansing, dilution of noxious materials. Aids solution of foods therefore promotes taste sensation; aids swallowing.
Glycoproteins	Lubrication for articulation, bolus formation and swallowing.
Amylase	Limited digestion of starch and glycogen in mouth, but continued in stomach within food bolus.
Sodium bicarbonate	Buffering, particularly at high flow-rates.
Calcium and phosphate ions	Maintenance of supersaturated solution restricting acid dissolution of enamel. Phosphate can act as a buffer.
Lysozyme	Antibacterial.
Peroxidase	Antibacterial.
Immunoglobin IgA	Uncertain role against oral antigens.
Blood clotting glycoproteins	Protective.
Statherin	Binds to calcium ions, maintains supersaturation.
Sialin	pH raising factor.

MASTICATION
(See also Vol. 1, Book 2, p. 331)

Definition

Mastication may be defined as the process by which food in the mouth is rendered suitable for swallowing. The way in which food is taken into the mouth is excluded from this account.

Today, in the so-called developed countries, more of this processing actually takes place in the kitchen and on the plate than in the mouth, to the general detriment of the dentition. However, the way food is dealt with in the mouth and the time needed to prepare it for swallowing depend on both its consistency and particle size. The preparation process may involve tearing, chopping, squashing, chomping, cutting or even grinding the food between the upper and lower teeth. In practice, the action of the teeth depends on their shape, the movements of the jaws and the forces generated by the jaw muscles (Fig. 12.42). These are not the only elements involved. The tongue controls the position of the food with the assistance of the muscles of the lips and cheeks, particularly the buccinator. It also moves the food from one side of the mouth to the other as well as collecting the triturated food to form a bolus. Salivary secretions moisten the food, 'glueing' small particles together to form the bolus and then lubricating its passage into

the pharynx. Mastication depends on the synchronized activity of a number of different systems and organs, innervated by a bewildering variety of cranial nerves.

The actions of the teeth

Food is broken up by the convergent movements of upper and lower teeth: lumps of all but the softest foods are first 'squashed' and, with the addition of saliva, softened by pounding between the cusps of the cheek teeth. This action, 'puncture-crushing', eventually blunts or abrades the tops of the cusps (cf. abrasion and attrition). Some foods, such as peanuts, are only 'chewed' in this way: successive impactions comminute the nuts and the resulting fragments can be swallowed. Most foods are, however, first crushed and then 'cut' or 'ground' to make a 'mush' from which a bolus is formed. At first the resistance of the food prevents the cusps of upper and lower teeth from interdigitating and then, later, from completely occluding. But as the food is softened, the teeth come progressively closer to full occlusion. As soon as the cusps can interdigitate, the ridges on their slopes shear the food as the teeth move past each other and the cusps grind it as they traverse the basins in opposing occlusal surfaces (the 'pestle and mortar action'). This type of mastication, true

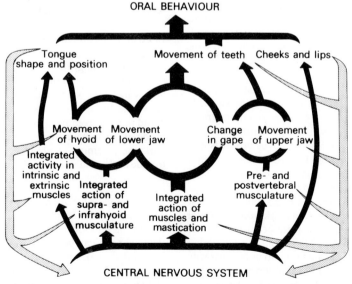

Fig. 12.42. The chain of events which results in oral behaviour such as suckling, chewing and the oral component of speech. The solid arrows show the order in which the components of the effector system, come into action (for clarity, the salivary glands have been omitted). The dotted arrows indicate the sensory pathways transmitting proprioceptive, general and special sensory information to the central nervous system from each structure.

chewing, produces attrition facets on the slopes of the cusps.

As mastication proceeds, the nature of the food is changed until it is 'fit' for swallowing. How that 'fitness' is determined is not yet clear but must, in large part, be based on sensory information from the oral mucosa of both the palate and the tongue as well as from the peridontium.

The movements of the jaws

All chewing movements are rhythmic: the same basic pattern or 'cycle' of movement is repeated until the food is ready for swallowing. As the nature of the food changes so, usually, does the amplitude of the cycle, its duration or both, although the direction of movement normally stays the same. The chewing cycle of all mammals, including man, has three main movements or 'strokes'. These are, first, an upwards closing stroke which brings the teeth into contact with the food. In man, the mouth is rarely opened more than the minimum needed to accommodate the bite between upper and lower teeth: the closing stroke is therefore a rapid movement over a short distance (Figs. 12.43 & 12.47). In other mammals, particularly carnivores and insectivores, the mouth is opened much more widely and the jaws converge very rapidly over a long distance. The closing stroke is followed by the power stroke in which, as its name implies, the food is reduced. During the power stroke the teeth continue to converge but much more slowly, due to the physical resistance of the food. If the food is soft, the teeth will come into contact at the end of the power stroke. If it is hard, they may not.

The mouth is not opened at a constant rate: at first the lower jaw moves very slowly downwards in the 'slow open' phase of the opening stroke (Figs. 12.43, 12.45 & 12.47). During this slow movement, the hyoid bone moves upwards and forwards (Figs. 12.5 & 12.44). When the hyoid has reached its most forward position the jaws begin to open more rapidly. The rapid movements of opening are distinguished as the 'fast open' phase of the chewing stroke. Many dental authorities use either 'centric occlusion' or the 'rest position' (p. 577) to define the beginning of a cycle. However, the teeth do not necessarily pass through centric occlusion during early mastication nor does the lower jaw have a specific and measurable 'rest point'; it actually 'hovers' about the rest position. Descriptions of the masticatory cycle based on work on experimental animals use widest mouth opening or 'maximum

gape' to define the point at which the cycle begins (Fig. 12.43).

Although the movements of the mandible are the most important movements during mastication, they are not the only ones. The expressions 'masticatory movement' and 'mandibular movement' are not synonymous. Animal studies have shown that if the mouth is to be opened widely, both jaws are moved: as the lower jaw is depressed the upper jaw is simultaneously elevated by extension of the cranium on the cervical vertebral column at the atlanto-occipital joints. Closing from the wide open position depends on a combination of cranial flexion and mandibular elevation. The exact contribution made by cranial movement to the cycle in man is not yet known. Since social convention dictates that the mouth be opened the smallest possible amount consistent with successfully chewing the food, it is likely to be minimal save when the food is particularly tough. Hyoid movement is, however, a constant feature of the cycle and is closely integrated with that of the mandible (Figs. 12.44 & 12.47). In all animals so far studied, and in man, the hyoid has a roughly elliptical orbit during chewing: it moves forwards and backwards as well as upwards and downwards (Fig. 12.44). These movements can be correlated with the actions of the tongue in positioning the food. For instance, the movement of the hyoid during the 'slow open' phase serves to raise and bring forward the base of the tongue. This assists it in collecting fully triturated material and in repositioning inadequately masticated food in readiness for the next power stroke. This integration of hyoid and jaw movement does not mean that their individual movements have the same amplitude in all feeding activities. In lapping or licking, the tongue and hyoid apparatus move a great deal but the amplitude of jaw movement is minimal. On the other hand the jaw moves a great deal in chewing but tongue and hyoid movements are much reduced.

The envelope of motion

The anatomy of the jaw apparatus, particularly that of the temporomandibular joint is such that the lower jaw can be moved in the sagittal plane (up and down), the transverse plane (side to side) and the anteroposterior plane. Normal chewing movements involve a smooth and fluid combination of movement in all three planes. Even during the apparently simple movement of closing the mouth from the wide open position, a point on the lower jaw moves through a sinuous

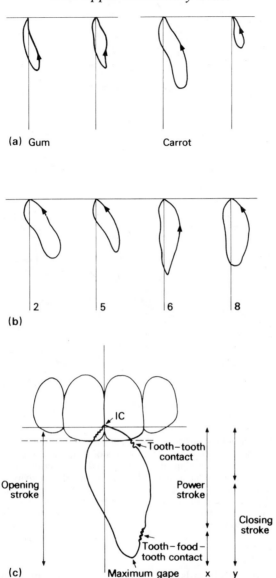

(a) Gum   Carrot

(b)   2   5   6   8

(c)   Opening stroke   IC   Tooth–tooth contact   Power stroke   Closing stroke   Tooth–food–tooth contact   Maximum gape   x   y

Fig. 12.43. 'Profiles' or 'loops' showing the path of movement of a marker point on the lower jaw during a single chewing cycle seen from in front. The position of the point is either recorded directly, for example by using a light source on the chin, or by analysing filmed records of the subject chewing. In analysing such films the position of the marker point in each frame is plotted against two reference planes: usually the midline (vertical plane in a, b and c; and a second plane perpendicular to it, drawn through the position of maximum intercuspation (horizontal line in a, b and c). Alternatively the edge of the upper incisors can be used as a horizontal plane (dotted line, c). However obtained, these profiles only show the *direction* and *amplitude* of movement in the two included dimensions, in this form they give no information as to the rate of movement or the duration of any part of the cycle. (a) Variation in cycle profile when feeding on gum (chewing) and carrot (puncture-crushing, then chewing). (b) Variation in cycle profile in a single individual chewing a single bite. The numbers refer to the number of the cycle in the sequence. (c) Illustrating the possible variation in the amplitude of the three strokes: the closing stroke ends at tooth–food–tooth contact when the power stroke begins. The level of this transition depends on the dimensions of the bite. In puncture crushing (x), a large bite results in a very short closing stroke and a long power stroke but the teeth may not reach the intercuspal position. In chewing (y), the smaller particle size of the food means that the teeth are almost in contact before the power stroke begins.

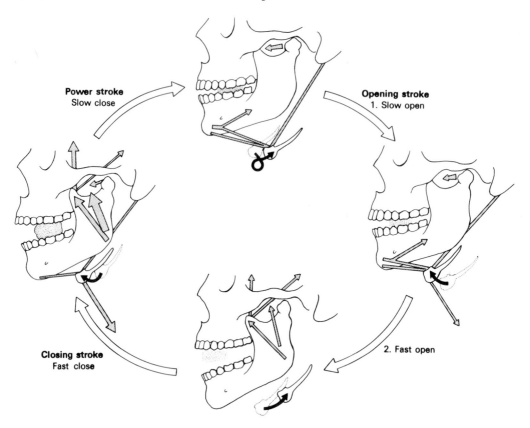

Fig. 12.44. *The chewing cycle.* The hollow outlines of the upper and lower jaws and the hyoid show their position as each stage of the cycle begins. The stippled hyoid outline shows the position of that bone at the beginning of the previous stage so the solid black arrow shows the path of hyoid movement during the part of the cycle just completed. The hollow arrows indicate which muscles are electrically active during each stage: for example the anterior and posterior fibres of temporalis, the masseter and medial pterygoid are all active during the closing stroke. In the power stroke their activity increases, reflected in the size of the arrows, and in addition, the anterior and posterior bellies of digastric and the infrahyoid muscles are also active (compare with Fig. 12.47).

path. This results from the backwards and upwards slip (translation) of both the mandibular condyle and the articular disc from the articular eminence into the articular fossa combined with the upward swing (rotation) of the condyle on the disc. Protrusion of the mandible involves a slight preliminary lowering of the jaw so that the lower incisor teeth clear the upper, but it is almost a pure sliding movement. The lateral pterygoids pull the condyles and discs forwards on to the articular eminence (Figs. 12.44, 12.45 & 12.46).

The complexity of the actual patterns of jaw movements in both feeding and speech, which depend on the shifting axes of rotation at the temporomandibular joints, led Posselt to develop the concept of an 'envelope of motion' (Fig. 12.45).

The envelope is 'the volume of space within which all movements of (a point on) the lower jaw take place'. The limits or 'borders' of the envelope are anatomical. Once the teeth have occluded the jaws cannot be closed further but the teeth can slide across each other in both the anteroposterior and transverse planes. These 'contact' or 'gliding movements' have a vertical (downwards) component which depends on the cuspal profile of the cheek teeth and the extent of the incisor overbite (Fig. 12.45). Normal jaw movements utilize very little of the possible range of movement in each plane and so little of the envelope.

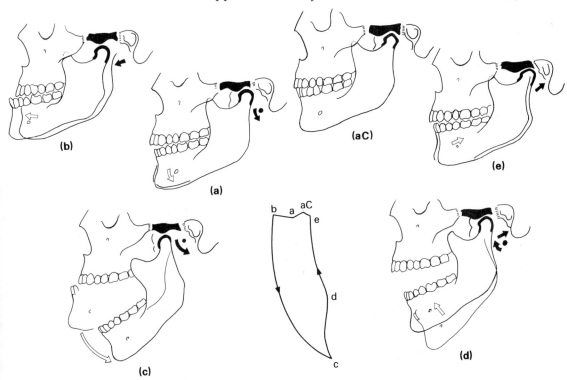

Fig. 12.45. The 'envelope of motion' in lateral view. *Contact movements* define the upper border of the envelope: the jaw can be retruded from the intercuspal position (aC) to position e or protruded from aC to position b. To reach the extreme protruded position b, the lower jaw has first to be slightly depressed to 'unlock' the occlusion (aC to position a) then slid forwards (position a to position b). *Border movements* occur between positions b and c (extreme protrusive opening) and positions c and e (extreme retrusive closing). Normal closing would bring the jaws from position c to the intercuspal position. The movements of the mandibular condyle relative to the upper articular surface are shown by solid black arrows: straight arrows indicate a sliding movement (translation); curved arrows round a point illustrate a swinging movement (rotation). Both types of movement occur as the jaw passes through position d. The change in the position of the front of the jaw (e.g. the anterior teeth or mental foramen) does not necessarily parallel that of the condyle, for example the shift between positions a and b, and c and d (shown by the hollow arrows).

The cycle profile

The amplitude of movement, and therefore the actual profile (as seen from in front or the side), varies during a single chewing sequence, varies between sequences in the same person feeding on different foods and also between individuals eating the same foods (Fig. 12.43). Much of this variation can be attributed to the effect of food consistency and particle size on the regulation of jaw movement. Some of the differences between individuals can be related to the idiosyncracy of the cycle pattern. It appears that most individuals establish a characteristic profile related to their occlusion and chewing habits. Once the pattern is disturbed, as may happen when the teeth are replaced by dentures, a 'new' pattern may have to develop: this involves a period of adjustment which can lead to discomfort and complaints.

There have been attempts to classify the forms of cycle profile found in chewing and to correlate them with occlusal and facial types in the hope of establishing 'norms' against which disturbances can be assessed. This approach has not been very successful. There is, however, evidence that in individuals with the 'temporomandibular joint syndrome' (painful or clicking joints) the movement becomes jerky and the profile jagged.

Profiles have usually been obtained by filming the head of the subject, whilst chewing, from in front. The position of a marker point on the lower jaw (often lower central incisor) is then plotted against a reference point on the upper

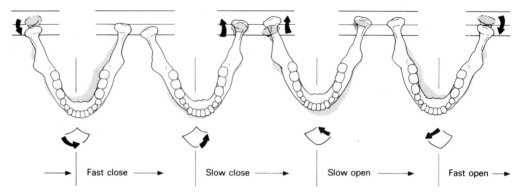

| → Fast close → | Slow close → | Slow open → | Fast open → |

Fig. 12.46. The transverse movements of the lower jaw during a chewing cycle with the working side on the right of the figure (left side of jaw). Compare with Fig. 12.44. The movements of a point on the front of the jaw are 'lozenge' shaped, each of the four stages broadly corresponding to one side of the lozenge (hollow arrows). Movements of the condyles on the upper articular surface (fossa, stippled; eminence, clear) are shown by the black arrows and the change in condylar position. The clear outline shows the position of the condyle at the beginning of each labelled stage (at the head of the arrow); the hatched outline shows the position of the condyles at the beginning of the previous stage (the tail of the arrow). In the closing stroke (fast close) the working side condyle translates slightly backwards; in the power stroke (slow close) the medial swing of the jaw involves the backwards translation of the balancing side condyle, followed by the forwards translation of the working side condyle as the lower jaw swings downwards and away from the midline in the first part of the opening stroke (slow open).

jaw (often the edge of an upper incisor) in each frame of film (Fig. 12.43c). Sample loops are shown in Fig. 12.43. In normal individuals, the power stroke is always directed upwards and medially towards the centric position. Unfortunately frontal cinefilms, unlike cinefluorographs, do not clearly show the position or the size of the bite in the mouth. (A 'bite', which is the ingested portion of food, is sometimes wrongly referred to as a bolus. The bolus is the chewed food collected on the tongue and swallowed as a unit.)

The pattern of movement in chewing can also be demonstrated by plotting gape (the angular or linear distance between upper and lower teeth) against time (Fig. 12.47). Time can be measured in msecs or in frames of film. The latter is a convenient unit since the camera speed of the recording is known (usually 30 or 60 frames per second). The actual duration of a single cycle in man varies around 600–1100 msec depending on the subject and the food. The closing movements take about 300 msec and opening somewhat longer, but the time taken for the opening stroke is more variable than for closing. Very sophisticated devices for recording jaw movements have recently been developed. These include accelerometers, telemetric devices and systems based on photocells. All give recordings of jaw displacement in at least one of the three possible planes. They are used in synchrony with the electromyograph (EMG) to obtain simultaneous recordings of jaw movement and jaw muscle activity.

The actions of the muscles
The movements of the mandible and hyoid are produced by a complex pattern of activity in either the 'elevators' (the closing and power strokes) or in the 'depressors' including the 'hyoid musculature' (the opening stroke). At no time during a chewing cycle is activity confined to one muscle or pair of muscles. There is even some activity of depressor muscles during closing and, in at least some mammals, activity of elevator muscles during opening.

There have been several electromyographic studies of mastication in man, the most important of which was carried out on dental students in Copenhagen. This study showed that the pattern of electrical activity in the jaw muscles alters when a subject switches from natural chewing to unilateral chewing. In natural chewing the bite is randomly shifted from side to side in the mouth: the working side changes with the position of the bite. In EMG studies unilateral chewing is often used deliberately as differences in the behaviour of the muscles on the working and balancing sides are much clearer. A natural pattern of unilateral chewing is considered to be pathological. It can develop if a tooth on one side is painful, loose or missing, or if a partial denture is

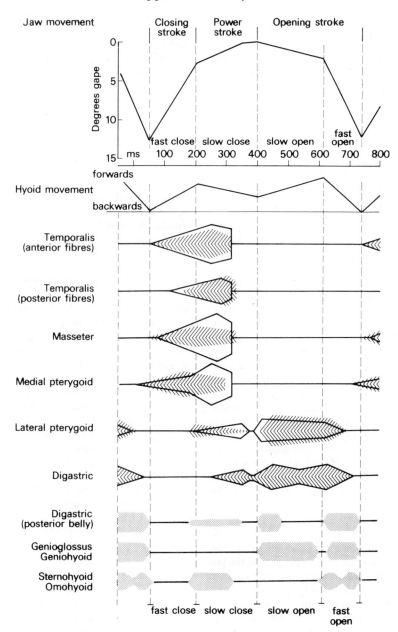

Fig. 12.47. *Jaw movement.* The vertical axis (degrees gape) is a measure of the separation between tooth rows. The horizontal axis records time. The slope of the gape/time plot therefore measures the *rate* of jaw movement in °/msec). This changes in the four stages of the cycle. *Hyoid movement.* The hyoid actually moves in both the vertical and horizontal planes but only the latter is shown. The distinctive forwards (and upwards) movement of the hyoid during slow opening has been observed in every mammal so far studied. It is associated with elevation of the tongue and repositioning the food in the mouth. *Jaw musculature.* The timing and scale of the electrical activity (EMG) in the jaw muscles during a chewing cycle is shown as the 'envelope' of the EMG signal. Data in bold is based on human studies, that in faint (stippled) is from animal experiments. 'Hollow envelopes' show the activity of the muscles on the working side, cross-hatched lozenges, the activity in the balancing side muscle. Compare with Fig. 12.50.

badly fitted. It can also be a habit acquired as a result of such past experiences.

The EMG activity of the muscles on the working and balancing sides differs (Fig 12.47). The following detailed description is based mainly on EMG data from the Copenhagen study, but includes some information from experimental work with animals.

Jaw closure

When the mandible approaches maximum gape the medial pterygoid is the first of the major elevators to show activity, some 10–40 msec ahead of temporalis (Fig. 12.47). The greater activity in the balancing side muscle assists the lateral pterygoid of that side in pulling the mandible towards the working side (Figs. 12.44 & 12.46). As the mandible reaches maximum gape, the balancing side masseter starts firing, followed by the anterior fibres of the temporalis of both sides. In the closing stroke, the greater activity in the working side of the masseter and temporalis and in the balancing side of the medial pterygoid, ensures that the mandible continues to move towards or retain its position on the working side. The anterior temporalis is considered to have a primary function in moving the mandible rather than in generating force for the comminution of food. This muscle is electrically active for about 300 msec, that is throughout both the closing stroke and most of the power stroke, although it only shows powerful activity for about the last 140–180 msec, i.e. during the power stroke. The posterior and near horizontal fibres of temporalis behave rather differently: the working side muscle comes into action some 30–40 msec ahead of the muscle on the balancing side and also fires synergistically with the lateral pterygoid of the balancing side. These two muscles form a couple pulling the jaw upwards and laterally towards the working side. As can be seen in Fig. 12.43, the point of maximum lateral excursion towards the working side can vary widely, from just above maximum gape to the beginning of the power stroke. The timing of activity in the posterior temporalis and the lateral pterygoid reflects this. Significant activity is seen in the masseters as upward movement continues into the power stroke against the resistance of the food. The balancing side muscle is the first to fire, reaches its maximum activity early and declines slowly. In contrast, the working side masseter shows a slower increase in activity but reaches a much higher peak level (Fig. 12.47). The masseter and medial pterygoid are considered to be the main 'power' muscles

for chewing, generating most of the force, about 5–15 kg, required to break up food. In the very last stages of the power stroke, the balancing side posterior temporalis and the working side lateral pterygoid act together to pull the mandible medially and into occlusion (Fig. 12.46). This medial movement is the reverse of that described previously for the temporalis–lateral pterygoid couple and is the more important as shown by the levels of activity in the muscles (Fig. 12.47).

Jaw opening

As the main elevators reach their peak levels of activity in the power stroke, the 'depressor' muscles begin to fire. The actual firing order in man is mylohoid, digastric and then lateral pterygoid. These are the only muscles for which detailed information based on human studies is available. The data on the hyoid muscles given in Fig. 12.47 is based on the results of animal experiments. Although the lateral pterygoid fires during closing, this is its secondary burst of activity. Its main, primary, activity is found in opening: the working side muscle begins to fire followed by the balancing side muscle in which the maximum level of activity is considerably higher. During the opening stroke, the lower jaw is not only being pulled downwards, it is also moved away from the working side (Fig. 12.43). This movement towards the balancing side is reversed as maximum gape approaches and a new cycle commences. The lateral pterygoids of both sides with the assistance of the digastric, which becomes active some 80–100 msec earlier, are pulling the condyles forward and also, in the case of the working side condyle, medially (Fig. 12.46). The mylohoid is active throughout the power stroke and continues to fire during opening.

The exact pattern of activity in the other hyoid muscles is not yet known for man. However, it is unlikely to prove very different from that recorded in animals particularly as the hyoid bone has a cyclical movement in man which is comparable to that of other mammals (Figs. 12.44 & 12.47).

It is not possible to give more than the most generalized account of the actions of the jaw muscles during a chewing cycle since the actual pattern of movement alters as the food is reduced. In eating an apple, the mouth has to be opened widely at first to get the large lump between the cheek teeth and the muscles have to generate more force to crush it than will be necessary when it has been reduced almost to a mush. The electrical activity in a single muscle and the pattern of activity in all the muscles change as mastication proceeds, reflecting the changing cycle profile and the diminishing resistance of the food.

The EMG only records the level and duration of electrical activity in part or all of a contracting muscle; it provides no direct information on the force generated by or degree of shortening of muscle following the sarcolemmal action potential.

The forces of mastication

There is a delay of 40–80 msec between the onset of electrical activity in the elevators and the generation of measurable force. This delay is attributable to the contractile behaviour of skeletal muscle (p. 338) and accounts for the observation that the elevator force is sustained and the teeth remain in occlusion for about 70 msec after all electrical activity has ceased (Fig. 12.47). In theory, and demonstrably in the laboratory, muscles can contract either isotonically or isometrically (p. 337). No such clear distinction can be demonstrated in normal chewing. The only time in a masticatory cycle at which the jaws can be alleged to be stationary (so 'fixing' both attachments of the elevators) is for the few milliseconds in which the mandible is believed to hold the intercuspal position on completion of the power stroke. But this is the period in which, as might be expected, all electrical activity in the elevators has ceased! It is, however, true that on occasion the convergent movements of the teeth are momentarily halted as they contact resistant food. At this time the muscles could be considered to be acting isometrically but only until the effect of their force on the food is shown by the resumption of the closing movement.

The force exerted on the food in chewing (often called the 'bite pressure') has been measured in two ways. The actual force exerted on the occlusal surface of a lower molar during mastication has been recorded using strain gauges mounted in inlays and found to be of the order of 5–15 kg, depending on the individual and the food. The force of a static 'bite' can be measured using a gnathodynamometer. This is an instrument with a pressure-sensitive pad on which subjects bite using one or more pairs of teeth or the whole dentition. The actual values obtained vary considerably from about 10 kg on the incisors to 50 kg on the first molars. This difference reflects both the different size and shape of these teeth as well as their position in

the jaws; the first molar is the stoutest tooth and is closest to the line of action of the powerful elevator muscles and to the root of the zygomatic process through which forces are allegedly dissipated.

These bite pressures were recorded in young adult males; values in the female are normally smaller. Values also decrease with age. The generally ennervated state of the jaw apparatus in 'civilized' populations is indicated by the results of two different investigations. Bite pressure has been found to increase with exercise: an hour's 'chewing practice' a day for 30 days produced an average increase of static molar bite pressure from about 59 kg to 70 kg in males and from about 35 kg to 50 kg in females. This improvement could not be sustained without continued exercise. By way of contrast, Eskimos, who have to chew their hard tough food over long periods, generated gnathodynamometer readings of the order of 150 kg in males and only slightly less in females. It is also perhaps significant that the bite forces produced by subjects with full dentures are very much lower than those recorded in their dentate compatriots. The reasons for this are not clear. The 'load threshold', above which touch/pressure sensations are appreciated as pain, could well be lower for oral mucous membrane than for periodontal ligament but the actual area of contact and load transmission under a lower denture may be less than the area afforded by the sum of the surface areas of the roots of the teeth it replaced. It may be that the average denture wearer finds it extremely difficult to bite hard on any material, not least a dynamometer pad, without the dentures slipping.

Various measurements have been made of 'masticatory efficiency' to assess the effectiveness of mastication in reducing the particle size of the food and increasing the surface area for exposure to digestive enzymes. Little clinically applicable information has been obtained. It does however appear that each individual tends to have a habitual number of chewing movements so that the chewing sequence is made up of almost the same number of cycles. In contrast, in experimental animals the number and the type of the cycles (whether puncture-crushing or chewing) in the sequence can be correlated with the original size and consistency of the food. Investigations of the mechanics and control of mastication in man are not helped by the extent to which normal 'civilized' chewing behaviour is as much, if not more, a function of habit and custom rather than of biological necessity.

Control of mastication

The intake of nutrients in virtually all vertebrates is associated with a rhythmic activity of the mouth and jaws which may be called chewing, biting, grinding, gnawing, drinking, licking, lapping or suckling. The name of the activity immediately suggests something about the consistency of the nutrient. The characteristics of the activity are in fact matched to the consistency of the substance ingested. This suggests that food consistency may control the activity.

The various activities for dealing with solid, semi-solid and liquid food may differ from each other in at least three ways; in the amplitude and duration of the cyclical opening and closing movement of the jaws; in the extent of tongue movement; and in the number of associated swallowing movements. The amplitude and duration of the jaw open and close cycle is not however fixed for each activity but varies for example during the course of chewing as the size and consistency of the food is changed by mastication. There are therefore three different aspects of ingestive behaviour to explain:

1 The origin of the rhythmic opening and closing movement.

2 The nature of the control modifying the amplitude and duration of the cyclical jaw movements.

3 The nature of the control initiating swallowing.

The origin of the rhythmic opening and closing movement

Most theories of oral function that have been advanced in the past have concentrated upon explaining the origin of the rhythmic jaw function alone. The ideas advanced fall into those which treat mastication as a conscious act, even as a 'learnt' activity, and those which treat it entirely as a series of reflexes. A third suggestion which was largely ignored until recently is that rhythmic activity originates in the brain stem under the command of signals from high centres and from stimulation of oral receptors.

There is a widely held view, representative of the first group of explanations, that the normal pattern of jaw movement is due to the activity of the higher centres of the brain, in particular the motor cortex. This view derives support from the experimental work of a number of investigators who have reported that electrical stimulation of fairly localized regions in the motor cortex of experimental animals or in man (in the course of neurosurgery) produces movements of the jaw, face or limbs (Fig. 12.48a).

Furthermore, it is well established that lesions of the same areas in the human brain produce corresponding defects in voluntary action. However, it has been found that animals, including primates, are able to feed following removal of the entire motor area of the cerebral cortices. Consequently, the centres subserving rhythmic jaw activity cannot be in the cortex although the cortex may normally exercise some control over them.

Electrical stimulation of a number of cephalic structures, such as the internal capsule, limbic system and hypothalamus, has been shown to elicit rhythmic jaw movements, but even these structures are not essential as similar movements can also be elicited reflexly in the decerebrate animal. There are reports of decerebrate rabbits chewing and of the human equivalent, the anencephalic infant, suckling. One is therefore left with the inescapable conclusion that rhythmic oral activity does not necessarily arise in the higher centres although it may be influenced by them.

Another view, representative of the second group of explanations, is the very opposite of the 'cortical' concept and is based on the general theory of movement originating in interacting chains of reflexes. The basic idea is that activation of reflex arc A produces a movement which gives rise to a sensory input. This sensory input then activates a reflex arc B which in turn produces a contrary movement giving rise to a sensory input that elicits the original reflex A. This sequence of reflexes therefore becomes self perpetuating. This general concept was first applied to oral function by Sherrington in 1917. The hypothesis relied upon the existence of a jaw opening reflex, elicited by mechanical stimulation of oral structures when food is taken into the mouth, which was then said to be followed by a 'central rebound phenomenon' producing closure. Closure upon food in the mouth resulted in mechanical stimulation of the teeth or mucosa so that reflex jaw opening followed and the cycle was repeated. It was subsequently suggested that, instead of closure being produced by the rebound of some unspecified neuronal system, it might be brought about by the jaw 'jerk' reflex. In this case it was argued that reflex jaw opening stretched the muscles which close the jaw so that their muscle spindles would be activated, causing a reflex closure via the monosynaptic reflex arc (p. 468). The reflex closure would then result in force being exerted on food so that oral

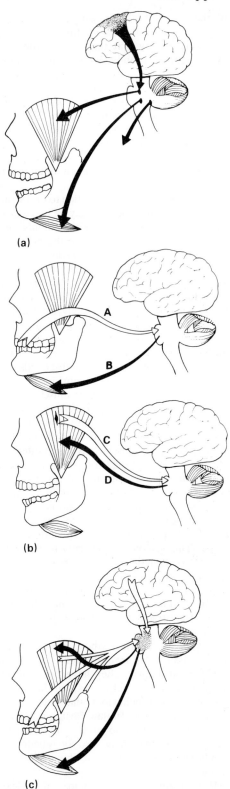

(a)

(b)

(c)

structures would be stimulated once more to initiate reflex opening (Fig. 12.48b). The attraction of these hypotheses is that they apparently explain the rhythmic jaw movement seen in decerebrate animals where little more than reflex action is present. One of the main objections to the 'reflex chain' concept is that reflex activation of muscle tends to be brief and of abrupt onset, whereas the regular bursts of muscle activity in mastication are of much longer duration and of gradual onset.

A third explanation was proposed by Bremer many years ago but is only now receiving the attention it deserves. The basic idea is that there is a centre for generating rhythmic activity in the brain stem. This 'rhythm generator' has at times also been referred to as a 'pattern' generator as it must generate the various rhythmic activities in the sequence in which the masticatory muscles have to be activated. The centre is considered to receive sensory inputs from the mouth (the nature of these is discussed later) and impulses from higher centres, either of which is seen as capable of driving the generator into rhythmic activity (Fig. 12.48c). Whilst there is no doubt that there is an area close to the motor nucleus of the trigeminal nerve that has such inputs, it has yet to be proved that it is in fact a 'pattern' generator. The hypothesis does however explain why rhythmic activity can be obtained on the one hand in the decerebrate animal by suitable intra oral stimulation and on the other hand in the intact animal by stimulation of the motor cortex.

Fig. 12.48. (a) The 'cerebral hemispheres' theory of the origin of rhythmic jaw activity. A more or less patterned set of instructions originates in some higher centre or centres, e.g. motor cortex, limbic system, and descends to drive the trigeminal, facial, and hypoglossal motoneurons directly. (b) The 'reflex chain' theory of the origin of rhythmic jaw activity. A given sensory input 'A' (force exerted on mucosa or teeth) elicits a reflex jaw-opening movement 'B', which in turn produces a sensory input 'C' from the temporalis muscle stretch receptors; this second input then elicits another reflex movement 'D' (jaw closing), which itself produces a sensory input of the type 'A' to elicit the original reflex. (c) The 'rhythm generator' theory of the origin of jaw activity. Any set of signals to the 'rhythm generator' causes oscillatory activity, whether those signals are volleys of action potentials arising from higher centres or from sensory receptors in the periphery. The pattern of the rhythmic activity, once elicited, may also be quite separately modified by the activity of specific sensory afferents acting upon other neurons in the system, e.g. upon motoneurons.

The ability of nerve impulses to drive a neuronal circuit into rhythmic activity, so that reciprocating movement of an anatomical structure is then obtained, is however the crucial issue. In general, to obtain cyclical movement of a jaw or limb, the motoneurons innervating the agonist and antagonist muscles must themselves alternate rhythmically in their activity. Neuronal circuits capable of making motoneurons behave in this way have now been identified in the spinal cord; computer models with similar general characteristics have also been constructed. The mechanism usually suggested to explain how a group of neurons produces rhythmic bursts of activity is that the group gradually becomes unable to respond to continuing excitation, then recovers and goes through the whole cycle again. It has been suggested that the periodic failure to respond to excitation is due to the development of a prolonged refractory period. The group of neurons may thus be looked upon as firing, 'tiring' and reviving. Alternatively, it has been suggested that afferent volleys originating in sensory receptors stimulated by one of the phases of movement (e.g. in jaw opening it might be the muscle spindles in the jaw closing muscles), assist in depressing the activity of the group of neurons producing that movement (in the example given it would be in a group of neurons activating, say, the digastric motoneurons). It is however still a matter of debate whether it is the accumulation of prolonged refractory periods or the inhibition generated by sensory feedback, that is more important in producing the rhythmic fluctuations in activity in the groups of neurons in a pattern generator. If a periodically active group of nerve cells has the power to inhibit another similar group of cells, rhythmic alternating firing will take place, i.e. when one group is firing, the other is having its activity depressed, is 'tiring' or is recovering. If the two groups of neurons control the motor units of pairs of antagonistic muscles, then rhythmic movements will occur.

The only prerequisite for rhythmic oral activity in the Bremer hypothesis is sufficient excitation of the rhythm or pattern generator, i.e. sufficient sensory input from oral receptors or sufficient descending excitation from higher centres. The student should note that, in the explanations advanced above, afferent volleys in sensory pathways are seen as producing two quite separate central effects. Although these effects may be produced simultaneously, there is no evidence yet as to whether sensory fibres coming from one particular set of receptors can have both the effects of (a) increasing general excitation centrally and, at the same time, (b) operating in such a way that they can temporarily inhibit neuron groups within the pattern generator.

The nature of the control over the profile of the jaw cycle and the initiation of swallowing

In order to understand the controls which modify the profile of jaw movement and initiate swallowing, it is necessary to consider some reflex responses that have been obtained in experimental animals.

If mechanical stimuli are applied to oral structures, a variety of responses may be elicited. In each case the characteristics of the stimulus and the site of application determine the nature of the response. For example, the reflexes elicited by stimulating the mucosa of the hard palate depend upon rate of application of force, its peak value, its duration, and the total area over which it is applied. Not surprisingly, brief stimuli elicit brief responses and prolonged stimuli elicit longer lasting responses. For example, in an experimental situation, a force rising to a few hundred grams in about ten milliseconds and applied to an area of a few mm² elicits brief reflex activation of the elevator muscles of the jaw and therefore produces transient jaw closure. If however the peak pressure is raised above a few hundred grams, the reflex is different. Not only is the elevator muscle activity inhibited but the anterior belly of digastric is also activated, resulting in reflex jaw opening. A vigorous jaw opening response is also elicited by any stimulus that causes tissue damage. In contrast, a slowly applied force (a few hundred grams or so) results solely in reflex inhibition of elevator muscle activity. This response is particularly marked if that force is applied over a large area of mucosa. In this case an additional response involving the tongue may also appear; this is a rhythmic movement of the dorsum of the tongue in which waves of contraction pass backwards towards the pharynx.

The reflexes described above are just a few that may be elicited from the oral cavity of an experimental animal. They have been chosen simply because they help to explain how some controls of oral behaviour may operate. It should be noted that the jaw closing reflex and the jaw opening reflex do not have to be elicited from mucosa, they may also be elicited by stimulating teeth or at least the periodontal membrane.

Mention must also be made of reflexes

originating in the muscles of mastication, i.e. reflex contraction produced by stretching muscle spindles and reflex inhibition produced by stimulating Golgi tendon organs. Both spindles and tendon organs seem to be absent from the submandibular muscles of the jaw in most species, but are found regularly in the elevator muscles of the jaw. It is not clear precisely what part is played by the Golgi tendon organs. It can be argued that high threshold periodontal receptors subserve the function of signalling the 'overload' state that, in other sites in the body, would be signalled by the Golgi tendon organs.

In whatever way all the above reflexes function, they should not be considered by the student as functioning simply to initiate particular movements of the jaw but rather in terms of the excitatory and inhibitory influences that they have upon the interneurons or upon the motoneurons that are involved in the various reflex arcs. If the excitability of any of those neurons is already being altered by rhythmic drive from a neuronal circuit making up the pattern generator, then the reflex inputs will undergo a form of algebraic summation with those existing influences.

The reflexes described above have all been elicited by experimental mechanical stimulation, but mechanical stimuli with similar characteristics probably arise during chewing and exert the equivalent influences on interneurons or motoneurons.

Closure upon hard food produces more rapidly rising forces than closure upon soft or masticated food. Furthermore, soft food deforms so that contact areas are large, whereas hard food tends to make localized contacts with oral structures. Since rapidly rising localized forces tend first to excite jaw closing motoneurons and then, as the forces rise further, excite jaw opening motoneurons, the effects produced when masticating hard food would tend to support any simultaneous alternating activity from a rhythm generator. Conversely contact with soft or masticated food, by eliciting only inhibition of elevator activity, would tend not to facilitate rhythmic jaw movement; by eliciting rhythmic waves of tongue activity it would however tend to elicit responses that are ultimately related to swallowing (p. 578). It therefore seems likely that oral contact with food initiates or facilitates those responses that are most appropriate to its consistency at the time.

The foregoing hypothesis concerns automatic oral activity. It remains to be proven whether in man, mastication of solid food falls into this category of activity. As stated before, there is evidence that automatic oral activity can occur in the human anencephalic (where little more than brain stem exists) but there is little information available concerning the relationship between such brain stem centres and the cerebral cortex in man. The fact that the constraints of Western culture result in less obvious displays of gustatory enjoyment than is customary in some other cultures, suggests that the cortical control of basic rhythmic oral activity may be considerable. Finally, the fact that there is direct control of the motoneurons from the cortex so as to produce sustained non-rhythmic activity is a matter of common experience. Anyone who has held his mouth open for half an hour in a dental surgery should know this.

At least in animals the level of activity in the various muscles of mastication, as shown by their EMG, reflects the nature of oral behaviour. For example, the elevator muscles of the jaw show very little activity in licking and lapping whereas during mastication their activity is considerable. When masticating solid food, this activity is not shown to a great extent during the initial fast closing phase of the jaw movement cycle but appears in the power stroke, i.e. as the jaws contact the bite and meet resistance (Fig. 12.47). This increase in activity may be explained by sensory feedback from a variety of oral structures (e.g. from mucosal receptors, from periodontal receptors, from muscle spindles, etc.) which facilitates further reflex closure. In man the increase may, of course, also be produced by voluntary effort.

Rest position
During the period that the jaws are not functioning in mastication (or in speech) the dental arches are separated by a few mm in what is known as the rest position. There is not complete agreement as to what constitutes the 'rest' position since it appears to be more of a range of possible positions or area of space that is occupied rather than one single fixed position. The student can test this for himself by relaxing and then alternately flexing and extending his neck; this alters the separation of the maxillary and mandibular arches. Since 'rest' position implies that the muscles of mastication are minimally active, the 'position' may be defined with reference to the level of electromyographic activity in these muscles, i.e. rest position is the 'position' at which there is minimal (or no) activity in elevators and depressors of the jaw. This

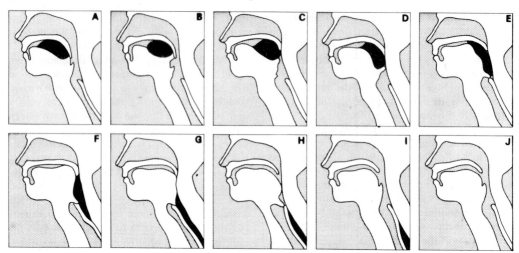

Fig. 12.49. The sequence of events during swallowing. A, The soft palate forms a partition extending to the base of the tongue; B, C, the soft palate is elevated to obstruct the nasopharynx as the bolus moves backward over the tongue; D, E, the bolus tilts the epiglottis backward; E, F, G, the bolus passes smoothly over the epiglottis, and the tongue moves backward with a cam-like action; H, I, the soft palate relaxes and the epiglottis ascends whilst the bolus moves down the oesophagus. The entire sequence takes just over a second. (Adapted from Rushmer, R. F. & Hendron, J. A. (1951): *Journal of Applied Physiology* **3**, 622–630.)

'position' can however change with head or neck posture. Factors affecting the level of activity in antigravity muscles of the body in general also affect jaw position by influencing trigeminal motoneuron activity. An example of this would be the level of reticular activity which influences γ-motoneuron discharge and so affects the 'sensitivity' of muscle spindles (p. 469). However there is now evidence that at least in some animals the 'rest position' is the result not of any reflex contraction in the antigravity (jaw closing) muscles but of a balance between gravity and the elastic forces in the jaw closing muscles and their associated fascial sheaths, etc.

SWALLOWING

Since swallowing occurs with only moderate frequency, the oropharynx spends most of the time in the 'non-swallowing' state. This state is associated with maintained respiration, i.e. the air entering the nose passes back into the pharynx and then proceeds on a ventral path through the larynx to the trachea. During swallowing, food from the mouth also passes into the pharynx but then proceeds dorsal to the larynx and trachea, down the oesophagus (Fig. 12.49). The two pathways therefore cross in the pharynx. The function of the pharynx as an air passage or a food passage is established by clos-

ing either its oral and oesophageal openings or its nasal and glottal openings. The controls ensuring that the airway alone is patent must be suspended during swallowing, which means that the respiratory movements of the thorax must be interrupted. In contrast it should be noted that when the respiratory drive is strong the act of swallowing is inhibited.

In the non-swallowing state, levator palati, tensor palati and the superior constrictor of the pharynx are relaxed to maintain an open nasal airway and an oral seal is produced by contracting orbicularis oris and by placing the tongue forward in contact with the anterior palatal mucosa. At the same time the inter-arytenoid muscles are relaxed to provide an open glottis whilst the constricted cricopharyngeus muscle acts as a sphincter to prevent the oesophagus being inflated during inspiration. The way in which the oral seal is produced is of dental importance since abnormal tongue and lip postures influence the shape and relationship of the anterior segments of the dental arches.

First stage
During mastication, food is mechanically broken down and mixed with saliva. The end product is the bolus of softened food for swallowing. Alternatively, if one of the modern proprietary convenience foods is involved it will probably

have that consistency to start with. The food consistency appropriate for swallowing is signalled to the central nervous system by a particular spatiotemporal pattern of activity from oral receptors. For example, closing the jaw deforms a soft bolus so that contact is made with a large area of mucosa and the force exerted, per unit area of mucosa, is low; it seems possible therefore that the sensory input produced (i.e. the spatiotemporal pattern) might be characterized by a relatively low frequency of firing of afferent impulses in a large number of afferent fibres.

It has been pointed out (p. 576) that a reflex tongue movement can be elicited by diffuse mechanical stimulation of the oral mucosa, and it has been suggested that closure on soft food would preferentially produce such stimuli. In response to this stimulus the tongue is repeatedly elevated with a movement like that of a cam which is capable of transporting food towards the fauces. The neural circuits (or centres) controlling this behaviour are located in the brain stem. In addition, the movement of the bolus towards the fauces is under a measure of voluntary control. However, there is disagreement about the relative importance of the reflex and voluntary components in man. This initial movement of the bolus is traditionally known as the first or oral stage of swallowing (Fig. 12.49A & B). It seems likely that in most swallowing the first stage is in fact reflex, contrary to the traditional view, but that the subject is conscious of this act and that the extent of the voluntary control is limited to facilitation of that reflex (p. 307). One can therefore swallow at will, providing there is at least saliva in the mouth to elicit the reflex, but, if the mouth is completely empty, it is almost impossible. In some cases, as when called upon to swallow a large pill, considerable facilitation of the swallowing reflex is required to get the object past the pillars of the fauces. Such 'deliberate' swallows tend to be associated with elevation of the jaw and firm tooth contact. Normally, swallowing of solid foods tends to be associated with only light tooth contact whereas liquids are frequently swallowed with the teeth slightly apart. The commonest liquid in the mouth is of course saliva, which is being continuously produced. Periodic 'idle' swallows clear the mouth of saliva and are actions of which we are rarely conscious.

Second stage

Whereas there is a measure of voluntary control over the initial stage of swallowing, as soon as the bolus reaches the fauces the act becomes totally reflex. The afferent pathway for the reflex is formed by branches of the glossopharyngeal and vagus nerves supplying the back of the tongue, fauces, uvula and posterior wall of the pharynx. Once the network of neurons in the medulla comprising the 'swallowing centre' is sufficiently aroused by the afferent input, a complete sequence of bilaterally symmetrical contractions is elicited in the striated muscles of the pharynx, tongue and hyoid apparatus. The pattern of activity spreads over the motor nuclei of cranial nerves V, VII, IX, X, XII, and lasts about 0.5 s. Since the muscles involved are poorly supplied with proprioceptors and since individual muscles can be denervated without affecting the rest of the sequence of activity, it would appear that swallowing is the expression of a complete and stereotyped pattern which exists as a network of neurons within the CNS. Classically, the passage of the bolus from the fauces through the pharynx to the upper end of the oesophagus is known as the second stage (Fig. 12.49C to G). The wave of activity which propels the bolus down the pharynx consists of relaxation of successive segments of muscle followed by their contraction (Fig. 12.50); the second stage of swallowing ends with a slight relaxation of the cricopharyngeus muscle (sphincter) followed by its firm contraction as the bolus passes into the oesophagus.

Throughout the second stage of swallowing the larynx is elevated and the glottis is closed to protect the airway. Using cineradiography it has also been shown that, as the bolus passes back, the epiglottis flexes and descends to form a 'cap' over the laryngeal opening; in addition there is some evidence that the epiglottis acts to divert food laterally rather like a rock sticking up in a stream. However, as it has been found that removal of the epiglottis does not impair swallowing, even of fluids, its exact role is something of a mystery. It would seem that the upwards and forwards movement of the larynx coupled with a posterior movement of the tongue is the major mechanism for protecting the airway whilst the glottal closure acts as an important second line of defence. The above movements of the larynx during swallowing can be clearly seen in some individuals (especially thin males) as movement of the 'Adam's apple'.

Third stage

The oesophagopharyngeal or third stage of swallowing takes several seconds. The bolus, together with a bubble of air which precedes it,

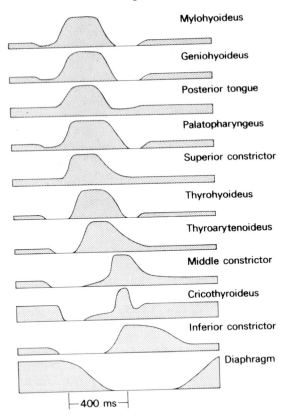

Mylohyoideus

Geniohyoideus

Posterior tongue

Palatopharyngeus

Superior constrictor

Thyrohyoideus

Thyroarytenoideus

Middle constrictor

Cricothyroideus

Inferior constrictor

Diaphragm

|— 400 ms —|

Fig.12.50. Summary of outflow of the swallowing centre of the dog shown diagrammatically. Height of line for each muscle indicates the relative intensity of activity. The upper three muscles represented affect tongue position; they contract almost simultaneously. The next two muscles take part in creating pressure in the pharynx. At the same time, the lower five muscles shown which belong to the hypopharynx and hypopharyngeal sphincter, relax. After the bolus has passed, these muscles contract, firmly shutting the sphincter. The diaphragm relaxes while the bolus is passing through the hypopharynx. (Modified from Doty R. W. & Bosma J. F. (1956) *Journal of Neurophysiology* **19**, 44–60.)

passes down the oesophagus in accordance with the pressure gradient generated by the contractions of successive segments of the muscle. The striated muscle in the upper part of the oesophagus is innervated by the vagus with motor end-plates, like those in the striated muscle of limbs, whereas the smooth muscle in the lower portion, though again supplied by the vagus, has a parasympathetic type of innervation, i.e. the vagal axons synapse with ganglion cells in a myenteric plexus. Neither continuity of the muscle coat nor intact afferent nerves are essential for propagation of the wave of contraction in the upper oesophagus. This implies that the pattern of activity is largely generated in the CNS and conveyed via vagal motor fibres, a control which is very different from the situation elsewhere in the gut where peristalsis is wholly dependent upon the myenteric plexus.

Although vagal afferents are unnecessary for the primary oesophageal peristalsis of swallowing, they are necessary for the secondary peristalsis, i.e. if any food remains in the lumen of the oesophagus after swallowing, the afferents are stimulated and a secondary peristalsis is reflexly and unconsciously initiated to clear the remaining particles. In contrast to the purely 'reflex' afferents, other afferents carry information which reaches consciousness and these fibres travel with the sympathetic nerves. At rest, the oesophagus, below the cricopharyngeus muscle, is relaxed except for the lowest eighth which forms a functional sphincter and prevents reflux from the stomach. This region relaxes slightly as soon as food enters the upper end of the oesophagus and contracts after the bolus has passed into the stomach.

Fluids

The foregoing description refers largely to the propulsion of a solid bolus down the oesophagus. In contrast, fluids pass down the oesophagus largely by gravity and arrive at the stomach ahead of the peristaltic wave that has also been elicited. Fluids are also actively propelled into the oesophagus by the pharyngeal phase of swallowing. It must be remembered that, prior to swallowing, the fluid can be ingested either by sucking or by filling the mouth from a vessel. In the first type of ingestion a subatmospheric pressure is developed, e.g. in suckling and when drinking through a straw. This is accomplished by retracting the tongue without breaking the posterior seal of the tongue against the palate. The posterior aspect of the tongue is subsequently depressed; the tongue is then raised and, with a sweeping movement backwards, fluid is propelled into the pharynx. In drinking from a cup gravity is used to assist in filling the mouth.

REGURGITATION AND RETCHING

Paralysis or cleft of the soft palate allows substances to be regurgitated into the nasopharynx during swallowing.

The transmural or transpharyngeal pressures produced by muscular contraction during swallowing in man are of the order of 100 mmHg. However experimental measurements of the net force actually propelling an artificial bolus along the tract suggests that this only comes to about 10 g. If swallowing is initiated by stimulating the fauces and pharynx but the bolus is prevented from moving, a rejection response follows. The mouth is held wide open and the back of the tongue acts to expel the bolus. This is known as the 'retching' or 'gag' reflex. It is all too easily elicited in some patients and may make it difficult to take impressions and construct satisfactory dentures.

If a gag reflex is unsuccessful in removing the source of an offending stimulus (as can be seen when a cat gets a fish bone stuck in its pharynx) the central excitation continues to build up so that the intensity of the responses increases until eventually it involves the vomiting centre (p. 607).

Finally it should be noted that whilst swallowed air may be regurgitated spontaneously (in less than polite society), its regurgitation may also be controlled to produce oesophageal speech. In some patients when the larynx has been surgically removed, this controlled regurgitation of air can be developed for communication.

FURTHER READING

EMMELIN N. & ZOTTERMAN Y. (Eds.) (1972) *Oral Physiology,* Pergammon Press, Oxford. Chapters by Emmelin, Petersen, Funakoshi, Schneyer and Schneyer, Garret, Young and Martin.

KERR A.C. (1961) *Salivary Secretions in man,* Pergammon Press, Oxford.

KLEINBERG I., ELLISON S.A. & MANDEL I.D. (Eds.) (1979) *Saliva and dental caries.* Information Retrieval Inc., New York.

MANDEL I.D. (1974) Relation of saliva and plaque to caries. *Journal of Dental Research* **53**, 246.

MASON D.K. & CHISOLM D.M. (1975) *Salivary Glands in health and disease.* W.B. Saunders, London.

OAKLEY B. & BENJAMIN R.M. (1966) Neural mechanisms of taste. *Physiological Reviews* **46**, 173.

PFAFFMANN C. (Ed.) (1969) *Olfaction and taste III.* Rockerfeller University Press, New York.

SCHNEYER L.H., YOUNG J.A. & SCHNEYER C.A. (1972) Salivary secretion of electrolytes. *Physiological Reviews* **52**, 720.

THORN N.A. & PETERSEN O.M. (Eds.) (1974) *Secretory mechanisms of exocrine glands.* Munksgaard, Copenhagen.

CHAPTER 13

The Remainder of the Alimentary Tract

ANATOMY

The rest of the alimentary tract is an elongated tube with certain local structural modifications, both gross and histological, which can be related to the functions of the different parts (Fig. 13.1).

Oesophagus

This is a tubular structure 25 cm long which begins at the level of the body of the sixth cervical vertebra in the neck, passes into the thorax and through the diaphragm at the level of the tenth thoracic vertebra, and ends by joining the stomach at the cardiac orifice (Fig. 13.2). It lies in front of the vertebral column but is separated from the lowest thoracic vertebrae by the thoracic aorta which is on its left in the middle part of the thorax. The aorta moves towards the

midline as the oesophagus passes to the left in front of it. In the neck and upper part of the thorax the trachea is anterior to the oesophagus. Lower down, the oesophagus lies behind the left atrium and left ventricle. The abdominal part of the oesophagus is about 2 cm long and lies in a notch of the left lobe of the liver.

The oesophagus is related to a number of important structures. In the neck the recurrent laryngeal nerve lies in the groove between it and the trachea; on the left side the recurrent laryngeal nerve has this relation in the upper part of the thorax. The thoracic duct runs upwards behind the right border of the oesophagus in the lower part of the thorax, passes to the left behind it at about the level of the fifth thoracic vertebra, and runs upwards into the neck behind the left border of the oesophagus until it arches forwards and joins the beginning

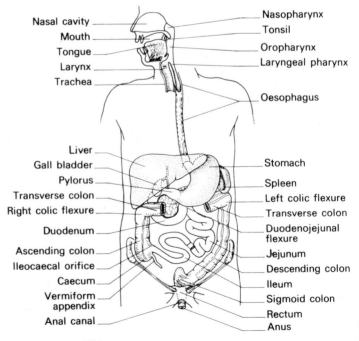

Nasal cavity — Nasopharynx
Mouth — Tonsil
Tongue — Oropharynx
Larynx — Laryngeal pharynx
Trachea

Oesophagus

Liver — Stomach
Gall bladder — Spleen
Pylorus — Left colic flexure
Transverse colon — Transverse colon
Right colic flexure — Duodenojejunal flexure
Duodenum — Jejunum
Ascending colon — Descending colon
Ileocaecal orifice — Ileum
Caecum — Sigmoid colon
Vermiform appendix — Rectum
Anal canal — Anus

Fig. 13.1. The different parts of the alimentary tract.

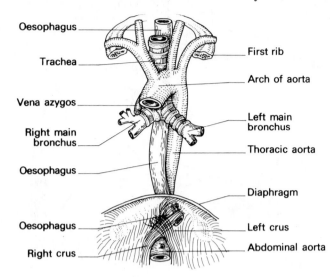

Fig. 13.2. The oesophagus.

of the left brachiocephalic vein. In the neck the lobes of the thyroid gland usually extend sufficiently backwards to lie lateral to the oesophagus where the carotid sheath and its contents are found. The vagus nerves below the level of the root of the lung form a plexus round the oesophagus and pass through the diaphragm with it as the anterior (mainly left vagus) and posterior (mainly right vagus) gastric nerves. The left bronchus lies anterior and lateral to the oesophagus more or less at the division of the trachea and the arch of the aorta has a similar relation to the oesophagus just above the left bronchus. The hemiazygos veins and the right posterior intercostal arteries from the thoracic aorta pass behind the oesophagus to the right.

The oesophagus is narrowed (a) at its beginning, just inferior to the cricoid cartilage, (b) where the arch of the aorta and (c) the left bronchus are related to it, and (d) where it passes through the diaphragm. Among the factors responsible for delaying the entry of food from the oesophagus into the stomach and thereby having a sphincteric action, are the following:
1 The right crus of the diaphragm through which the oesophagus passes.
2 Circular muscle at the junction of the oesophagus and stomach.
3 Some nervous mechanism in this region.
4 The oblique nature of the entry of the oesophagus into the stomach.
5 Folds of mucous membrane in the region of the cardiac orifice.

The motor and sensory nerve supply of the oesophagus in its upper part is from the recurrent laryngeal and sympathetic nerves; the rest of the oesophagus is innervated by the vagus and sympathetic nerves. It is probable that the sensory fibres come from the vagus although some may travel with sympathetic nerves. The blood supply comes from the inferior thyroid artery, the thoracic aorta, and the inferior phrenic, a branch of the abdominal aorta. The left gastric artery also supplies the lowest part of the oesophagus. This region provides a venous anastomosis between the portal and systematic venous systems.

Stomach

This is a dilated part of the alimentary tract and lies in the upper left quadrant of the abdominal cavity (Fig. 13.3). The cardiac orifice, where the oesophagus enters the stomach, is about 2 cm to the left of the midline at the level of the tenth thoracic vertebra and the pylorus where the stomach continues into the duodenum, the first part of the small intestine, is about 2 cm to the right of the body of the first lumbar vertebra. Between these relatively fixed points, the body of the stomach is very variable in size and position.

The stomach is described as having two borders, a right border called the lesser curvature and a left border called the greater curvature.

The stomach is divided into the fundus, that part above the level of entry of the oesophagus, the body which is inferior to the fundus, and a smaller pyloric part leading to the pyloric orifice (Fig. 13.4). At the pylorus, there is a consider-

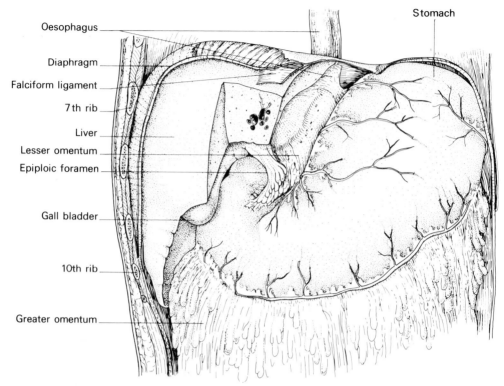

Oesophagus

Diaphragm

Falciform ligament

7th rib

Liver

Lesser omentum

Epiploic foramen

Gall bladder

10th rib

Greater omentum

Stomach

Fig. 13.3. The stomach (most of the liver has been removed).

able thickening of the circular muscle called the pyloric sphincter which is marked externally by the pyloric groove.

From above downwards the anterior surface of the stomach is in contact with the diaphragm, the left lobe of the liver and the anterior abdominal wall. Behind the stomach are structures which collectively form what is known as the stomach bed. This includes the pancreas passing to the left across the left kidney, and the transverse colon as it passes to the left colic flexure lying on the lower pole of the left kidney next to the spleen.

The arteries of the stomach come from the coeliac trunk (of the abdominal aorta) either directly (left gastric) or from one of its branches (the common hepatic and the splenic). The arteries run along the curvatures. The nerve supply is sympathetic from the plexus round the coeliac trunk and parasympathetic from both vagus nerves through the anterior and posterior gastric nerves. The parasympathetic when stimulated increases gastric motility and gastric secretion, and the sympathetic when stimulated

causes vasoconstriction. Sensory (pain) fibres are said to be mainly sympathetic.

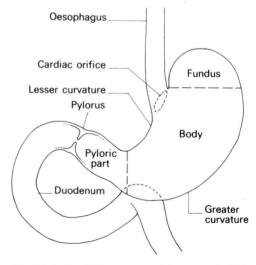

Oesophagus

Cardiac orifice

Lesser curvature

Pylorus

Pyloric part

Duodenum

Fundus

Body

Greater curvature

Fig. 13.4. The different parts of the stomach (This shape is regarded as average and is called a 'J-shaped' stomach).

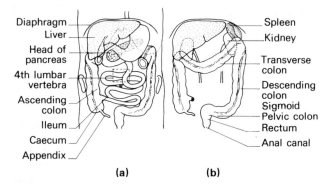

Diaphragm
Liver
Head of pancreas
4th lumbar vertebra
Ascending colon
Ileum
Caecum
Appendix

Spleen
Kidney
Transverse colon
Descending colon
Sigmoid
Pelvic colon
Rectum
Anal canal

(a) **(b)**

Fig. 13.5. (a) The position of the stomach, small and large intestines, liver and pancreas. (b) The main relations of the large intestine.

Small intestine

This extends from the pylorus to the ileocaecal orifice where the small intestine joins the large intestine (Figs. 13.1 & 13.5). It is about 6 m long, but there is considerable variation and it may be anything from 3.5–8 m in length. Its mean length is less in women than in men. The small intestine is divided into the duodenum (about 25 cm long), the jejunum and the ileum. The duodenum is fixed to the posterior abdominal wall. The rest of the small intestine is suspended from the wall by a double fold of peritoneum called the mesentry whose line of attachment runs from the left of the second lumbar vertebra downwards and to the right and ends at the right sacro-iliac joint.

The duodenum is C-shaped and is related to the first, second and third lumbar vertebrae with the second in the hollow of the C (Fig. 13.6). It has four parts. The first (superior) passes upwards to the right, the second (descending) downwards, the third (inferior) to the left and the fourth (ascending) upwards. The duodenum embraces the head of the pancreas and is deep to the liver. More particularly, the first part is related anteriorly to the neck of the gall bladder, with the bile duct passing behind it. The bile duct and main pancreatic duct have a common opening on a papilla (the duodenal papilla) in the posteromedial part of the wall of the second part. This part lies in front of the hilum of the right kidney and is crossed by the transverse colon. The portal vein passes upwards to the liver behind the first part. The third part crosses a number of structures including the inferior vena cava and abdominal aorta and some of their branches. It is crossed anteriorly by the superior mesenteric vessels which supply and drain the small intestine and a large part of the large intestine. The fourth part lies to the right of the left kidney and ureter, next to the abdominal aorta, and turns forwards at the duodenojejunal flexure. The jejunum and ileum form the rest of the small intestine. The division into a proximal two-fifths (jejunum) and distal three-fifths (ileum) of its length is arbitrary since the jejunum only changes gradually in structure. Characteristically the jejunum has a thicker wall and is more vascular than the ileum. The circular folds of the jejunal lining are larger and can be felt. The villi in the jejunum are larger. Lymph follicles, which can be found almost anywhere along the alimentary tract from the mouth to the anus, become aggregated only in the ileum and form patches of a considerable size, up to 10 cm long (Peyer's patches).

The loops of small intestine lie more or less framed by the large intestine with the ascending colon on the right and the descending colon on the left. The jejunal loops tend to lie above and to the left and the ileal below and to the right. This is influenced by the oblique attachment of the mesentery to the posterior abdominal wall. Loops of ileum hang downwards into the pelvis

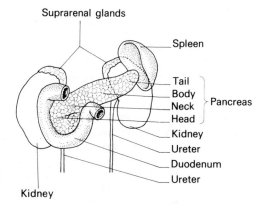

Suprarenal glands

Spleen
Tail
Body
Neck
Head
Pancreas
Kidney
Ureter
Duodenum
Ureter

Kidney

Fig. 13.6. The relations of the organs on the posterior abdominal wall. (Apart from the spleen they are all retroperitoneal.)

and lie on top of the bladder (and uterus in the female). The terminal part of the ileum always passes upwards to the right out of the pelvis and joins the left border of the upper end of the caecum.

The arteries of the jejunum and ileum (midgut structures) come from the superior mesenteric artery and run in the mesentery. The veins form the superior mesenteric vein which joins the splenic vein to form the portal vein passing to the liver. The nerve supply is both sympathetic and parasympathetic (vagus) and they pass from the coeliac plexus to the jejunum and ileum along the blood vessels.

Large intestine

The large intestine is about 150 cm long and extends from the ileum to the anus (Figs. 13.1 & 13.5). It is divided into several parts. The part inferior to the ileocaecal orifice is called the caecum. The vermiform appendix is attached to the lower part of the posteromedial wall of the caecum. Passing upwards from the caecum above the entry of the ileum is the ascending colon which turns to the left at the right colic (hepatic) flexure and becomes the transverse colon. The transverse colon runs slightly upwards as well as to the left until it reaches the spleen where it turns downwards and becomes the descending colon at the left colic (splenic) flexure. The descending colon continues as a loop which hangs into the pelvis. This is the sigmoid (pelvic) colon which passes towards the midline. In the cavity of the sacrum it turns downwards as the rectum which bends backwards and becomes the anal canal at the anorectal junction. The anal canal opens on to the exterior at the anus.

The caecum (meaning 'blind') hangs downwards in the right iliac fossa above the lateral half of the inguinal ligament. Anteriorly it is related to the anterior abdominal wall. It is usually completely surrounded by peritoneum and is relatively mobile. In 80–90% of subjects the (vermiform) appendix arises from the posteromedial wall and lies, in about 65% of subjects, behind the caecum or colon. In a further 30% the appendix points downwards into the pelvis. The caecum is about 7 cm wide and 7 cm long but the latter is variable.

The ileocaecal orifice is the site of the opening of the ileum into the large intestine. It is said to have a valve which consists of two horizontal projections into the lumen of the large intestine. These projections mark the junction of the caecum with the ascending colon. They contain circular smooth muscle which may act as a sphincter but there is some doubt about how this valve functions. The opening of the appendix is usually about 2 cm below the ileocaecal orifice.

The ascending colon, about 15 cm long, passes upwards on the right side of the posterior abdominal wall and lies immediately deep to the anterior abdominal wall until it passes deep to the right lobe of the liver where it turns to the left at the right colic (hepatic) flexure. This flexure lies on the lower lateral part of the right kidney and is here related to the gall bladder and duodenum. Usually both the ascending colon and right colic flexure have peritoneum only anteriorly so that they are relatively fixed to the structures on which they lie.

The transverse colon, about 50 cm long, is the longest of the subdivisions of the large intestine because it hangs downwards from the posterior abdominal wall in the form of a loop and ascends to the left where it turns downwards at the left colic (splenic) flexure. The transverse colon is suspended from the posterior abdominal wall by a double fold of peritoneum, called the transverse mesocolon, which is attached along a line passing over the middle of the head of the pancreas. It is usually described as lying behind the liver, the lower part of the stomach and the lower part of the spleen. It lies on the second part of the duodenum, the head of the pancreas, coils of small intestine and the duodenojejunal flexure. The left colic flexure lies on the lower part of the left kidney behind the spleen and is higher and deeper (more posterior) than the right colic flexure.

The descending colon passes downwards on the left side of the posterior abdominal wall as far as the inlet of the true (lesser) pelvis, where it becomes continuous with the sigmoid colon. It is about 20 cm long. At its start, the descending colon lies in front of the lower part of the left kidney. It is covered by loops of small intestine but its lower part may be in contact with the anterior abdominal wall.

The sigmoid (pelvic) colon is suspended from the posterior pelvic wall in the region of the pelvic inlet, sacroiliac joint and upper part of the sacrum by the sigmoid (pelvic) mesocolon. The sigmoid colon is of variable length (about 45 cm) and position and hangs down into the pelvis forming an S-shaped loop in front of the rectum. The bladder is anterior in the male and the uterus is anterior in the female.

At the level of the body of the third sacral vertebra, the sigmoid colon becomes the rectum which lies in the hollow of the sacrum and coccyx and is therefore curved backwards.

Just below the level of the tip of the coccyx and about 2.5 cm in front of it, the rectum bends backwards acutely at the anorectal junction and becomes the anal canal. Usually coils of ileum and the sigmoid colon lie in front of the rectum between it and the bladder in the male and the uterus and upper part of the vagina in the female.

The anal canal (about 4 cm long) passes downwards and backwards and opens externally at the anus. The anal canal develops partly from the hindgut and partly from a depression from the surface called the proctodeum. The anal veins may become varicose, forming haemorrhoids (piles).

The sphincters of the anal canal are important and complicated. There are two main sphincters, the internal which is a thickening of the circular smooth muscle of the alimentary tract round the upper half of the canal and an external sphincter round the whole of the canal. The external sphincter consists of skeletal muscle. The levator ani where it passes round the anorectal junction is thought to exercise a sphincteric action.

The large intestine has certain external features which distinguish it from the small intestine. On the whole it is of a larger diameter. (The caecum and lower part of the rectum tend to be of a larger diameter than the rest of the large intestine.) The obvious exception is the vermiform appendix. The longitudinal muscle of the large intestine is in the form of three bands called taeniae coli. These are easily seen on the exterior of the wall. The appendix, however, has a complete coat of longitudinal muscle (the three taeniae of the caecum converge and lead to the attachment of the appendix to the caecum), and the rectum has an almost complete layer of longitudinal muscle deficient only at its lateral edges. Since the taeniae are shorter than the circular muscle coat the large intestine shows characteristic sacculations. Small projections of fat covered by peritoneum, called appendices epiploicae, are found over the surface of the large intestine. They are not seen over the caecum, appendix and rectum.

The artery of the midgut, the superior mesenteric, supplies those parts of the large intestine derived from the midgut, the caecum, appendix, ascending colon, right colic flexure and most of the transverse colon. The inferior mesenteric artery (the artery of the hindgut) supplies the rest of the transverse colon, the descending and sigmoid colons, the rectum and the anal canal as far as the anal valves.

The veins from the large intestine correspond with the arteries and therefore go to the superior mesenteric and inferior mesenteric veins, both of which go to the liver via the portal vein. The veins of the rectum and anal canal link the systematic with the portal system of veins.

The nerves of the large intestine, as far as the terminal part of the anal canal, are autonomic. The parasympathetic nerves are motor to the muscle, causing the longitudinal muscle to contract and the circular muscle to relax. From the caecum to the left colic flexure the parasympathetic nerves are derived from the vagus nerves. The rest of the large intestine receives its parasympathetic nerves from the pelvic splanchnics (second, third and fourth sacral nerves). The sympathetic nerves are mainly motor in function. The sensory nerves are both sympathetic and parasympathetic but sensations of distension are said to be mediated entirely by the parasympathetic nerves. The external sphincter of the anal canal has a somatic nerve supply which also gives a sensory supply to the lining of the terminal part of the anal canal.

This means that the terminal part of the anal canal responds to different modalities of sensation, for example touch, pain and changes of temperature, as compared with the upper part which reacts to tension and distension.

Peritoneum

This is the serous membrane of the abdominal cavity and organs, and is comparable with the pleura of the lungs and the serous pericardium of the heart. All three are derived from the same structure in the fetus and in the course of development become separated from each other. They have the same basic arrangement, that is, organs are invaginated into them, with the result that they become two-layered; an outer layer lines the cavity (parietal) and an inner layer more or less covers the organ (visceral). The serous membranes have a cavity or potential cavity between these two layers. Histologically they are all similar and consist of loose connective tissue with a layer of flattened cells (mesothelium) on the adjacent surfaces of the two layers. The peritoneum, however, is much more complex in its arrangement than the pleura and pericardium. The complications are due to (a) the way in which the liver develops, (b) the presence of a diverticulum from the peritoneal cavity extending to the left behind the stomach and then upwards behind the liver and

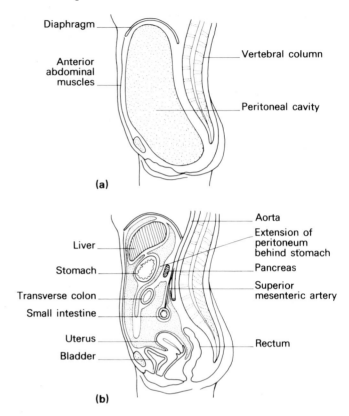

Fig. 13.7. (a) A simple concept of the peritoneal cavity. (b) The actual arrangement of the abdominal organs to the peritoneum. (The arrangement behind the liver has been simplified.)

downwards below the stomach, and (c) the adhesion of adjacent layers to each other.

The following description is very simplified: an examination of Fig. 13.7 enables one to follow the peritoneum in a longitudinal section of the abdominal cavity to the left of the midline, that is through the diverticulum referred to. The main cavity is called the greater sac or simply the peritoneal cavity, and the diverticulum the lesser sac or omental bursa. The following points should be noted:

1   The liver to the right and left is invaginated into the greater sac.

2   A considerable area of the liver, to the right of the midline and on its posterosuperior aspect, is devoid of peritoneum— the bare area of the liver. The inferior vena cava is almost embedded in the liver on the left part of this area, (**1**, and **2** are not seen in the figure).

3   There is an apron of peritoneum which hangs downwards below the stomach and usually lies directly behind the anterior abdominal wall. This is the greater omentum (Figs. 13.3 & 13.7).

4   The adjacent surfaces of the peritoneum behind the stomach and in front of the transverse colon have fused and form the transverse mesocolon. The line of attachment of this mesocolon is approximately along the body of the pancreas.

5   The bladder is below and anterior to the peritoneum. When it enlarges it strips the peritoneum off the anterior abdominal wall and lies immediately deep to the wall (Fig. 13.7).

6   The duodenum, ascending and descending colons and rectum are described as retroperitoneal because they have peritoneum only on their anterior surface and therefore no mesentery.

A transverse section at the level of the opening of the greater sac into the omental bursa (epiploic foramen) is seen in Fig. 13.8. Note that (a) the arrangement of the peritoneum of the spleen permits the splenic artery to pass on the posterior abdominal wall from the coeliac trunk to the spleen and brànches of the splenic artery to go to the stomach, and (b) because the structures going to and from the liver lie in front of the diverticulum, they become enclosed in a double fold of peritoneum passing between the lesser curvature of the stomach and the liver.

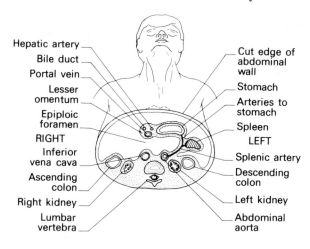

Hepatic artery
Bile duct
Portal vein
Lesser omentum
Epiploic foramen
RIGHT
Inferior vena cava
Ascending colon
Right kidney
Lumbar vertebra

Cut edge of abdominal wall
Stomach
Arteries to stomach
Spleen
LEFT
Splenic artery
Descending colon
Left kidney
Abdominal aorta

Fig. 13.8. Transverse section through the upper part of the abdomen to show the arrangement of the peritoneum. (The upper segment is looked at from below.)

The relation of the peritoneum to the gonads is of considerable importance. The gonads in both sexes are outside the peritoneum as are all other abdominal organs. In the male the testis passes down the posterior abdominal wall, across the pelvis to the anterior abdominal wall and through the muscles just above the inguinal ligament into the scrotum. It is accompanied by a process of peritoneum which also passes into the scrotum (Fig. 13.9). The testis is invaginated into the lower end of this process which forms a double layer of peritoneum round the testis. The process normally disappears from the upper pole of the testis to the deep ring in the anterior

Anterior abdominal wall
Peritoneum
Scrotum
Testis
Peritoneum
Ductus (Vas) deferens

Normally disappears
Peritoneal covering of testis
Peritoneum

Fig. 13.9. The peritoneal relations of the testis.

abdominal wall through which it came. It may not disappear in which case a hernia may form. A hernia is defined as the protrusion through the wall of the lining of any body cavity together with some of the contents of the cavity. The hernia just described would be a congenital inguinal hernia, in that it is due to the persistance of a peritoneal process seen at one stage of development in all normal males and females. A hernial sac of this type without something in its cavity is not visible. The commonest structure to enter the sac is a loop of small bowel.

In the female, the ovary also develops outside the peritoneum on the posterior abdominal wall. It moves downwards into the pelvis where it remains. It invaginates the posterior layer of the peritoneum at the side of the uterus and acquires a mesentery, the mesovarium. The peritoneum covering the ovary disappears so that an ovum is shed into the abdominal cavity. The ovum then finds its way into the uterine tube which develops as an evagination of the peritoneal cavity. The uterine tube leads to the cavity of the uterus and vagina. In this way the peritoneal cavity in the female communicates with the exterior, and the spermatozoa can reach the ovum.

Liver

The liver, which is the largest gland in the body, weighs about 1.5 kg. It lies in the upper right part of the abdominal cavity and extends to the left of the midline for about 7 cm (Figs. 13.1 & 13.5). It is dark red in colour due to the large amount of blood in it, but it is easily torn. The normal human liver has a colour and texture similar to that of the fresh liver of animals seen in a shop.

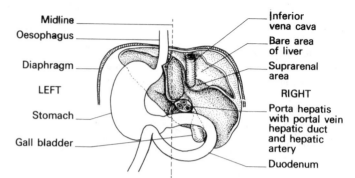

Fig. 13.10. The postero-inferior surface of the liver seen from behind.

The liver is described as having a diaphragmatic surface and a visceral surface. The former is usually subdivided into superior, posterior, right and anterior surfaces all of which are in contact with the diaphragm. The superior surface is separated by that muscle from the right pleura and lung, the pericardium and heart and a small part of the left pleura and lung. The heart often produces a slight concavity on this surface. The posterior surface corresponds with the bare area referred to above, and has the inferior vana cava on its left side. The right surface is related to the right pleura and lung and lower right ribs. The anterior surface has similar relations but its lower border extends beyond the rib cage for about 2 cm and comes in contact with the anterior abdominal wall especially inferior to the xiphoid process of the sternum. This is more marked on deep inspiration in which the liver can move down 3–4 cm.

The visceral surface faces inferoposteriorly, is related to a number of abdominal organs and is subdivided by grooves, unlike the diaphragmatic surface which is on the whole uniformly smooth. The organs which are related to the inferior surface of the liver are shown in Figs. 13.10 & 13.11. The right side is in contact with the right colic (hepatic) flexure. Above that area is the right kidney, its hilum being separated from the liver by the second part of the duodenum. The right suprarenal is related to the upper part of this renal area and to the bare area; both are to the right of the inferior vena cava. The gall bladder is related to the visceral surface medial to the hepatic flexure (Fig. 13.11). The oesophagus produces a groove to the left of the midline. This groove continues downwards into an area of the left lobe which is in contact with the stomach.

The middle of the visceral surface contains the porta hepatis into which go the hepatic artery and portal vein and out of which comes the common hepatic duct. Two grooves pass upwards and downwards from the left end of the porta hepatis. These are more or less in the midline and divide the liver into a large right and small left lobe. The right lobe is further subdivided by the left edges of the inferior vena cava and gall bladder. The division of the liver into lobes determined by these surface structures does not correspond with the subdivisions of the hepatic duct, hepatic artery and portal vein. These divide in such a way that their left subdivisions pass to or from a considerable part of the right lobe. Apparently there are a number of segments each having its own branch of the hepatic artery, portal vein and hepatic duct. The

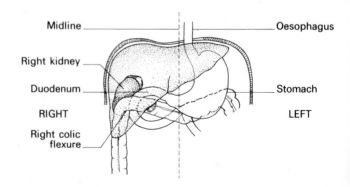

Fig. 13.11. The main relations of the postero-inferior surface of the liver. (The position of the liver is indicated by dots.)

hepatic veins are not segmental in arrangement but tend to lie between segments and any one large hepatic vein drains several segments.

The portal vein and hepatic artery enter the liver at the porta hepatis and the common hepatic duct leaves the porta. The portal vein is posterior to the other two and the hepatic duct is to the right of the hepatic artery. If followed into the liver the vessels and duct are found to divide and subdivide but remain together as a portal triad consisting of a branch of the hepatic artery, portal vein and hepatic duct. The hepatic veins run separately from the triad and their tributaries join up and form several veins which open into the inferior vena cava as it lies next to the liver. The liver receives autonomic nerves, both sympathetic and parasympathetic. Apart from the effect of the sympathetic on the blood vessels, the role of the nerves is not very clear.

The histology and biochemistry of the liver are described on p. 619.

Gall bladder and bile ducts

The gall bladder is a pear-shaped structure about 8 cm long and 3 cm wide at its fundus and has a capacity of about 50 ml (Fig. 13.12). It lies to the right of the midline on the visceral surface of the liver and projects beyond the inferior margin at the level of the tip of the right ninth costal cartilage, where the lateral edge of the rectus abdominis crosses the costal margin. It is attached by connective tissue to the liver and its inferior surface is covered by peritoneum. The neck leads into the cystic duct which joins the common hepatic duct near the porta hepatis and together they form the bile duct. The body and

neck of the gall bladder are related to the first part of the duodenum and the fundus to the transverse colon. The lining of the neck and duct has a series of folds which look like a spiral, hence its name, the spiral fold or valve.

The bile duct passes downwards behind the first part of the duodenum then behind the head of the pancreas. It enters the posteromedial aspect of the second part of the duodenum together with the main pancreatic duct and forms a common duct which opens into the duodenum.

The gall bladder receives its arterial blood supply from the hepatic artery through the cystic artery. The origin of the cystic artery is very variable. The nerve supply of the gall bladder is both sympathetic and parasympathetic but contraction of the gall bladder is thought to be largely under hormonal control.

Pancreas

This is a mainly exocrine compound racemose gland which lies on the posterior abdominal wall and extends from the hollow of the duodenum to the left and upwards as far as the spleen (Figs. 13.6 & 13.13). Scattered throughout the exocrine tissue are clumps of cells called the islets of Langerhans which are endocrine in function. The pancreas is described in terms of a head (the large part in the concavity of the duodenum), a neck, a body and a tail. From right to left it lies in front of the bile duct, portal vein, inferior vena cava, aorta and left kidney. The splenic artery and vein lie transversely behind the pancreas, the vein being inferior to the artery. Anterior to the pancreas are the stomach and the attachment

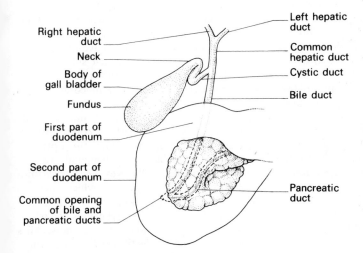

Right hepatic duct
Neck
Body of gall bladder
Fundus
First part of duodenum
Second part of duodenum
Common opening of bile and pancreatic ducts

Left hepatic duct
Common hepatic duct
Cystic duct
Bile duct
Pancreatic duct

Fig. 13.12. The gall bladder and biliary ducts. (The gall bladder has been pulled to the right.)

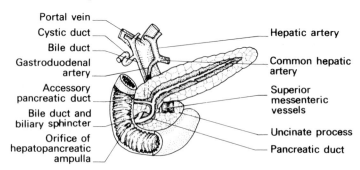

Portal vein
Cystic duct
Bile duct
Gastroduodenal artery
Accessory pancreatic duct
Bile duct and biliary sphincter
Orifice of hepatopancreatic ampulla

Hepatic artery
Common hepatic artery
Superior messenteric vessels
Uncinate process
Pancreatic duct

Fig. 13.13. The bile and pancreatic ducts.

of the two layers of the transverse mesocolon. The tail of the pancreas lies posterior to the hilum of the spleen and the splenic vessels entering and leaving the hilum.

The main duct of the pancreas runs from left to right and receives along its course the ducts of the lobules of the gland (Fig. 13.13). Near the neck the main duct turns somewhat downwards as it passes towards the duodenum. The bile duct passing downwards behind the head of the pancreas joins the main pancreatic duct in the wall of the second part of the duodenum. There is a dilatation, the hepatopancreatic ampulla before the common opening into the duodenum. This ampulla is surrounded by a thickening of circular smooth muscle called the sphincter of Oddi or the ampullary sphincter. This sphincter extends upwards round the terminal parts of the bile and main pancreatic ducts. The sphincter round the bile ducts is much thicker and more extensive than that round the pancreatic duct.

The arterial blood supply of the pancreas is derived from the coeliac trunk (splenic and superior pancreaticoduodenal arteries) and the superior mesenteric artery (inferior pancreaticoduodenal artery). Its veins go to the hepatic portal system of veins. The islets of Langerhans have a particularly rich blood supply with fenestrated capillaries of a sinusoid structure which have a larger diameter than the small vessels leaving the islets. The nerve supply of the pancreas is both sympathetic (splanchnic nerves) and parasympathetic (vagus nerves). The exocrine cells have non-myelinated axons ending on their base. These are thought to be vagal. The endocrine cells have both adrenergic (sympathetic) and cholinergic (vagal) fibres closely related to them. The role of these nerves is not known because it is generally accepted that pancreatic secretion depends largely on hormones from the gastro-intestinal tract.

The spleen is described on p. 660.

HISTOLOGY

General features

The alimentary tract is a fibromuscular tube extending from the mouth to the anus. Its wall surrounds a sample of the external environment and prepares it for use by the body. Preparation involves a series of steps which follow each other in a regular order, the gut wall being divided up into lengths each of which is specialized to deal with one of these steps. Food entering the alimentary tract is effectively entering a one-way traffic system and is normally propelled through it from mouth to anus by peristaltic contraction of the muscles of its wall. In this way anarchy is avoided and the food is processed in an orderly manner.

Variations associated with specialization are superimposed on a general plan. The gut wall consists of four concentric layers; beginning at the inside of the tube and progressing outwards, these are: mucosa (mucous membrane), submucosa, muscularis externa, and tunica adventitia or serosa (peritoneum). Fig. 13.14 shows these layers diagrammatically.

The mucosa consists of a surface epithelium with glands opening on to its free surface; a lamina propria of loose connective tissues, well supplied with capillaries, which supports and nourishes the epithelium; and a thin layer of smooth muscle, the muscularis mucosae (absent from some parts of the gut).

The submucosa underlies the mucosa, as its name indicates, and consists of connective tissues somewhat denser than the lamina propria. It contains many blood and lymphatic vessels, lymphatic nodules, and nerves. The nerves form a plexus (Meissner's plexus) which includes parasympathetic ganglion cells which are secretomotor to the epithelial glands and which also cause contraction of the muscularis mucosae and the muscle fibres of the villi (where

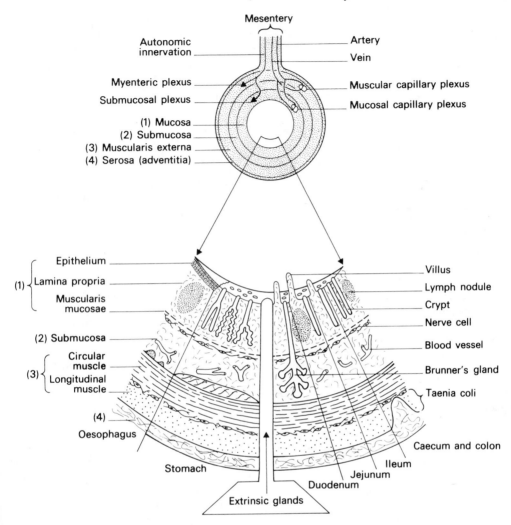

Fig. 13.14. The wall of the alimentary tract.

present), and sympathetic fibres which stimulate contraction of the smooth muscle of the blood vessels. Where there is no muscularis mucosae there is a gradual transition from the lamina propria to the submucosa.

The muscularis externa generally has two layers of smooth muscle: an inner circular and an outer longitudinal layer, with a nerve plexus, the myenteric or Auerbach's plexus, sandwiched between them. The plexus contains parasympathetic ganglion cells which are motor to the smooth muscle cells of the muscularis externa, and sympathetic fibres which stimulate vasoconstriction. The main function of the plexus is to coordinate movement of the various parts of the gut wall.

Some regions of the gut, such as the pharynx and most of the oesophagus, have a tunica adventitia as their external coat. This is a layer of fairly dense fibrous connective tissue continuous with that of the adjacent organs, yet not so dense as to prevent the tube expanding as food is passed through it. The attachment is sufficently lax to allow the gut to move independently of its neighbours, yet strong enough to ensure that they retain their relative positions. The rest of the gut loops out to varying degrees into the abdominal and pelvic cavities and, since these cavities are lined by peritoneum, the gut they contain is covered by peritoneum (or serosa as it is called here). In some zones, such as the small intestine, the loops of gut are attached to the

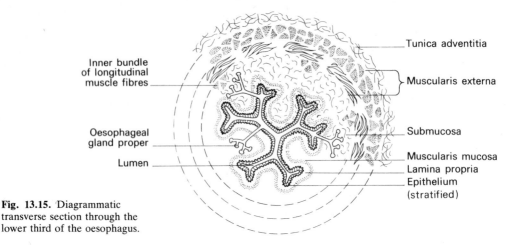

Inner bundle
of longitudinal
muscle fibres

Oesophageal
gland proper

Lumen

Tunica adventitia

Muscularis externa

Submucosa

Muscularis mucosa
Lamina propria
Epithelium
(stratified)

Fig. 13.15. Diagrammatic
transverse section through the
lower third of the oesophagus.

body wall via a thin mesentery of loose connective tissue covered on its free surface by peritoneal epithelium continuous with that surrounding the alimentary tract and lining the body wall, whereas elsewhere, for example the rectum, the attachment is broad and is effectively an adventitia continuous with a serosa. The peritoneum consists of a deep layer of fibrous connective tissue covered by a simple squamous epithelium (mesothelium), the cells of which are moistened by a film of serous fluid (peritoneal fluid) which seems to act as a lubricant, allowing the mobile gut to glide over the other viscera without damage.

Oesophagus

This has specializations which enable it to convey food, which may be rough or infected, from the pharynx to the stomach.

The mucosa or mucous membrane is generally between 0.5 and 0.8 mm thick. A thick stratified non-keratinized epithelium lines its inner surface (Fig. 13.15). As the superficial cells are worn away by friction, they are replaced by cells from the deeper layers, which in turn are replaced by the products of division of the basal cells. The lamina propria contains clusters of macrophages, lymphocytes and plasma cells, which collectively form a first line of defence against any pathogens which invade the wall of the oesophagus. The ducts of a variety of oesophageal glands extend through the lamina propria and open on to the surface of the epithelium. They can be grouped into two types: oesophageal glands proper, and oesophageal cardiac (or gastric) glands. The mucus they secrete helps to reduce friction as food passes down the oesophagus. The oesophageal glands proper are compound tubuloalveolar glands, whose secretory portions lie in the submucosa. The oesophageal cardiac glands are simple branched tubular glands, whose secretory portions lie in the lamina propria, and which closely resemble the cardiac glands of the stomach (p. 596). There are generally two groups of oesophageal cardiac (gastric) glands, one near the pharynx and one near the stomach. The surface epithelium near their openings is often of the simple columnar type, like that of the stomach, and it has been suggested that this ectopic gastric epithelium, which may contain oxyntic and chief cells as well as mucus-secreting cells, may be the site of origin of oesophageal ulcers and cancerous growths. The mucous membrane is completed externally by the muscularis mucosae. It consists of longitudinal smooth muscle fibres interspersed with thin elastic fibres. When it contracts, the mucosa is thrown temporarily into horizontal folds.

The submucosa is a layer of dense irregular fibrous connective tissue containing collagen, elastin, and clusters of lymphoid and reticuloendothelial cells surrounding the oesophageal glands proper which, since they open on to the surface of the oesophagus, are prone to infection. Except when swallowing, the mucosa and submucosa are longitudinally pleated, so that the lumen of the oesophagus is irregular in transverse sections (Fig. 13.15).

The muscularis externa is important in swallowing. Its upper third consists of voluntary striated muscle, which in the middle third is gradually replaced by involuntary smooth

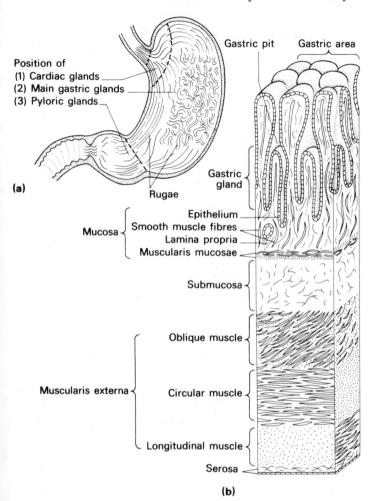

Position of
(1) Cardiac glands
(2) Main gastric glands
(3) Pyloric glands

(a)

Rugae

Gastric pit

Gastric area

Gastric gland

Mucosa
- Epithelium
- Smooth muscle fibres
- Lamina propria
- Muscularis mucosae

Submucosa

Oblique muscle

Muscularis externa
- Circular muscle
- Longitudinal muscle

Serosa

(b)

Fig. 13.16. Histology of the stomach. (a) Longitudinal section of whole stomach. (b) Wall structure in the body of the stomach.

muscle, while in the lower third only smooth muscle fibres are present. This change-over of muscle type is related to the mechanism of swallowing (p. 578) which begins as a voluntary act but then becomes involuntary. The circular fibres of the muscularis externa are continuous superiorly with the inferior constrictor muscle of the pharynx, and inferiorly with the oblique fibres of the stomach. The longitudinal muscle coat is thicker than the circular and completely invests the oesophagus apart from a V-shaped notch beginning about 3 or 4 cm below the cricoid cartilage, where the longitudinal fibres diverge, thus allowing the circular fibres to emerge and join up with those of the inferior constrictor muscle. At its lower end the muscularis externa acts as a sphincter between the oesophagus and the stomach, although it shows no structural specialization in this region, and is

therefore sometimes referred to as a 'physiological' rather than an 'anatomical' sphincter. The myenteric plexus of nerve cells and fibres lying between the two layers of muscularis externa helps to control sphincteric action and the involuntary part of the act of swallowing, mainly through local reflexes.

The cervical and thoracic parts of the oesophagus are completed by a layer of dense irregular fibrous connective tissue continuous with that of the surrounding structures and called the tunica adventitia, while the rest of the oesophagus, that is, the abdominal part, is covered by peritoneum.

Stomach

This region is lined by a mucosa which has an even surface when the stomach is distended with

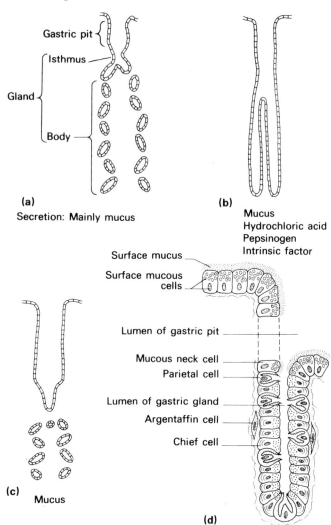

Fig. 13.17. Histology of the gastric glands. (a) Cardiac gland. (b) Gastric gland proper. (c) Pyloric gland. (d) Cell arrangement in a gastric gland proper.

food, but is thrown into longitudinal folds or rugae by the contraction of the muscularis mucosae when it is empty. Each ruga consists of a number of irregular zones about 5 mm wide called gastric areas, and which are grooved by gastric pits (Fig. 13.16).

The surface epithelium of the mucosa lines the gastric pits and covers the ridges between them. It is of the simple columnar type, and each cell secretes mucus. The cells generally live for about 3 days, and as each dies it is replaced by a younger cell in a systematic manner.

There is an abrupt transition from the stratified squamous epithelium of the oesophagus to the simple columnar epithelium of the stomach at the cardia, the entrance to the stomach, although the lower end of the oeso-

phagus contains isolated cardiac glands. The transition to intestinal epithelium is less abrupt and occurs at the pylorus.

Opening into the pits are the gastric glands, which are of three types: cardiac glands, found near the cardia; gastric glands proper or fundic glands, found throughout most of the fundus and the body of the stomach; and pyloric glands, generally restricted to the distal third, that is, the pyloric end of the stomach.

The gastric glands proper are the most numerous and the most important in the secretion of gastric juice. They are simple, branched, tubular glands which extend through the full thickness of the lamina propria and which consists of four types of cells: chief or zymogenic cells, parietal or oxyntic cells, mucous cells, and

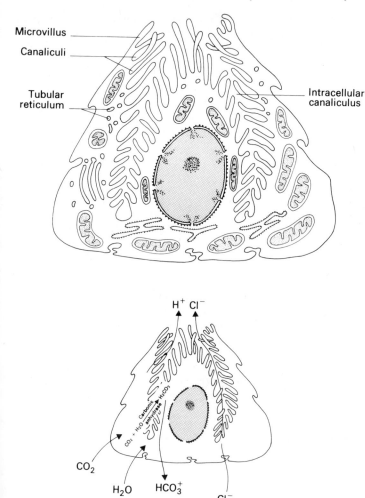

Microvillus

Canaliculi

Tubular reticulum

Intracellular canaliculus

H^+ Cl^-

CO_2

H_2O HCO_3^+

Cl^-

Fig. 13.18. Diagrammatic representation of the ultrastructural features and activity of a parietal (oxyntic) cell (see p. 606).

argentaffin or enterochromaffin or APUD cells (Fig. 13.17). The basophilic chief cells contain 'zymogen' granules, that is, enzyme-generating granules containing precursors of the proteolytic enzyme pepsin and other gastric enzymes. The acidophilic parietal cells, so called because they lie on the wall of the gland, or oxyntic cells, are the acid-producers of the stomach. They are unique in that the cytoplasm is penetrated by an extensive system of intracellular canaliculi leading to the luminal surface of the cell. Active cells are lined by microvilli which provide them with a vast surface area across which H^+ can be secreted (Fig. 13.18). It has been suggested that these microvilli appear as a tubular reticulum within the cytoplasm in resting cells. To visualize the change which takes place, in an over-simplified way, consider the fingers of a rubber glove, first infolded into the hand (resting) and then blown out straight again (active). A high density of mitochondria, characteristic of cells which are capable of rapid metabolic activity, is a prominent feature of these cells.

It is intriguing that although the activity of the parietal cells makes the stomach contents highly acidic, there is virtually no diffusion of H^+ back into the mucosa; if, however, the mucosa is damaged, by drugs such as aspirin, for example, H^+ can no longer be held back but diffuses into the subepithelial tissues where it aggravates the ulceration. Little is known about the nature of this mucosal barrier; gastric mucus is not responsible. Mucous cells are most common in the neck of the gland; they generally contain so many granules of mucinogen (the precursor of mucus) that in haematoxylin and eosin preparations they appear frothy.

The cardiac glands are compound, branched,

tubular glands consisting mainly of mucous cells between which are scattered a few argentaffin cells of uncertain function.

The pyloric glands are simple, branched, tubular and coiled. They open into deep gastric pits which are as long as the glands themselves (Fig. 13.17). These glands consist of mucous, parietal and argentaffin cells.

The argentaffin cells, so called because they can be stained with silver salts, lie between the bases of the other secretory cells. Some argentaffin cells manufacture and store serotonin or 5-hydroxytryptamine (p. 688); others which abound in pyloric glands produce the hormone gastrin; a third type, which resembles a pancreatic alpha cell (p. 604), probably secretes enteroglucagon. These various functions have been ascribed to these cells because of their reactions to specific immunofluorescence staining.

The lamina propria shows no particular specializations. Strands of smooth muscle extend through it from the muscularis mucosae towards the epithelium, and their contraction aids the emptying of the gastric glands. The submucosa is also unspecialized.

The muscularis externa is triple-layered, consisting of inner oblique, middle circular and outer longitudinal layers. In the pyloric region the middle layer forms the anatomical sphincter of the pylorus.

The stomach wall is completed by the peritoneum, a layer of loose connective tissue covered by peritoneal mesothelium continuous with that of the omenta.

Small intestine

This comprises the duodenum, jejunum and ileum. Fluids poured into it from the gall bladder and pancreas, and from the glands in its wall, are mixed with the chyme and propelled through it by peristalsis. During the progress of this mixture through the small intestine digestion is completed and the products of digestion are absorbed into the blood and lymph capillaries. The structural specializations of the various parts of the small intestine reflect these activities.

As a result of the following modifications the mucosa of the small intestine has an absorption surface area of about 40 m^2.
1   The mucosa and submucosa are folded transversely into many crescentric plicae circulares.
2   The surface of the entire mucosa is covered by fingerlike villi which project into the lumen of

the gut. Each is about 1 mm high and as there are up to 40/mm^2, the inside of the small intestine has a 'velvety' appearance.
3   The simple columnar epithelium covering the villi has a brush border of microvilli on its luminal aspect.
4   The epithelium dips down into the lamina propria between the villi forming the crypts of Lieberkühn (Fig. 13.19).

The epithelium of the mucosa consists of three types of cells: absorptive, goblet and argentaffin.

ABSORPTIVE CELLS

These are columnar cells with a prominent striated or brush border composed of microvilli (Fig. 13.20). A coat of glycoprotein rests on the tips of the microvilli. This coat, which resists proteolytic agents, protects the epithelial cells from digestion, and helps in the intraluminal digestion of food by carrying an adsorbed layer of specific digestive enzymes, and ensuring that the products of digestion are formed at the site of absorption, i.e. the microvilli. To reach the capillaries, digested materials must pass through the epithelial cell cytoplasm by one means or another (p. 611). The energy required for these processes is provided by the many mitochondria the absorptive cells contain. The absorptive cells are tightly packed together forming a single layer and each is encircled at its luminal aspect by a junctional complex which seals it off from its neighbours and stops material from the gut passing between the cells (p. 174).

The absorptive cells also synthesize lipids and transport the products of fat digestion from the lumen into the lacteals. This is outlined in Fig. 13.20.

GOBLET CELLS

These are mucus-secreting flask-shaped cells found scattered among the absorptive cells (Fig. 13.21). The mucus they secrete helps to lubricate and protect the surface of the epithelium.

ARGENTAFFIN OR APUD CELLS

These lie between the bases of some of the columnar cells of the epithelium. They are particularly common in the duodenum, and some at least have an endocrine function (p. 616). All the epithelial cells rest on a basement membrane, through which absorbed materials and endocrine secretions pass to reach the capillaries.

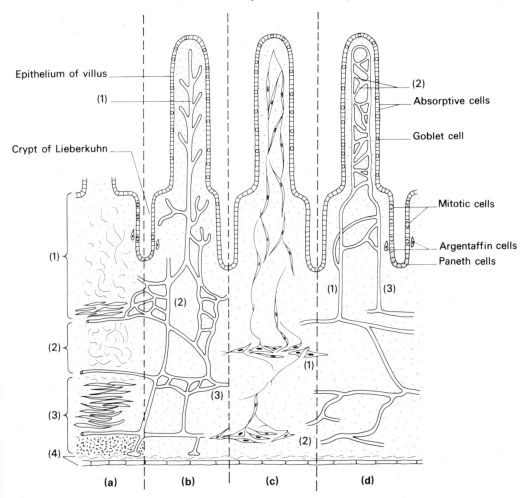

Fig. 13.19. The wall of the small intestine. (a) Wall structure: 1, mucosa; 2, submucosa; 3, muscularis externa; 4, serosa. (b) Lymphatic supply: 1, lacteal of villus; 2, mucosal and submucosal vessels; 3, muscular plexus. (c) Nerve supply: 1, submucosal plexus; 2, myenteric plexus. (d) Blood supply: 1, arteriole from mesenteric artery; 2, capillaries of villus; 3, venule.

EPITHELIUM OF THE CRYPTS OF LIEBERKÜHN (INTESTINAL CRYPTS)

The simple columnar epithelium covering the villi continues down into the crypts. Each crypt is really a simple tubular gland whose walls are lined by the cell types mentioned above. The epithelial cells in the bases of the crypts are less differentiated than those elsewhere, and by their repeated mitotic divisions they provide a source of new cells to replace those lost from the rest of the epithelium by wear and tear. Millions of damaged cells are shed from the human small intestine every day and are replaced by cells displaced from the crypts. On their way upwards the cells differentiate into absorptive, goblet or argentaffin cells.

Not all the cells in the bases of the crypts can divide. There are also scattered groups of cells called Paneth cells (Fig. 13.22). These are pyramidal cells filled with secretory granules of glycoprotein and possibly some other materials. Incredibly, despite years of investigation, it is still not clear what the function of the Paneth cells is. They are known to concentrate zinc, a component of a number of enzymes, but it has not been proved that they secrete the enzymes they make. One interesting suggestion is that their granules contain lysozyme, a substance

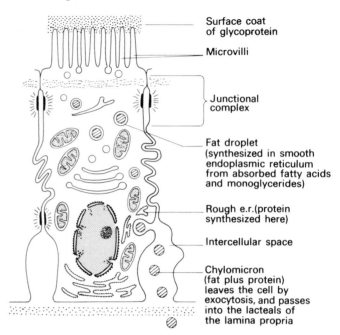

Surface coat of glycoprotein

Microvilli

Junctional complex

Fat droplet (synthesized in smooth endoplasmic reticulum from absorbed fatty acids and monoglycerides)

Rough e.r.(protein synthesized here)

Intercellular space

Chylomicron (fat plus protein) leaves the cell by exocytosis, and passes into the lacteals of the lamina propria

Fig. 13.20. Absorptive cell.

which lyses bacteria, in which case they may help to protect a part of the gut prone to attack from infection.

LAMINA PROPRIA

This fills the spaces between the crypts and forms the cores of the villi. Its only specialization is that it is rich in lymphoid tissue, the cells of which form nodules which may aggregate into oval masses coextensive with similar masses in the submucosa, and collectively called Peyer's

patches. These are most commonly found in the ileum.

The connective tissue fibres of the lamina propria support the central lacteal (lymph capillary) and the plexus of blood capillaries in each villus into which absorbed materials pass. Passing around them, and arranged longitudinally, that is, parallel to the longitudinal axis of the villus, are fine strands of smooth muscle continuous with the muscularis mucosae. Their contraction 'milks' the lacteals of lymph and thus aids the transport of nutrients.

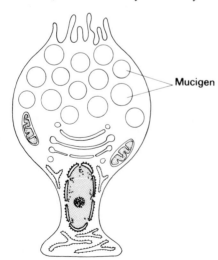

Mucigen

Fig. 13.21. Goblet cell.

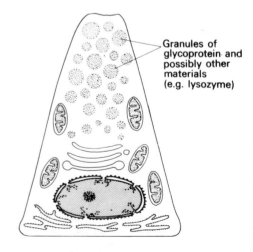

Granules of glycoprotein and possibly other materials (e.g. lysozyme)

Fig. 13.22. Paneth cell.

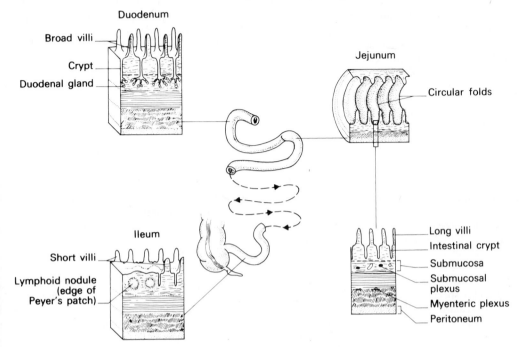

Fig. 13.23. Small intestine showing regional variations. The circular folds and the height and numbers of villi all diminish towards the ileum.

Aggregated lymphoid nodules characterize the lower ileum.

MUSCULARIS MUCOSAE, SUBMUCOSA, MUSCULARIS EXTERNA AND PERITONEUM

These show no particular specializations, with the exception of the submucosa of the duodenum which contains mucus-secreting duodenal glands or Brunner's glands (Fig. 13.14). These are compound tubuloalveolar glands whose ducts penetrate the muscularis mucosae and open between the bases of the duodenal villi. The fluid they secrete is alkaline and contains bicarbonate salts which have a buffering action. Its main function is to protect the duodenal mucosa from the action of the acidic chyme.

In the above description the small intestine has been considered as a whole. However, its structure varies along its length. The variations which characterize the duodenum, jejunum and ileum are listed below and illustrated in Fig. 13.23.

1 Duodenum
  (a) Broad, leaf-shaped villi.
  (b) Submucosal Brunner's glands present.
2 Jejunum
  (a) Villi elongated and closely packed (the

bulk of absorption occurs here).
  (b) Prominent transverse folds throughout its length.
3 Ileum
  (a) Villi shorter and less closely packed than in the jejunum.
  (b) Fewer absorptive cells but more goblet cells than in the jejunum.
  (c) Lymphoid tissue (e.g. Peyer's patches) most prominent here.

Large intestine

This extends from the ileocaecal junction to the anus, and includes the appendix. With the exception of the appendix, which in man is primarily a lymphoid organ, the rest of the large intestine is concerned with absorption of water and electrolytes (the proximal half) and with the temporary storage of faeces (the distal half), and as elsewhere in the gut, it shows specializations reflecting these functions.

APPENDIX

This is a blind ended worm-shaped tube opening out from the caecum. Its wall is thickened by lymphoid tissue to such an extent that its lumen is virtually obliterated. There are no villi but crypts are present, containing absorptive cells, goblet cells, argentaffin cells, and relatively undifferentiated cells capable of mitosis. The muscularis mucosa and muscularis externa are thinner than elsewhere in the gut, while the submucosa forms a thick, supporting layer. The peritoneum is similar to that covering the rest of the intestine.

CAECUM AND COLON

Unlike the small intestine, these lack plicae circulares and villi. The crypts (Fig. 13.24) resemble those of the small intestine but contain more goblet cells and usually no Paneth cells. The absorptive cells have fewer microvilli than do those of the small intestine. The lamina propria, muscularis mucosae and submucosa show no particular specializations. The circular coat of the muscularis externa is complete, while the longitudinal coat is thickened in places to produce three taeniae coli and may be absent between them. The peritoneum has fat-filled appendages called appendices epiploicae scattered over it.

RECTUM AND ANAL CANAL

The rectum resembles the caecum and colon except for the longitudinal layer of the muscularis externa which is again complete and regular as elsewhere in the gut. Over the whole of the rectum and the upper third of the anal canal the lining epithelium is of the colonic type, i.e. simple columnar. The mucosa of this upper part of the anal canal is thrown into longitudinal folds or anal columns which are joined at their

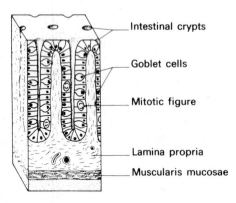

intestinal crypts

Goblet cells

Mitotic figure

Lamina propria

Muscularis mucosae

Fig. 13.24. Colon. The mucosa has a flat surface and simple mucous glands.

lower ends by anal valves. Then follows a transitional zone where the epithelium is stratified columnar, and then, just below an irregular line about 2 cm above the anal opening, the canal is lined by keratinized stratified squamous epithelium continuous with that of the skin. The change over from mucosa to skin takes place at the level of the external muscular sphincter.

Pancreas

The fluids secreted into the small intestine come not only from its intrinsic glands but also from two extrinsic glands, the pancreas and the liver. The exocrine secretions of the pancreas pass directly to the intestine via the pancreatic ducts, while those of the liver are first concentrated in the gall bladder.

The pancreas has an exocrine component which manufactures and secretes over a litre of digestive juice each day, and an endocrine component, comprising about 1% of its volume, which produces hormones that help to control carbohydrate metabolism, notably insulin.

THE EXOCRINE PANCREAS

This is a compound acinar or alveolar gland (p. 416) enclosed in a delicate layer of connective tissue continuous with that of the peritoneum, behind which the gland lies against the prevertebral fascia. Septa of even more delicate connective tissue extend into the gland, dividing it up into lobules. Each lobule consists of secretory units drained by ducts, and 'life support systems' in the form of blood vessels, lymphatics and nerves, together with connective tissue giving them mechanical support.

The secretory units are grape-shaped acini, the cells of which surround a central lumen into which they release an enzyme-containing fluid which, before secretion, is stored within the cells as zymogen granules. The lumen of each acinus opens into a duct bounded proximally by a single layer of clear centroacinar cells, so called because they extend into the centre of the acinus (Fig. 13.25).

The ducts of several acini converge on a wider intralobular duct lined by cells differing from the centroacinar cells only in that they take the form of a simple columnar epithelium. Centroacinar and intralobular duct cells never contain zymogen granules and so are readily distinguished from the acinar cells proper.

Groups of intralobular ducts open into larger interlobular ducts which are lined by a columnar

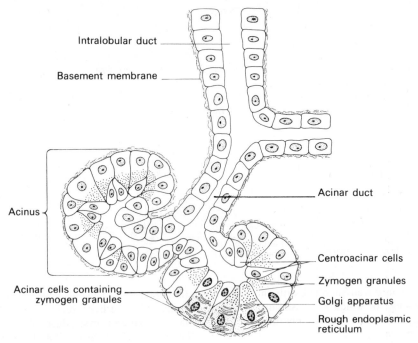

Intralobular duct

Basement membrane

Acinus

Acinar cells containing zymogen granules

Acinar duct

Centroacinar cells

Zymogen granules

Golgi apparatus

Rough endoplasmic reticulum

Fig. 13.25. Pancreatic acini.

epithelium containing scattered mucus-secreting goblet cells. The interlobular ducts converge, in turn, on one of the two pancreatic ducts, whose epithelium is covered by connective tissue containing many elastic fibres.

The roughly pyramidal acinar cells vary in appearance according to their activity. The apical zymogen granules contain enzymes elaborated in the rough endoplasmic reticulum and packaged by the supranuclear Golgi apparatus. They are most numerous just before a meal and least numerous just after one when their membranes fuse with the apical plasma membrane and their contents are released into the acinar lumen, activities which are under the influence of secretin and cholecystokinin-pancreozymin (CCK-PZ). These controlling hormones are probably produced by cells at the tips of the intestinal villi. The acini are supplied by nerve fibres from the coeliac plexus.

THE ENDOCRINE PANCREAS

The hormone-secreting cells of the pancreas are grouped into scattered, well-vascularized units, called islets of Langerhans of which there are generally over a million in an adult pancreas. Each islet which, in marked contrast to the basophilic acini, is palely stained in a routine haematoxylin and eosin preparation consists of irregular cords of hormone-secreting cells separated by and secreting into blood capillaries (Fig. 13.26). There are at least three types of granular secreting cell, designated α, β and δ.

The α-cells, also termed A2 cells, contain numerous, dense, membrane-bound bodies, and are the source of the hormone glucagon. The β-cells, or B cells, have secretory granules in which are crystalline bodies and are the source of the hormone insulin. Glucagon and insulin cooperate in the control of carbohydrate metabolism (p. 794). The δ-cells (D or A1) cells) are the probable source of pancreatic gastrin, somatostatin and serotonin. They have a similar ultrastructure to the argentaffin cells of the alimentary tract and belong to the same cell class, the APUD group of cells. APUD is an acronym for 'amine precursor uptake and decarboxylation', activities which are characteristic of these very important cells. As well as synthesizing biologically-active amines by the decarboxylation of precursors, probably in their copious smooth endoplasmic reticulum, their main function is polypeptide synthesis, and in view of this it is surprising that they have a relatively sparse rough endoplasmic reticulum.

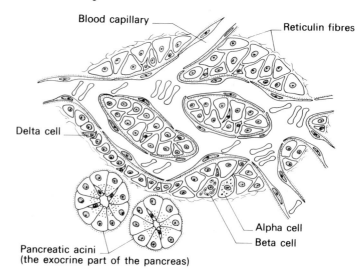

Fig. 13.26. Islet of Langerhans.

Pancreatic acini
(the exocrine part of the pancreas)

The islets are well supplied with cholinergic neurons, most of which are vasomotor to the blood vessels, while others supply the secretory cells themselves.

Gall bladder

This is a pear-shaped sac, closely applied to the posterior surface of the liver, which collects, concentrates and stores bile, releasing it into the duodenum when stimulated to do so by the entry of fat and amino acids into this part of the alimentary tract. The bile, which is secreted continuously by the liver, reaches the gall bladder via the hepatic and cystic ducts, and is forced into the duodenum via the cystic and bile ducts when the smooth muscle fibres in the wall of the gall bladder contract. The muscle is thickened into a biliary sphincter where the bile duct joins the main pancreatic duct.

The gall bladder is lined by a mucous membrane, which rests on a fibromuscular layer. Those surfaces which project into the peritoneal cavity are covered by peritoneum, and the rest

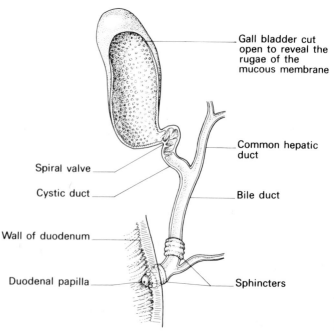

Fig. 13.27. The gall bladder and the bile ducts.

by an adventitia of loose irregular connective tissue.

The mucous membrane is folded into tiny rugae in such a way that the inside of the gall bladder looks rather like a honeycomb (Fig. 13.27). It consists of a simple columnar epithelium and a thick, highly vascular lamina propria; there is no muscularis mucosae. The epithelium concentrates the bile by resorbing salts and water from it. Its luminal surface is covered with microvilli and although adjacent cells are sealed together apically by tight junctions, they are separated elsewhere by dilated intercellular spaces. Some of the surface cells, particularly those near the cystic duct, are mucus-secreting. The mucosa also contains simple tubuloalveolar mucous glands which extend into the lamina propria.

The fibromuscular layer consists of loose bundles of smooth muscle fibres interspersed with fibrous connective tissue. The fibre bundles are arranged longitudinally, circularly and obliquely, but not in distinct layers.

The peritoneum and adventitia are thick, and contain many large vessels and nerves, including vagal and splanchnic sympathetic fibres. Sensory nerve endings monitor the degree of distension of the gall bladder when for some pathological reason it becomes overdistended.

PHYSIOLOGY

In this section, the functions of the various parts of the alimentary tract, namely the processes of secretion, digestion and absorption, are each considered in a descriptive way; control mechanisms are alluded to where necessary but not explained in detail until the whole scene has been set.

From a biochemical viewpoint, digestion involves primarily hydrolytic reactions. Digestive enzymes called hydrolases are secreted into the tract and are responsible for catalysing the hydrolysis of the food macromolecules—the proteins, carbohydrates, lipids and nucleic acids. Hydrolysis is a breaking-down of chemical bonds by water molecules, e.g.

$$R_1 - R_2 + H-O-H \quad \rightarrow \quad R_1 - H + HO-R_2$$

The stomach

ENTRY OF FOOD

Pressure in the oesophageal lumen is normally very low if the muscles in its wall are at rest.

However, at the cardiac sphincter a steady tonic contraction of the circular muscle causes the intraluminal pressure to be about 5–10 mmHg higher than the pressure in the stomach, and higher still than the intraluminal pressure cranial to it, since this reflects the negative intrathoracic pressure.

The sphincter normally prevents reflux of acidic gastric contents into the oesophagus. It relaxes and opens ahead of a peristaltic wave and the arrival of a bolus. If reflux occurs, it often causes pain, commonly known as 'heartburn'.

FUNCTIONS

Reservoir
The stomach relaxes to accept a large meal then releases it slowly into the small intestine. Probably the stomach's most important function is to act as a reservoir. The loss of this function is of the greatest importance to the patient whose stomach has been surgically removed and causes inconvenience and discomfort.

Formation of chyme
Within the stomach, food is only partially digested. It may enter as lumps in a coarse suspension and if so, by the time it passes into the duodenum, it has been softened and pulped to a well-lubricated suspension (known as chyme) which does not abrade the delicate intestinal mucosa too severely.

The stomach secretes hydrochloric acid, pepsinogen, mucus, and a carrier protein, known as intrinsic factor, which binds vitamin B_{12} (p. 675).

Acid. The hydrochloric acid secreted by parietal cells produces a pH of 1–2 in gastric juice and has several functions. It is bactericidal or bacteriostatic (i.e. it kills or inhibits the growth of bacteria), acting as a barrier to infection and preventing the gastric contents from fermenting into a horrible broth culture of miscellaneous bacteria. It aids hydrolysis of disaccharides and it activates the enzyme precursor pepsinogen, to the active form, pepsin.

Parietal cells (Fig. 13.18) undergo profound ultrastructural changes when they are stimulated to secrete acid but the mechanism by which acid is secreted is not yet completely understood. It involves active transport of both H^+ and Cl^-, i.e. the movement of these ions against their electrochemical gradients by the controlled expenditure of energy. The Cl^- is derived (indirectly) from the plasma and during secretion Cl^-

leaving the plasma is replaced by HCO_3^- formed within the parietal cells. A high concentration of the enzyme carbonic anhydrase is present in parietal cells and catalyses the reaction:

$$CO_2 + H_2O \xrightarrow[\text{anhydrase}]{\text{Carbonic}} H_2CO_3$$

$$\rightleftharpoons H^+ + HCO_3^-$$

In mammals it is this hydration of CO_2 and subsequent dissociation within the parietal cells which produce the H^+ for secretion.

Intrinsic factor. Parietal cells in man also secrete the intrinsic factor required for the active absorption of vitamin B12 (p. 675).

Pepsin. The proenzyme pepsinogen, is a polypeptide released from zymogen granules in the peptic cells. Under the action of acid it loses a terminal peptone fragment to become pepsin; the pepsin can then activate more pepsinogen. Several pepsins from human gastric samples have been separated by electrophoresis.

Although pepsin attacks proteins anywhere in the length of their chains (i.e. it is an endopeptidase) it seeks out particular peptide bonds, preferring those which leave a phenylalanine, tryptophan, or tyrosine residue on the N-terminal side of the point of cleavage. It is interesting to note that it is these aromatic amino acids which are most active, whether free or still attached to peptones, in stimulating pancreatic enzyme output following the passage of chyme into the duodenum. Gastric pepsin is not an essential enzyme for digestion, but because of this unmasking action it facilitates intestinal digestion. Whole proteins (e.g. egg albumin) placed directly in the duodenum initially evoke little or no pancreatic enzyme secretion.

The pH optimum for pepsin is 1.5–2.0 but the gastric contents approach this optimum only in the pyloric region of the stomach. If a large meal has been eaten much of it will not be mixed with gastric juice for some time.

The stomach eventually 'titrates' all the food to a low pH (pH 2–3) immediately before the chyme passes into the intestine. This process can justly be called titration, because the mechanism regulating the secretion of gastric juice is first stimulated by food (especially protein) in the pyloric region and then inhibited by the negative feedback effect of a low pH (3 or less). The amount of acid secreted is therefore related to the buffer capacity of the meal. As protein is by far the most important buffer in food, it follows that large volumes of gastric juice are secreted only if a high protein meal is eaten (Fig. 13.28).

Mucus. Gastric mucus, derived from mucinogen, lubricates the milling processes undergone by food in the stomach. It has a consistency like the nasal mucus secreted during a cold.

Sampling mixed gastric juice. Samples of gastric juice may be obtained quite easily from man by passing a narrow tube (Ryle's tube) through the nasopharynx and swallowing until it enters the stomach. The samples obtained vary in composition according to the conditions under which they are collected.

Absorption

The stomach is not designed as an absorptive organ; it has a small surface area:volume ratio and is really of no importance in this respect although some movement of water by osmosis helps to equilibrate the tonicity of the gastric contents with blood. A few drugs are thought to be absorbed in significant amounts from the otherwise empty stomach (e.g. alcohol, aspirin).

Regulation of chyme entering the intestine

The rate of gastric emptying is controlled by a number of factors. The intestine is not able to handle large volumes of highly acid, hypertonic, or fatty chyme, and by one means or another

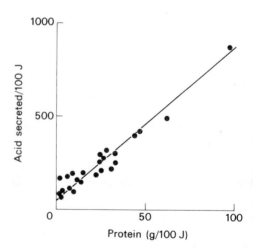

Fig. 13.28. Relationship between acid secretion and protein content of meals containing 100 J of energy fed to dogs. (Redrawn from Davenport H. W. (1966) *Physiology of the Digestive Tract*, 2nd edition. Year Book Medical Publishers, Chicago.)

each of these factors acts as a signal to limit the rate of gastric emptying. Controlled emptying, together with neutralization of the chyme by pancreatic juice, bile and intestinal electrolyte secretion brings the pH in the jejunum to about 6.

The behaviour of the mechanisms regulating gastric emptying has been found to be surprisingly predictable when foods containing different concentrations of energy-producing substrates (fat or carbohydrate) are placed in the stomach. The volume of chyme entering the duodenum in 30 minutes is inversely related to the energy content of the meal (Fig. 13.29), the relationship following the curve of a parabola.

VOMITING

The existence of a reservoir holding most of a meal makes the rejection of bad food a relatively simple matter. The ingestion of toxins, produced for example, by staphylococci or other food-poisoning bacteria, is followed by the absorption of a small fraction of the toxin. This is detected in the central nervous system. The victim feels nauseated, vomiting is triggered, and the whole meal is rejected. Vomiting is a complex movement usually composed of two elements in the adult although each may occur separately; retching, sometimes described as 'heaving' because of the movements which cause reduced intra-thoracic pressure, and projectile vomiting which involves sudden contraction of the abdominal

muscles with ejection of the gastric contents and is often seen in infants with no preliminary retching. The cardiac sphincter is either relaxed, or pushed into the thoracic cavity, where it can be forced open by raised intra-abdominal pressure. The stomach muscles themselves may be profoundly relaxed during vomiting although they are not invariably so.

The control of vomiting is coordinated by a group of neurons in the medulla of the brain. It is worth noticing that this 'centre', lying close to the areas for respiratory and cardiovascular control, is not readily depressed by general anaesthesia unless this is sufficiently deep to impair breathing and the other vital centres. Vomiting is a primitive mechanism, and it can be induced during surgical anaesthesia.

When toxins cause vomiting, they usually act on the chemosensitive triggering zone in the medulla, close to the vomiting centre. However, other receptors also cause vomiting, notably stretch (or touch) receptors in the pillars of the fauces, and pain receptors anywhere in the body. Vomiting may also be provoked by emotional distress.

For man, with an adventurous diet, vomiting provides a valuable safety mechanism; for the dentist, the possibility of provoking vomiting is a significant hazard (to the patient!). It is very dangerous to inhale vomit; many people still die either of the asphyxia caused by blocked bronchi, or of inhalation pneumonia caused by lung damage.

Prolonged vomiting results in severe dehydration and (usually) in metabolic alkalosis due to loss of gastric acid (p. 751).

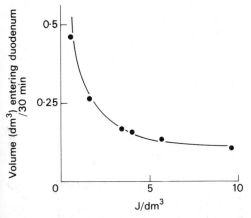

Fig. 13.29. Relationship between the rate of gastric emptying (volume/30 min) and the energy density of stomach contents (Joules/volume). The rate of emptying is much greater when meals of high volume but low energy content, are ingested. (Redrawn from Hunt J. N. (1975) In *Functions of the Stomach and Intestine*. Editor, M. H. F. Friedman. University Park Press, Baltimore.

DISTURBANCE OF GASTRIC FUNCTION

Man can survive surgical removal of the stomach (gastrectomy) but:
1   Loss of intrinsic factor leads to deficient absorption of vitamin B_{12}.
2   The protective action of HCl in limiting the growth of ingested microorganisms is lost, and an abnormal bacterial flora may develop in the small intestine.
3   Food may be presented to the intestinal digestive juices too rapidly for its digestion to be completed.

The small intestine

The small intestine is designed to digest and to absorb food.

DIGESTION

The gall bladder, pancreas and mucosal cells and glands in the intestine each add their contribution to the chyme which has entered the duodenum from the stomach and these will be considered in turn.

Bile

Bile is a faintly alkaline, yellowish or brown fluid formed in the hepatocytes of the liver. The organic matter in bile consists of bile salts, bile pigments, neutral fat, phospholipids and cholesterol. The primitive bile is stored in the gall bladder until required in the intestine and as this storage organ is able to reabsorb salt and water but not the organic constituents to which the cell membranes of its lining epithelium are highly impermeable, the concentration of organic matter is increased by a factor of about tenfold during an overnight fast. The HCO_3^- concentration in bile varies with flow rate, being highest at high rates of secretion and lowest after storage.

Bile does not contain enzymes. Its main contribution to digestion is to provide bile salts which emulsify the dietary lipids. Bile salts are structurally related to cholesterol from which they are formed in the liver by a series of reactions. The rate of the first step is regulated by the concentration of the final products by a direct negative feedback. There are only two bile salts produced by the human liver, cholate and chenodeoxycholate, and the reaction sequences which produce them are very similar. Following conjugation with glycine or taurine they become glycocholate and taurocholate, glycochenodeoxycholate and taurochenodeoxycholate. Taurocholate and glycocholate are present as their sodium salts in a ratio of about 1:3.

Bile salts have a structure which attracts them to the interface between lipid and aqueous phases. They are an odd shape, with their polar hydrophilic hydroxyl groups facing predominantly one way, leaving the 'back' of the molecule a hydrophobic area of hydrocarbon rings. This ambivalent attitude towards water (a mixture of sympathy and antipathy) is ideal, particularly when a second species of polar lipid is present in solution, for the formation of minute, highly charged particles called micelles, the centre of which contains the lipid element of the mixture while the outside is bristling with hydrophilic polar groups (Fig. 13.30). In the intestine, micelles are formed, composed of bile salts with monoglyceride as the principal polar lipid. Micelles are also formed in bile itself, between polar phospholipids such as lecithin and bile salts. In either case the solution formed, if the various species of molecule are present at balanced levels, is a stable, collidial suspension of particles so minute that the solution is optically clear. One of the important features of micelles is that once formed, a lot of non-polar lipid, such as cholesterol or triglyceride can absorb into them and these too are then held in a stable colloidal solution. In bile this solubilizes the cholesterol allowing it to be excreted into the intestine. Intestinal bacteria reduce any unabsorbed cholesterol to coprostanol which is then excreted in the faeces. In the intestinal lumen, bile salts bring the coarse emulsion of dietary fat to a fine level of subdivision exposing the lipids to close contact with pancreatic lipase, a water-soluble enzyme. Micelles are then formed again, containing the monoglyceride and free fatty acids released by lipolysis.

The other organic components of bile have no obvious function. Bile pigments are simply excretory products of degraded haemoglobin (p. 676).

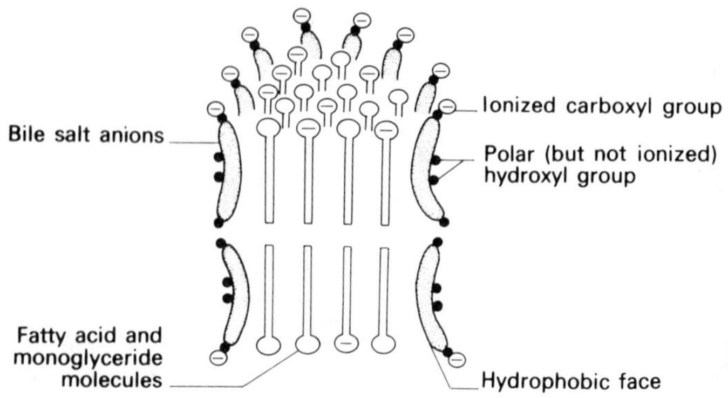

Bile salt anions

Ionized carboxyl group

Polar (but not ionized) hydroxyl group

Fatty acid and monoglyceride molecules

Hydrophobic face

Fig. 13.30. A possible form (in section) for mixed micelles in the intestinal lumen. (Redrawn from Hoffman A. F. (1968) In *Medium Chain Triglycerides.* Editor, J. R. Senior. University of Pennsylvania Press.)

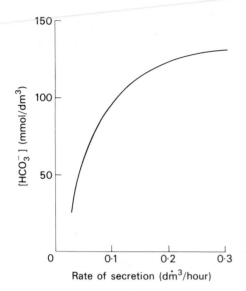

Fig. 13.31. Relationship between the bicarbonate ion concentration of human pancreatic juice and the rate of secretion. (Redrawn and simplified from Dreiling D. A. & Janowitz H. D. (1959) *American Journal of Digestive Diseases* **4**, 137–144.

Pancreatic exocrine secretions

The pancreatic secretion is a watery alkaline juice in which is dissolved a variable amount of enzyme-rich, viscid juice produced by the acinar cells of the exocrine pancreas. The watery juice is of uncertain origin. Its composition is affected by the actions of the duct cells of the gland and it may be that these contribute directly to the secretion, or that they modify a primary secretion (as in the salivary glands) produced by centroacinar cells. Whichever hypothesis is correct, HCO_3^- concentration varies greatly with flow rate (Fig. 13.31). The other principal electrolytes are Na^+ and Cl^-.

While the stomach is emptying, the pancreatic juice provides the greater part of the neutralizing fluid which brings the pH up towards the optimal level for the activity of intestinal enzymes. The mechanisms controlling pancreatic secretion behave as though they were titrating the duodenal contents to pH 4.5. This is soon raised further by the intestinal electrolyte secretion and bile, making the jejunal pH about 6.0. The output of pancreatic bicarbonate is closely related to the rate at which acid enters the duodenum (Fig. 13.32).

Among the many pancreatic enzymes and enzyme precursors secreted are amylase, lipase, trypsinogen, chymotrypsinogen, proelastase, and the carboxypeptidases.

Carbohydrate digestion. Pancreatic amylase, which is very much like salivary amylase (p. 556), continues the digestion of polymeric carbohydrates (e.g. starch and glycogen) to disaccharides (principally maltose, the glucose dimer) in the lumen of the small intestine. Some common dietary carbohydrate polymers remain undigested by amylase and these make up the greater part of the crude fibre found in faeces. Examples of these are:

1 Celluloses—a major constituent of green plants, digested by bacterial cellulase in ruminants.
2 Lignin—found in 'woody plants'; not a simple polysaccharide.
3 Hemicelluloses—which differ from cellulose in that hydrolysis yields monosaccharides other than glucose (e.g. xylose). These may be broken down by microorganisms in the colon.
4 Pectins—complex polysaccharides (not fibrous) containing galacturonic acid—found in plant cell walls.

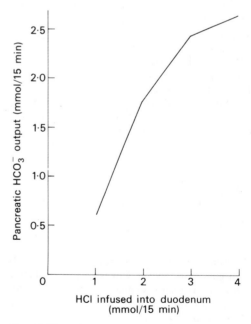

Fig. 13.32. In dogs, the output of pancreatic HCO_3^- is almost linearly related to the rate that acid enters the duodenum. Pancreatic juice plays the major role in raising the pH of chyme when gastric contents enter the duodenum. (Simplified and redrawn from Grossman M. I. (1971) In *The Exocrine Pancreas.* Editors, I. T. Beck & D. G. Sinclair. Longman, London.

Lipid digestion. After the dietary lipids have been emulsified and, to some extent, dissolved into micellar solution by bile, pancreatic lipase adsorbs to the surface of emulsified fat droplets 0.5–1.0 μm in diameter. Triglycerides are preferentially hydrolysed at positions 1 and 3 to produce the 2-monoglyceride.

$$H_2C-O-CO.R_1 \quad \xrightarrow[+\ 2H_2O]{lipase} \quad H_2C-OH + R_1COOH$$
$$HC-O-CO.R_2 \longrightarrow HC-O-CO.R_2$$
$$H_2C-O-CO.R_3 \qquad\qquad H_2C-OH + R_3COOH$$

| Triglyceride | 2-monoglyceride + fatty acids |

However, some are completely broken down to glycerol and fatty acids while others are hydrolysed only to diglycerides. These reactions are quantitatively less important than hydrolysis to monoglyceride. Mono and diglycerides and fatty acids dissolve into micelles and so are carried to the brush border of the mucosal cells for absorption.

Protein digestion. The proteolytic endopeptidases chymotrypsin, trypsin, and elastase are all secreted as inactive precursors. Like pepsin, they are only activated in the lumen of the gut. In this case the initial activation is by an enzyme called enterokinase. This is found on the surface of the mucosal cells of the intestine, and splits off the masking fragment from trypsinogen. Active trypsin then activates more trypsinogen, and also liberates active chymotrypsin and elastase.

Each of these three endopeptidases has its own preferred peptide bonds for hydrolytic attack within the peptide chain; they are fairly specific enzymes.

$$\underset{\text{Point of cleavage}}{NH_2 \cdots\cdots NH.CH.CO \overset{R_1}{\underset{\uparrow}{|}} NH.CH.CO \overset{R_2}{\underset{}{|}} \cdots\cdots COOH}$$

Trypsin is active against peptide bonds where R_1 is arginine or lysine. Chymotrypsin is active where R_1 is phenylalanine, tyrosine or tryptophan and elastase is active where R_1 is a neutral amino acid.

Carboxypeptidases are end-peptidases or, as they are better termed, exopeptidases because they strip off single amino acids at the end of a polypeptide chain, working from the C-terminal end (–COOH). They are of low specificity; i.e. they are able to dislodge a wide variety of amino acids.

This battery of proteolytic enzymes is capable of breaking down 70–80% of the food protein to di- and tri-peptides and free amino acids by the time the food residue enters the ileum.

RNA and DNA digestion. Ribonuclease and deoxyribonuclease begin the breakdown of RNA and DNA (Table 13.1).

Intestinal glands and mucosa

Although bile and pancreatic juice are both very important for intraluminal digestion of the chyme, the intestine itself participates in several ways.

The secretions of mucosal glands in the small intestine are thought to have a mainly protective function, keeping the mucosal surface well lubricated. They also contribute to neutralizing the acidic chyme which leaves the stomach.

The mucosal cells carry enzymes bound to the microvilli of their free surface, the brush border. These cells are continually being shed from the tips of the villi into the lumen. They contain a rich variety of enzymes, including the powerful lysosomal enzymes, which are liberated after cell death and autolysis (self-digestion). Some textbooks describe a whole battery of enzymes in the intestinal juice (succus entericus), but many of these are only present in the juice because of cell desquamation.

The digestive enzymes may be classified by their mode of action as follows:
1 Peptidases
   Aminopeptidases
   Dipeptidases
   Tripeptidases
   Enterokinase

Short peptides are liberated from proteins by tryptic digestion in the lumen and then diffuse into the brush border of intestinal cells. There they are hydrolysed to their constituent amino acids.

2 Carbohydrases
   (a) α-Dextrinase (isomaltase). This is capable of hydrolysing γ- (1–6) bonds in branched dextrins (Fig. 12.38).
   (b) Disaccharidases which catalyse the following reactions:

$$\text{Maltose} \xrightarrow{\text{maltase}} \text{2 glucose molecules}$$

$$\text{Lactose} \xrightarrow[\substack{\text{(also known} \\ \text{as lactase)}}]{\beta\text{-galactosidase}} \text{glucose + galactose}$$

Sucrose $\xrightarrow[\text{(also known as sucrase)}]{\text{invertase}}$ glucose + fructose

Like the peptidases these enzymes are found within the brush border of epithelial cells from the mid-jejunum down to the upper ileum.

Two rare inborn errors of metabolism are worth considering here:

(i) β-Galactosidase deficiency. Individuals who lack this enzyme are incapable of hydrolysing the milk sugar lactose. This leads to milk intolerance and hence milk avoidance. This in turn can result in a low dietary intake of calcium.

(ii) Invertase deficiency. Subjects lacking invertase in their intestinal mucosa cannot tolerate sucrose. If sucrose is fed it is metabolized to lactic and fatty acids in the intestine and these are excreted in the stool. One incidental benefit of sucrose avoidance in these individuals is a very low incidence of dental caries. Normally digestion and absorption of these sugars is about 95% complete.

3 Nucleases and phosphatase

Nucleic acids occur in foods as nucleoproteins. The protein portion is hydrolysed in the stomach and small intestine by pepsin and the pancreatic proteolytic enzymes. Nucleic acids are then broken down to polynucleotides by pancreatic nucleases. Further breakdown is shown in Table 13.1.

ABSORPTION

It is in the small intestine that all nutrient substances are absorbed, the upper two-thirds of the small intestine being responsible for almost all the absorption of hexose, pentose, amino acid, free fatty acid, and monoglyceride molecules. The final third of the small intestine is particularly important for performing two special functions; the reabsorption of bile salts and the active absorption of vitamin B_{12}.

The absorption of salt and water is an important function of the whole small intestine. The volume of fluid passing along the jejunum daily is of the order 7–8 dm^3 but only about 0.5–1.0 dm^3 finally passes through the ileocaecal valve into the large bowel. Of this, 80–90% is conserved, leaving about 100 cm^3 in the faeces. Salt is absorbed first, to be followed passively by water throughout the intestine. Ca^{2+} and Fe^{2+} are also absorbed in the small intestine (pp. 761, 674).

The products of the hydrolytic digestion of carbohydrates and proteins become attached to carrier proteins in the intestinal mucosal cell membranes during absorption. Although hexose and pentose sugars and free amino acids are all much smaller than ingested polymeric carbohydrates and proteins, they are still too large and too polar to diffuse through the very small aqueous pores in the lipid of the cell mebrane. The carrier proteins create preferential channels through the cell membranes. Within this group of substances, some such as fructose, sorbose, and L-glutamic acid, enter the cells by passive diffusion down a concentration gradient. This form of carrier-mediated diffusion is known as facilitated diffusion. Many other substances, like glucose, galactose and most amino acids, are even taken up against a concentration gradient. This requires the expenditure of energy and is an example of active transport.

A popular hypothesis proposes that sugars and amino acids are carried into the intestinal mucosal cell by binding to carriers which also carry Na^+ into the cell. Sodium is travelling down an electrochemical gradient, and this provides the energy required to carry the nutrient molecules into the cell against their own concentration gradients. The sodium gradient is

Table 13.1. Enzymes of intestinal mucosa in the breakdown of nucleic acids (p. 102).

Process of nucleic acid break-down	Enzymes of intestinal mucosa
Nucleic acids	
$\downarrow$(1)	(1) nuclease
Polynucleotides	
$\downarrow$(2)	(2) phosphodiesterase
Nucleotides	
$\downarrow$(3)	(3) nucleotidase
Nucleosides	
$\downarrow$(4)	(4) nucleosidase
Purine + pyrimidine bases + pentose-1-phosphate	
$\downarrow$	
Xanthine, uric acid	

maintained by the active transport of sodium out of the cell, across its lateral and serosal borders, the energy for this process being provided by hydrolysis of ATP.

Like enzyme catalysis, the rate of absorption is proportional to 'substrate' concentration. The rate of absorption is therefore limited when all the hypothetical carrier molecules are thought to be functioning. The carriers involved in either active transport or facilitated diffusion processes are, at least in part, proteins. They exhibit a degree of specificity, but closely related molecules (e.g. glucose and galactose) may complete for the same carrier (p. 253).

After absorption, most of the sugars and amino acids pass into the portal blood to be carried to the liver without undergoing any metabolic changes within the mucosal cells.

Partially digested fats are presented to the brush border of the mucosal cells in the upper small intestine as elements of a micelle. Because they are fat-soluble, molecules of monoglycerides, fatty acids and cholesterol can diffuse from micelles through liprotein membranes of epithelial cells. There is a diffusion gradient of monoglycerides and free fatty acids from lumen to cell, because once inside the cell their concentration is reduced as triglycerides are resynthesized. Bile salts, however, are not absorbed in the upper small intestine, remaining available in the lumen to produce more micelles. Within the mucosal cells, some monoglyceride is hydrolysed to free glycerol and fatty acid, but most of the fatty acid is built up into triglyceride again. Cholesterol is also esterified with fatty acids. The mucosal cells also use some fatty acid in synthesizing phospholipid. Some lipid particles known as chylomicrons, about $0.2\ \mu$m diameter, are then secreted by a process of exocytosis from the lateral borders of the cells. Chylomicrons consist very largely (90%) of triglyceride, with a small fraction of cholesterol and a surface coat of phospholipid. They enter the lymphatic vessels of the villi, making the lymph appear milky. Because of this appearance, lymphatic vessels from the villi are often known as lacteals. The triglyceride is thus carried away in the lymph, not in the portal blood. It enters the bloodstream through the thoracic duct and right lymph duct.

Some fats do not follow the same absorptive route, however. Medium and short chain fatty acids (less than twelve carbon atoms) such as are present in milk fat, are absorbed from mucosal cells directly into the portal circulation.

Bile salts are reabsorbed in the distal small intestine by a highly efficient active transport mechanism. After absorption and passage into the portal blood, some 90% is then extracted from the blood on the first passage through the liver, and secreted again into bile. Because bile salt is conserved in this way, and used repeatedly, this recycling of bile salts is known as the 'enterohepatic circulation'. Only about 3–5% of bile salt is lost during a single cycle of the bile salt pool.

The large intestine

The major functions of the large intestine in man are limited to the absorption of salt and water, and to bacterial fermentation, both of which reduce the volume of faeces. There may be a connection between these two processes. A considerable volume of gas, mainly CO_2, is produced during fermentation. It is possible that CO_2 is partly used to assist in the reabsorption of salt and water. The mucosa of the mammalian large intestine contains much carbonic anhydrase which promotes the formation of $H^+ + HCO_3^-$ in the cells. There is evidence that H^+ and HCO_3^- move out of the cells into the lumen in exchange for Na^+ and Cl^-.

The absorption of water is necessary to preserve the osmotic balance, because in the lumen, the $H^+ + HCO_3^-$ would again revert to $CO_2 + H_2O$. By a mechanism which is not entirely clear, K^+ also enters the lumen of the large intestine, so that eventually very little Na^+ is lost in faeces, while rather more K^+ is excreted.

Control mechanisms in the digestive tract

Control mechanisms include nervous reflexes and hormones and possibly also local mechanisms involving either substances which are not found circulating in systemic blood or short nervous reflexes contained within the intramural plexus.

Nerves
Parasympathetic and sympathetic autonomic nerves provide the extrinsic supply to the gut. Of the parasympathetic division, the vagus nerves are by far the most important, as they influence the stomach, pancreas, biliary system, and upper small intestine. The sacral parasympathetic flow is mainly involved in the control of defaecation.

The adrenergic sympathetic nerves are distributed widely to the gut and its accessory organs, but they do not usually play an important role during the digestion of a meal. Their function is to hold up digestion at times of crisis, when the blood supply usually demanded by an active alimentary canal must be diverted for more pressing needs elsewhere. They reduce glandular

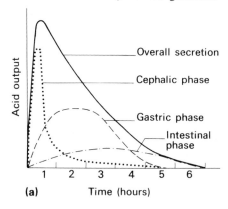

(a)

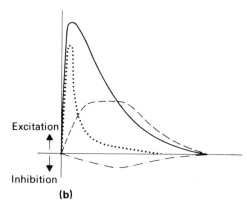

(b)

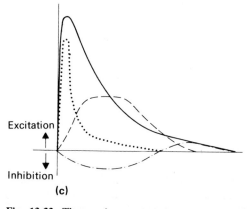

(c)

Fig. 13.33. The gastric secretory response to a meal, described in terms of three phases which contribute to the overall response. (a) Traditional diagram. (b) A possible situation; inhibitory influences throughout the intestinal phase. (c) Another possibility; inhibitory influences shown early in the intestinal phase, but excitatory effect later.

secretions, principally by discontinuing the essential blood flow, and they inhibit motility. They are also known to regulate motility in the interdigestive period (see below).

Hormones

At present, four hormones are known to be involved in the control of digestion. These are: gastrin, secretin, cholecystokinin-pancreo-zymin (CCK-PZ), and gastric inhibitory poly-peptide (GIP). During the search for these hormones in extracts of mucosa, other pure poly-peptides (e.g. motilin, vasoactive intestinal pep-tide (VIP), somatostatin) have been isolated which also affect digestive processes under experimental conditions. It would be premature to go into detail about these as many more discoveries will be made about the functions and mode of action of these biologically active substances.

All the gastrointestinal hormones are poly-peptides, some of which are related to one another structurally.

GASTRIC SECRETION

After a meal is eaten, gastric secretion reaches a peak in 30–60 minutes and declines slowly over a period of 3–4 hours. The time course is affected by the nature of the food, being longest after a fatty meal. The process of secretion is usually described in terms of a sequence of three phases, the cephalic, gastric, and intestinal phases (Fig. 13.33), but these overlap considerably. Diagrams give no more than an inspired guess about the relative contributions made by the three phases of control.

Under ordinary circumstances, the cephalic phase, due to the anticipation and enjoyment of eating a meal has scarcely begun before the gastric phase begins, the latter being defined as secretion due to the effects of food in the stomach. It is sometimes not appreciated that the cephalic phase continues throughout eating a meal.

The cephalic phase

The thought of food, the smell of good cooking and most particularly the enjoyment of tasting a delicious meal, all stimulate the vagal motor nuclei to promote in several different ways gastric secretion and motility.

The first description of the cephalic phase of secretion was given by the great Russian physiologist, Pavlov, following his experiments on dogs with a gastric and oesophageal fistula

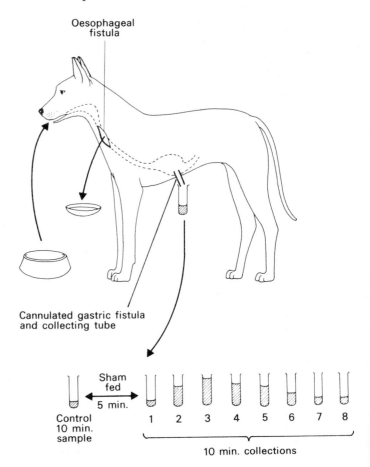

Oesophageal
fistula

Cannulated gastric fistula
and collecting tube

Fig. 13.34. Pavlov's simple
experiment to study the effect of
sham-feeding in the conscious
dog. These experimental dogs
could be kept alive for long
periods by feeding them through
the gastric fistula. Following
sham-feeding, a brisk secretion
occurred which tailed off to
control levels in about 1 hour.

Sham
fed

5 min.

Control
10 min.
sample

1   2   3   4   5   6   7   8

10 min. collections

(Fig. 13.34). A fistula is an abnormal hole connecting two regions, in this case the gut lumen
with the surface of the animal. When the dogs
were fed, food did not enter the stomach but fell
out of the fistula in the oesophagus. The secretory response to sham feeding was brisk but
tailed off within an hour (Fig. 13.34). When
Pavlov sectioned the vagus nerves to the
stomach the secretory response was abolished.

Although the vagus nerves directly stimulate
the gastric glands, resulting in a mixed secretion
of acid and enzymes, they also provoke the
release into the blood stream of the hormone
gastrin from the pylorus. The very high initial
secretory response seen in the cephalic phase is
undoubtedly due to the combined influence of
gastrin and direct vagal activity on the fundic
gastric glands.

The gastric phase
Food in the stomach is the principal stimulus for
gastric secretion (Fig. 13.33). Again, there are

both nervous and hormonal mechanisms.
Experimental evidence for these comes mainly
from studies on dogs with pouches which have
been surgically constructed from various parts of
the stomach; two such pouches are illustrated in
Fig. 13.35

Food acts on two distinct areas of the stomach
(a) the fundus and body, and (b) the pyloric
antrum.

The fundus. In the fundus, food enhances secretion in several ways:

1   It distends the stomach and so (a) activates
local reflexes which increase motility and secretion, and (b) stimulates stretch receptors which
may trigger long vago-vagal reflexes (up to the
brain and back again) with the same effect as
local reflexes.
2   Digested proteins or free amino acids act
directly on the secretory mucosa to cause secretion.

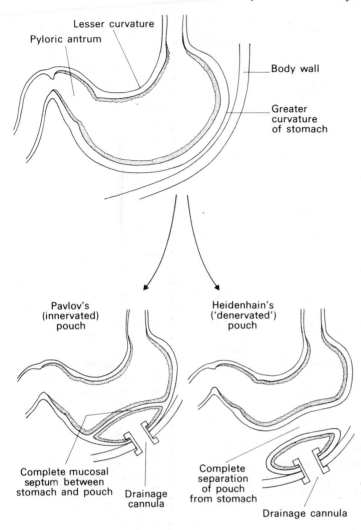

Lesser curvature

Pyloric antrum

Body wall

Greater curvature of stomach

Pavlov's (innervated) pouch

Heidenhain's ('denervated') pouch

Complete mucosal septum between stomach and pouch

Drainage cannula

Complete separation of pouch from stomach

Drainage cannula

Fig. 13.35. Experimental stomach pouches which have been used for the study of gastric function. In a Pavlov pouch, the vagal nerve supply to the mucosa in the pouch is intact. In a Heidenhain pouch this main nerve supply is interrupted, but a few sympathetic fibres may reach it along with its blood vessels; so too may a few vagal fibres passing via the coeliac ganglion. Stimuli which cause gastrin release from the pyloric antrum cause gastric juice to flow from the isolated Heidenhain pouch.

The pyloric antrum. In the antrum, food promotes the release of gastrin which in turn stimulates gastric secretion. Gastrin is produced by scattered specialized mucosal endocrine cells (G cells or argentaffin) which border the lumen of the pyloric glands (Fig. 13.17). It is released by the following three stimuli if the pH is greater than 3: (a) vagal excitation; (b) moderate distension and motility of the pyloric antrum; (c) proteins, peptones and a number of amino acids.

If the pH falls to 3 the release of gastrin in response to all of these stimuli is greatly depressed and it stops completely if the pH falls further. Somatostatin appears to be involved in preventing gastrin secretion in these circumstances.

Gastrin acts on some other tissues besides the secretory mucosa of the fundus and body of the stomach, but it is difficult to decide which of the responses, which are demonstrable under experimental circumstances, actually occur under physiological conditions. It seems likely that gastrin, in normal circulating amounts, can stimulate enzyme secretion from the pancreas and can increase gastric antral motility, so increasing gastric emptying.

The presence of food in the stomach buffers gastric acid to an extent which depends upon its protein content (p. 606). Protein is therefore both the primary stimulus for acid secretion by the stomach and the principal supporter of its continuation (Fig. 13.28).

The intestinal phase

As chyme enters the duodenum the intestinal phase of gastric secretion begins. Again, the overlap with other phases is obvious (Fig. 13.33). Cells containing gastrin are found, in small numbers, in the intestine of man. Although the number in the duodenum is only one-tenth that in the pyloric antrum of the stomach, these may release sufficient gastrin to enhance gastric secretion.

The original description of the intestinal phase, made at the turn of the century, was based on experimental evidence obtained from fasting dogs. It was observed that if food, or a suspension of nutritious substances, was placed in the intestine of fasting dogs this resulted in gastric secretion. Under more normal conditions it has been found, again in dogs, that a peptone solution of reasonable pH, say 4.5, when placed directly into the small intestine, augments gastric secretion, even while the gastric phase is in full-swing. It is not possible to say at present whether this finding is applicable in man because the actions of intestinal hormones are known to differ in different species. The best one can say is that a case can be made for suggesting that each of the four well-established hormones of the gut would influence the intestinal phase of gastric secretion.

CCK-PZ is released into the bloodstream from specialized cells in the mucosa of the duodenum and jejunum. Release is best stimulated by either peptone solutions and amino acids (p. 606) or by fatty acids in chyme.

Within the structure of CCK-PZ is a tetrapeptide C-terminal sequence which alone possesses high gastrin-like biological activity and is identical to the sequence in gastrin. When administered intravenously to fasting animals, CCK-PZ stimulates gastric secretion although less efficiently than gastrin. In experiments in which CCK-PZ has been given to man during a gastric secretory response to gastrin, a partial inhibition of acid secretion was observed. This suggests that during the intestinal phase, CCK-PZ may sometimes exert a negative influence on gastric secretion, at least while the gastric phase is still being driven by gastrin from the pyloric antrum (Fig. 13.33b).

Secretin is also released from specialized endocrine cells in the mucosa of the duodenum and jejunum. The principal stimulus is acid chyme (pH 4.5). In experiments similar to those described above in man, it has been shown that secretin also inhibits acid secretion, though only possibly by delaying its secretion, not by reducing the eventual yield. It is not known whether this is a physiological effect, but if so, it might contribute to the intestinal phase.

GIP (gastric inhibitory polypeptide) is released into the circulation from specialized endocrine cells in the duodenal and jejunal mucosa in response to the presence of glucose or fat in the upper small intestine. It has an inhibitory effect on gastric secretion.

In summary, it seems that the intestinal phase of gastric secretion can be demonstrated under certain conditions, but the nature of this phase may well vary with meals of differing composition (Fig. 13.33).

GASTRIC EMPTYING

The stomach contracts regularly, three times a minute, due to an intrinsic pacemaker region located near the cardia (p. 595). Extrinsic nerves do not greatly influence the rhythm but have a considerable effect on the depth and vigour of contractions. The vagus nerves increase these while sympathetic activity renders the stomach flaccid.

If vagal tone is high, the wave of gastric peristalsis gathers strength as it approaches the pylorus, and chyme is pushed into the duodenum. During contractions the pylorus constricts, preventing the escape of large pieces of food. However, between contractions the pylorus is not a closed sphincter with sustained tone in its walls (like, for example, the anus) but is simply a muscular, partially folded, valve. Regurgitation of bile-stained duodenal contents into the stomach is by no means uncommon. As the chyme enters the duodenum and jejunum, receptors sensitive to its acidity, osmolarity and fat act by either hormonal or neural means, to regulate the emptying of the stomach.

Under physiological circumstances it is likely that CCK-PZ, secreted in response to peptones, amino acids and fatty acids, decreases the tone of the body of the stomach and slows emptying. It is also likely, although conclusive evidence is not yet available, that GIP, secreted in response to fat and glucose, inhibits gastric motility and emptying. Injected secretin has also been shown to have an inhibitory effect on gastric motility, but so little secretin is released during a meal that it is uncertain whether this effect is of physiological importance in regulating emptying. Finally, somatostatin may perform this inhibitory function.

Nervous reflex inhibition of gastric emptying may also contribute to the overall control. This reflex, with afferents stimulated by acid in the duodenum, was described many years ago and given the name 'the enterogastric reflex', but its status will have to be re-examined in the context of more recent discoveries of hormonal feedback upon the stomach.

Although the details of the mechanisms involved are still confused, gastric emptying is delicately controlled in relation to the energy-density of the food (Fig. 13.29).

PANCREATIC SECRETION

Like gastric secretion, pancreatic secretion is also stimulated by vagal impulses at the beginning of a meal. These cause a scanty, enzyme-rich flow of viscid juice which is probably further stimulated by gastrin. However, the hormone CCK-PZ is still considered to be the most important in this respect. It is released from the mucosa of the duodenum and jejunum. While partially digested protein in chyme stimulates the release of both gastrin and CCK-PZ, the receptors for each differ. The release of gastrin is strongly stimulated by glycine and alanine, while that of CCK-PZ is apparently greatest in response to aromatic amino acids and also to fatty acids.

The release of secretin in response to chyme of low pH in the duodenum is believed to be the essential stimulus for the secretion of a copious flow of the watery alkaline component of pancreatic juice. This is the principal mechanism by which the duodenal pH is raised to 4.5

BILE RELEASE AND SECRETION

The gall bladder and biliary sphincter (Fig. 13.27) are innervated by the vagus nerves, and some bile is quickly released by vagal action if an enjoyable meal is eaten. Subsequently hormonal control through CCK-PZ becomes important. The name 'cholecystokinin' means 'bile-bladder movement'. After the initial spurt of bile due to vagal action, the fat and protein content of the meal determine the release of CCK-PZ as described previously. It is actually the free fatty acid released from fat which ensures adequate bile release through its action on the receptors of the CCK-PZ secreting cells of the mucosa. This action of CCK-PZ is not shared with gastrin. It depends upon a feature in the CCK-PZ amino acid sequence which is absent from gastrin.

The volume of bile secreted by the liver is determined mainly by the rate at which recirculating bile salts are taken up from portal blood, but secretin, under experimental conditions at least, exerts a minor stimulating effect on the volume produced.

INTESTINAL MOTILITY

There is a marked difference in the pattern of motor activity in the gastrointestinal tract during fasting and following feeding. In the fasting state the gut is quiescent for a time, followed by a burst of propulsive activity. This wave of activity moves slowly down the gut, taking 1–2 hours to pass along the entire intestine. It is known as an 'interdigestive migratory myoelectric complex'.

On feeding, this pattern of activity is completely lost; there are no longer periods of quiescence between periods of contractions. It is the motility of the postprandial period with which we are most concerned, and which is described below.

The basic electrical rhythm of smooth muscle is myogenic; i.e. it is intrinsic to the muscle. This activity is initiated by an unstable membrane potential. Intracellular recordings, even in isolated denervated cells, have shown that the membrane potential 'wanders' (this wandering is known as the 'slow wave') and that if the potential falls to a critical threshold level, a spontaneous action potential is generated and the cell contracts (Fig. 13.36). These muscle cells act in synchrony, communicating with their neighbours by direct electrical transmission. Specialized regions of membranes of adjacent cells, known as nexuses (Fig. 6.12), which are blunt abutments or bulbous interdigitations between the two surfaces, serve to transmit the impulse.

The slow, more or less synchronous, waves of

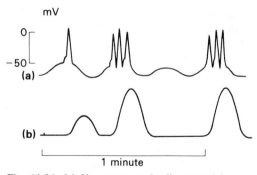

Fig. 13.36. (a) Slow waves and spike potentials (action potentials) as recorded by an intracellular microelectrode in a smooth muscle cell. (b) The tension developed. The pace of the slow waves shown here, 3/min., is that found in the stomach. Contractions occur during the first. second and fourth slow waves, coincident with the spike potentials.

changing membrane potential develop in groups of cells at a rate which is characteristic for any given level of the gastrointestinal tract. As the membrane potentials of many individual cells fall to the threshold and fire action potentials, these cells contract. Action potentials are also discharged in adjacent cells due to the spreaad of current from cell to cell across the nexuses. In this way, the partially synchronous slow wave of electrical activity results in a coordinated wave of contraction.

The intestine, like the stomach, has its own pace of contractile activity. In the duodenum, this is quite high, about eleven contractions per minute, but this slows down as some waves die out while going down the intestine.

The intestine exhibits polarity; i.e. waves of contraction always pass from above to below, away from the oesophagus. This is caused by the same phenomon as that which ensures that the heart does not beat 'backwards' (p. 702). The natural pace of intrinsic activity declines steadily as one moves down the gut; consequently, segments of intestine tend to be driven by those upstream. Eventually, the action potentials in the driving segment meet a lower segment whose electrical potential is still so far from threshold that they are unable to excite it. This wave of contraction then drops out.

It is upon this intrinsic activity of the smooth muscle that controlling influences act. When stimulated to release their acetylcholine, cholinergic nerve fibres, whether from the vagus or from the cells of Auerbach's plexus (p. 593), have the effect of reducing the membrane potential of smooth muscle towards the threshold and so increases contractile activity. Distension also increases motility, either by its direct effect on smooth muscle cells, or through local cholingeric reflexes, while sympathetic activity relaxes smooth muscle by hyperpolarizing the cells.

The principal object of intestinal motility is to redistribute the intestinal contents and so facili-tate digestion and absorption. Along most of the intestine, simple annular contractions (segmentation) predominate. The idea that the contents are continually being moved on is incorrect. Many peristaltic waves are rather inefficient so that onward movement is slow.

It is now believed that both peristalsis and segmentation are forms of contraction which are determined by the characteristics and anatomical arrangements of the longitudinal and circular layers of smooth muscle in the intestinal wall. No nervous reflexes, local or distant, are needed. Peristalsis is usually more evident in the duodenum and jejunum, and segmentation in the ileum.

Local hormones do affect the motility of the intestine, but their place in the normal regulation of this function remains obscure. This is partly because the subject is very difficult to study quantitatively.

One approach to measuring motility is to study the transit time of marker substances from the lumen of the stomach to the rectum. This is delayed on a highly refined carbohydrate diet, and accelerated on a high fibre diet. There are many good reasons for preferring a high fibre diet, which may be partly related to intestinal transit time. For example, fibre tends to trap and carry away bile salt, reducing the efficiency of bile salt reabsorption thereby stimulating synthesis of bile salt from cholesterol, resulting in a fall in blood cholesterol level. This is almost certainly a good thing; in experimental animals it reduces the incidence of gall stones, diabetes, and atherosclerosis.

FURTHER READING

BURTOFF, A. (1976) Myogenic control of intestinal motility. *Physiological Reviews* **56**, 418–434.

GREGORY, R.A. (1979) The gastrointestinal hormones: A review of recent advances. *Journal of Physiology* **241**, 1–32.

CHAPTER 14

The Liver

HISTOLOGY

This is the largest gland in the body, weighing about 1.5 kg, and is also one of the most vascular, about 20% of its volume being occupied by blood. Its most numerous cells, the liver parenchymal cells or hepatocytes, are unique because they combine excretory, exocrine, and endocrine functions. The hepatocytes produce bile which can be regarded both as an excretory product, because it contains detoxified waste destined for elimination via the alimentary tract, and as an exocrine secretion, because it leaves the liver through ducts and is an important digestive juice. The endocrine functions of the liver are less obvious but equally important; endocrine glands were originally defined as structures which secrete useful substances, not necessarily hormones, directly into the blood, and since hepatocytes do this (p. 623) the liver is thus an endocrine gland. It is also part of the reticulo-endothelial system, and contains many cells specialized for phagocytosis. If the various functions of the liver are borne in mind, the significance of its structure will be more readily understood.

Gross features

The liver is a roughly wedge-shaped organ, whose upper convex surface fits snugly against the underside of the dome-shaped diaphragm. It has two main lobes, the right being much larger than the left. Its inferior or visceral surface lies against part of the alimentary tract, the gall bladder, the right adrenal and the right kidney. A liver which has been fixed 'in situ' shows the impression of these structures. The visceral surface is also marked by a short but deep transverse fissure, the porta hepatis (door of the liver), through which the hepatic artery, portal vein and the hepatic plexus of nerves enter, and the hepatic ducts and some lymph vessels leave. Blood leaves the liver through the hepatic veins,

which emerge from its posterior surface and immediately enter the inferior vena cava.

The liver is attached to the abdominal wall and to the diaphragm by ligaments, but is held in place mainly by the intra-abdominal pressure due to the tonus of the abdominal muscles. It is covered by a thin connective tissue capsule, which in turn is covered by peritoneum, except for that part of its surface which is in direct contact with the diaphragm, the 'bare area' of the liver.

Fresh liver tissue has the consistency of a table jelly, and is very vascular. It is therefore easily damaged, bleeds profusely, and is difficult to repair surgically; provided that bleeding can be staunched it has excellent powers of regeneration.

Basic organization of the liver

About 70% of the cells of the liver are hepatocytes arranged in sheets or laminae, one cell thick, rather like the bricks of a wall. Although the laminae tend to be arranged in groups radiating from branches of the hepatic veins called central veins, they branch and anastomose, forming a continuous wall-like structure or muralium (Fig. 4.3, p. 164).

Adjacent laminae are separated by hepatic lacunae, consisting of liver sinusoids surrounded by perisinusoidal spaces (often called spaces of Disse). The sinusoids are lined by endothelial cells and phagocytic Kupffer cells, the latter being part of the reticulo-endothelial system. Discontinuities in the endothelium allow plasma to pass through into the perisinusoidal space and bathe the lacunal surfaces of the hepatocytes. The sinusoids carry blood from branches of both the hepatic portal vein and hepatic artery to the central veins and thence to the hepatic veins and inferior vena cava. Fat storage cells are generally present in the perisinusoidal spaces.

Between contiguous hepatocytes are minute bile canaliculi into which the bile produced by the cells drains. These canaliculi are simply a series of anastomosing cylinders formed by grooves in adjacent hepatocytes. If a lamina is sectioned tangentially, they appear as a network of hexagonal meshes, each mesh outlining a hepatocyte (Fig. 4.3). The bile canaliculi unite to form ductules (canals of Hering) which open into bile ducts; these in turn unite to form the left and right hepatic ducts which leave the liver at the porta hepatis.

Liver lobules and acini (Fig. 14.1)

CLASSICAL LOBULES

In some animals, the pig for example, the liver consists of a series of clearly defined polyhedral lobules, about 1 mm in diameter, and separated from their neighbours by a capsule consisting of connective tissue septa (Glisson's capsule). Passing through the centre of each lobule is a central vein from which radiate sinusoids which separate the hepatic laminae. At the corners of the lobules are the portal triads, each composed of an interlobular bile duct, a branch of the hepatic portal vein, and a branch of the hepatic artery. Each portal triad is enclosed within a portal canal bounded by a sheath of connective tissue.

In man there are no clearly marked connective tissue septa between the lobules—the laminae appear to extend from one lobule into neighbouring lobules with the result that 'classical' lobules are not defined.

PORTAL LOBULES

The liver can also be visualized as a collection of portal lobules. In sections, these are triangular units centred on a portal triad, and limited by imaginary lines constructed between the central veins of the three 'classical' lobules which are in part drained and supplied by it. This definition of a liver lobule is consistent with the lobular organization of other exocrine glands in that the secretion (here bile) drains towards a duct (here the 'interlobular' bile duct) situated at the centre of the lobule. (The bile duct is described as 'interlobular' because of its position between the classical lobules.)

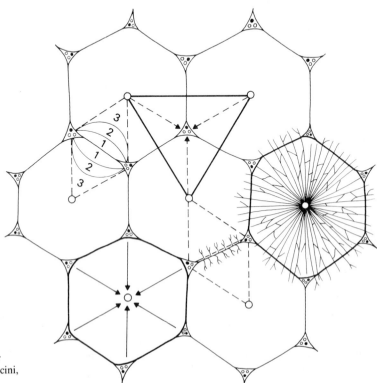

Fig. 14.1. Diagram of liver showing liver lobules and acini, also blood supply.

ACINUS

This is the smallest unit of functional organization of the liver. It consists of a group of hepatocytes and the terminal branches of the hepatic portal vein, hepatic artery and bile ductule which supply them. These branches leave the portal triads at intervals, and run at right angles to them along the sides of the classical lobule. In a section, a hepatic acinus is a diamond-shaped region with two adjacent portal triads at one pair of opposite corners, and two central veins occupying the other pair (Fig. 14.1). The blood vessels which supply the acinus extend out from a plane drawn between the adjacent portal triads. The cells nearest to this plane, the so-called 'zone 1' cells, receive blood first. Cells in 'zone 2' and then in 'zone 3' (the latter being at the edge of the acinus), receive blood sequentially. These zones, introduced by Rappaport and others in 1954, correspond to three zones of differing activity which can be identified cytologically. It is interesting that some thirty years earlier Noel introduced a similar type of zonation based on activity, describing a zone of permanent function, equivalent to zone 1, a zone of varying activity, equivalent to zone 2, and a zone of permanent repose, equivalent to zone 3. This gradation in activity is related to the distance of the cells from their source of oxygen and nutrients, those in zone 1 being in the nearest, and therefore most favourable, position, while those in zone 3 are furthest away. Zonation is most obvious in liver tissue which has been subjected to noxious blood-borne conditions, when the first cells to be affected are those in zone 1, then those in zone 2 and finally those in zone 3.

Vessels, ducts and nerves of the liver

VESSELS

These are the hepatic portal vein, hepatic artery, hepatic veins and lymph vessels.

Most of the blood reaching the liver is carried to it from the alimentary tract by the hepatic portal vein. With the exception of fats, all the materials absorbed from the gut pass into tributaries of the hepatic portal vein and are transported directly to the liver. A smaller supply of blood rich in oxygen reaches the liver by way of the hepatic artery. Both vessels enter at the porta hepatis, branch repeatedly and enter the portal canals. There are no anastomoses between the terminal branches of the hepatic artery, each of which is thus an end artery (p. 650).

Using 'classical' terminology, the branches of the hepatic portal vein and hepatic artery within the portal canals are 'interlobular'. At intervals along their length they give rise to tributaries, finer branches of which enter the radially disposed liver sinusoids which converge on the central vein of each lobule.

Each central vein has very delicate walls, perforated at intervals for the entry of blood from the sinusoids. As it passes along the length of the lobule it naturally widens. On leaving the lobule it becomes a sublobular vein. Numbers of sublobular veins converge and unite, eventually leaving the liver at the porta hepatis as one of the two or more hepatic veins that drain into the inferior vena cava. On its way through the sinusoids the contents of the blood are monitored and modified by hepatocytes, endothelial cells and Kupffer cells.

The lymphatic drainage of the liver consists of superficial and deep vessels which eventually communicate with the thoracic duct. Since the liver manufactures many plasma proteins, the lymph leaving it has a high protein content.

DUCTS

These remove bile from the hepatocytes and convey it to the gall bladder.

The bile first collects in the bile canaliculi, cylindrical spaces between adjacent hepatocytes. Encircling each polygonal cell, they form a continuous network with polygonal meshes which extend from lobule to lobule throughout the liver. The canaliculi are bounded by the plasma membranes of the hepatocytes between which they lie, and short microvilli extend into them from the hepatocyte surfaces (Fig. 14.2). Each is simply a local enlargement of the intercellular space between adjacent hepatocytes, and is sealed off from the rest of the space by tight junctions.

The bile canaliculi unite to form bile ductules (canals of Hering) which converge on the portal canals, where they fuse to form interlobular bile ducts. Both bile ductules and bile ducts have a small lumen surrounded by cuboidal epithelium resting on a basement membrane. As the porta hepatis is approached, the bile ducts fuse to form a hepatic duct, and their epithelium changes from cuboidal to columnar. The hepatic duct leaves the liver and joins the cystic duct, through which bile passes to the gall bladder for storage and modification. The hepatic duct and cystic duct are linked by the common bile duct (ductus choledocus) to the duodenum.

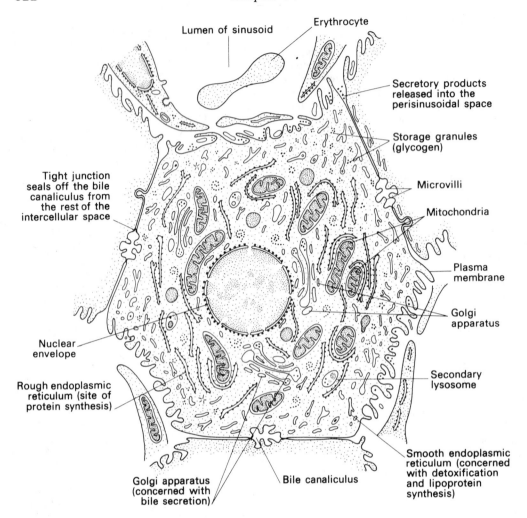

Fig. 14.2. Ultrastructure of hepatocyte showing bile canaliculi.

The hepatic, cystic and common bile ducts are lined by a mucous membrane deep to which is a layer of smooth muscle surrounded by a sheath of connective tissue. The muscle layer is thickest at the opening of the common bile duct into the duodenum, where it forms a sphincter which regulates the flow of bile (Fig. 13.27).

NERVES

These control the contraction of the smooth muscle in the vessels and ducts of the liver and, to some extent, its secretory activity.

Sympathetic and parasympathetic (vagal) nerves enter the liver at the porta hepatis. A few nerves run between the hepatocytes but their

terminations are unknown; the rest accompany the blood vessels and bile ducts. Some nerve fibres also reach the liver from nerves in its peritoneal folds.

The hepatocyte

Hepatocytes are polyhedral cells. Unlike the majority of the somal cells, which are diploid, hepatocytes frequently show varying degrees of polyploidy, and their size varies accordingly. They contain many mitochondria, and much smooth as well as some rough endoplasmic reticulum. Their cytoplasm is acidophilic (it stains pink with eosin). The detailed cytology of the hepatocyte is related to the level of its activity, and this varies with its distance from the edge of the classical lobule (Fig. 14.1), that is, from the source of the nutrient-bearing blood vessels. The ultrastructure of a typical hepatocyte from zone 2 is shown in Fig. 14.2. The multifarious and complex activities of the cell—protein synthesis, bile secretion, detoxification, storage, and so on, are reflected in its ultrastructure.

The hepatocyte has about fourteen surfaces. Of these, some border on bile canaliculi and are in contact with adjacent hepatocytes, while others are exposed to the perisinusoidal space. That part of the surface bordering on a bile canaliculus is covered with microvilli, as are the surfaces adjacent to the perisinusoidal spaces. The endothelial cells lining the sinusoids rest on the tips of these microvilli, and since the endothelium is discontinuous, the hepatocytes have direct access to the blood plasma and can exchange materials with it. Adjacent hepatocytes are linked by tight junctions, gap junctions and desmosomes.

The cytoplasm contains scattered basophilic bodies. Each of these is a unit of rough endoplasmic reticulum, a site of protein synthesis. Fasting causes a decrease in the number of basophilic bodies. Also present is a considerable amount of smooth endoplasmic reticulum, taking the form of a plexus of branching and anastomosing tubules. It often contains globules of serum lipoprotein, which is synthesized here and then released into the blood. The amount of glycogen in the cytoplasm depends on the nutritional state and position of the hepatocyte within the lobule. During digestion, the glycogen content increases first in the cells at the edges of the lobules and then progressively in cells nearer their centres. During fasting, it disappears first from the cells at the centres of the lobules and then progressively outwards. There are several stacks of Golgi saccules, each one usually situated near a bile canaliculus, suggesting that they are concerned with bile secretion. Lysosomes and peroxisomes are also present.

Fat storing cells

These are located in the perisinusoidal spaces, between the hepatocytes and the endothelial cells. Their origin is unknown.

Liver sinusoids

These lie between adjacent hepatic laminae, and are separated from them by the plasma-filled perisinusoidal spaces of Disse. They are lined by a discontinuous endothelium consisting of two cell types: typical endothelial cells and fixed macrophages or Kupffer cells. The latter are cells of the reticulo-endothelial system (p. 663).

ENDOTHELIAL CELLS

Many of the endothelial cells are fenestrated and there are discontinuities between adjacent cells. The pores so formed are big enough to allow plasma to pass through, but sufficiently small to hold back the erythrocytes. There is no basal lamina beneath the endothelium, and so plasma penetrating the pores can reach the surface of the hepatocytes.

KUPFFER CELLS

These are stellate, phagocytic cells, lying on the luminal aspect of the endothelium, with some of their processes extending between its cells. They show all the features of typical reticulo-endothelial cells (p. 360), being rich in rough endoplasmic reticulum, Golgi saccules, and primary and secondary lysosomes. One of their main functions is to digest effete erythrocytes, the remains of which are often to be found in the secondary lysosomes. The number of Kupffer cells varies, and it is likely that they can be recruited when required from the bone marrow. They may also develop from monocytes (p. 678) but this is still a matter of some controversy.

BIOCHEMISTRY

The liver plays a crucial role in the metabolism of carbohydrates, lipids and amino acids. It is an important site for the synthesis of plasma proteins. The liver protects the body from toxic metabolites by converting them to non-toxic substances before they enter the systemic blood. It is the principal tissue in the body where hormones and drugs, including alcohol, are detoxified.

Carbohydrate metabolism

Glucose-6-phosphate provides a key to an understanding of hepatic carbohydrate metabolism.

FORMATION OF GLUCOSE-6-PHOSPHATE

This can occur by four main routes:

Phosphorylation of glucose
After a carbohydrate-containing meal glucose is absorbed from the small intestine and transported to the liver via the hepatic portal vein. The liver enzyme glucokinase then catalyses its phosphorylation to glucose-6-phosphate.

Interconversion of sugars
The liver possesses enzymes which are able to interconvert different phosphorylated monosaccharides, for instance:

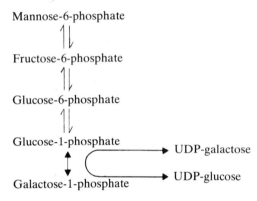

Mannose-6-phosphate

Fructose-6-phosphate

Glucose-6-phosphate

Glucose-1-phosphate

Galactose-1-phosphate

UDP-galactose

UDP-glucose

By this means fructose and galactose, obtained from dietary sucrose and lactose respectively, can be channelled into the liver's major metabolic pathways, via glucose-6-phosphate.

Glycogenolysis (p. 189)
A number of hours after a meal liver stores of glycogen are broken down in order to maintain blood levels of glucose. Glucose-6-phosphate is an important intermediate in this pathway.

Gluconeogenesis (p. 187)
When liver stores of glycogen are depleted, blood glucose homeostasis still can be achieved by synthesis of glucose from lactate, glycerol, or from glucogenic amino cells (e.g. alanine, aspartate or glutamate). Formation of glucose-6-phosphate is the penultimate step in this gluconeogenic pathway.

METABOLISM OF GLUCOSE-6-PHOSPHATE

This also occurs via four main routes:

Hydrolysis
Glucose-6-phosphate can be hydrolysed to free glucose and inorganic phosphate when blood glucose needs to be replenished. This reaction cannot occur in muscle which lacks the necessary glucose-6-phosphatase enzyme.

Glycogenesis
Glucose-6-phosphate may be converted via glucose-1-phosphate to UDP-glucose (p. 192). This is then used in the synthesis of glycogen (and to a lesser extent, glycoproteins). Reported values for the glycogen content of the liver of a 70kg normal fed adult range from 70–110g. This compares with 120–240g glycogen stored in muscle.

Glycolysis
Approximately 70% of glucose which is oxidized flows through the glycolysis pathway. Glucose-6-phosphate can be considered the common starting molecule, whether the original substrate is free glucose or glycogen.

Pentose phosphate pathway (p. 210)
Some 30% of glucose-6-phosphate which is oxidized follows the pentose phosphate pathway, with production of CO_2 and H_2O. One benefit is that $NADP^\oplus$ is reduced to $NADPH + H^\oplus$ in this pathway. The reduced form of this coenzyme is needed for fatty acid and steroid biosynthesis. A second advantage is that this route provides a source of pentose sugars, needed in synthesis of nucleotide bases.

Amino acid metabolism and protein biosynthesis (p. 215)

The liver is the major site for the deamination and transamination of amino acids. It is also the only tissue where urea is synthesized from the surplus of amino acids not required for protein synthesis (p. 215). The action of bacterial and intestinal digestive enzymes on food proteins produces some ammonium ions. These are carried to the liver in a bound form.
For example:

$NH_4^\oplus + \alpha$ ketoglutarate $\rightleftharpoons$ glutamate
$NH_4^\oplus +$ glutamate $\rightleftharpoons$ glutamine.

In the liver these two reactions are reversed and most of the toxic ammonium ions are removed via urea synthesis so that when the liver is functioning normally the blood concentration of ammonium ions is kept low.
    The liver is also important in the biosynthesis of various plasma proteins. Hepatocytes are the only site for the synthesis of fibrinogen and

serum albumin, and the main site for the synthesis of α- and β-globulins (γ-globulins are synthesized by plasma cells in lymph nodes). Albumin, the major protein of plasma has a molecular weight of about 65 000 daltons. It is important in maintaining the osmotic pressure of blood, and also binds and transports a variety of small molecules including fatty acids and bile pigments (see below).

Other proteins synthesized in hepatocytes include prothrombin and other blood clotting factors and various enzymes including transaminases, dehydrogenases and phosphatases.

Lipid metabolism (p. 205)

Free fatty acids and chylomicrons containing triglycerides reach the liver from the small intestine. Triglycerides are hydrolysed to glycerol and fatty acids. The liver itself can synthesize more fatty acids. There are then six routes fatty acids can follow:

1   Triglycerides can be synthesized and incorporated into plasma very low density lipoproteins (VLDL). The VLDL deliver fatty acids either to skeletal and cardiac muscle for oxidation, or to adipose tissue for storage as triglycerides. The latter may subsequently be hydrolysed by a hormone sensitive lipase (activated via the cyclic AMP mechanism) releasing free fatty acids and glycerol into the bloodstream.

2   Fatty acids can be oxidized to CO_2 and H_2O. Under basal conditions this reaction provides some 75% of the energy liberated in the liver.

3   Fatty acids can be broken down to ketone bodies which are transported by the blood to peripheral tissues where they may be oxidized by the citric acid cycle. Ketone bodies provide an important source of energy, for example, in heart muscle.

4   Fatty acids can be incorporated into phospholipids.

5   Cholesterol is esterified, principally by unsaturated fatty acids, and cholesterol esters are incorporated into lipoproteins. The synthesis of cholesterol is considered below.

6   Fatty liver. The liver is infiltrated by fat (steatosis) in several disorders including alcoholism and kwashiorkor oedematous protein energy malnutrition). Administration of choline or other lipotropic factors can cure fatty liver, as these combine with phosphatidic acid forming lecithin and other phospholipids which may then be removed from the liver, and transported in blood to other tissues.

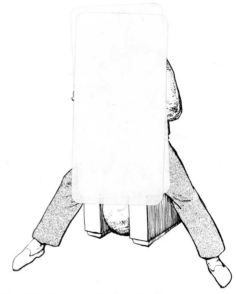

Fig. 14.3. 'Le gavage'—force feeding a goose.

The French have made use of the ability of goose liver to convert excess carbohydrate to fat, in their 'pâté de foie gras'. A typical 'foie gras' weighs about 800 g and contains 60% of fat. Before 'le gavage' (Fig. 14.3) a goose liver normally only weighs about 100 g.

While vertebrates are able to convert carbohydrate into lipid via acetyl CoA, they are unable to reverse the reaction:

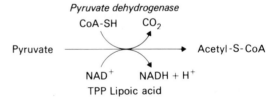

This is the reason that a diet high in lipid and low in carbohydrate leads to ketosis.

Bile formation

The three major components of bile are cholesterol, bile pigments and bile salts. Cholesterol and the bile pigments are excretory products, but bile salts have the important function of emulsifying dietary lipids in the small intestine. This detergent-like action assists fat digestion by producing a greater surface area of substrate for the pancreatic lipase to hydrolyse. Bile salts together with some cholesterol are resorbed from the terminal ileum and transported back to the liver, circulating in this way about twice during the digestion of an average meal.

CHOLESTEROL

Cholesterol is synthesized in hepatocytes from acetate units (in order to construct plasma membranes, for example), and the liver is also the major site of cholesterol catabolism (to form bile acids). Exactly how these processes are controlled is not yet known but the observation of an association between the incidence of coronary heart disease and raised blood cholesterol levels means that this is an important subject for research.

BILE PIGMENTS

These result from the breakdown of aged erythrocytes. Macrophages of the bone marrow, spleen and liver (i.e. Kupffer cells) catabolize haemoglobin releasing iron, globin and biliverdin. Most of the liberated globin and iron are reutilized, but the porphyrin residue of haem is not. Its derivative, biliverdin, is reduced to bilirubin which is then transported in plasma (bound to albumin) to hepatocytes. Hepatocytes remove bilirubin from the blood stream and conjugate it with glucuronic acid to form water-soluble bilirubin diglucuronide which passes in bile to the gall bladder. The liver excretes about 0.3 g of bilirubin daily in this way. In the terminal ileum and large intestine intestinal bacteria reduce bilirubin to urobilinogen which may subsequently be oxidized to urobilin and stercobilin, the normal pigments of faeces. Serum bilirubin levels are raised (jaundice) if there is a defect in this pathway (see below).

BILE SALTS

These are synthesized in the liver from cholesterol (p. 608).

Metabolism of hormones and detoxication of drugs

The liver is responsible for the metabolism of various hormones. In general steroid hormones are inactivated by conjugation with either sulphate or glucuronic acid. These conjugated derivatives are less metabolically active than the steroids from which they are derived, and their water solubility increases their rate of excretion in bile. They may also be inactivated by reduction, for example: progesterone $\longrightarrow$ pregnane

diol. Failure to metabolize aldosterone in liver disease can contribute to water retention and the accumulation of fluid in the peritoneal cavity known as ascites. Thyroxine is metabolized by the liver and so are polypeptide hormones. Liver extracts have been shown to inactivate oxytocin initially by reducing a disulphide bond, followed by proteolytic attack on the peptide chain.

DETOXICATION

Several chemical reactions which take place predominantly in the liver are collectively known as detoxication processes. Just as a number of normal intermediary metabolites are converted to less toxic substances and eliminated (for example, bilirubin to bilirubin diglucuronide) so too similar reactions assist in the disposal of drugs and other compounds foreign to the organism. The two major detoxication reactions are oxidation and conjugation.

Examples of drugs inactivated by oxidation include pentobarbital (a barbiturate), amphetamine (a monoamine oxidase inhibitor), and halothane (an anaesthetic).

The mechanism of oxidation is as follows. Oxygenases have been found in association with endoplasmic reticulum together with two haem proteins, cytochrome B_5 and cytochrome P-450 (so called because of the strong light absorption at 450nm produced when microsomes are exposed to carbon monoxide). Cytochrome B_5 is involved in electron transport, and cytochrome P-450 acts as a mixed function oxygenase which, like mitochondrial cytochrome, reduces molecular oxygen but at the same time oxidizes an organic substrate. The overall reaction can be written as:

$$\text{substrate} \quad + O_2 + NADPH + H^+$$
(e.g. amphetamine)

$$\longrightarrow \text{Oxidized} + H_2O + NADP^+$$
substrate

The metabolism of the organic fluorine-containing anaesthetic gases halothane and methoxyflurane is complex, but one surprising finding is that after anaesthesia, patients' sera contain elevated levels of ionic fluoride.

Conjugation reactions
Conjugation reactions in the endoplasmic reticulum of hepatocytes can also serve to detoxify foreign compounds. The principal types of conjugation are:

Glucuronide formation. For example, benzoic acid:

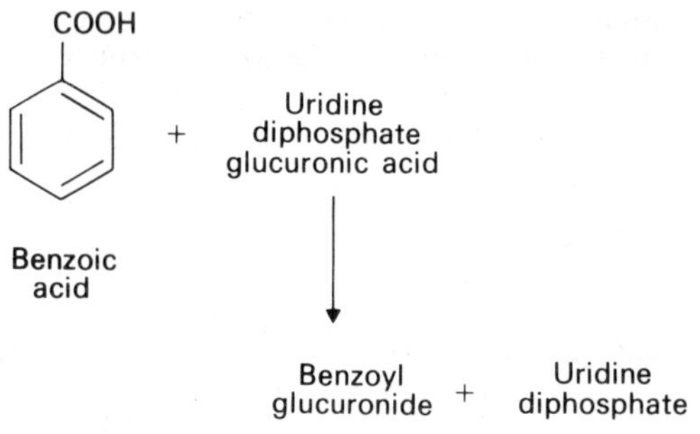

COOH

Benzoic
acid

+ Uridine
diphosphate
glucuronic acid

↓

Benzoyl
glucuronide + Uridine
diphosphate

Conjugation with amino acids. Benzoic acid can also be rendered water soluble by conjugation with glycine. Measurement of hippuric acid excretion following an oral dose of sodium benzoate is one method of assessing the liver's ability to perform conjugation reactions.

COOH

Benzoic
acid

+ H₂NCH₂COOH

Glycine

↓

CONHCH₂COOH

Hippuric
acid

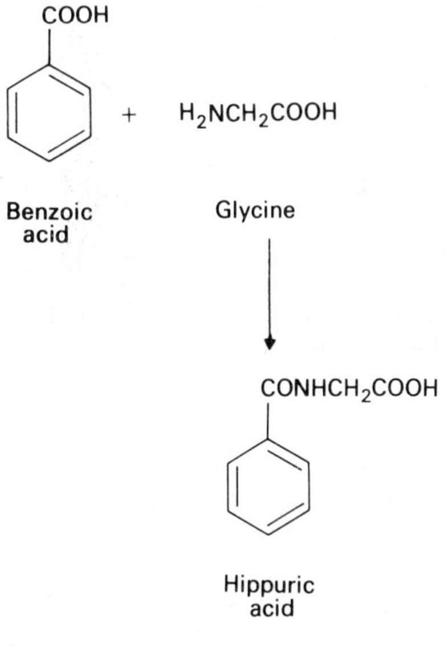

Other conjugation reactions occur by sulphate ester formation, methylation, dealkylation, mercapturic acid formation, and acetylation.

Liver metabolism of carcinogens

Oxidation and conjugation reactions by the liver generally have an important function in protecting man from various toxic substances. How-

ever, it is possible for metabolism by the liver to increase the toxicity of certain chemicals. This is the case with aflatoxins, among the most potent carcinogens known, produced by the fungus *Aspergillus flavus* which can grow on poorly stored food. When testing new drugs, the possibility that the resultant liver metabolites may have dangerous side-effects must therefore be investigated.

Microsomal enzyme induction

A further point to be borne in mind when considering hepatic drug metabolism is that more than two hundred compounds, when administered to animals, enhance the activity of oxidative microsomal enzymes. For example, by this process caffeine, cigarette smoke and ethanol all alter the duration and the intensity of the action of other drugs. The potential therapeutic implications are serious. Patients treated with say phenobarbital may require larger than normal doses of other drugs; if phenobarbital is discontinued and the enzyme induction disappears the large doses of the other drug may now be toxic. Drugs which have been implicated in enzyme induction fall into three major groups:

1 The phenobarbital type;
2 The polycyclic hydrocarbon type; and
3 Anabolic steroids.

Hepatitis following halothane anaesthesia

A rare complication of repeated exposure to halothane is the development of unexplained hepatitis. With the recognition of the possible toxic side effects of halothane, more precautions are being taken to reduce pollution of the atmosphere in operating theatres. Various suggestions have been made regarding the pathogenesis of this type of hepatitis.

One suggestion that has been made is that a metabolite of halothane may behave as a hapten—that is a small molecule which by itself cannot stimulate antibody synthesis, but which can combine with liver macromolecules which then do stimulate an immune response (p. 680). Hence repeated exposure to halothane could induce a hypersensitivity reaction. Halothane anaesthesia should not be repeated if there is suspicion of an adverse reaction after the first administration.

Metabolism of ethanol

The cytoplasm of hepatocytes contains the enzyme alcohol dehydrogenase, which converts ethanol to acetaldehyde:

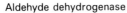

$$CH_3CH_2OH \xrightarrow[\substack{NAD^+ \quad NADH + H^+}]{\text{Alcohol dehydrogenase}} CH_2CHO$$

Acetyl-S-CoA is then produced from the acetaldehyde in the following manner:

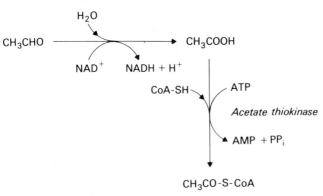

$$CH_3CHO \xrightarrow[\substack{NAD^+ \quad NADH + H^+}]{\substack{\text{Aldehyde dehydrogenase} \\ H_2O}} CH_3COOH$$

$$CH_3CO\text{-}S\text{-}CoA$$

(with CoA-SH, ATP, Acetate thiokinase, AMP + PP$_i$)

Formation of acetaldehyde may be partly responsible for the 'hangover' following excessive alcohol consumption. Alcohol is hepatotoxic. In one investigation ultrastructural changes were observed in liver biopsy specimens taken from volunteers who consumed about one bottle of spirits each day for ten days, despite the fact that the subjects were not obviously intoxicated! Ingestion of about two-thirds of a bottle of whisky daily, for a number of years, can lead to severe alcoholic liver damage (cirrhosis). The chronic alcoholic frequently suffers from malnutrition as a result of bad eating habits, particularly deficiencies in protein and vitamins. In France between 1941 and 1947, rationing of wine from five to one litre per week led to an 80% reduction in mortality from cirrhosis.

Storage of nutrients in the liver

The liver is the principal site for storing fat-soluble vitamins. Under normal conditions the liver in a well-fed person contains sufficient vitamin A to meet his needs for 1–2 years. Hepatocytes synthesize a specific retinol-binding protein, which helps to maintain a fairly constant level of vitamin A in the circulating blood. Vitamin B_{12} (a water-soluble vitamin) is stored in a similar way.

Minerals also accumulate in the liver, this being the predominant tissue store of iron, copper and several trace elements including zinc, cobalt, manganese, molybdenum and selenium.

Liver disorders

JAUNDICE

Jaundice arises from excessive amounts of bilirubin in blood, and can be caused by several mechanisms:
1 Haemolytic jaundice is caused by an increased rate of turnover of erythrocytes.
2 Cholestatic jaundice arises as a result of the failure of bile to reach the duodenum. This can be caused by a defect within hepatocytes, or else by mechanical bile duct obstruction for example by a pancreatic tumour or gall-stones.
3 Hepatocellular jaundice can be caused by inflammation of the liver (hepatitis) or cirrhosis (see below).

VIRUS HEPATITIS

There are two major types of virus-induced liver inflammation termed virus A (infective) hepatitis, and virus B (serum) hepatitis. Virus A hepatitis is usually spread by the faecal–oral route, school children being the group most affected. The more dangerous, virus B hepatitis, can be spread by blood, for instance from contaminated dental instruments, or equipment used by drug addicts. Special care must be taken in handling all blood samples, especially those coming from patients with hepatitis.

CIRRHOSIS

This is an irreversible chronic liver disease in which liver tissue is replaced by collagenous scar tissue and also formation of nodules occurs. There are a number of possible causes including alcoholism, virus hepatitis, and some forms of metabolic disease.

INHERITED DISORDERS AFFECTING THE LIVER

1 In Wilson's disease, due to a genetic defect in the structure of a plasma protein (caeruloplasmin) manufactured by the liver and used for transporting copper in the blood, toxic levels of the ion accumulate and produce degenerative effects in the liver and brain.
2 In idiopathic haemachromatosis increased quantities of dietary iron are absorbed leading to toxic damage of the liver.
3 Several glycogen storage diseases arise from the absence of enzymes involved in glycogen metabolism. This can lead to hypoglycaemia because the liver fails to convert glycogen to blood glucose in times of need.

MISCELLANEOUS LIVER DISORDERS

The liver can be destroyed by cancer. The most common form arises from metastases—secondary tumours spreading through the bloodstream from primary cancers elsewhere in the body. The liver can also be infected by a variety of organisms, ranging from liver flukes, tapeworms and a species of amoeba to several different species of bacteria.

Liver function tests

Since it has such a central role in metabolism, disturbances of the liver can have diverse clinical consequences. Over 100 chemical tests of liver function have been devised, though no single set is ideal. Pathology laboratories usually have a battery of hepatic function tests, and a typical group is summarized below:
1 *Bilirubin*. In jaundice the serum level of bilirubin is elevated. If the rise is due to an increase in conjugated bilirubin, it can be deduced that the hepatocytes are probably functioning normally. The condition may be due to obstructive jaundice for instance. An increase in unconjugated bilirubin arises either from increased destruction of red cells (haemolytic jaundice) or a failure of hepatocytes to conjugate the bilirubin normally.
2 *Alkaline phosphatase*. The serum level of (liver) alkaline phosphatase is increased in liver damage. Its presence can be distinguished from that of bone alkaline phosphatase, a different protein, by electrophoresis.
3 *Serum albumin and globulin*. Biosynthesis of serum albumin is reduced in chronic liver disease such as cirrhosis. In hepatitis there is also an increase in antibody production, hence a greater proportion of γ-globulin in serum.
4 *Blood clotting factors* (p. 689). Failure of the liver to produce the proteins involved in blood clotting may be an indication of liver disorders. An increase in the prothrombin time from about 15 seconds to a minute or more which is not corrected by administration of vitamin K suggests such a disorder.
5 *Serum transaminases*. When hepatic cells are damaged asparate aminotransferase and alanine aminotransferase leak into the blood. Serum levels of the latter are especially high in active chronic hepatitis.
6 *Serum cholesterol*. A common finding in obstructive jaundice is that serum cholesterol levels are increased above normal because of a failure to excrete cholesterol in bile.
7 *Glucose tolerance test*. In the absence of other abnormalities in glucose metabolism (for example diabetes), this test may reveal a failure of the liver to convert excess glucose to glycogen.

FURTHER READING

BITTAR E. (Ed.) (1969) *The Biological Basis of Medicine* Volume 5, Chapters 5–9. Academic Press, London.

EDDLESTONE A., WEBER J. & WILLIAMS R. (Eds.) (1979) *Immune Reactions in Liver Disease*. Pitman Medical Press, London.

KAPPAS A. & ALVARES A. (1975) How the liver metabolizes foreign substances. *Scientific American*, June 1975, **232**, 22.

LIEBER C.S. (1976) The metabolism of alcohol. *Scientific American*, March 1976, **234**, 25.

SHERLOCK S. (1981) *Diseases of the Liver and Biliary System*, 6th Edition. Blackwell Scientific Publications, Oxford.

CHAPTER 15

Cardiovascular System

ANATOMY

The heart pumps blood through a series of vessels so that all cells can both receive the substances they require, and, where necessary, dispose of the products of their metabolism. The structure of the blood vessels varies according to their function. Arteries conduct blood from the heart, capillaries allow exchanges to take place and veins return the blood to the heart. There are, however, intermediate vessels between the arteries and capillaries, called arterioles and between capillaries and veins, called venules.

It is easy to see the main arteries and veins, but the microscopic nature of small arterioles, capillaries and small venules makes it difficult to appreciate their quantity and relationships. For example almost half the volume of the liver consists of sinusoids (a special type of capillary). It has been estimated that there are about 2000 capillaries in 1 mm³ of skeletal muscle. However, the number open at any one time varies with the functional state of the organ. For this reason histological sections can be very misleading with regard to the vascular relationships in any tissue.

ARTERIES

These consist of the basic three layers in all blood vessels (Fig. 15.1) with the exception of capillaries and sinusoids.

1 The tunica intima consists of the endothelium and some delicate subendothelial connective tissue.
2 The tunica media consists of an internal elastic lamina, a layer of smooth muscle cells and elastic fibres and an external elastic lamina.
3 The tunica adventitia is mainly collagenous with the fibres arranged longitudinally.

The thickness of the wall and the proportion of elastic and muscular tissue, especially in the tunica media, vary considerably in different types of blood vessels. Large arteries such as the

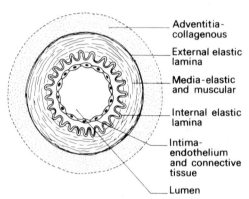

Fig. 15.1. Transverse section through medium-sized artery.

aorta and its main branches contain many layers of elastic tissue in the tunica media. These arteries are called elastic arteries, which enlarge when the heart contracts and recoil when the heart relaxes so assisting the propulsion of the blood during diastole.

As the arteries divide and diminish in size the elastic fibres decrease and the smooth muscle increases in quantity. As a result the internal and external elastic laminae become more distinct and the tunica media consists largely of spirally arranged smooth muscle fibres. These smooth muscle cells are smaller than those found in viscera. They contain dense bodies, closely related to myofilaments, which are attached to the plasma membrane of the cell. The muscle cells are connected to each other and also to the endothelial cells by tight junctions. These junctions become more frequent and longer as the vessels decrease in size. This type of artery is called a muscular artery. It can vary the size of its lumen thus individually controlling the volume of blood reaching the tissues served and collectively influencing blood pressure, since they and the arterioles are the 'resistance vessels' making the greatest contribution to the peripheral vascular resistance (see p. 697).

ARTERIOLES

Small muscular arteries divide to become arterioles. Arterioles may have a diameter up to 500 μm. When they are about 50 μm in diameter they have only one layer of muscle cells in their wall. Their branches, which lead to the capillaries, are less than 20 μm in diameter. At their origin the smallest branches have a specialized sphincter of smooth muscle, or precapillary sphincter. In the smallest arterioles there is no internal elastic lamina and the tunica adventitia is reduced to a very thin layer of collagen and a few fibroblasts.

CAPILLARIES

These are usually defined as vessels with walls one-cell thick consisting of longitudinally arranged endothelial cells (Fig. 15.2). Since cells with contractile properties (Rouget cells) form an incomplete layer outside the endothelium, it has been suggested that capillaries have the three basic layers of blood vessels (Fig. 15.1). The nature of the capillary wall, namely the cells and their junctions, allows the exchange of materials between the lumen and tissues.

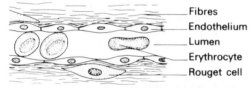

Fibres
Endothelium
Lumen
Erythrocyte
Rouget cell

Fig. 15.2. Longitudinal section through capillary.

Capillaries have a diameter of about 8 μm, similar to the diameter of a red blood corpuscle. The nuclei of the flattened endothelial cells bulge into the lumen. Capillaries are either continuous or fenestrated. The continuous type, in which there are tight junctions between the cells, is found for example in all varieties of muscle, the lungs and the brain. There is a continuous basal lamina on the non-luminal surface and invaginations on the cell surface and vesicles in the cytoplasm which may be part of a mechanism for the transport of fluids across the cell (pinocytosis). Fenestrated capillaries on the other hand, for example as seen in the renal glomeruli, endocrine glands and gastrointestinal tract, have pores which may contain a diaphragm.

Pericytes or Rouget cells lie on the outer surface of the endothelial cells of capillaries and in some ways resemble smooth muscle cells, although there is doubt as to whether they play a role in controlling the size of the lumen of capillaries. Similarly there is still some controversy regarding the contractility of the endothelial cells themselves; in some lower animals these are capable of altering the diameter of the capillary. The true capillaries have at their entrance a sphincter-like arrangement of a few muscle cells. These aid the control of the blood flow through the capillary.

Sinusoids are found in the liver, spleen, red bone marrow and suprarenal gland and are similar to capillaries in structure but have a larger irregular diameter. They have little or no connective tissue round the endothelium and often have phagocytic cells in their walls. The large lumen slows the rate of blood flow thereby permitting a longer time for contact between their contents and the surrounding tissues and therefore for phagocytosis of particulate matter in the blood in their lumen. Some sinusoids, for example those of the liver, have relatively large spaces between the cells.

VEINS

Venules are said to be formed when the capillaries increase in size and acquire a thin but distinct coat of connective tissue. The smallest venules, about 30 μm in diameter, like the capillaries and sinusoids permit the exchange of substances through their walls. As the venules become larger their walls become thicker but the three distinct coats of arterioles and arteries are difficult to differentiate (Fig. 15.3). This is because the tunica media is mainly collagenous with fibroblasts and a few elastic fibres and muscle cells. The tunica adventitia in large veins is much thicker than the tunica media and contains longitudinal muscle fibres.

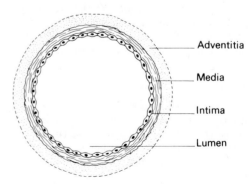

Adventitia
Media
Intima
Lumen

Fig. 15.3. Transverse section through medium-sized vein.

The veins of the brain and spinal cord, the intracranial venous sinuses, and the veins of the retina and red bone marrow have no muscle fibres in their wall. The lumen of a vein is larger than that of a comparable artery and is able to accommodate a larger volume of blood at a lower pressure. Many veins have valves, made of two crescentic cusps each consisting of two layers of endothelium separated by a very small amount of loose connective tissue (Fig. 15.4). Valves are arranged so that they prevent back-flow of the blood; their proximal free edges come together when the blood they contain flows away from the heart. Valves are most commonly found in a tributary vein close to its termination and in a main vein just beyond the entry of a tributary. There are no valves in some veins, for example cerebral veins, and also large veins such as the superior and inferior venae cavae.

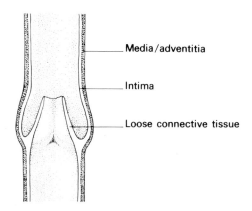

Fig. 15.4. Venous valves.

The presence of valves is related to the intermittent pressure to which some veins are subjected; during walking for example, intermittent pressure due to the contraction of the surrounding large muscles is an important factor in returning venous blood from the legs to the heart.

VASCULAR ARRANGEMENTS

Not all blood travels in sequence through arteries, arterioles, capillaries, venules and veins. The term 'anastomosis' is used in this context to indicate connections between blood vessels which allow changes in this sequence.

Arterial anastomoses
These refer to connections between arteries before they form arterioles. These anastomoses provide alternative channels for the blood supply of an organ or part of the body. They are seen in the base of the brain where large vessels join to form the arterial circle of Willis, in the mesenteries of the gastrointestinal tract, and round the joints of the limbs where movements may compress one arterial channel and open another. Anastomoses also provide a means of smoothing out changes of pressure in the vascular territories which are linked in this way.

Sometimes the anastomotic channels enlarge and become the main artery supplying a part, and the normal vessel is reduced. These are called aberrant arteries, and unless looked for, can easily be cut in surgical operations. On the other hand a knowledge of the possibility of anastomotic channels being present enables a surgeon to tie a main vessel because a collateral circulation will be established. However, it is important to know how long it will take for this circulation to be opened up.

The term end arteries is used to describe arteries which have no anastomotic connections with other arteries. If such an artery is occluded, the organ or part of the organ supplied by it will die. The central artery of the retina is an artery of this type. Many other arteries are included in this category although they may have small anastomotic connections. The large arteries entering the brain, the splenic and pulmonary arteries, the main branches of the renal artery and the large branches of the coronary arteries of the heart come into this category.

Arteriovenous anastomoses
These are connections between arterioles and venules, about 300 μm in diameter, which enable the blood to short-circuit the capillaries. They arise from terminal arterioles and go directly to a venule. Characteristically the wall of these anastomotic channels is thick due to an increase in smooth muscle which has a rich sympathetic innervation. These anastomoses close under sympathetic stimulation and also show a rhythmic contractility. They are found in organs which are intermittently active such as the mucous membrane of the gastrointestinal tract. They are closed during digestion and absorption so that the blood must pass through the capillaries. Similar anastomoses are also found in the skin where they are associated with temperature regulation (p. 725); they are especially numerous in the fingers, toes, nose, lips and ears. Other sites include the nasal mucosa (possibly related to changes in the temperature of inspired air),

the carotid and coccygeal bodies, sympathetic ganglia and the erectile tissue of the sexual organs.

The term 'portal system' of blood vessels refers to an arrangement in which blood passes through two sets of capillaries before returning to the heart. The hepatic portal system is a good example. Arterial blood supplying the gastro-intestinal tract and spleen passes through one set of capillaries and after collecting in the portal vein passes through another set of capillaries (sinusoids) in the liver, before entering the inferior vena cava. A similar arrangement is found between the vessels of the hypothalamus in the base of the brain and the anterior lobe of the hypophysis cerebri (pituitary gland). The capillaries in the region where the hypophysis is attached to the hypothalamus form portal vessels which are the main source of blood to the anterior lobe of the pituitary where they break up and form a second set of capillaries.

BLOOD AND NERVE SUPPLY OF BLOOD VESSELS

All arteries and veins larger than about 0.5 mm in diameter have in their tunica adventitia small blood vessels called vasa vasorum. They come from either the main artery or adjacent branches. In the adventitia they form capillaries and venules which drain into nearby venules or in the case of a vein, into the lumen of the vein itself.

Blood vessels have a nerve supply consisting of small myelinated (probably sensory) and non-myelinated nerves, almost all of which are postganglionic sympathetic and on stimulation produce vasoconstriction, thus playing an important part in the control of both the blood pressure and peripheral circulation. There is some evidence that stimulation of the nerves to the coronary and pulmonary arteries produces vasodilation. Two groups of sympathetic nerves supply the vessels in skeletal muscle; the majority produce vasodilation but some cause vasoconstriction. The parasympathetic may supply vasodilator fibres to the coronary vessels. The parasympathetic nerves which are secretomotor also cause vasodilation of the blood vessels of the glandular tissue.

The way in which the postganglionic fibres reach the blood vessels varies. The blood vessels supplying the abdominal viscera have a periarterial plexus round the proximal part of the vessel, extending along the main trunk and continuing along all its branches. Elsewhere in the body, although the sympathetic ganglia supply the proximal parts of the main trunks, peripheral nerves running close to the vessels supply them along the whole of their course.

The myelinated fibres of the blood vessels may mediate impulses interpreted as pain. Their collaterals to the skin form the anatomical basis for the axon reflex. There are, however, special sensory mechanisms related to some blood vessels, for example the aorta and the beginning of the common carotid, right subclavian and pulmonary arteries. These sensory nerves respond to changes in blood pressure (baro- or pressoreceptors: p. 711) and/or changes in the carbon dioxide and oxygen tensions of the blood (chemoreceptors). There are also sensory nerve endings in the walls of the superior and inferior venae cavae which respond to changes in venous pressure.

The thorax

PERICARDIUM

The heart and beginning or ends of the large blood vessels lie in the pericardium, which consists of an outer tough membranous part, the fibrous pericardium and an invaginated layer of serous membrane, the serous pericardium (Fig. 15.5). The outer (parietal) layer of the serous pericardium is firmly adherent to the inner surface of the fibrous pericardium and the inner (visceral) layer (also called the epicardium) is attached to the surface of the heart with a potential space between the two layers. The fibrous pericardium has been compared to a paper bag with its mouth superiorly. The heart is said to be dropped into the bag from above and the edges of the opening fuse with the walls of the large vessels entering and leaving the upper part of the heart. Inferiorly the fibrous pericardium is attached over a variable area to the tendinous part of the diaphragm, anteriorly to the upper and lower ends of the sternum and superiorly to the pretracheal fascia. Since the heart is invaginated into the serous pericardium, the parietal and visceral layers are continuous with each other round the large vessels, behind the heart.

HEART

General
The heart, approximately conical in shape, is about 12 cm long, 9 cm wide and 6 cm anteroposteriorly. The apex is below and to the left, the base is posterior and to the right. Its

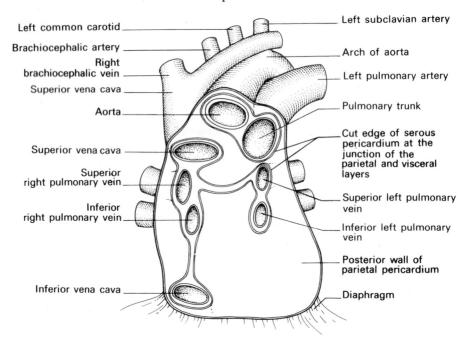

Left common carotid

Brachiocephalic artery

Right brachiocephalic vein

Superior vena cava

Aorta

Superior vena cava

Superior right pulmonary vein

Inferior right pulmonary vein

Inferior vena cava

Left subclavian artery

Arch of aorta

Left pulmonary artery

Pulmonary trunk

Cut edge of serous pericardium at the junction of the parietal and visceral layers

Superior left pulmonary vein

Inferior left pulmonary vein

Posterior wall of parietal pericardium

Diaphragm

Fig. 15.5. The reflection of the serous pericardium.

projection on to the surface of the body is shown in Fig. 15.6. It weighs about 300 g in the male and 250 g in the female.

The heart has four chambers, the right and left atria, and the right and left ventricles. The atria are separated from the ventricles by the coronary sulcus (atrioventricular groove) in which lie the coronary arteries (Fig. 15.7). This almost vertical groove is partly covered where the pulmonary artery arises from the right ventricle.

Certain terms are used in describing the heart. The apex, that part which is furthest inferior,

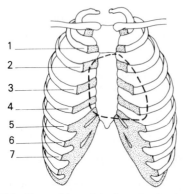

Fig. 15.6. The position of the heart in the thorax.

anterior and to the left, is part of the left ventricle. The base, which is posterior and to some extent superior, is formed mainly by the left atrium. The right border, formed by the right atrium, is the edge where the sternocostal surface meets the right surface. The left border, which is between the sternocostal and left surfaces, is formed by the left ventricle. The inferior border is between the sternocostal and diaphragmatic surfaces.

Posterior to the heart are the oesophagus, thoracic aorta and the fifth to the eighth thoracic vertebrae (Fig. 15.8). Anteriorly are the sternum and the third to the sixth costal cartilages. To the right and left the heart is related to the lungs and pleurae both of which extend over the sternocostal surface to some extent. The phrenic nerves, one on each side, pass downwards between the heart and the lung.

Passing upwards from the heart are the aorta and pulmonary trunk. The aorta is posterior to, and to the right of, the pulmonary trunk and is somewhat overlapped by it. The superior and inferior venae cavae enter the right atrium, the superior to the right of the aorta. The inferior vena cava enters the lowest part of the right atrium posteriorly. Two pulmonary veins on each side pass horizontally into the left atrium on the posterior surface of the heart.

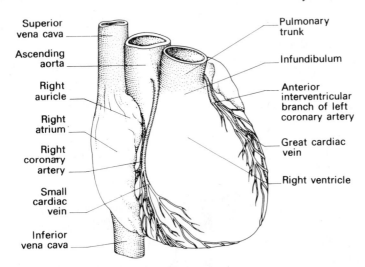

Fig. 15.7. The anterior surface of the heart.

Chambers of heart

The heart is divided into right and left halves by a septum and each side is divided into an atrium and a ventricle. The interatrial septum between the right and left atria is almost in the coronal plane so that the right atrium is anterior as well as to the right of the left atrium.

The right atrium. This chamber is roughly rectangular with the long axis vertical but has a projection superiorly and to the left, in front of the beginning of the aorta, the right auricle ('auricle' means 'ear-shaped'). The interior of the atrium can be divided into the smooth posterior part into which the venae cavae open (sinus venarum) and a ridged anterior part. The ridges extend into the auricle, contain muscle and are called musculi pectinati ('pecten' means a 'comb'). The opening of the inferior vena cava has an anterior fold called the valve of the inferior vena cava. The fossa ovalis is a depression on the interatrial septum which marks the site of a fetal opening between the right and left atria, the foramen ovale (Book 2). The valve of the inferior vena cava directed the blood from the inferior vena into the left atrium through the

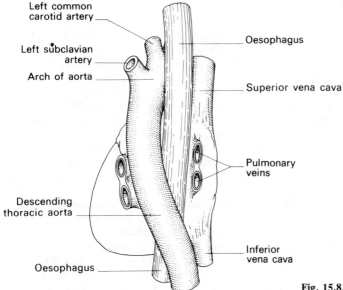

Fig. 15.8. The posterior surface of the heart.

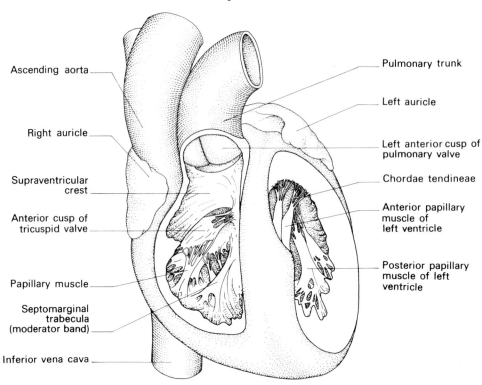

Ascending aorta

Right auricle

Supraventricular crest

Anterior cusp of tricuspid valve

Papillary muscle

Septomarginal trabecula (moderator band)

Inferior vena cava

Pulmonary trunk

Left auricle

Left anterior cusp of pulmonary valve

Chordae tendineae

Anterior papillary muscle of left ventricle

Posterior papillary muscle of left ventricle

Fig. 15.9. The interior of the right and left ventricles.

foramen ovale in the embryo. The right atrioventricular opening is about 3 cm in diameter. Between this opening and the fossa ovalis there is the opening of the coronary sinus which returns most of the blood from the heart wall to the right atrium. This opening has a semilunar fold inferiorly, the valve of the coronary sinus, which covers the opening and prevents blood being forced into the coronary sinus during atrial systole.

The right ventricle. The triangular interior of the right ventricle leads upwards into the smooth-walled, cone-shaped, infundibulum or conus arteriosus which itself leads into the pulmonary trunk. The ventricular wall is markedly ridged by columns of muscle called trabeculae carneae (Fig. 15.9). Some of these muscular columns are attached along their whole length, some only at both ends and others only at one end. These latter pass into the cavity of the ventricle and become attached to the chordae tendineae of the cusps of the atrioventricular valve.

The interventricular septum is oblique so that it forms the posterior left wall of the right ventri-

cle. This septum could be regarded as part of the left ventricle insofar as it bulges into the right ventricle and is as thick as the much thicker wall of the left ventricle.

The right atrioventricular opening is on the right side of the cavity of the ventricle and is guarded by the right atrioventricular valve, also known as the tricuspid valve. It consists of three triangular cusps — anterior, posterior and septal (to the left) (Fig. 15.10). The bases of the cusps are attached to the fibrous ring surrounding the opening and are joined to each other. The cusps consist of a double layer of endothelium, the lining of the heart, with a small amount of fibrous tissue between the two layers. Except for the part next to the atrium, the cusps are almost avascular. When the valve is closed during ventricular contraction, systole, the cusps overlap each other and are prevented being pushed into the atrium by the chordae tendineae attached to the contracting papillary muscles.

Chordae tendineae are fibrous cords which are attached to the apices and edges of the cusps and to the wall of the ventricle by the papillary muscles. The anterior papillary muscle is

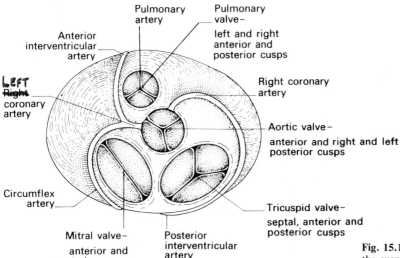

Labels on figure:
Pulmonary artery
Pulmonary valve – left and right anterior and posterior cusps
Anterior interventricular artery
Right coronary artery
LEFT ~~Right~~ coronary artery
Aortic valve – anterior and right and left posterior cusps
Circumflex artery
Tricuspid valve – septal, anterior and posterior cusps
Mitral valve – anterior and posterior cusps
Posterior interventricular artery

Fig. 15.10. The arrangement of the cusps of the valves.

attached to the anterior and posterior cusps and the posterior muscle to the posterior and septal cusps. The moderator band or septomarginal trabecula (Fig. 15.9) is the name given to a muscle which passes from the interventricular septum to the base of the anterior papillary muscle. It contains part of the conducting tissue of the heart.

The opening into the pulmonary trunk lies at the upper end of the infundibulum and is about 3 cm in diameter. During diastole, it is closed by the pulmonary valve which consists of three semilunar cusps (Fig. 15.10). Each cusp is attached to the wall of the pulmonary trunk and has a free border projecting upwards into the lumen of the vessel. In the adult heart there are two anterior (right and left) and one posterior cusp. In the middle of the free border of each cusp is a thickened nodule which helps to close the central region.

The left atrium. The left atrium is roughly rectangular with its long axis horizontal. It lies behind the right atrium and the beginnings of the pulmonary trunk and aorta, and an appendage extends forwards as the left auricle to the left of the pulmonary trunk. The wall is smooth internally except for the lining of its auricle which is ridged. Two pulmonary veins on each side open into the left atrium posterosuperiorly. The left atrioventricular opening, 2 cm in diameter, lies below and to the left.

The left ventricle. The cavity of the ventricle

appears circular when sectioned and the wall is about 1 cm thick, three times the thickness of the right ventricular wall. In other respects the interior of the left ventricle is similar to that of the right ventricle. The anterior papillary muscle is attached to the sternocostal wall and the posterior to the diaphragmatic wall. The left atrioventricular opening is guarded by the left atrioventricular (bicuspid or mitral) valve. It has two triangular cusps, an anterior lying adjacent to the aortic opening, and a posterior, which is smaller, behind, and to the left (Fig. 15.10). The bases of the cusps are attached to a fibrous ring round the left atrioventricular opening and their free edges are attached to chordae tendineae which in turn are attached to the papillary muscles.

The aortic opening is about 3 cm in diameter, lies anterior and to the right of the atrioventricular opening and is guarded by the aortic valve. This has three semilunar cusps with nodules (Fig. 15.10). There are marked sinuses at the beginning of the aorta opposite the cusps which are anterior, and right and left posterior in position.

Structure of heart wall
The heart wall consists of an outer layer, the epicardium which is the visceral serous pericardium, a middle layer of muscle, the myocardium and the endocardium. There are rings of fibrous tissue related to the aortic and pulmonary openings and the atrioventricular openings. The ring around the pulmonary opening is joined by

fibrous tissue to the fibrous ring round the aortic opening. The rings round the atrioventricular openings form a figure eight and are joined by fibrous tissue to the ring round the aortic opening which lies anterior to and between them (Fig. 15.10). The cusps of all the valves are attached to the fibrous rings, as already described. The cardiac muscle fibres are attached to the rings, the atrial and ventricular fibres being completely separate. The arrangement of the atrial fibres is the simpler. The superficial layer encircles the two atria but the deeper muscle fibres of each atrium are separate. Some of the deeper circular fibres extend into the venae cavae. The arrangement of the ventricular muscle fibres is much more complex. Most of the fibres pass in a series of spiralling layers round both ventricles.

Blood supply and innervation of heart

The coronary arteries supplying the heart come from the ascending aorta just above its origin (Figs. 15.10 & 15.12). There are two coronary arteries. The right comes from the anterior aortic sinus and passes forwards and to the right between the pulmonary trunk and the right

auricle. It then turns downwards in the coronary sulcus between the right atrium and right ventricle to the lower border of the heart where it passes on to the back of the heart. It continues to the left as far as the posterior interventricular groove where it anastomoses with the left coronary artery. The right coronary artery supplies the right atrium and gives off a marginal branch at the inferior border of the heart. This branch runs to the left towards the apex of the heart and supplies both ventricles. At its termination the right coronary artery gives off the posterior interventricular artery which passes towards the apex and supplies both ventricles and the posterior part of the interventricular septum. A branch of the right coronary artery near its origin forms a plexus round the beginning of the superior vena cava. From this plexus in more than half the hearts studied, a branch is given to the sinoatrial node.

The left coronary artery arises from the left posterior aortic sinus and passes forwards between the pulmonary trunk and the left auricle in the coronary sulcus. It divides into an anterior interventricular branch and a circumflex branch

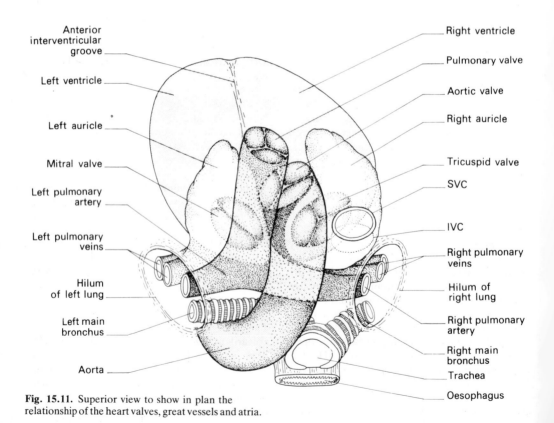

Fig. 15.11. Superior view to show in plan the relationship of the heart valves, great vessels and atria.

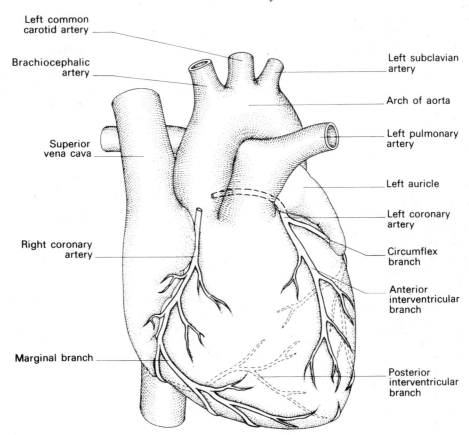

Fig. 15.12. The arteries of the heart.

which winds round the left border of the heart on to its posterior surface where it passes to the right and anastomoses with the right coronary artery. The left coronary artery supplies the left atrium. The large anterior interventricular artery passes downwards in the anterior interventricular groove towards the apex of the heart and supplies both ventricles and the interventricular septum. The circumflex artery gives off a branch which runs along the left border of the heart. In less than 50% of hearts the sinoatrial node is supplied by an early branch of the left coronary artery. Although the ends of the left and right coronary arteries anastomose they are functional end arteries. Most of the veins draining the heart wall end in the coronary sinus which lies in the posterior part of the coronary sulcus between the left atrium and left ventricle.

There are two cardiac nerve plexuses, a superficial which lies inferior to the arch of the aorta and a deep which lies on the bifurcation of the trachea behind the arch of the aorta. The superficial receives branches from the sympathetic trunk and vagus nerve on the left side of the neck. It gives branches to the deep plexus and to the right coronary artery. The deep plexus is much larger than the superficial and receives branches from the sympathetic trunk and vagus of both sides. Some of these nerves arise in the neck and some in the thorax. The left recurrent laryngeal nerve also gives a branch to the deep plexus. The thoracic sympathetic branches come from the first to the fifth thoracic ganglia. The branches from the deep plexus go to the heart mainly as a coronary plexus accompanying the coronary arteries. Some fibres go directly to the atria.

The preganglionic parasympathetic efferent fibres have their cell bodies in the dorsal nucleus of the vagus in the medulla oblongata and they synapse mainly in the deep cardiac plexus. Some fibres synapse with ganglion cells near the nodes of conducting tissue in the walls of the atria. The preganglionic sympathetic efferent fibres have their cell bodies in the first to the fifth thoracic spinal segments and they synapse in the upper five thoracic sympathetic ganglia and the cervical ganglia. The postganglionic fibres go to the cardiac plexuses and continue from there to the heart.

There are both sympathetic and parasympathetic afferent fibres from the heart. The former are associated with the painful sensations in the condition called angina pectoris in which reduced blood supply to the heart muscle results in pain. The afferent parasympathetic fibres are associated with cardiac reflexes. The sinoatrial node is the structure controlling the rate and rhythmicity of the heart beat; the activity of the node is modulated by autonomic nerves.

Conducting system of heart
Cardiac muscle fibres in the form of nodes and bundles coordinate the contraction of the atria and ventricles. The various parts of the conducting system are the sinoatrial (or sinuatrial) node, the atrioventricular node and bundle (bundle of His) which divides into two, and the Purkinje fibres which form subendocardial plexuses in the ventricles. Purkinje fibres usually have a larger diameter than the rest of the myocardial fibres. They have extensive contact with one another, numerous desmosomes and relatively few myofibrils. They are not found in the atria.

The sinoatrial node, a pacemaker of the heart, is about 10 mm long and 4 mm wide, is situated on the right of the junction between the superior vena cava and the right atrium, in the upper part of the sulcus terminalis, and occupies the whole thickness of the wall. Its cells are smaller than cardiac muscle fibres and are arranged in a network. Many non-myelinated nerve fibres terminate in the node, both sympathetic and parasympathetic. Impulses from the former make the heart beat faster, and from the latter makes the heart beat more slowly. Nerve cells are found adjacent to the node but not in it. The impulses from the node controlling the frequency of the heart beat are conveyed to the atrioventricular node by the atrial myocardial fibres with which the nodal fibres are in close contact, there being no other conducting tissue in the walls of the atria.

The atrioventricular node, about 5 mm long and 3 mm wide, is situated in the interatrial septum just above the opening of the coronary sinus. The node is continuous with the atrioventricular bundle (of His) which passes towards the interventricular septum in which, after a short

course, it divides into two, the right and left limbs of the bundle. These pass downwards on the right and left sides of the septum to reach the apex. The right limb passes into the moderator band to the anterior papillary muscle where it becomes a plexus of Purkinje fibres which spread over the whole of the right ventricle deep to the endocardium and establish close contact with the muscle fibres of the ventricle. The left limb breaks up into several branches as it passes towards the apex of the heart. The cells of the atrioventricular node and bundle and first part of the limbs are similar to those of the sinoatrial node. They gradually change into the larger Purkinje cells which are found dispersed throughout the whole left ventricle deep to the endocardium in close contact with the myocardial fibres.

The atrioventricular node has a large number of non-myelinated nerve fibres, both sympathetic and parasympathetic, and a number of nerve cells closely related to it. Impulses reaching the node via the atrial muscle are then conveyed to all parts of the ventricular muscle by the atrioventricular bundle. Nerve fibres are not responsible for the propagation of the impulse beyond the sinoatrial node. If the atrioventricular bundle is interrupted, the result is a condition known as total heart block in which the ventricles beat slowly and rhythmically at their own rate independently of the atria which beat at the rate determined by the pacemaker of the heart.

ARTERIES OF THE THORAX

Pulmonary trunk (Fig. 15.13)
Passing upwards from the right ventricle, the pulmonary trunk (artery) lies at first to the left and in front of the aorta and then to its left. It is about 5 cm long and 2.5 cm wide and, inferior to the arch of the aorta, divides into the right and left pulmonary arteries. The fibrous layer of the pericardium fuses with the tunica adventitia of the pulmonary trunk. The right pulmonary artery passes to the right lung behind the ascending aorta, superior vena cava and upper right pulmonary vein and in front of the oesophagus and right main bronchus. The left pulmonary artery goes to the left lung in front of the descending aorta and left main bronchus. The ligamentum arteriosum, the fibrous remnant of the ductus arteriosus of the fetus, is attached to the upper border of the left pulmonary artery and the concave inferior surface of the arch of the aorta. The recurrent laryngeal nerve lies to the left of the ligamentum arteriosum.

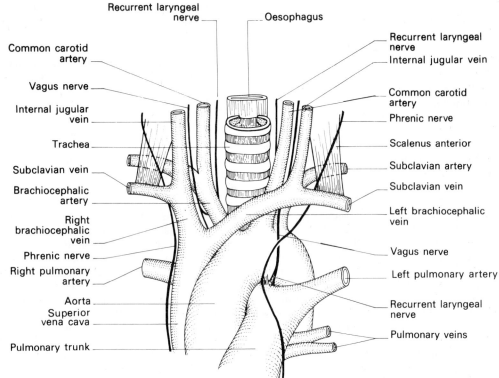

Fig. 15.13. The superior mediastinum.

Aorta

The aorta begins at the upper end of the left ventricle where it lies to the right and behind the pulmonary trunk. It starts as the ascending aorta passing upwards and to the right, then arches backwards and to the left where it is called the aortic arch, and continues downwards on the left side of the thoracic vertebrae as the descending aorta which inclines towards the midline and enters the abdominal cavity behind the diaphragm at the level of the twelfth thoracic vertebra through the aortic opening. That part of the descending aorta in the thorax is called the thoracic aorta to distinguish it from the abdominal part (abdominal aorta) which lies to the left of the anterior surface of the lumbar vertebrae. The abdominal aorta divides at the level of the fourth lumbar vertebra into the common iliac arteries. The ascending aorta is about 3 cm wide and 5 cm long. It lies behind the left part of the body of the sternum at the level of the third costal cartilage and, since it next passes to the right, behind the lower part of the manubrium sterni nearer the midline. Near the heart it is enclosed in the pericardium, and the pulmonary trunk and right auricle lie in front of it. Higher up

the right pleura and lung together with the remains of the thymus separate it from the sternum. The right pulmonary artery and right main bronchus pass to the right lung behind the ascending aorta. The superior vena cava lies to the right posteriorly, and the pulmonary trunk lies to the left.

Arteries of head, neck and arm

The arch of the aorta passes mainly backwards and its upper border is normally no higher than the middle of the manubrium of the sternum. It begins anteriorly at the level of the sternal angle and ends posteriorly at the level of the body of the fourth thoracic vertebra. The left brachiocephalic vein lies in front of the three great branches of the arch, the brachiocephalic, the left common carotid and the left subclavian arteries, from right to left. Inferior to the arch are the bifurcation of the pulmonary trunk and the left bronchus.

A small inconstant artery, the thyroidea ima artery, may arise from the aortic arch (to supply the thyroid gland) in addition to the three large branches named above.

Branches of arch of aorta

The branchiocephalic (innominate) artery is the first and largest branch. It arises behind the manubrium sterni and runs upwards, backwards and to the right. At the level of the right sterno-clavicular joint it divides into the right sub-clavian and right common carotid arteries. At its beginning the left brachiocephalic and the right inferior thyroid veins lie in front of the artery, which is anterior and then lateral to the trachea (Fig. 15.13). The right brachiocephalic vein is on the right of the artery and the left common carotid artery is on its left.

Common carotid artery. The right common carotid artery lies only in the neck. The left has its origin in the thorax from the arch of the aorta and has a short course in the thorax before reaching the level of the left sternoclavicular joint and passing into the neck. The left brachiocephalic vein passes downwards and to the right in front of the left common carotid artery. As it passes upwards the artery becomes more posterior so that it is related to the left side of the oesophagus.

As the common carotid artery (and internal carotid artery) passes upwards in the neck it lies lateral to the trachea and oesophagus and then lateral to the larynx and pharynx. Posteriorly the artery lies on the transverse processes of the cervical vertebrae and the muscles attached to them anteriorly. Anterolaterally the common carotid artery is covered by the sternocleidomas-toid muscle. Only the anterior border of this muscle overlaps the artery at the level of the sixth cervical vertebra against which the artery can be compressed.

The common carotid artery (and internal carotid artery) lies in the carotid sheath with the internal jugular vein lateral to it and the vagus nerve between the artery and vein posteriorly (Fig. 15.14). Posterior to the sheath is the sym-pathetic ganglionated trunk embedded in the prevertebral fascia. The superior and middle thyroid veins pass laterally anterior to the com-mon carotid artery as they go to the internal jugular vein. The common carotid artery usually divides into the internal and external carotid arteries at the level of the upper border of the thyroid cartilage. At its division there is a dilata-tion called the carotid sinus, where there is a thickening of the tunica adventitia and a thin-ning of the media. The adventitia contains sen-sory endings of the sinus nerve, a branch of the glossopharyngeal nerve. These react to changes in blood pressure, that is they are baroreceptors. Behind the division of the common carotid artery there is a small structure called the carotid body. This has sensory nerve endings which respond to changes in the oxygen and carbon dioxide content of the blood, i.e. they are chemoreceptors. Normally there are no branches from the common carotid artery apart from its two terminal divisions.

Subclavian artery. The left subclavian artery is the third of the large branches arising from the aortic arch. The right subclavian is a branch of

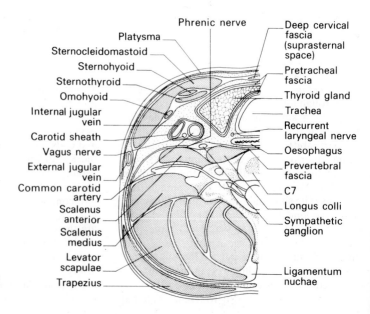

Fig. 15.14. Transverse section through the neck at the level of the seventh cervical vertebra.

Phrenic nerve

Platysma

Sternocleidomastoid

Sternohyoid

Sternothyroid

Omohyoid

Internal jugular vein

Carotid sheath

Vagus nerve

External jugular vein

Common carotid artery

Scalenus anterior

Scalenus medius

Levator scapulae

Trapezius

Deep cervical fascia (suprasternal space)

Pretracheal fascia

Thyroid gland

Trachea

Recurrent laryngeal nerve

Oesophagus

Prevertebral fascia

C7

Longus colli

Sympathetic ganglion

Ligamentum nuchae

the brachiocephalic. The left therefore has a short thoracic course before entering the neck. As it passes upwards the left subclavian artery grooves the mediastinal surface of the lung which is lateral to it, and is related medially to the trachea and oesophagus. The further course of the two subclavian arteries, i.e. beyond the level of the sternoclavicular joint, is the same on both sides.

From the sternoclavicular joint to the lateral border of the first rib where it becomes the axillary artery, it is customary to describe the subclavian artery as being divided into three parts by the scalenus anterior muscle lying anterior to it. The first part is medial to, the second behind and the third lateral to the muscle (Fig. 15.14). The internal jugular vein is in front of the medial part of the artery where the vein joins the subclavian vein to form the brachiocephalic vein: this region is covered by the sternocleidomastoid. The subclavian vein is below and in front and is separated from the middle part of the artery by the scalenus anterior. Lateral to this muscle a number of veins lie in front of the artery, the most important of which is the external jugular vein which joins the subclavian vein. The subclavian artery is anterior to and grooves the apex of the lung in front of the pleural dome and suprapleural membrane. The subclavian artery can be marked in the living subject by an upward arching band about 1 cm wide, beginning at the sternoclavicular joint and ending medial to the middle of the clavicle. It rises about 3 cm above the level of the clavicle. Laterally the artery is relatively superficial and can be pressed downwards and medially against the first rib, lateral to the edge of the sternocleidomastoid.

This is a pressure point well known to first-aid workers. The subclavian artery has a number of large important branches.

1 The vertebral artery arises from the most medial part of the subclavian artery, and passes upwards and medially to enter the foramen transversarium of the sixth cervical vertebra. In this region it lies in a triangular area (Fig. 15.15) bounded laterally by the scalenus anterior, medially by the longus colli and inferiorly by the transverse process of the seventh cervical vertebra.

The vertebral artery passes vertically upwards in the foramina transversaria of the cervical vertebrae until it reaches that of the second. The artery then has to pass laterally and enters the foramen transversarium of the atlas from where it winds medially behind the lateral mass of the atlas on to the adjacent area of its posterior arch. It enters the vertebral canal by going deep to the posterior atlanto–occipital membrane and passes into the skull through the foramen magnum. Along its course the vertebral artery is accompanied by a plexus of sympathetic nerves and veins. The latter forms the vertebral vein in the region of the lower cervical vertebrae. The first cervical spinal nerve lies between the vertebral artery and the posterior arch of the atlas and the ventral rami of the second to the sixth cervical spinal nerves pass behind the artery.

The vertebral artery gives off spinal branches to supply both the spinal cord and the vertebrae. There are also muscular branches in the suboccipital triangle. Within the skull it gives off meningeal, spinal and cerebellar branches. The intracranial distribution is described on p. 892.

2 The internal thoracic (mammary) artery

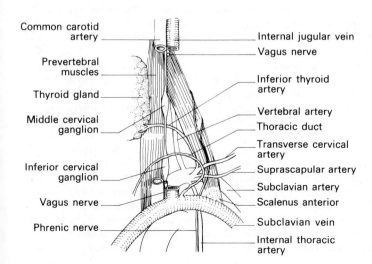

Common carotid artery
Prevertebral muscles
Thyroid gland
Middle cervical ganglion
Inferior cervical ganglion
Vagus nerve
Phrenic nerve

Internal jugular vein
Vagus nerve
Inferior thyroid artery
Vertebral artery
Thoracic duct
Transverse cervical artery
Suprascapular artery
Subclavian artery
Scalenus anterior
Subclavian vein
Internal thoracic artery

Fig. 15.15. The main relations of the left subclavian artery.

arises medial to the scalenus anterior, passes downwards into the thorax and lies 1 cm lateral to the lateral border of the sternum (Fig. 15.15). At the sixth intercostal space it divides into the musculophrenic and superior epigastric arteries. The internal thoracic artery gives branches to the mediastinum, pericardium, anterior parts of the intercostal spaces and perforating branches which accompany the anterior cutaneous branches of the intercostal nerves. In the female the branches going to the breast are fairly large and increase in size during pregnancy. The peri-cardiophrenic artery accompanies the phrenic nerve. The musculophrenic artery passes some-what laterally as it descends and perforates the diaphragm near the ninth costal cartilage ending in the abdominal wall, where it anastomoses with the other arteries of that region. The superior epigastric artery passes between the sternal and costal attachments of the anterior part of the diaphragm and enters the rectus sheath posterior to the rectus abdominis muscle in the anterior abdominal wall to which it is distributed. It anastomoses with the inferior epigastric artery.

3   The thyrocervical trunk arises from the sub-clavian artery at the same level as the origin of the internal thoracic artery, runs upwards for about 1 cm and it divides into three branches, the inferior thyroid, suprascapular and transverse cervical arteries. The inferior thyroid artery runs upwards and medially to enter the lower part of the thyroid gland. It is closely related to the recurrent laryngeal nerve near the gland and usually lies behind the nerve. This relationship is somewhat variable especially on the right side.

The inferior laryngeal artery accompanies the recurrent laryngeal nerve. A large branch runs upwards behind the carotid sheath. The branches to the thyroid gland supply the lower pole and most of its posterior part as well as both the parathyroid glands. The suprascapular and transverse cervical arteries pass laterally and backwards superficial to the scalenus anterior and phrenic nerve behind the internal jugular vein (Fig. 15.15). The suprascapular artery has a wide distribution to the muscles and joints related to the scapula and clavicle as well as to the bones themselves. The transverse cervical artery is distributed in the region deep to the trapezius by ascending and descending branches.

4   The costocervical trunk is the most lateral of the branches of the subclavian artery and, as its name suggests, is distributed to areas associated with the ribs and the neck. The deep cervical branch passes upwards and ascends among the deep muscles of the back of the neck, whilst the superior intercostal artery, passes downwards on the neck of the first and second ribs and gives off the posterior intercostal arteries of the first and second intercostal spaces.

The distribution of the subclavian artery is difficult to summarize. It supplies:
1   The upper limb.
2   The anterior and upper posterior regions of the thorax and the upper anterior part of the abdominal wall.
3   Part of the thyroid gland.
4   Many of the muscles of the neck and scapula, and
5   Parts of the spinal cord and brain.

Through some of its branches it provides arterial anastomotic channels between the medial part of the subclavian artery and its con-tinuation, the axillary artery, especially through the scapular branches of both these arteries. There are also anastomoses between the thoracic and abdominal aortae through their thoracic and abdominal branches.

Arteries of the head and neck

Internal and external carotid arteries
(Fig. 15.16)
The common carotid artery usually divides at the upper border of the lamina of the thyroid cartil-age (about the level of the third or fourth cervi-cal vertebra) into the internal and external carotid arteries. The internal carotid continues upwards in the carotid sheath in the line of the common carotid artery to the base of the skull. The internal jugular vein is lateral to it but at the base of the skull it is posterior (cf. carotid canal and jugular foramen). The vagus nerve is pos-terior to and between the vein and artery. Pos-terior to the carotid sheath are the transverse processes of the upper three cervical vertebrae; medially there is the pharyngeal wall. The exter-nal carotid artery is at first medial to the internal but soon becomes lateral and superficial. The sternocleidomastoid covers the internal carotid artery along almost its whole course. The next set of relations are important (Fig. 15.16). The superior laryngeal nerve is deep to both carotid arteries. The glossopharyngeal nerve, pharyngeal branch of the vagus nerve and stylopharyngeus muscle are usually the only structures passing between the arteries. The hypoglossal nerve, the posterior belly of the digastric, and the stylohyoid muscles are superfi-cial to both arteries. At the base of the skull the

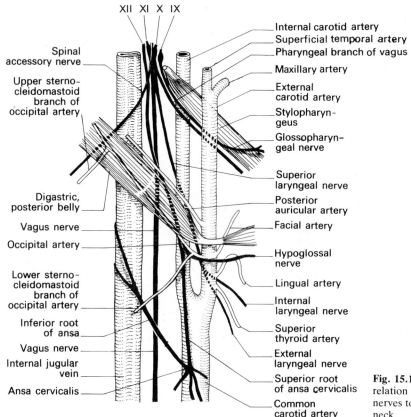

XII XI X IX

Spinal
accessory nerve

Upper sterno-
cleidomastoid
branch of
occipital artery

Digastric,
posterior belly

Vagus nerve

Occipital artery

Lower sterno-
cleidomastoid
branch of
occipital artery

Inferior root
of ansa

Vagus nerve

Internal jugular
vein

Ansa cervicalis

Internal carotid artery
Superficial temporal artery
Pharyngeal branch of vagus

Maxillary artery

External
carotid artery

Stylopharyn-
geus

Glossopharyn-
geal nerve

Superior
laryngeal nerve

Posterior
auricular artery

Facial artery

Hypoglossal
nerve

Lingual artery

Internal
laryngeal nerve

Superior
thyroid artery

External
laryngeal nerve

Superior root
of ansa cervicalis

Common
carotid artery

Fig. 15.16. A diagram of the relation of the last four cranial nerves to the large vessels of the neck.

last four cranial nerves lie between the internal carotid artery and the internal jugular vein.

Internal carotid artery (Fig. 15.17)
The internal carotid artery enters the skull through the carotid canal in the petrous part of the temporal bone (follow its subsequent course with the aid of a skull). At first it passes upwards, but it then becomes horizontal, turning medially and forwards, lying on the fibrocartilage in the foramen lacerum. In the carotid canal the artery is anterior to the middle and internal ears and then inferior to the trigeminal ganglion. It is separated by thin bone from these structures. The artery then turns forwards into the cavernous sinus and lies in a groove on the side of the sella turcica. It turns upwards again and somewhat backwards medial to the anterior clinoid process, pierces the dura mater and runs inferior to the optic nerve. It divides lateral to the optic chiasma into its terminal branches, the anterior and middle cerebral arteries. The internal carotid artery is accompandied by a plexus of postganglionic sympathetic nerves.

There are no branches from the internal carotid artery in the neck. In the petrous temporal it gives off branches to the middle ear and the upper part of the pharynx, and in the cavernous sinus it gives small but important branches to the hypophysis cerebri. Before dividing, the internal carotid artery has a large branch, the ophthalmic artery which enters the orbit through the optic canal. In the orbit it lies within the cone of muscles formed by the four recti muscles, and runs forwards on the medial side of the orbit at the front of which it divides into the supratrochlear and dorsal nasal arteries. These are distributed to the region of the forehead and the skin of the nose respectively.

The ophthalmic artery has a number of important branches. As it lies inferior to the optic nerve it gives off the central artery of the retina which continues inferior to the optic nerve and, about 1 cm posterior to the eyeball, enters the nerve and runs forwards in its centre to the retina where it divides into two terminal branches each of which divides into two. This artery is a true end artery. Other branches supply the lacrimal

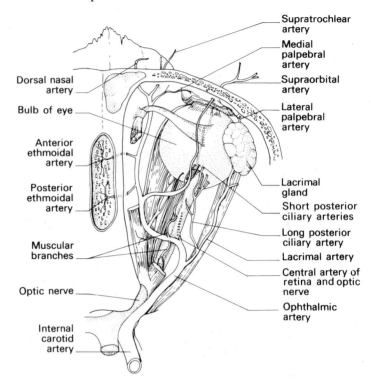

Supratrochlear artery

Medial palpebral artery

Dorsal nasal artery

Supraorbital artery

Bulb of eye

Lateral palpebral artery

Anterior ethmoidal artery

Posterior ethmoidal artery

Lacrimal gland

Short posterior ciliary arteries

Long posterior ciliary artery

Muscular branches

Lacrimal artery

Central artery of retina and optic nerve

Optic nerve

Ophthalmic artery

Internal carotid artery

Fig. 15.17. The ophthalmic artery and its branches.

gland, the scalp, the frontal and ethmoidial sinuses, the skin of the side of the nose and the eyeball.

The remaining branches of the internal carotid artery to the brain are considered with the blood supply of that organ (p. 892).

External carotid artery. The external carotid artery begins at the level of the upper border of lamina of the thyroid cartilage and at first lies medial and anterior to the internal carotid artery. As it runs upwards it passes backwards and becomes lateral to that artery. It then enters

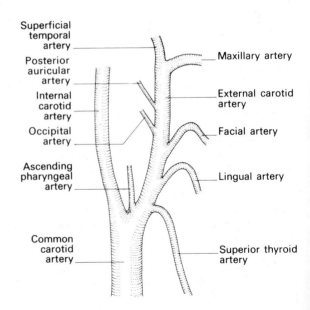

Superficial temporal artery

Maxillary artery

Posterior auricular artery

Internal carotid artery

External carotid artery

Occipital artery

Facial artery

Ascending pharyngeal artery

Lingual artery

Common carotid artery

Superior thyroid artery

Fig. 15.18. A diagram of the branches of the external carotid artery.

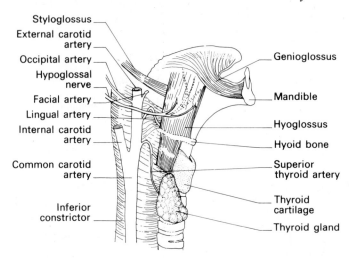

Styloglossus
External carotid artery
Occipital artery
Hypoglossal nerve
Facial artery
Lingual artery
Internal carotid artery
Common carotid artery
Inferior constrictor

Genioglossus
Mandible
Hyoglossus
Hyoid bone
Superior thyroid artery
Thyroid cartilage
Thyroid gland

Fig. 15.19. The superior thyroid and lingual arteries.

the parotid gland in the substance of which it divides, deep to the neck of the mandible, into its terminal branches, the superficial temporal and maxillary arteries.

Many of its relations have already been given in the description of the internal carotid artery. In the parotid gland the facial nerve and its branches pass forwards superficial to the retromandibular (posterior facial) vein which is superficial to the external carotid artery. Apart from its two terminal branches the external carotid artery has three branches passing anteriorly, one medially and upwards and two posteriorly (Fig. 15.18).

1 The superior thyroid artery arises below the level of the hyoid bone and runs forwards and downwards to reach the upper pole of the lobe of the thyroid gland (Fig. 15.19). It is accompanied by the external laryngeal nerve. Its terminal branches supply mainly the upper pole and anterior surface of the thyroid gland. It supplies the adjacent muscles as well as the sterno-cleidomastoid, and gives off the superior laryngeal artery which accompanies the internal laryngeal nerve into the interior of the larynx through the thyrohyoid membrane. In this region the inferior thyroid and superior laryngeal arteries and internal laryngeal nerve are comparatively superficial because they are not covered by the sternocleidomastoid. The inferior thyroid artery also supplies the exterior of the larynx below the hyoid bone and above the cricoid cartilage.

2 The lingual artery arises from the external carotid at the level of the hyoid bone (Fig. 15.19). It loops upwards on the middle constrictor of the pharynx and passes forwards deep to

the hyoglossus muscle. It then follows a tortuous course on the inferior surface of the tongue as far as its tip. Beyond the hyoglossus the artery runs lateral to the genioglossus with the lingual nerve. The terminal part is called the deep artery of the tongue. The other large branches are the dorsal lingual arteries which arise deep to the hyoglossus and pass to the posterior part of the tongue, the palatoglossal fold, the soft palate and the tonsil. The sublingual artery is a branch which supplies the sublingual salivary gland and the mucous membrane of the floor of the mouth and the gingivae.

3 The facial artery (Fig. 15.20) arises just above the level of the hyoid bone and arches upwards on the middle constrictor of the pharynx, deep to the posterior belly of the digastric and stylohoid muscles and deep to the mandible. It descends to reach the lower border of the mandible where it lies between the medial pterygoid muscle and posterior part of the sub-mandibular salivary gland. It then runs forwards between the gland, which it grooves, and the mandible. The facial artery winds round the lower border of the mandible at the anterior border of the masseter and enters the face. In the face it lies anterior to the facial vein and runs towards the angle of the mouth, then towards the junction of the ala of the nose with the face, and finally towards the inner angle of the eye. In the face the facial artery runs in a plane between several of the facial muscles. The facial artery is markedly tortuous. This is thought to be associated with the frequent movements of the muscles close to which it runs. As it crosses the lower border of the mandible just in front of the masseter it can be felt pulsating. The branches of

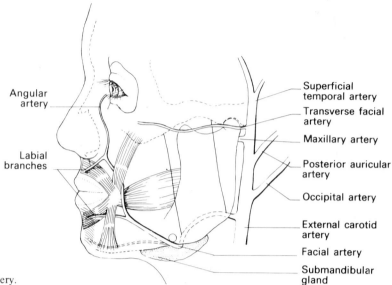

Angular artery

Labial branches

Superficial temporal artery

Transverse facial artery

Maxillary artery

Posterior auricular artery

Occipital artery

External carotid artery

Facial artery

Submandibular gland

Fig. 15.20. The facial artery.

the facial artery have a large number of anastomotic connections with the branches of other arteries, for example, the maxillary, the ascending pharyngeal, the ophthalmic and the facial artery of the opposite side. Not infrequently the facial and lingual arteries arise by a common trunk from the external carotid. Occasionally the facial artery loops upwards on to the superior constrictor of the pharynx and becomes a lateral relation of the tonsil, where it may be inadvertently cut in tonsillectomy.

Along its course the facial artery supplies the submandibular gland and muscles of the neck and face. Its named branches include the ascending palatine artery which passes upwards on the side of the pharynx lateral to the superior constrictor. It usually gives off a tonsillar branch which passes through the superior constrictor and supplies the tonsil. The ascending palatine artery reaches the palate by passing, with the levator veli palatini, along the upper border of the superior constrictor. The main tonsillar artery is an important branch of the facial artery and may arise from the ascending palatine. It runs upwards on the pharynx and perforates the superior constrictor to reach the tonsil. The submental artery, as its name implies, runs medially inferior to the chin and arises from the facial artery before it crosses the lower border of the mandible. It runs on the inferior surface of the mylohyoid muscle towards the midline. It anastomoses with a number of arteries—the sublingual branches of the lingual, the mylohyoid

branch of the inferior alveolar, the inferior labial branch of the facial and the mental branch of the inferior alveolar. On the face the branches to the lips are given names, the inferior and superior labial arteries. The branch of the latter to the septum of the nose is important. Both labial arteries run near the edge of the lips. The terminal part of the facial artery (from the ala of the nose to the medial angle of the eye) is called the angular artery.

4   The ascending pharyngeal artery is a comparatively small branch with a long course. It arises at the origin of the external carotid and passes upwards lateral to the wall of the pharynx and medial to the carotid sheath. It supplies the pharyngeal muscles and also gives off a branch to the palate which reaches that structure by accompanying the levator veli palatini. When the ascending pharyngeal artery reaches the base of the skull it divides into small branches which pass through different foramina and supply the meninges.

5   The occipital artery arises at the lower border of the posterior belly of the digastric and runs backwards with that muscle towards the mastoid process. It therefore is superficial to the internal carotid artery, the internal jugular vein, and the last three cranial nerves. The occipital artery lies in a groove on the petrous temporal bone medial to the mastoid notch to which the posterior belly of the digastric is attached. Here it lies deep to the muscles attached to the mastoid process and as it passes to the apex of the

posterior triangle it runs superficial to the muscles of the suboccipital triangle. It ends in the superficial fascia of the scalp. One further important relation should be mentioned. The hypoglossal nerve hooks round the occipital artery inferiorly as the nerve becomes superficial to the two carotid arteries (Fig 15.19). The branches of the occipital artery are indicated by its course. They go to the sternocleidomastoid and other muscles, the auricle and the scalp. There is a large descending branch which anastomoses with the arteries of the deep muscles of the neck. It also has meningeal branches which enter the cranial cavity through the mastoid and jugular foramina and condylar canal.

6 The posterior auricular artery runs backwards along the superior border of the posterior belly of the digastric deep to the parotid gland towards the groove between the auricle and mastoid process. It is distributed to the auricle, scalp, parotid gland and neighbouring muscles. It has an important branch, the stylomastoid artery which enters the stylomastoid foramen and is distributed to the middle ear, mastoid air cells and antrum, and semicircular canals. It also supplies the facial nerve.

Terminal branches of the external carotid artery. The superficial temporal artery, one of the two terminal branches of the external carotid, passes upwards out of the parotid gland and then lies superficial to the posterior end of the zygomatic arch before entering the scalp where it divides. The auriculotemporal nerve is posterior to it as it crosses the zygomatic arch. In the parotid gland some of the branches of the facial nerve pass forwards superficial to the artery. As the artery crosses the zygomatic arch it can be felt pulsating. This site is frequently used by anaesthetists for counting the pulse and is also a pressure point.

The superficial temporal artery is distributed to the auricle and external acoustic meatus, to the temporalis muscle and fascia, and the scalp in which it divides into anterior and posterior branches. There is a large transverse facial artery (Fig. 15.20) which arises while the artery is in the parotid gland and passes forwards between the zygomatic arch and the parotid duct on the masseter. This artery supplies the parotid gland, masseter and skin. Another named branch is the zygomatico-orbital artery which passes forwards along the upper border of the zygomatic arch towards the orbit.

The distribution of the superficial temporal, posterior auricular and occipital arteries to the scalp (there are also branches from the ophthalmic artery) results in its blood supply being rich enough to permit the successful replacement of the scalp if it has been pulled off in an accident. Bleeding from injuries is profuse and comes from both ends of the cut vessels because of the anastomoses. There is a similar situation in relation to wounds of the face; bleeding is profuse but because of the rich blood supply facial wounds heal readily.

The maxillary artery is the other terminal branch of the external carotid. It begins posteromedial to the neck of the mandible in the parotid gland and passes forwards, medially and upwards either deep to the inferior head of the lateral pterygoid or between its two heads. If the artery passes deep to the inferior head, it may bulge laterally between the two heads. It lies between the sphenomandibular ligament and the mandible and lateral to the inferior alveolar nerve. It is medial to the temporalis muscle at the lower border of the lateral pterygoid muscle. The artery enters the pterygopalatine fossa through the pterygomaxillary fissure. The mandibular and maxillary nerves and their branches are closely related to the maxillary artery and its branches. With this in mind, it is easier to remember at least some of the fourteen or fifteen branches of the artery.

Two branches, the deep auricular and anterior tympanic arteries, pass behind the temporomandibular joint (where the auriculotemporal nerve runs). The deep auricular goes to the external acoustic meatus and the anterior tympanic to the middle ear via the petrotympanic fissure.

One of the most important branches is the middle meningeal artery which passes upwards between the two roots of the auriculotemporal nerve to enter the skull through the foramen spinosum with the nervus spinosus, a branch of the mandibular nerve. Within the skull the artery runs laterally and forwards on the squamous temporal and divides into an anterior (frontal) and posterior (parietal) branch. This artery is frequently torn in skull injuries (the result is an extradural haemorrhage): trephination over part of its course, removing the blood and stopping the haemorrhage can be a lifesaving operation. The surface marking of the foramen spinosum is the posterior end of the zygomatic arch. (This marking is often erroneously given as the middle of the arch, which is where the artery turns upwards.) The artery divides about 2 cm above the middle of the arch and the surface marking of the pterion, where the anterior branch is frequently torn, is 4 cm above. The anterior branch runs upwards to the midpoint between the nasion and inion. The posterior branch of the middle meningeal artery passes backwards towards the lambda which is 6–7 cm directly posterior to the zygomatic arch.

The accessory meningeal artery enters the skull through the foramen ovale but is distributed mainly to the pterygoid muscles and the mandibular nerve. The inferior alveolar (dental) artery accompanies the nerve of that name and passes between the sphenomandibular ligament and mandible. The artery and nerve enter the mandibular foramen and run in the mandibular canal as far as the midline and slightly beyond. The mylohyoid branch of the artery pierces the sphenomandibular ligament and runs in the mylohyoid groove, inferior to the mylohyoid muscle. At the level of the first premolar tooth the inferior alveolar artery gives off a mental branch which leaves the body of the mandible through the mental foramen and supplies the chin. Both the mylohyoid and mental branches are accompanied by nerves of the same name.

The deep temporal, masseteric and pterygoid arteries go to the appropriate muscles and a buccal artery accompanies the buccal nerve passing between the two heads of the lateral pterygoid muscle then forwards between temporalis and medial pterygoid muscles and on to the buccinator where it is distributed to the cheek. Note that unlike the branches of the first and last parts of the maxillary artery, all these middle branches are named after, and supply, muscles.

The posterior superior alveolar artery is given off as the maxillary artery enters the pterygopalatine fossa. It passes downwards on the posterior surface of the maxilla and supplies the molar and premolar teeth, gingivae and also the lining of the maxillary sinus. The infra-orbital artery is given off at about the same point. It enters the orbit through the inferior orbital fissure, runs on the floor of the orbit and enters the infra-orbital canal. It ends on the face after it emerges from the infra-orbital foramen. The infra-orbital artery gives off the anterior superior alveolar artery, which enters the wall of the maxilla, divides and runs through canals to the canine and incisor teeth. It also supplies the wall of the maxillary sinus. All these arteries and their branches are accompanied by nerves of the same name (p. 896).

Within the pterygopalatine fossa the descending palatine artery which forms the greater and lesser palatine arteries, the artery of the pterygoid canal and the long and short sphenopalatine arteries are given off. The long sphenopalatine artery may be regarded as the terminal part of the maxillary artery. It enters the nasal cavity with the nasopalatine nerve through the sphenopalatine foramen. The descending palatine passes downwards in the palatine canal, and divides. Its branches are seen at the posterolateral angle of the hard palate.

The thoracic aorta

The thoracic aorta begins on the left of the fourth thoracic vertebra and passes downwards and slightly medially until it reaches the diaphragm in the midline behind the oesophagus. The vertebral column is posterior. The thoracic aorta gives off branches to the viscera of the thorax — bronchial, oesophageal and pericardial arteries. The branches to the oesophagus supply its middle part and anastomose with branches from the inferior thyroid artery at its upper end and branches from the left phrenic and left gastric arteries at its lower end.

The largest branches are the posterior intercostal arteries of which there are nine pairs (p. 434).

Arteries of abdomen and pelvis

After passing behind the diaphragm, the thoracic aorta becomes the abdominal aorta (Fig. 15.21) which runs downwards slightly to the left of the midline on the bodies of the lumbar vertebrae as far as the fourth lumbar vertebra where it divides into the right and left common iliac arteries. The inferior vena cava lies to the right of the abdominal aorta which is crossed by the pancreas, third part of the duodenum and the mesentery of the small intestine. At its upper end the aorta lies between the crura of the diaphragm and to its right are the cisterna chyli and azygos vein. The left sympathetic trunk lies just behind the left border of the aorta and there are autonomic ganglia and plexuses on its anterior surface related to and named after the arteries supplying the gastrointestinal tract. They are usually referred to as the preaortic ganglia and plexuses.

The branches of the abdominal aorta (Fig. 15.21) are either visceral or parietal. The visceral arteries are unpaired or paired. The unpaired arteries arise from the front of the aorta and go to the gastrointestinal tract, liver, pancreas and spleen (p. 584). They are the coeliac (the artery of the foregut), the superior

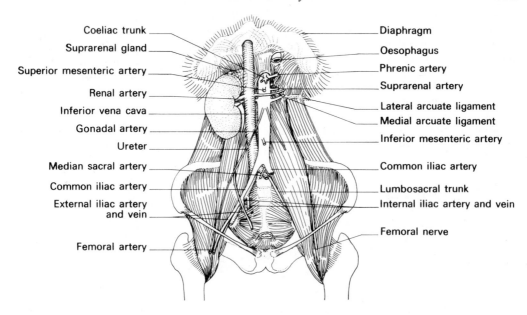

Coeliac trunk
Suprarenal gland
Superior mesenteric artery
Renal artery
Inferior vena cava
Gonadal artery
Ureter
Median sacral artery
Common iliac artery
External iliac artery and vein
Femoral artery

Diaphragm
Oesophagus
Phrenic artery
Suprarenal artery
Lateral arcuate ligament
Medial arcuate ligament
Inferior mesenteric artery
Common iliac artery
Lumbosacral trunk
Internal iliac artery and vein
Femoral nerve

Fig. 15.21. The abdominal aorta and its branches.

mesenteric (the artery of the midgut) and the inferior mesenteric (the artery of the hindgut). The coeliac supplies the stomach, part of the duodenum, and the liver, pancreas and spleen; the superior mesenteric supplies the rest of the duodenum, the whole of the jejunum and ileum, the caecum, appendix, ascending colon and most of the transverse colon; and the inferior mesenteric supplies the left colic flexure, descending and sigmoid colons and part of the rectum.

Arising more laterally are the paired visceral arteries — the middle suprarenal, renal and gonadal (testicular or ovarian). The suprarenal gland receives a superior branch from the inferior phrenic and an inferior branch from the renal artery. The coeliac trunk arises just below the opening in the diaphragm and the superior mesenteric about 1 cm below the coeliac. The inferior mesenteric comes off the aorta about 4 cm above its bifurcation; this is much lower in origin than the rest of the visceral branches. The other three arteries arise near the origin of the superior mesenteric artery.

The parietal branches are paired except for a small artery which continues in the line of the aorta into the pelvis, the median sacral; they are the inferior phrenic and four lumbar arteries which are segmental arteries and similar to the intercostal arteries. The common iliac arteries begin slightly to the left of the midline on the

fourth lumbar vertebra. The left is shorter than the right, about 4 cm as compared with 5 cm, and passes obliquely towards the left sacroiliac joint where it divides into the internal and external iliac arteries. The right has a similar course; it passes to the right and divides in a similar way. The common iliac veins are posterior to the arteries. The internal iliac artery is the artery of the pelvis and perineum. It therefore supplies visceral and parietal branches to both these regions. The viscera include the bladder, rectum, anal canal and genitalia. The parietes include the bones and muscles of the pelvis and perineum, and the gluteal region (the buttock). The external iliac artery is the artery of the lower limb but before passing into the thigh it gives off two branches to the abdominal wall. The external iliac runs along the brim of the pelvis lateral to the psoas muscle and enters the thigh about midway between the symphysis pubis and the anterior superior iliac spine.

Veins

Very frequently veins do not run with their corresponding arteries. This, which is the usual arrangement in the embryo, can be illustrated in the limbs. In the embryo the artery of a limb is axial in position and the veins marginal and superficial.

Chapter 15

Internal jugular vein
Almost all the blood from the head and neck drains into the internal jugular vein. The exceptions are the anterior and external jugular, the vertebral and inferior thyroid veins. Inside the skull the veins draining the blood from the brain eventually end in channels which lie between the inner (true) dura mater and the outer (endosteal) dura mater. These are called sinuses and they are described with the central nervous system (p. 891). The sigmoid sinus on each side passes through the jugular foramen (Fig. 15.22a) and becomes the internal jugular vein which passes vertically downwards in the neck lateral to the internal and common carotid arteries with the vagus nerve posterior to and between the artery and vein. The vein is posterior to the artery at the base of the skull and the last four cranial nerves lie between them. As the vein enters the thorax behind the sterno-

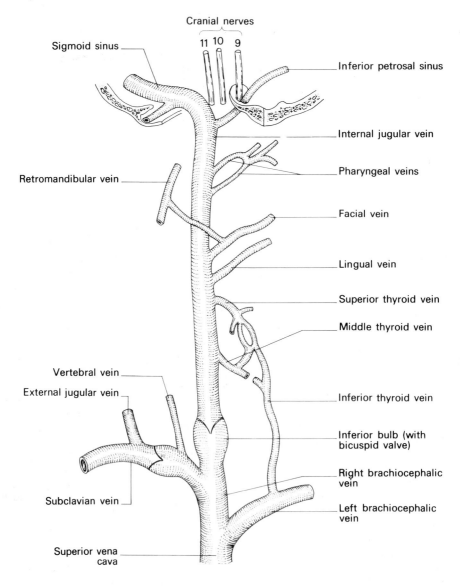

Fig. 15.22. The main tributaries of the internal jugular vein.

clavicular joint it tends to lie in front of the artery on its lateral side. At the level of the joint the subclavian vein joins the internal jugular vein and forms the brachiocephalic vein. The vein is more or less deep to the sternocleidomastoid and is crossed anteriorly by the posterior belly of the digastric and the intermediate tendon of the omohyoid. Above the digastric the parotid gland and styloid process are anterior to the vein, the posterior auricular and occipital arteries cross the vein with the digastric and more inferiorly the accessory nerve passes backwards anterior to the vein. Posterior to the vein are the transverse processes of the cervical vertebrae. The vein is more lateral than the artery and therefore lies on the cervical plexus and the origin of the phrenic nerve.

The internal jugular vein is dilated at its beginning and end forming a superior and inferior bulb. Above the inferior bulb is a valve consisting of two cusps. The superior bulb is joined by the inferior petrosal sinus which leaves the skull through the medial part of the foramen (Fig. 15.22). The other large tributaries are the veins from the tongue, the veins from the pharynx, and the facial and occipital veins. The veins from the back of the tongue run deep to the hyoglossus and form the lingual veins which join the internal jugular vein. The veins from the anterior part of the tongue and the sublingual salivary gland join and run superficial to the hyoglossus. Because it runs with the hypoglossal nerve this vein is called the vena comitans of the hypoglossal nerve. It ends eventually in the internal jugular vein either directly or by joining either the facial or lingual vein. The superior and middle thyroid veins, which drain the gland and the larynx and trachea, cross anterior to the common carotid artery and join the internal jugular vein. Along the whole length of the vein there are lymph nodes (deep cervical). They lie anterior and lateral to the vein. The right lymphatic duct opens into the right brachiocephalic vein where it is formed by the union of the right subclavian and right internal jugular veins. On the left the thoracic duct opens into the beginning of the left brachiocephalic vein in a similar manner.

Subclavian vein

This vein is the medial continuation of the axillary vein which changes its name at the outer border of the first rib. The subclavian vein arches over the first rib in front of the scalenus anterior which separates it from the subclavian artery. On the superior surface of the first rib in front of the scalene tubercle there is usually a shallow groove in which the vein lies. The phrenic nerve on the right side runs downwards between the vein and the muscle (Fig. 15.13). On the left side the nerve is more medial and lies between the artery and vein. The vein is behind the clavicle. Medial to the scalenus anterior the vein is separated from the lung by the subclavian artery and joins the internal jugular vein to form the brachiocephalic vein. Its main tributaries are the external jugular vein, which receives a large amount of the blood from the superficial parts of the head and neck, and the dorsal scapular vein.

SUPERFICIAL VEINS OF HEAD AND NECK

The veins draining the anterior part of the scalp are the supratrochlear and, lateral to it, the supraorbital. These veins join at the medial angle of the eye and form the angular vein which passes downwards and laterally between the facial muscles to become the facial vein (Fig. 15.23). Unlike the artery the vein is not tortuous. The facial vein becomes separated from the artery and passes more posteriorly over the lower part of the masseter and enters the neck superficial to the submandibular gland. It continues in a backward direction where below and behind the angle of the mandible it is joined by the anterior branch of the retromandibular (posterior facial) vein. The facial vein (formerly called the common facial vein beyond this union) continues downwards and backwards superficial to the internal and external carotid arteries and hypoglossal nerve and joins the internal jugular vein.

The facial vein receives a large number of branches corresponding with the branches of the artery, from the external nose, lips, submandibular gland, submental region, palate and tonsil. In addition it receives veins from other structures such as the eyelids, pterygoid region (deep facial vein), parotid gland and buccinator and masseter muscles. Through the orbital ophthalmic veins which drain into the (intracranial) cavernous venous sinus the veins of the scalp and face are connected with the intracranial veins. The deep facial vein, through the veins of the pterygoid region, also provides a communication with the cavernous sinus through the foramina in the greater wing of the sphenoid bone. In addition the veins of the scalp communicate with the intracranial venous sinuses through the diploic veins within the skull bones. These connections between the veins outside the skull with those inside the skull are important

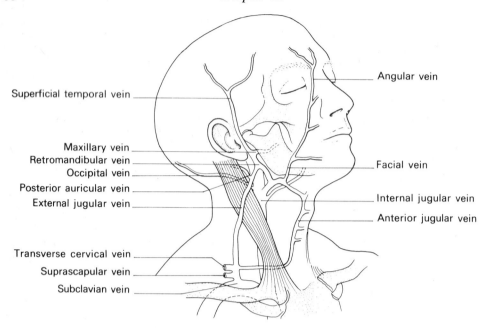

Fig. 15.23. Superficial veins of the head and neck.

because of the possibility of the spread of infection from the face or scalp to the intracranial region.

The superficial temporal vein drains the lateral aspect of the scalp and communicates with the anterior and posterior veins (supraorbital and supratrochlear, posterior auricular and occipital). The definitive vessel begins above the zygomatic arch and crosses its posterior end. The vein passes downwards and enters the parotid gland where it is joined by the maxillary vein, which lies behind the neck of the mandible, and forms the retromandibular (posterior facial) vein. As would be expected the superficial temporal vein receives tributaries from the parotid gland, temporomandibular joint and auricle. It also receives the transverse facial vein from the face, and veins from the eyelids.

The maxillary vein is a short vein draining the pterygoid plexus of veins which lies between the temporalis and pterygoid muscles. This is a large plexus which receives a number of tributaries corresponding to the branches of the maxillary artery—sphenopalatine, pterygoid, masseteric, buccal, alveolar and middle meningeal. The pterygoid plexus of veins communicates with the venous sinuses inside the skull and also the facial vein through the deep facial vein.

The retromandibular vein runs downwards in the parotid gland and divides into an anterior

branch which joins the facial vein and a posterior branch which joins the posterior auricular vein to form the external jugular vein. In the parotid gland the retromandibular vein is deep to the facial nerve and superficial to the external carotid artery.

The back of the scalp is drained by the posterior auricular vein which passes downwards behind the auricle and joins the posterior branch of the retromandibular vein to form the external jugular vein in the lower part of the parotid gland. The occipital vein drains the back of the scalp and may join (a) the vertebral vein, (b) the internal jugular vein or (c) the posterior auricular vein. The veins of the scalp are linked with the intracranial venous sinuses through emissary veins, and have connections with the diploic veins which in turn are connected with the intracranial sinuses.

The external jugular vein runs downwards more or less vertically over the sternocleidomastoid muscle. The vein therefore crosses from the anterior to the posterior border of the muscle from about the angle of the jaw to about the middle of the clavicle. It is deep to the platysma and superficial to the superficial fascia until just before its termination at the antero-inferior angle of the posterior triangle where it perforates the deep fascia and joins the lateral part of the subclavian vein. The main tributaries of the external jugular vein are the two veins from which it is formed at the angle of jaw, the retromandibular and the posterior auricular. Before it joins the subclavian vein, the external jugular receives tributaries which correspond with branches of the subclavian artery—the transverse cervical and the suprascapular. In addition, the anterior jugular vein from the front of the neck passes laterally deep to the sterno-cleidomastoid just above the sternum and clavicle and joins the external jugular vein.

The anterior jugular vein begins below and posterior to the mental protuberance and runs downwards near the midline superficial to the deep fascia to the region of the jugular notch, where it is usually described as lying in a space formed by a split in the deep fascia. The vein then passes laterally and joins the external jugular vein. There are several cross-anastomoses between the two anterior jugular veins including a large one above the jugular notch.

Both the external and anterior jugular veins become filled from below if the pressure in the right atrium is increased. They are distended in respiratory obstruction and surgical attempts to open the trachea (tracheostomy) are complicated by the distended anterior jugular veins and their cross-anastomoses. Most of the veins described in this section are quite superficial, except the pterygoid plexus and the vertebral vein which also lies deeply in the neck. The latter is a single channel only at the level of the fifth cervical vertebra. A plexus of veins, communicating with the suboccipital region, accompanies the vertebral artery through the foramina of the transverse processes from the atlas to the fifth cervical vertebra and emerges from the foramen transversarium of the sixth cervical vertebra as the vertebral vein which passes behind the internal jugular vein and joins the brachiocephalic vein.

VEINS OF THORAX

Brachiocephalic veins (Fig. 15.13). Each brachiocephalic vein is formed by the union of the internal jugular and subclavian veins posterior to the sternoclavicular joint. The left brachiocephalic vein is superior to the arch of the aorta and anterior to its three large branches (the left subclavian, left common carotid and brachiocephalic arteries) and the trachea. It passes obliquely to the right behind the upper half of the manubrium of the sternum where it joins the right brachiocephalic vein to form the superior vena cava.

Each brachiocephalic vein receives the vertebral, internal thoracic and inferior thyroid veins of its own side. The internal thoracic drains the breast and abdominal wall and forms one of the connections between the superior and inferior venae cavae. The left and right inferior thyroid veins also draining the oesophagus, trachea and larynx descend on the trachea to open into the left brachiocephalic vein although the right may join the right brachiocephalic vein.

Superior vena cava. This vein formed by the union of the two brachiocephalic veins returns the venous blood of the head, neck, upper limbs and thorax to the heart. It enters the right atrium at the level of the third costal cartilage. The superior vena cava has one large tributary, the azygos vein, and a few small tributaries from the mediastinum.

Azygos and hemi-azygos veins (Fig. 15.24). These veins drain most of the posterior parts of the intercostal spaces. The azygos vein is usually said to begin inferior to the diaphragm to the right of the abdominal aorta (the cisterna chyli lies between them). At the level of the fourth thoracic vertebra it arches forwards over the root of the right lung and enters the superior vena cava.

The azygos and hemi-azygos veins, because they begin inferior to the diaphragm, provide another important connection between the blood returning to the heart through the superior and inferior venae cavae. If the inferior vena cava is blocked the blood from the lower limbs, abdomen and pelvis may be able to return to the heart via the venous anastomoses on the posterior and anterior abdominal walls.

Pulmonary veins. There are four pulmonary veins, two from each lung. They leave the hilum of the lung and pass horizontally to the left atrium.

VEINS OF THE LIMBS

In both the upper and lower limbs there are superficial and deep veins, all of which possess valves. The superficial veins run in the superficial fascia along the borders of the limbs. They are connected with the deep veins and also have cross-anastomoses with each other. The superficial veins of the upper limb begin as a plexus on the dorsum of the hand. The cephalic vein runs upwards along the lateral border of the forearm, elbow and upper arm, and ends in the axillary

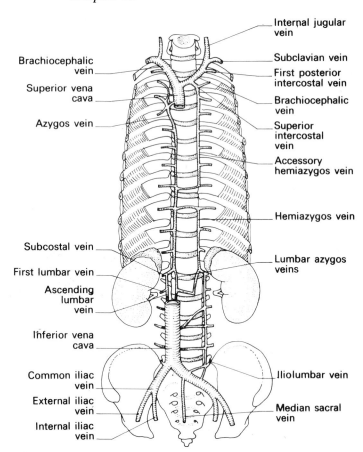

Fig. 15.24. The veins of the thorax.

vein. The basilic vein runs up the medial side of the upper limb and about the middle of the upper arm passes deeply to join the brachial vein. In front of the elbow a large vein passes upwards and medially from the cephalic to the basilic (the median cubital) vein. This vein is used frequently for venepuncture and intravenous injection. The arrangement of the superficial veins at the elbow is subject to considerable variation.

The superficial veins of the lower limb arise from the venous plexus on the front of the foot. The great (long) saphenous vein runs upwards in the superficial fascia on the medial side of the limb and ends by perforating the deep fascia in the groin and joining the femoral vein. Its position anterior to the medial malleolus at the ankle is important in that it is often used at this site for giving a blood transfusion. The small (short) saphenous vein runs upwards on the lateral side of the leg and passes backwards behind the knee where it ends by perforating the deep fascia and joining the popliteal vein which becomes the

femoral vein. Varicose veins are seen mainly in the great saphenous vein. Deep veins accompany the main arteries and finally end as the femoral vein which passes upwards deep to the inguinal ligament and becomes the external iliac vein.

VEINS OF THE PELVIS AND ABDOMEN (Fig. 15.25)

The inferior vena cava is formed by the union of the right and left common iliac veins at the level of the fifth lumbar vertebra (Fig. 15.24). It lies in front of the lumbar vertebrae to the right of the midline and at its upper end is behind the liver in which it may be almost embedded. The inferior vena cava passes through the central tendon of the diaphragm about 2 cm to the right of the midline and ends in the lower posterior part of the right atrium. As it passes up the posterior abdominal wall it receives:

(a) the lumbar veins, (b) the right gonadal vein, (c) the renal veins, (d) the right suprarenal vein,

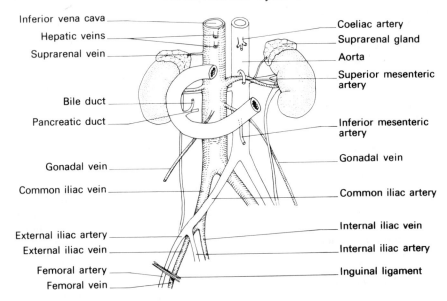

Fig. 15.25. The veins of the abdomen and pelvis.

(e) the right and sometimes the left phrenic vein, and (f) the hepatic veins.

The hepatic portal venous system refers to the veins which convey the blood from the alimentary tract, its glands and the spleen to the inferior vena cava via the liver (Fig. 15.26). The word 'hepatic' is usually omitted but it is important to realize that there are other portal systems in the body. The hepatic portal system drains the capillaries in the intestinal wall, pancreas and spleen, and subsequently the sinusoids of the liver. The portal vein is formed behind the neck of the pancreas by the union of the splenic and superior mesenteric veins.

The sites of anastomoses between the portal system and systemic system are important as they constitute an alternative route for the return of blood from the alimentary tract to the general circulation if the portal vein is obstructed. The most important site is the rectum in which the veins from the upper part go to the inferior mesenteric vein and those from the lower go to the internal iliac vein directly or indirectly. Enlargement of this venous anastomosis produces varicosities called haemorrhoids (or piles). This condition most commonly occurs without any evidence of portal obstruction, and may be due to the lack of support for the veins in the wall of the rectum. Another important site of a portal-systemic anastomosis is the lower end of the oesophagus.

LYMPHATIC SYSTEM

Lymphatic vessels form alternative channels to the veins for the return of fluid (lymph) from the tissues to the blood. The fluid passes through lymph (lymphatic) nodes on its way to the large veins in the neck. The nodes used to be called glands but they do not produce any secretion, hence the change in name, although the idea of a glandular structure is retained in clinical terms

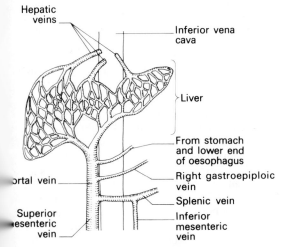

Fig. 15.26. The hepatic portal system of veins.

such as 'lymphadenitis' meaning inflammation of a lymph gland. The nodes contain among other structures aggregations of lymphocytes.

Aggregations of lymphocytes are also found as separate organs as in the spleen and thymus and in various parts of the alimentary tract in the form of tonsils, and in the ileum and vermiform appendix. These aggregations are often referred to as lymphoid tissue. It is therefore necessary to be able to define what is meant by (a) lymphatic vessels, (b) lymph, (c) lymph nodes, (d) lymphocytes, and (e) lymphoid tissue.

Lymphatic vessels

Their structure and arrangement can be compared with those of venules and veins. Lymphatic vessels, however, begin as blind-ending capillaries whose walls are one cell thick. They have no pericytes and the basement membrane is either deficient or absent. Fluid containing particulate matter and dissolved substances of large molecular size passes from the tissues into the lumen of the lymphatic capillaries either by transport across the cells (pinocytosis) or between the cells. Such substances cannot re-enter the vascular capillaries. The small lymphatic capillaries join together and form larger vessels which acquire the basic structure of all blood vessels namely an inner endothelial lining, a middle connective tissue coat containing some smooth muscle, with a sympathetic innervation and elastic fibres, and an outer adventitial coat consisting of connective tissue. Lymphatic vessels, however, are never large (the diameter of the largest is classically compared with that of a quill pen) and never have a thick wall. There are valves inside the vessels and these are similar to, but more numerous than, the valves in veins and they point in the direction of the flow of lymph. These valves give a beaded appearance to the lymphatic vessels when they contain lymph. The larger lymphatics are not contractile and depend upon the massaging action of skeletal muscle contractions for the movement of lymph. Lymphatic capillaries can bud and form new capillaries in special conditions such as inflammation and the presence of abnormal amounts of fluid. These new capillaries disappear when conditions return to normal. Some tissues and organs have no lymphatic vessels, e.g. bone, cartilage and the central nervous system. The lymphatic vessels form plexuses in the tissues which they drain and are usually divided into superficial and deep vessels. For example in the limbs there is a super-ficial plexus in the deeper layer of the skin and a deep plexus within the deep fascia. A similar arrangement is found in the body wall and frequently in various viscera. For example, the lungs and liver have a superficial plexus deep to their covering tissue and a deep plexus in the tissues of the organ itself.

In the small intestine the lymphatic vessel in the villus is called a lacteal because when filled with the products of the digestion of fat it contains a milky looking fluid, called chyle.

Lymphatic obstruction results in the accumulation in the tissues of fluid containing a large amount of protein. Absorption by lymphatic capillaries and the flow of lymph are increased in different ways by mechanical irritation, inflammation and movement. It is now accepted that substances such as soluble dyes can pass directly from blood capillaries into lymphatic vessels in contact with them. In addition phagocytic cells can pass through the wall of a lymphatic vessel. The relation of the spread of infection and cancer to the lymphatic system is very important. Both spread along lymphatic channels and reach lymph nodes. All the lymph, as has already been mentioned, finally joins the circulating blood by means of relatively large lymphatic vessels which join the beginning of the right and left brachiocephalic veins. These larger vessels are called trunks or ducts and fortunately only a few have been given definitive names. The largest is called the thoracic duct (Fig. 15.27). This begins as the cisterna chyli which is about 5 cm long and 0.5 cm wide and lies in front of the bodies of the first and second lumbar vertebrae. The cisterna chyli receives a number of intestinal trunks (from the stomach, small intestine, large intestine) and the lumbar trunks (draining the posterior abdominal wall, including the organs lying in it, e.g. the kidneys, the pelvis and the lower limbs). The cisterna chyli when followed upwards becomes the thoracic duct.

It generally enters the junction of the subclavian and internal jugular veins where they form the brachiocephalic vein. The thoracic duct drains the lymph from the whole body except the right side of the head and neck, right upper limb and right side of the thorax including the right lung and right side of the heart. These are drained respectively by the right jugular, subclavian and bronchomediastinal trunks which frequently end separately in the beginning of the right brachiocephalic vein. These trunks may unite near the lower end of the scalenus anterior and form the right lymphatic duct which joins the right brachiocephalic vein.

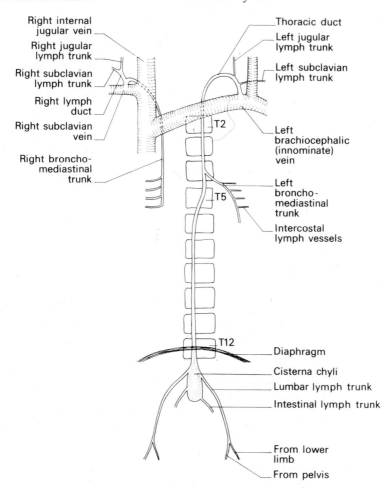

Right internal jugular vein

Right jugular lymph trunk

Right subclavian lymph trunk

Right lymph duct

Right subclavian vein

Right broncho-mediastinal trunk

Thoracic duct

Left jugular lymph trunk

Left subclavian lymph trunk

T2

Left brachiocephalic (innominate) vein

Left broncho-mediastinal trunk

T5

Intercostal lymph vessels

T12

Diaphragm

Cisterna chyli

Lumbar lymph trunk

Intestinal lymph trunk

From lower limb

From pelvis

Fig. 15.27. The main lymphatic trunks and ducts.

Lymph

This is the fluid found in lymph vessels. Its composition is similar to that of blood plasma but has a much more variable amount of fat and protein. The fat content is high after a fatty meal, as would be expected. The protein content varies with the site from which the sample of lymph is taken but an average figure could be about half that of plasma, although lymph from the liver contains much more. Although lymph percolates through lymph nodes which contain and form lymphocytes, the number of these cells in a sample of lymph is very variable and may be between 500 and 70 000 mm³(the average figure for blood is about 2000).

Lymph nodes

Lymph nodes have already been described as lying in groups along the lymphatic vessels and consisting of masses of lymphocytes in a connective tissue framework surrounded by a capsule (Fig. 15.28). Typically lymph nodes are bean-shaped and about 2–10 mm in length. Because of their size and consistency they are not usually palpable, although those in the groin can be felt quite frequently. If infected, nodes become enlarged, painful, firm and therefore readily palpable.

A lymph node receives a number of afferent vessels which enter along its convex border. The concave border has a hilum from which emerges

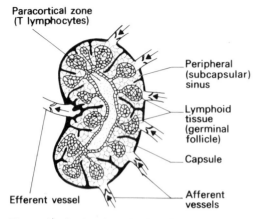

Paracortical zone
(T lymphocytes)

Peripheral
(subcapsular)
sinus

Lymphoid
tissue
(germinal
follicle)

Capsule

Afferent
vessels

Efferent vessel

Fig. 15.28. Section through a lymph node.

one efferent vessel. The lymph node also has an arterial blood supply and venous drainage which enters and leaves at the hilum. The veins provide a pathway for the entry of lymphocytes into the blood. There are valves in the afferent and efferent vessels. The capsule of the node sends in to its interior a number of trabeculae or partitions which divide the periphery of the node into sections which contains masses of lymphocytes in the form of follicles. These trabeculae fade out as they pass towards the hilum. Within the node itself there is a fine network of reticulin fibres in which there are channels called sinusoids. Their walls are incomplete and contain phagocytic cells. There is also a peripheral sinus (marginal, subcapsular) deep to the capsule into which the lymph flows before passing into the sinusoids. In the reticulin meshes are masses of lymphocytes. Near the centre of the node the lymphocytes are arranged as cords along the reticulin fibres. This different arrangement of the lymphocytes is used to distinguish an outer part of the node, the cortex, from an inner part, the medulla. The functions of lymph nodes are the production of lymphocytes and to act as filters of the lymph.

The lymph circulates slowly through the nodes from the afferent vessels into the marginal sinus, into the sinusoids, towards the hilum, and finally into the efferent vessel. During its course the lymph is brought into close contact with the phagocytic cells in the walls of the sinusoids and these cells ingest particulate matter and organisms. In the latter case the nodes usually limit the spread of the infection. Not infrequently the first sign of infection is a painful enlargement of the lymph nodes to which the vessels drain from the site of infection; for example the submandibular lymph nodes are enlarged in association with a

dental abscess. In addition the superficial lymph vessels may become visible as red streaks in the skin (lymphangitis) because absorbed inflammatory substances pass through the walls of the lymph vessels and cause hyperaemia of the adjacent blood capillaries.

The second function of lymph nodes is related to their production of lymphocytes. These cells are involved with the immune reactions of the body and will be dealt with more fully elsewhere (p. 679).

Lymphocytes

The peripheral part of the follicle of the lymph node contains mature lymphocytes. These consist almost entirely of a nucleus with a very thin layer of cytoplasm. The cells in the centre of the follicle are lymphoblasts which develop from the lymphocytes and have much more cytoplasm. This explains why the centre appears much paler than the periphery. Lymphoblasts can develop into plasma cells, which are the source of antibodies and are characterized by the presence in their cytoplasm of a large amount of rough endoplasmic reticulum associated with the elaboration of a protein secretion. The lymphocytes in the peripheral part of the follicle are called B lymphocytes because in certain animals they are produced by a structure in the abdomen called the bursa of Fabricius which is not present in man. There are also T lymphocytes in the follicles, situated between the cortex and medulla, the paracortical zone (Fig. 15.28). These lymphocytes have matured in the thymus, hence the 'T' (see p. 680).

It can be seen that the lymph nodes are important in the defence mechanisms of the body, both locally and generally. However, they are unevenly distributed. Apart from one or two nodes near the elbow and knee, the only nodes draining the limbs are either in the axilla (armpit) or in the groin. In addition the lymphatic vessels of almost the whole of the body wall go to either the axillary or inguinal lymph nodes. There are lymph nodes along the carotid sheath and a collar of nodes more superficially round the neck. There are also many nodes in the mediastinum, especially at the hilum of the lung, and in the abdomen and pelvis.

Other lymphoid tissue

THE SPLEEN

This organ is the largest single mass of lymphoid tissue in the body. It lies along the line of the tenth rib, against the diaphragm in the upper left quadrant of the abdominal cavity behind the stomach and in front of the left kidney. Its lower intestinal surface is related to the left colic (splenic) flexure of the large intestine. The spleen is about 12 cm long, 6 cm wide and 3 cm thick, and weighs about 150 g. The splenic artery comes from the coeliac trunk; the vein, inferior to the artery, joins the superior mesenteric and forms the portal vein behind the head of the pancreas. The spleen has a thick capsule from which trabeculae pass into its substance, but it is not lobulated. The cut surface of the spleen shows a large number of white dots about the size of a pin head. These are called splenic lymphatic follicles (Malpighian bodies) and constitute the white pulp as distinct from the rest of the interior of the spleen which is called the red pulp. The functions of the spleen can be summarized as follows:

1 The production of lymphocytes and monocytes.

2 Storage of red blood corpuscles.

3 Phagocytosis of exhausted red and white blood corpuscles and blood platelets.

4 Haemopoiesis in the fetus from the fourth month onwards (this function may be resumed in pathological conditions in the adult).

THYMUS

This organ is present at birth, grows until puberty and begins to atrophy from that time until in the adult it is almost entirely replaced by fat and connective tissue. It weighs about 15 g in the newborn and may double in weight before degenerating. It consists of two lobes each of which develops in the neck from the third pharyngeal pouch. As the neck develops the thymus comes to lie in the upper anterior part of the thorax behind the manubrium of the sternum and in front of the arch of aorta, its large branches and the left brachiocephalic vein. It is related to the front and sides of the trachea and extends upwards into the neck to a variable extent sometimes reaching the thyroid gland. Its largely pinkish colour changes to yellow due to the deposition of fat.

The thymus has a capsule from which septa pass into the substance of the gland and divide it into interconnecting lobules which have an outer dark, densely cellular cortex and an inner, paler, less cellular medulla.

There are two main types of cells in the thymus, the lymphocytes and the epithelial cells. The densely packed cortical lymphocytes have a very high mitotic rate, estimated as seven times greater than that of lymphocytes elsewhere. The medullary lymphocytes do not divide but have mitochondria, rough endoplasmic reticulum and nucleoli, none of which are seen in the cortical lymphocytes. These lymphocytes originate from stem cells which come from the bone marrow. Some of the lymphocytes produced in the thymus pass into the blood and contribute to the circulating pool of lymphocytes which pass into the circulation and enter and leave the lymph nodes, spleen and other lymphoid tissues. They do not return to the thymus. Surprisingly most of the lymphocytes produced by the thymus are destroyed in the thymus itself by phagocytes within 5 days of their formation.

The epithelial cells of the thymus are derived from the endoderm of the third pharyngeal pouch. These cells are stellate, the processes of one cell sometimes contacting those of another. In both the cortex and medulla these cells form fenestrated sheets.

They are thought to produce a hormone which acts on the lymphoid precursor cell from the bone marrow to produce one group of immunologically competent lymphocytes (T lymphocytes). A Hassall's corpuscle develops following the degeneration of an epithelial cell and its encirclement by concentric layers of other epithelial cells. The degenerated centre increases in size by the addition of adjacent epithelial cells and of dying macrophages which have phagocytosed some of the lymphocytes and found their way into the centre of the corpuscle. Hassall's corpuscles increase in number and size from birth.

The thymus is now recognized to be an essential organ for the generation of T lymphocytes which are passed to lymphoid tissues. If the thymus is removed during fetal life or shortly after birth, lymphoid tissue is largely depleted of its lymphocytes and the circulating lymphocytes are greatly reduced in number. Death usually results from a viral or fungal infection because of the lack of defensive cell-mediated immunity.

After puberty, because the lymphoid tissue of the body has become populated with lymphocytes, removal of the thymus does not produce the same effects as removal at birth.

LYMPHOID TISSUE OF THE ALIMENTARY TRACT

Areas of lymphoid tissue can be found all along the alimentary tract. There are, however, special sites where relatively large masses of this tissue

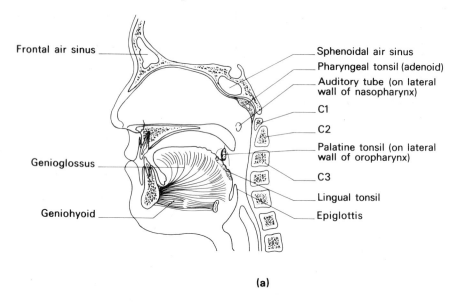

Frontal air sinus

Genioglossus

Geniohyoid

Sphenoidal air sinus

Pharyngeal tonsil (adenoid)

Auditory tube (on lateral wall of nasopharynx)

C1

C2

Palatine tonsil (on lateral wall of oropharynx)

C3

Lingual tonsil

Epiglottis

(a)

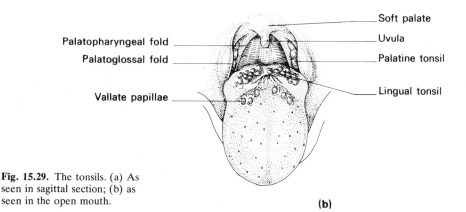

Palatopharyngeal fold

Palatoglossal fold

Vallate papillae

Soft palate

Uvula

Palatine tonsil

Lingual tonsil

Fig. 15.29. The tonsils. (a) As seen in sagittal section; (b) as seen in the open mouth.

(b)

are found. These are the tonsils in the region of the mouth and naso- and oropharynx, the aggregated lymph follicles of the small intestine, especially the ileum (Peyer's patches), and the vermiform appendix.

The different tonsils (Fig. 15.29) have already been described (p. 484). The pharyngeal tonsil is on the posterior wall of the nasopharynx. It extends laterally and can reach the medial opening of the auditory tube, or there may be a separate tubal tonsil posterior to the opening. This tonsil is often referred to as the adenoid. The palatine tonsil lies on the lateral wall of the nasopharynx between the palatoglossal and palatopharyngeal folds. This is the structure usually referred to as the tonsil and it may extend

upwards and medially into the soft palate or downwards and medially into the posterior third of the tongue. There are small masses of lymphoid tissue on the posterior third of the tongue collectively known as the lingual tonsil. All the tonsils form a ring known as Waldeyer's ring, and are said to protect the entrance to the respiratory and alimentary tracts. Structurally all the tonsils consist of masses of lymphocytes often in the form of follicles with germinal centres. It is now accepted that the tonsils and the rest of the endotheliolymphoid tissue become populated by T lymphocytes from the thymus and B lymphocytes probably from the bone marrow. It was once thought that the lymphocytes actively destroyed invading organisms.

However, any phagocytosis is due to macrophages in the lymphoid tissue. The lymphocytes react by secreting immune bodies to the invading antigens if they are B lymphocytes, and cell-mediated responses if they are T lymphocytes.

Reticuloendothelial system

This system of vessels and cells is difficult to describe because it appears in very different parts of the body. It is often but not always associated with lymphoid tissue. It is helpful to remember that the vessels involved consist of a network of reticular fibres whose meshes contain cells which, unlike other endothelial cells, are phagocytic. Because they are phagocytic the system is often called the macrophage system. The sites of and structures constituting this system were discovered by injecting into the animal vital dyes such as trypan blue and vital red and subsequently examining all the tissues of the body. In this way the sinusoids of the lymph nodes, spleen and tonsils were shown to have endothelial cells which ingested the vital dyes and stored them in their cytoplasm. The sinusoids of the red bone marrow and those of the liver, lined by Kupffer cells, although not associated with lymphoid tissue, are included as well as the sinusoids of the suprarenal gland and anterior lobe of the hypophysis cerebri. Certain phagocytic cells circulating in the blood also contain the dye and may be derived from the endothelial cells of the sinusoids of the macrophage system.

Included in this system are cells such at the microglial cells of the central nervous system, the alveolar phagocytes of the lung and the monocytes of the blood, because all of them are phagocytic and play an important part in the defence mechanisms of the body. In certain conditions some of the cells of the pia mater and arachnoid, the two inner membranes surrounding the brain and spinal cord, are set free and become phagocytic.

The functions of the reticuloendothelial system, although associated with phagocytosis, are more complex. First, the cells directly ingest organisms, including protozoa such as those causing malaria and trypanosomiasis, and particulate matter, e.g. dust in the lungs. Second, although it is usually said that moribund red blood corpuscles are broken down in the spleen and probably the liver, they are also dealt with by the circulating macrophages with the formation of bilirubin from the broken-down pigment of haemoglobin, and the freeing of the iron

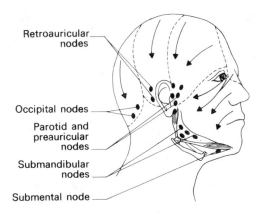

Fig. 15.30. The collar of superficial lymph nodes of the neck.

which can be re-used. Third, the macrophages ingest and act on antigenic substances so that they can stimulate the lymphocytes to produce the appropriate immune reactions.

Lymph nodes and lymphatic drainage of the head and neck (Table 15.1)

Information about this drainage has been obtained from clinical observations in relation to the spread of cancer and infections while more recently the injection of radio-opaque material into a distal lymphatic vessel has given information about the main channels and lymph nodes. Alternatively, dyes such as Prussian blue, or particulate matter such as Indian ink, are injected into the loose connective tissue of a part of the body. In a subsequent dissection the dye is seen in the vessels and nodes. The lymph nodes of the head and neck are arranged in two groups, superficial and deep. The superficial nodes (Fig. 15.30) form a sort of collar at the junction of the head and neck and are divided into the following groups. The submental lie posterior to the lower border of the mandible on the inferior surface of the mylohoid muscle (i.e. in the neck) on either side of the midline. They receive vessels from the tip of the tongue the anterior part of the mouth including the lower incisor teeth and the central part of the lower lip. Some of their efferent vessels go to the deep cervical nodes but most pass to the next group on both sides, the submandibular lymph nodes which lie near or even in the submandibular salivary gland between the mandible and mylohyoid muscle. The afferent vessels to these nodes come from an extensive area including the major part of the cheek and lips, the anterior part of the scalp, the upper and lower teeth and periodontium, the side of the tongue, the posterior part of the floor of the mouth, the medial halves of the eyelids and the vestibule and the anterior part of the nasal cavity. The efferent vessels from the submandibular nodes go to the deep cervical nodes (see below).

Continuing in a circular manner round the junction of the head and neck, the next group of nodes is the parotid or preauricular. These nodes are usually superficial to the parotid gland but one or two may be embedded in the gland itself. Their afferent vessels come from the side of the scalp, the anterior parts of the external ear (both the pinna and the external acoustic meatus), the middle ear and the lateral halves of the eyelids. Their efferent vessels go to the deep cervical nodes. There are nodes behind the auricle (retroauricular) and along a line corresponding with the superior nuchal line (occipital). The afferent vessels to these nodes come from the posterior part of the external ear and the back of the scalp. Their efferents go to the deep cervical nodes.

Included with the superficial nodes are those behind the nasopharynx—the retropharyngeal nodes. These lie in the space between the pharyngeal wall and the prevertebral fascia. They receive vessels from the nasopharynx and auditory tube and may receive efferent vessels from the back of the nasal cavity and paranasal sinuses. Their efferent vessels go to the deep cervical nodes. Occasionally solitary lymph nodes are found on the face—over the body of the mandible laterally, in the cheek over the buccinator and below the orbit. They drain the tissues nearby and their efferent vessels go to the submandibular nodes. There are superficial cervical lymph nodes which lie on the superficial surface of the sternocleidomastoid along the external jugular vein. There may also be superficial nodes in the midline of the neck anteriorly along the anterior jugular vein and in the posterior triangle along the line of the accessory nerve. These nodes receive afferent vessels from the skin overlying them and their efferents pass to the deep cervical nodes.

The deep cervical nodes are arranged longitudinally along the internal jugular vein and are sometimes divided into superior and inferior cervical nodes. All the superficial nodes already described send efferent vessels to these deep nodes directly or indirectly and the vessels from the deep nodes pass downwards and finally form the jugular lymph trunk. On the right this often joins the subclavian trunk from the upper limb to become the right lymph duct, which ends in the beginning of the right brachiocephalic vein. The jugular lymph trunk may end independently in the vein. On the left the jugular lymph trunk usually joins the thoracic duct. There are also a few lymph nodes deeply placed in front of and at the sides of the larynx and trachea. These nodes receive vessels from the nearby structures (larynx, trachea and thyroid gland) and efferents pass to the deep cervical

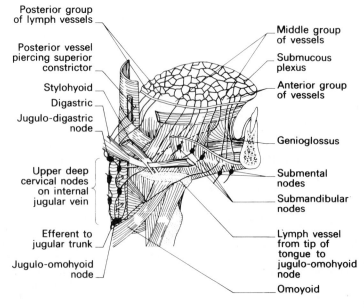

Posterior group of lymph vessels

Posterior vessel piercing superior constrictor

Stylohyoid

Digastric

Jugulo-digastric node

Upper deep cervical nodes on internal jugular vein

Efferent to jugular trunk

Jugulo-omohyoid node

Middle group of vessels

Submucous plexus

Anterior group of vessels

Genioglossus

Submental nodes

Submandibular nodes

Lymph vessel from tip of tongue to jugulo-omohyoid node

Omoyoid

Fig. 15.31. Lymphatic drainage of the tongue. Lateral view.

Table 15.1. Lymphatic drainage of the head and neck

Structure	Nodes
Middle ear	⟶ parotid ⟶ deep cervical
Neck superficial	⟶ superficial cervical (either anterior, lateral or posterior) ⟶ deep cervical
deep	⟶ deep cervical
Floor of mouth (anterior) and lower incisors Tip of tongue	⟶ submental ⟶ submandibular ⟶ deep cervical or submental ⟶ deep cervical
Floor of mouth (lateral) Teeth and periodontium (except lower incisors) Side of tongue	⟶ submandibular ⟶ deep cervical
Palatine tonsil	⟶ jugulodigastric (deep cervical)
Pharyngeal tonsil Nasopharynx Paranasal sinuses Soft palate	⟶ retropharyngeal ⟶ deep cervical

Nasal cavity
  anterior
  posterior
	⟶ submandibular ⟶ deep cervical
	⟶ retropharyngeal ⟶ deep cervical

Oropharynx, laryngeal pharynx and cervical part of oesophagus Back and central part of tongue Larynx (above vocal folds)	⟶ deep cervical
Larynx (below vocal folds) and trachea Upper part of thyroid gland	⟶ laryngeal and tracheal ⟶ inferior deep cervical
Lower part of thyroid gland	⟶ tracheal ⟶ deep cervical
	or ⟶ deep cervical
	or ⟶ superior mediastinal

nodes. Some of the deep cervical nodes have been given special names. The jugulodigastric nodes lie where the posterior belly of the digastric crosses the carotid sheath, and the jugulo-omohyoid node lies where the sheath is crossed by the inferior belly of the omohyoid. Both of these named nodes receive afferents from the tongue.

THE LYMPHATIC DRAINAGE OF THE TONGUE

There are two plexuses of lymphatics in the tongue, a plexus of vessels in its mucous membrane and also an intramuscular plexus (Fig. 15.31). The deeper vessels pass to the more superficial. Those from the tip of the tongue pierce the mylohyoid muscle and go to the submental nodes. The vessels from the submental nodes drain into the submandibular and deep cervical nodes on both sides. The vessels from the side of the tongue go mainly to the submandibular nodes. The vessels from the back of the tongue go directly to the deep cervical nodes.

It has been said that there is a sharp

Table 15.2. Lymphatic drainage of the walls and organs of the thorax.

Structure	Nodes
Superficial chest wall	$\longrightarrow$ axillary $\longrightarrow$ subclavian trunk
Deep chest wall anterior posterior	 $\longrightarrow$ parasternal $\longrightarrow$ bronchomediastinal trunk $\longrightarrow$ intercostal $\longrightarrow$ right lymph or thoracic duct
Diaphragm anterior lateral and posterior	 $\longrightarrow$ parasternal $\longrightarrow$ bronchomediastinal trunk $\longrightarrow$ posterior mediastinal $\longrightarrow$ thoracic duct
Heart and pericardium	$\longrightarrow$ mediastinal $\longrightarrow$ bronchomediastinal trunk
Pleura parietal visceral	 $\longrightarrow$ parasternal, intercostal and phrenic $\longrightarrow$ (with lungs)
Oesophagus	$\longrightarrow$ posterior mediastinal $\longrightarrow$ thoracic duct
Lungs	(see text p. 495)

anteroposterior division between the two halves of the tongue and that lymph vessels do not cross the midline. If they do, only a few near the midline cross to the opposite side. Again one must emphasize that lymph vessels can go directly to a second group of nodes and by-pass the first group. There are always one or two vessels which go from the tip of the tongue directly to the deep cervical (jugulo-omohyoid) nodes. Another characteristic of lymph vessels from the tongue is that they frequently pierce muscles, for example those from the tip pierce the mylohoid muscle and some from the back of the tongue pierce the superior constrictor muscle.

THE LYMPHATIC DRAINAGE OF THE
THYROID GLAND

The main features of the lymphatic drainage of the thyroid gland are fairly obvious. Vessels from the upper part go to the laryngeal nodes and from the lower part to the tracheal nodes. Some vessels, however, may pass downwards following the inferior thyroid veins to nodes related to the left brachiocephalic vein in the superior mediastinum. Some vessels pass directly to the deep cervical nodes.

The lymphatic drainage of the head and neck is shown in Table 15.1.

Lymph nodes and lymphatic drainage of the rest of the body

THORAX (see Table 15.2)

ABDOMEN AND PELVIS

The lymph nodes are arranged along the main blood vessels and are named accordingly. The nodes related to the aorta (pre-aortic in front, and para-aortic at the sides) are now called lumbar. The pre-aortic are related to the large single branches of the aorta supplying the gastro-intestinal tract, liver and pancreas and are named after these vessels. Their afferent vessels drain from the nodes along their branches and efferent vessels go to the cisterna chyli. There are nodes along the branches of the three single vessels and near the wall of the organ itself. Their afferents come from the organ and their efferents go to the lumbar nodes. In the organ itself there are superficial and deep plexuses. In a hollow organ, for example the stomach, there is a submucous plexus which passes to an intramuscular plexus. The intramuscular plexus passes to the nodes along the border of the stomach, vessels then drain to the nodes along the arteries supplying the stomach, and from there vessels pass to the lumbar nodes. The liver also has a superficial and deep plexus and these plexuses drain into different groups of nodes related to the liver. There are important lymphatic connections between the liver and the thorax.

The urinary system, suprarenal glands and gonads are drained by lymphatic vessels which go to the para-aortic nodes from which vessels pass to the cisterna chyli. The pelvic organs except for the female gonads and lower part of the rectum have efferent vessels which go to nodes along the internal iliac vessels and thence to nodes along the common iliac vessels. The latter nodes also receive the efferent vessels running along the external iliac vessels which receive the vessels from the inguinal nodes. The nodes along the common iliac vessels are drained by efferent vessels which go to the para-aortic nodes.

BLOOD AND BODY FLUIDS

Body fluids

The two major constituents of blood can be separated from each other by standing some blood in a vertical tube containing anticoagulant. After a period of some hours the red blood cells sink, leaving a clear straw-coloured fluid, plasma, above. This may be achieved more rapidly by centrifugation and if carried out in a graduated tube (Fig. 15.32) it can be seen that the red cells (erythrocytes) occupy about 45% of the volume of whole blood, which is termed the haematocrit or packed cell volume (PCV). The other particulate components of blood are the white cells (leucocytes) which form a thin 'buffy'

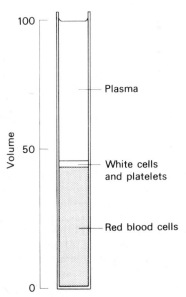

Fig. 15.32. Separation of the constituents of blood after centrifugation in a haematocrit tube.

coat on top of the cell column in the haematocrit tube (Fig. 15.32) and the platelets. They are dealt with in greater detail later.

The fluid remaining after blood has been allowed to clot is called serum. It is similar to plasma but contains less protein.

Red blood cells and plasma serve as an example of how cells differ greatly from the fluid which surrounds them in terms of their content of water, inorganic ions and organic molecules (see Table 15.3). For example, red cells have a high intracellular potassium concentration and a low sodium concentration whilst plasma is high in sodium and low in potassium. Plasma is 93% water but red cells are only some 65% water.

Units of concentration given in this chapter refer to those found in either plasma or in red blood cells, not to those in whole blood. Obviously, as there are wide differences in the composition of the two phases, an overall concentration for cells plus plasma is meaningless. Nevertheless, sometimes in clinical practice, concentrations of some substances are given in whole-blood, e.g. calcium and iron. They have a limited meaning because the molecules are confined almost exclusively to one compartment (to plasma and cells respectively in the above cases) so that changes in whole-blood content reflect changes in one compartment. Care should be taken, therefore, to distinguish between values in the literature represented as levels in whole-blood or in plasma or in red blood cells.

In this chapter we shall first consider how water and ions are distributed throughout the body and then discuss the physiological processes that maintain the constant composition of cells and their environment.

Total body water
The water in the body contributes some 50–75% of total body weight; the proportion varies widely between individuals—mainly as a function of the amount of adipose tissue present. Storage fat contains only some 10% water so that the greater the amount of fat cells the less, in proportion, is the amount of water per unit body weight. An alternative approach giving a clearer indication of the state of the body water is to consider the body to be made up of a 'lean mass' or the mass of the functional tissues (muscles, liver, kidney, etc.) together with a variable amount of adipose tissue. This latter proportion can be determined by measuring the specific gravity (SG) of the body. A low specific gravity indicates a high adipose tissue content whilst a high SG corresponds to a low fat content

because storage fat has an SG of 0.940 compared to an average of 1.060 for other cells. If the amount of adipose tissue determined in this way is subtracted from the total body weight then a value for the lean body mass is obtained. The water content expressed as a function of the lean body mass is much more consistent between individuals and is some 73% or 50 dm³ in our standard 70 kg man.

The total volume of body water can be estimated by the dye or indicator dilution method (which can also be applied to measuring the volumes of other compartments discussed below). If a known quantity (Q) of dye or marker is added to an unknown volume (V) and the resulting concentration (C) measured after complete mixing, then the three parameters are simply related by the equation

$$V = \frac{Q}{C}$$

This is only valid if the marker used satisfies the following criteria:

1 It is freely diffusible within the compartment.
2 It is not lost from the compartment.
3 It is neither excreted nor metabolized.
4 It does not itself alter the distribution being measured (for example by increasing the osmotic pressure in the compartment into which it is injected).
5 It should also be non-toxic and its concentration easily estimated.

It must be remembered that the volumes measured by the dye dilution method are volumes of distribution of that marker, and may not represent a physiological entity if any of the above criteria are not met. Examples of markers that can be used to measure total body water are the drug antipyrene or the isotope of water, deuterium oxide (D_2O).

The total body water can be envisaged as being in two main compartments, the intracellular fluid and the extracellular fluid (Fig. 15.33). Water is distributed evenly throughout the body, and most membranes, with the exception of some in the kidney and bladder, are freely permeable to water. The osmotic pressure is the same, about 300 mosmol/dm³, in both compartments. Thus if the osmotic pressure is increased in one compartment, for example by increasing the solute concentration (decreasing the concentration of water), then water tends to move from the other compartment to lower the

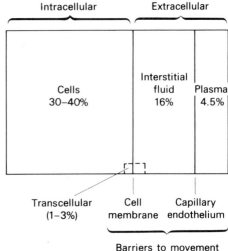

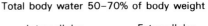

Fig. 15.33. Distribution of body water. (Modified from Pitts R. F., *Physiology of the Kidney and Body Fluids* (1963) Year Book Medical Publishers, Chicago).

pressure. This has important consequences in altering the volume of the compartments.

Intracellular fluid
The water content of cells (intracellular) can range from 10% in adipose tissue through 70–75% for muscle and red blood cells to 83% in the kidney. The actual amount of water in each tissue varies with cell type. Overall, however, the intracellular water contributes some 30–40% of total body weight (Fig. 15.33). In cells the main cation is potassium and the main anions are proteins and organic phosphates such that their total osmotic pressure is 300 mosmol/dm³ (see Table 15.3).

Extracellular fluid
The extracellular fluid (ECF) compartment is some 16–22% of body weight or approximately 11–16 dm³ depending on the method of measurement and comprises (as a percentage of body weight) interstitial fluid (16%), plasma (4.5%) and lymph (<2%) (Fig. 15.33).

Extracellular fluid volume may be assessed using a number of markers such as inulin, thiocyanate, sulphate or mannitol—all of which distribute into slightly different parts of the extracellular fluid space according to their per-

Table 15.3. Concentrations of cations and anions in plasma, interstitial fluid and intracellular fluid of erythrocytes and skeletal muscle.

	Ion	Plasma* (mEq./dm³)	Interstitial fluid† (mEq./dm³)	Erythrocytes (mEq./dm³ intracellular water)	Skeletal Muscle (mEq./dm³ intracellular water)
Cations	Na⁺	142	145.1	19	12
	K⁺	4.0	4.1	136	150
	Ca²⁺	5.0	3.5	$<10^{-6}$	34
	Mg²⁺	2.0	1.3	6	4
	Total	153.0	154.0	161	200
Anions	Cl⁻	102.0	115.7	78	4
	HCO₃⁻	26.0	29.3	18	12
	PO₄³⁻	2.0	2.3	4	40
	Other	6.0	6.7		
	Protein	17.0	0.0	36	54
	Total	153.0	154.0	136	110
Total mosmol/dm³		306.0	308.0	310	310

*A plasma water content of 93% was used in the calculation.
†Gibbs-Donnan factors used are 0.95 for monovalent anions and 1.05 for monovalent cations.
Modified from Ruch & Patton (1965), *Physiology and Biophysics*, 19th edition.

meability properties and consequently give varying volumes of distribution (p. 668). Plasma volume is usually taken as the volume of distribution of the plasma protein albumin, either by combining it with a dye (Evans blue) or with a radioactive marker (^{125}I). Over the experimental period albumin is considered to remain within the vasculature.

The interstitial fluid is that which surrounds cells. It forms the true environment of cells—the 'mileu interieur' discussed by the French physiologist Claude Bernard in 1885. Development of physiological controls maintaining a constant composition of this environment has enabled higher organisms to lead a 'free-life' as he expressed it. The interstitial fluid surrounds cells in thin films some 1 μm thick and does not normally form 'pools' of fluid. However, under pathological conditions this may happen and is termed oedema. Plasma forms the other compartment of the ECF and is that part confined within the vasculature (Fig. 15.33). It is normally some 3 dm³ or 4.5% of the total adult body weight. Lymph can be viewed as forming an alternative route for transport of fluid from the interstitial space to the vasculature. This is not its only role, however.

The composition of extracellular fluid differs markedly from intracellular fluid, the former being high in sodium (142mM) and low in potassium (4 mM) with the ratio reversed in intracellular fluid (Table 15.3).

In some inacessible parts of the body, such as in bones, little is known about the composition of interstitial fluid. The activity of the bone cells may affect this. The membrane which separates interstitial fluid from plasma is the capillary endothelium. Its properties will be dealt with in more detail later (p. 686) but its most important characteristic is its relative impermeability to plasma proteins. Plasma contains protein in the region of 70 g/dm³ but interstitial fluid has virtually none (Table 15.3). This has two effects. First, and most important, the osmotic pressure on the side containing protein is some 25 mmHg higher than that of the interstitial fluid. This extra 'pressure' is proportional to the protein (particularly the albumin) concentration. Fluid would therefore tend to flow from the interstitial fluid into the vasculature if it were not opposed by the hydrostatic forces across the capillary. This view was first put forward by Starling and is known as 'Starling's hypothesis' (p. 685).

The second effect of the unequal distribution of proteins between plasma and interstitial fluid is that diffusible cations are at a slightly higher concentration and anions at a slightly lower concentration in plasma (Table 15.3). The effect is explained by the Gibbs-Donnan rule (Appendix 1). When a freely diffusible solute (NaCl in this case) is separated by a membrane (the capillary endothelium) impermeable to another molecule (the plasma proteins—negatively charged at physiological pH), then in order to reach electrical equilibrium, more diffusible cations are needed on the side with protein to balance the negative charges on the protein, and correspondingly fewer diffusible anions. Conversely, the ratio on the side not containing protein is reversed (Table 15.3) because the total number of positive and negative charges in the whole system must balance. It is really the ion concentrations in plasma water which ought to be compared to interstitial fluid because 1 dm³ plasma contains only 930–940 g water, since 60–70 g is protein. It is these ion concentrations in plasma water which are in dynamic equilibrium with those in interstitial fluid.

Transcellular fluid
The last compartment to be discussed (Fig. 15.33) is really neither intracellular nor strictly extracellular. Certain specialized areas of the body contain fluid, such as the cerebrospinal fluid, intraocular fluid, synovial fluid and pleural fluid and these are termed 'transcellular' compartments. They are generally characterized by being separated from blood not only by a capillary endothelium but also by epithelial (or mesothelial) cells which modify the composition of the fluid. The transcellular fluids constitute some 1–3% of total body weight.

Plasma proteins
The plasma proteins can be separated into the following major components (with their approximate molecular weight): fibrinogen 3 g/dm³ (mw 460 000), globulins 24 g/dm³ (mw 150 000) and albumins 45 g/dm³ (mw 69 000). Fibrinogen is a single protein, whereas globulins and albumins comprise many different proteins. The capillary membrane is relatively impermeable to plasma proteins by virtue of the fact that they are larger than the size of the 'pores' in the membrane (p. 686). The osmotic pressure of an impermeable solute on one side of a semipermeable membrane is proportional to the number of particles present. Albumins forming the largest amount of protein and being the smallest molecular weight contribute the highest number of molecules. They are therefore the most important species in determining the colloid osmotic or oncotic pressure of the plasma. Fibrinogen, on the other hand, has a very high molecular weight and, being present only in low concentrations, contributes very little to the col-

loid osmotic pressure. Globulins contribute a little to the colloid osmotic pressure. They are primarily concerned with the immune system of the body, blood clotting and with the transport of various molecules in plasma such as copper, iron and many hormones. The globulins can be separated by electrophoresis (p. 62) into α, β and γ fractions. The β-fraction contains the IgA and IgM immunoglobulins, whilst the γ-fraction contains the IgG immunoglobulins. The main functions of the albumins are to provide the major colloid osmotic constituents of plasma, as discussed above, and to participate in the buffering action of the plasma by virtue of their free amino and carboxyl groups. Plasma proteins are synthesized almost exclusively by the liver. the γ-globulins are the exception; they are produced in the reticuloendothelial system of the body.

The capillary endothelium is not completely impermeable to protein. Any plasma albumin entering the interstitial space is rapidly taken up into the lymphatic system, from where it is transported back to the vasculature (p. 658).

Control of ECF osmolarity and volume
The osmolarity of the ECF is kept at 300 mosmol/litre, despite wide variations in fluid intake, by the regulation of water excretion through the kidneys and by the thirst mechanisms (p. 741). The major osmotic constituent of the ECF is sodium chloride, and water loss and gain is controlled such that the sodium concentration is kept within very narrow limits of its mean value (142 mM). Alterations in the concentration of sodium chloride in the ECF cause water to be redistributed between the intracellular and extracellular compartments. If the sodium concentration rises, for example, water is withdrawn from the cells and the volume of the intracellular water compartment is reduced. Assuming that the sodium concentration is maintained at a constant value by water excretion and conservation, how is the ECF volume regulated? The volume is a function of the amount of sodium present in the ECF. If, for example, a high salt diet is given, the NaCl concentration in ECF rises and water is taken in to restore osmolarity to 300 mosmol/kg. Thus there must follow an increase in the ECF volume. Increasing the NaCl content of the body expands both the plasma and interstitial compartments as salt is freely diffusible within the ECF, but is effectively barred from entering the intracellular compartment.

On the other hand, severe salt loss, such as might occur in sweating caused by maximal exercise in a humid environment, results in a reduction in body salt content, and a corresponding reduction in ECF volume. The volume changes are monitored by 'volume' receptors in the walls of the atria; when the ECF volume is reduced these reflexly activate sodium reabsorption by the kidney and when ECF volume increases they cause increased sodium excretion (p. 744). Other receptors involved in controlling ECF volume are sensitive to changes in arterial blood pressure. These are in the carotid artery and afferent arterioles of renal glomeruli (p. 745).

The cell membrane

The barrier separating intracellular from extracellular fluid is the cell membrane. Large concentration gradients of ions exist across this membrane and these need to be maintained (Table 15.3). We have seen that the cell membrane behaves osmotically as if it were impermeable to NaCl. Changes in ECF sodium concentration will change cell volume. However, if radioactive sodium is added to the ECF it is found that it slowly penetrates into cells down its concentration gradient. Conversely, if cells are loaded with radioactive sodium then it is extruded from them.

We have a picture therefore of a dynamic equilibrium of sodium diffusing slowly into cells and being pumped out again, maintaining a constant low intracellular sodium concentration. Pumping sodium out of cells up a concentration gradient is an energy requiring process known as the sodium pump and is mediated by an enzyme, located in the cell membrane, which derives its energy from the hydrolysis of ATP. The sodium pump makes cell membranes 'effectively' impermeable to sodium and thus directly controls cell volume. Cessation of the sodium pump (during anoxia for example) allows sodium to leak into cells, increasing the osmotic pressure and therefore making cells swell. At the same time as the pump extrudes sodium it also takes up potassium from the ECF into the cells, so helping to maintain the high intracellular potassium content.

The cell membrane itself is thought to have a lipid-bilayer structure with proteins situated on the surfaces and penetrating into the hydrophobic regions (p. 167). Lipid soluble molecules (O_2, CO_2) can diffuse rapidly through the lipid regions, whilst polar molecules probably penetrate along protein lined 'pores', some 0.3–0.4 nm in radius. Water and urea permeate rapidly through these. The membrane is more permeable to potassium ions than to sodium ions. Cells have therefore both a low permeability to sodium, as well as having a sodium pump to extrude any sodium ions which may have leaked in. Charged molecules larger than the monovalent ions such as proteins and organic phosphates cannot cross the membrane at all or penetrate only slowly unless they have specific 'carriers' which allow them to cross very rapidly. Many vital molecules such as glucose and amino acids fall into this category.

Red blood cells

CHARACTERISTICS OF RED CELLS IN THE CIRCULATION

When mixed with sodium citrate (an anticoagulant) and allowed to stand in a vertical graduated tube, erythrocytes sediment slowly. The erythrocyte sedimentation rate (ESR) thus measured is usually less than 10 mm in 1 hour in healthy males, slightly more in females. In some diseases, probably as the result of an increase in certain plasma proteins, notably the γ-globulins and to a smaller extent, fibrinogen, the red cells have an exaggerated tendency to clump together (rouleaux formation) and the rate of sedimentation is increased. An increase in the viscosity of plasma accelerates rouleaux formation. Although not specific for any particular disease, the ESR is useful clinically; repeated estimates, for example, are valuable in assessing the progress of chronic diseases.

An accurate measure of the proportion of red cells to plasma is obtained by measuring the packed cell volume (Fig. 15.32). The PCV is obviously related to both the number of red blood cells in a unit volume of blood and the volume of each cell. It may differ in the same individual in different parts of the circulation, for example 'capillary' blood from a finger-prick has a lower PCV than blood taken by venepuncture (Fig. 15.45) and also may be altered by changes in posture.

A red blood cell count (usually expressed as cells/mm³) is obtained by counting under the microscope the number of cells in a specimen of diluted blood, spread in a layer of known uniform thickness on a specially ruled slide known as a haemocytometer. The red cell count (RBC) is normally $4.5–6.5 \times 10^6$ cells/mm³ in males and $3.9–5.6 \times 10^6$/mm³ in females.

Red cells owe their colour to their high content of haemoglobin. If placed in a hypotonic solution, red cells take up water, swell and rupture. The haemoglobin is released from the cells, and the previously turbid suspension suddenly becomes optically clear. This phenomenon is known as haemolysis. The haemoglobin concentration (Hb) of whole blood may be measured by haemolysing the red cells in a hypotonic solution containing sodium cyanide, and comparing the stable colour of the resulting cyanmethaemoglobin solution with that of a standard of known concentration in a colorimeter or spectrophotometer. The concentration of haemoglobin in blood is high, being about 135–180 g/dm³ in adult males and 115–164 g/dm³ in females.

Microscopic examination of a stained smear of blood by a trained observer is a useful procedure. The diameter of the red cell averages 7.2 μm (range 6.7–7.7 μm) on a flat slide. Floating freely in plasma its characteristic biconcave shape becomes apparent. Abnormalities, such as an overall reduction in size of the cells (microcytosis), an increase in size (macrocytosis), inequalities in size (anisocytosis), or abnormalities in shape, may suggest the presence of various disorders. In addition, a reduction in the haemoglobin concentration in the cell may be suggested by pallor of the cell (hypochromia), especially in the thin central area.

Quantitative estimates of some of these changes may be obtained by calculating three red cell indices from the RBC, Hb and PCV:

1   Mean corpuscular volume (MCV):

$$MCV = \frac{PCV}{RBC} \text{ (normal range: 76–96 μm}^3\text{)}$$

2   Mean corpuscular haemoglobin (MCH):

$$MCH = \frac{Hb}{RBC} \text{ (normal range 27–32 pg per cell)}$$

3   Mean corpuscular haemoglobin concentration (MCHC):

$$MCHC = \frac{Hb}{PCV} \text{ (normal range 32–38\% or g/100 cm}^3 \text{ red cells)}$$

For example, in a patient with marked iron deficiency anaemia, the red cells are usually small and pale (microcytic and hypochromic). This could be confirmed by finding a low concentration of haemoglobin in the red cells.

FORMATION OF RED CELLS (ERYTHROPOIESIS)

In the developing fetus, red cells are first formed in the yolk sac, later on in the liver and spleen, and finally in the marrow cavities of the bones. For the first few years after birth, erythropoiesis occurs in the red marrow of most bones, but by adult life much of the red marrow contains fat cells and erythropoiesis tends to be confined to the cavities of the bones of the skull, the ribs, sternum, vertebrae and pelvis. The earlier sites of red cell production including the liver and spleen may become reactivated when there is an increased demand for red cells, for example after persistent haemorrhage or haemolysis, or the loss of bone marrow due to disease.

Biopsies may be obtained by aspirating bone marrow from the sternum or iliac crest and examining stained smears under the microscope. In addition to primitive cells of the red cell or erythroid series, primitive white cells of the myeloid (granular white cell) series and megakaryocytes (precursors of blood platelets) are also to be found in the bone marrow. Because of the shorter lifespan of cells of the myeloid series compared with that of the erythroid series, the former usually outnumber the latter; the myeloid:erythriod ratio is usually 3–4:1.

It is probable that there is a common undifferentiated parent cell for the myeloid and erythroid series (Fig. 15.34, Plate 1), from which are formed partially committed stem cells. Bone marrow contains a line of these primitive, partially differentiated, 'stem' cells which divide in order to maintain the stock of stem cells and also to give rise to proerythroblasts, the most immature cells definitely belonging to the erythroid series.

The proerythroblast then enters an irreversible process of cell division and maturation to produce mature erythrocytes (Fig. 15.34). An average of three cell divisions takes place over a period of approximately 4 days. At each stage the cells become smaller, the nuclei more dense and the cytoplasm more pink-staining due to the increasing haemoglobin content. Once the normoblast stage has been reached, the cell is incapable of further division. The nucleus either disintegrates or is extruded and the cell becomes a reticulocyte. After a further 1 or 2 days the reticulocyte escapes into the circulation by its own active movement (diapedesis), and after a further day or so it loses its reticular appearance and becomes a mature erythrocyte with a lifespan of about 120 days. The synthesis of haemoglobin commences in the proerythroblast stage and is complete by the end of the reticulocyte stage.

There is a close connection between the microscopic appearance of the erythroid cell and the biochemical processes taking place in it. During the period of cell division DNA synthesis is

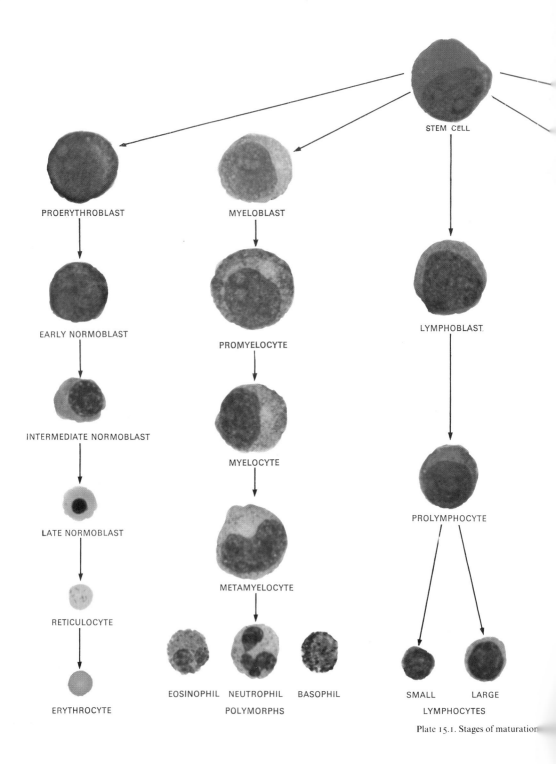

STEM CELL

PROERYTHROBLAST

MYELOBLAST

LYMPHOBLAST

EARLY NORMOBLAST

PROMYELOCYTE

INTERMEDIATE NORMOBLAST

MYELOCYTE

LATE NORMOBLAST

PROLYMPHOCYTE

RETICULOCYTE

METAMYELOCYTE

ERYTHROCYTE

EOSINOPHIL   NEUTROPHIL   BASOPHIL
POLYMORPHS

SMALL   LARGE
LYMPHOCYTES

Plate 15.1. Stages of maturation

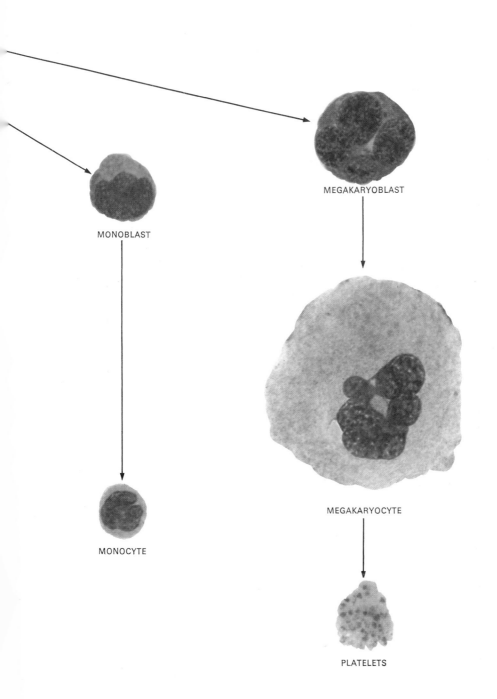

MEGAKARYOBLAST

MONOBLAST

MEGAKARYOCYTE

MONOCYTE

PLATELETS

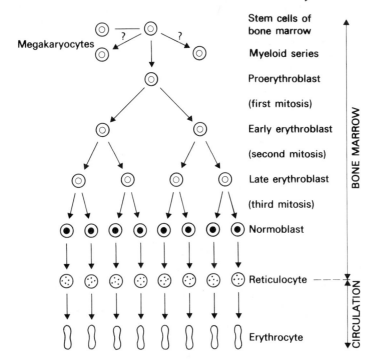

Fig. 15.34. Probable sequence in erythropoiesis. Terminology may vary, but the terms 'proerythroblast', 'normoblast' and 'reticulocyte' are common to most classifications. On average there are three mitoses but this may vary from two to four.

active: mitochondria, ribosomes and other organelles are plentiful, reflecting the synthesis of haemoglobin as well as the enzymes and biochemical systems that will be required during the life of the red cell for energy production, synthesis of 2,3-diphosphoglycerate, repair of the cell membrane and so on. The loss of the nucleus from the normoblast marks the end of DNA synthesis. The disappearance of all mitochondria, ribosomes and other organelles at the end of the reticulocyte stage reflects the end of protein synthesis. For the rest of its lifespan in the circulation, the red cell is a highly specialized cell 'remnant', packed with haemoglobin and other materials required to fulfill its physiological functions.

HAEMOGLOBIN

The chief functions of haemoglobin are to transport oxygen and carbon dioxide and to buffer the changes of $[H^+]$ in the red cell. The structure of haemoglobin is described on p. 73 Iron is essential for the synthesis of haem molecules and iron deficiency is the commonest cause of anaemia seen in clinical practice. Protein supplies the amino acids required for globin synthesis but, as haemoglobin has a high priority for available protein, anaemia due to protein deficiency is exceptional. Iron in haemoglobin is in the ferrous (reduced) state. Trace amounts are continually being oxidized to the ferric state, converting the normal oxyhaemoglobin into methaemoglobin, but an enzyme system in the red cell normally converts methaemoglobin back into oxyhaemoglobin. Methaemoglobin does not combine with oxygen. It must be emphasized that haemoglobin becomes oxygenated when it combines with more oxygen and deoxygenated when it loses oxygen—it is not oxidized and reduced (p. 505).

Haemoglobin has a greater affinity for carbon monoxide than for oxygen, and carboxyhaemoglobin is formed. This may be produced for example in coal-gas poisoning (but not 'natural' gas poisoning) and causes a reduction in the oxygen-carrying capacity of the blood.

IRON METABOLISM

Iron is an essential constituent not only of haemoglobin but also of myoglobin in muscle cells, and of a number of enzymes such as the cytochromes and catalase. Iron, surplus to the above requirements, is stored mainly in the liver and spleen.

The approximate amounts of iron present in the various body compartments, and the esti-

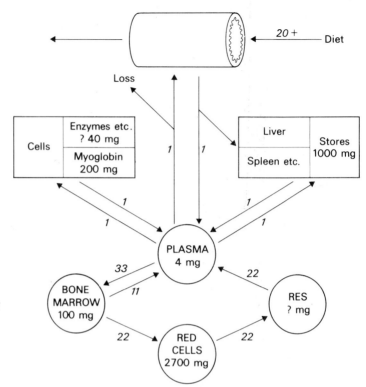

Fig. 15.35. Theoretical stores of iron in various body compartments of an adult man (mg), with possible rates of movement of iron between compartments (italicized numerals, in mg/day).

mated rates of movement of iron from one location to the other are shown in Fig. 15.35. There are three striking features:

1 Only about 1 mg of iron per day is absorbed to replace normal iron losses, compared with the total iron content of the body of about 5000 mg, most of which is in haemoglobin.

2 The iron movement from plasma to bone marrow to reticuloendothelial system (RES) and back to plasma is very large in comparision with the relatively minor movements of iron in and out of stores, enzymes and myoglobin.

3 Although plasma contains only a small amount of iron there is a rapid turnover of this iron, most of it moving to the bone-marrow for haemoglobin synthesis.

In healthy adults the loss of iron from the body is very small and most of this occurs by desquamation of cells, particularly the mucosal cells of the intestine. This loss amounts to 0.5–1.0 mg per day. In addition, women during their reproductive years lose iron in menstrual blood, to the placenta and fetus during pregnancy, and in milk during lactation; their total iron requirements may thus amount to 2–3 mg per day. As the iron intake in the average western diet is 20–30 mg per day, the absorption of only 5–10% of this

amount is sufficient to replace the daily iron loss.

Ferrous iron is more readily absorbed than ferric, and hence absorption is enhanced by ascorbic acid and other reducing substances. The conversion from the ferric form in foods to the ferrous form is aided by hydrochloric acid in gastric juice. It is common for persons with a partial gastrectomy to have iron deficiency anaemia. Dietary phytic acid and phosphates bind iron rendering it unavailable for absorption. It has also become clear in recent years that a considerable proportion of absorbed iron is derived from haemoglobin and myoglobin in the diet, the iron from the porphyrin ring being liberated within the mucosal cell. Intestinal mucosal cells contain the protein apoferritin which combines with some of the iron entering the cell to form ferritin. This remains in the cell and is lost to the body when the mucosal cell is shed after its lifespan of about 4 days. The iron which is not trapped passes through the mucosal cell into plasma and all of this is bound to a β-globulin called transferrin. Normally, this protein is only about 35% saturated with iron. The usual plasma iron concentration is about 0.8–1.3 mg/dm³.

When body iron stores are depleted and under

hypoxic conditions when erythropoiesis is increased, iron absorption is usually increased and is decreased when these conditions are reversed. It has been suggested that iron absorption is regulated by the proportion of iron which is retained as ferritin in the mucosal cell. For example, in iron overload when the body has more than sufficient iron, the mucosal cell might contain more apoferritin and hence would bind more of the iron entering the cell which in turn reduces the quantity entering the plasma.

Under normal conditions iron is not present in the body in the free state but is attached to carrier proteins such as apoferritin inside cells, and transferrin in plasma.

Iron stores in the liver and spleen are usually sufficient to make good the iron lost during a moderate haemorrhage, such as a blood donation. Iron deficiency is found most commonly in children (due to growth and hence an increase in total body haemoglobin), and in women during the reproductive period.

Increased iron stores (iron overload) may also be encountered, either as haemochromatosis, a disorder in which there is persistent increase in iron absorption above the body's requirements or, perhaps surprisingly, as a result of repeated blood transfusions.

VITAMIN B_{12} AND FOLIC ACID (p. 816)

Vitamin B_{12} (cyanocobalamin) is required in very small quantities for the normal development of red cell precursors. In vitamin B_{12} deficiency, the morphology of these cells in the bone marrow is altered and they are larger than normal, being described as megaloblasts. They give rise to erythrocytes called macrocytes, as they vary considerably in size and have a mean corpuscular volume of 110–150 μm^3, well above the normal MCV of 76–96 μm^3. There is reduced production of cells and their lifespan in the circulation is shortened. Folic acid deficiency is another cause of megaloblastic anaemia.

Almost all cases of vitamin B_{12} deficiency arise from defective absorption: the reason for this lies in the unique mode of absorption of vitamin B_{12}. The clues to the absorption of vitamin B_{12} came from studies of patients with pernicious anaemia. These patient have a megaloblastic anaemia due to vitamin B_{12} deficiency, together with atrophy of the gastric mucosa. The anaemia cannot be overcome by giving vitamin B_{12} by mouth, but if it is administered together with normal gastric juice, the vitamin is absorbed and the anaemia responds. This fact led to the discovery that the parietal cells of the stomach secrete intrinsic factor, a glycoprotein which binds with dietary vitamin B_{12}, and which enables the large B_{12} molecule to be absorbed at specific receptor sites situated on the mucosal cells of the terminal ileum. This is the explanation of the fact that vitamin B_{12} deficiency may also result from disease or surgical removal of the ileum.

Pernicious anaemia and other anaemias due to vitamin B_{12} deficiency are usually treated by parenteral injections of pure vitamin B_{12} at intervals of a month or so, thus avoiding the problems of absorption.

REGULATION OF ERYTHROPOIESIS

When plasma from anaemic or hypoxic animals is injected into normal animals, erythropoiesis is stimulated. This is due to the presence of increased amounts of a circulating factor, erythropoietin, which has been convincingly demonstrated as the main day-to-day physiological regulator of normal red cell production. Erythropoietin levels are increased following haemorrhage, under hypoxic conditions, and when there is increased destruction of red cells in the circulation. On the other hand, when the red cell count is increased above normal levels, for example by overtransfusion of red cells, erythropoietin levels fall and the rate of erythropoiesis decreases.

The evidence suggests that as blood oxygen falls a precursor of erythropoietin is produced, usually in the kidney. This behaves as an enzyme and acts on a substrate present in plasma to produce erythropoietin itself. The latter acts mainly by increasing the production of proerythroblasts from primitive stem cells in the bone marrow, thus increasing the number of 'production lines' of red cell precursors. It is also possible that erythropoietin may lead to an earlier release of reticulocytes from the bone marrow under these conditions.

LIFESPAN OF RED CELLS

The normal red cell has a fairly constant life span in the circulation of about 120 (100–130) days. In the investigation of the cause of anaemia in a patient, it may be necessary to determine whether the red cells have an inherently shortened lifespan, or whether they are being destroyed at a faster rate than normal.

There are two main methods of measuring red cell survival. The first is to label the red cells with a single 'pulse' of a radioactive substance such as ^{15}N or ^{59}Fe which is incorporated into the cell or the haemoglobin while it is being synthesized in the bone marrow, and to note the time taken for the radioactivity in the resulting red cell population to drop at the end of their lifespan. This method cannot be used clinically.

To measure the lifespan of a patient's red cells, a sample of the patient's circulating cells is labelled with ^{51}Cr and then reinjected into the circulation. The decline in radioactivity in blood samples as successive age groups of red cells reach the end of their lifespan is measured (correction having been made for radioactive decay and the constant but small leakage of ^{51}Cr from the cells). The ^{51}Cr is bound to Hb in the red cell and does not appear to affect the lifespan or function of the cell. It is not necessary to collect samples for the whole 120 days; the time taken for the radioactivity to fall to half its original level ($t_{\frac{1}{2}}$) is the result usually reported.

DESTRUCTION OF RED CELLS

As a red cell ages its metabolic activity alters and structural changes develop in its cell membrane. For example, the cells become more fragile, the rate of glycolysis decreases, the activity of certain enzymes decreases and K^+ ions are lost at an increasing rate, but the final changes which lead to the destruction of the cell are not known. After about 120 days the old red cells are either haemolysed or, more commonly, are engulfed and digested by phagocytic cells of the reticuloendothelial system, particularly in the liver and spleen. The haemoglobin molecule is broken down, liberating amino acids from the globin chains, and the haem rings are opened, releasing the ferrous atoms which are taken up by transferrin in the plasma. The residue of the porphyrin ring becomes first biliverdin and then bilirubin, the so-called bile pigments, both of which are excreted (p. 626).

White blood cells (leucocytes) (Plate 1)

For many years, five kinds of leucocytes have been described; the three granulocytes (neutrophil, eosinophil, basophil), lymphocytes, and monocytes. Recently it has become widely accepted that there are two kinds of lymphocyte, the T and B cells. With traditional stains, these are indistinguishable, but there are functional and ultrastructural differences between them (see below).

All the leucocytes share two important characteristics:
1 They are all involved in defence of the body against material which is recognized as 'foreign' or 'not-self'.
2 They are all cells which leave the bloodstream and spend most of their lives wandering about in the tissues on 'perpetual patrols of immunological surveillance'.

Total and differential leucocyte counts
To find the total number of white blood cells in a measured volume of blood, a small sample is diluted with a solution which stains the white cells and disrupts the red cells. A suitable diluting fluid is 2% acetic acid coloured slightly with gentian violet. The diluted sample is then observed on a haemocytometer slide through a microscope, for direct counting of the cells. The total number of white blood cells in blood from a healthy adult is 4000–15 000/mm³. Higher levels are described as leucocytosis; lower levels as leucopenia. In children, there are always more leucocytes than in adults.

The relative contribution of different cell types towards the total white blood cell population, a differential count, can be derived by merely counting the number of different cell types in a stained blood smear.

The five cell types are recognized by a few simple characteristics in the stained preparation, such as cell size, the size and shape of the nucleus, and the presence and character of coloured granules in the cytoplasm. Although in life all of these cells are highly irregular in shape, in smears they are sufficiently well rounded to allow their diameters to be estimated. It is useful to remember that the red blood cells, which are present in large numbers in the smear, have a diameter of just over 7 μm.

The salient features involved in identifying cells in a smear stained with one of the traditional Romanovsky stains can be summarized as follows:
1 Neutrophils: 10–12 μm diameter, nucleus lobed (two to five lobes) arranged in an irregular way (hence the alternative name, polymorphonuclear leucocytes); nucleus darkly stained; small lightly stained granules in cytoplasm which appear pale mauve or reddish purple.
2 Eosinophils: 10–15 μm diameter, nucleus usually bilobed, darkly stained. Granules in cytoplasm are bright red or orange red and may be densely packed.
3 Basophils: 10–12 μm diameter, nucleus of very irregular shape occupying about half the

cell, and staining less darkly than that of other granulocytes. Large blue granules in cytoplasm (which may dissolve during the staining procedure). This cell is seldom seen in class practicals, despite claims to the contrary!

4 Lymphocytes: mostly small, 5 μm diameter, some larger, up to 8 μm diameter. These give the impression at first that they are composed of little more than a darkly stained nucleus, but careful inspection reveals a thin rim of slightly less darkly stained blue cytoplasm around the nucleus. They usually appear to be oval rather than circular.

5 Monocytes: 12–15 μm diameter. Distinctly larger than lymphocytes. The cytoplasm stains pale blue and is almost agranular; a few small granules may be seen, which are azure in colour (blue).

The differential count reveals that the five kinds of leucocyte are usually present in the following proportions in the adult:

55–70%	neutrophils
25–30%	lymphocytes
2–10%	monocytes
1– 6%	eosinophils
< 1%	basophils

Leucopoiesis—the stem cells

There is little doubt that the original source of all blood cells is an undifferentiated stem cell which resides in the bone marrow. However, it seems that in the adult these primitive stem cells are not dividing (i.e. they are in the G_0 phase of the cell cycle (p. 257)) and that there exists a rather complicated hierarchy of partially differentiated stem cells. Some cell lines, especially lymphocytes, are more self-contained than others; monocytes and granulocytes, on the other hand, seem to be quite closely related.

Granulocytes and monocytes in the adult are exclusively produced in the bone marrow but lymphocytes are derived partly from dividing populations of cells in the peripheral lymphoid tissues. The bone marrow ceases to be the active source of fresh T lymphocyte cell lines once these are well established elsewhere. Many short-lived lymphocytes, probably B lymphocytes, are produced by the bone marrow throughout adult life (see below).

PRODUCTION, SUPPLY AND FUNCTIONS OF WHITE BLOOD CELL TYPES

Neutrophils

The earliest cell type recognizably committed to neutrophil production in the bone marrow is known as a myeloblast. This probably undergoes five further mitotic divisions before the neutrophils finally mature; the fully differentiated cells do not divide. A large pool of mature or nearly-mature neutrophils, perhaps 15–20 times the number present in the circulation, is held in reserve in bone marrow.

The circulating neutrophil pool consists of two populations; those cells in free-flowing blood and actually counted in a blood sample, and those which are marginated, i.e. loosely stuck on to the inner walls of the vascular endothelium. This tendency to stick to vessel walls is greatly increased in regions of traumatic damage and is the first step in emigration from the blood vessels into the tissues. However, in the absence of trauma, margination is often a temporary 'rest' which is followed by a return to the flowing stream of blood.

The entire pool of circulating neutrophils is renewed every 9 hours, known as the turnover time. After entering the interstitial fluid the average life of these motile, phagocytic cells is only a few days (perhaps a week). They do not return to the circulation in significant numbers. Like all circulating white cells, neutrophils are 'birds of passage'; their functions normally begin after emigration into the tissues. The turnover time for the pool in blood being so short, it is not surprising to find that the number of circulating cells can be changed quickly, by alterations in the degree of margination, the rate of emigration, or the rate of release from the storage pool in bone marrow. It is well known that severe exercise transiently doubles the leucocyte count. Adrenaline causes a similar response. In these instances much of the increase is due to the temporary return of marginated neutrophils to the free flowing stream of blood.

Sustained increases in the number of neutrophils in the circulation are probably associated with increased secretion of the adrenal hormone, cortisol, and similar corticosteroids. These hormones apparently decrease the rate at which neutrophils leave the circulation, as well as increasing the rate at which they leave the bone marrow. Neutrophil levels are often doubled by the effects of infection, e.g. a severe cold, and inflammatory conditions, e.g. pneumonia. It is probable that some of the products of tissue and bacterial breakdown stimulate neutrophil production. Mature neutrophils contain many lysosomes. Among the many enzymes contained within these lysosomes is lysozyme, which disrupts the cell walls of some bacteria.

The neutrophil is an extremely valuable

trooper; not very bright, but willing to die for the cause. It plays a major role in the inflammatory response by migrating to the site of damage or infection and engaging in 'hand-to-hand' combat (if phagocytosis, which is engulfing and digesting the opposition, can be adequately described by such a metaphor). Neutrophils are attracted to these sites by substances released there; a process known as chemotaxis. Even in the absence of oxygen a neutrophil can undertake phagocytosis by virtue of the glycolytic use of its glycogen reserves. This is especially valuable during the acute phase of inflammatory responses when the supply of blood may be impaired by oedema or trauma. Neutrophils are particularly effective against pyogenic (pus-forming) bacteria. Indeed these bacteria are really named after them, for pus is largely made up of the dead, autolysed bodies of neutrophils which have been expended during the battle against a focus of infection.

Monocytes

The bone marrow produces monocytes at a much slower rate than that of neutrophils. The monocyte, like the neutrophil, is migrating to the tissues through the bloodstream. In man, the entire blood monocyte pool is renewed about twice daily. Circulating levels are raised during infectious diseases, and depressed by the administration of cortisol.

After leaving the bloodstream, the monocytes mature to become avidly phagocytic tissue macrophages. All tissue macrophages originate in this way. These may continue to wander about or may settle as 'fixed' macrophages, especially in the sinusoidal vascular channels of the bone marrow, liver (as Kupffer cells), spleen, and in the lymphatic sinuses of lymph nodes. High concentrations of macrophages are also found in the peritoneum and in between the alveoli of the lungs. There is also evidence that osteoclasts are formed by fusion of tissue macrophages.

The very large number of tissue macrophages makes it certain that at least some of these cells are long-lived, some living for a year or longer.

In many texts macrophages are regarded as part of the 'reticuloendothelial system'. This name was introduced to describe what was believed to be a functionally unified system, diffusely scattered throughout the body, concerned with the protection of the body by the phagocytic destruction of particular antigens and worn-out cells. It included not only the tissue macrophages, but also reticular cells, endothelial cells and fibroblasts, because these cells, like the macrophages, ingest vital-dye particles injected into animals. However, these other cells are not related to macrophages either in origin or in their normal function; in particular, they are not usually phagocytic. A new name, the 'mononuclear phagocyte system' has been proposed, but the original name remains in common use at present (p. 663).

Macrophages participate in both inflammatory and immune responses to foreign material. They work in close collaboration with lymphocytes, particularly with T lymphocytes. Foreign antigens cannot be recognized and phagocytosed with maximum efficiency by macrophages working alone; the presence of T lymphocytes is required to provide the recognition and to supply the instructions to macrophages which make them real killers. The T lymphocytes, on the other hand, have no powers of phagocytosis. The activation of macrophages by lymphocytes results in a demonstrable increase in motility, metabolic rate, phagocytosis and effective digestion of the ingested material. This process takes up to 2 days. The 'angry macrophage' becomes, to extend the simile, 'blind with rage'. It will ingest and destroy quite unrelated antigenic material without any delay.

After antigen has been phagocytosed, the information required for the production of specific antibody is transferred, in an unknown way, to the B lymphocytes and their derivatives, the plasma cells. It is interesting that it is the most insoluble antigens, held for long periods in the macrophages, which have the strongest immunogenicity and evoke the greatest antibody production.

Macrophages are clearly tough customers; if neutrophils are to be thought of as troopers, macrophages bear more resemblance to tanks. Their destructive power is, however, tempered by a useful restraint, for antigenic material is not rendered unrecognizable in the onslaught, but survives to guide the immunogenic cells (B lymphocytes) in the creation of specific antibodies and to be filed away in the immunological memory.

Eosinophils

The total number of eosinophils in circulating blood is quite small; there are about 300–900/mm^3 of blood. They do not stay long in the circulation, emigrating into the tissues at very much the same rate as neutrophils. Blood levels are subject to very rapid changes. Glucocorticoid hormones reduce the levels of eosinophils (this is known as eosinopenia).

High levels of eosinophils are a well-known feature of immune responses to the presence of a foreign protein in the body; this increased release of eosinophils from bone marrow may be a response to the release of histamine. Persistently raised eosinophil counts are often indicative of parasitic infestations by various worms. The gut mucosa is rich in mast cells containing histamine, and the burrowing worm heads presumably provoke the release of this histamine.

Eosinophils are less motile, less avidly phagocytic, and less effective as bactericidal cells than neutrophils, although they do possess many of the lysosomal enzymes found in neutrophils. It has been suggested that their prime function is to inactivate histamine; they certainly arrive in large numbers at any site infiltrated with histamine, or containing basophils which have discharged their granules (of which histamine is a major component). Several factors in addition to histamine are chemotactic for eosinophils.

Basophils

Very little is known about these cells. In some respects they resemble tissue mast cells; for example both contain heparin and histamine, but differences between them make it seem unlikely that circulating basophils mature to form tissue mast cells; for example, the tissue mast cell has a single oval nucleus, whereas the circulating basophil has a bilobed or trilobed nucleus. As lobulation of the nucleus represents a degenerative change in other granulocytes, it seems unlikely that the nucleus of the basophil could be rejuvenated to the unlobed form in the mast cell. However, the similarities between the two cells are sufficient to make it necessary to remain open-minded about the possibility that they are related.

There are no data on the lifespan or transit time of basophils in blood. Basophils are only sluggishly motile, and although capable of phagocytosis, this is probably not their major function. There are only scanty reserves of glycogen in basophils, indicating that they could not work for long under anaerobic conditions.

Lymphocytes

Some crucial animal experiments have established that lymphocytes have several different functions, amongst which are a group collectively described as 'cell-mediated immunity'. Surgical removal of the thymus from neonatal rabbits or mice prevents the development of this group of responses although antibody secretion, another function of lymphocytes, is not seriously impaired. It is now known that immature cells pass from the bone marrow to the thymus, where they mature to become those lymphocytes responsible for cell-mediated immunity. They are called T lymphocytes to remind us of the role of the thymus in the induction of their functional competence.

In chicks, extirpation of a small lymphoid organ of the hindgut (called the bursa of Fabricius) prevents the development of another subpopulation of lymphocytes, capable of secreting humoral antibodies (immunoglobulins). This operation does not prevent the development of the T lymphocytes. Clearly, there is a different subpopulation of cells, again maturing to functional competence in a peripheral lymphoid organ. These cells are usually known as B cells (B for bursa). The B prefix is probably also apt for mammalian lymphocytes, since the functional equivalent of the bursa in mammals is now thought to be the bone marrow.

The applicability of this fundamental animal research work to man is well illustrated by the recognition of two rare inherited diseases which appear in children with incompetent lymphocytes. In one of these there is inadequate development of the thymus. Affected children are particularly susceptible to fungal infections, to viruses, to tuberculosis, and to a variety of organisms which rarely cause disease in normal people. The children have a normal capacity for synthesizing immunoglobulins.

The other condition is infantile sex-linked agammaglobulinaemia. Boys with this disease almost completely lack B-cell function; their plasma is almost devoid of immunoglobulin and no increase in concentration is seen in response to illness. Cell-mediated immunity is not seriously impaired and these children usually cope adequately with childhood viral diseases (e.g. measles, chicken pox, mumps and rubella) which are dealt with by this system.

The two populations of lymphocytes do not normally function in isolation from each other, but cooperate closely both with each other and with the phagocytic cells in the various forms of the immune responses.

In the adult, lymphocytes are produced in bone marrow and in germinal centres or peripheral lymphoid tissues. Fully differentiated T cells are able to change to a cell type which can divide mitotically and so produce peripheral colonies of competent T cells. Similarly, B cells may divide in the peripheral lymphoid tissue to form competent daughter B cells. Bone marrow production of lymphocytes continues throughout life but in later life, as the thymus dwindles in size and finally atrophies, cells leaving the bone marrow cannot become differentiated into new T cells. At this stage only peripheral T cell colonies can sustain the supply of T cells.

The lymphocytes in the circulation leave the bloodstream quite quickly; some enter the tissue interstices, while many others migrate directly into the lymph nodes from blood capillaries which perfuse these organs. The pool of functionally differentiated lymphocytes in blood is renewed several times each day. The T cells are known to be actively recirculated for many years, re-entering the blood with thoracic duct lymph. In man, the mean lifespan of these cells is estimated to be 4.4 years, with some surviving for at least 20 years. There is also a pool of short-lived cells in blood; these are probably mainly B lymphocytes, which have a 'lifespan' in the blood of 2–3 days, followed by a period of uncertain duration outside the bloodstream. B lymphocytes differentiate into plasma cells in lymphoid tissues. These cells are highly specialized for antibody production and probably survive for only a few days or weeks.

T-cell functions
1   The delayed hypersensitivity reaction. This is a localized reaction to certain antigens, usually described in skin. The most common cause is probably contact-allergy to substances such as soaps, cosmetics, and so on. The reaction is seen as a slowly formed, rather hard, painful itchy, red swelling, Microscopically, the tissue is seen to be invaded by lymphocytes and macrophages.
2   Immunity to intracellular parasites (especially fungi, viruses, the bacilli of tuberculosis and leprosy). Macrophages make good hosts for such parasites unless the immunological surveillance due to T cells has alerted and 'angered' them, whereupon the macrophages attack and destroy them.
3   Tumour rejection. It is calculated that there are several thousand mutant cells produced every day in the body. Those that do not die spontaneously must be killed; both must be disposed of by macrophage activity. T cells are believed to be important in preventing colonization by mutant cells (tumour formation).
4   Allograft rejection. Tissues bearing antigens which are 'not self' are rejected.
5   Autoimmune disease. Sometimes T cells fail to recognize a particular tissue as 'self' and they destroy it. This destruction may be very limited and specific, e.g. thyroid cells. It is not known how this reaction begins.

How do T cells act? It has already been mentioned that lymphocytes are not phagocytic and that the T cell is unable to secrete immunoglobulins. There is no doubt that T cells 'recognize' foreign antigens and activate macrophages, but it is uncertain what the activating molecule is. Amongst a number of factors secreted by T-cells are:
1   Large amounts of 'interferon', a protein which conveys enhanced resistance to viral infection upon previously virus-susceptible cells.
2   Toxins called 'lymphokines', which can kill bacteria.
3   Chemotactic agents which attract macrophages, other lymphocytes and neutrophils.

In addition to these active functions, T cells constitute a part of the memory system which allows the body to make a more prompt response on subsequent encounters with those antigens which it has experienced at least once before.

B-cell function (see also p. 77)
It is now generally accepted that B cells secrete imm--- globulins. They may do so while still recognizable as lymphocytes but, if antibody production is active, many B cells become highly differentiated to form plasma cells.

The immunoglobulin antibodies are a family of protein molecules and for each antigen there is a specific antibody which binds it. This may directly damage the antigen-bearing surface by, for example, altering the permeability of bacterial cell walls or the antibody may simply act as a marker molecule guiding the phagocytosis of the antigen by neutrophils or macrophages (opsonization).

A single lymphocyte produces a single type of antibody. If this cell is stimulated to divide, a clone of cells develops, all of which secrete this particular antibody. This fact underlies the recent development of monoclonal antibody production *in vitro*, using cultured cells, a technique which will certainly have far-reaching consequences in science and medicine.

Blood groups

Blood groups have acquired an important place in many fields of study:
1   In *genetics* they are excellent examples of genetically inherited characters.
2   In *immunology* they are systems of antigens and antibodies.

3 In *clinical medicine*. Because of the vast scale on which blood transfusions are given, certain blood group systems, notably ABO and Rh, cannot be disregarded when choosing blood for transfusion. In addition they have important associations with certain diseases. A blood group incompatability between mother and fetus is the underlying cause of haemolytic disease of the newborn.

4 In *anthropology* there are marked racial differences in the frequency of blood group characters.

5 In *forensic science* they are useful tools for investigating problems of doubtful paternity and for the identification of blood stains.

The end product of a blood group gene is an antigen situated on the red cell surface while blood group antibodies exist in the immunoglobulin fraction of the plasma. Agglutination tests of various kinds are the essence of blood group investigations. Each blood group anti-gen has a specific antibody with which it reacts, thereby causing agglutination of the cells possessing the antigen.

Blood group antigens are said to belong to the same system if they are shown to be allelomorphs. Also included in the same system are genes situated so close to each other on the chromosome that they are inherited together as a complex (e.g. the Rh genes).

BLOOD GROUP ANTIBODIES AND THEIR DETECTION

Blood group antibodies are plasma globulins (p. 77) and on suitable fractionation of the plasma are principally found either with the IgM macromolecules or with the IgG fraction which contains smaller molecules (of lower mw).

Most blood group antibodies of the IgM type are able to agglutinate red cells containing the corresponding antigen (Fig. 15.36b) in a simple

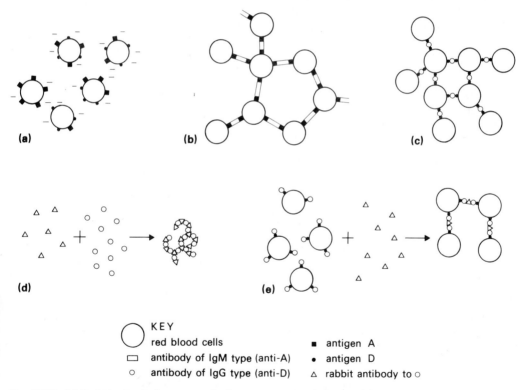

KEY
◯ red blood cells
▢ antibody of IgM type (anti-A)
○ antibody of IgG type (anti-D)

■ antigen A
• antigen D
△ rabbit antibody to ○

Fig. 15.36. (a) Red blood cells have a negatively charged surface which keeps them apart; (b) when added to a suspension of red cells, IgM antibodies attach to the corresponding antigenic sites on the cells and cause agglutination; (c) if the negative charges are reduced, e.g., by adding bovine serum albumin, the red cells draw closer together, and IgG antibodies then cause agglutination; (d) rabbits can be induced to form antibodies to human IgG immunoglobulins. Note that in this case the IgG antibody has acted as an antigen in the rabbit; (e) when added to red cells with a blood group antibody of the IgG type attached, the rabbit anti-human IgG agglutinates the red cells.

test using a saline suspension of the cells. Although IgG antibodies can also attach to the surface of the red cell, they cannot cause agglutination without assistance. This assistance may take the form of creating an environment which reduces the negative charge which normally keeps red cells apart, so that the smaller antibody molecules can span the gap between cells and cause agglutination (Fig. 15.36c). The use of a high protein medium such as bovine albumin does this, as does treatment of the cells with certain proteolytic enzymes. Alternatively, the anti-human globulin or Coombs technique is very often used. This exploits a different principle. When antibodies to human globulin are produced in a suitable animal (e.g. rabbit or goat) they will form a precipitate with human globulin (Fig. 15.36d). However, if the human globulin is an IgG antibody which has been allowed first to combine with its corresponding antigen on the red cells, mixture with the anti-human globulin causes the cells to agglutinate (Fig. 15.36e). The agglutination caused by anti-human globulin does not depend upon reducing the distance between sensitized red cells but on spanning the gaps by bridges in which anti-human globulin molecules serve as links between antibody molecules on adjacent red cells. This technique is one of the most important in blood group serology.

It is proposed to deal briefly with the ABO and Rh systems since these are clinically the most important. However, all blood group systems are basically alike in their structure.

The ABO system

There are four common ABO groups and these are determined by the presence or absence on the red cells of antigens A and B so that the group of an individual is either A, B, AB or O. The O gene is considered to be silent since it does not give rise to a specific O antigen. A remarkable feature of the system and one of great clinical importance, is the constant presence of anti-A and/or anti-B antibodies in the sera of people who lack the corresponding antigen (agglutinogen) on their red cells. Thus, as can be seen in Table 15.4, the serum of group A contains anti-B, while that of group B contains anti-A; group O individuals, who lack both antigens, have both antibodies and those whose red cells have both A and B antigens lack both anti-A and anti-B in the plasma.

One theory to explain the presence of these antibodies is as follows. Some common bacterial proteins have antigenic properties similar to the A and B antigens on red blood cells. Exposure of the infant to these bacteria probably leads to the development of appropriate antibodies. A host already having agglutinogen A clearly does not produce anti-A antibodies.

ABO grouping is carried out on a suspension of red blood cells using sera containing anti-A (prepared from the serum of group B) and anti-B (prepared from group A serum). The tests are not considered adequate without the inclusion of a test for the corresponding antibodies. Thus serum also is tested using standard group A and group B red cells. The results of both tests which give a characteristic pattern of agglutination reactions for each of the four groups are set out in Table 15.5.

The A and B genes are dominant characters (i.e. they give rise to the corresponding antigen on the red cell even when inherited from one parent only) but because the O gene is silent and has no corresponding antibody, the difference between the genotypes AO and AA and also BO and BB cannot be determined by serological tests but may sometimes be resolved by family studies, e.g. if a group A person is known to have a group O parent or child, his genotype must be AO.

Although group O cells lack the product of an

Table 15.4. The red cell antigens and serum antibodies of the ABO groups.

Blood group	Red cell antigens	Antibodies in serum	Percentage in British population
A	A	Anti-B	42
B	B	Anti-A	8
AB	A and B	Neither anti-A nor anti-B	3
O	Neither A or B	Both anti-A and anti-B	47

Table 15.5. ABO grouping results.

Blood group	Reaction of red cells with:		Reaction of serum with:	
	Anti-A serum	Anti-B serum	A cells	B cells
A	+	−	−	+
B	−	+	+	−
AB	+	+	−	−
O	−	−	+	+

+ indicates agglutination.

O gene they do possess an antigen called H, which has been shown to be a precursor substance necessary for the production of the antigens A and B. In fact the red cells of all four groups contain some H but when the A and B genes are present these give rise to A and B transferase enzymes which convert some of the H to A and B. Most H antigen is in group O where it remains, unconverted, in the absence of A and B transferases. In group AB there is maximum conversion owing to the presence of both transferases.

A, B and H in body fluids and tissues. A, B and H antigens are not confined to the red cell but can be detected in almost all tissue cells; they also occur as soluble substances (glycoproteins) in body fluids. Although all individuals have their appropriate ABH antigens in tissues, 24–30% of people in the British Isles have only trace amounts in the body fluids; they are called 'non-secretors'. It has been established that the ability to secrete ABH substance is determined by two allelic genes, 'Se' and 'se'. Individuals homozygous 'SeSe' or heterozygous 'Sese' are secretors, whereas those who are homozygous 'sese' are non-secretors. Secretors of group A secrete both A and H and similarly group B secretors secrete B and H. The fluids of AB secretors contain A and B but only small quantities of H. Group O secretors of course secrete only H.

The fluid that is commonly tested to establish secretor status is saliva and the tests consist of mixing saliva with anti-A, anti-B and anti-H. If the corresponding substance is present in the saliva it binds to the specific antibody and inhibits the activity of the antibody. The addition to the tests of a red cell suspension of the appropriate group determines whether or not specific inhibition of the activity of the corresponding antibody has taken place because the

expected agglutination either fails to occur or is greatly reduced.

Only serological tests can distinguish between secretors and non-secretors. Biochemically the saliva of secretors and non-secretors is essentially similar and both contain glycoproteins although higher protein levels have been recorded for secretors. The role of the secretor gene is unknown except that it appears to act as a regulator gene which provides the right environment for the appearance of blood-group-specific glycoproteins in the secretions. It does not control the appearance of A, B and H on red cells. The frequency of occurrence of the secretor gene shows racial variation and is even significantly different in various parts of the British Isles.

The Rh or D system
This blood group system was discovered by Landsteiner and Wiener in 1940 through the immunization of guinea pigs and rabbits with blood from the Macacus rhesus monkey. The antibody thus formed, not only agglutinated rhesus monkey (Rh) red cells but also the red cells of about 85% of a panel of blood samples from the white population of New York. The enormous clinical significance of the anti-rhesus antibody became apparent when it was shown that the 15% of individuals who are Rh-negative could themselves form similar anti-Rh antibodies if stimulated by a transfusion from an Rh-positive donor or, after a challenge by the Rh antigen possessed by a fetus *in utero*. Moreover in the first instance the antibodies produced were capable of causing a severe haemolytic transfusion reaction and in the second, a haemolytic process beginning in the fetus *in utero* and leading at birth to an infant suffering from haemolytic disease of the newborn.

It was not long before it was realized that the simple division of the human population into Rh-positive and Rh-negative phenotypes was only the beginning of the Rh story and over the years a very complex blood group system has been disclosed consisting of many subgroups and a number of Rhesus anitbodies of differing specificities.

Haemolytic disease of the newborn. The following serological picture is associated with haemolytic disease of the newborn. The Rh-negative mother forms an antibody to an antigen present in the fetus which has been inherited by the infant from its father. This antigen enters the maternal circulation through a transplacental haemorrhage occurring at delivery or because of small bleeds from fetus to mother during pregnancy. The antibodies produced by the mother, being IgG and therefore small, cross the placenta and cause damage to the fetal red cells. The first Rh-positive (D positive) infant in a family usually escapes haemolytic disease, but once the mother is immunized there is a greater risk to the subsequent Rh-positive fetus. It is usual in treating haemolytic disease to replace approximately 90% of the infant's own cells with Rh-negative cells which are compatible with the maternal antibody. The child of course produces its own Rh-positive cells slowly, but meanwhile the concentration of maternal antibody in its circulation has been greatly diluted and what remains continues to fall rapidly.

The diagnosis, treatment and finally the prevention of haemolytic disease of the newborn, all within a span of 30 years, is one of this century's medical success stories.

Prevention stems from the comparatively recent finding that passively administered anti-Rh (anti-D) has the effect of suppressing an immune response to the Rh antigen and it is now standard practice to protect Rh-negative women giving birth to an Rh-positive child by injection with concentrated purified anti-D. The procedure is initiated immediately after delivery of the first Rh-positive child.

CHOICE OF BLOOD FOR TRANSFUSION AND CROSS-MATCHING

Not for some time after the discovery of the ABO system at the turn of the century was it generally accepted that blood grouping and cross-matching were prerequisites for successful blood transfusion.

Today blood transfusion is medicine's most successful tissue transplant, since compatible donor red cells are eliminated at the rate of only 1% per day, which is similar to the normal rate at which the recipient's own red cell population is eliminated.

With the discovery of numerous blood group systems and the possible differentiation of hundreds of blood group combinations it is necessary to decide which systems have to be considered in choosing blood for transfusion. Experience has shown that it is essential to type donors and recipients for ABO and Rh (D) but a more detailed analysis is required only in special cases.

The ABO system is potentially the most dangerous hazard in blood transfusions because over 95% of all recipients have anti-A and/or anti-B in their plasma.

The antibodies in the plasma of the donor can usually be ignored as they are very much diluted by the large volume of plasma in the recipient. It follows that the antigens on the recipient's cells are of little concern. In blood transfusion it is the antibodies in the plasma of the recipient and the antigens on the cells of the donor which are of paramount importance (but see below).

When incompatible blood is tranfused in error, the red cells (usually those of the donor) are agglutinated and haemolysed. Haemoglobin is released into the plasma and is degraded by cells in the spleen and liver producing a rise in the circulating bilirubin level and jaundice. If the transfusion reaction is more severe an excess of free haemoglobin in the plasma causes it to be precipitated in the renal tubules leading to anuria (lack of urine production).

Except in great emergencies when group O blood (lacking A and B antigens) may have to be given, patients receive at all times blood of their own ABO group. This minimizes possible danger to the patient from receiving incompatible agglutinins (antibodies) present in the donor serum. Occasionally very high titres of anti-A or anti-B present in the plasma of group O donors cause transfusion reactions in recipients who have A and/or B antigens.

Typing with anti-D is a routine procedure for all recipients and ideally all D (Rh) negative individuals receive D-negative (i.e. Rh-negative) blood. When Rh-negative blood is in short supply priority must be given to the claims of (a) patients who already have anti-Rh antibodies, (b) Rh-negative women of child-bearing age and (c) infants with haemolytic disease due to anti-D. It is exceedingly important that girls and young women who are Rh-negative never receive Rh-positive blood because of its possible adverse effect on their future pregnancies. A transfusion of Rh-positive blood to a Rh-negative recipient almost invariably primes them for the production of antibodies at the next stimulus, which in women may well be that afforded by an Rh-positive fetus.

A cross-matching test is a routine procedure before a transfusion is given. This consists of testing the recipient's plasma against the red cells of each proposed donor by a number of techniques designed to detect all possible antibodies in the recipient which may react with the donor red cells and subsequently cause a haemolytic transfusion reaction. The test also has to be geared to the detection of IgG antibodies so the anti-human globulin technique (Fig. 15.36e) is never omitted from the cross-matching procedure.

TISSUE FLUID

Formation

In 1896 Starling proposed that fluid is exchanged between the intravascular and extravascular compartments across the capillary wall, as a result of changes in the magnitude of two opposing forces. His suggestion that hydrostatic pressure moves fluid out into the interstitial spaces and that the osmotic pressure created by plasma protein moves it back into the capillaries has come to be known as the Starling hypothesis. In man, the mean pressure at the arterial end of skin capillaries is about 32 mmHg. Starling obtained a value of 25 mmHg for the osmotic pressure exerted by human plasma proteins—a value which has since been repeatedly confirmed. Although the magnitude of these pressures varies considerably with the site of the tissue beds, the degree of constriction within the arterioles, and species, the principle enunciated by Starling still holds.

Blood entering the capillary from its arterial end has a hydrostatic pressure considerably in excess of the total absorptive force, i.e. plasma colloid (plasma protein) osmotic pressure, sometimes called oncotic pressure, plus the tissue fluid pressure (usually 1–4 mmHg in most tissues). As a result, there is a net outwardly directed force across the capillary wall from the lumen to the interstitial space. Water and small molecules in solution are driven out through the selectively permeable wall of the vessel. The interstitial (tissue) fluid so formed has a composition similar to plasma freed of most of its protein, because although the plasma proteins are larger than most of the pores in the capillary wall, some do escape even from normal capillaries and must be returned to the circulation. Filtration proceeds, and the hydrostatic driving force becomes progressively reduced along the length of the capillary until a point is reached where the total outward force is equal to the total inward force and there is no net force across the capillary wall. Beyond this point there is a net absorptive force because the osmotic pressure of the plasma proteins plus the tissue fluid pressure now exceed the capillary hydrostatic pressure. Consequently, fluid is absorbed from the interstitial space into the capillary and adds

to the venous blood returning to the heart. Sodium and chloride ions are distributed in equal concentrations on both sides of the capillary wall so that the large osmotic pressures created by these are equal and opposite and hence do not influence this model.

By this process a volume of fluid equal to about 70% of the blood volume is filtered and reabsorbed each minute. Dissolved in this fluid are the substrates for, and the products of, metabolism. Some of the fluid does not return to the capillaries but passes instead into the lymphatic capillaries which ramify through nearly all tissues together with the blood capillaries. Lymph only flows when the exchange of fluid and protein across the capillary is out of balance. In man, some 2–4 litres of tissue fluid are returned to the circulation via the thoracic and right lymph ducts each day and in it are transported proteins, lipids and particulate matter from the interstitial space. Dysfunction of the lymphatic system therefore leads to the accumulation of fluid in interstitial spaces. The lymphatic drainage of the small intestine is specialized and carries fat in the form of chylomicrons from the intestinal mucosa.

Oedema

When excess fluid is retained in the extravascular compartment, for whatever reason, oedema is said to be present. Oedema, which may be caused by a large number of widely differing factors, may be local or general and may be restricted to surface structures or to body cavities and internal structures. It forms part of the inflammatory response to injury (p. 687). The accumulated fluid in oedema can be classified either as exudate or as transudate. Exudates are formed when the oedema is caused by a condition which alters capillary permeability. Such fluids are characterized by a large quantity of protein which has come from the plasma, by their high specific gravity and by the presence of numerous cells. With transudates, the capillary permeability remains normal and the composition is similar to normal tissue fluid. Pulmonary oedema acompanying congestive heart failure, for example, is due to raised venous pressure and the fluid is a transudate. Acute inflammatory oedema is usually accompanied by the accumulation of an exudate containing numerous plasma factors which protect and repair. This form of oedema is frequently seen in hypersensitivity and in infections.

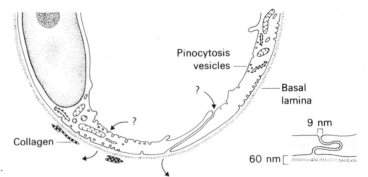

Fig. 15.37. Cross-section through capillary wall. (From Davson, *Textbook of General Physiology* (3rd edition); Churchill Livingstone, London).

Permeability and structure of capillary

To gain access to the interstitial space, plasma constituents must pass through the endothelial cell layer, a basal lamina and an outermost incomplete layer, the adventitia (Fig. 15.37). The question arises as to whether the capillary is a 'porous membrane' which acts as a passive filter under the influence of hydrostatic, osmotic and Gibbs–Donnan forces. Water and crystalloids are filtered through the capillary rapidly while the large plasma proteins are retained. It has been shown, however, that the barrier to albumin, one of the smaller plasma proteins, is such that the equivalent of 0.1% of the total plasma protein leaves the circulation every minute which means that more than the total weight of plasma protein is 'turned-over' every 24 hours. The vascular permeability to proteins is not uniform throughout the body; the differences in protein concentrations in lymph drained from different tissues are probably related to variations in the permeability of different vascular beds. This implies that capillary walls are not purely passive filters, as the Starling hypothesis would suggest, and that their structure may vary.

Solutes with molecular weights of up to 5000 appear to pass readily out of capillaries. Above this limit there are increasing restrictions. Some molecules probably travel by aqueous intercellular routes, in which case the junctions between cells, the basement membrane or adventitia are selective. A route through the cells would require the existence of pores and active mechanisms such as vesicular transport; both of which have been observed. In addition there is likely to be exchange by simple diffusion through the layers comprising a capillary. Vesicular transport cannot, by virtue of its very limited capacity, account for more than a small proportion of the total transcapillary fluid movement, but may be important in the transfer of large molecules of up to 500 000 mw for which no other route would be available.

The structure of capillaries is not uniform throughout the body. In the 'fenestrated' type, the cytoplasm and cell membranes are thinned to about 4 nm over restricted parts of the cell to give the appearance of holes of about 40 nm diameter. These fenestrations should not be confused with the pores previously mentioned. Such vessels are found in the capillary beds of the intestine, renal glomeruli and tubules, ciliary body, choroid plexus and endocrine glands—in situations where large volumes of fluid are moved. The liver has the most permeable vascular bed with a protein concentration in hepatic lymph which is close to, but does not reach, that of plasma.

The predominant type of capillary in mammals, however, is the 'continuous' type in which the passage of material is confined to the transcellular route and subject to its restraints. There is evidence for two types of pores within the cells; small pores with effective diameters of 6–9 nm through which dissolved particles could pass unless restricted by their size, charge and other physical parameters; and a smaller number of large pores about 26 nm in diameter through which larger molecules such as albumin can pass. Water movement does not appear to depend on the nature of the pore system.

TISSUE INJURY AND HAEMOSTASIS

Degrees of injury

The physiological response to injury very much depends upon its severity. For convenience, four separate grades of injury and associated

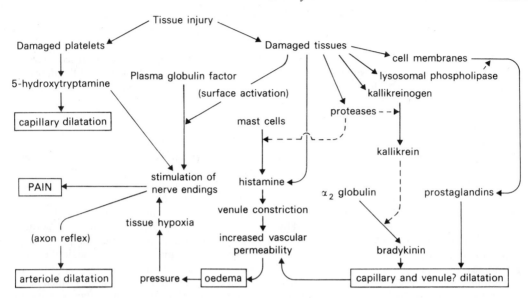

Fig. 15.38. Some of the principal reactions which occur in the acute inflammatory response. The physiological consequences of these processes are shown in boxes (it is best to work backwards from each of these in turn in order to appreciate their development).

responses can be recognized, though it should be noted that the most damaging injuries include all the responses to some degree.

1 Minimal injury, with unbroken vessels and no blood loss. This covers a wide assortment of assaults varying from the effect of mechanical trauma, pressure, heat, minor burns and insect bites to pathological defects in the endothelial lining of the vessels. Within this group there are differences in response.

2 Microtrauma, with bleeding from capillaries, as when a finger is pricked by a needle.

3 Tissue damage and bleeding from small vessels. An injury of this type would be presented after tooth extraction where there is a cavity lined by bone, connective tissue and damaged gingiva with saliva and bacteria gaining immediate access.

4 Severe bleeding with extensive tissue trauma as in surgery or where large arteries are severed in major accidents. In this case we have also to consider the systemic responses to injury and haemorrhage (p. 727).

The overall response in (2)–(4) is aimed first at minimizing blood loss by encouraging haemostasis (the main concern in this section) and preventing invasion by bacteria; second, at confining the area of injury; and third, at repairing damaged tissue.

ACUTE INFLAMMATION

Provided they retain their vitality, all tissues react to irritation and damage by a complex local vascular, lymphatic and cellular response known as acute inflammation. The four cardinal signs of acute inflammation and the reactions which produce them are summarized in Fig. 15.38. They are heat (due to arteriole dilatation), redness (due to capillary dilatation), pain, and swelling (oedema).

Platelets (or thrombocytes as they are more appropriately termed) are smaller than the circulating blood cells, having a diameter of 2–4 μm and a life span of about 8–11 days. They participate in many of the responses in tissue injury and haemostasis. These granular cells are metabolically active and contain high concentrations of ATP. They do not contain a nucleus. Their importance derives from the ease with which they adhere to damaged surfaces and because of the substances which they contain and readily release such as phospholipid, 5-hydroxytryptamine, catecholamines and histamine. Platelets are produced from giant cells lying outside the sinusoids in the bone marrow—the megakaryocytes. It is thought that cytoplasmic processes of these parent cells protrude through the blood sinusoids; the platelets are really just pinched-off portions of this cytoplasm.

Histamine is derived from the amino acid histidine and has a widespread distribution in plant and animal cells: it is responsible for the pain, itch and swelling which result from being stung by nettles and wasps. There are large species differences in the source and actions of histamine. When injected subcutaneously in man histamine causes dilatation of arterioles and capillaries and probably constriction of venules leading to increased capillary permeability and oedema. It also stimulates some sensory nerve endings directly and others indirectly by virtue of the dilatation of peripheral blood vessels. Even the most trivial injury such as is caused by rubbing the skin firmly, releases histamine.

5-hydroxytryptamine, also known as 5HT or serotonin, is in high concentrations in platelets but is found also in many other cells in the gastrointestinal tract and in the brain. It is synthesized from tryptophane and inactivated by the enzyme monoamine oxidase. In many aspects 5HT is similar to histamine, e.g. it is widely distributed in nature and is found in nettle stings and wasp venom. The physiological responses to it show marked variations. It is a potent stimulant of pain nerve endings in the skin; it is rapidly destroyed by enzyme action after its release from tissues; and in high concentrations it can cause increased blood flow in capillaries. As the name serotonin suggests, it stimulates smooth muscle and in low concentrations causes vasoconstriction, particularly of veins.

Other substances which participate either individually or in concert in the inflammatory response are sometimes collectively called the plasma kinins. These are; the decapeptide, kallidin; the nonapeptide, bradykinin, which can, but need not, be derived from kallidin; and a pain-producing plasma globulin. The common stimulus for the formation of these active compounds is the release of proteases from damaged tissues which then act on several plasma protein precursors that have leaked into the tissue spaces through the dilated, permeable capillaries and venules. Many of the properties of these substances are similar to those of 5HT and histamine.

The recently discovered group of substances, the prostaglandins, are synthesized and released by damaged tissues. They have been found in inflammatory exudates and interstitial fluid of inflamed human skin and are known to be potent vasodilators. Anti-inflammatory agents, such as aspirin, indomethacin and corticosteroids inhibit the synthesis of prostaglandins.

The sequence in which each reaction occurs in relation to the others involved in tissue injury and haemostasis has yet to be discovered, it probably depends on the nature of the damage. For example, it has been argued that an immediate dilatation of arterioles and capillaries to the injured part, which constitutes part of the inflammatory response, would be helpful in providing adequate amounts of those factors required in defence and in the subsequent haemostasis: but might this increased blood flow not make it more difficult to stop the bleeding? In many injuries the inflammatory response persists long after haemostasis has been effected.

The increase in vascular permeability permits large, osmotically active, plasma proteins to enter the interstitial fluid and some, in the presence of damaged tissue, cause the deposition of fibrin (see later) in the tissue spaces which helps to form a barrier around the inflamed area. In certain sites this is aided by the natural cohesiveness of the tissues. In addition to the fluid and macromolecules, cells also invade the tissue spaces. The surface of the damaged endothelium causes passing neutrophils and monocytes to become attached and these later migrate between the cells and move by chemotaxis into the inflamed tissue spaces.

HAEMOSTASIS

This composite term means cessation of blood flow. It involves first, constriction of injured vessels; second, formation of a platelet plug; and finally, if much bleeding has occurred, coagulation of blood around and behind the plug. This sequence was worked out about 100 years ago and since then much effort has been expended in trying to elucidate the mechanisms involved. Even so, there remain many unanswered questions. Recently the use of high-speed cine-photography has allowed some of the very rapid cellular changes which follow injury to vessels to be studied in the tissues of living animals (for example, the hamster cheek-pouch).

Constriction of vessels

Most vessels respond to injury by constricting or by retracting away from the injured point. This is due to contraction of muscle in the walls of arterioles, arteries and veins, but in capillaries, which are devoid of muscle except at the precapillary sphincter, the mechanism is still uncertain. The apposed endothelial walls of a con-

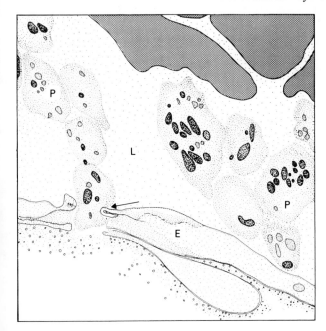

Fig. 15.39. Earliest stages of platelet aggregation. One platelet (arrowed) occupies a gap between the endothelial cells (E) lining the vein. Such a gap can be created by very mild trauma. L is the lumen of vessel and P represents platelets. (From French J. E. (1967) *British Journal of Haematology* **13**, 595).

stricted vessel adhere to each other to maintain a seal. In some circumstances, fluid oozing out into tissue spaces helps to compress small vessels. Traces of 5-hydroxytryptamine, when released from damaged platelets, cause constriction, most probably of the pre-capillaries.

Platelet plug

Platelets adhere within seconds to damaged endothelial cells, subendothelial tissue and the rim of connective tissue at the opening of the vessels; they then aggregate around this focal point (Fig. 15.39). The primary adhesion must be considerable to withstand the flow of blood, but as this soon becomes reduced by the accompanying constriction of the vessels, the plug stands less chance of being dislodged.

It has been suggested that platelets adhere due to changes which are induced in their surfaces by ADP released from damaged tissues. The ADP causes them to change shape and bind to any exposed collagen and to the vascular basement membrane (Fig. 15.40a). Platelets too contain ADP and this is released during adhesion to cause more of them to collect together. This aggregation is aided by 5HT, thrombin (see later) and catecholamines. The latter finding is important clinically since raised plasma levels of adrenaline are found in people during stress.

Part of the explanation of gastrointestinal bleeding frequently observed in persons on pro-longed aspirin treatment is a failure of platelets to participate in haemostasis following small mucosal lesions because their aggregation is inhibited by acetylsalicylate.

A defect in platelet function or a reduction in their number (thrombocytopenia) retards both vascular spasm and platelet aggregation. As these stages in haemostasis are all that are required to stop bleeding from a small injury such as a pin-prick, the deficiency in platelet activity can be conveniently detected by measuring the time required for bleeding to cease after such an injury. This test is the well-known 'bleeding-time'. Depending upon local conditions such as temperature, the normal bleeding time is from 1½–3 minutes.

The plug formed by the platelets (Fig. 15.40b) may be subsequently strengthened by threads of fibrin, the formation of which we shall now consider. There are, however, many factors which keep this process in check so that persistence of the plug is not a foregone conclusion.

Blood clotting

When blood is drawn from the body with minimal damage to tissues, as for example by a careful venepuncture, on being transferred from the syringe to a clean, dry glass tube at room temperature it forms a solid mass within 5–10 minutes (the coagulation time). The tube can then be inverted without displacing its contents.

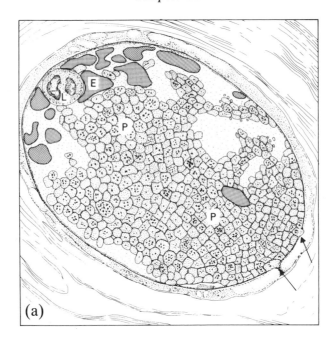

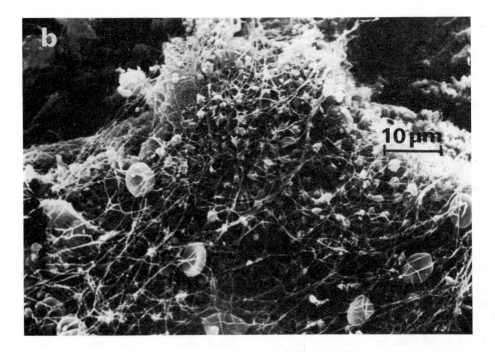

Fig. 15.40. (a) An experimental thrombus in a small artery, produced by local injury (arrowed) of the vessel. (E, erythrocyte; L, leucocyte; P, platelets.) (From French J.E. (1967) *British Journal of Haematology* **13**, 595). (b) Scanning EM picture of an experimentally produced thrombus formed on a plastic surface in the heart of a rabbit. Erythrocytes are tangled in a mass of fibrin threads in which are also embedded platelets. This is similar to the appearance of a blood clot. (By courtesy of D. A. McGowan).

Much later the clot retracts away from the sides of the tube and serum is separated. The retraction is due to a contractile protein within the platelets, thrombosthenin, which pulls on the fibrin threads within the clot. At the onset of visible clotting, these threads of fibrin suddenly appear and as the meshwork becomes more dense it entangles red and white blood cells (Fig. 15.40b). Fibrin is derived by an enzymatic process from circulating fibrinogen, its inactive precursor. The enzyme thrombin is also derived from an inactive precursor, prothrombin. These clotting factors, in common with all the others to be described, are plasma proteins, manufactured in the liver. In a test-tube, clotting is prevented by adding sodium citrate, oxalates or EDTA, all of which in different ways reduce the free calcium ions which are essential for clotting. These findings were accounted for in a scheme suggested in 1905 (Fig. 15.41), but it was not until the 1940s that it became obvious that many observations could not be reconciled with this simple scheme, and that additional, complex reactions precede the activation of prothrombin. Some of the difficulties which prevented the acceptance of this scheme are now described.

To derive a measurement known as the 'one stage prothrombin time', tissue extract (usually of the brain, lung or thymus) containing 'thromboplastin' is added to plasma (from which the Ca^{2+} ions have been removed by 'citration'). To start the reaction, a calcium chloride solution is added and the time for fibrin to form is noted. The norm for this test at 37°C is about 11–20 seconds. It was formerly thought that a delay indicated a deficiency of prothrombin or, more rarely, fibrinogen (Fig. 15.41). It was then found that the prolonged prothrombin time obtained with plasma of patients receiving anticoagulant coumarin drugs was shortened by adding normal

serum in the test. As serum does not contain prothrombin or fibrinogen, it must have contributed a factor or factors missing from the patient's plasma. Next it was observed that although plasma from haemophiliacs gives a normal prothrombin time, their blood is very slow to coagulate: yet, with the addition of tissue extract to a blood sample the coagulation time is greatly accelerated. Tissue extract is acting as a substitute for a clotting factor or factors which are missing in the blood of a haemophiliac. Further, if blood is contained in a very smooth walled tube lined with polythene or silicone, clotting is delayed: a 'contact factor' seems to be necessary for normal clotting. For the present we must omit the various lines of evidence which have been painstakingly collected and merely try to summarize the story. It is all too easy to lose sight of the overall principles in haemostasis by concentrating on isolated, rather academic points, about which there is considerable controversy. With that note of caution in mind we can examine the probable sequence of chemical reactions in clotting in Figs. 15.42 and 15.43.

The clotting of blood is usually described as involving extrinsic and intrinsic systems. 'Intrinsic' describes the reactions which take place in blood or plasma free of contamination from damaged tissues; those which occur in a clean glass tube when measuring the coagulation time. The extrinsic scheme describes the sequence of reactions initiated by factors which originate in damaged tissues. Both mechanisms are necessary for normal haemostasis and are interrelated in practice. It must be emphasized that these terms 'intrinsic' and 'extrinsic' are rather artificial and are used only as a convenience.

When blood comes into contact with damaged tissues these release factor III (thromboplastin) which sets in motion the so called 'extrinsic' scheme of clotting (Fig. 15.42). Several steps lead to traces of thrombin (IIa) being formed which act autocatalytically at several of the preceding stages to increase thrombin production. Thrombin also aids platelet aggregation. The small friable clot which is thus rapidly formed around the damaged area slows down blood flow and allows accumulation of other clotting factors required in the supporting 'intrinsic' clotting scheme.

The intrinsic clotting mechanism (Fig. 15.43) involves the sequential activation of a whole train of factors; the scheme is aptly called the 'waterfall' or 'cascade theory'. This complexity is not unexpected when one thinks how important

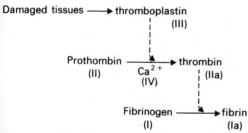

Fig. 15.41. The basic scheme of blood clotting as described by Morawitz. Activation by an enzymatic process is shown as a broken line. The new nomenclature (roman numerals) for the various factors has been included.

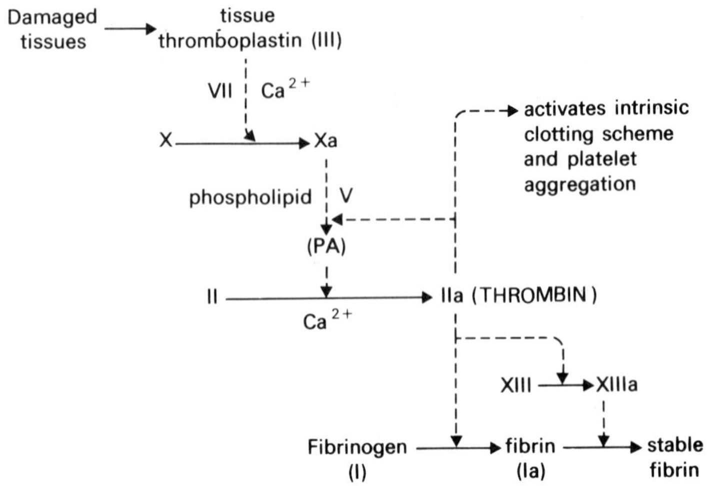

Damaged tissues
tissue thromboplastin (III)
VII
Ca 2+
X
Xa
phospholipid
V
(PA)
activates intrinsic clotting scheme and platelet aggregation
II
Ca 2+
IIa (THROMBIN)
XIII
XIIIa
Fibrinogen (I)
fibrin (Ia)
stable fibrin

Fig. 15.42. A summary of the main reactions in the clotting of blood or plasma in the presence of damaged tissue. Activation by an enzymatic process is shown as a broken line. The important position occupied by thrombin (11a) is clear. The symbol (a) is used to denote the activated form of a previously inactive precursor. The intermediary complex, prothrombin activator, is designated as PA.

it is both to maintain fluidity of blood in the absence of haemorrhage and to prevent an established clot from spreading too far upstream from a damaged area. There is no doubt that in a test-tube the Hageman factor (XII) is activated by the glass surface and that this triggers the intrinsic clotting mechanism. The initiator *in vivo* is still uncertain, but the principal contenders are collagen and long chain saturated fatty acids; there is also evidence that platelets can activate factor XI *in vivo* and that activation of factor XII is by-passed.

Several safeguards lower the deadly risk of intravascular clotting. Amongst these are the dependence of the clotting mechanism on the activation of inactive precursors, and the presence in plasma of natural anticoagulants and fibrinolytic agents which have to be 'neutralized' before clotting can occur. Some antithrombins interfere with the thrombin-fibrinogen reaction,

Surface contact?
XII
XIIa
XI
XIa
IX
IXa
VIII
VIIIa
?
? phospholipid
Ca2+
X
Xa
V
platelets
phospholipid
(PA)
XIII
XIIIa
II
IIa (THROMBIN)
Ca2+
I
fibrin
stable fibrin

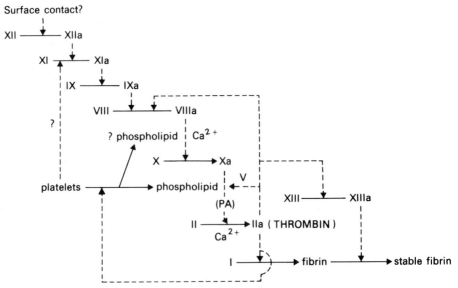

Fig. 15.43. A summary of the main reactions in the clotting of blood or plasma in the absence of damaged tissue. One or two stages in this scheme are still questionable and these are denoted by (?). The dominant role of thrombin is again very obvious. (If you think these schemes are complex consider what they would be like if all the naturally occurring inhibiting agents were included. Certainly the life of a student was easier in the days of Morawitz!)

others irreversibly destroy thrombin. Anti-IXa, anti-Xa, and anti-XIa substances have also been demonstrated. Fibrin adsorbs and inactivates 85–90% of the thrombin and prevents excess clotting. Heparin, released from mast cells, is a cofactor for antithrombin which prevents the production of thrombin and inhibits its activity. Fibrinolysin, or plasmin, causes lysis of fibrin and also breaks down factors I (fibrinogen) VII and VIII. Endothelial damage is one of many agents such as exercise, emotional stress, major surgery, adrenaline and bacterial pyrogens, which activate the precursor plasminogen from which plasmin is derived. An understanding of these processes is vital in clinical medicine not just because of their importance in stopping bleeding, but also in relation to the prevention and treatment of thrombosis—a condition in which a thrombus or aggregation of platelets in a fibrin meshwork develops in a vessel as a result of a degenerative condition in the walls or due to stasis of blood, for example, following major surgery.

Defects in haemostasis and coagulation (also considered in Volume 2)

It is a reflection of our times that acquired co-agulation disorders are now seen more often than are inherited defects. Oral anticoagulants, widely used in the treatment of coronary disease and thrombosis, reduce the activity of factors VII, IX, X and also prothrombin (II).

FUNCTIONS OF THE CARDIOVASCULAR SYSTEM

General principles

The cardiovascular system is required to transport and exchange heat, gases, nutrients, waste products, water, electrolytes, hormones and other chemical messengers. The heart is the pump, the major blood vessels are conduits, and the capillaries are the sites of exchange. The capillary surface in a mammal has the same exchange function as the cell membrane of a protozoan. It has been estimated that man has a theoretical maximum capillary surface area of about 500–1000 m², rather more than the size of a tennis court, which can be expressed as 7000–9000 mm²/g of body weight. For a uni-cellular organism whose radius is 0.5 mm, the calculation is 6000 mm²/g of body; a very similar figure. However, an important difference between the simple organism and a mammal is that

6000 mm²/g is the unvarying surface area of the protozoan, but in mammalian muscle for example, only a relatively small proportion of the total capillary bed has blood flowing through it during resting conditions. During exercise many more capillaries are opened up in muscles and the surface area increases accordingly. The limiting factor on the rate of steady exercise is largely determined by the rate at which oxygen and nutrients can be delivered to the muscles by the circulation rather than the area for exchange. The requirements of the increased demand necessitated by exercise must have had an important role in determining the evolution of our circulatory system.

PHYSICS OF BLOOD FLOW

Pressure

In order to fulfil its functions blood has to be made to flow around the body. Therefore, we need to briefly consider the physics of flow.

Fluids tend to flow when a force is applied to them, but flow is resisted by friction between the molecules of the fluid and between the fluid and the wall of the containing vessel. The amount of the force per unit area is known as the pressure and this is opposed by the resistance. Pressure, flow and resistance are related simply thus:

$$\text{Flow} = \frac{\text{pressure}}{\text{resistance}} \tag{1}$$

This can be translated as 'the harder you push, the faster it flows'. An analogy is afforded by the flow of water out of the domestic hot water tap. The tap provides a variable resistance which is infinite when the tap is turned off so the flow is zero. As the tap is opened, reducing the resistance, flow starts and increases until the tap is fully open when the flow is maximal. The flow rate now depends on the resistance provided by the piping and the pressure head determined by the height of the reservoir above the tap. The greater the height, the higher the pressure head and, from (1), the greater the flow.

Pressures are often given as centimetres or inches of water or some convenient liquid, e.g. mercury. Pressure is force per unit area, so a denser liquid produces a higher pressure for a given column height. The relationship is:

$$\text{Pressure} = \text{h} \, \rho \, \text{g} \tag{2}$$

where h = height of column, ρ = density and g = the acceleration due to gravity. Although they are not SI units, mmHg or cmH₂O are accepted as units of pressure but it is as well to be familar with the fundamental unit: Newtons/m² or Pascals. A Newton is the force necessary to accelerate 1 kg through $1m/s^2$. Gravity exerts a force of 9.8 kg m/s^2, in other words it can accelerate 9.8 kg to a speed of 1 metre per second in one second. Force = mass × acceleration, so if the pressure of the atmosphere can support a column of liquid of a given height, knowing the density of the liquid we can determine the pressure in the atmosphere.

Typically, atmospheric pressure can sustain a column of mercury 760 mm high. The density of mercury is 13.6 times that of water, i.e. 13.6×10^3 kg/m³. Thus the mass of a column of mercury 0.76 m high is:

$$0.76 \times 13.6 \times 10^3 \times \pi r^2$$

where r = radius of column
so the force on the column (mass × acceleration) is

$$0.76 \times 13.6 \times 10^3 \quad = \quad 10.1 \times 10^4 \text{ Nm}^{-2}$$
$$\times \pi r^2 \times 9.8 \text{ kg m}^{-2} \qquad \times \pi r^2$$

Atmospheric pressure is exerted over an area of πr^2, so atmospheric pressure per unit area (m²) = 10.1 N × 10^4/ m².

The radius of the column cancels out. The atmospheric pressure is thus

$$10.1 \times 10^4 \text{ N/m}^2 \text{ or Pa (Pascals. } 1Pa = 1N/m^2)$$

Thus 1 mmHg is equivalent to

$$\frac{10.1 \times 10^4}{760} = 133 \text{ N/m}^2 \text{ or } 133 \text{ Pa}$$

Flow

Poiseuille's Law states that in rigid straight tubes:

$$\text{Flow = pressure drop} \times \frac{\pi r^4}{8\eta l} \qquad (3)$$

where η = viscosity of the fluid (see below), l = the length of the tube, r = radius of the tube. ($\pi/8$ is a constant which comes from the mathematics of the situation and need not concern us here.)

It is not pressure as such that determines flow, of course, but the pressure gradient. Flow occurs from a region of higher pressure to one of lower, just as water flows downhill from a region of higher potential energy to one that is lower. It is important to distinguish between velocity of flow and volume of flow. For a given flow-rate, velocity decreases as cross sectional area increases. This is clearly shown by comparing the velocity of flow in the aorta and in the capillaries. The cardiac output is about 5 dm³/min (5×10^6 mm³/min) and the aorta is 20 mm in diameter; so in the aorta, flow velocity per second is:

$$\frac{\text{flow/min}}{\pi r^2 \times 60} \quad \text{or} \quad \frac{5 \times 10^6}{\pi \times 10^2 \times 60} \text{ mm/s} = 265 \text{ mm/s}$$

The total cross sectional area of open capillaries is approximately 1×10^6 mm². Velocity in these capillaries therefore will be:

$$\frac{5 \times 10^6}{1 \times 10^6 \times 60} = 0.8 \text{ mm/s}.$$

This calculation assumes that only 5–10% of all capillaries at rest are open at any one time.

From (1) it is clear that the term on the right of (3) must represent the reciprocal of the resistance to flow. Now consider each factor in this equation in turn.

Viscosity (η). Unlike the plunger in a syringe, liquid does not flow uniformly through the cross-section of a tube. Friction is greatest at the walls and an infinitesimally thin layer of molecules next to the wall is almost stationary. Because of the friction between adjacent molecules the outer layers flow less rapidly than the inner layers and as we move progressively in towards the centre the fluid flows more rapidly. During flow a liquid may be considered to consist of concentric layers or laminae which slide over each other (Fig. 15.44). The viscosity of a liquid is a measure of the difficulty which these layers or laminae encounter in sliding over each other and Newton described viscosity as a lack of slipperiness between layers of the liquid. The greater the viscosity, the less the flow for a given pressure drop.

Viscosity can be measured in a number of ways but one of the simplest, in theory if not in practice, is to pass a known volume of fluid through a fine capillary tube by applying different pressures to it. If the time is measured and 1/t is plotted against pressure, the slope is proportional to the viscosity of the liquid. Relative viscosity may be determined by comparing the slopes of different liquids with that of water. Plasma is about 1.6 and whole blood 4–5.

The viscosity of the blood is obviously influenced by the number of red cells. It is surprising that at high haematocrits blood is able to flow at all through capillaries, because red cell diameters are similar to or only slightly smaller than that of the capillaries through which they pass. There are several explanations for this, amongst which is the observation that red cells are sufficiently flexible to distort as they squeeze through in single file.

As they pass through a wider tube, red cells move towards the centre of the flowing stream

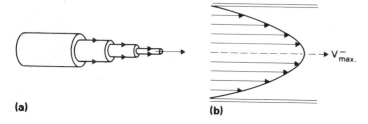

Fig. 15.44. (a) A representation of flow in a liquid with thin layers sliding over each other; (b) an illustration of the velocity profile obtained by taking a longitudinal section through the vessel.

(Fig. 15.45). The reasons for this axial accumulation are still not fully understood but the consequences are that the apparent viscosity is reduced in small tubes compared with large ones. From Fig. 15.44 it can be seen that the greatest change in velocity occurs at the edge of the tube. Since there are fewer red cells towards the edges, the viscosity is less here. In large vessels the reduced haematocrit near the edge becomes smaller in proportion to the total vessel diameter and thus not significant. Due to axial accumulation the red cell-rich blood in the centre of the vessels travels faster than the plasma-rich fluid at the edge. Overall this means that red cells pass through the circulation faster on average than plasma. It also follows that at branching points in a vessel more plasma than red cells may enter a branch vessel (Fig. 15.45) so that the dynamic haematocrit of blood from small vessels is less than that of blood drawn from a main vessel. The term 'plasma skimming' is used to describe this phenomenon.

The increased viscosity with increased haematocrit is important clinically in the disease polycythaemia. Here there is excessive production of red blood cells and unless this is treated the increased blood viscosity increases the work of the heart and eventually leads to heart failure.

Length (l). Resistance increases linearly in proportion to vessel length. The anatomy of the bed determines the length of the major vessels. Although nerve stimulation reduces vessel diameter, it has no significant effect on length.

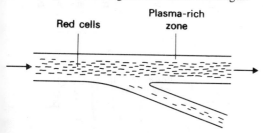

Fig. 15.45. Plasma skimming is shown at the branch which receives plasma-rich fluid from the periphery of the vessel.

Radius (r). For a given pressure head, the 4th power relationship in Poiseuille's Law (3) means that the radius has to increase only by 20% to double the flow; doubling the radius increases flow sixteen-fold. Although blood does not circulate through straight and rigid tubes, Poiseuille's relationship shows that tube radius is the single most important variable controlling blood flow.

When a vessel branches, what happens to the resistance to flow? In Fig. 15.46 the vessel AB, whose radius is 1, divides into 2 identical vessels whose total cross-sectional area equals that of the parent vessel (radius of each branch vessel is thus 0.707 of AB).The resistance to flow is proportional to $1/r^4$, i.e. $R = k/r^4$. The resistance in the parent vessel is $k/1^4 = k$. The resistance in each daughter vessel is $k/0.707^4 = k/0.25 = 4k$. If individual resistances in parallel are R_1, R_2, etc. and total resistance is Rt then

$$\frac{1}{Rt} = \frac{1}{R_1} + \frac{1}{R_2}$$

or $\quad Rt = \dfrac{1}{\dfrac{1}{R_1} + \dfrac{1}{R_2}}$

Since there are two daughter vessels the total resistance Rt is

$$Rt = \frac{1}{\frac{1}{4} + \frac{1}{4}} = 2;$$

that is, twice the resistance in the parent vessel. Flow = P/R (1). Since the flow between A and B must be the same as that between B and C, and yet the resistance is doubled, the pressure drop between A and B can only be half the pressure drop between B and C. This is true when the cross sectional area is constant and the parent vessel divides into two. Generally daughter vessels are about 0.7 of the parent diameter but there are usually more than 2 branches from each parent. If there were 4 branches in the above example the pressure drop AB would equal tht of BC, and if 8 branches the pressure drop AB would be twice that of BC. Thus although each individual vessel may have a high resistance, if they are arranged in parallel the total resistance through that bed will

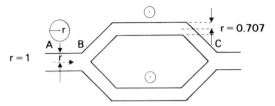

Fig. 15.46. The effect of bifurcation on resistance to flow. Cross-sectional area at A is the same at the total cross-sectional area of two branches at B.

be reduced.

In the circulation the biggest drop in pressure and hence the main peripheral resistance is sited in the arterioles (Fig. 15.47). This is discussed later in more detail. The smallest arterioles have a diameter similar to that of capillaries but capillaries only make a small contribution to the peripheral resistance as there are many capillaries arranged in parallel for each arteriole.

PRESSURES IN THE CARDIOVASCULAR SYSTEM

Fig. 15.48 shows representative values for pressures in the circulation. It is important to stress here that pressure is a dependent variable, being determined by the two independent variables, cardiac output which is synonymous with flow in this context and total peripheral resistance (see (1) again). Other variables which influence but do not control arterial pressure are blood volume, elasticity of vessels, and the viscosity of blood (p. 710).

The pressure at any point in the circulation may be determined from knowledge of the central pressures and the resistances up to and beyond that point. At the point B in Fig. 15.46 we determine the resistance of BC to be twice that of AB. If the total pressure drop across A–C is 100 units then the pressure at B is 66% that at A.

Capillary pressure
If the mid-capillary pressure is taken to be 20–25 mmHg and the total pressure drop from aorta to vena cava about 100 mmHg, we can calculate the ratio of precapillary resistance, R_a (resistance from aorta to mid-capillary measuring point) to post-capillary resistance, R_v (resistance from mid-capillary to vena cava), i.e.

$$25 = 100 \left(1 - \frac{R_a}{R_a + R_v}\right)$$

from which it can be calculated that $R_a/R_v = 3$. Similarly for 20 mmHg when R_a would be 4 times R_v. This confirms our previous statement that arterioles constitute the main site of the peripheral resistance.

Changes in the precapillary: post-capillary resistance ratio thus affect capillary pressure. An increase in the diameter of arterioles (arteriolar vasodilation) reduces R_a and hence increases capillary pressure. Capillary pressure could also be increased by an increase in R_v and when considering changes in capillary pressure both pre- and post-capillary resistances need to be borne in mind.

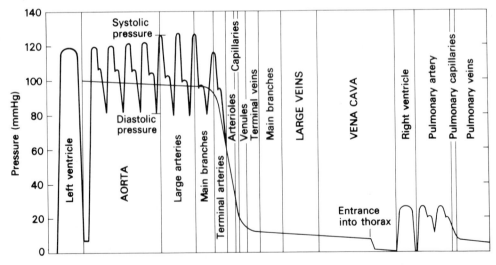

Fig. 15.47. Blood pressure in various parts of the systemic circulation. The most rapid fall in pressure, associated with loss of the pressure pulse, occurs in the arterioles.

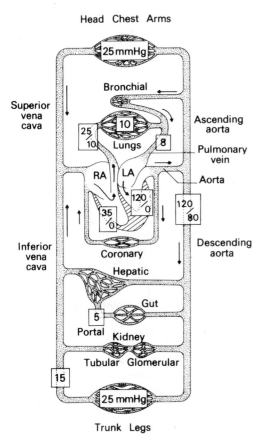

Head Chest Arms

25 mmHg

Bronchial

Superior
vena
cava

Ascending
aorta

25/10 10 Lungs 8

Pulmonary
vein

RA LA

Aorta

120/0 120/80

35/0

Inferior
vena
cava

Coronary

Descending
aorta

Hepatic

Gut

5

Portal Kidney

Tubular Glomerular

15

25 mmHg

Trunk Legs

Fig. 15.48. Diagrammatic representation of the circulation together with typical pressures in mmHg.

Control of blood flow and peripheral resistance
It will be recalled from (1) that the flow through a system is determined by the pressure head available divided by the resistance (F = P/R). Therefore in order to vary flow, pressure or resistance is varied. The vascular system is interesting in that both pressure and resistance are determined to a substantial extent by changes in the diameter of the arterioles. The total peripheral resistance (which is the algebraic summation of the resistance in all the arterioles), together with the cardiac output, determine the arterial blood pressure (i.e. BP = CO × TPR) and local resistance regulates the local blood flow. These statements will now be examined more fully.

Of the three main factors determining resistance to flow, namely blood viscosity, vessel length and vessel radius, it is the fourth power relationship of vessel radius which dominates

the situation. The arterioles largely determine the peripheral resistance and can have their diameters altered by nervous activity. The sympathetic nervous system innervates the arteriolar smooth muscle and normally is in a state of tonic activity. An increase in this activity reduces the diameter of the arterioles and hence increases the resistance, thus raising arterial blood pressure and reducing capillary pressure, as long as other factors such as cardiac output and post-capillary resistance stay constant. Conversely, a fall in sympathetic firing rate (a reduction in sympathetic 'tone') reduces resistance and arterial blood pressure and raises capillary pressure. Arterioles are often referred to as 'resistance' vessels.

The capacitance vessels
About 2/3 of the blood in the body is in the venous system at any one time. The veins and venules are known as capacitance vessels and act as a sort of reservoir. When blood leaves the capillaries it passes into the relatively thin-walled distensible venules and veins. The nearer the venous reservoir volume is to the total blood volume the more improbable it is that blood leaving the capillaries could reach the heart before the heart would stop because of lack of blood. In this situation, decreasing the volume of the venous reservoir (i.e. decreasing the venous capacitance) would mean that some blood would now reach the heart, but still at a reduced pressure; a low filling pressure means a low cardiac output and a correspondingly low arterial blood pressure (p. 710). If the capacitance were reduced still further, blood would enter the heart from the vena cava at a higher pressure and thereby be able to increase cardiac output correspondingly. The capacitance vessels, like the resistance vessels, are innervated by the sympathetic nervous system, but unlike the arterioles, changes in the diameter of the veins lead to only small changes in pressure and large changes in volume. The term 'vasomotor' applies to the sympathetic control of the smooth muscle in arteries, arterioles (precapillary vessels) and veins. Sometimes a distinction is made by referring to the control of veins as 'venomotor.'

The peripheral vasculature can thus be divided into resistance vessels and capacitance vessels. A fall in circulating blood volume from haemorrhage or severe burns leads to a fall in cardiac output and hence a reduced systemic arterial blood pressure. From the relationship BP = CO × TPR, it follows that this fall in blood pressure can be minimized or prevented by increasing arteriolar resistance, but at the expense of reducing perfusion of the micro-vascular bed. Contraction of the smooth muscle in the capacitance vessels by contrast raises ven-ous pressure, increases the return of blood to the heart and so increases cardiac output, thereby increasing blood pressure without any reduction in microvascular perfusion.

Venous return and central venous pressures

The pressure gradient between capillaries and central (great) veins is the main factor deter-mining the return of blood from the tissues to the heart. The venous capacitance vessels can accommodate a large fraction of the blood volume and on standing up a significant pooling of blood in venous vessels may occur. This would reduce the central venous pressure and hence cardiac output and blood pressure. In order to compensate for these changes various reflex mechanisms occur including a reduction in venous capacitance.

Inspiration may also aid venous return by increasing the pressure gradient in the veins. During inspiration the intrapleural pressure (intrathoracic) becomes more sub-atmospheric (p. 500). The pressure in the great veins in the thorax is decreased and thus the venous pressure gradient is increased. Vena caval blood flow is correspondingly increased. The fluctuating ven-ous pressure may be well seen in the jugular veins of the neck if a subject reclines at about 45°.

A very important mechanism for ensuring the adequacy of venous return is the skeletal muscle pump. Peripheral veins are equipped with one-way valves (Fig. 15.4), so arranged that they allow blood to flow only in the direction of the heart (Fig. 15.49). When standing still, blood distends the veins in the legs and the venous pressure rises. If the leg muscles are rhythmically contracted, this forces blood upwards and lowers the venous pressure in the legs.

THE NEED FOR MONITORING SYSTEMS

Muscular exercise

We have already seen that a fall in local resis-tance increases local flow if central arterial blood pressure remains constant. If the resistance in muscle blood vessels all over the body were halved during mild exercise then, since the muscle vasculature contributes about half the total peripheral resistance, blood pressure would fall by 25 % unless the peripheral resis-

tance in other parts of the body were simultan-eously increased. In order to allow for the big increases in muscle blood flow during exercise there are systems for monitoring arterial blood pressure so that it can be maintained constant. These baroreceptor reflexes (baro = pressure) are dealt with on p. 711.

The effect of gravity

Another example of the need for monitoring systems is that of the effect of gravity. When one stands up quickly from a sitting or lying position, a feeling of faintness or dizziness is sometimes experienced for a moment or two. This is due to a reduced blood flow to the brain consequent upon a reduced central arterial blood pressure. On standing up, blood tends to collect in the distensible capacitance vessels of the lower limbs and abdomen due to the force of gravity. Return of blood to the heart is thus reduced, cardiac output falls and hence blood pressure falls and cerebral blood flow is reduced. The faintness is usually only temporary as the fall in blood pres-sure is detected by the baroreceptors (situated between the heart and brain) in the aortic arch and carotid sinus, whose change in activity leads to vasoconstriction of both the resistance and capacitance vessels, tending to restore blood pressure and cardiac output.

Guardsmen standing 'to attention' on parade for prolonged periods in hot weather have a reputation for fainting. Here too the explanation lies in excessive pooling of blood in the capaci-tance vessels. The tendency to pool blood in the veins of the limbs is normally restricted by reflex vasoconstriction and the muscle pump. Standing still with little muscle movement in the limbs reduces or removes the contribution of the muscle pump to venous return (Fig. 15.49). In hot weather the skin receives a high blood flow to promote body cooling and this causes a low-ered overall peripheral resistance. If this is com-bined with a gradual fall in venous return due to pooling in the veins of the limb and lower abdo-men, cardiac output and blood pressure fall with the result that cerebral blood flow also falls and the guardsman faints.

Intrathoracic pressure

Several activities such as coughing, straining and lifting heavy weights, result in an increase in intrathoracic pressure which in turn reduces flow of blood to the heart. The effects (Fig. 15.66) are similar to those just described for a person who suddenly stands up.

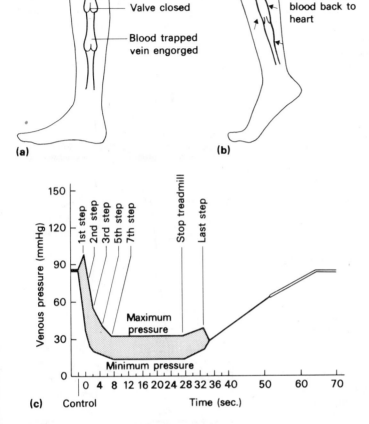

Fig. 15.49. (a) One-way valves in the veins of the leg distended in the standing position during muscle relaxation; (b) contraction forces blood back to the heart; (c) effect of muscle contraction on pressures in the foot vein in human volunteers walking on a treadmill.

The cardiac cycle

The human heart normally beats at between 60 and 80 beats/min but the rate may fall as low as 30 under pathological conditions or rise as high as 200 in extremes of exertion. Each event which takes place during what is termed the 'cardiac cycle' is thus repeated once every 2 seconds to once every 0.3 seconds. It is found that changes in the length of the cardiac cycle are achieved largely by changes in the duration of relaxation (diastole); the duration of the heart contraction (systole) is only slightly affected by rate changes.

MECHANICAL EVENTS

The myocardium contracts in an orderly sequence and the consequential pressure changes determine the opening and closing of the heart valves. The accurate coordination of these events, which is effected by the conducting sys-

tem of the heart, enables the blood to be pumped into the pulmonary and systemic circuits. Even so, the mechanical efficiency, i.e. work done/energy used is only 15–20%, which is roughly comparable to many man-made machines.

Both atria contract simultaneously as do both ventricles: the onset of atrial systole precedes the onset of ventricular systole by 0.1–0.2 seconds. Through most of the cardiac cycle, when one pair of chambers is contracting the other is relaxed, but there is a short period following ventricular and preceding atrial systole when all chambers are in diastole. During atrial diastole (and at the onset of ventricular diastole) blood flows from the great veins into the atria under a motive force provided by the pressure gradient between the veins and atria. The factors affecting central venous pressure have been briefly discussed above. While blood is flowing into the atria, the ventricular pressure is falling as the ventricles relax. Eventually atrial pressure exceeds ventricular pressure, and the atrioventricular valves open (Fig. 15.50). Blood flows into the ventricles rapidly at first, but as each ventricle becomes distended, filling slows.

Contraction of the atria follows and causes most of their contents to be expelled into the ventricles; this is the final 'topping up' phase of ventricular filling. The contribution made by atrial systole to ventricular filling is only some 20% of the total. There are no valves guarding the orifices through which the blood enters the atria. As a result there is a tendency during atrial systole for blood to regurgitate into the veins. Although this is limited by the narrowing of these orifices through contraction of the atrial musculature around them, it is sufficient in some pathological situations to give rise to visible pulsation in the neck veins—the jugular venous pulse (JVP).

At the onset of ventricular systole, the ventricular pressure exceeds that in the atria and the atrioventricular (AV) valves close. The sounds made by the mitral and tricuspid valves as they close may be heard (as a 'lub' sound) by listening with a stethoscope over the heart and together are called the first heart sound (Fig. 15.50).

After the AV valves have closed, the contraction of the ventricles is at first isovolumetric since both inflow and outflow valves are closed. This means that the myocardium contracts and the ventricular pressure rises, although the contained volume remains unchanged. The ventricular pressure rises very rapidly (0.05 sec) until it exceeds the pressure in the aorta and pulmonary arteries, thus forcing open the aortic and pulmonary outflow valves and causing blood to flow into the arteries. Ejection is at first rapid, but becomes slower as the contraction begins to weaken.

During ventricular systole, ventricular volume falls from its initial or end-diastolic volume to its final or end-systolic volume, the difference between the two being the amount of blood ejected during contraction — the stroke volume. As the ventricles start to relax the ventricular pressure falls. When it has fallen below that in the aorta and pulmonary arteries, the aortic and pulmonary valves close, so producing the second heart sound ('dup'). This is frequently heard as two separate sounds, particularly on taking a deep breath, when the aortic component precedes the pulmonary component by a short interval. Once again the ventricles become closed chambers and during this second isovolumetric phase the

ventricular pressure falls rapidly (0.1 sec). When it is less than that in the atria, the atrioventricular valves re-open and the cycle is repeated.

Not infrequently other sounds of cardiac origin may be heard. The commonest of these are 'murmurs' which are caused by turbulence of blood flowing through a narrowed valve orifice

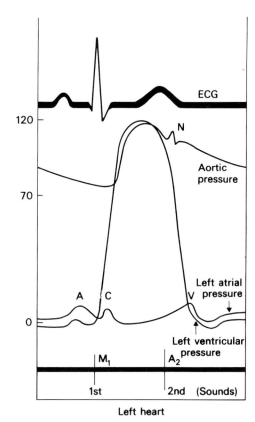

Fig. 15.50. The relationships between atrial, ventricular and arterial pressure changes during one heart beat are shown for the left side of the heart. Atrial systole is denoted by a rise in atrial pressure (A) which produces a small increase in ventricular pressure. Following closure of the atrio-ventricular valves, the ventricular pressure rises, and when it exceeds that in the arteries, forces open the arterial valves. Thus the ventricular pressure leads the arterial pressure on the upstroke. When the ventricular pressure passes its peak, the arterial pressure becomes greater and thus the lines cross. A small amount of blood regurgitates into the ventricles before the arterial valves close. The dicrotic notch (N) is a vibration which can be detected in the aortic pressure waveform and is caused by closure of the aortic valve. The atrial pressure reaches a peak (V) as it becomes distended with venous blood before the atrioventricular valves open and allow blood to enter the ventricles. The electrical activity (ECG) is described later in the text.

(stenosis) or leakage of blood past a poorly closed valve (incompetence).

The changing pressures in the aorta, atrium and left ventricle during one cardiac cycle are shown in Fig. 15.50. The form of those in the right ventricle and pulmonary artery are similar but have a peak pressure of some 35 mmHg (4.7 kPa) as compared to about 120 mmHg (16 kPa) in the systemic circulation.

ELECTRICAL EVENTS

Myocardial action potential
The shape of the myocardial action potential differs markedly from that of a nerve (Fig. 15.51), and it follows that the ionic movements which cause it must also differ.

The depolarization phase is similar to that in nerve, as is the over-shoot, and the ionic movements consist principally of Na^+ entering the cells. Repolarization is initially also similar, but soon differs, as a plateau is formed at about zero potential. This lasts for some 100 msec before the cell continues to repolarize and returns to resting potential. What causes the plateau is not completely clear, but a second rise in Na^+ permeability is certainly one factor, together with a rise in Ca^{2+} permeability. As these two ions

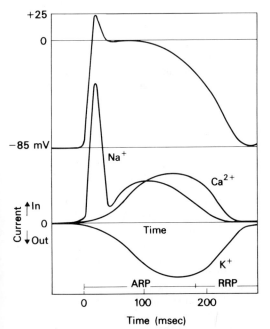

Fig. 15.51. Form of myocardial action potential. Note the plateau phase during which the transmembrane potential changes only slowly. The duration of the absolute (ARP) and relative (RRP) refractory periods is indicated.

enter the cell, K^+ leaves and the net result is that the transmembrane potential undergoes little change (plateau). However, eventually the K^+ efflux swamps the Ca^{2+} and Na^+ influx and repolarization is effected. (Fig. 15.51).

The prolonged action potential means that the refractory period of cardiac muscle is much longer than that of nerve and skeletal muscle. The myocardial cell is absolutely refractory until the final phase of repolarization and this state lasts until the mechanical contraction has passed its peak, thus making it impossible under normal circumstances to elicit sustained (tetanic) contraction in cardiac muscle. This special feature is important since tetanus of the myocardium would prevent any effective pumping by the heart.

Conduction system
The complexity of the cardiac cycle makes it necessary for the relationship between the various events to be synchronized. Thus there must be a means both for initiating regular contractions of the myocardium at a rate that is appropriate to the immediate requirements of the body and for co-ordinating the activation of all the chambers of the heart in relation to this signal.

The anatomical components of the excitatory and conducting system of the heart have been considered (p. 640). The electrical impulse originates in the SA node, and passes through the atrial myocardium causing it to contract (Fig. 15.52). The impulse passes on to the AV node where it is delayed by the low rate of conduction in this tissue. This allows the atria sufficient time to expel their contents into the ventricles before the ventricles start to contract.

The impulse leaves the AV node via the bundle of His and then passes along the bundle branches to the ventricles. This initiates a contraction which starts at the apex of the heart and moves towards the base of the ventricles at the atrioventricular fibrous ring. Relaxation then begins in the ventricles spreading upwards from the apex towards the base of the heart.

There is no specialized conducting pathway supplying each individual cell yet the electrical impulse moves throughout each cell (intracellular conduction) and from one cell to its neighbours (intercellular conduction).

Intracellular conduction. In the region of a depolarization the transmembrane potential is reversed. Since the fluid media on both sides of the membrane are conductors, an electrical

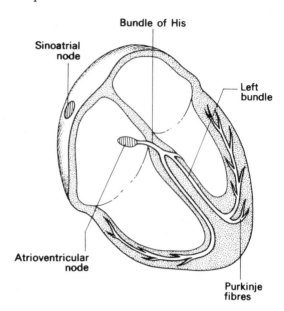

Fig. 15.52. The conducting system of the heart.

gradient is created between the adjacent oppositely charged regions of the membrane which causes charged particles to move (Fig. 15.53). These ion movements are sometimes called 'local currents'. They cause the transmembrane potential of the region from which these ions come to be reduced until this neighbouring segment reaches its firing potential. Once the impulse is moving it always proceeds unidirectionally since the region from which it has just come is refractory and thus temporarily inexcitable. In this way the depolarization spreads across the whole surface area of the membrane, whatever its shape.

Intercellular conduction. Each myocardial cell must be stimulated by a neighbour. Intercellular transmission takes place in the heart because the cells are joined to each other by special structures called intercalated discs. These junctions allow the cells to be structurally separate but provide pathways of very low resistance so that

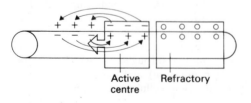

Active centre   Refractory

⟵——————— Movement of action potential

Fig. 15.53. Constraint in movement of charged particles around the active centre caused by the presence of a refractory zone. This keeps the active centre moving always in the same direction.

ions may pass freely. Thus the action potential is propagated from one cell through the discs to its neighbours. Since electrical impulses can travel freely throughout the myocardial mass the heart is often described as being a functional syncytium.

Although there is extensive cell to cell conduction in the heart the presence of the anatomical conduction system in the mammalian ventricle enables many points in the myocardium to be stimulated simultaneously in a precisely synchronized sequence. By this means the impulse is propagated throughout the heart and the necessary time delays are introduced. But how does the impulse arise in the first place?

Pacemakers

If the heart is removed from an animal immediately after death it continues to beat as long as it is kept in a physiological solution and supplied with oxygen. Even if dissected into its component parts, each part continues to beat separately although only one section contains the SA node or pacemaker. We can say, therefore, that cardiac tissue possesses an inherent or intrinsic rhythmicity which means that in the absence of any driving impulse it continues to generate its own electrical stimuli. In fact it seems that this property resides not in any heart muscle cell but chiefly in those that constitute part of the conduction network, although some atrial myocardial fibres around the SA node may also show intrinsic activity.

Microelectrodes inserted into isolated cells of

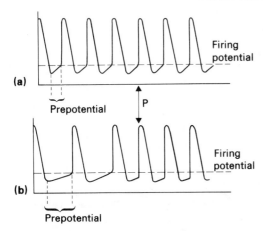

Fig. 15.54. The form of the pacemaker potential showing the regular action potentials, prepotential and firing potentials, and the result of connecting together two pacemakers (a) and (b) of different rates. At P they are connected and the slower pacemaker (b) is then triggered by the faster (a) thus synchronizing the two. The different prepotential slopes are retained but the effective firing potential of (b) is reduced.

the conduction system show that they undergo a sequence of changes which results in regular depolarizations. It can be shown that their resting membrane potential is unstable and decays progressively until it reaches its firing potential. Following each depolarization it returns to its resting potential but once again this is unstable and decays: thus the cycle repeats itself (Fig. 15.54). The phase between the end of one action potential and the start of the next is termed the pre-potential and it is the sloping nature of this that endows the cell with intrinsic rhythmicity. The slope of the pacemaker prepotential defines its intrinsic rate, since the steeper the slope, the sooner the firing potential is reached. The slope of the pacemaker pre-potential is affected by many factors such as temperature, catecholamines and acetylcholine (Fig. 15.55) but its origin is not known for certain.

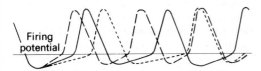

Fig. 15.55. The effects of the transmitters acetylcholine and adrenaline on the form of the pacemaker potential. Acetylcholine (– –) reduces the prepotential slope thus reducing the discharge frequency and adrenaline (— —) increases it so increasing the discharge frequency.

Although many potential pacemakers are present in the heart, a synchronous rate of firing is achieved. This can be explained if we consider two pacemaker cells with unequal firing rates connected to one another. The one with the faster rate will cause the slower one to depolarize prematurely and the two cells will thereafter continue to depolarize at the same rate (Fig. 15.54). The SA node, which is the pacemaker with the fastest intrinsic rate of depolarization and repolarization, will control the heart unless for any reason another group of pacemakers start to depolarize at a faster fate.

Alternative pacemakers. If conduction between the atria and the ventricles is prevented, such as in the clinical condition of complete heart block, these alternative pacemakers take over and drive the ventricles although at a much slower rate. Sometimes, because of disease, but more often than not for no apparent reason, additional pacemakers may take over control of the heart for a period. Any such pacemaker is termed an 'ectopic' focus.

Length-tension relationships
The contractile elements and processes of excitation–contraction coupling in cardiac muscle do not differ materially from those described for skeletal muscle (p. 337). However, in skeletal muscle all the fibres are orientated with their long axes in the same direction, but in cardiac muscle the fibre axes vary through some 180° between the endocardium and epicardium. Thus tension is not generated in any one plane but in all directions throughout the myocardium. It also follows that stretching the muscle in one plane only stretches those sarcomeres which have their long axes in that plane.

When cardiac sarcomere length is increased the active tension generated at first increases, but after the peak is reached the tension declines with further extension of the sarcomeres. Thus on the rising part of the curve, stretching the muscle causes it to contract more strongly when stimulated, but over-stretching causes the myocardium to 'fail' and the tension declines. We can now see why an increase in central venous pressure, which aids ventricular filling and leads to a rise in the end-diastolic volume, affects myocardial performance (p. 698). To start with, the additional stretching of the myocardial fibres increases the force of contraction and so increases the cardiac output if all other factors remain constant (e.g. peripheral resistance). Beyond a certain point, however, further increase in the venous pressure, and hence the myocardial fibre stretch, fails to augment performance and may, in fact, be detrimental to myocardial function. This is part of the explanation for the falling output and disordered myocardial dynamics seen in heart failure.

THE ELECTROCARDIOGRAM (ECG)

Skeletal muscle contracts as a result of the asynchronous depolarization of many muscle fibres. There is no definable time relationship between the depolarization of individual fibres so that the surface recording (electromyogram–EMG) consists of a multitude of spikes in an apparently random pattern (p. 342).

The electrical events of the heart differ since large groups of myocardial cells depolarize in a sequential fashion and an organized wave of depolarization sweeps through the myocardium in a particular direction. This electrical activity is intense enough to be detected at any point on the surface of the body since the body fluids act as suitable conductors.

The leads

The form which the ECG assumes depends on whether the waves of depolarization and repolarization are sweeping towards or away from the recording electrode and the angle which the plane of depolarization makes with it. The electrocardiogram may be detected as a potential difference between any two points on the body surface, and displayed on a paper trace using suitable amplification and recording equipment. The standard limb leads are as follows:

Lead I; Left arm (+ ve), Right arm (− ve).
Lead II; Right arm (− ve), left leg (+ ve).
Lead III; Left arm (− ve), left leg (+ ve).

Let us see how the electrical activity of the heart may appear when viewed by these electrode arrangements. By convention, when an electrical wave is moving towards an electrode it produces a deflection of the same polarity as that electrode. Thus for example in lead I, as the atria depolarize from the SA node towards the apex, the wave is moving towards the left arm and away from the right arm so producing a positive deflection. Similarly in lead III as the ventricles depolarize from the apex towards the base of the heart, the wave is moving towards the left arm and away from the left leg so producing a negative deflection, and so on.

The classical form of the ECG for descriptive purposes is taken from lead I (Fig. 15.56). The

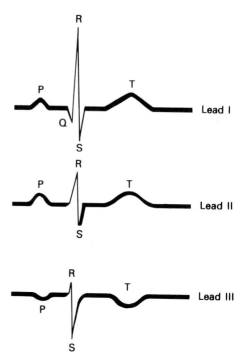

Fig. 15.56. Electrocardiogram traces from the standard limb leads (see text).

various peaks and troughs which may be seen on this diagram are labelled by convention P, Q, R, S and T, although all of these are not necessarily present in any particular ECG lead. The P-wave which develops shortly before the large easily identified QRS complex, is produced by atrial depolarization. The interval between this wave and the positive peak of the QRS complex (R-wave) is called the PR interval and is normally 0.12–0.2 secs in duration. This delay stems mainly from the long conduction time at the AV node: excitation of the bundle of His and bundle branches is rapid. The QRS complex results from depolarization spreading to different parts of the ventricular myocardium and may assume a wide variety of forms in pathological conditions. During the S–T interval, all parts of the ventricles remain depolarized, and the consequent absence of net movements of charged ions should normally cause this segment to be 'isoelectric', which means that following the S wave the trace should return to the baseline from which it started. The T-wave which follows is generally of low amplitude and long duration and of the same polarity as the P-wave. It represents the process of ventricular repolarization.

In order to provide additional information about the heart it is customary to use a different system of leads. A chest lead is positioned at one of six sites so that it overlies different parts of the ventricles. The potential difference is recorded between this and a zero reference electrode which is connected to all of the limbs. The chest lead is therefore really unipolar and by convention it is made positive. Relative positivity of the chest electrodes gives an upward deflection in the record. Since each lead is recording the same electrical event, why is there a need for multiple leads? The answer is that the contribution of each segment of heart muscle to a particular lead varies, being greatest in the lead overlying that segment. One lead can show up a disorder in a particular part of the myocardium better than another.

Uses of the ECG

Many abnormalities of cardiac function may be detected by analysis of the ECG. These include variations in rate or rhythm, the order and temporal relationship of atrial and ventricular contraction and in the electrical events occurring in specific areas of the myocardium. This last group embraces a wide variety of pathological disorders including myocardial infarction (local tissue death), intraventricular conduction defects and many others.

Cardiac output

Cardiac output is the volume of blood flowing through the circulation in unit time. In the absence of abnormal communications (shunts) between the pulmonary and systemic circulations, cardiac output is thus the output of either the right or the left ventricle, or the flow through the pulmonary or systemic circulations. In the healthy adult at rest, this amounts to about 5 dm³/min (litres per minute), and during severe exercise may increase to 25 dm³/min or more.

Cardiac output = stroke volume × heart rate

Changes in cardiac output may thus be produced by changes in either stroke volume or heart rate, or both.

While there is considerable individual variation, the average resting cardiac output of 5 litres per minute is achieved with a stroke volume of about 70 cm³ and a heart rate of about 70 beats per minute. During exercise, heart rate may increase to a maximum of 180 per minute, with an increase in stroke volume up to about 120

cm³. This would allow a four to five fold increase in cardiac output.

MEASUREMENT OF CARDIAC OUTPUT

A number of methods are in clinical use, and each has its advantages and disadvantages.

One of the first reliable methods to be developed was based on the Fick principle, which states that the blood flow through an organ is equal to the quantity of a substance added to or removed from the blood in unit time by the organ divided by the difference in the arterial and venous concentrations of that substance.

For example, in measuring pulmonary blood flow (cardiac output), one can measure the oxygen consumption and the concentrations of oxygen in blood entering and leaving the lungs. Oxygen consumption is usually measured with a spirometer (Fig. 18.1a); a sample of arterial blood may be collected from any convenient artery to measure the oxygen concentration of blood leaving the lungs, while that of blood entering the lungs requires the insertion of a catheter along a peripheral vein into the right atrium or preferably the pulmonary artery to collect 'mixed venous blood'. Then:

$$\frac{\text{Cardiac}}{\text{output}} = \frac{\text{oxygen consumption}}{\text{arterio-venous oxygen difference}}$$

Some typical figures for a healthy individual are:

$$\frac{0.25 \text{ dm}^3\text{min}^{-1}}{(0.20 - 0.15) \text{ dm}^3.\text{dm}^{-3}} = 5 \text{ dm}^3\text{min}^{-1}$$

or in other units

$$\frac{(250 \text{ cm}^3/\text{min})}{(5 \text{ cm}^3/100 \text{ cm}^3)} = (5 \text{ l/min})$$

The advantage of the Fick principle is its simplicity and accuracy. Its disadvantages are that it is applicable only under steady-state conditions and hence cannot follow rapid changes in cardiac output, and that it is necessary to catheterize the pulmonary artery. For this reason, it is usually only used when there are other reasons for cardiac catheterization, such as the measurement of pressures in the right side of the heart, and the detection of shunts in patients with suspected congenital heart disease.

The indicator dilution technique is another method of measuring cardiac output. A known quantity of a suitable substance such as a coloured dye or radio-isotope is injected rapidly into a large systemic vein, and its concentration on reappearance in a large systemic artery is plotted against time.

$$\text{Flow (cm}^3\text{/sec)} = \frac{I \ (\text{mg})}{C \ (\text{mg/cm}^3) \ \times \ t \ (\text{sec})}$$

where I = the quantity of indicator injected, C = the mean concentration of the indicator and t = the time under the curve. Ct may be measured graphically as the area under the curve. The advantages of this method are that it is necessary to puncture only a peripheral artery and a vein, and that several rapid successive measurements of cardiac output can be made.

Other techniques of measuring cardiac output (such as ultrasound and doppler flow velocity sensors) are being developed, and these may soon lead to non-invasive measurements of cardiac output in man.

FACTORS DETERMINING CARDIAC OUTPUT

The main mechanisms which are usually considered to determine cardiac output are summarized in Fig. 15.57. Of these, the heart rate, arterial (aortic) pressure, and the filling pressures of the ventricles (central venous and pulmonary venous pressures) can all be measured in the intact animal or man, but the size of the two ventricles at the end of diastole and at the peak of systole can as yet only be directly measured in the experimental heart preparation.

The 'distensibility' of the relaxed ventricle, and its subsequent 'contractility' are terms which have proved difficult to define, let alone measure. As a result, much of the evidence on the control of cardiac output depends on studies of anaesthetized animals or isolated heart preparations. While much information has been obtained from such experiments, there is considerable controversy over the applicability of

some of this to cardiac control in conscious, intact man.

The experimental evidence will be briefly described and an attempt made to achieve some synthesis.

Factors affecting stroke volume
In the heart-lung preparation of the dog (Fig. 15.58) the heart beats at a constant rate, being deprived both of its nerve supply and sources of adrenaline and noradrenaline. The volume changes of the two ventricles are measured and hence their average stroke volume is determined.

On raising the venous reservoir and hence increasing the filling pressure of the right ventricle, Starling found an increase in both end-diastolic and end-systolic volumes of the ventricles, but the overall result was an increase in stroke volume. A greater diastolic volume of the heart thus resulted in the ejection of a larger volume of blood, against a fixed resistance in the arterial system. In other experiments, the venous pressure was kept constant while the outflow resistance was increased; i.e. the blood pressure against which the ventricle had to eject its blood was increased. This resulted in increased diastolic and systolic volumes of the ventricles but little change in stroke volume. In both these situations, the increased diastolic volume resulted in either an increase in the volume ejected, or in the load being overcome; that is, an increase in the work done during that contraction. Starling concluded: 'The law of the heart is thus the same as the law of muscular tissue generally–that the energy of contraction, however measured, is a function of the length of the muscle fibre.'

Starling's findings have been repeatedly confirmed by other workers. Sarnoff and Mitchell have demonstrated that the output of the isolated heart is also increased by infused

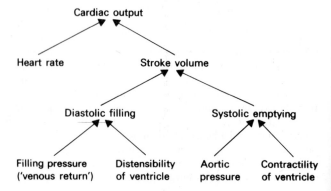

Fig. 15.57. Some factors influencing cardiac output.

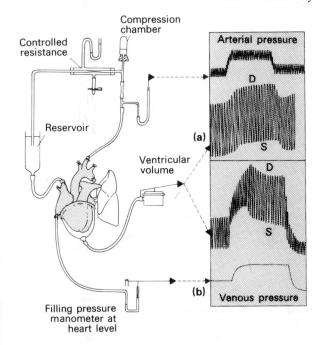

Fig. 15.58. Diagram of the heart-lung preparation (left), and on the right, typical changes in the ventricular volume (D=diastolic; S=systolic) during (a) increased output resistance and (b) increased venous filling pressure. (After Starling E. H. from R. F. Rushmer (1972) *Structure and function of the Cardiovascular System.* Saunders, Philadelphia.

adrenaline. However, these workers did not apportion the contribution made to the overall change in cardiac output to changes in stroke volume and heart rate.

In the intact circulation the performance of the heart is affected by the autonomic nerve supply to the heart and the presence of circulating adrenaline. Adrenaline enhances cardiac output at all levels of filling pressure by enhancing the 'contractility' of the myocardium.

Adrenaline or noradrenaline increases the speed and shortens the duration of contraction of isolated heart muscle. It is possible, at least in an isolated heart, to achieve the same stroke volume by a more complete emptying of a relatively small ventricle (in which case the end-

systolic size is reduced) or a small contraction of a dilated ventricle (Fig. 15.59).

Factors affecting heart rate
In the intact individual, both divisions of the autonomic nervous system exert a continuous influence (tone) on heart rate. Increase in vagal activity liberates more acetylcholine which slows the heart rate, while sympathetic stimulation liberates noradrenaline which increases heart rate. Thus the heart rate at any moment depends on the balance between the slowing effects of vagal discharge and the accelerating effects of sympathetic discharge (Fig. 15.60).

The sympathetic fibres accelerating heart rate have their origin in poorly localized sites in the

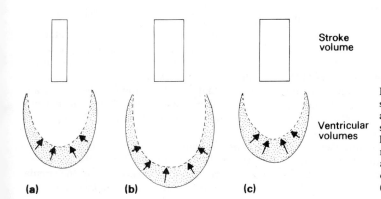

Fig. 15.59. Two ways by which stroke volume can be increased above the normal (a); a relatively small degree of contraction of a large dilated ventricle (b) may result in a stroke volume as large as that from more complete contraction of a smaller ventricle (c).

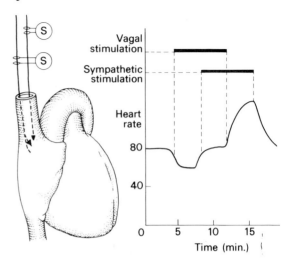

Fig. 15.60. Vagal stimulation produces slowing of the heart rate, which is counteracted by sympathetic stimulation. The heart rate thus depends on the balance between the effects of the sympathetic and parasympathetic on the pacemaker. (After R. F. Rushmer (1972) *Structure and function of the Cardiovascular System.* Saunders, Philadelphia.

medulla close to the motor nucleus of the vagus nerve; these areas are often collectively termed the 'cardio-regulatory or cardiac centre' of the medulla. Because of the widespread distribution of the sympathetic supply to the heart, increased sympathetic activity not only increases the heart rate, but has a direct effect on improving the performance of the heart as a whole. These effects include an increase in the rate of conduction of the impulse from SA node to AV node and hence to ventricular muscle, and also an increase in the rate and force of contraction of the ventricles. However, increased sympathetic activity tends to reduce the size of the ventricle just before contraction so that despite the ventricle emptying itself more completely under sympathetic stimulation, the two effects tend almost to cancel out and there may be little change in stroke volume. Hence the increase in cardiac output on sympathetic stimulation is mainly effected by the increase in heart rate.

The vagus nerves supply the SA and AV nodes and atrial muscle; there is no clear evidence of parasympathetic nerve supply to the ventricles. Parasympathetic stimulation does not affect the force of ventricular contraction. At rest, vagal control of heart rate predominates, resulting in a slow rate. In trained athletes, vagal tone may be particularly marked, accounting for resting heart rates as low as 50 per minute in some persons. Interruption of vagal activity by cutting the vagus nerves in experimental animals, or blocking the action of the vagus with atropine, releases the heart from vagal restraint and the rate rises to approach the inherent rhythm of the SA node.

The 'cardiac centres' in the medulla have numerous connections with other parts of the brain. Fear, anxiety, depression, excitement and the anticipation of exercise may all affect heart rate (and cardiac performance) without any direct relation to the metabolic requirements of the body. There are also connections with the vasomotor centre, and with afferent nerves from aortic and carotid baroreceptors (p 711); a fall in blood pressure, for example, results not only in peripheral vasoconstriction but also in increased heart rate (tachycardia) and hence cardiac output. Conversely, a rise in blood pressure results in a reduction in heart rate (bradycardia) and cardiac output, brought about by decreased sympathetic activity and increased vagal activity.

Heart rate can also be altered by factors acting directly on the SA node rather than through the CNS. Temperature and circulating adrenaline act in this way.

CONTROL OF CARDIAC OUTPUT IN MAN

Having discussed some of the factors determining cardiac output it now remains to assess their relative contributions in the control of cardiac output in man. A useful approach is to examine changes that have been found in heart rate and stroke volume first during changes in posture, and second during exercise.

Posture. When a subject lies down, there is a considerable shift of blood from the periphery, into the central 'capacitance' part of the circulation, namely the large abdominal veins, the pulmonary veins and the heart; all of these dilate to hold this increased volume of blood which may be 500 cm³ or more. The ventricles are stretched and eject more blood with each heart beat, i.e. stroke volume is increased. In addition, vagal control of the heart now preponderates over the sympathetic, and the heart rate slows.

On standing up, blood tends to accumulate in dependent parts of the circulation under the influence of gravity, especially the lower limbs, and the capacity of the heart shrinks. Venous return is temporarily reduced and there is a tendency for cardiac output and hence blood pressure to fall. This is monitored by low pressure receptors in the great veins and by arterial baroreceptors (p. 711) which reduce their rate of firing and hence reduce their inhibition of the vasomotor centre. Sympathetic activity thus increases, causing (a) reflex venoconstriction, so restoring venous return to the heart, (b) increased overall peripheral resistance, (c) increased heart rate and (d) increased degree of emptying of the ventricles. Thus in these ways blood pressure is maintained at a normal level. The stroke volume is decreased in the upright posture because of the smaller capacity of the ventricle, despite its greater degree of emptying during systole. As a result of the increased heart rate, however, cardiac output is only slightly reduced. All of these responses reflect greater sympathetic activity in the upright posture.

Exercise. The extent to which changes in cardiac output during exercise are dependent on changes in heart rate or stroke volume appears to depend largely on the posture in which it is performed. During moderate exercise in the supine position, the increase in cardiac output is due almost entirely to an increase in heart rate, stroke volume remaining almost constant. However, during even mild exercise in the erect position stroke volume increases to the level found in the supine state. Thereafter, increasing amounts of exercise in the normal untrained individual produce little change in stroke volume, most of the increased cardiac output being due to increased heart rate. On the other hand, trained athletes, who have larger diastolic volumes at rest and accompanying slow heart rates, are more able to increase their stroke volume during exercise and hence do not develop such high heart rates for a given level of exercise.

There is, however, still much controversy about this subject. Each of the several schools of thought places emphasis on a different mechanism of cardiac control. Included in these are: (a) those who emphasize the venous return to the heart and suggest that when this increases, the heart increases its output by the Starling-type mechanism because of the increased filling and hence stretching of the ventricles just prior to contraction. (b) The key role of the baroreceptors is stressed by some workers. For example, a fall in arterial blood pressure induced by local dilatation of skeletal muscle blood vessels during exercise is monitored, and through the baroreceptor reflex changes in heart rate are initiated in order to maintain blood pressure at a normal level. (c) Another group emphasizes the importance of the central nervous system in controlling the rate and force of contraction of the heart.

It is perhaps unwise at this stage to emphasize any single viewpoint to the detriment of others.

Arterial blood pressure

Arterial pressure wave
With each beat the heart pumps blood into the arterial system and creates a pressure wave which moves much faster than blood, just as a ripple on a pond may travel rapidly over still water. As the wave passes each point its energy distends the arterial wall as the 'pulse', but when it has passed, the elastic wall recoils.

Near the heart, the pressure wave (Fig. 15.61) shows a sharp upstroke. Its fall is interrupted by a small rise in pressure due to vibrations set up when the aortic valve snaps shut, the dicrotic wave. This wave is not seen more distally because the wave form is modified by reflections set up as the arteries branch.

The character of the pulse wave is useful clinically (Fig. 15.62). For example, if the aortic valve is narrowed (aortic stenosis) blood can only be pumped into the aorta slowly and the pulse wave is small with a slow upstroke. If the

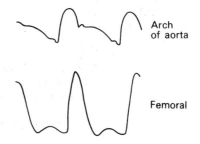

Fig. 15.61. Pulse waves recorded by high frequency catheter-tip manometer in dog. Upper trace: arch of aorta. Lower trace: femoral artery.

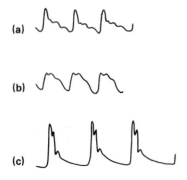

(a)

(b)

(c)

Fig. 15.62. Arterial pulse in aortic valve disease. (a) Normal radial pulse; (b) pulse in aortic stenosis; (c) 'water-hammer pulse', aortic incompetence.

aortic valve allows blood to leak back into the left ventricle during diastole (aortic incompetence) arterial pressure rises sharply and falls away rapidly; the difference between the peak (systolic) and minimum (diastolic) pressures, the pulse pressure, is much greater than normal and the excursions of the artery wall can be felt as a 'water hammer pulse'. When the elasticity of the arterial wall is reduced as in the degenerative condition of atherosclerosis, there is less 'give' in the vessels during systole and also less recoil in diastole; both the upstroke and the dicrotic wave are reduced in size.

ARTERIAL BLOOD PRESSURE

Arterial blood pressure is the force per unit area that the blood exerts on the artery wall. It depends upon (a) the volume of blood forced into the arteries (cardiac output) and reflects the energy imparted by the heart to drive the blood round the circulation, and (b) the 'total peripheral resistance', that is the state of all the arterioles of the body which together control the flow of blood to the tissues. Without a certain level of peripheral resistance blood pressure falls too low to perfuse the tissues. In some forms of shock there is generalized dilatation of resistance vessels and blood pressure falls precipitously, sometimes to lethal levels. Usually organs have high blood flows only when active and indeed there is not enough blood in the body to fill all the capillaries if these were to be opened up at the same time.

Figs. 15.47 and 15.48 show the pressure gradients in the circulation. Pressure (energy) is lost as blood flows, chiefly because work is needed to move the viscous fluid against vessel walls.

It has already been mentioned that blood flow near the heart is intermittent or 'pulsatile'. The walls of the aorta and larger arteries are elastic and are expanded by blood ejected at each beat of the ventricles. In diastole, pressure falls and flow slows, and the elastic recoil of the vessel walls helps to force blood along. The elasticity gradually evens out the pulsatile flow through the more peripheral parts of the arterial system so that flow in the arterioles is almost steady.

Measurement of blood pressure in man

During operation on the cardiovascular system and in the intensive therapy unit, blood pressure may be measured directly through a catheter inserted into an artery, but in other circumstances an indirect method is used. The sphygmomanometer is the most important instrument for measuring blood pressure clinically (Fig. 15.63). A pressure cuff is wrapped around the upper arm and inflated until the radial pulse disappears and all blood flow to the limb is stopped. The pressure in the cuff is then slowly reduced while listening with a stethoscope over the brachial artery at the elbow. Nothing is heard until the cuff pressure falls just below systolic pressure. Blood then begins to flow under the cuff at systole only and its turbulent spurts are heard as the Korotkov sounds. The cuff pressure is read on the sphygmomanometer scale. Flow finally becomes continuous and smooth as the cuff is deflated below diastolic pressure and as it does these sounds become first muffled and then finally disappear. The point of disappearance of the sounds is often slightly nearer true diastolic pressure (measured by arterial catheter) but many clinicians prefer to take the point of muffling because in a few people the sounds do not disappear until well below the true diastolic pressure. The sphygmomanometer measures brachial artery pressure relative to atmospheric with an accuracy of $\pm$ 5 mmHg. Measurements are altered by the position of the arm relative to that of the heart.

The mean arterial blood pressure is not simply the mean of the systolic (SP) and diastolic pressures (DP). The shape of the arterial pressure tracing (Fig. 15.62a) shows that it is more complicated. The descending limb of the curve has a longer duration than the rising limb so that the mean pressure is best described by the approximate equation

$$\text{mean BP} = \text{DP} + \frac{(\text{SP} - \text{DP})}{3}$$

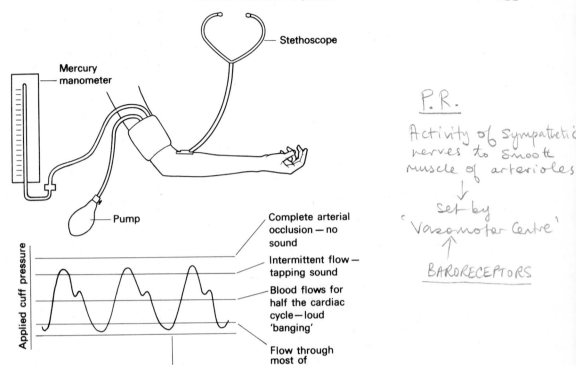

Fig. 15.63. Sphygmomanometer.

Factors affecting systolic blood pressure

The most important physiological variable affecting systolic arterial pressure is the stroke volume. The more blood the heart pumps into the arterial tree at each beat the higher the pressure rises. Increased stroke volume is an important cause of the high pressures often associated with exercise (see below). The stiffness of the arterial wall also determines the systolic rise, but this is not a physiological variable. Arterial walls tend to 'harden' with increasing age.

Maintenance of diastolic blood pressure

Because the blood pressure falls steadily between beats, it follows that the interval between beats, i.e. the heart rate, within certain limits is an important factor determining diastolic pressure. The other major factor is the ease with which blood can 'run-out' of the arterial system into the tissues. This depends upon both the viscosity of the blood and the total peripheral resistance. If the arterioles are constricted, diastolic pressure remains high, but if they are dilated, pressure falls.

Peripheral resistance is principally regulated by the activity of sympathetic nerves to the smooth muscle of arterioles. The level of sympathetic activity is set by the vasomotor centre, an area of the brain stem which integrates the activity of many afferent pathways, particularly those from the arterial baroreceptors.

Baroreceptors and chemoreceptors in the control of blood pressure

Arterial blood pressure is influenced from moment to moment by reflexes acting on heart rate and peripheral vascular tone. In addition, hormonal responses, acting over longer periods, regulate renal salt and water loss and hence indirectly, blood pressure.

Blood pressure reflexes depend on groups of stretch receptors in the arterial walls of which the most important are in the carotid sinus (Fig. 15.64) where they sense the pressure of blood circulating to the brain. Other important arterial stretch receptors are in the aortic arch and subclavian vessels.

The carotid sinus is a highly specialized organ. Its tunica media has relatively little smooth mus-

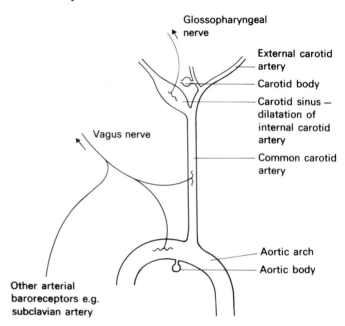

Fig. 15.64. Arterial baroreceptors and chemoreceptors.

Other arterial baroreceptors e.g. subclavian artery

cle but is rich in elastin fibres so that it is more distensible than a normal artery and therefore a more sensitive stretch receptor. Its adventitia has three layers. From the inner layer (rich in elastin) and the middle layer (rich in collagen) arise afferent nerve fibres which are predominantly myelinated. From the outer layer which is also rich in collagen, but has scattered smooth muscle cells in addition, arise afferent nerve fibres which are predominantly unmyelinated.

For technical reasons, only myelinated fibres have been studied in most experiments. At low blood pressures they are silent but they discharge rhythmically once the carotid sinus pressure exceeds a threshold value (Fig. 15.65). Frequency of firing increases with increasing pressure until a maximum frequency is reached. Impulses pass to the brain stem in the glossopharyngeal nerve while other baroreceptor afferents join the vagus. Activity caused by increased blood pressure acts on the brain stem 'centres' controlling blood pressure so that it

falls (depressor reflex). The afferents of this feedback loop are sometimes termed 'buffer nerves' by analogy to the system that minimizes change of plasma pH.

Stimulation of several areas in the brain stem alters arterial blood pressure. A pool of neurons has been found in the dorsal motor nucleus of the vagus nerve (or in the nucleus ambiguus in some species), often for convenience referred to as the 'cardioinhibitory or cardiac centre', but this is a misleading term. When the baroreceptor nerves are stimulated these neurons are activated; the heart is slowed and blood pressure falls. Another larger diffuse region in the medulla and pons has both pressor and depressor areas. The name vasomotor 'centre' has been applied to this. When isolated from afferent activity these 'centres' fire spontaneously giving rise to the tonic sympathetic vasoconstrictor activity that underlies peripheral vascular tone. If the sino-aortic afferents are cut this tonic activity increases and blood pressure rises partly because of tachy-

Fig. 15.65. Baroreceptor afferent discharge. Single fibre recording from carotid sinus nerve (bottom trace) shown with femoral arterial pressure (middle trace). Upper trace: 50 cycles per second.

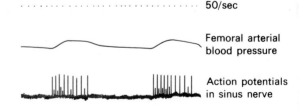

50/sec

Femoral arterial blood pressure

Action potentials in sinus nerve

cardia due to decreased vagal tone and also because of peripheral vasoconstriction. If the baroreceptors are stimulated by a rise in blood pressure, vasomotor tone is decreased. It seems then that the inherent activity of the vasomotor centre is normally kept in check by afferent nerve stimulation from baroreceptors which are responding to the 'normal' arterial pressure.

The circulatory changes on moving from the supine to the upright position are chiefly due to baroreceptor reflexes. On moving from the horizontal to upright posture the pressure in the carotid sinus and the aortic arch falls because of venous pooling and reduced cardiac output. At once, baroreceptor nerve activity is reduced and a pressor reflex is induced in which the brain stem centres restore arterial pressure by bringing about generalized sympathetic vasoconstriction and by increasing heart rate.

Some diseases, for example, diabetes mellitus and chronic lead poisoning, cause degeneration of autonomic nerve fibres. Baroreceptor reflexes may then be reduced leading to a fall in blood pressure on standing up — 'postural hypotension'. If this is severe there may be insufficient cerebral blood flow which causes feelings of faintness or even collapse.

Mild postural hypotension is usually present for a few days after a prolonged period of bed rest; the pressor reflex is sluggish at first but soon revives. The changes in strength of the baroreceptor reflex under these circumstances develop very gradually, but there is evidence that other mechanisms can adjust its responsiveness more quickly. For example, blood pressure falls a little in sleep but the body does not respond with tachycardia and vasoconstriction. Similarly the higher blood pressures associated with exercise do not cause bradycardia and generalized vasodilation. The way by which the body alters the sensitivity of the baroreceptor reflex is the subject of current research. One possibility is that the properties of the reflex are changed within the central nervous system; another is that the sensitivity of the stretch receptors is altered by sympathetic nerves causing contraction of smooth muscle fibres near these receptors in the artery walls.

Low pressure or volume receptors are located in the atria at the junction with the great veins. These discharge in response to filling of the atria. When venous return is increased a depressor reflex is induced; there is bradycardia and vasodilatation which cause a fall in blood pressure and venodilation which reduces venous return. When blood volume is reduced, for example after a haemorrhage, these atrial receptors are no longer stretched and their tonic depressor effect is removed with the result that there is less vagal restraint on the heart rate and less inhibition on vasoconstrictor tone.

Receptors which sense the chemical composition of blood also have actions on the cardiovascular system. The inherent activity of the vasomotor centre is probably explained by the direct influence of the carbon dioxide tension of its blood supply. The centre responds to raised carbon dioxide levels (hypercapnia), causing generalized vasoconstriction (p. 516). This is in contrast to the local vasodilator effects of hypercapnia on most resistance vessels. Chemical stimuli also exert effects through peripheral chemoreceptors. Hypoxia and hypercapnia (and especially the combination of these stimuli) act directly on the carotid bodies to produce reflex bradycardia, vasoconstriction and the release of adrenal catecholamines. Such carotid body stimulation however, also causes hyperventilation by acting on the respiratory centres. The increased frequency of breathing induces strong pulmonary reflexes which outweigh most of the direct cardiovascular effects, so that peripheral chemoreceptor stimulation in the intact animal in fact causes tachycardia and generalized vasodilation. The bradycardia produced by carotid body stimulation when respiratory movement is inhibited may be important in life, for example in people swimming underwater. If they have hyperventilated, either deliberately or unconsciously in excitement before submerging, the $P\text{CO}_2$ in the arterial blood is reduced. Under the water hypoxia develops, but the swimmer is able to continue holding his breath because the $P\text{CO}_2$ is low. The reflex bradycardia induced by the chemoreceptors may become so intense that occasionally there is sudden cardiac arrest.

The brain-stem centres which regulate blood pressure respond to stimuli other than baroreceptor and chemoreceptor afferents. For example emotions and pain change blood pressure, the direction of the change depending on the precise nature of these stimuli. Nervous connections which might be responsible can be traced from many parts of the central nervous system.

Valsalva manoeuvre
Forced expiration against the closed glottis causes a sharp rise in intrathoracic pressure, and this reduces venous return to the heart and thus stroke volume and systolic blood pressure. This 'Valsalva manoeuvre' (Fig. 15.66) serves clini-

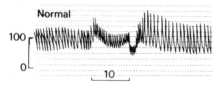

Fig. 15.66. Valsalva manoeuvre on arterial blood pressure of a normal subject. Time in seconds; blood pressure in mmHg. (From *Journal of Physiology* London (1956) **134**, 2.).

cally as a useful test of baroreceptor function. It is not restricted to the clinical environment, however, as similar effects are produced when lifting or pulling a heavy object, during vigorous coughing and during defaecation.

When intrathoracic pressure rises the pulmonary veins are compressed and there is an initial increased filling of the left ventricle and an increase in stroke volume. However, because venous return to the thorax is greatly reduced there quickly follows a decrease in stroke volume, a fall in systolic pressure, and decreased baroreceptor activity. This causes reflex tachycardia and vasoconstriction leading to an elevation of diastolic blood pressure. When the glottis is re-opened intrathoracic pressure falls. Venous return increases suddenly, cardiac output is restored and systolic blood pressure rises. The baroreceptors respond to this and cause bradycardia. Normal pressures are then quickly restored (see Fig. 15.66).

Baroreceptor responses to vasoactive drugs
Baroreceptor reflexes help to explain some apparently puzzling effects of drugs on the cardiovascular system. In the intact animal, as opposed to the isolated perfused heart, adrenaline causes marked tachycardia yet the closely related noradrenaline causes bradycardia. The explanation lies in the fact that noradrenaline has a great affinity for the α-receptors on peripheral resistance vessels so causing intense peripheral vasoconstriction. Because of this, noradrenaline increases blood pressure and the consequent baroreceptor stimulation leads to bradycardia. Adrenaline, however, has a greater affinity for β-receptors than α-receptors, so that, although causing tachycardia by a direct action on the heart it leads to relaxation of skeletal muscle arterioles. The net result is that diastolic blood pressure changes very little; often there is a slight fall; the baroreceptors are therefore not stimulated. Use

can be made of these differences when one needs to stimulate the heart without endangering blood flow to the tissues or alternatively to increase blood pressure without causing excessive cardiac work.

Venous pressure waves
When the atria contract flow into them momentarily stops and central venous pressure rises; when they relax and begin to fill, venous pressure falls. The normal venous pressure wave is however more complicated than a simple rise and fall because movements of the heart pull on the relatively thin-walled veins (Fig. 15.67). These waves can be recorded over the neck veins close to the right atrium.

The 'a wave' is the rise in venous blood pressure due to contraction of the right atrium. When the ventricles contract, the atria are pulled downwards towards the cardiac apex so that the atria are stretched and venous pressure falls ('x descent'). The 'c' wave interrupts the x descent; it is caused by the tricuspid valve being pushed upwards into the right atrium as the right ventricle begins to contract. The fall in pressure continues into the very early part of ventricular diastole, then as blood fills the atrium and the ventricle relaxes and moves upwards, pressure again rises ('v wave') until the tricuspid valve opens and blood rushes into the right ventricle ('y descent'). Abnormal venous pressure waves may be of value in the diagnosis of heart disease. In heart failure, for example, not all the blood returning to the heart is pumped into the arteries. It accumulates in the heart and in the veins so that the heart enlarges and venous pressure rises. If the pressure within a vein rises beyond a certain level it becomes distended. Veins therefore become distended higher up the venous tree above the heart as the central venous pressure (CVP) rises. Normally the mean CVP is less than 5 cm H_2O and the veins are only distended to about the level of the clavicle.

The level of the CVP is in part determined by

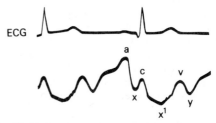

ECG

Fig. 15.67. Jugular venous pulse during the cardiac cycle.

how efficiently the heart accepts blood from the veins and so the height of the column of blood in the jugular veins provides a simple index of the degree of heart failure and the effectiveness of treatment. CVP may be measured by a catheter slipped up a vein to the superior vena cava.

Regional blood flow

GENERAL CONSIDERATIONS

Need for variable blood flow

It is generally true to say that the blood flow to an organ is related to, and determined by, its needs. Increased metabolic activity causes striking increases in flow in muscle, salivary glands and intestine for example. There are organs however, such as skin, kidney and lung in which blood flow is not related to the metabolic needs. In the skin, flow is mainly regulated according to the needs of heat conservation or loss; in the kidney the blood flow is much greater than would be expected for metabolic reasons alone.

To what extent is it necessary to increase blood flow to certain metabolically active regions? This question can be answered by a simple quantitative assessment. For example, the P_{O_2} in interstitial fluid bathing muscle cells is in equilibrium with that in the vessels supplying the muscle; initially about 100 mm Hg. An average value for oxygen consumption is about 2 cm^3/min/kg muscle which increases to about 100 cm^3/min/kg during maximal exercise. Extracellular fluid volume in muscle is about 20% of total tissue volume and solutions of salts in water generally absorb about 0.2 cm^3 O_2/mmHg P_{O_2}/dm^3. In our situation, therefore, muscle ECF holds

$$0.2 \times 100 \times \frac{20}{100} = 4 \text{ cm}^3 O_2/\text{kg}$$

During the resting state the ECF could theoretically sustain oxygen consumption for only about 2 minutes so that replenishment from the blood is necessary. As fully oxygenated blood carries 200 cm^3 O_2/dm^3, and the blood flow at rest is about 30 cm^3/min/kg, this can supply

$$30 \times \frac{200}{1000} = 6 \text{ cm}^3 O_2/\text{min/kg}$$

At rest there is thus about 30% extraction of the oxygen from the blood flowing through the muscle. In order to provide the 100 cm^3 O_2/min required during maximal activity, assuming the same extraction rate, the blood supply would have to be increased to

$$\frac{100 \times 100}{200 \times 30} \times 1000$$

or about 1.3 dm^3/kg/min. However, the extraction rate of oxygen is also increased to 85%, so it follows that

$$\frac{100 \times 100}{200 \times 85} \times 1000$$

or 0.58 dm^3/min/kg will satisfy the muscle's requirements—an increase over the resting flow of some twenty fold.

How is blood flow increased when required?

Control of local blood flow

The smooth muscle of resistance vessels is maintained in a state of partial contraction by tonic activity of sympathetic nerves and by vasomotor humoral agents. Increased sympathetic activity increases vascular resistance and reduces flow while a reduction in tonic firing induces an increase in flow. However, even in the absence of any such nervous or hormonal activity, smooth muscles are partially contracted. This

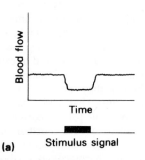

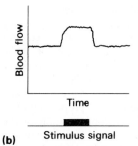

Fig. 15.68. The effect of sympathetic stimulation on blood flow through an organ is seen to be reduced by sympathetic stimulation. Between (a) and (b) the sympathetic nerves have been cut and it can be seen that blood flow increases due to the lack of

vasoconstrictor tone. 'Active' vasodilation is produced in (b) by appropriate nervous or humoral means (depending on the situation, e.g. activation of sympathetic vasodilator pathway in muscle) and blood flow increases still further.

tone can be reduced by vasodilator nerve activity and vasodilator substances (Fig. 15.68). Most active tissues appear to release such agents and this is discussed in more detail later.

Blood flow to an organ or tissue is therefore seen to be regulated by an interplay of nervous and chemical influences and these will now be dealt with in turn.

Nervous mechanisms. Changes in sympathetic tone have an important influence on the blood flow through most organs. The constrictor fibres come close to the smooth muscle cells in the outer layers of the blood vessel but the nerves do not penetrate through to the inner layers. Noradrenaline is released from varicosities along the nerves and diffuses to the muscle cells where it activates receptors and causes vasoconstriction. Sympathetic constrictor fibres supply virtually all of the body.

Vasodilator nerves have a restricted distribution. Muscle blood vessels of the limbs of some species appear to be supplied with sympathetic vasodilator nerves whose chemical transmitter is acetylcholine. Such fibres are known as sympathetic cholinergic fibres to distinguish them from the adrenergic fibres, whose transmitter is noradrenaline. The erectile tissue of the external genitalia and certain areas supplied by some of the cranial nerves, including the salivary glands and parts of the gastrointestinal tract, are supplied with parasympathetic cholinergic vasodilator nerves.

Sensory fibres may also be able to elicit vasodilation via the 'axon reflex' which will be considered in the section on cutaneous circulation (p. 723).

Chemical influences. A number of hormones and humoral factors affect vascular resistance.
1   The adrenal medulla secretes adrenaline and noradrenaline, the relative amounts varying from species to species. Noradrenaline activates α-receptors and causes vasoconstriction while adrenaline activates both α- and β-receptors. β-receptor activation leads to relaxation of vascular smooth muscle. The overall effect in any region depends on the relative proportion of α- and β-receptors and the concentration of the hormone. Adrenaline released *in vivo* generally causes vasodilatation of skeletal muscle blood vessels, but constricts cutaneous and splanchnic vessels. It has the affect of redistributing the blood.
2   Angiotensin, a peptide produced from a

plasma globulin by the action of renin from the kidney (p. 745), is one of the most potent vasoconstrictors known, but the conditions in which it is released in sufficient quantity to increase overall vascular resistance directly, remain to be clarified. It certainly seems to influence vascular tone indirectly by its ability to release aldosterone from the adrenal cortex. This steroid alters the electrolyte content and/or environment of the vascular smooth muscle and this in turn affects both its resting tone and its response to other constrictor agents.
3   Vasopressin (ADH). In large doses ADH causes vasoconstriction. Its main role, however, is to control water resorption from the distal nephron (p. 744) but it also appears to be released after haemorrhage in sufficient quantity to cause vasoconstriction.
4   Vasoactive Intestinal Polypeptide (VIP). As its name suggests, this vasodilator peptide was discovered in the intestine. More recently it has been found to be present in post-ganglionic parasympathetic nerve endings in a number of organs and an important role in mediating atropine resistant parasympathetic phenomena has been postulated. There is evidence, for example, that it may play a part in mediating functional hyperaemia in the salivary gland (p. 552).
5   Prostaglandins (p. 799) are a group of lipid-soluble unsaturated hydroxy acids. They are found in a wide variety of tissues and have an equally wide variety of actions. They are synthesized when the need arises. Some prostaglandins can cause contraction and others relaxation of vascular smooth muscle. They also have regulatory effects on blood flow in that they modify sympathetic transmission.
6   Kinins. All exocrine glands produce enzymes which leak into interstitial fluid and act on a globulin substrate from plasma to release small peptides, the kinins. In the salivary gland, for example, the enzyme is kallikrein and the kinins are kallidin and bradykinin (which are closely related). The kinins are powerful vasodilators and are clearly involved in certain pathological situations such as inflammation (p. 688) but, although they have been implicated in the hyperaemia that accompanies salivary gland activity, their role in normal physiology is still subject to debate. Further information about prostaglandins and kinins will be found in a standard pharmacology textbook.

Vasodilator metabolites. As mentioned previously, the increased metabolism that accompanies activity in many organs leads to the release of vasodilator metabolites. Many substances have been cast in the role of vasodilator metabolites but no single candidate has entirely fulfilled all the relevant criteria for it to be considered as the natural agent. Low P_{O_2}, high P_{CO_2}, raised H^+, adenosine compounds, lactic acid, kinins, prostaglandins, K^+, histamine, phosphate and local hyperosmolality, among others, have all been shown to be vasodilators. However, no single agent brings about hyperaemia like that seen during increased metabolic demand when given at concentrations similar to those found in the blood during such a state. It seems likely that more than one agent is involved and it is also likely that interactions between such agents may give rise to a more powerful dilator response than would be expected by simple addition of the dilator properties of the individual agents—an example of synergism.

Reactive hyperaemia and autoregulation. Before considering details of some vascular circuits, two general phenomena will be described—reactive hyperaemia and autoregulation. Reactive hyperaemia is an increased blood flow that follows a period of restricted arterial inflow. Fig. 15.69 shows that forearm blood flow increases several fold immediately after release of a pressure cuff which occluded the brachial artery: the increase over the basal value is related to the duration of the occlusion. The most important factor controlling this is the release of vasodilator metabolites by the tissues and their accumulation during the period of restricted blood flow. As pointed out above, the agents responsible remain to be clarified.

If the pressure applied to fluid in a rigid tube is increased, flow increases in proportion, as expected from Poisueille's Law (p. 694). If the tube is distensible, flow increases in greater proportion because the greater pressure distends the tube and since flow is proportional to the fourth power of the radius, a substantial increase in flow may be achieved with quite small increases in pressure. The vasculature of the lung behaves in this way as it is very compliant and the large increase in pulmonary blood flow during exercise is accommodated with only a small increase in pulmonary blood pressure. This is important as otherwise transmural capillary pressure could exceed plasma colloid osmotic pressure and excess tissue fluid filtration would lead to pulmonary oedema and death.

In many other organs, resistance actually increases when blood pressure is increased so the expected rise in flow is minimized and may be almost abolished. This is because smooth muscle in arteries is normally stretched by the pressure of blood within them and tends to resist this stretch by contracting. This is known as autoregulation of blood flow and it is notably developed in the kidney and brain (p. 719) although other organs demonstrate the phenomenon to a variable extent.

Methods of measuring blood flow
Blood flow (i.e. the quantity of blood flowing past a point in the circulation in a unit of time) to parts of the body such as the hand or forearm can be measured indirectly by a technique known as venous occlusion plethysmography (Fig. 15.70). When venous drainage is temporarily blocked by applying a sphygmomanometer cuff around a limb at a pressure above venous and below diastolic blood pressure there is an increase in volume of the limb which is proportional to the inflow of arterial blood. In the hand, blood flow is mainly to the skin whereas in the forearm or thigh it is principally to muscle. It is customary to express blood flow as $cm^3/min/100g$ tissue (or $100cm^3$, as it is usually volume which is measured by displacement of water).

Other indirect methods of measuring blood

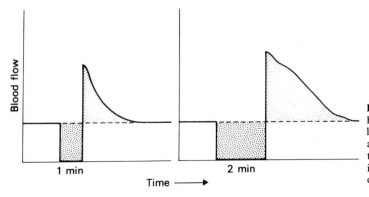

Fig. 15.69. Reactive hyperaemia. Arterial occlusion leads to an increased blood flow after the occlusion is released and the post-occlusion hyperaemia is in proportion to the length of the occlusion.

flow to organs depend on the clearance of a variety of substances from plasma as the blood flows through particular organs. This principle is used to measure blood flow to the kidney, brain, and lungs. Electromagnetic flowmeters are now used experimentally and can be implanted in an animal. The blood vessel is exposed and placed between the poles of the magnet and the voltage induced by the flow of blood through the magnetic field is recorded. Very rapid changes in flow can be measured by this technique.

In addition to these methods there are other techniques which apply particularly to cutaneous blood flow. These involve measurements of the heat given out by blood flowing to the skin by means of sensitive temperature sensors. It is assumed that the skin temperature is largely due to the amount of warm blood brought from the body core to the surface, therefore changes in this volume flow alter the skin temperature.

The rate at which blood flows along a vessel (velocity of flow) which is not the same as the volume flow, can be measured by conductivity and ultrasonic methods.

CEREBRAL CIRCULATION

The brain is one of the most active organs of the body and obtains its energy by the oxidative phosphorylation of glucose. Although the average adult brain comprises about 2% of body weight (1400 g) it consumes approximately 20% of the total oxygen requirements of the whole body at rest. The blood flow to the brain is regulated to supply its metabolic requirements and as a consequence has an average blood flow

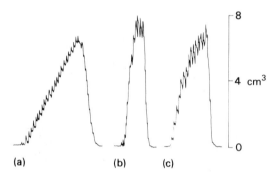

(a)   (b)   (c)

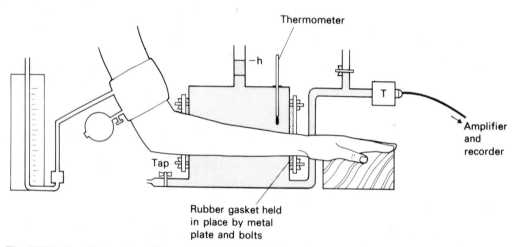

Fig. 15.70. Simplified version of fore-arm plethysmograph. The arm is put through a tight-fitting rubber sleeve and placed in a water-tight container. Water maintained at a constant temperature fills this container, the pressure head (h) of the water varies with changes in volume of the fore-arm and is monitored by a transducer (T). The apparatus is calibrated by adding known volumes to the water tank. (a) The record obtained here was for a subject at rest, water temperature 24°C, fore-arm volume 610 cm³. With paper speed of 1 mm/sec, the blood flow was calculated:

$$\text{Change in volume} = \frac{8}{44} \times 34 \text{ cm}^3$$

$$\text{Change in volume/min} = \frac{8}{44} \times 34 \times \frac{60}{18} \text{ cm}^3/\text{minute}$$

$$\text{Change in volume/min/ 100 g fore-arm} = \frac{8}{44} \times 34 \times \frac{60}{18} \times \frac{100}{610} \text{ cm}^3$$

$$= 3.4 \text{ cm}^3$$

(b) this record was for the same subject as in (a) 1 minute following repeated vigorous movement of the fingers and hand.

Change in volume/min/100 g fore-arm = 11.0 cm³

(c) 1½ minutes following the above exercise:

Change in volume/min/100 g fore-arm = 5.1cm³ (Note small variations due to pulse.)

of about 54 cm³/min/100 grams of tissue in the adult. Interruption of the cerebral circulation brings about loss of consciousness within 8–10 seconds and the onset of irreversible changes within one or two minutes. To ensure a constancy of the blood supply to the brain is one of the most important physiological objectives.

Control of blood supply

The cerebral circulation is rigidly encased in bone. For this reason the brain, blood and cerebrospinal fluid, being incompressible, together have a constant volume, and changes in volume or pressure in one are reflected by the others. The calibre of small vessels can be changed slightly by redistributing fluid between the vascular and CSF compartments, but such changes do not significantly alter the cerebral blood flow. Several factors are responsible for this constancy. A myogenic mechanism for autoregulation has been proposed; the smooth muscles in the cerebral arteries relax in response to a reduced perfusion pressure and contract when the stretching force is increased. However, when arterial pressure falls below about 50% of normal, cerebral blood flow falls precipitously to very low levels, producing cerebral hypoxia.

A relatively constant arterial–venous pressure gradient is maintained in the cerebral circulation during acceleration, in postural adjustment and some other situations. For example, if you suddenly stand up there is a fall in arterial perfusion pressure but this is accompanied by a reduction in cerebral venous pressure and intracranial pressure so that the change in arterial–venous pressure gradient is small. A sub-atmospheric pressure exists in the CSF and venous sinuses in the cranium, but because the whole system is within a rigid structure these channels do not collapse. The CSF pressure has little effect on cerebral blood flow until it rises above 33 mmHg, when flow is significantly reduced. The resultantt ischaemia stimulates the medullary vasomotor centre and causes a rise in systemic arterial pressure which serves to maintain the cerebral circulation.

A third factor which influences cerebral circulation is the tension of the blood gases.

Blood gases

Carbon dioxide is the most potent factor in the control of cerebral flow. An increase in the arterial P_{CO_2} produces a marked increase in flow which is aided by an accompanying rise in arterial blood pressure. A decrease in flow occurs with hypocapnia. Hypoxia induces an increase but the effect is smaller than that seen with CO_2.

The mechanism producing vasodilatation in response to hypercapnia is uncertain. It has been suggested that the local pH of the brain extracellular fluid is changed by the freely permeable CO_2 and that pH affects the calibre of vessels. In support of this it has been observed that local microinjections of pH buffers in the vicinity of pial vessels alter their calibre.

Autonomic innervation

An extensive autonomic innervation to the cerebral blood vessels has been demonstrated histologically. In addition, it has been shown in experimental animals that marked vasoconstriction with a fall in cerebral blood flow can be elicited by stimulating the stellate (sympathetic) ganglion. In contrast, cerebral flow in a resting, recumbent man is not altered after either sympathectomy or stellate ganglion blockade.

Circulating catecholamines have little effect on cerebral flow but this may be due to their inability to reach the smooth muscle of the cerebral blood vessels through the blood–brain barrier formed by the endothelial cells in the intact animal.

Cerebral blood flow increases when the distal end of a sectioned seventh cranial nerve is stimulated. Local changes can also be elicited by topical application of cholinergic drugs to the surface vessels of the brain in experimental animals.

All these experiments indicate the ability of the cerebral blood vessels to respond to nervous stimuli but do not elucidate the role of the autonomic nervous system in the control of cerebral blood flow. Cerebral innervation in man does not appear to participate in baroreceptor reflexes, but there remains the possibility that its effect is to alter the response of the vasculature to such factors as CO_2.

THE CORONARY CIRCULATION

The maintenance of an adequate blood supply to the myocardium is essential for the viability of the heart and thus of the individual. The distribution of the coronary arteries is described on p. 639).

The density of the capillary network (number per unit cross-sectional area) is at least five times that in skeletal muscle. The greater density of capillaries and significantly shorter diffusion distance is due to the fibres in cardiac muscle being thinner than those in skeletal muscle rather than because of a higher capillary to fibre ratio.

The myocardial blood flow differs in different

parts of the heart; the flow to the left ventricle exceeds that to the right, consistent with the greater mass of the left ventricle. The epicardium is richly perfused whereas the endocardium is relatively poorly supplied and is thus most at risk when perfusion pressure is low, as in circulatory collapse. Perhaps the most striking feature of coronary blood flow is its complex phasic nature during one cardiac cycle (Fig. 15.71). Most blood flows during diastole, and in the left coronary artery it is reduced almost to zero in early systole. Such alterations in blood flow during the cardiac cycle do not occur in other organs and tissues, where changes in post-arteriolar perfusion pressure take place slowly and blood flow is virtually constant for minutes or hours at a time. The dramatic fall in coronary flow during early systole is a result of the large rise in ventricular wall pressure during isovolumetric contraction and the early ejection phase. Thus although the pressure head for the coronary circulation rises in systole it is counteracted by an impedance to blood flow as the vessels are compressed by contraction of the cardiac muscle. This feature is particularly marked in the blood supply to the left ventricle; by contrast the blood flow to the right ventricle falls only slightly below the mean value in early systole. Venous outflow from the myocardium is accelerated by the compression and aided by the low atrial pressure during ventricular systole.

Coronary blood flow claims about 4% of the cardiac output at rest (200 cm³/min) but the heart has an oxygen consumption equal to about 11% of total body uptake. The oxygen extraction per unit volume of blood by the myocardium (the arterial–venous difference) is thus very high. Even when the subject is at rest, coronary sinus blood has an oxygen content of only 5 cm³/100 cm³ blood compared with about 14 cm³ in mixed venous blood.

The two unique features of the coronary circulation, namely high oxygen extraction and predominantly diastolic flow, have important consequences on the manner of the response to the increased demands of the heart in exercise.

First, since coronary venous blood is almost exhausted of oxygen even under resting conditions, it is clear that increased oxygen supply can result only from increasing coronary blood flow. Second, since there is commonly a tachycardia with exercise, total diastolic time is reduced both because there are more systoles per unit time and also because diastole is reduced proportionately more than systole as heart rate increases. Thus there is less perfusion time. In addition,

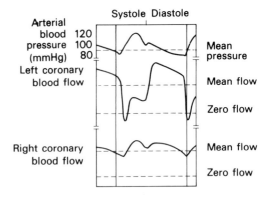

Fig. 15.71. Relationship between arterial blood pressure and coronary blood flow.

increased cardiac sympathetic nerve activity, which augments the force of ventricular contraction, serves only to decrease flow during systole. To some extent, these restrictions on perfusion of the myocardium in exercise are offset by the small rise in mean arterial pressure, but principally, coronary blood flow increases because of a fall in the impedance during diastole. Total coronary flow increases 3–4 fold to about 700 cm³/min.

The mechanism responsible for this fall in coronary vascular resistance is not clear. It appears unlikely in humans that neural control is significant and circulating hormones such as the catecholamines do not have consistent effects. Most workers believe that the major factor controlling coronary blood flow is a local metabolic one; adenosine is probably the principal vasodilator. Myocardial hypercapnia (increased CO_2) and fall in pH do not appear to be involved, but it remains possible that local hypoxia could cause coronary vasodilation.

MUSCLE BLOOD FLOW AND EXERCISE

Because muscle constitutes 40–50% of the total body weight and is very vascular, it follows that large changes in muscle blood flow have profound consequences for the circulation. Abolition of sympathetic nervous drive to muscle arterioles approximately doubles skeletal muscle blood flow (see Fig. 15.68). The maximal discharge of 10–20 impulses per second reduces flow to 25% or less of the resting value. Such changes in flow are part of reflex responses concerned primarily with whole-body needs and which include changes in cardiac output, blood pressure and distribution of flow to the different vascular beds. These cardiovascular adjustments are integrated centrally. A different situation arises during exercise. The needs of the rest of the body remain but the increased work of the skeletal musculature demands an increased blood flow far in excess of that produced by a decrease in sympathetic tone.

Histochemically, mammalian skeletal muscle can be seen to consist of two fibre types, red (slow or tonic) and white (fast or phasic) and these are present in different proportions in different muscles. Red fibres, which constitute perhaps 15–20% of the muscle bulk are used mainly during periods of steady prolonged activity such as is required in the maintenance of posture. The soleus muscle, for example, is composed largely of red fibres. Red muscle has rather more capillaries per fibre than white and has a higher resting blood flow which increases relatively little during activity. It contains more myoglobin (p. 72) than white muscle. These properties are to be expected of a muscle which has to keep in oxygen balance. In contrast, white muscle fibres can temporarily utilize the anaerobic glycolytic pathway for energy supply, which leads to the formation of lactic acid. This property is extremely useful because it enables the muscle to produce a greater output of work for limited periods than could be sustained by the oxygen supply at a steady state. The 'oxygen debt' incurred is repaid later by a maintained increase in blood flow after the exercise is finished.

Muscle blood flow increases just prior to exercise and this is effected by the sympathetic cholinergic vasodilator pathway. The hypothalamus is responsible for integration of this anticipatory response along with other aspects of the 'flight or fight' reaction, and it does not appear to involve the vasomotor centre in the medulla.

The sympathetic vasodilator pathway is activated in another situation worth mentioning here. During the common type of fainting (vasovagal) attack, there is an increase in sympathetic vasodilator drive and a consequent fall in total peripheral resistance (p. 729). In exercise, an increase in cardiac output accompanies the increased muscle blood flow, so blood pressure remains at an adequate level, but in fainting, cardiac output does not rise (in fact it usually falls) so blood pressure falls and loss of consciousness ensues.

Once exercise starts, metabolic products from the active muscle play the dominant role in increasing flow. So powerful are these agents that this vasodilatation can be sustained experimentally in the presence of maximal sympathetic vasoconstrictor nerve activity. It appears that the combined effects of low P_{O_2}, increased K^+ and increased osmolality of the venous blood due to the release of small molecular-weight metabolic products, are sufficient to explain exercise hyperaemia. This does not deny other possibilities.

Adrenaline is released into the circulation by the adrenal medulla in times of sudden crisis and this too dilates the arterioles of skeletal muscles. Since a muscle and its blood vessels are enclosed within a fascial compartment, contraction tends to compress both artery and vein so that arterial inflow is impeded and venous outflow temporarily increased. During sustained isometric contraction, blood flow is reduced or abolished, but afterwards, there is a post-contraction hyperaemia. In rhythmically exercising muscle there is increased blood flow during the relaxation periods and at the end of exercise.

PULMONARY CIRCULATION

General characteristics

Unlike the systemic circulation, the vascular bed of the lungs offers only a small resistance to flow. The precapillary vessels in the lungs are thin-walled, distensible tubes and most contain little smooth muscle. The larger arteries contain smooth muscle but this is arranged mainly to prevent too much distension rather than to narrow their calibre. If the cardiac output from the right ventricle increases several fold, as in exercise for example, the pressure in the pulmonary arteries rises only slightly, if at all. The pulmonary arteries expand and accommodate the extra blood pumped into them. The system is a low pressure (low resistance) high capacitance system.

Like the cutaneous circulation, the pulmonary circuit is not designed to serve the metabolic needs of the tissues; its prime function is to ensure optimal gaseous exchange across the capillaries in the alveoli. The combined surface area of these capillaries is enormous—about 90 m² in man.

The mean pressure in the pulmonary artery is about 15 mmHg, the peak systolic pressure in the right ventricle being about 25 mmHg and the pulmonary arterial diastolic pressure around 10 mmHg (Fig. 15.48). The transmitted pressure in the pulmonary vein is about 5 mmHg. There is thus only a relatively small A–V pressure gradient but this suffices to force blood through the short system of vessels. The fall in pressure occurs as blood passes through the capillary network; this is quite unlike the situation in the systemic circulation (Fig. 15.47).

Effects of transmural and hydrostatic pressures
The pulmonary vessels are exposed indirectly to the effects of changes in intrathoracic and intra-alveolar pressures. On inspiration, the intra-thoracic pressure is reduced and the lungs are stretched; more blood is drawn into the great veins and so into the right ventricle and the pulmonary circuit. The pulmonary vessels accommodate this. Conversely, in expiration, particularly a forced expiration against a resist-ance, there is a reduction in the lung blood volume. Variations from over 1000 cm³ on inspiration to 200 cm³ on a forced expiration are possible (Fig. 15.72). Normal variations in alveolar pressures from −3 to +3 mmHg in quiet breathing have little effect on capillary blood flow, but if air is forced into the lungs (as in some methods of artificial respiration) the capil-laries can become compressed. In the upright posture there is more blood and a greater flow in the base of the lungs below the level of the heart than in the apices of the lungs. However, the capacity of the pulmonary system is greater in the recumbent position: most of the blood is in the very distensible veins. In lung tissue, which, for one reason or another, is underventilated, it appears that the small precapillary vessels adja-cent to the respiratory bronchioles are sensitive to the hypoxia. Their smooth muscle contracts so that blood is shunted from poorly ventilated alveoli (or even an entire lung if it has collapsed) to other parts which are adequately oxygenated.

Fluid movement across pulmonary capillaries
It was formerly thought that the tissue space around lung capillaries did not contain any filtered fluid under normal conditions. This reasoning stemmed from the finding that the capillary blood pressure averaged only about 10 mmHg in the recumbent position whereas the plasma colloid osmotic pressure drawing fluid into these spaces immediately reduces the osmotic pull and minimizes further fluid move-determines the overall filtration pressure, is probably smaller than was supposed and some fluid exchange takes place between capillaries and tissue spaces. The reason seems to be that there is a small amount of a protein rich fluid in the narrow tissue spaces and that this exerts an osmotic influence. Movement of any transudate into these spaces immediately reduces the oss-motic pull and minimizes further fluid move-ment. The most usual cause of an increase in capillary pressure is pressure transmitted back from the left side of the heart in the pulmonary veins, as in mitral stenosis. This results in pul-monary oedema.

Functional significance of the innervation of pulmonary vessels
The arteries and veins receive sympathetic vaso-constrictor nerve fibres but have a minimal tone. Stimulation causes a reduction in the capacities of both the arterial and venous sides of the pul-monary system so that there is little change in pulmonary capillary pressure. These fibres are probably activated as part of the pressor reflex in response to a fall in arterial pressure in the carotid sinus. The overall effect of this decrease in capacitance is that blood is driven from the pulmonary system, particularly the veins, into

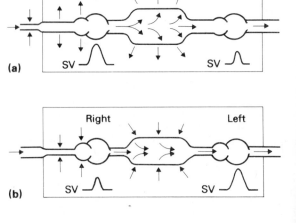

Fig. 15.72. Diagrammatic representation of the immediate effects of changes in intrathoracic pressure during (a) inspiration and (b) expiration on cardiac filling, stroke volume (SV), pulmonary blood flow and pulmonary blood volume. (From Folkow & Neil (1971) *Circulation.* Oxford University Press).

the left ventricle. Thus extra blood required to increase cardiac output is rapidly obtained. This is a particularly important adjustment on suddenly assuming the upright posture after lying down.

SKIN BLOOD FLOW

Blood flow through the skin contrasts with that in skeletal muscle in several respects. In particular, it is mainly controlled by activity of the sympathetic nervous system and the flow has little to do with the metabolic activity of the skin.

Serving as the boundary between the body and its environment, the skin has many functions, among them that of heat exchanger (p. 726).

The white reaction and the triple response

If skin is stroked lightly with a blunt instrument, such as the edge of a ruler, after about 20 seconds a vasoconstrictor response can be observed along the line of stroking. This lasts for about a minute and for obvious reasons is known as the 'white' reaction. It seems to be a direct response of the subpapillary venules and is independent of nervous connections. If the ruler is pressed more firmly into the skin, a red line appears under the ruler track due to a direct response of the venules beneath (the 'red' reaction). Following this, a patchy reddening of the skin appears and spreads several millimetres on either side of the red line. This 'flare', which may last many minutes, is not seen when the circulation is occluded, and it is thus assumed to be due to dilatation of the arterioles and/or venules.

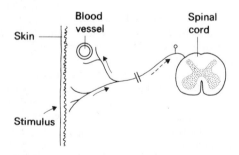

Fig. 15.73. The axon reflex. The sensory nerve fibre passing to the dorsal root of the spinal cord not only sends impulses centrally when an injurious stimulus excites the skin, but an antidromic impulse passes to the skin blood vessels. A vasodilator substance is released that is responsible for the flare of the triple response. The flare persists after acute nerve section but disappears if the nerves are given time to degenerate.

The flare response develops in patients who have had sympathectomy and occurs even if the sensory nerves are cut acutely, but it is not obtainable after they degenerate. This suggests it is an 'axon reflex' due to antidromic stimulation of sensory fibres (Fig. 15.73). With a sufficiently strong stimulus the initial red reaction gives rise to a raised pale wheal. This appears to be a secondary reaction due to the release of substances from the damaged skin that increase permeability of the vessels beneath, thus causing transudation of fluid. Histamine or histamine-like substances, kinins, prostaglandins and ATP have all been suggested as the mediator. The sequence, red reaction, flare and wheal is known as the 'triple response'. A similar response occurs in all cases of cutaneous inflammation whatever the initial cause (p. 687).

SPLANCHNIC BLOOD FLOW

The circulation to the alimentary tract, liver and spleen is known as the splanchnic circulation. The vessels are coupled together and arranged in parallel (Fig. 15.74).

Liver blood flow, 70% of which comes from the portal vein and 30% from the hepatic artery, is about 1500 cm³/min; 25% of the total cardiac output at rest. The architecture of the blood supply to the liver is described elsewhere (p. 620). Under experimental conditions the splanchnic blood flow can be increased 3-fold, but during digestion flow increases by about 50% because the different regions of the splanchnic bed are affected one after the other, rather than all at once. Only about 25% of the O_2 is extracted from splanchnic blood during resting conditions so the flow can be substantially reduced before there is any danger of hypoxia. This is important because the splanchnic bed, like that of skeletal muscle, provides a large reservoir of blood for cardiovascular adjustments. During heat loss, for example, sympathetic vasoconstriction in the splanchnic and skeletal muscle beds leads to a redistribution of blood to the skin. During exercise more blood can be passed to active muscles because of vasoconstriction in the splanchnic bed and inactive muscles. Both the pre-capillary arterioles and post-capillary venules and veins of the whole splanchnic bed are richly supplied with sympathetic vasoconstrictor nerves: both resistance and capacitance vessels can be constricted.

The adjustments in splanchnic blood flow are particularly important following severe haemorrhage (p. 727).

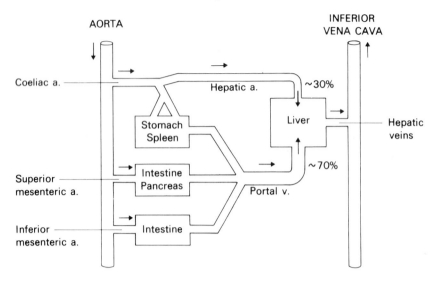

AORTA

INFERIOR
VENA CAVA

Coeliac a.

Hepatic a.

~30%

Stomach
Spleen

Liver

Hepatic
veins

Superior
mesenteric a.

Intestine
Pancreas

~70%

Portal v.

Inferior
mesenteric a.

Intestine

Fig. 15.74. Diagrammatic representation of splanchnic vascular bed. Note parallel coupling.

arrangement and that all the intestinal, pancreatic, stomach and splenic venous blood passes to the liver.

Temperature control

LIMITS OF OPERATION

Only mammals and birds are homoeotherms, in the sense that they maintain deep body temperature within narrow limits in spite of wide variations in external temperature. Virtually all animals, however, have the ability to detect temperature and to move towards the environmental temperature that they prefer. In homoeotherms this behavioural type of temperature regulation remains important. If we include in this the means that man has developed to modify his environment, such as clothes, buildings and artificial heating, it is the dominant means of regulation even in man.

Nevertheless, internal physiological mechanisms provide the fine control that keeps the temperature of the deep body tissues such as the heart and brain within approximately 1°C of 36.5°C under normal circumstances. The importance of this is that the enzyme systems of the body, particularly those of the brain and heart, are enabled to operate at optimal level. A large rise in temperature is an immediate threat to life, since some tissue proteins start to undergo irreversible denaturation at approximately 44°C. A body temperature approaching that level as a result of simple exposure to heat, or of operations on the hypothalamus, is therefore an emergency calling for immediate steps to lower temperature. A fall in body temperature below

34–35°C causes progressive lethargy, confusion and finally unconsciousness, with slowing of the heart and respiration, and finally cardiac arrest.

TEMPERATURE RECEPTORS

The initial sensory information that is provided on exposure to a hot or cold environment is given by temperature receptors in the skin. Although various structures in the skin have been tentatively identified as these receptors, they are now believed to be simply the bare terminals of specific nerve fibres, specialized so that either warming or cooling depolarizes them. The rapidly adaptive behaviour of the receptors accounts for the familiar observation that water feels much less cold after swimming in it for a minute or two than at first.

After 'warm' and 'cold' fibres enter the cord they relay, and the temperature pathway then ascends in the lateral part of the spinothalamic tract to the hypothalamus. The hypothalamus contains two temperature-regulating centres; the anterior, which extends forward into the preoptic region, is itself the main temperature sensing region for deep body temperature. Some of its neurons have been shown to increase, and others to decrease, their rate of firing when local temperature is increased. Some of these neurons are believed to be the deep temperature receptors. The importance of the deep receptors is that they detect even small, slow deviations of

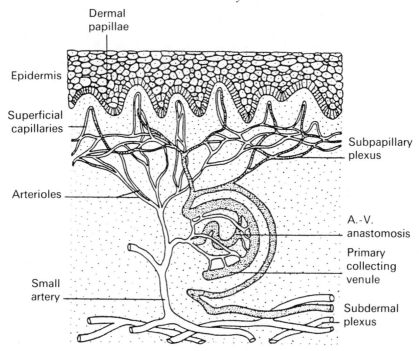

Fig. 15.75. Schematic drawing of main vessels in a digital glomus. (Reproduced by permission from Mescon H., Hurley J. H. Jr. and Moretti G. (1956) *Journal of Investigative Dermatology* **27**, 133–145.

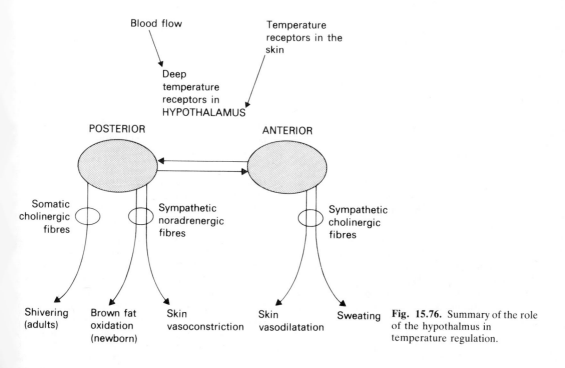

Fig. 15.76. Summary of the role of the hypothalmus in temperature regulation.

deep body temperature from the optimal level. Other deep temperature receptors exist, in the posterior hypothalamus, in the cervical part of the spinal cord, and in the abdominal viscera, but they are in general much less sensitive and contribute less to the body's overall response to temperature change.

CONTROL OF HEAT LOSS (Figs. 15.75 and 15.76)

Apart from acting as a temperature sensing region, the anterior hypothalamic area also acts as the heat loss centre. It activates mechanisms that increase heat loss from the body whenever combined sensory information indicates heat exposure and a rise in body temperature. These can be recruited experimentally by stimulating the heat loss centre electrically. Destruction of the area prevents heat loss mechanisms being activated when required, and can lead to a rapid and fatal increase in body temperature.

The first heat loss mechanism to be recruited on exposure to heat is vasodilatation in the skin. This is due partly to reduced vasoconstrictor tone, but also to active dilatation brought about by sympathetic nerve fibres that release acetylcholine on the blood vessels. Much of the increased skin blood flow in the extremities takes place through arteriovenous anastomoses (AVAs), which allow very rapid flow and transfer of heat. AVAs connect arteries directly to veins in the dermal region (Fig. 15.75). They contain a thick wall of smooth muscle which is innervated by the sympathetic nervous system and is under the control of the hypothalamus. AVAs are present in the skin of the fingers, toes, ears and nose and when they open they bring large amounts of warm blood close to the skin surface. If the increase in skin blood flow fails to stabilize body temperature, a second mechanism, sweating, is activated. This is also brought about by cholinergic sympathetic fibres that supply the sweat glands. Secretion of sweat is accompanied by bradykinin production by the glands, and this further increases skin blood flow. The main importance of sweating, though, is that the latent heat of evaporation of the fluid cools the skin even when the temperature of the surrounding air is near to, or even above, that of the body core. It is therefore essential to enable heat produced in the body to be dissipated under these conditions. Sweat is of course only effective if it can evaporate: if the air is already saturated with water vapour at near body tempera-

tures, as it may be in a tropical rain forest, sweating does not assist body heat loss. Adrenaline released by the adrenal medulla in the 'fight or flight' reaction stimulates some sweat glands directly, causing a paradoxical 'cold sweat' in the absence of any increase in body temperature.

CONTROL OF HEAT GAIN

Responses to body cooling are integrated in the heat gain centre, which is in the posterior hypothalamus. When sensory information from surface and deep receptors indicates body cooling, the first mechanism activated by the centre is vasoconstriction in the skin. This is brought about by sympathetic nerve fibres that release noradrenaline on the arterioles and AVAs. Some blood flow is always maintained to provide nutrition and remove waste products, but in the limbs a countercurrent exchange system allows this to be done with very little transfer of heat. The explanation for this is that the deep arteries in the distal part of the limbs are closely accompanied by venae comitantes. When there is vasoconstriction, flow in the cutaneous veins ceases and blood returning from the cold extremities flows slowly up the venae comitantes and is warmed by the blood flowing in the adjacent artery in the opposite direction. By the time the venous blood returns to the heart it is nearly at heart temperature, while the arterial blood reaches the extremity at near skin temperature, so that little heat is transferred.

Direct effects of cold on blood vessels also play an important part. Moderate cooling constricts skin vessels, reinforcing the neurogenic vasoconstriction in the cold. However, severe local cooling below about 12°C causes paralysis of the muscles in the blood vessels with consequent increase in blood flow and heat loss. This is described as cold vasodilatation and usually follows a cyclical pattern. If a finger is put into ice water there is first vasoconstriction. The finger cools to near 0°C, the blood vessels become paralysed and dilate, and a high blood flow returns and warms the finger. The vessels then become responsive again and a further wave of constriction and cooling follows.

Cold vasodilatation has some beneficial effect by warming severely chilled extremities and so protecting them against freezing, but it increases body heat loss. This is most serious during whole body immersion in cold water. As long as vasoconstriction is maintained heat is lost largely by physical conduction through the surface tissues,

ANT
HYPOTHAL

and in people with a thick layer of subcutaneous fat this loss is very small, so that fat people survive almost indefinitely in water at 15°C. In water below 12°C cold vasodilatation allows blood flow to carry enough heat through the fat to the skin, from which it is lost to the water, so that even the fattest man cannot survive for long.

If vasoconstriction is for any reason insufficient to stabilize body temperature, mechanisms to increase body heat production are brought into action. In adult man the most important of these are shivering and other forms of striated muscle contraction, such as tensing of muscles and increased voluntary movement. Shivering can increase heat production as much as fivefold for short periods, although this is offset to some extent by associated increase in blood flow to the muscles, with increased heat loss.

The full-term newborn infant does not shiver; instead it has a special mechanism for keeping warm. This is 'brown' fat (p. 360), so called because of its rich blood supply. It is located mainly between the scapulae. These fat cells are unusual in having a sympathetic nerve supply which releases noradrenaline, induces oxidation of the fat and releases large amounts of heat.

Haemorrhage, shock and fainting

Patients may faint in a dental surgeon's chair through fear and apprehension, particularly when receiving a local anaesthetic by injection. Sometimes fear is associated with the sight of blood.

Occasionally the lingual, inferior dental, or palatine arteries are severed during surgical operations and the resultant haemorrhage may be sufficiently severe to contribute to fainting and even to shock. Incorrect management of a patient who has fainted or who is in shock could be fatal.

HAEMORRHAGE

Accidents which cause bleeding are common and animals have evolved powerful mechanisms to stop bleeding, to cope with what blood is left, and to replace the loss. In sudden, rapid haemorrhage, powerful mechanisms help to maintain blood pressure in the face of a severe fall in blood volume. Almost all the responses to a severe haemorrhage are related to maintaining an adequate oxygen supply to the brain.

If bleeding is less severe, blood pressure is not threatened because the small fluid losses are readily corrected but persistent haemorrhage has other dangers, in particular, iron losses may be large.

Immediate responses

In an acute severe haemorrhage it might be expected that arteries would bleed most. However the smooth muscle of injured arteries contracts strongly and this 'traumatic arterial spasm' effectively reduces arterial bleeding so that often most of the blood lost from cut tissues oozes from veins. Platelets soon begin to clump together in the lumen of cut vessels and an important benefit of arterial spasm is that flow is so reduced that platelets are not washed away (Fig. 15.77). Platelet aggregation initiates the sequence of reactions which leads to clotting (p. 689).

As well as these local reactions there are reflex responses to haemorrhage. Bleeding reduces venous return to the heart so that cardiac output falls. Baroreceptor and volume receptor reflexes cause generalized sympathetic activity with tachycardia and vasoconstriction (p. 713). Pain and fear augment this activity and together with the effects of catecholamines released from the adrenal medulla by sympathetic activity, help to maintain blood pressure. Sympathetic venocon-

Baro + Volume receptors

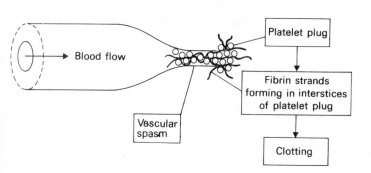

Fig. 15.77. Summary of haemostatic mechanisms.

striction reduces venous capacitance and aids blood return to the heart. The vasoconstricted skin is pale and feels characteristically cold and clammy (sympathetic fibres are sudomotor i.e. they supply the sweat glands).

Vasoconstriction of arteries by sympathetic activity brings about a useful re-distribution of the body fluids. Capillary hydrostatic pressure is reduced as the arterioles constrict so that the osmotic attraction of the plasma oncotic pressure is less opposed and tissue fluid is drawn into the vessels, thus the blood becomes diluted within a few hours after a haemorrhage and the haematocrit falls. Blood volume is thus raised.

Sympathetic nerves constrict the arterioles of the kidney glomeruli and cause the release of renin so that angiotensin II is produced in the blood (p. 745). Its pressor action helps to maintain blood pressure directly and its action on the adrenal cortex leads to the release of aldosterone which stimulates renal tubular sodium reabsorption so raising the osmolality of ECF (extracellular fluid) and drawing fluid from cells, hence raising the blood volume and pressure.

ADH is also released in this situation because of the reduced stretch on atrial wall receptors when blood volume falls; a reflex which is mediated by afferent vagal fibres. Antidiuretic hormone acts on the kidney to produce a concentrated urine so that water loss is minimized.

The desire to obtain water is stimulated after a haemorrhage, thirst is probably chiefly due to the central effects of angiotensin II and possibly also to the effects of aldosterone in raising the osmotic pressure of the extracellular fluid. As water is drunk, blood volume increases, but the blood is diluted further and the haematocrit falls even more.

All the responses described so far help to maintain perfusion of the brain. However, haemorrhage may precipitate the fainting reflex in which blood pressure suddenly falls. This apparently paradoxical situation is discussed in detail later.

Because the body cannot 'afford' to perfuse every organ when blood volume is reduced, severe blood loss inevitably causes stagnant hypoxia. This together with the anaemic hypoxia due to the reduced number of red cells causes the hypoxic tissues to respire anaerobically with the result that acidosis develops. To compensate, the release of oxygen at the tissues is improved. This is because acidosis and stagnant hypoxia increase levels of 2–3 DPG inside red blood cells so that the haemoglobin-oxygen dissociation curve is displaced to the right (p. 507).

Delayed responses

After the blood volume has been restored the composition of blood is more gradually brought back to normal. Plasma proteins are restored by hepatic synthesis over several days.

Renal hypoxia causes the release of the hormone erythropoietin which stimulates red cell synthesis in the bone marrow. In its haste the marrow releases reticulocytes as well as mature red cells. The reticulocytosis reaches its peak at approximately the tenth day, and the original red cell mass is restored in 4–8 weeks.

Compensatory mechanisms may be inadequate after sudden severe haemorrhage and tissues may be badly damaged by hypoxia, resulting in acute renal failure or even permanent brain damage. If the tissues of the body remain hypoxic for too long, generalized damage leads to the shock syndrome (see later).

Treatment

The treatment of haemorrhage is to:
1 Stop the bleeding,
2 Maintain the circulation,
3 Replace fluid which has been lost.

Bleeding is quickly stopped by local pressure with the thumb or by encouraging the patient to bite on a gauze pad placed over a bleeding tooth socket. If bleeding has been severe, the patient should rest on his back with his legs up on a chair or if in hospital on a bed tilted feet up. He will feel better because the brain is better perfused when lying flat. He should be kept at a temperature which is comfortable but not warm because heating the skin causes vasodilation and blood is diverted from more important organs. Fluid must be replaced either by encouraging drinking, or if a great deal has been lost, by an intravenous infusion to expand blood volume thereby directly raising blood pressure. The oxygen carrying capacity must be restored by blood transfusion.

SHOCK

Signs and Causes

Shock is an example of a 'syndrome'; a clinical state brought about in several different ways. Treatment therefore is aimed both at the shock state itself and at the underlying condition.

The term 'shock' is used clinically in a quite specific way. To the laymen shock may simply mean a dazed reaction to a piece of bad news, but to a clinician it signifies a very serious physiological disturbance. Shock occurs when the cardiac output is insufficient to meet the

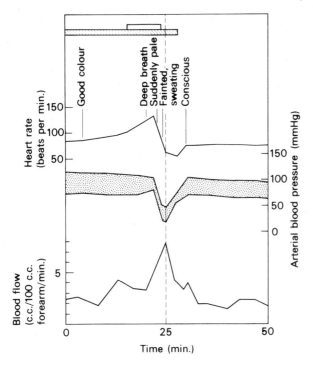

Fig. 15.78. Post-haemorrhagic fainting. Typical symptoms and changes in heart rate, arterial blood pressure, and fore-arm blood flow. Plain rectangle, venesection; shaded rectangle, venous torniquets applied to both thighs (dams in legs to simulate haemorrhage).

oxygen requirements of all the tissues of the body. Common causes are:

1 Decreased blood volume, 'hypovolaemic shock', due to severe bleeding, either internally or externally or to loss of plasma as in severe burning.

2 A sudden reduction in cardiac output, due to myocardial infarction.

3 Cardiac output becoming insufficient because of widespread vasodilation. Injection of penicillin for instance, in a person made hypersensitive by previous exposure, may trigger a massive allergic reaction; the vasodilator substances which are released cause a sudden fall in blood pressure causing 'anaphylactic shock'. In 'endotoxic shock' similar vasodilation results from endotoxin released in severe infections caused by Gram-negative bacteria.

The body attempts to counter the reduced cardiac output and fall in arterial perfusion pressure in shock by increased sympathetic activity as described for the response to haemorrhage. The reduced cerebral blood flow means that the patient is unable to help himself. Prompt specific treatment for the underlying condition is essential.

Shock which fails to respond to such treatment is termed 'irreversible shock'. Probably in such cases tissue hypoxia and resulting acidosis affect cell membranes and gradually potassium ions and other intracellular substances leak into the blood. As heart muscle is among the tissues so affected, the condition rapidly worsens. The fluid environment of the cells becomes more and more abnormal so that simple replacement of blood volume may not be enough.

FAINTING

Signs and causes

Fainting is a reflex event often resulting in loss of consciousness. Many circumstances, for example haemorrhage or standing still for prolonged periods (so that blood pools in leg veins) may cause fainting. Usually these are situations in which it is difficult to maintain blood pressure and such cases can be recognised initially by the signs of reflex sympathetic activity such as tachycardia and cutaneous vasoconstriction as the body attempts to maintain the blood supply to the brain. Paradoxically however, the body then responds by suddenly lowering blood pressure.

Sympathetic vasodilator nerves cause the resistance vessels of skeletal muscles to open so that blood pours into them (Fig. 15.78). Blood pressure drops rapidly, the brain becomes hypoxic with the result that the person falls to the ground unconscious. However, once horizontal there is a quick recovery; first because only a very low blood pressure is then needed to perfuse the brain and second, because baroreceptor reflexes soon cause intense sympathetic vasoconstriction.

The most common type of fainting occurs, however, when cerebral blood flow is not threatened at all, for example, after an unpleasant emotional experience. This type of fainting is referred to as vaso-vagal syncope. The vagal component is inhibition of the heart rate caused by increased vagal activity. This, with the accompanying vasodilation in skeletal muscle arterioles, causes a large fall of blood pressure. Faints do not last long and require no treatment if the person is allowed to lie flat. In the dental chair a person is usually told to lean forward so that the head is low and below the level of his

heart — or the chair is tilted right back with the same effect. These remedies may raise the blood pressure to the brain sufficiently for consciousness to be regained. However, if a person who has fainted is prevented from falling, say by being propped up in a crowd, then cerebral hypoxia may cause convulsions and even death.

Further reading

Blood Group Topics by B. E. Dodd and P. J. Lincoln (1975). Edward Arnold, London. This is a handy paperback appearing in the *Current Topics in Immunology* series. It offers a short survey of the blood grouping field very much from the antibody point of view and could be read with profit by those who do not wish to become involved in works that may go more deeply into the subject than their needs require.

CHAPTER 16

The Urinary System

URINARY SYSTEM

Anatomy and histology

The urinary system is usually regarded as primarily associated with excretion but it is equally important for the maintenance of water and acid/base balance in the body. The kidneys are the organs which carry out these functions and the rest of the system, the ureter, bladder and urethra are the means whereby the urine produced by the kidneys is passed to the exterior.

KIDNEYS

A coronal section passing through the kidney shows the following features on the cut surface (Fig. 16.1). The hilum leads into a space, the renal sinus, where the renal vessels and the expanded upper part of the ureter, the pelvis can be seen. The pelvis of the ureter is formed by the union of two or three major calices which in turn are formed by the union of three or more minor calices. The cut surface of the kidney shows pyramidal structures the renal pyramids, which project at their narrow ends (renal papillae) into the cup-shaped minor calices. The collecting ducts open on the papillae into the minor calices. The pyramids are darker than the rest of the cut

surface. A line indicated by the outer edge of the pyramids divides the renal substance into an outer cortex and inner medulla. The cortex appears to extend into the medulla between the pyramids as the renal columns, and the pyramids appear to extend outwards into the cortex as the medullary rays.

The nephron

The structural and functional unit of the kidney is a complicated tubule called the nephron (Fig. 16.2a). There are said to be about one million nephrons in each kidney and that at least one third of these have to be functional for normal health; thus it is easily appreciated that an individual can function with only one kidney. The nephron, about 30 cm long, consists of a renal (Malpighian) corpuscle and a renal tubule. The renal tubule joins a collecting tubule which joins a collecting duct.

The renal corpuscle consists of a vascular glomerulus (Fig. 16.2b) surrounded by a glomerular (Bowman's) capsule. An afferent glomerular arteriole enters the glomerulus (from the Latin glomus, a ball of thread) and splits into a tuft of capillary vessels from which arises an efferent glomerular arteriole. The entry and exit of the arterioles are adjacent to each other and are called the vascular pole. The

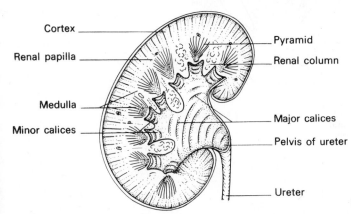

Fig. 16.1 Coronal section of kidney.

Cortex — Pyramid
Renal papilla — Renal column
Medulla — Major calices
Minor calices — Pelvis of ureter
Ureter

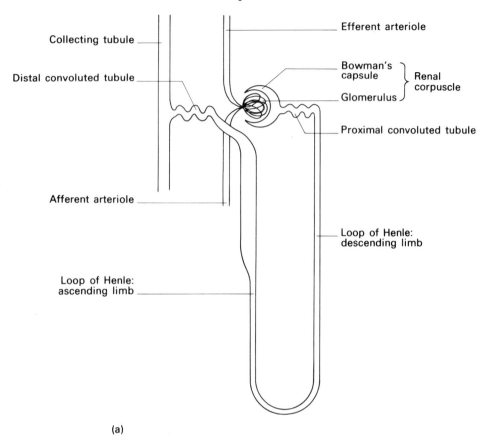

Collecting tubule

Distal convoluted tubule

Afferent arteriole

Loop of Henle: ascending limb

Efferent arteriole

Bowman's capsule ⎱ Renal corpuscle
Glomerulus ⎰

Proximal convoluted tubule

Loop of Henle: descending limb

(a)

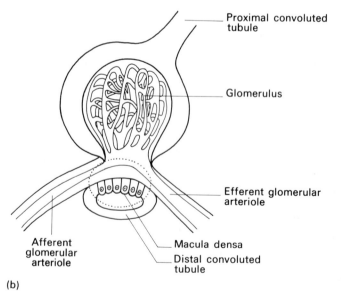

Proximal convoluted tubule

Glomerulus

Efferent glomerular arteriole

Afferent glomerular arteriole

Macula densa

Distal convoluted tubule

(b)

Fig. 16.2 (a) Diagram of the nephron. (b) Diagram of the renal corpuscle and juxtaglomerular apparatus (indicated by a dotted circle).

capillaries form an anastomosing plexus and are of the fenestrated type. The capsular layer next to the capillaries consists of cells called podocytes (from the Greek pous, a foot) because they have a large number of footlike processes which are related to the capillary wall but are separated from it by the glomerular basement membrane about 300 nm in thickness. The outer capsular layer consists of a single layer of flattened cells continuous with the cells of the first part of the renal tubule.

The glomerular capsule continues into the proximal convoluted tubule which is in the cortex. The cells have microvilli on their luminal surface and contain a large number of basal mitochondria. Their lateral and external surfaces are very much folded so that neighbouring cells interdigitate with each other.

The proximal convoluted tubule leads into the loop of Henle which has a descending (thin) and ascending (thick) limb lying in the medulla. The first part of the loop is really the termination of the proximal convoluted tubule and there is an abrupt transition to the flattened squamous cells of the descending loop. These cells have no special features. The ascending limb consists of cells similar to those of the proximal convoluted tubule but they have no microvilli. The length of the loop of Henle is variable. It may extend into the outer part of the medulla in which case the change from the thin to the thick part is at the bend of the loop, or they may reach almost to the papilla in which case a considerable part of the ascending limb is thin.

The ascending loop of Henle leads into the distal convoluted tubule which is in the cortex and is much shorter (about 5 mm long) than the proximal (about 15 mm long). The cells of this part of the renal tubule have numerous basal mitochondria and the cells interdigitate with each other laterally and basally. The distal convoluted tubule approaches its own glomerulus and is attached to the efferent arteriole at the vascular pole. A structure called the juxtaglomerular apparatus (Fig. 16.2b) is formed (juxta means next in Latin) consisting of specialized cells of the tunica media of the arteriole and the macula densa of the distal convoluted tubule. The cells forming the macula densa are more columnar than the cells of the rest of the distal convoluted tubule and their base is separated from the specialized cells of the afferent arteriole by only a thin basement membrane. The specialized cells of the arteriole have rough endoplasmic reticulum, a well marked Golgi complex, and a number of granules all of which

indicate that these cells have a secretory function. Their secretion is renin (p. 745).

The collecting tubules receive the distal convoluted tubules in the cortex and pass into the medulla towards the papillae of the pyramids. In the pyramid, collecting tubules join together and form the terminal collecting ducts (of Bellini) which open at the papillary apex into a minor calyx. The single layer of cells lining the smaller collecting tubules are cuboidal with a clear cytoplasm. These cells become columnar in the larger tubules and in the ducts.

URETERS

These are tubular structures, one on each side, about 25 cm long and 0.5 cm in diameter. They pass downwards on the posterior abdominal wall from the hilum of the kidney to the bony pelvis where they join the bladder. The ureter enters the posterosuperior angle of the bladder at an oblique angle and runs through its wall for about 1.5 cm before opening into the bladder. This obliquity results in the closure of the ureter when the bladder contracts in micturition so that reflux of urine into the ureter is prevented. When the urine leaves the kidneys, it is propelled along the ureters by slow peristaltic waves towards the bladder.

BLADDER

The urinary bladder is a hollow, muscular organ lying in the pelvis behind the symphysis pubis from which it is separated by fat. The bladder, in front of the uterus and vagina in the female (Fig. 13.7), and the rectum in the male, is usually described as having a triangular pyramidal shape with the apex of the pyramid anterior and superior and the base posterior. Of the remaining three sides one is superior and the other two are inferolateral. The position of the bladder varies with age and its state of distension. In the infant it is elongated anteriorly and upwards so that it extends into the abdominal cavity, but by the age of six years the bladder is in the pelvis although its final position depends on the development of the reproductive organs at puberty. As the bladder distends it enlarges upwards between the peritoneum and the anterior abdominal wall, i.e. the bladder lies outside the peritoneum.

The bladder has three coats, an outer serous formed by the peritoneum, a middle muscular and an inner epithelial. The serous coat is restricted to the superior surface and a small part of the posterior surface. The muscular coat has three layers, an outer and inner longitudinal and middle circular. The detailed arrangement of the muscle is complex especially in the region of the beginning of the urethra, where some of the circular muscle may form a sphincter. The muscle is so arranged that the opening into the urethra is kept closed until micturition takes place. The bladder muscle as a whole then contracts (it is often referred to as the detrusor muscle) and at the same time alters the shape of the beginning of the urethra converting this region of the bladder from a closed flat plate into an open funnel-shaped structure. The bladder is lined by transitional epithelium which has six or eight layers when the bladder is empty. As the bladder is filled the epithelial layers are reduced in number. The other main property of transitional epithelium is that it does not absorb the dissolved substances in the urine.

Micturition
The adult urinary bladder has the special property of being able to increase its size in order to accommodate increasing amounts of urine. As the bladder fills, there is at first a gradual build up of pressure within it. However when a volume of about 200 cm³ is reached, further filling is accompanied by relaxation of the bladder and so there is little further increase in pressure. Eventually, a point is reached at about 400 cm³ when further entry of urine causes a rapid increase in pressure. The sensation of bladder distension is apparent once the volume is greater than about 300 cm³ and gradually becomes stronger as the volume increases. This sensation can be temporarily suppressed, but when the volume reaches about 650 cm³ it ultimately becomes so strong that micturition must follow.

The bladder is supplied with both sympathetic and parasympathetic motor and sensory nerve fibres. The sympathetic sensory fibres are associated with sensations of pain. The preganglionic sympathetic motor nerve fibres come from the eleventh and twelfth thoracic and first lumber segments of the spinal cord. The preganglionic parasympathetic fibres come from the second, third and fourth sacral segments of the spinal cord (the nervi erigentes or pelvic parasympathetic nerves).

Micturition is essentially a reflex response to a full bladder, as seen in babies and in adults with a complete transection of the spinal cord. Normally however, from the age of about 2 years, there is a considerable degree of voluntary control over the reflex.

The exact mechanism is a complicated interaction of many factors. In the resting state, the detrusor muscle is relaxed and the opening into the urethra is closed due to the action of the sympathetic nervous system. The external (voluntary) sphincter urethrae is also closed. As the pressure in the bladder increases, stretch receptors in the walls of the bladder are stimulated and sensory parasympathetic fibres convey the information to the spinal cord, from where it is relayed to the sensory cortex. When a critical level of sensory stimulation is reached in either the uncontrolled reflex state, or in a normal and socially convenient situation allowing inhibition to be removed, the detrusor muscle contracts, the sphincters relax and urine is expelled. These events are brought about by the stimulation of the parasympathetic motor nerves and inhibition of the sympathetic nerves. It is important to realize that in this respect, the parasympathetic nervous system is by far the more important of the two; when sympathetic innervation to the bladder is destroyed, there is minimal interference with micturition. During micturition, the activity of the external sphincter urethrae is inhibited and it relaxes. Once started, urine flow can be temporarily interrupted by the voluntary closure of the external sphincter.

It is possible to bring about micturition voluntarily even though the bladder is not full enough to produce any sensation. In these circumstances the initiation of micturition requires an increase in intra-abdominal pressure by fixation of the thorax and contraction of the anterior abdominal muscles. The areas of the brain which are associated with this voluntary control of micturition lie in the pons and midbrain and stimulation of, or lesions affecting, these areas (and the hypothalamus) produce dramatic effects on micturition.

URETHRA

This is the tube leading from the bladder to the exterior. In the female it is about 5 cm long and passes downwards and slightly forwards close to and in front of the vagina. It opens into the vestibule immediately in front of the vaginal opening, about 2.5 cm behind the clitoris, the homologue of the penis.

The female urethra is lined by stratified squamous epithelium, except near the bladder where the epithelium is transitional, and has an inner longitudinal and outer circular layer of muscle. There is a sphincter of skeletal muscle round the urethra (sphincter urethrae) about halfway between the bladder and the external opening. Although this is very important in controlling voluntary micturition the muscular floor of the pelvis is equally important in preventing the involuntary expulsion of small quantities of urine.

In the male the urethra is about 20 cm long and is divided into three parts, prostatic, membranous and spongy (penile). The prostatic part passes through the prostate, is about 3 cm long and is the widest and most dilatable part. The ducts of the glands of the prostate and the common ejaculatory ducts open into this part of the urethra.

The membranous part of the urethra about 2 cm long is the narrowest part. It is called the membranous part because it passes through two layers of fascia which are attached laterally to the ischiopubic rami. The sphincter urethrae (skeletal muscle) surrounds the membranous urethra.

The spongy part passes through the corpus spongiosum of the penis and is about 15 cm long. It opens on to the exterior at the external urethral orifice which is as narrow as the membranous urethra.

FUNCTIONS OF THE KIDNEY

The obvious function of the kidney is the elimination of the nitrogenous waste products of protein metabolism, mainly as urea, but there are other functions that are equally important to the body and contribute to homeostasis. Among these are the maintenance of the body's water and electrolyte balance and the regulation of its acid/base balance. These functions are all achieved by the production of urine, the composition of which can be varied according to the state of the body.

In addition, the kidney acts as an endocrine gland. It secretes three hormones. Erythropoeitin is released under conditions of chronic hypoxia and increases red blood cell production (p. 675). Renin converts angiotensinogen in plasma to angiotensin and is concerned in the maintenance of arterial blood pressure (p. 716) and the control of aldosterone production by the adrenal cortex (p. 745). A third hormone, 1,25-dihydroxycholecalciferol is produced from a less active precursor and brings about the actions associated with vitamin D_3 (p. 766).

Under normal conditions, the kidneys produce about 1.5 dm³ of urine each day. Urine is usually slightly acid, although its pH can vary between 4.7 and 8.2. It has a specific gravity between 1.015 and 1.025 and contains about 49 constituents, the chief of which are urea (20 g/dm³ or about 30 g/day), chloride (6.0 g/dm³ or about 9 g/day) and sodium (3.5 g/dm³ or 5 g/day).

The formation of urine

The process of urine formation comprises (a) filtration, (b) selective absorption and (c) selective secretion.

GLOMERULAR FILTRATION

The kidneys receive about one quarter of the cardiac output at rest, 1200 cm³/minute. In the renal (Malpighian) corpuscle (Fig. 16.2b) there is a very close relationship between the walls of the capillaries of the glomerulus and the Bowman's capsule. Together they create a filter which allows only particles below a critical size to pass through. It has been found by injecting a series of proteins of different molecular weights that this size corresponds to a molecular weight of about 68,000. This means that all the constituents of blood except cells, platelets and plasma proteins can pass into the Bowman's capsule.

The process of filtration requires a driving force and this is provided by the blood pressure within the capillaries of the glomerulus. Due to the anatomical arrangement of the blood vessels to and from the glomerulus, the pressure in the glomerular capillaries is about 70 mm Hg which is higher than is usually found in capillaries. However, all of this pressure is not used to drive the constituents through the filter as it is opposed by the colloid osmotic pressure of the blood (about 25 mm Hg) and the back pressure within the Bowman's capsule (about 10 mm Hg). Thus:

Effective filtration pressure = Glomerular capillary pressure − (Colloid osmotic pressure + Back pressure)

= 70 − (25 + 10)

= 35 mm Hg.

By this process 120 cm³ of filtrate is produced from the 1200 cm³ of blood passing through the kidneys in each minute (170 dm³/day). This figure, 120 cm³/min, is the glomerular filtration rate (GFR) and can be measured by a method that will be discussed later. Although glomerular filtration is considered to remain relatively constant under normal conditions, the equation giving the effective filtration pressure shows that the GFR can be altered by anything that changes the glomerular capillary pressure, the hydrostatic pressure in the Bowman's capsule, and the osmotic pressure of the plasma proteins. In addition, any pathological condition which alters the permeability of the filter or reduces the total surface area of the filter will also affect the glomerular filtration rate.

Control of renal blood flow (RBF) and glomerular filtration rate (GFR)

In order to function normally the kidney requires an adequate blood supply at the correct glomerular capillary pressure, which in turn is dependent on the arterial blood pressure.

Though the renal arteries and arterioles are constricted in generalized pressor reflexes and participate in the redistribution of blood from the viscera to active muscles, it is not thought that the renal nerves exert a tonic influence on the renal vessels or for that matter have any significant role in normal renal function. Nevertheless renal arterioles can be constricted by stimulation of the sympathetic nerves and by circulating adrenaline. Since it is mainly the afferent (preglomerular) vessels which are affected, both RBF and GFR are much reduced under conditions of stress such as heavy exercise, shock and haemorrhage, with a resultant reduction in urine flow.

A remarkable feature of RBF and GFR is their relative constancy over a wide range of mean arterial blood pressure or renal arterial perfusion pressures (from 80–180 mm Hg), a phenomenon which can be demonstrated in a denervated isolated kidney. Only two of several mechanisms which have been proposed for this autoregulation will be considered, as only these two are supported by sufficient evidence.

The principal mechanism is the myogenic response of the renal arterioles. The smooth muscle of the arterioles entering the glomerulus contracts in response to distension caused by a raised perfusion pressure thereby increasing the preglomerular resistance and holding in check the glomerular flow and pressure. Conversely, when perfusion pressure falls slightly below normal, the smooth muscle in the afferent arteriole relaxes and glomerular flow is maintained. If the perfusion pressure falls further (corresponding to a mean arterial pressure of below 80 mm Hg) the response is insufficient to maintain the steady state and there is a fall in

RBF and GFR. This theoretically might be made worse in the whole body situation where vasoconstriction of the renal arterioles would be part of a pressor reflex resulting from the fall in mean arterial pressure. However, if the pressure in the renal artery falls, renin is somehow released by the juxtaglomerular apparatus (Fig. 16.2b); this converts angiotensinogen in the blood to angiotensin. This causes generalized vasoconstriction, which tends to raise the arterial blood pressure but, in addition, it causes constriction of the renal arterioles, particularly the efferent, which, although reducing glomerular blood flow restores pressure and therefore helps to maintain some glomerular filtration.

TUBULAR REABSORPTION

The filtrate from the Bowman's capsule passes into the proximal convoluted tubule (PCT) (Fig. 16.3) at a rate of 120 cm³/min. Here the volume of the filtrate is reduced by about 85%. This reabsorption is known as obligatory reabsorption. It does not vary under normal physiological conditions. The remaining 20 cm³/min enters the descending limb of the loop of Henle which passes down through the medulla and then rises up again in the ascending limb to the cortex. The volume of fluid is only slightly reduced when it enters the distal convoluted tubule. It then passes into the collecting duct, which dips down again through the medulla and out to the bladder by way of the ureters. In these distal regions of the nephron, reabsorption is varied according to the electrolyte or water balance in the body and this is known as facultative reabsorption. Under normal conditions the urine flow is about 1 cm³/min, which gives the usual daily urine volume of about 1.5 dm³, but under conditions of extreme dehydration and hydration urine flow can vary from about 0.3 to about 20 cm³/min respectively.

Obligatory reabsorption

The main feature of reabsorption in the PCT is that there is no change in the tonicity of the filtrate although its volume is reduced by 85%. One of the major net changes to occur in the composition of the fluid is the removal of all glucose from the glomerular filtrate along the PCT. Obligatory reabsorption involves the movement of substances from the filtrate into the tubular cells and back into the blood against concentration gradients. Thus sodium diffuses into the tubule cells and is then pumped out of the cells into the plasma. Metabolic energy is

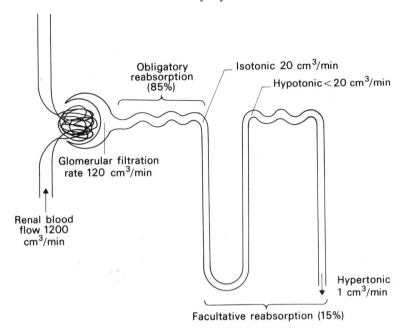

Fig. 16.3 A diagrammatic summary of the flow and tonicity of the filtrate in the various regions of the nephron.

necessary for this, as indicated by the kidney's high oxygen consumption. In different ways glucose and potassium reabsorption also depend on cellular metabolism. Chloride is reabsorbed in conjunction with sodium in order to maintain electrical balance, and bicarbonate ions are reabsorbed by a complicated mechanism which is associated with the reabsorption of sodium and the secretion of hydrogen ions into the tubule, in order to regulate the body's acid–base balance (p. 750).

In this way about 85% of the solutes of the filtrate are reabsorbed and water follows them. It is probable that this reabsorption of water is a passive process, being governed by the concentration gradients of plasma proteins and electrolytes between the blood and the filtrate. This reabsorption does not participate in the normal osmotic regulation of the body. If however, there is an increase in the concentration of osmotically active substances in the glomerular filtrate, obligatory reabsorption can alter dramatically (see osmotic diuretics, p. 741). As a result of active reabsorption of certain substances and passive reabsorption of water, some other substances in the filtrate, for example urea, become more concentrated in the filtrate

than in the blood and are to some extent passively reabsorbed by simple diffusion.

The mechanisms for actively transporting glucose and sodium out of the tubule into the blood have a maximum rate at which they can operate. Normally this rate is sufficient to handle all the reabsorption that is required, but under certain conditions the mechanism may be swamped. If the concentration of glucose in plasma rises to about 180 mg/100 cm^3, so that about 220 mg glucose is filtered each minute, the cell cannot deal with all the glucose presented to it and as a result some glucose appears in the urine (glycosuria). The full capacity of the 'pump' (tubular maximum or Tm) is not reached however until the filtration rate approaches 360 mg/min.

Facultative reabsorption

The amount of facultative reabsorption is varied so that the composition of the urine is adjusted in order to minimize changes in electrolyte or water balance of the body. This variable reabsorption occurs in the loop of Henle, the distal convoluted tubule (DCT) and the collecting duct (Fig. 16.3).

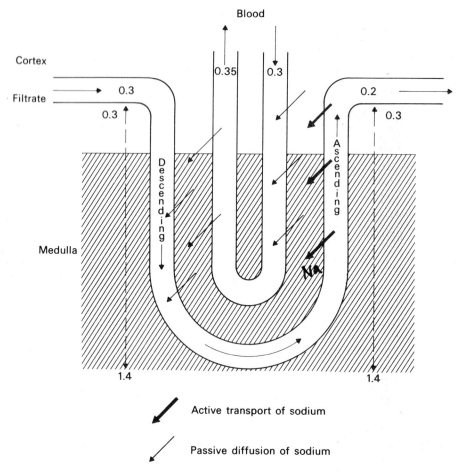

Fig. 16.4 A simple diagram illustrating the movement of sodium in the counter current multiplier system which occurs in the loop of Henle. Figures indicate the osmolarity in osmoles.

Loop of Henle. Only animals which produce a hypertonic urine (birds and mammals) have well developed loops of Henle, and those mammals which produce the most concentrated urine generally have the longest loops of Henle. Thus there would appear to be a definite role for the loop in the production of a concentrated urine.

This region of the nephron has recently been the centre of much work and a complicated mechanism has been formulated. The details of it however, are by no means certain and there are many different versions. It will only be dealt with in general terms in this account. The key fact is that when the filtrate enters the descending limb at about 20 cm³/min it is isotonic with the non-protein fraction of plasma and when it leaves the ascending limb to enter the DCT the volume is only slightly altered but it is now

slightly hypotonic (Fig. 16.3). The reason for this is that during its passage through the loop the filtrate retains almost all its water since the walls are only slightly permeable to water but there is a net loss of sodium and chloride. Although a small amount of sodium moves passively into the tubule from the blood in the descending limb, on the way up the ascending limb sodium or chloride is actively pumped out, and overall more is lost than was gained. This movement of sodium is not involved in the control of electrolyte balance; it has a particular significance because of the way in which it occurs (Fig. 16.4). The loop of Henle and the accompanying blood vessels (vasa recta) are arranged in such a way that the flows are in the opposite directions. Sodium is actively pumped out of the ascending limb of the tubule into the tissue fluid so that it is more concentrated than the blood in the capillary. Sodium therefore diffuses into the capillary and is carried deep into the medulla again. As the capillary climbs up towards the cortex on the other side its contents are more concentrated than the surrounding tissue, so sodium diffuses out again. Alongside is the descending tubule which dips down into the medulla. Sodium tends to diffuse in to the tubule and again is carried deep into the medulla. As a result of these events, sodium tends to be trapped deep in the medulla around the base of the loop and the osmolality is about 1.4 osmoles. As the depth into the medulla decreases, so the osmolality decreases until in the region of the cortex it is less than 0.3 osmoles, which is hypotonic to the fluids in the PCT and DCT. The mechanism of this movement of sodium and the establishment of the sodium concentration gradient, is known as the counter-current multiplier system.

All this activity has caused the filtrate to become hypotonic but otherwise has had little effect on its volume and composition. This appears to be a step in the wrong direction as the objective is to make it hypertonic. The establishment of the high osmolality in blood and tissue fluid in the medulla is however, of great importance in the final process of concentrating the urine. Recent evidence suggests that urea also becomes concentrated in this region and makes a small contribution to the osmotic gradient.

Distal tubule and collecting duct
The hypotonic filtrate entering the DCT at slightly less than 20 cm³/min is now subjected to the final processes of reabsorption. The chief substances reabsorbed are water, sodium, chloride and bicarbonate.

During its passage through the DCT and collecting duct some 19 cm³/min of water are reabsorbed, the bulk of it in the collecting duct, which is permeable to water. The duct dips down through the medulla and thus passes through the area of increasing sodium concentration established by the processes occurring in the loop of Henle. Water is drawn out of the duct into the interstitial fluid and then into the blood and the final concentration and volume of the urine are achieved. However, as urine flow can be very variable, it follows that the permeability of the collecting duct must be regulated in some way. Variation is controlled by antidiuretic hormone or ADH (vasopressin) which is secreted from the posterior pituitary according to the body's

water load. Under conditions of dehydration the secretion of ADH is maximal and under its influence the pores between the cells of the collecting duct are fully open and the maximum amount of water passes back into the blood. In the opposite situation, when the body is overloaded with water, the secretion of ADH is stopped, the pores are sealed, and water passes straight through the collecting duct and out as urine. The exact way in which ADH controls the pore size is not known but it has been described as a process of 'dissolving the cell cement'. The control of ADH secretion is considered later (Fig. 16.8).

The reabsorption of sodium is against the concentration gradient and is therefore active. Here, unlike the PCT, it is a variable process, stimulated by aldosterone from the adrenal cortex. As in the PCT, chloride ions are absorbed in association with the sodium ions. Certain substances are actively secreted into the DCT, among which are potassium and hydrogen ions and it seems that in some way the reabsorption of sodium is linked with this. Bicarbonate is also reabsorbed in the DCT so that under normal circumstances there is little or no bicarbonate in the urine. This process is dependent on many factors, for example, the secretion of potassium, hydrogen and ammonium ions, and will be considered in more detail when the body's acid–base balance is discussed (p. 750).

TUBULAR SECRETION

Substances which actively secreted into the PCT and DCT fall into two categories; first, those that are naturally present in the body such as potassium, hydrogen and ammonium, and second those foreign to the body such as p-aminohippuric acid (PAH), various contrast media used in renal radiography and many drugs or their derivatives like penicillin, histamine and some sulphonamides. The kidney's handling of potassium should be emphasized since potassium ions are reabsorbed in the PCT but then actively secreted into the DCT. In addition creatinine, from the breakdown of muscle creatine, is secreted in very small amounts.

RENAL CLEARANCE

Renal clearance is a mathematical concept which in the past has been widely used to study renal function in both animals and man. Modern techniques have to a large extent replaced those measurements, but clearance is still worth considering as it illustrates a number of basic points in renal physiology.

The best way to understand the idea of renal clearance is to work through an example from first principles: if a substance X is present in urine at a concentration of say 2 mg/cm³ and the urine flow is 1 cm³/min. Then:

Rate of excretion of X = 2 × 1 mg/min
= 2 mg/min

This substance X is derived entirely from the blood passing through the kidneys.

If the simultaneous concentration of X in the blood plasma is 1 mg/100 cm³, it follows that the 2 mg excreted must have come from 200 cm³ of plasma. Thus, the renal clearance of substance X (C_x) is 200 cm³/min. In other words, the renal clearance of a substance is the volume of plasma that would contain the amount of that substance excreted in urine in one minute. Mathematically:

$$C = \frac{UV}{P}$$

where U = concentration of the substance in urine
      P = concentration of the substance in plasma
      V = Urine (volume)/minute

For the example worked out above,

$$C_x = \frac{200 \text{ mg}/100 \text{ cm}^3}{1 \text{ mg}/100 \text{ cm}^3} \times 1 \text{ cm}^3/\text{min}$$

$$= 200 \text{ cm}^3/\text{min}$$

The measurement of renal clearance is a fairly simple procedure, which involves the injection of the test substance and the collection of the urine formed over a timed period. Arterial blood samples must be taken at appropriate times throughout the urine collection period to give a mean plasma concentration.

Clearance measurements are valuable in the study of renal physiology because a substance that is freely filtered by the kidney and which passes straight through the tubule without loss by reabsorption or gain by secretion, has a clearance equal to the GFR. Additionally, such a substance must not be toxic, metabolized, taken into any cells or bound to plasma proteins. One foreign substance, inulin (a polysaccharide, mw 5200) satisfies these conditions, and its clearance of 120 cm³/min can be taken as a measure-

ment of the GFR. Although creatinine gives a slightly higher value than inulin because it is secreted into the kidney tubule in very small amounts it has the advantage of being present naturally, which means that its clearance can be measured without having to inject it. Although it is known to be slightly inaccurate, creatinine clearance can be used as an acceptable measurement of GFR and is used in the clinical investigation of renal function.

Now that GFR has been established, it follows that any substance having a lower clearance value is being partially reabsorbed and any substance having a higher value is being actively secreted. The limits of the clearance value are set at one end by glucose, which is normally completely reabsorbed (U glucose = 0) and therefore C glucose = 0. The upper limit is fixed by any substance that is totally cleared from the blood in one passage through the kidneys. Strictly speaking, there is no such substance as about 10% of the renal plasma flow does not pass through tissue participating in the formation of urine. However, p-aminohippuric acid (PAH), nearly fulfils this condition, and it's clearance of about 650 cm³/min is a good indication of the renal plasma flow.

Fig. 16.5 illustrates the use of renal clearances in determining how a substance is handled by the kidney. It must be remembered however, that substances that are actively reabsorbed or secreted can swamp such mechanisms if the blood concentration rises too high. Thus if the blood glucose level rises to such an extent that the reabsorptive mechanism in the PCT cannot cope, as in diabetes mellitus for example, then glucose starts to appear in the urine. In the clearance formula therefore, $U_{glucose}$ no longer equals zero and there is now a glucose clearance value. Similarly, if the PAH level in the blood is so high that the secretory mechanism cannot remove it all, then its clearance value begins to fall. Only inulin, which is neither secreted nor reabsorbed, has a clearance that is completely independent of blood concentration.

The ratio of GFR to renal plasma flow is known as the filtration fraction (FF).

$$FF = \frac{GFR}{\text{Renal plasma flow}}$$

$$= \frac{C_{inulin}}{C_{PAH}}$$

$$= \frac{120}{650} = \frac{1}{5.4}$$

Thus, approximately one fifth of the plasma

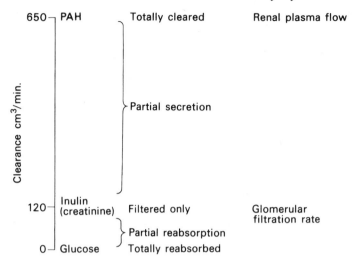

Clearance cm³/min.

650 — PAH | Totally cleared | Renal plasma flow

Partial secretion

120 — Inulin (creatinine) | Filtered only | Glomerular filtration rate

Partial reabsorption

0 — Glucose | Totally reabsorbed

Fig. 16.5. The use of renal clearance to indicate how a substance is handled by the kidney.

entering the kidney in the renal artery passes into the kidney tubule as glomerular filtrate.

DIURESIS

The condition of increased urine flow is known as diuresis, and any substance causing it is a diuretic. Water is the natural diuretic in the body and when ingested in excess may produce urine flows of up to about 20 cm³/min. The mechanism of this diuresis and also that of alcohol diuresis will be discussed in the next section. Urine flow can however also be increased by quite a different method. The volume of urine is to some extent governed by the concentration of solutes in the renal tubule. Substances that are filtered but then poorly reabsorbed in the PCT will, when present in excess, act as diuretics because by raising the osmotic pressure in the tubule there is reduced water reabsorption and therefore increased urine flow. Osmotic diuretics which can be given orally are mannitol, urea and sulphates. Osmotic diuresis can sometimes occur naturally, the best example being in diabetes mellitus (p. 799). The increased amount of glucose in the PCT results in an increase in the daily urine volume (polyuria). It is difficult to give a maximum figure for urine flow achieved by these types of diuretics, but certainly figures around 35 cm³/min have been reported.

CONTROL OF RENAL FUNCTION —FLUID BALANCE

It was seen in the previous section that the urinary flow-rate can vary from about 0.3 to 20.0

cm³/min, according to the state of hydration. This large physiological variation is aimed at the preservation of a constant body water volume and is achieved by a change in reabsorption rather than a change in the glomerular filtration rate.

The control of reabsorption can be considered as a humoral process comprising the control of water reabsorption and the control of electrolyte reabsorption, which is effectively the control of sodium reabsorption. These two processes participate in regulating the body's water balance and electrolyte balance.

Water balance

The average water loss by the body is normally taken as about 2.6 dm³ per day. It must be realized that this is the water lost by a person living a sedentary life, on a normal balanced diet, and in a climate that puts no stress on the body's temperature regulation. The routes by which water is lost under these conditions are shown in Fig. 16.6.

Now the body contains about 50 dm³ of water (p. 668), so if this daily loss of about 2.6 dm³ is not replaced, this would amount to a daily deficit of about 5% of the total body water. This degree of water loss can be tolerated, but is approaching the 'danger level' at which the body's physical condition would start to deteriorate. Under these conditions the body conserves water. It is only by reducing the daily urinary flow that this can be achieved, as water loss through the other three routes cannot be effectively controlled. Even so, the control over the kidney is limited as

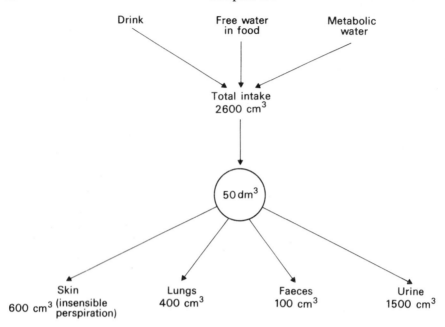

Fig. 16.6. The daily water balance of the body, showing the amounts of water lost by the various routes under basal conditions.

there must be a minimum daily urine volume of between 300 and 500 cm³, depending on the diet, in order to keep some urinary constituents in solution. Thus, under conditions of dehydration, the minimum daily total water loss can only be reduced by about 1 dm³.

To counteract normal water loss, water is taken in by drinking (see p. 744, thirst) and by ingesting the substantial amounts of free water in many foods. In addition, the body produces a small amount of water by metabolism (p. 200) which must be taken into consideration in the overall water balance of the body.

DEHYDRATION

So far, only the body's 'minimum water loss' has been considered. As soon as the body is required to lose excess heat, an additional strain is placed on the body's water balance for this involves the loss of considerable quantities of water in sweating. It is important to realize that sweating and insensible perspiration are completely different. Insensible perspiration is the passive loss of water through the skin which goes on all the time irrespective of the condition of the body or the environment. It is simply due to the fact that the skin is not quite water-tight. Sweating on the

other hand is an active process controlled by the sympathetic nervous system (p. 726).

Conditions that cause high rates of sweating present massive problems to the water balance of the body. When heat is produced by occupational activities or by the occurrence of severe fever, it is quite possible for 10–15 dm³ of sweat to be produced in a day when fluids are ingested. If there is no water replacement the situation is very serious. Haemoconcentration occurs and the temperature rises further as the rate of sweating declines. Normally about 400 cm³ water/day is lost through the lungs. Conditions which cause prolonged hyperventilation, such as high altitude, will increase this loss of water up to a maximum of about 6 dm³/day. Diarrhoea and vomiting cause water and electrolyte depletion. Loss of water in the faeces is normally about 100 cm³/day.

Since a minimum daily volume of urine (300–500 cm³) must be excreted, this means that the body can only conserve about a litre of water a day. When water loss is severe this is an insignificant saving and the body's only defence is to register the sensation of thirst (Fig. 16.7). If water is not available the physical condition of the body starts to deteriorate (with more than a 5% water loss (about 2.5 dm³)) and it gets pro-

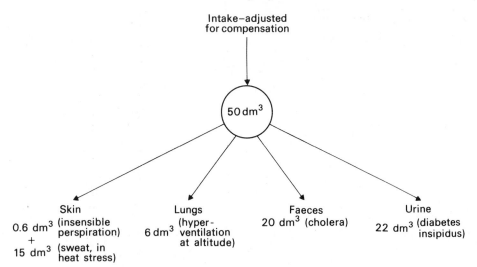

Fig. 16.7. An indication of the problem that various abnormal conditions of water loss can impose on the water balance of the body. The values represent maximum loss in extreme conditions.

gressively worse until the individual becomes delirious (when the loss reaches about 14% (7 dm³)).

EXCESS WATER INTAKE

If the body's water content is greater than normal, the excess is quickly and accurately removed by increasing the urine flow. The body is therefore very well equipped to counter hydration, in contrast to being so inadequately protected against dehydration.

CONTROL OF WATER REABSORPTION

Variations in urine flow are due to the action of antidiuretic hormone (vasopressin) on the collecting duct of the kidney (p. 739). It must be remembered that ADH is normally exerting an antidiuretic action to produce the low basal urine flow of about 1 cm³/min. If the secretion of ADH is increased under conditions of severe dehydration, more water is reabsorbed and this results in a reduction of urine flow to a minimum of 0.3 cm³/min. If the release of ADH is reduced or abolished when the body is overloaded with water, reabsorption of water in the collecting duct is reduced or stopped and the urine flow increases towards its maximum of about 20 cm³/min.

Alteration of the body water content results in a change in volume and a change in the osmotic pressure of the body fluids. It is possible to distinguish between the effects of these two by a simple experiment in which one drinks a litre of water on one day and on another a litre of 0.9% saline. The mechanisms involved in the two responses are quite different. In response to the water, the urine flow increases rapidly to a maximum of about 16 cm³/min in an hour and then starts to decline until it is back to normal in three hours. With the isotonic saline however, the increase in urine flow is much less, the maximum being about 3 cm³/min, but it is much longer lasting. Even four hours after drinking, the urine flow is still above the control level.

Response to osmotic changes

When water is ingested, the extracellular fluid is diluted and its osmotic pressure reduced. Conversely, when the body is dehydrated the ECF is concentrated. It is therefore reasonable to postulate some type of receptor that is sensitive to changes in osmotic pressure and which would control the release of ADH. Changes in osmotic pressure are detected by osmoreceptors in the hypothalamus, in the region of the supra-optic nucleus, and their activity modifies the release of ADH. The mechanism of this control is summarized in Fig. 16.8.

When the secretion of ADH is reduced or stopped, the existing ADH in the circulation is slowly metabolized and this accounts for the delay of about half an hour between drinking fluid and the onset of diuresis. The ingestion of a

MIN 0·3 mℓ/min
MAX 20 mℓ/min

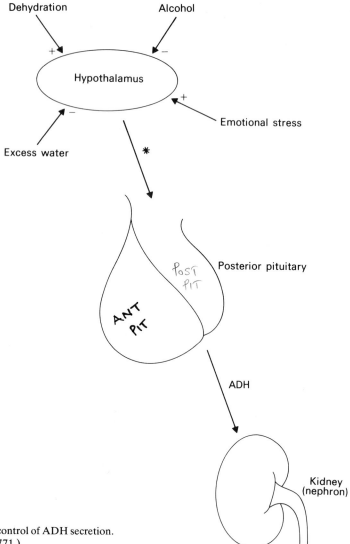

Fig. 16.8. Summary of the control of ADH secretion. (*Details on pp. 769 and 771.)

small volume of alcohol produces a diuresis that is almost identical with that produced by a larger volume of water. This diuretic action is explained by the depressant action of alcohol on the central nervous system, in this case the hypothalamus, with the resultant reduction in antidiuretic hormone secretion. The net result of the ingestion of alcohol is that the body loses more water than it ingests with the alcohol. This dehydration partly accounts for the 'hangover'.

Response to volume changes

The body responds to the ingestion of a litre of isotonic saline by a small but prolonged increase in urine flow over a period of several hours. The mechanism of this response is currently being investigated and there is still much to be clarified. It seems certain that there are 'volume receptors' in the walls of the pulmonary vein and left atrium and that stretching of these results in a degree of diuresis. It has been claimed that the cause of this diuresis is a reduction in the secretion of ADH, but other mechanisms may also be involved. ANATURIC PERTIDE?

THIRST

The sensation of thirst is difficult to explain satisfactorily. One explanation is that under conditions of dehydration the secretion of saliva stops and the dry mucous membranes of the mouth and pharynx result in the sensation of thirst. This appears to be a reasonable explanation and is supported by the common observation that drugs such as atropine, which are given for various reasons, cause drying of the mouth and result in thirst. This, however, is not the complete explanation. If an experimental animal such as dog, with an oesophageal fistula (Fig. 13.34), is deprived of water and then given free access to it, it will start drinking and go on and on. The water is moistening the mucous membranes, but none is being ingested. It therefore seems that some mechanism that monitors the electrolyte concentration of body fluids is also involved in thirst. An obvious candidate for this is the osmoreceptor control of ADH. There is definite evidence for an area in the hypothalamus being concerned with thirst. Lesions of the appropriate part cause a reduction or even abolition of fluid intake, while electrical stimulation causes drinking; in addition, the injection of hypertonic saline into this region in conscious animals causes drinking.

This combination of dryness of the mucous membranes and osmotic pressure of the body fluids still leaves much that is not understood about the regulation of water intake. If for example, a 10 kg dog is deprived of water until it has lost 5% of its body weight (a 500 cm³ water deficit) and is then given access to unlimited water, it drinks for a while and then stops. When the volume of water drunk is measured, it is about 500 cm³! The water deficit has been accurately replaced although most of this water is still in the stomach and has not come into contact with either the osmotic pressure sensors or the volume sensing mechanism. This experiment is more dramatic when carried out with a camel, when the volume involved is 20–30 gallons and is drunk in a few minutes!

It seems therefore that animals have some mechanism which tells them when the correct amount of water has been drunk; maybe it is simply 'instinct'. This ability seems to have been lost in man, for if a man is deprived of water, he will seldom make up his full deficit by drinking.

Electrolyte balance

All the normal constituents of urine, with the exception of creatinine, are reabsorbed to some extent in the kidney tubules. About 600 g sodium are filtered each day of which some 85% is reabsorbed in the PCT. This means that about 90 g reach the parts of the nephron where facultative reabsorption occurs, but of this only about 5 g is normally excreted in the urine. Any failure in facultative sodium reabsorption will rapidly cause a major upset in the sodium balance of the body. Chloride presents a quantitatively similar problem but it is now generally thought that the reabsorption of chloride passively follows the active reabsorption of sodium.

Regulation of the sodium balance of the body is by a group of adrenal cortical hormones, the mineralocortoids. The principal one is aldosterone from the zona glomerulosa.

THE ACTION OF ALDOSTERONE *ZONA GLOMERULOSA*

The structure and the site of secretion of aldosterone and its role in tissues other than the kidney are discussed elsewhere (p. 780). Its importance is illustrated by the simple observation that when the adrenal cortex is secreting reduced amounts of aldosterone, there is an increased loss of sodium in the urine and a corresponding reduction in the body sodium. Coupled with this is a retention of potassium. Aldosterone promotes the reabsorption of sodium in the DCT of the kidney by carrying out an exchange of sodium and potassium ions.

The most likely explanation of the control of aldosterone secretion with respect to the sodium–potassium balance of the body, is that the zona glomerulosa in some way monitors the composition of its blood supply and adjusts the secretion of aldosterone accordingly. It is probable that sodium concentration is the primary factor involved, but potassium may also play a part. There is still much detail of this mechanism to be worked out, but experimental evidence from work with perfused adrenal glands supports the general idea of this method of control.

THE JUXTA-GLOMERULAR APPARATUS AND ALDOSTERONE

Changes in the systemic blood pressure and the blood volume also affect the rate of aldosterone secretion. One site which is involved is the juxta-glomerular apparatus (JGA) in the kidney (Fig. 16.2). It seems that there is some mechanism, possibly within the renin-secreting cells themselves, which is sensitive to changes in pressure within the afferent arterioles and varies the secretion of renin accordingly. Thus, when for any reason there is a fall in the pressure within the glomerular afferent arterioles the secretion of renin is increased. A reduction in blood

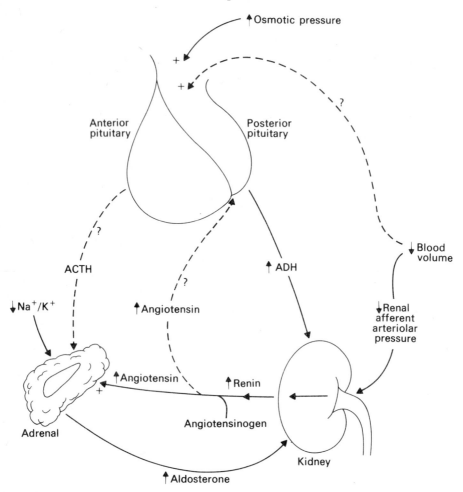

Fig. 16.9. A summary of the interactions between mechanisms which occur in the maintenance of the body's water and electrolyte balance. The dotted lines indicate possible mechanisms.

volume probably stimulates the secretion of renin in this way although volume receptors in the great veins have also been implicated in aldosterone release.

In addition to detecting changes in renal perfusion pressure, the JGA in some way responds to the sodium balance in the body. The macula densa appears to monitor the amount of sodium entering it from the DCT and the secretion of renin is inversely related. In this way the macula densa is indirectly monitoring plasma sodium levels.

Renin is an enzyme, secreted into the blood, which converts the plasma protein angiotensinogen into angiotensin I. This form of angiotensin is relatively inactive, but is converted into angiotensin II by a converting enzyme which is present in the blood and is particularly active in the lungs. The active form of angiotensin then stimulates the secretion of aldosterone by the adrenal cortex. As mentioned earlier, angiotensin, being a very powerful vaso-constrictor, increases glomerular filtration both by its local constrictor action on the efferent arteriole and also by its generalized effect in raising the systemic blood pressure. In this way the fall in GFR in response to decreased arterial blood pressure or blood volume is minimized.

In this account, the controls of water and sodium excretion have been considered as completely separate mechanisms. It must be realized that in the intact animal there is a very complex inter-relationship between the two because the alteration of one is likely to affect the other. For example, when sodium excretion is increased by giving an aldosterone antagonist, there is a concomitant diuresis. In addition, the specific actions of the hormones described in the preceding account are probably gross simplifications of the actual picture. There is now evidence that angiotensin affects the release of ADH and that ADH affects the secretion of renin. A summary of the interactions which occur in the maintenance of water levels and electrolyte balance occurs in Fig. 16.9.

SALT APPETITE

Just as the body signals a water deficit by the sensation of thirst, there is some mechanism, which, although not a conscious one, indicates that the body is in need of sodium (chloride). Animals (including man) tend to eat salt by choice whether the body needs it or not. It is well known that wild animals tend to move to areas where salt occurs naturally and lick it. Pets frequently lick sweat from one's skin and man tends to flavour his food with liberal additions of salt. Thus there is normally an excessive intake of salt and the surplus is excreted.

Having introduced this idea of a salt appetite, it must be said that although taste seems to be involved, our understanding of it is minimal. In addition, an area in the hypothalamus appears to be implicated as its destruction affects the salt drive. There is however much to be discovered before a satisfactory explanation can be given.

CONTROL OF PLASMA pH

The need for control

The limits of pH tolerated by the adult human are 7.0–7.8, with the normal pH at 7.4 (7.36–7.44). This is deceptive, because pH is a logarithmic scale (pH = $Log_{10} 1/[H^+]$). The $[H^+]$ corresponding to the lowest, normal, and highest values of pH are 100, 40 and 16 $nmol/dm^3$. The body clearly tolerates acid loads better than the loss of acids; this is appropriate since acid loads are more commonly experienced (e.g., during exercise).

It is essential that $[H^+]$ should be kept reasonably constant for the following reasons:
1 The ionization and the tertiary structure of proteins (p. 60) are greatly affected by $[H^+]$. This is particularly important in enzymes, whose optimal activity is often seen only within a narrow range of pH.

2 Transmembrane potentials are affected by pH. Both the degree of ionization of calcium and the distribution across the membrane of K^+ are altered, which in turn affects the excitability of nerve and muscle cells.
3 The binding and transport of oxygen by haemoglobin is influenced by pH.

Although the pH of plasma is not typical of the whole body pH, it is usual to measure the pH in blood since it is easily sampled and handled. Intracellular fluid is considerably more acid (estimated average pH is 7.0) and the interstitial fluid has an intermediate value. Even the red cells in blood have an intracellular pH which is 0.2 unit below that in plasma. There is also a difference between arterial and venous blood such that in mixed venous blood taken from a resting man, the pH in plasma is slightly lower. Associated with this difference is the higher P_{CO_2} (about +6 mm Hg) and higher $[HCO_3^-]$ (about +1 $mmol/dm^3$).

In the absence of disease, the principal threats to the constancy of the $[H^+]$ of the plasma come from acids generated during metabolism. The acids formed are of two kinds:
1 Those formed *de novo* during metabolism, e.g., carbonic acid, lactic acid and acetoacetic acid. These are usually excreted entirely as carbon dioxide and water, since lactic acid and acetoacetic acid are further metabolized to release more of their potential chemical energy, but in untreated diabetes mellitus or during starvation some acetoacetic and β-hydroxybutyric acids are wasted in the urine.
2 Those mineral acids (phosphoric, sulphuric) released from dietary constituents which are surplus to requirements and found in the diet in amounts in excess of counterbalancing cations such as Na^+ and K^+. Phosphoric and sulphuric acids are predominantly observed in the plasma as their bases, HPO_4^{2-} and SO_4^{2-} but they must be excreted through the kidneys accompanied by an equivalent molar quantity of (buffered) protons.

A general idea of the relative turnover rates of acids through the blood stream can be gained from the following figures:
1 CO_2 transport from tissues to lungs; CO_2 excretion from a 70 kg man at rest amounts to about 200 cm^3, or 9 mmol/min, of which 90% is carried in forms such as carbamino compounds and HCO_3^- (see later) whose formation involves the transient release of protons.
2 Lactic acid is produced continually, by many tissues, but in particular by red blood cells, white blood cells, and the renal medulla. The turnover

is about 1 mmol/min in a 70 kg man at rest. In severe exercise, in tissue hypoxia associated with haemorrhagic shock, and in a number of other conditions, lactic acid production is increased considerably.

3   Urinary acid output averages about 50–100 mmol/day. This figure is very variable as it depends on the diet consumed. Total renal failure with oliguria or anuria (little or no urine production) will result in the accumulation of acid.

Mechanisms controlling plasma pH

The body responds to the challenge of a change in its content of acid in the following ways:
1   By buffering H^+
2   By adjusting ventilation; this alters CO_2 excretion, so effectively altering the content of H_2CO_3, or of $H^+ + HCO_3^-$.
3   By altering the rate of renal excretion of H^+.

BUFFERS IN THE BODY

The physical chemistry of buffering is discussed in the Appendix. Protons are buffered in blood, interstitial fluid, cells and bone. Blood and interstitial fluid play the greatest part in short-term responses to acid-base disturbances and rely on proteins and bicarbonate to different degrees, depending on circumstances, for regulating pH. If an acid load is added to blood it takes about 2 minutes for it to be buffered and for a new equilibrium to be reached. If all the interstitial fluid is included, equilibration would take about 10 minutes.

When there are long-term changes in the acid-base balance, as in prolonged illness, intracellular proteins and various phosphates assume importance as buffers, even though H^+ diffuse only slowly across cell membranes. In addition, bone can be resorbed by acid and the phosphate and carbonate in the mineral can act as buffers by accepting hydrogen ions. This form of long-term buffering may seriously weaken the skeleton in such conditions as chronic renal failure.

Buffers in relation to CO_2 transport
Proteins play the major role in buffering protons derived from the continuous dissociation of carbonic acid. They accept the protons onto the side chains of their basic amino acids.

A resting 70 kg man produces about 9 mmol/min CO_2 for excretion and this is carried to the lungs in the volume of cardiac output (5 dm³/min). Therefore each litre of blood carries

$9/5 = 1.8$ mmol CO_2 for excretion, the arteriovenous difference in the total content of CO_2 (p. 509). It is known that 10% of this CO_2 (0.18 mmol/dm³) is unchanged CO_2 carried in simple solution; the remaining 90% is carried by proteins and as HCO_3^-.

During the uptake of CO_2, protons are produced in the following ways:

$$HbNH_2 + CO_2 \rightleftharpoons HbNHCOO^- + H^+$$
(haemoglobin)   (carbamino
                          haemoglobin)

$$CO_2 + H_2O \underset{\text{anhydrase}}{\overset{\text{carbonic}}{\rightleftharpoons}} H_2CO_3 \rightleftharpoons HCO_3^- + H^+$$

Thus, as the CO_2 is bound to form either carbamino groups or bicarbonate ions, there is release of an equivalent amount of protons (i.e., $1.8 - 0.18 = 1.62$ mmol/dm³). Despite the release of 1.62 mmol H^+ ions/dm³, the difference between $[H^+]$ in arterial blood (36 nmol/dm³) and venous blood (40 nmol/dm³) is only 4 nmol/dm³. Since 1 nmol is 1×10^{-6} mmol this means that for every million protons released during the transport of CO_2, only about 2 remain free in solution during the journey. There is obviously a remarkably efficient buffering system.

It is important to realise that the protons released during the formation of bicarbonate cannot be buffered by the bicarbonate itself. Haemoglobin base accepts about 80% of these protons (p. 508) while the plasma proteins accept about 20%. The imidazole ring of the histidine residues in haemoglobin is most important in this reaction.

The nature of the reaction with haemoglobin is extremely complex because the buffering capacity varies with the configuration of the molecule, which is influenced by several factors. Of particular significance is the change from HbO_2 to Hb when O_2 is released to the tissues. Deoxygenated haemoglobin is the stronger buffer. Each mole of oxyhaemoglobin which becomes converted to the deoxy form accepts 0.3 mol H^+ with no change in the pH of the medium. Since there are 9 mmol of Hb per litre of blood in a normal adult; and since arterial Hb is 97% saturated with O_2 and mixed venous Hb only 75% saturated (p. 509), then the amount of H^+ ions accounted for by merely changing HbO_2 to Hb is

$$\frac{97 - 75}{100} \times 9 \times 0.3 = 0.6 \text{ mmol}$$

This corresponds to about one third of the protons produced by the entry of CO_2 into the capillaries. The remaining 1 mmol H^+/dm^3 is buffered by the titration of other base (proton-accepting) sites on the haemoglobin molecule and on the plasma proteins and only a slight change of pH occurs.

Bicarbonate as a 'buffer'

Whenever an acid other than carbonic acid is formed in the tissues or lost from the body the pH change is minimized by the CO_2–carbonic acid–bicarbonate system. This is a three-stage system which may be expressed as:

$$H_2O + CO_2 \rightleftharpoons H_2CO_3 \rightleftharpoons HCO_3^- + H^+$$

If protons are added to the blood, $[HCO_3^-]$ is lowered, CO_2 is excreted and the sum of $[H_2CO_3] + [HCO_3^-]$ is lowered. This is possible because carbonic acid is in equlibrium with dis-solved CO_2 which is itself in equilibrium with the P_{CO_2}. The excretion of CO_2 is normally set so that ventilation maintains P_{CO_2} in arterial blood at 40 mm Hg. Carbonic acid is therefore effec-tively a volatile acid, easily displaced from solu-tion. In other circumstances, if the body needs more acid, it is possible to store this volatile acid in its dissociated form (as $H^+ + HCO_3^-$) by reducing ventilation and so raising the P_{CO_2}. The protons formed are then available to bind on to the basic sites of other buffers (e.g. protein).

It is possible to apply the Henderson–Hassel-balch equation to this buffer system provided that the P_{CO_2} is constant; the equation would be:

$$pH = pK + \log \frac{[HCO_3^-]}{[H_2CO_3]}$$

As we are not able to measure the undissociated $[H_2CO_3]$ directly, it is sensible to substitute the (much larger) value for the amount of dissolved CO_2 in this equation. This is given by the product of the solubility coefficient, S, and the P_{CO_2}, and it is directly proportional to the unknown value $[H_2CO_3]$. We must then make an adjustment to pK; remembering that $[HCO_3^-]$ in plasma is normally 24 mmol/dm^3; the values in the mod-ified Henderson–Hasselbalch equation may be set out as:

$$pH = pK' + \log \frac{(HCO_3^-)}{S \times P_{CO_2}}$$

$$S \times P_{CO_2} \times 0.03 \times 40 = 1.2 \text{ mmol } CO_2/dm^3$$

$$7.4 = pK' + \log \frac{24}{1.2} = pK' + 1.3$$

Therefore $pK' = 6.1$

The Henderson–Hasselbalch equation with its modified pK' value is infallible as a description of the interrelationship between the three vari-ables pH, P_{CO_2} and $[HCO_3^-]$, but it cannot be used to predict the change in, let us say, P_{CO_2}, when an acid load is added to the body. A com-mon and very misleading error made by students is to predict that the following reactions:

$$CO_2 + H_2O \rightleftharpoons H_2CO_3 \rightleftharpoons H^+ + HCO_3^-$$

reach a state of equilibrium and result in an elevated P_{CO_2} if they are driven to the left by raising the $[H^+]$. The error stems from forgetting that CO_2 is escaping all the time in expired air and that the principal factor regulating P_{CO_2} is the ventilation. P_{CO_2} is in fact the most sensi-tively regulated variable in the modified Hen-derson–Hasselbalch equation, and it is not fixed by simple application of the Law of Mass Action but by control of the level of ventilation. The body is excreting 9 mmol/min of CO_2 produced by metabolism, and it can certainly excrete a little more CO_2 derived from HCO_3^- which has taken up protons, without losing control of the P_{CO_2}. There is after all nothing unusual about varying the level of CO_2 excretion; this varies according to the level of exercise or other forms of metabolic activity (e.g. during digestion). Unless specific fresh instructions reach the respiratory centre, ventilation will maintain the normal P_{CO_2}.

RESPIRATORY COMPENSATION FOR A CHANGE IN pH

Under normal circumstances, ventilation is regu-lated to maintain the P_{CO_2} (and thus carbonic acid content) of the body constant whatever the rate of CO_2 production and excretion. In doing so, it helps to maintain a normal pH and a nor-mal balance of acid and base in the body.

However, if an acid other than carbonic acid enters the blood, the increased $[H^+]$ increases ventilation by stimulating the peripheral chemoreceptors which further increase the ven-tilatory drive. The hyperventilation caused by this stimulus actually reduces the P_{CO_2} below normal, despite the fact that far more CO_2 may be produced from HCO_3^- and excreted each

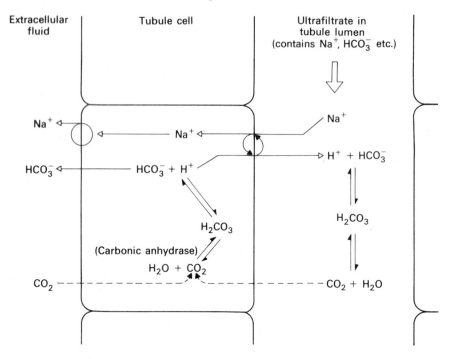

Fig. 16.10. Proton secretion and the reabsorption of sodium bicarbonate by kidney tubules. The luminal border of the cell is impermeable to HCO_3^-, but permeable to the diffusion of carbon dioxide (down its concentration gradient; indicated by broken lines).

minute than under normal circumstances. The observed P_{CO_2} is therefore lowered under precisely those conditions which may lead an incautious student to anticipate a rise. Beware!

In the modified Henderson–Hasselbalch equation it is the ratio HCO_3^-/P_{CO_2} which really determines the pH. It follows that the consequences of reducing $[HCO_3^-]$ following the buffering of H^+ is to reduce the numerator. If the P_{CO_2} is now reduced by increasing ventilation, the denominator becomes smaller too, so that the ratio and pH return towards normal. The change in ventilation which makes this possible is known as respiratory compensation for a change in pH. If, on the other hand, the original disturbance is a loss of acid (e.g., by vomiting) ventilation is reduced. This has the effect of conserving CO_2, so returning the pH towards normal. In this case, the absolute values of both $[HCO_3^-]$ and P_{CO_2} are increased.

Excretion of acid or alkali in urine

The glomerular filtrate contains HCO_3^- at the same concentration as that in plasma but the nephron is unable to reabsorb HCO_3^- directly. Instead, the cells of the PCT, DCT and collecting duct secrete H^+ into the tubular lumen. The secretion involves a linked carrier system; as each H^+ enters the tubular lumen, a Na^+ ion moves into the tubule cell, down its concentration gradient. In the PCT, the secreted H^+ are trapped by the HCO_3^-, and the carbonic acid formed reverts to the unhydrated form as dissolved CO_2 which diffuses into the tubule cells. The H^+ secreted throughout the nephron are derived from the catalysed hydration of CO_2 and the dissociation of H_2CO_3 within the cells (Fig. 16.10). The HCO_3^- formed here is returned to the blood in the peritubular capillaries. The overall effect of these manoeuvres is the 're-absorption', during H^+ secretion, of equal amounts of Na^+ and HCO_3^- (as CO_2) from the primitive urine.

The glomerular filtration rate (GFR) is about $0.125 \ dm^3/min$ and the $[HCO_3^-]$ in plasma is about $24 \ mmol/dm^3$. The load of HCO_3^- filtered and present in the ultra filtrate entering the PCT is $0.125 \times 24 = 3 \ mmol/min$. However, each day urine contains $50–100 \ mmol \ H^+$ ($0.035–0.07 \ mmol/min$) so that the total H^+ secreted into urine along all the tubules is about $3.05 \ mmol//min$. Normally there is an almost perfect balance

HCO₃⁻ is 24mmol/L

between the secretion of H⁺ and the filtration of HCO₃⁻ by the glomerulus.

When the [HCO₃⁻] in plasma reaches about 27 mmol/dm³, HCO₃⁻ spills into the urine. This is the renal threshold for HCO₃⁻. Since the normal plasma level of HCO₃⁻ is 24 mmol/dm³ there is a narrow margin between the HCO₃⁻ load and the H⁺ secretory capacity of the nephron. If HCO₃⁻ does appear in the urine, it contains an equivalent amount of Na⁺ and the urine is alkaline. This is how the body corrects an alkali load or an acid deficiency through the renal excretion of alkaline urine. On the other hand if a normal or diminished load of HCO₃⁻ is filtered while H⁺ secretion is not diminished to the same degree, the HCO₃⁻ is completely reabsorbed before the primitive urine has reached the end of the nephron. Subseqently, H⁺ secretion results in an accumulation of H⁺ in the urine; the urine becomes acid. Its capacity for accepting H⁺ is greatly increased by the presence of buffers.

URINARY BUFFERS

The two buffers of importance in urine are phosphate and ammonium.

Primitive urine normally becomes acidified while travelling from the Bowman's capsule (pH 7.4) to the collecting ducts (pH 6.0–5.5), so that almost every phosphate ion (predominantly HPO₄²⁻) in the glomerular filtrate accepts a H⁺ and changes to the dihydrogen phosphate form. This accounts for the buffering of some 20–30 mmol of the H⁺ secreted by the renal tubule each day. The limitation of this system is its inflexibility. The amount of phosphate in urine is not varied in response to the needs of the body to secrete acid: it is merely a surplus, derived from the diet, which has to be excreted.

The other buffer is far more flexible. The cells of the distal tubules can produce free ammonia. This diffuses out of the cells and into the tubular lumen where it traps a proton to become an ammonium ion. Ammonia production is mainly due to the action of the enzyme glutaminase using glutamine as the substrate. The activity of this mechanism is increased and enzyme synthesis is induced by a low pH in blood and primitive urine, with the result that the capacity to buffer an excreted acid load increases when acid urine is being produced. Several days of excreting a large acid load (e.g., during severe diabetes mellitus) may result in a tenfold increase in NH₄⁺ excretion. The basal rate is usually 25–50 mmol/day, while in exceptional cases it may reach 250 mmol/day. The pH of urine in these circumstances reaches a limit of 4.5.

RENAL COMPENSATION FOR pH DISTURBANCES OF RESPIRATORY ORIGIN

Suppose that there is inadequate ventilation in a disease such as bronchial asthma, so that the P_{CO_2} rises markedly. This leads inevitably to a small rise in plasma HCO₃⁻, just as it would when transporting extra CO_2 from the tissues in venous blood. If the P_{CO_2} were to be doubled, the pH of plasma would drop to about 7.2. The extent of this change has been limited by titration of the non-bicarbonate buffers (haemoglobin, plasma protein), but buffers cannot, of course, remedy the situation.

In these circumstances the kidneys temporarily sacrifice their usual role of maintaining normal acid-base stores in the body to the urgent need for pH regulation. The raised P_{CO_2} increases the secretion of H⁺ into the urine and the production of HCO₃⁻ in the tubule cell. Extra H⁺ excretion occurs and the plasma HCO₃⁻ is raised. Such a response is known as renal compensation for a disturbance in pH. When the asthmatic attack is over and the pH is returning to normal the excess HCO₃⁻ will have to be excreted again.

CLINICAL CONDITIONS AND TERMINOLOGY

It is usual to consider a disturbance of acid–base balance in terms of its cause (respiratory or metabolic) and its primary result (acidosis or alkalosis). Acidosis is a condition in which there is an excess of acid (either carbonic acid in respiratory acidosis, or a stronger acid in metabolic acidosis) or a deficit of base. Alkalosis is a condition in which there is a deficit of acid or an excess of base.

With respiratory acidosis (e.g., bronchial asthma) or with respiratory alkalosis (e.g., hyperventilation at high altitudes or induced by a mechanical ventilator) renal compensation will occur. With metabolic acidosis (e.g., diabetes mellitus, starvation or severe exercise) or metabolic alkalosis (vomiting) respiratory compensation will occur.

FURTHER READING

American Physiological Society (1964) *Handbook of Physiology, Section 4,* Adaptation to the Environment.

VANDER Arthur J. (1975) *Renal Physiology.* McGraw Hill Book Co., New York.

CHAPTER 17

The Endocrine and Associated Organs

GENERAL PRINCIPLES

The secretion of an endocrine gland passes from the cell in which it is manufactured or stored directly into the circulation. In exocrine glands the secretion passes into a duct and thence into a hollow viscus. The active substance produced by an endocrine gland is called a hormone; this circulates to all parts of the body. Its actions may be exerted on many tissues or on a specific target tissue or organ.

The endocrine system complements the nervous system in the control and regulation of body function, and there are numerous interactions between the systems. A hormone usually exerts its effect by influencing cellular activity. It may increase the size of the cell or stimulate cell division, thus giving rise to growth either of the whole body or of a specific tissue. On the other hand it may affect a specific function of a cell. By exerting these effects on cellular activity the hormones are able to carry out one of their most important functions, the maintenance of the constancy of the internal environment.

It is usual in a chapter on the endocrine system to discuss only the major endocrine organs (the pituitary, thyroid, parathyroids, pancreas, adrenals and gonads), but many other tissues and organs are known to produce hormones which have either local or general effects:

1   The secretion of digestive juices into the gastrointestinal tract and also the motility of the tract are partly controlled by hormones released from the gastric and intestinal mucosae in response to the presence of food within the gut (p. 613).

2   The kidney secretes a substance, renin, which may be considered both as an enzyme and as a hormone (p. 745).

3   The production of red blood cells is partly under the control of erythropoietin, a hormone produced from the kidney (p. 675).

4   The main function of the thymus is the production of lymphocytes and the development of immunity within the body (p. 661). It has also been suggested that the thymus secretes a hormone, tentatively named thymosin.

5   Throughout pregnancy the fetus and the placenta produce hormones which influence maternal physiology. 793).

ACTIVE SUBSTANCES OF WIDESPREAD OCCURRENCE IN THE BODY

There are many substances present in tissues which, if released into the circulation in large amounts, exert powerful pharmacological effects throughout the body. Normally, under physiological conditions, only small amounts are released which have mainly local effects. This group of substances includes (a) the neurotransmitters of the autonomic nervous system, acetylcholine and noradrenaline, (b) 5-hydroxytryptamine which may be a neurotransmitter of the intrinsic nerve plexuses in the intestine, (c) histamine which is stored in mast cells and in the intestinal wall, and (d) bradykinin which is a powerful vasodilator that may be released from salivary and sweat glands. These substances cannot be classed as hormones since their large-scale release into the circulation occurs only under pathological conditions.

Other substances of almost universal occurrence in the body are cyclic 3,5-AMP and the prostaglandins. These probably act as intracellular transmitters and modulators of hormone activity (p. 193 & 799).

FACTORS INFLUENCING THE ACTIVITY AND METABOLISM OF HORMONES

The biological effect of a hormone depends on its concentration in the interstitial fluid which in turn is determined not only by the rate at which it is secreted but also by the rate at which it is broken down or excreted (Fig. 17.1). Small quantities of hormone may be excreted in the urine, but most hormones are metabolized to

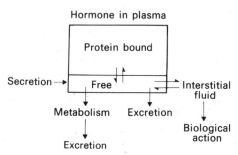

Fig. 17.1. Factors determining the concentrations of a hormone in the body fluids and its biological activity.

less active forms which are then excreted. An important factor influencing the activity and metabolism of some hormones is their reversible binding with plasma proteins. There is an equilibrium between the bound portion of the hormone and the smaller (usually less than 10%) free portion. Only the free portion can diffuse through the capillary wall into the interstitial fluid to influence cellular activity and only this portion can be filtered through the glomerulus or enter the liver and be metabolized. Where hormone secretion is controlled by a negative feedback mechanism, it is the unbound fraction which exerts this effect. Hormones may be bound to specific binding proteins which are usually α- or β-globulins, or non-specifically to plasma albumin.

ESTABLISHING HORMONAL ACTIVITY

The classical criteria for establishing a suspected hormonal mechanism are as follows:

1   The suspected endocrine gland is removed in an experimental animal and any changes in the body are noted.

2   These changes can be prevented by the administration of a cell-free extract of glands from other animals. If an excess of extract is given then a different set of changes may be induced in the body, corresponding to over-activity of the gland.

It is necessary to eliminate the possiblility that substances in an extract may mimic a hormone action where none exists. For example, histamine, present in many tissue extracts, is a potent stimulant of gastric secretion.

3   The hormone is purified, and its chemical structure is elucidated. Attempts are then made to synthesize the hormone in the laboratory. The final stage in the characterization of a hormonal mechanism is the demonstration that the synthetic hormone mimics the actions of the endogenous hormone.

ESTIMATION OF HORMONE LEVELS IN BODY FLUIDS

To investigate a patient who may be suffering from an endocrine disease, or to perform research into endocrine mechanisms, it is clearly necessary to be able to measure levels of hormones in plasma or urine. The determination of many hormones, whose concentrations in plasma are exceptionally low (of the order of picograms, i.e. 10^{-12}g/cm³) presents a real challenge to the analyst.

The earliest assays of hormones in tissue extracts were biological assays based on a physiological action of the hormone. Thus adrenaline and vasopressin were assayed by comparing the pressor effect (blood pressure-raising effect) of crude extracts of glands with those of known quantities of the pure compounds (Fig.17.2).

Some hormones may be determined spectrophotometrically but the methods used often lack specificity and are usually too insensitive for use with biological material. Much greater sensitivity may be achieved by converting the hormones to fluorescent derivatives, and estimating the

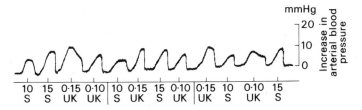

Fig. 17.2. (a) Assay of the vasopressin content of an extract of the posterior pituitary gland on the blood pressure of an anaesthesized rat. S indicates doses of standard solution as milliUnits of international standard. UK indicates volumes of tissue extract. An approximation of the potency of the extract can often be obtained merely by inspecting the record obtained. Thus the response to 0.10 cm³ extract is similar to that of 10 milliUnits of the standard vasopressin.

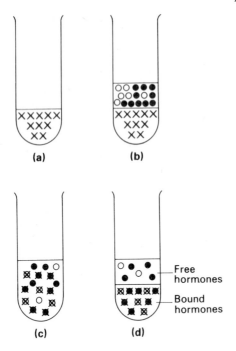

(a)   **(b)**

(c)   **(d)**

Free
hormones

Bound
hormones

Fig. 17.3. The principles of radioimmunoassay.
Unlabelled hormone (○) contained in biological fluids
is mixed with labelled hormone (●) and with the
antibody (×). Both forms of the hormone are bound to
antibody (⊠ and ✖) according to their relative
concentrations. The bound and unbound hormones
are then separated.

amount of fluorescence. If the hormone can be
converted into a volatile derivative, then it may
be assayed by gas-liquid chromatography.

The methods most widely used involve binding hormones to protein. In immunochemical
assays an antibody to a protein or peptide hormone is raised in a suitable animal. If solutions of
hormone and antibody are mixed *in vitro* the
hormone binds to the antibody (Fig. 17.3). In a
mixture of radioactively labelled hormone and
natural hormone each will compete for binding
sites; the greater the quantity of labelled hormone which binds to the antibody, the less of the
natural hormone was present in the original
mixture.

CONTROL OF SECRETION

The simplest type of control is one in which the
body function which is being controlled exerts an
influence on the endocrine gland. For instance,
insulin regulates the level of glucose in the blood
by stimulating the uptake of the sugar into cells.
An increase in blood glucose level, as occurs
after a meal, stimulates the pancreas to secrete
more insulin and when the blood sugar level is
low the secretion of insulin is suppressed (Fig.
17.4a). This type of control is a form of 'negative
feedback'.

The secretion of some hormones is controlled
by trophic hormones from the pituitary gland.

Fig. 17.4. The control of
endocrine function. (a) The rate
of secretion of the hormone is
determined by the level of a
metabolite of the target tissue
(e.g. insulin and glucose); (b)
The secretion of the hormone is
stimulated by a trophic hormone
from the pituitary. The level of
the hormone in turn controls the
secretion of the trophic
hormone; (c) The hypothalamus
controls the secretion of trophic
hormone from the pituitary.
Feedback may occur at both
hypothalmic and pituitary levels
(e.g. thyroid). (d) Hormone
production may show temporal
variations with periods of a day,
several days or even a year (e.g.
sex hormone); it may be
influenced by changes in the
external environment (e.g.
cortisol).

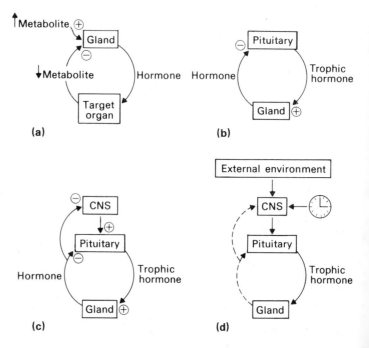

For example, adrenocorticotrophic hormone (ACTH) stimulates the secretion of cortisol from the adrenal cortex. The raised plasma levels of cortisol in turn may suppress ACTH secretion (Fig. 17.4b) but a simple negative feedback hypothesis does not completely explain the control of ACTH secretion. The hypothalamus also modifies the release of this and other pituitary hormones (Fig. 17.4c). The CNS can induce regular cyclical fluctuations in ACTH release which produce a marked circadian rhythm of cortisol secretion and can also induce a sudden increase in ACTH secretion in response to stress (Fig. 17.4d).

The CNS may cause rhythmical variations in endocrine activity of longer period. For instance in women the secretion of gonadotrophins which control the menstrual cycle has a periodicity of 25–35 days and in animals which have a short breeding season the cycle of gonadotrophin secretion may be repeated only once a year.

In the case of adrenaline secretion from the adrenal medulla, control is effected directly through the sympathetic nerve supply.

THYROID

Anatomy and histology

The thyroid gland is a horseshoe-shaped, brownish-red, highly vascular organ lying in the lower part of the neck, where it embraces the front and sides of the upper part of the trachea. It consists of right and left lobes connected across the midline by a narrower part, the isthmus, from the superior border of which a small pyramidal lobe sometimes arises. Each lateral lobe is about 5 cm long and extends upwards from the level of the sixth tracheal cartilage as far as the oblique line of the thyroid cartilage of the larynx while the isthmus lies in front of the second and third tracheal cartilages. The thyroid usually weighs 25–40 g being slightly heavier in women, in whom it enlarges during pregnancy and menstruation.

The thyroid has a rich blood supply. The superior thyroid artery, a branch of the external carotid, enters the superior part of each lateral lobe while the inferior thyroid artery, a branch of the thyrocervical trunk of the subclavian artery, enters the inferior part of each lobe. Venous blood is removed by three sets of veins, the superior and middle which drain into the internal jugular veins, and the inferior which drain into the left brachiocephalic vein after passing in front of the trachea.

The thyroid gland is enclosed within the pretracheal fascia. In front of the thyroid are the sternohyoid and sternothyroid muscles. Lying posterior and lateral to each main lobe is the carotid sheath, containing the internal jugular vein, the vagus and the carotid artery. The four parathyroid glands (p. 759) lie posterior to the thyroid, usually embedded within its outer capsule (the pretracheal fascia).

Sometimes small accessory thyroid glands are found above the lobes and isthmus of the main gland.

The thyroid is the only endocrine gland to store its main product extracellularly before it is released into the blood. Each secretory unit is a hollow sphere of cells termed a follicle, and the secretion of these cells, colloidal thyroglobulin, fills the space within the sphere (Fig. 17.5). The follicles range in diameter from about 0.02 to 0.9 mm. In some follicles the colloid has a 'motheaten' appearance which may indicate that some has been absorbed by adjacent follicular epithelial cells.

FOLLICULAR EPITHELIAL CELLS

These are arranged as a single layer of cuboidal cells forming the wall of each follicle. In underactive glands they are squamous instead of cuboidal, while in overactive glands they are columnar. The follicular cells secrete thyroglobulin and digest it to release thyroid hormones (T_3 and T_4).

The ultrastructure of the follicular epithelial cells reflects these activities (Fig. 17.6). They have a copious basal rough endoplasmic reticulum, a central euchromatic nucleus with an eccentrically-placed nucleolus, supranuclear or perinuclear Golgi apparatus, transfer and secretory vesicles (the latter containing colloidal thyroglobulin), microvilli on the luminal part of the plasma membrane, numerous lysosomes, and relatively few mitochondria. Adjacent cells are united by junctional complexes.

The follicular epithelium rests on a basal lamina about 50 nm thick. Beyond this, in the spaces between the follicles, is a little reticular connective tissue, through which run nerves, lymphatics and blood vessels. The blood capillaries are of the highly porous fenestrated type; the raw materials needed for hormone synthesis and the completed hormones can pass readily through their walls.

PARAFOLLICULAR CELLS

About 2% of the secretory cells of the thyroid synthesize another hormone, the polypeptide

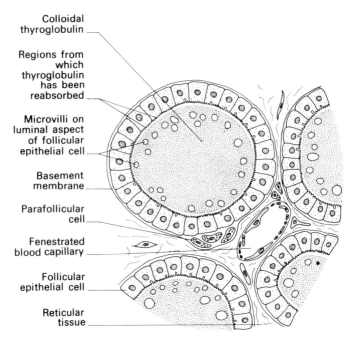

Colloidal
thyroglobulin

Regions from
which
thyroglobulin
has been
reabsorbed

Microvilli on
luminal aspect
of follicular
epithelial cell

Basement
membrane

Parafollicular
cell

Fenestrated
blood capillary

Follicular
epithelial cell

Reticular
tissue

Fig. 17.5. The fine structure of the thyroid gland.

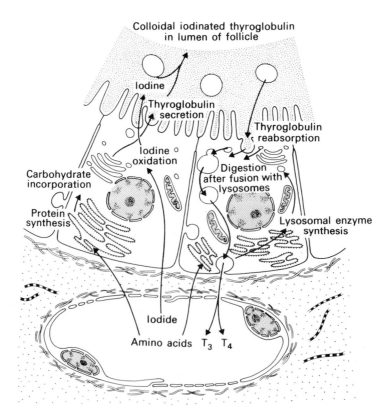

Colloidal iodinated thyroglobulin
in lumen of follicle

Iodine

Thyroglobulin
secretion

Thyroglobulin
reabsorption

Iodine
oxidation

Carbohydrate
incorporation

Digestion
after fusion with
lysosomes

Protein
synthesis

Lysosomal enzyme
synthesis

Iodide

Amino acids T_3 T_4

Fig. 17.6. The mechanisms of production of
thyroglobulin and T_3 and T_4 by the thyroid.

calcitonin (p. 765). These cells have been called 'parafollicular' cells, 'clear' cells or C-cells, and 'ultimobranchial' cells. The term parafollicular refers to their position, either between the follicles or between the follicular cells and their basal laminae. The term 'ultimobranchial' refers to their origin; they arise from cells in the last pair of pharyngeal pouches which in fish, amphibia, reptiles and birds become ultimobranchial bodies located in the neck and the mediastinum, and which in mammals are incorporated into the thyroid. The hormone is sometimes referred to as thyrocalcitonin to distinguish it from calcitonin produced elsewhere in the body.

Ultrastructurally the parafollicular cells have the characteristics of APUD (amine precursor uptake and decarboxylation) cells (p. 603). They contain membrane-bound dense bodies that are probably hormone storage granules, a little rough endoplasmic reticulum, a well-developed Golgi apparatus, numerous mitochondria and an eccentrically placed nucleus.

Physiology of the thyroid gland

The thyroid secretes the hormones thyroxine (T_4), triiodothyronine (T_3) and calcitonin. Thyroxine and triiodothyronine are important regulators of metabolism and growth. Calcitonin affects the equilibrium between the calcium in extracellular fluid and that in bone.

SYNTHESIS OF THYROXINE AND TRIIODOTHYRONINE

The manufacture of the thyroid hormones depends upon both an adequate intake of iodide into the body and its uptake by the gland. The follicular cells have an avid uptake mechanism for circulating iodide, and are able to concentrate the ion more effectively than any other tissue. If a radioactive isotope of iodide (^{131}I) is injected intravenously, some 25% of the injected radioactivity becomes trapped in the thyroid within about 4 hours. Within the follicular cells the iodide ion (I^-) is first oxidized to iodine (I_2) by peroxidase (Fig. 17.8).

The next stage involves the iodination of some of the tyrosine molecules in thyroglobulin (TG) which has already been synthesized and later secreted into the lumen of the follicle where it is stored. This iodination probably takes place at the brush borders of the follicular cells and

Monoiodotyrosine — MIT

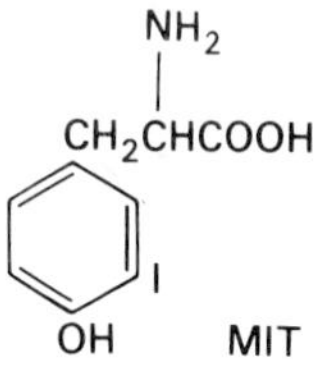

Diiodotyrosine — DIT

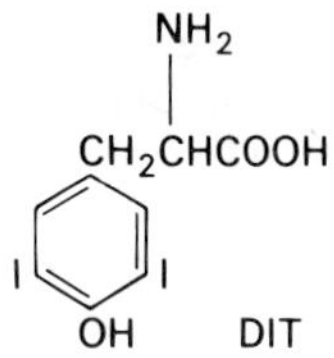

Tyrosine

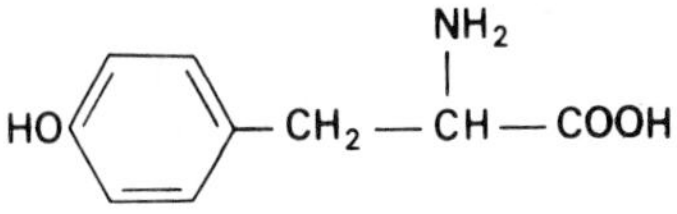

Thyroxine (T_4)

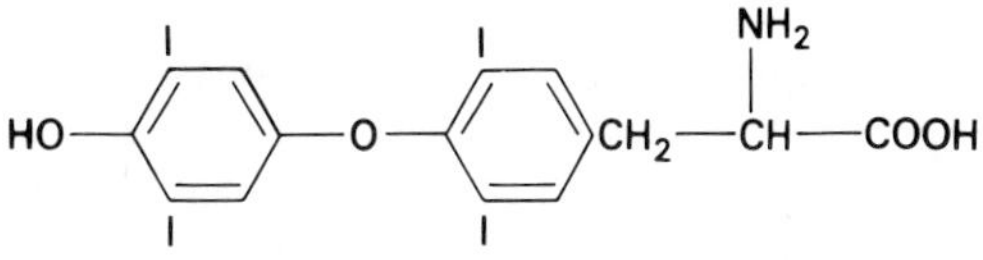

Triiodothyronine (T_3)

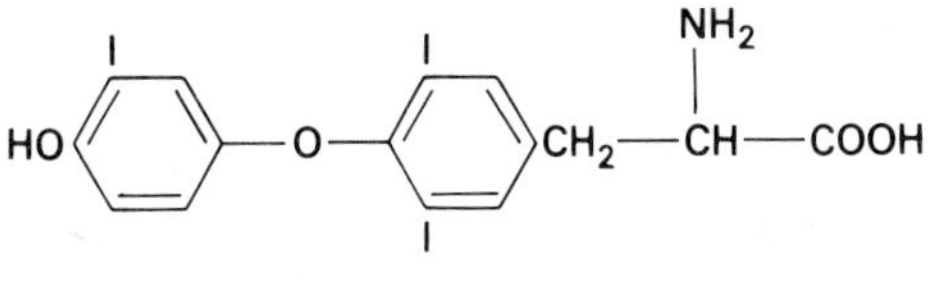

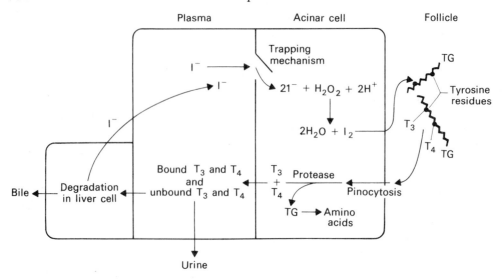

Fig. 17.7. The synthesis and metabolism of thyroid hormones.

results in the formation of some mono-iodotyrosine (MIT) and some diiodotyrosine (DIT), both bound to TG. In the fourth stage some DIT is coupled with MIT to give T_3 and some with DIT to give T_4. This coupling requires an enzyme which is activated by thyroid stimulating hormone (TSH) from the anterior pituitary. The T_3-TG and T_4-TG molecules are stored in the follicles of the thyroid. To release the hormones from thyroglobulin, small droplets of colloid are taken in by pinocytosis to the follicular cells where a lysosomal proteolytic enzyme then splits off the active hormones which are discharged into the plasma and lymph (Figs. 17.6, 17.7).

METABOLISM OF THYROID HORMONES

In the plasma the thyroid hormones are again bound to a protein (thyroxine binding globulin, TBG), leaving only small amounts of the free, physiologically active hormones. T_3 is more loosely bound than T_4 and is therefore more readily available to the tissues. The hormones are broken down in the liver and the residues excreted in the bile, whilst the iodide is recycled. Small amounts of thyroxine are excreted in the urine (Fig. 17.7).

FUNCTIONS OF THYROID HORMONES

Oxidative metabolism. Removal of the thyroid

gland from the experimental animal leads to a marked reduction of the metabolic rate and of the breakdown of both carbohydrates and fats. If excessive amounts of hormones are administered oxygen consumption is raised above normal, with increased breakdown of carbohydrates and fats. If inadequate amounts of these substrates are available in the diet then body proteins are broken down and there is a marked loss of weight.

Growth. Removal of the thyroid gland early in life, or its congenital absence, impairs growth and development. Bone growth and tooth eruption are retarded; the individual is stunted and secondary sex characteristics do not develop; the tongue is enlarged; mental development may be very backward.

Molecular mechanism of action. Since changes in metabolic rate do not appear for several hours after the injection of thyroid hormones, it is likely that the stimulus to increase metabolism is the result of enzyme synthesis. This view is confirmed by the swelling of the mitochondria and increased levels of enzymes within them. It is likely that the hormones stimulate the production of messenger RNA in the cell nucleus, leading to synthesis of protein by the ribosomes and endoplasmic reticulum. This accounts for both the metabolic and growth-promoting actions of the hormones.

Effects on organs and systems. The effects of under-or overactivity of the thyroid are reflected in the functioning of many tissues and organs. In hypothyroidism the pulse rate is slowed, whereas in hyperthyroidism it is increased. The cardiac output and bloodflow to specific organs are also affected by the thyroid state. These changes are in part due to the direct action of thyroxine on the heart and in part secondary to changes in tissue metabolism. Some of the effects may be due to an increased sensitivity of the vessels and heart to adrenaline and noradrenaline and may be alleviated by sympathetic blocking agents.

In hypothyroidism the motility of the gastro-intestinal tract is impaired, leading to constipation, whereas in hyperthyroidism there may be increased motility, which causes diarrhoea.

In hyperthyroidism increased protein catabolism causes muscular wasting and subsequent weakness. The mental state is abnormal in patients with both underactivity and overactivity of the thyroid. Those with underactivity are sluggish and apathetic and often show intellectual deterioration. Because of their lowered heat production they characteristically prefer warm conditions. Patients with overactive thyroids are tense and excitable. Because of their increased heat production they sweat profusely and prefer a cooler environment.

CONTROL OF THYROID FUNCTION

The secretion of the thyroid hormones is partly controlled by thyroid stimulating hormone (TSH, thyrotrophin) which is produced and released by the anterior pituitary. Hypophysectomy (removal of the pituitary) causes a marked reduction in thyroid activity but does not completely abolish it. Thyroid activity in the hypophysectomized animal may be increased by the administration of an extract of the pituitary gland.

It has been found that removal of the thyroid gland is followed by hypertrophy of those cells which secrete TSH, and that this hypertrophy is prevented by injecting thyroid extract in quantities sufficient to mimic normal thyroid function. Thus it has been postulated that the secretion of TSH is modulated by the level of circulating thyroid hormones; a fall in the plasma concentration of thyroid hormones leading to an increase in TSH secretion, whereas an elevation of plasma thyroxine depresses TSH secretion (Fig. 17.4b). It is by means of this negative feed-back loop that constant plasma levels of T_3 and T_4 are maintained.

The secretion of TSH and hence of thyroid hormones is also under the control of the central nervous system. Section of the pituitary stalk leads to a marked reduction of TSH secretion, and it is now known that the hypothalamus produces thyrotrophin releasing factor (TRF) which passes to the pituitary along the hypothalamohypophyseal portal vessels (p. 767). By this means, emotion, stress and environmental changes may affect thyroid function. The feedback mechanism described above probably acts at both pituitary and hypothalamic levels (Fig. 17.4c).

Diseases of the thyroid gland

SIMPLE GOITRE

The term 'goitre' indicates an enlargement of the thyroid. A dietary deficiency of iodide produces a simple goitre because of an increased secretion of TSH in response to decreased circulating thyroxine which causes the acinar cells to hypertrophy. The increased mass of thyroid tissue enables the gland to extract more iodide from plasma and the patient does not usually suffer from hypothyroidism.

HYPERTHYROIDISM

The thyroid is also enlarged when the gland is overactive but in this case there is no oversecretion of TSH. Instead the gland appears to be stimulated by long-acting thyroid stimulator (LATS) which is an immunoglobulin produced in lymphoid tissue. The condition may therefore be an immune disorder.

HYPOTHYROIDISM

Underactivity of the thyroid gland may be congenital (cretinism) or it may be acquired during adult life (myxoedema).

Myxoedema may result from autoimmune destruction of the thyroid gland or it can be due to pituitary failure.

PARATHYROID GLANDS

Anatomy and histology

These glands are yellowish-brown, ovoid structures, each weighing about 50 mg, and measuring about 6 mm by 4 mm by 1 mm. There are

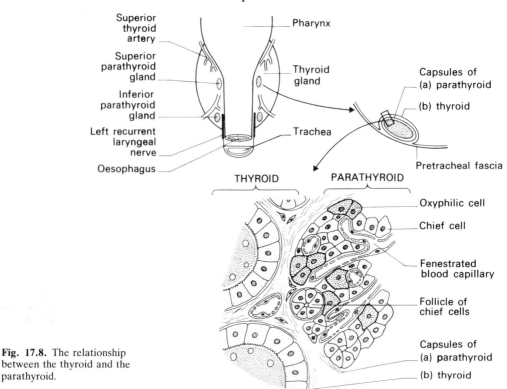

Fig. 17.8. The relationship between the thyroid and the parathyroid.

usually four parathyroids, and they lie at the back of the thyroid, generally between the posterior borders of its lateral lobes and its outer capsule, although they are sometimes embedded in the substance of the gland itself (Fig. 17.8). Although most parathyroids lie within the capsule of the thyroid, they are always separated from that gland by their own thin connective tissue capsule. Trabeculae extend from this into the substance of the parathyroid and support the main blood vessels, nerves and lymphatics of the gland. Delicate reticular tissue ensheathes and supports the secretory cells of the parathyroid and the rich capillary networks which serve them.

The parathyroid glands receive blood from either the inferior thyroid arteries or from the anastomoses between these and the superior thyroid arteries.

GLANDULAR EPITHELIAL CELLS

These collectively form the parenchyma of the glands. They are generally packed together in either compact masses of branching cords, although occasionally a few cells are grouped

into small follicles (Fig. 17.8). Each cell has direct access to a blood capillary, into which its secretions pass. The glandular epithelial cells are of two types: (a) chief or principal cells and (b) oxyphilic cells.

Chief cells. Most of the glandular epithelial cells are of this type. They produce parathyroid hormone, secreting it directly into the blood. Each chief cell is polygonal and about 7–10 μm in diameter. The single nucleus is central in position. The cytoplasm is faintly acidophilic, and contains a little rough endoplasmic reticulum where parathyroid hormone is manufactured, a small Golgi apparatus lying close to the nucleus, and numerous elongated mitochondria. Also present are irregular secretory granules about 200–400 nm in diameter; they are assumed to store parathyroid hormone awaiting release, and are scattered throughout the cytoplasm, being particularly numerous at the vascular pole of the cell (that is, at the end nearest to a blood capillary). Secretory granules can be demonstrated by treating sections of parathyroid with iron-haematoxylin stain. Chief cells contain histochemically detectable levels of glycogen particularly when 'resting'. There is generally a single cilium extending from the surface of each chief cell.

The organelle content of the cytoplasm of the chief cells varies with the state of their secretory activity and affects their staining properties; this has led to a classification of dark cells (having the most acidophilic cytoplasm), light cells (less acidophilic), and clear cells (in which the cytoplasm is not readily stained).

Oxyphilic cells (oxys=acid). These first appear early in childhood and increase in number at and around puberty. They are found singly or in small, scattered groups and are most common at the periphery of the glands. They are larger than the chief cells and have strongly acidophilic cytoplasm. They have more mitochondria than the chief cells, have little rough endoplasmic reticulum, and only a small Golgi apparatus. Light microscopy reveals numerous acidophilic granules in the cytoplasm, but electron microscopy shows that these 'granules' are really mitochondria: no true secretory vesicles can be found in oxyphilic cells. The function of the oxyphilic cells is not yet known, but the presence of many mitochondria suggests that they are metabolically very active.

Calcium homeostasis

Until about 20 years ago it was considered that the control of plasma calcium was effected solely by the parathyroid hormone, but two additional factors are now known to be involved. These are calcitonin, and 1,25-dihydroxycholecalciferol $(1,25\text{-}(OH)_2D_3)$, a metabolite of vitamin D_3 which is formed in the kidney and released into the blood in order to reach its target organs—the intestinal mucosal cells and bone. So, by definition, $1,25\text{-}(OH)_2D_3$ is a hormone too.

A control system is necessary because of the potential variations in plasma calcium (Fig. 17.9).

CALCIUM ABSORPTION

The amount of calcium absorbed in the intestine is variable. Not only does the daily intake vary, but between meals there may be long periods when no calcium is entering the blood from the intestine.

From a daily intake of about 1 g calcium, only about 200–400 mg is absorbed. There are several reasons for this low efficiency. At the cellular level the absorptive process is rate-limited and involves two major components; a straightforward diffusion or facilitated diffusion

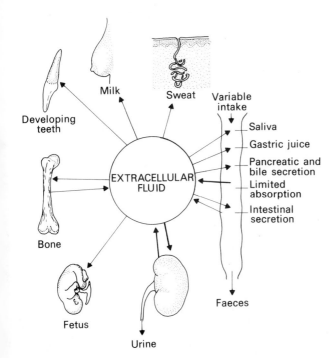

Fig. 17.9. Schematic representation of calcium balance. The important features are the variability of absorption and the pathways through which calcium is lost from the extracellular fluid.

at the luminal membrane, and a saturable, energy-dependent, active transport at the opposite membrane.

Local factors operating in the intestinal lumen can encourage or inhibit absorption. Thus the ingestion of phytic acid, in unrefined cereals such as porridge, wholemeal flour and chapatties, and in legumes, such as beans, peas and soya bean, can lead to a transient decrease in the absorption of calcium. Phytic acid, is a hexaphosphate of inositol, which readily combines with many calcium ions to form an insoluble and therefore non-diffusible calcium phytate. However, for two reasons this effect is usually of little consequence: wholemeal flour is fortified with calcium; and certain bacteria which colonize the intestine produce the enzyme phytase, promoting the breakdown of phytic acid and reducing its potentially harmful effects. This enzyme is also present in yeast and is activated during the bread-making process. Conditions leading to a more alkaline pH in the small intestine such as the ingestion of alkaline salts, also reduce calcium absorption since the solubility of many calcium salts, particularly calcium phosphate, is reduced by an increased pH. In old age the ability to absorb calcium is reduced. This is probably due to changes in the complex cellular mechanisms which are involved in absorption and in the reduced number of absorptive cells.

One particularly interesting finding is that of the adaptive capacity of the calcium absorptive process. It has been shown that, in both animals and man, a restricted intake of dietary calcium is followed within a few days by more efficient absorption with the result that the amount of calcium absorbed may remain almost unchanged. The converse situation is also true in that an increase in calcium intake above the nutritionally adequate level may not result in significantly more being absorbed. Adaptation is not dependent on the parathyroid gland, but does require an adequate intake of vitamin D_3.

PREGNANCY AND LACTATION

The demands which the developing fetal skeleton makes upon the mother's calcium supply are considerable and if the baby is breast-fed this withdrawal of calcium will be exaggerated and prolonged. Since the calcium concentration in milk is about 30 mg per 100 cm³, a daily loss of up to 250 mg calcium in milk is quite possible. These situations are bound to cause a potential decrease in plasma calcium levels.

In parts of the world the consequences of numerous pregnancies, prolonged lactation and inadequate nutrition can sometimes be seen in the abnormal histological structure of the maternal skeleton. The body attempts to maintain a constant plasma calcium level at the expense of the skeletal reservoir though this is minimized by increased intestinal absorption of calcium caused by the presence of increased amounts of $1,25(OH)_2D_3$ and certain hormones associated with pregnancy. In the developed countries it is customary for the diet to be supplemented with calcium and vitamin D and this, together with the spacing of pregnancies due to birth control, to some extent spares the physiological control systems from being called into action.

BONES AND TEETH

An equilibrium exists in the adult between bone mineral and calcium and phosphate ions in extracellular fluid. A decrease in the plasma concentration of either calcium or phosphate causes mobilization of bone mineral (the law of Mass Action). This concept of a bone-mineral–extracellular fluid equilibrium has given rise to the view that there is always a reciprocal relationship between plasma calcium and phosphate ions; if one of these increases then this causes a reduction in the other because the solubility product is exceeded and solid is formed. To a large extent this is true, but factors such as the activity of the metabolizing bone cells and the excretion of these ions by the kidney can upset this relationship.

The entire skeleton is not available for correcting disturbances of plasma calcium, it is only that which is accessible to bone tissue fluid. This is about 5% of the total adult skeletal calcium and is often described as 'exchangeable' calcium.

URINARY EXCRETION

Because calcium is actively reabsorbed by the kidney tubule only about 0.5–1.0% of the calcium in the glomerular filtrate is lost in the urine. The calcium concentration in the urine increases in proportion to that in the glomerular filtrate and plasma.

CALCIUM BALANCE

When the net intestinal absorption of calcium is equal to its urinary excretion, the person is said to be in calcium balance; but when urinary Ca^{2+} is in excess, the balance is negative. Some calcium (endogenous urinary calcium) is excreted even when no calcium is ingested.

From Fig. 17.9, which summarizes calcium balance, it is easy to guess the sites which might be susceptible to any controlling influences. These are:

1 Intestinal absorptive cells
2 Digestive glands
3 The interface between bone and tissue fluid
4 Osteoclasts and osteoblasts
5 Kidney tubule cells

Many vital physiological processes require a critical level of ionic calcium, some of these being sensitive to small changes within the physiological range whereas others seem only to be affected by gross changes made possible in the laboratory. Care should be taken to distinguish between these.

1 The excitability of neurons is increased by a small drop in calcium ion concentration because less depolarization is then necessary to initiate action potentials. Low amplitude, naturally occurring oscillations in membrane potential which are normally ineffective may, under these conditions, assume the proportions of action potentials. Such a condition of hyperexcitability of nerve causing muscle twitching or even sustained contraction is called hypocalcaemic tetany.

2 Calcium ions are also necessary for the synthesis and release of acetylcholine at synapses and neuromuscular junctions. A large decrease in the concentration of ionic calcium interferes with synaptic transmission.

3 The contractility (the amount of contraction in response to a standard stimulus) of all types of muscle is increased by an increase in calcium ions. Motility of intestinal muscle is augmented when plasma calcium levels are raised. The entry of calcium ions through smooth muscle cell membranes activates part of the contraction process (p. 343).

4 The mechanism coupling the release of transmitter substances to the secretory processes in both exocrine and endocrine glands is calcium-dependent. This may be more of academic interest rather than practical importance over the physiological range of calcium concentration.

5 Calcium is probably necessary for the structural integrity of many cell membranes. It is also necessary for the function of platelets.

6 The importance of calcium ions as cofactors for certain enzymatic reactions in blood clotting is well established, but it would be absurd to suggest that plasma calcium levels could ever be low enough to affect these reactions. Death from other causes would intervene!

STATE OF CALCIUM AND PHOSPHORUS IN PLASMA

The mean calcium concentration for healthy adults is about 10 mg/100 cm^3 plasma (2.5 mmol/dm^3) of which about 5.3 mg/100 cm^3 is in ionic form. Small amounts are combined with bicarbonate, citrate and phosphate as complex ions or undissociated molecules. The ionic fraction is more important physiologically and must be controlled. It diffuses readily through capillaries. This leaves about 2.7 mg/100 cm^3 combined with plasma albumin and 0.6 mg with globulin, both these non-diffusible fractions being largely confined to the plasma. Changes in plasma protein concentration and the charge carried by protein (because of pH changes) will alter these levels. Since negligible concentrations of calcium are present within the blood cells, the calcium in whole blood is only about 6 mg/100 cm^3.

Inorganic phosphate (Pi) is mainly present as the ions HPO_4^{2-} and $H_2PO_4^-$ in the ratio of 4:1 at the normal pH of plasma. The amount of PO_4^{3-} is infinitesimally small. The total Pi is about 3.8 mg/100 cm^3 plasma (1.2 mmol/dm^3) of which some 15% may be bound. Very small quantities of pyrophosphate may also be present.

CONTROL SYSTEMS

Parathyroid hormone (parathormone, PTH)

Characterization of hormone. The active principle of the glands, first properly isolated by Collip in 1925, has now been purified and its amino acid composition and sequence determined. Of the 84 amino acid residues which constitute parathormone only residues 1–29 are essential for its activity and this part of the molecule has recently been synthesized.

Actions of parathyroid hormone. Parathyroid hormone (PTH) is a calcium-raising factor, its release from the glands being increased in response to a fall in the concentration of Ca^{2+} in blood flowing through them and conversely being switched off when the concentration rises much above normal. This control is illustrated by Fig. 17.10, in which the circulating hormone has been assayed at various plasma calcium levels.

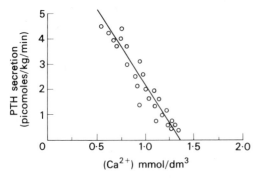

Fig. 17.10. Effect of variations in the calcium ion concentration in plasma on the rate of secretion of parathormone in the cow. (Taken from Copp D. H. (1970) *Annual Review of Physiology* **32**, 72.)

PTH is destroyed slowly by healthy kidney tissue.

The calcium-raising effect of injections of PTH is brought about in several ways. These take place in a sequence over several days.

1   The first observation is an increase in the phosphate concentration in urine (phosphaturia) due to reduced tubular reabsorption of phosphate. In consequence, the plasma phosphate level falls, upsets the equilibrium with bone mineral and causes the withdrawal of the phosphate, together with calcium, from the skeleton.

2   Following this by several hours there is an increase in the activity, and sometimes the number, of osteoclasts. These cells increase their synthesis of RNA and lysosomal enzymes. In tissue culture these cellular changes are accompanied by decreased activity of osteoblasts. Hyperparathyroidism of long-standing is characterized by the removal of mineralized tissue from bone and its replacement by poorly formed fibrous tissue, an appearance which is aptly termed 'osteitis fibrosa cystica'.

3   After some delay, calcium absorption from the intestine is increased, a response which probably involves the mediation of vitamin D_3 metabolites. There is also some evidence to suggest that the hormone reduces the amount of calcium in the digestive secretions.

4   Another action of PTH is its effect in conserving calcium by restricting its excretion in urine. In patients with hyperparathyroidism with elevated plasma calcium levels of 15–20 mg/100 cm^3, there is less calcium in the urine than is predicted from experimentally induced hypercalcaemia in healthy persons. This concept is made clearer by reference to the graph in Fig. 17.11.

By these mechanisms large increases in the levels of circulating PTH can bring about an increase in the plasma calcium level. But are these mechanisms characteristic of the normal physiological action of the hormone?

In some carefully designed studies in dogs, it

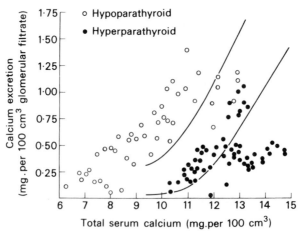

Fig. 17.11. Relationship between calcium excretion in urine and total serum calcium concentration in three groups of subjects. The normal limits for healthy controls whose blood calcium levels were experimentally altered by ingestion or infusion of calcium are between solid lines. The theoretical calcium threshold (the serum level above which calcium appears in the urine) falls from 9.0 mg/100 cm^3 serum to about 6.5 mg in hypoparathyroid patients similarly treated (○), whereas it is probably raised to about 12 mg/100 cm^3 in hyperparathyroid patients (●). (Adapted from Peacock M., Robertson W. G. and Nordin B. E. C. (1969) *Lancet* **i**, 385.)

has been possible to imitate the physiological actions of PTH. Instead of injecting the hormone it was continuously perfused into conscious dogs in amounts corresponding to those shown to be necessary to maintain normal plasma calcium levels in parathyroidectomized dogs. It was concluded that the main actions of the hormone are to promote intestinal absorption and renal tubular reabsorption of calcium.

Parathyroid hormone deficiency. The pronounced fall in plasma calcium to 6–7 mg/100 cm³ in hypoparathyroidism or after experimental parathyroidectomy is associated with decreased urinary phosphate excretion and because of the hypocalcaemia there is decreased calcium excretion also (Fig. 17.11). Bone resorption is reduced and presumably those responses which are activated by PTH will be absent. Sometimes a reasonably stable plasma calcium level of 6–7 mg/100 cm³ is seen in the absence of PTH and this suggests that the hormone is normally boosting the level to above that which could be achieved by the solubility of bone mineral in extracellular fluid (p. 394).

Tetany is either present and reveals itself as tingling, numbness or spasm of the forearm and hand muscles, or is latent. If latent, it can easily be induced by tapping the skin above the course taken by the facial nerve over the angle of the mandible, thereupon the muscles of the face twitch (Chvostek's sign).

Calcitonin

The infusion of calcium into an animal should switch off the release of PTH and allow the plasma level to fall gradually to normal levels by the excretion of calcium in the urine and its deposition in the bone. In 1962 Copp made what was then a surprising observation. He showed that if the thyroid/parathyroid complex had been removed from a dog (causing a complete absence of PTH) it took longer for high plasma calcium levels to fall to normal than if the thyroid/parathyroid complex was present (where there would be a switching off of PTH and destruction of circulating hormone) (Fig. 17.12). Copp explained his results by suggesting the existence of a calcium-lowering principle, calcitonin, which was released in response to raised levels of circulating calcium. This has been subsequently shown to be correct, but the source of the hormone in mammals is not in the parathyroids as originally thought, but in the then largely ignored parafollicular cells of the thyroid gland (Fig. 17.5).

The research and interest shown in calcitonin has been phenomenal. Its source, detailed chemical structure and physiological activity were discovered and even its synthesis achieved within the short space of some 10 years.

Release of calcitonin as a function of the plasma calcium concentration has been shown to complement that of PTH (Fig. 17.13). Injection of calcitonin depresses the plasma calcium to about 6–7 mg/100 cm³. A variety of experimental approaches has shown that this action is effected principally by a direct inhibition of bone resorption and that it is not due to an inhibition of either the action or release of PTH. Reports of increased urinary phosphate excretion after calcitonin administration are probably due to a pharmacological rather than a physiological effect. The level of circulating calcitonin in man is normally very low and this fact together with the finding that the response to calcitonin depends on a high rate of bone turnover has made some people relegate calcitonin to a position of less importance than PTH and vitamin D₃ in the delicate control of plasma calcium.

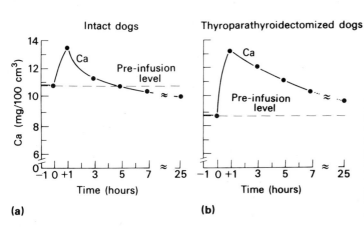

Fig. 17.12. Effect of thyroparathyroidectomy (right) on precise control of plasma calcium; unoperated control response on left. Recovery from hypercalcaemia induced by 1 hour infusion of calcium gluconate. (Modified from Copp D. H. (1970) *Annual Review of Physiology* **32**, 72.)

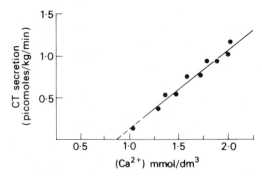

Fig. 17.13. Effect of variations in the calcium concentration in plasma on the rate of secretion of calcitonin in an adult sheep. (Adapted from Copp D. H. (1970) *Annual Review of Physiology* **32**, 72.)

VITAMIN D₃ METABOLITES (see also p. 819)

For many years it had been known that administration of vitamin D₃ to a vitamin D deficient animal is effective in increasing calcium absorption in the intestine, but only after some 20 hours or so. Much effort was expended in an attempt to unravel both the reason for the delay and the mechanism of action of this vitamin. With the development of a more sophisticated and sensitive analytical technique a new picture began to take shape although many details are continually being added.

In summary, vitamin D₃ is converted by the liver to a more active form, 25-hydroxycholecalciferol (25-(OH)D₃). This is released back into the circulation and carried to the kidney

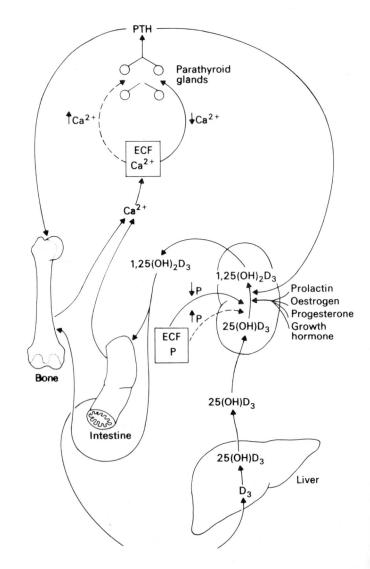

Fig. 17.14. Summary of vitamin D₃ metabolism and its possible interactions with parathyroid hormone in controlling plasma calcium levels. Broken arrows denote an inhibitory effect.

tubule cells where it is converted to the very active metabolite, 1,25-dihydroxycholecalciferol (1,25-$(OH)_2D_3$) under the influence of an enzyme 25-OHD$_3$ 1-hydroxylase. This key stage is probably sensitive to several factors including the plasma calcium levels and the amount of circulating 1,25-$(OH)_2D_3$ (at least in rats this is so), PTH, calcitonin, inorganic phosphate, prolactin and growth hormone. Providing that there is an adequate supply of the parent vitamin (D$_3$), a fall in plasma calcium could then induce an increase in the amount of 1,25-$(OH)_2D_3$ either by acting directly on the hydroxylase in the kidney or indirectly on this through the mediation of PTH. PTH could also act indirectly by decreasing intracellular phosphate in the tubules. (It will be remembered that PTH reduces the reabsorption of phosphate in the kidney tubule.)

The 1,25-$(OH)_2D_3$ released by the kidney in some way activates the mechanism of calcium absorption in the intestinal mucosal cells and the reabsorptive process in the kidney tubule cells. Fig. 17.14 is an attempt to summarize this story.

Other metabolites of 25-$(OH)_2D_3$ have been detected recently but their function is still a matter of debate. It seems probable that 24,25-$(OH)_2D_3$ is involved in bone mineralization. It is likely to be formed when the plasma calcium level is raised.

Numerous suggestions have been made as to the site of action of 1,25-$(OH)_2D_3$ in the intestinal absorptive process. Most prominent amongst these is the synthesis of an intracellular calcium-binding protein (CaBP), but also implicated are alkaline phosphatase, a Na-Ca dependent ATPase, structural changes in the glycocalyx or cell membrane, a change in membrane permeability and an interference with intracellular pump systems.

PITUITARY (HYPOPHYSIS)

Anatomy

This small gland, weighing only about 0.5 g, is one of the most important organs of the body. Suspended from the base of the brain, with which it has neural and vascular connections, it is in an ideal situation to link the activities of the nervous and endocrine systems.

The pituitary gland consists of a neurohypophysis—which develops as a downgrowth from the floor of the diencephalon and is effectively an outpost of the brain—and an adenohypophysis, which develops as an ectodermal upgrowth from the roof of the primitive buccal cavity or stomodaeum called Rathke's pouch (Book 2). The neurohypophysis and adenohypophysis unite, and the connection with the stomodaeum is lost while that with the hypothalamus (the floor of the diencephalon) is preserved. The anterior part of the adenohypophysis enlarges and the cavity of Rathke's pouch is reduced to a small continuous or discontinuous cleft (Fig. 17.15).

The neurohypophysis consists of two main regions: the infundibulum and the pars nervosa. The infundibulum consists of a neural stalk, the infundibular stem, through which nerve tracts pass from the hypothalamus to the pars nervosa, and the median eminence of the tuber cinereum (p. 868), the latter being continuous with the hypothalamus. The infundibular stem is continuous with the pars nervosa, a bulbous region which forms the posterior lobe of the pituitary gland.

The adenohypophysis consists of three parts: the pars anterior or pars distalis, the pars intermedia and the pars tuberalis. The pars anterior develops from the anterior wall of Rathke's pouch and is separated from the pars intermedia, which develops from the posterior wall, by vestiges of the cavity of the pouch. The pars tuberalis wraps around the infundibular stem and the median eminence, and is continuous with the pars anterior (Fig. 17.16).

The pituitary gland is surrounded by a capsule which is continuous with the cranial meninges (p. 885). It lies in the hypophysial fossa or sella turcica of the sphenoid bone beneath the diaphragma sellae, a circular fold of dura mater containing a small central hole through which the stalk of the hypophysis passes.

Blood supply (Fig. 17.17)

The pituitary gland is supplied with blood by branches of the internal carotid arteries—the superior and inferior hypophysial arteries—which anastomose freely in the gland substance. The branches give rise to tufts of capillaries which drain into the hypophysial portal veins which pass to the pars anterior where they open into sinusoids between the cords of glandular cells. The portal system of the pituitary gland has the important function of carrying hormones called releasing factors (p. 774) from the median eminence of the hypothalamus, where they are synthesized and secreted, to the pars anterior, where they stimulate the release of specific trophic hormones. The inferior hypophysial arteries supply the lower part of the

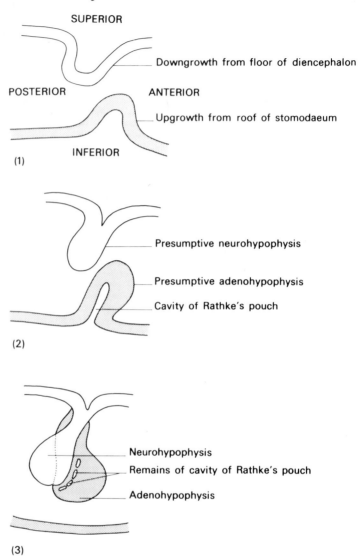

Fig. 17.15. The embryological origin of the neurohypophysis and the adenohypophysis of the pituitary gland.

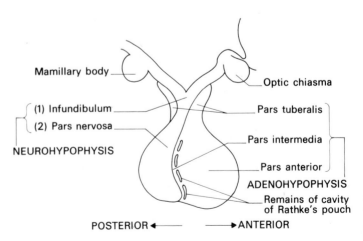

Fig. 17.16. The main regions of the pituitary gland.

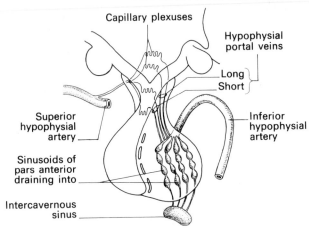

Fig. 17.17. The vasculature of the pituitary gland.

pituitary stalk and the posterior lobe of the gland. Together with the superior hypophysial arteries, they also give off small end arteries to the anterior lobe.

Blood leaves the pituitary gland through short veins which open into the intercavernous sinus which lies in the dura mater surrounding most of the gland.

Nerve supply (Fig. 17.18)
The neurohypophysis is supplied by sympathetic vasomotor nerves and neurosecretory cells whose bodies lie in nuclei of the hypothalamus, and whose axons run in the neural stalk. A few nerve fibres may enter the pars intermedia, but it is unlikely that any pass to the pars anterior. The neurosecretory cells manufacture the hormones vasopressin and oxytocin, storing them in granules in the swollen ends of their axons until stimulated to release them.

The adenohypophysis has no direct innervation apart from a few sympathetic vasomotor fibres.

NEUROHYPOPHYSIS

This is continuous with the floor of the diencephalon and in many respects resembles it histologically. It consists mainly of the unmyelinated axons of neurosecretory cells whose bodies lie in the hypothalamus, and a population of supporting cells called pituicytes (Fig. 17.19).

The axons reach the pars nervosa by way of the neural stalk. Once within the pars nervosa they fan out and end blindly in contact with the endothelia of its fenestrated blood capillaries, into which their secretions, manufactured in the rough endoplasmic reticulum of their cell bodies, are released. The two secretions are antidiuretic hormone (vasopressin) and oxytocin, each bound

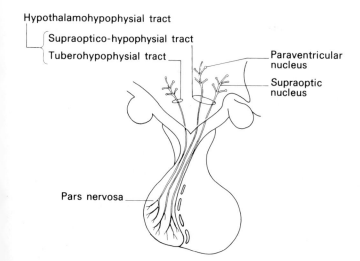

Fig. 17.18. The innervation of the pituitary gland.

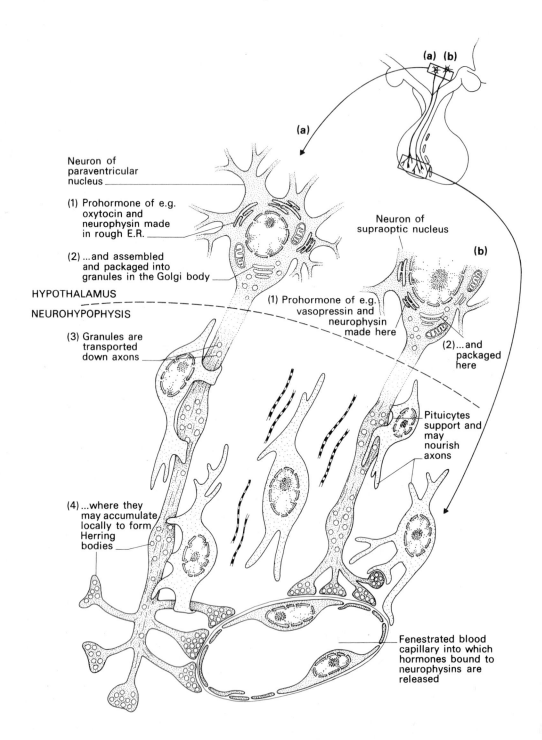

Neuron of paraventricular nucleus

(1) Prohormone of e.g. oxytocin and neurophysin made in rough E.R.

(2) ...and assembled and packaged into granules in the Golgi body

HYPOTHALAMUS

NEUROHYPOPHYSIS

(3) Granules are transported down axons

(4) ...where they may accumulate locally to form Herring bodies

Neuron of supraoptic nucleus

(1) Prohormone of e.g. vasopressin and neurophysin made here

(2) ...and packaged here

Pituicytes support and may nourish axons

Fenestrated blood capillary into which hormones bound to neurophysins are released

Fig. 17.19. The fine-structural relationship between the hypothalamus and the neurohypophysis, showing the mechanism of hormone transport.

to a specific protein carrier called a neurophysin, and are made primarily by cells of the supraoptic and paraventricular nuclei. After manufacture, each hormone is linked to its neurophysin in the Golgi apparatus and is packaged into a granule. These granules, about 100–300 nm in diameter, cannot be readily identified by light microscopy without special staining techniques.

The granules are transported actively along the axons toward their expanded terminations which, together with any other local accumulations of granules in the axoplasm, are called Herring bodies. The hormones are stored at the ends of the axons, ready for release into adjacent blood capillaries.

The hypothalamohypophysial axons (Fig. 17.18) have normal electrical properties and conduct action potentials in the usual manner. Release of hormones from the vesicles (Fig. 17.19) is brought about by the passage of a nerve impulse from the cell body.

The pituicytes are a special group of cells lying in the connective tissue between the axons of the neurosecretory cells. They are irregular, branched cells, often containing lipid droplets and pigment granules. They do not secrete hormones, as was once thought, but are a type of glial cell whose functions are to support and possibly nourish the axons of the neurosecretory cells.

ADENOHYPOPHYSIS

Pars anterior
This consists of glandular cells of the APUD type (p. 603) arranged in irregular cords and clumps, separated from each other by thin-walled vascular sinusoids, and supported by a delicate stroma of reticular tissue.

The glandular cells can be classified according to their affinity for stains into chromophobic cells, which do not stain readily, and chromophilic cells, which do. The latter used to be further subdivided into acidophilic and basophilic according to the staining properties of the granules they contain, those of acidophilic cells staining with acid dyes such as eosin and those of basophilic cells with basic dyes such as haematoxylin. In recent years the application of more informative staining techniques and electron microscopy has shown this classification to be inadequate. The terms 'chromophobic', 'acidophilic' and 'basophilic' have been retained, but each group is subdivided further. It is also now known that the glandular cells of the pars anterior produce six hormones, each secreted by a different cell type, and wherever possible each cell is named according to the hormone it produces. Table 17.1 lists the various glandular cells of the pars anterior, together with their functions, and the characteristic features of their granules. Each type is described briefly below.

Acidophilic cells (α-cells). These comprise about 40% of the glandular cells of the pars anterior. They are usually commonest towards the outside of the gland.

1   *Somatotrophic cells.* These secrete the proteinaceous growth hormone somatotrophin (STH). They are columnar cells arranged in groups along the sinusoids. They have a conspicuous rough endoplasmic reticulum consisting of cisternae arranged generally parallel to the surface of the cell, a well-developed juxtanuclear Golgi apparatus, and numerous rod-shaped mitochondria.

2   *Mammotrophic cells.* These secrete prolactin, also known as luteotrophic hormone or lactogenic hormone, which stimulates lactation. As befits cells manufacturing protein for export, their rough endoplasmic reticulum and Golgi apparatus are well-developed, and they contain many mitochondria. They also contain a moderate number of lysosomes. Mammotrophic cells increase in activity during lactation. Once suckling ceases, the synthetic activity of the mammotrophic cells decreases and excess stored hormone is destroyed by the lysosomes which fuse with the secretory granules and hydrolyse their contents.

Basophilic cells. These comprise about 10% of the glandular cells of the pars anterior. Their basophilia is due to the chemical composition of their granules, not to the presence of large numbers of ribosomes which is usually the case in basophilic cells. Hormones stored in their granules are all conjugated proteins containing periodic acid/Schiff-positive carbohydrates, and can thus be readily distinguished from the acidophilic cells described above.

1   *Thyrotrophic cells (β-cells).* These secrete thyroid-stimulating hormone (TSH) and are mainly found towards the centre of the pars anterior. Their irregular secretory granules stain selectively with aldehyde-fuchsin and are the smallest in the pars anterior.

2   *Gonadotrophic cells (δ-cells).* These are larger than the other basophils and usually lie

Table 17.1. Glandular cells of the pars anterior.

Type	General group	Secretion	Staining reactions of granules		Electron microscopic appearance of granules and size (diameter)
			Aldehyde fuchsin	Periodic acid Schiff	
Somatotrophic	Acidophilic	STH	− (Orange G +ve)	−	Granules spherical, 400 nm
Mammotrophic	Acidophilic	LTH	− (Erythrosin and carmine +ve)	−	Granules elliptical, 600 nm
Thyrotrophic	Basophilic	TSH	+	+	Granules irregular, 140 nm
Gonadotrophic	Basophilic	LH	−	+	Granules spherical, 250 nm
		FSH	−	+	Granules spherical, 200 nm
Corticotrophic	Chromophobic	ACTH	−	−	Granules sparse, 200–250 nm
Undifferentiated reserves	Chromophobic	−	−	−	Few granules, heterogeneous

(Modified from Bloom W. and Fawcett D. W. (1975) *A Textbook of Histology*, 10th ed., p. 513. London: W. B. Saunders.)

next to the sinusoids. They are scattered throughout the pars anterior but none can be found in young children or in women during the last two trimesters of pregnancy.

They are of two types: δ_1 cells and δ_2 cells. The δ_1 cells secrete luteinizing hormone or LH (called interstitial cell stimulating hormone or ICSH in males), while the δ_2 cells secrete follicle stimulating hormone or FSH. The rough endoplasmic reticulum of the δ_1 cells generally takes the form of flattened cisternae. In contrast in the δ_2 cells the cisternae are generally dilated.

Chromophobic cells. These poorly-stained cells form about 50% of the glandular epithelial cells of the pars anterior, and are generally grouped in clusters within the cell cords. They seem to be relatively undifferentiated, and most of them probably act as reserves which can be programmed to differentiate into any of the other glandular epithelial cells as required. The chromophobes are, however, a heterogenous group, and include cells which, although appearing to belong to it, are actually differentiated but contain only a few small granules which stain

poorly and cannot be resolved by the light microscope. The corticotrophic cells fall into this category.

Corticotrophic cells. These secrete adrenocorticotropic hormone (ACTH). They are stellate cells, the processes of which extend between adjacent cells to reach the sinusoids. Although ACTH is a protein, they contain only a little rough endoplasmic reticulum, and only a few secretory granules.

If the adrenals are removed, the numbers and activity of the corticotrophic cells increase, while if the adrenals are overactive (as in Cushing's syndrome), or if a patient is receiving cortisone therapy, the corticotrophic cells decrease in activity and may even degenerate.

Pars intermedia
This lies adjacent to the neurohypophysis, i.e. posterior to the remains of the cavity of Rathke's pouch (Fig. 17.16). Sometimes this cavity is encroached upon by cells of the pars intermedia and is replaced by a group of cysts filled with a colloidal fluid and lined by a ciliated epithelium.

Cells of the pars intermedia may also invade the tissue of the neurohypophysis. In terms of size it is relatively insignificant in man, comprising only about 2% of the total volume of the hypophysis.

The glandular cells of the pars intermedia are weakly basophilic. They secrete melanocyte-stimulating hormone (MSH or intermedin), a polypeptide which is stored in the cells bound to a proteoglycan within secretory granules. These are about 200–300 nm in diameter, and stain faintly with periodic acid/Schiff and with aldehyde-fuchsin. The function of the hormone MSH, which in amphibia is known to cause melanocyte expansion, is obscure in man, whose melanocytes appear to be only influenced by ultraviolet light. The glandular cells of the pars intermedia also secrete endorphin.

For a hormone-secreting region, the pars intermedia has a relatively poor blood supply.

Pars tuberalis
This is the part of the adenohypophysis which wraps around the neural stalk of the neurohypophysis. It is continuous with the pars anterior (Fig. 17.16).

The glandular cells of the pars tuberalis are arranged as longitudinal cords, between which lie longitudinally-running blood vessels. It is the most highly vascularized part of the pituitary gland. It contains basophilic, acidophilic, and chromophobic cells, but their functions are unknown.

Physiology of pituitary and hypothalamus

The hypothalamus is responsible for a wide range of regulations within the body and acts through both the nervous system and the endocrine glands. Within the hypothalamus are collections of neurons or 'centres' involved with the stimulation of hunger and thirst which, through cortical centres, control eating and drinking behaviour. The hypothalamus is the main centre controlling heat gain and heat loss of the body (p. 724). Most of this control is effected through the nervous system but the long-term control of heat production is regulated by thyroxine secretion.

Many of the regulatory mechanisms of the hypothalamus are mediated through the actions of the anterior and posterior pituitary glands.

THE ANTERIOR PITUITARY GLAND

This gland probably secretes seven hormones in man. They may be classified as: (a) growth hormone (GH), (b) prolactin (c), melanocyte-stimulating hormone (MSH) and (d) those expressing their effects on the body by stimulation of target glands, namely trophic hormones: thyroid-stimulating hormone (TSH, thyrotrophin), adrenocorticotrophic hormone (ACTH, corticotrophin), and two gonadotrophins—follicle-stimulating hormone (FSH) and luteinizing hormone (LH). In this section we will discuss in detail only growth hormone, prolactin and MSH; TSH has already been discussed in the section on the control of thyroid function (p. 759) and it will be more convenient to discuss ACTH and the gonadotrophins in the sections on the respective target organs.

Growth hormone. As the name suggests, growth hormone is involved in the regulation of growth. Removal of the pituitary in a young animal or impaired secretion in a young child results in failure to grow. On the other hand, excessive secretion of growth hormone in a child results in abnormally rapid growth and gigantism (p. 801).

Secretion of growth hormone continues after growth has ceased since the hormone has other actions: it stimulates the uptake of amino acids and synthesis of protein in most tissues, and lowers the excretion of nitrogen from the body, it raises the blood levels of both glucose and fatty acids thus making these available for metabolism and sparing the oxidation of protein. To this end, secretion is increased during muscular exercise and by a variety of stresses.

It is possible that growth hormone may exert its growth-promoting actions indirectly. Following the injection of labelled hormone, there is rapid uptake into the liver, kidneys and adrenals, but no uptake can be detected at the epiphyses of growing long bones. A group of peptides known as somatomedins, possessing growth-promoting activity is present in plasma: the concentration of these somatomedins is raised following injection of growth hormone. It is postulated that growth hormone stimulates the growth of bone through the release of somatomedins from other tissues, particularly the liver.

Prolactin. This hormone may be found in the plasma of both sexes. The highest levels are found in pregnant and lactating females since the most important actions of the hormone are the preparation of the breast for lactation and the stimulation of the synthesis of milk. The hormone may also be responsible for the adaptation of the body to lactation, since it appears to have an antidiuretic action thus lowering renal excretion of water and making water available for secretion in milk. There is evidence in the rat that the hormone increases blood flow to the mammary gland, gastrointestinal tract and liver.

Melanocyte-stimulating hormone. When released in excessive amounts, causes darkening of the skin by stimulating the formation of melanin. Its physiological role is unknown.

Control of secretions

There has already been a description of the ways in which TSH secretion is controlled and the role of a releasing factor (TRF) produced in the hypothalamus (p. 759). Releasing factors (RF) have been found which stimulate secretion of other pituitary hormones, namely growth hormone (GHRF), ACTH (CRF), MSH (MSHRF), LH (LHRF) and FSH (FSHRF). Prolactin secretion, on the other hand, is controlled mainly by an inhibitory factor (PIF), although marked elevation of prolactin secretion follows the injection of TRF.

There appear to be distinct areas of the hypothalamus associated with the control of each pituitary hormone (Fig. 17.20). Electrical stimulation of these areas causes increased secretion of the releasing factor; destruction of the areas depresses the secretion. The releasing factors pass from the hypothalamus to the pituitary along the hypothalamohypophyseal portal blood vessels. In addition to its portal system, the anterior pituitary has a direct arterial blood supply through the inferior hypophyseal artery.

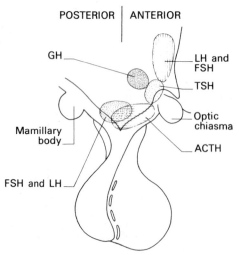

Fig. 17.20. The specific areas of the hypothalamus where releasing factors are produced.

The advantage of the portal system for transporting releasing factors is that only small quantities need be secreted from the hypothalamus to achieve a high level in the plasma reaching the pituitary. Subsequent passage of the factors into the general circulation leads to considerable dilution so that they are ineffective on recirculation.

The secretion of releasing factors (and PIF) is due to endogenous activity of the secretory neurons. The secretions may be altered by impulses from higher centres in the brain or by the effects of circulating hormones (Fig. 17.4). Thyroxine, cortisol and the sex hormones can suppress release of the respective trophic hormones although only in the case of thyroxine is this a major method of control. The secretion of growth hormone is influenced by circulating levels of amino acids and glucose, but these can have little effect on the long-term regulation of the hormone.

Diseases

Pituitary overactivity. Overactivity of the pituitary gland is normally due to a hormone-secreting tumour. Generalized oversecretion of all pituitary hormones does not occur.

Oversecretion of growth hormone occurring in the young, before fusion of the epiphyses of the long bones, leads to excessive growth of these bones and to a greater than normal stature. This condition is known as gigantism. When oversecretion of growth hormone begins after fusion of the epiphyses the condition of acromegaly occurs. There is broadening of the long bones, considerable thickening of the mandible, maxilla and temporal bones and a marked increase in the volume of soft tissues. Elevation of plasma glucose by growth hormone leads to increased secretion of insulin. If the pancreas is unable to meet and sustain this increased need for insulin, the patient becomes diabetic (p. 799).

Excessive secretion of ACTH causes overactivity of the adrenal cortex.

Pituitary underactivity. Hypopituitarism frequently involves several or all of the hormones. Pharmacological depression of a single pituitary hormone may be caused by prolonged administration of target organ hormones or their synthetic analogues (e.g. cortisol, oral contraceptives).

In children, insufficiency usually leads to infantilism or dwarfism. Infantilism is a condition in which both somatic growth and sexual development are retarded, whereas dwarfism implies a reduced stature without associated sexual immaturity.

The features of pituitary failure in the adult may be attributed to lack of TSH, ACTH and the gonadotrophins. Such patients are hypoglycaemic and hypothermic, and they are susceptible to stress and liable to collapse. Following surgical removal of the pituitary, thyroid or adrenal, hormones have to be administered.

THE POSTERIOR PITUITARY

The posterior pituitary secretes the hormones oxytocin—which has important actions on both the uterus during labour and the breast during lactation—and antidiuretic hormone. ADH increases water reabsorption from the renal tubules (p. 739) and at high concentrations elevates blood pressure (hence the alterative name–vasopressin).

Actions of posterior pituitary hormones
When plasma levels of antidiuretic hormone are raised, there is an increase in the amount of water reabsorbed from the distal convoluted tubules and collecting ducts in the kidney and the volume of urine is decreased (p. 739). This is the most important action of this hormone.

Injection into experimental animals causes marked vasoconstriction and elevation of arterial blood pressure, but the dose needed to exert measurable pressor effects is much greater than that needed for the antidiuretic action and it is unlikely that the release of posterior pituitary hormones contributes to the control of arterial blood pressure under physiological conditions.

Oxytocin causes contraction of the uterus during labour. During suckling in the lactating woman, myoepithelial cells in the breast contract and expel the milk (p. 794). Oxytocin is found in the pituitaries of males and of non-pregnant, non-lactating, females and small quantities are usually circulating in the blood. The function of the hormone in these people is unknown.

Control of secretion
Antidiuretic hormone. The main physiological factor controlling the release of ADH is the crystalloid (electrolyte) osmotic pressure of the extracellular fluid which is monitored by osmoreceptors in the hypothalamus, possibly within the supraoptic nucleus. Ingestion of water dilutes the plasma, decreases crystalloid osmotic pressure and inhibits ADH release with the result that the excess water is excreted as urine.

Severe haemorrhage causes release of large quantities of ADH which reduce water excretion (though the patient may already be anuric as a result of the lowered blood pressure) and may exert a pressor action. Large quantities of ADH are also released due to the effects of general anaesthetics and surgery, which may account for the period of low urine production following surgery. Other drugs such as morphine, nicotine and barbiturates also cause the release of ADH; ethanol is an exception and inhibits the release of ADH. Antidiuretic hormone secretion is increased during muscular exercise, when there is increased water by loss by evaporation, and during fear and other emotional stresses.

Oxytocin. Very little is known about the control of oxytocin secretion. The commonest factor which will raise the plasma level of oxytocin is sex play and coitus, though the function of the hormone in these circumstances is conjectural. Suckling causes a reflex release of oxytocin.

Diseases
The only important disease of the posterior pituitary is failure to secrete ADH, a condition known as diabetes insipidus which is characterized by the excretion of very large volumes of urine (up to 15 cm^3/min or 22 dm^3/ day).

ADRENALS (SUPRARENALS)

Anatomy

The adrenal glands are flattened structures lying just above the superior pole of each kidney (Fig. 17.21). They are surrounded by retroperitoneal areolar tissue containing a variable amount of fat. The right gland is roughly pyramidal in shape, while the left is semilunar. The size and shape of the adrenals vary with the age and physical condition of the individual, but in the average adult each measures about 50 mm by 30 mm by 10 mm and weighs about 5 g.

Each gland is supplied by branches of the inferior phrenic artery, abdominal aorta and renal artery. Venous blood from the right gland drains directly into the inferior vena cava while that from the left gland passes first to the left renal vein.

Each adrenal is a composite structure, consisting of an outer cortex and an inner medulla.

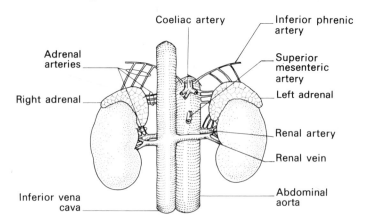

Fig. 17.21. The relationship of the adrenals with the surrounding structures. The right adrenal has been displaced laterally.

Although intimately related anatomically in that both share a common capsule, these two components differ in structure, function and developmental origin to such an extent that they are best considered as two separate glands.

ADRENAL CORTEX

If a fresh adrenal gland is cut transversely, the pale yellow cortex can be readily distinguished from the dark red medulla. The cortex, which is of mesodermal origin, developing from collections of coelomic mesothelial cells lying on the medial side of each mesonephros (Book 2), consists of large polyhedral secretory cells grouped into clusters and columns and separated by blood capillaries and sinusoids into which their secretions are released.

The arrangement of the cells is such that three concentric zones can be distinguished: (a) the zona glomerulosa—a thin superficial region, (b) the zona fasciculata—a thicker middle region and (c) the zona reticularis—a thinner region lying next to the medulla (Fig. 17.22).

Zona glomerulosa
The secretory cells of this region are arranged in closely-packed clusters, each surrounded by blood capillaries. They secrete the mineralocorticoid known as aldosterone.

Each cell has a single spherical nucleus and its cytoplasm contains basophilic secretory granules, the extensive smooth endoplasmic reticulum typical of cells manufacturing steroids, some rough endoplasmic reticulum, a well-developed Golgi apparatus, numerous filamentous mitochondria and lipid droplets.

Although the manufacture of steroids begins in the smooth endoplasmic reticulum, the recent finding of the enzymes needed for the conversion of some deoxycorticosterone to aldosterone in the mitochondria suggests that this part of the manufacturing process may take place in the mitochondria.

Zona fasciculata
Here the secretory cells are arranged in straight cords, one cell wide, running at right angles to the surface of the gland. Sinusoidal blood vessels lie between the cords and parallel to them. The secretory cells are larger than those of the zona glomerulosa, and may contain 1 or 2 spherical nuclei. The cytoplasm is so crowded with lipid droplets that it has a foamy, spongy appearance which led to the cells being named 'spongiocytes'. There is even more smooth endoplasmic reticulum in these cells than in the secretory cells of the zona glomerulosa, and the rough endoplasmic reticulum is also better represented; lysosomes, a well-developed Golgi apparatus and many mitochondria are present. Lipochrome, the yellow pigment which gives the cortex its characteristic colour, is also conspicuous and increases in amount with advancing age.

The cells of the zona fasciculata secrete sex hormones and the glucocorticoids cortisol and corticosterone.

Zona reticularis
Here the secretory cells are arranged in irregular cords forming a network or 'reticulum' with blood vessels lying between them. The secretory cells of this region are smaller than those of the rest of the cortex, although they resemble them in most other respects. Towards the medulla light and dark cells can be distinguished. The nuclei of the light cells stain very faintly, while

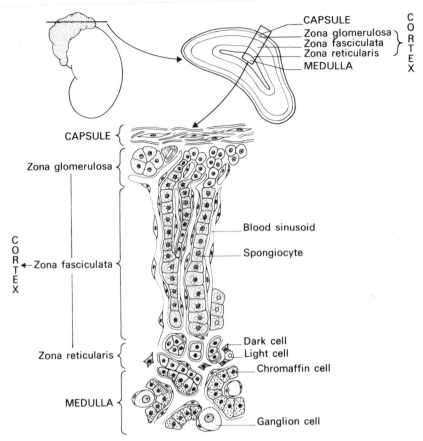

Fig. 17.22. The fine structure of an adrenal gland.

those of the dark cells stain deeply and are often shrunken and pyknotic. The role of these two cell types is not yet clear, but it has been suggested that the dark cells may be degenerative.

The secretory cells of the zona reticularis appear to manufacture the same hormones as do those of the zona fasciculata, that is, glucocorticoids and sex hormones. The histological differences between the two zones have not yet been satisfactorily explained in functional terms.

ADRENAL MEDULLA

The adrenal medulla consists of a parenchyma of large polyhedral secretory cells arranged in small clusters or short cords adjacent to blood capillaries and venules into which their secretions—the catecholamines adrenaline (epinephrine) and noradrenaline (norepinephrine)—pass directly. It also contains a few sympathetic ganglion cells. The parenchymal cells develop

from the same group of neural crest cells that give rise to the sympathetic ganglion cells of the coeliac plexus (Book 2). However, on reaching the adrenal only a few differentiate into ganglion cells proper; the rest become specialized secretory cells. Like the sympathetic ganglion cells they are innervated by preganglionic nerve fibres. Since the secretory cells of the adrenal medulla have the same developmental origin as the postganglionic neurons of the sympathetic part of the autonomic system (p. 929) and in many respects have similar functions, they are best regarded as specialized postganglionic neurons and the adrenal medulla as a specialized sympathetic ganglion.

If the medulla is treated with a fixative containing chromium salts, the chromaffin reaction occurs; the catecholamines within the granules of the secretory cells react with the chromium salts and turn brown. Because of this, the secretory cells of the medulla are often called chromaffin cells. Electron microscopy has shown that the granules are about 100–300 nm in diameter, and that those containing nor-adrenaline are more electron dense than those containing adrenaline. The cells have an exten-sive rough endoplasmic reticulum consisting of cisternae arranged parallel to each other in small groups. The Golgi apparatus is well represented and gives rise to the secretory granules. The membrane surrounding these granules is rich in ATPase and it is thought that this enzyme makes available the energy needed to transport the catecholamines to the granules and retain them there. In the absence of such a mechanism they would readily diffuse out of the granules because they have a low molecular weight. The secretory granules also contain a soluble protein, chromo-granin, which is manufactured in the rough endoplasmic reticulum, but the catecholamines are not bound to it.

The release of catecholamines from the sec-retory cells of the adrenal medulla is under direct neural control. Preganglionic sympathetic axons reach the secretory cells via the splanchnic nerves (p. 926). Arrival of a nerve impulse causes the release of acetylcholine from synaptic vesicles at the ends of the axons, and this changes the permeability of the plasma membranes of the secretory cells so that the catecholamine-containing granules can be liberated by exocytosis.

Physiology

The effects of total adrenalectomy
These have been widely studied in experimental animals and have been largely responsible for our present knowledge of the functions of the adrenal gland. Bilateral removal of the glands causes widespread metabolic upsets which may lead to death unless replacement therapy with adrenocortical hormones is given. Whereas a normally functioning adrenal cortex is essential for life, removal of the medulla alone (adrenal demedullation) causes only transient metabolic changes and it is now believed that the medulla is not essential for life. Observations on patients with atrophy of the adrenal gland suggest that the loss of the adrenocortical secretion in man may have similar effects to those of adrenalec-tomy in animals. These include:
1   A marked increase in sodium excretion which lowers plasma sodium concentration. At the same time, potassium excretion is reduced and the plasma potassium concentration may rise to toxic levels.

2   Reduction of plasma sodium concentration causes inhibition of ADH secretion, resulting in increased water excretion and reduction of extracellular fluid volume. Since plasma protein concentration is unchanged the plasma volume remains normal but the interstitial fluid volume is lowered.
3   Blood pressure and cardiac output are both reduced and there is a reduction in glomerular filtration rate.
4   There is a metabolic acidosis which may ini-tially be due to extrusion of hydrogen ions from cells because of their high potassium uptake. Later, impaired renal function results in a failure to excrete hydrogen ions. Finally, circulatory insufficiency may lead to anaerobic metabolism with production of lactic acid.
5   A reduced appetite together with failure to absorb glucose adequately (p. 797) leads to hypoglycaemia. This may be worsened by a failure to form glucose from protein and amino acids (p. 797).
6   Resistance to stress is reduced. Mortality fol-lowing surgery, during cold exposure, or as a result of exercise, is considerably increased.

THE ADRENAL CORTEX

The hormones secreted by the adrenal cortex are all steroids and may be considered in three classes based on their physiological actions; glucocorticoids, mineralocorticoids and sex hormones.

STRUCTURE OF THE STEROID HORMONES

The structure and details of the synthesis of the various hormones will be considered in the relevant sections. A word of introduction to the field of steroid chemistry is, however, necessary at this stage.

The parent compound of the very large number of steroids is cholesterol. This molecule, which contains 27 carbon atoms (designated C_{27}), is found in gallstones and has been known for many centuries. It is known that cholesterol is biosynthesized from the C_2 compound acetate by a complex series of reactions.

The parent hydrocarbon of cholesterol and all C_{27} steroids is cholestane ($C_{27}H_{48}$) which is derived, structurally at least, by reduction of the three ringed aromatic compound phenanthrene. Cholesterol contains a fourth ring fused to the three-ringed nucleus, two angled groups at C-10 and C-13, and a sidechain:

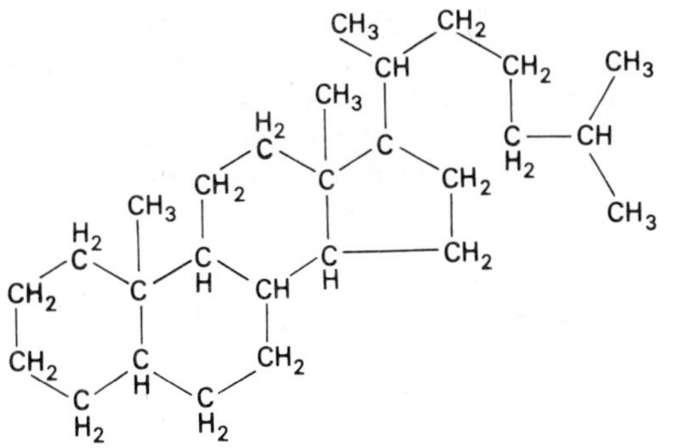

Cholestane

This C_{27} structure and its derivatives will be written in the following abbreviated form:

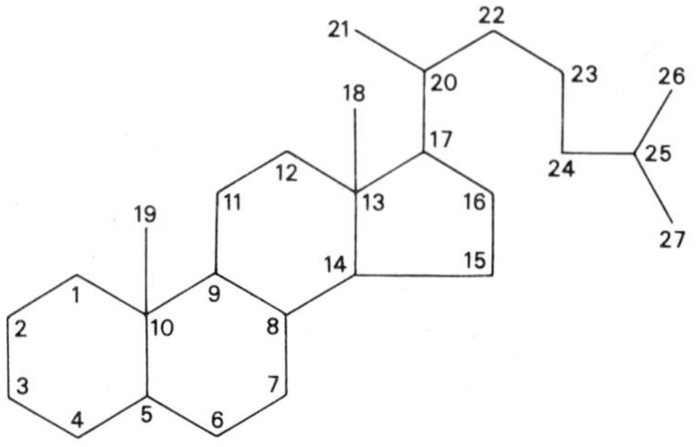

The C_{21} steroids, of which the hormones progesterone and cortisol are good examples, are derived from the parent hydrocarbon pregnane. This differs from cholestane in that the sidechain at C-17 is only 2 carbon atoms long.

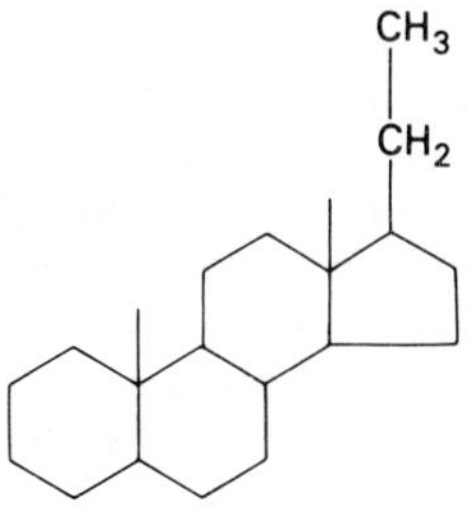

Pregnane

Complete removal of this sidechain leaves C_{19} steroids, the parent hydrocarbon being androstane:

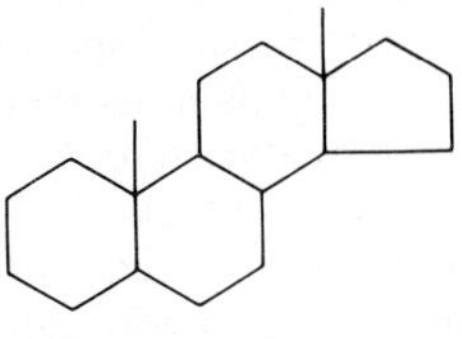

Androstane

Examples of steroid hormones derived from this are testosterone and 4-androstenedione.

The fourth group, the oestrogens, is derived from the hydrocarbon oestrane:

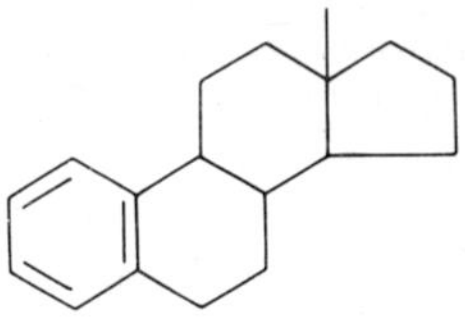

Oestrane

This C_{18} compound lacks the angular methyl group at C-10 and possesses an aromatic ring. The oestrogens, of which oestradiol-17β is the most well known example, bear a hydroxyl group at C-3.

Glucocorticoids. The main glucocorticoid secreted by the human adrenal is cortisol; small quantities of corticosterone are also secreted.

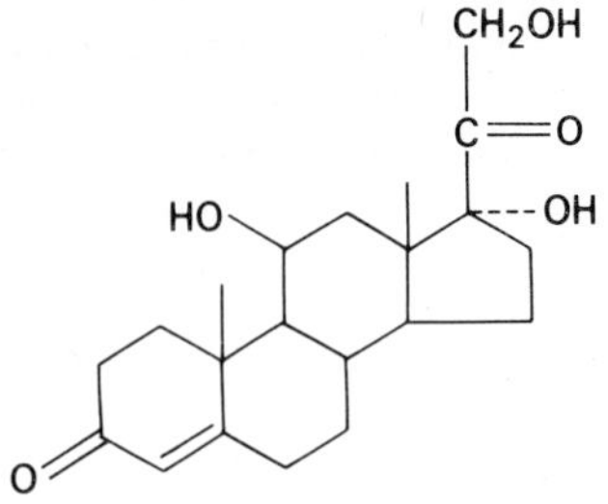

Cortisol

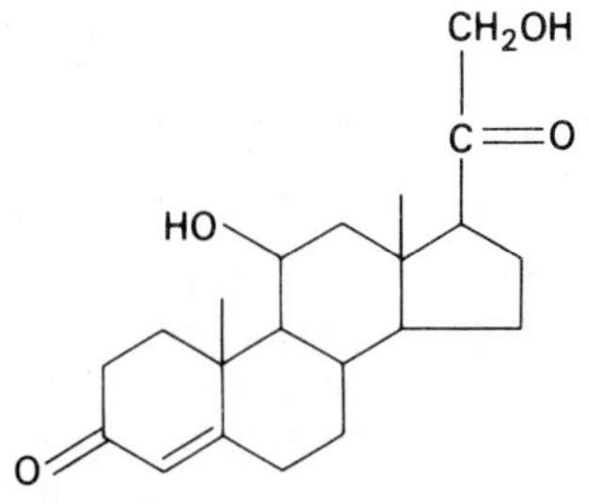

Corticosterone

They are synthesized in the zona fasciculata and zona reticularis.

The term glucocorticoid implies that the hormones affect glucose metabolism (p. 797). The overall effect is to raise the blood sugar level by inhibiting the uptake of glucose by tissues, thus antagonizing the action of insulin, and at the same time increasing the catabolism of protein to amino acids. They have pronounced stimulatory effects on aminotransferases and phosphatases with the result that gluconeogenesis is increased. Cortisol is needed for mobilization of fatty acids from fat depots (p. 150).

The catabolic effect of cortisol on protein may explain how cortisol has inhibitory effects on lymphoid tissue.

Some other actions of cortisol cannot be explained in terms of metabolic effects. These include the lowering of the eosinophil count, the maintenance of normal cardiac output and blood pressure and normal secretion of acid by the stomach. The mechanisms by which glucocorticoids protect the body against the effects of stress are also unexplained. They seem to maintain an adequate circulation by their actions on both the heart and microcirculation and ensure a favourable internal environment for the cells. At the subcellular level, glucocorticoids appear to stabilize the lysosomes and thus prevent autolysis which may occur during cellular hypoxia.

Mineralocorticoids. The only mineralocorticoid secreted by the adrenal cortex is aldosterone. This is a C_{21} steroid with an aldehyde group at position 13, which is secreted by the zona glomerulosa.

Aldosterone

The main site of action of aldosterone is on the renal tubule where it increases the reabsorption of sodium ions from glomerular filtrate. At the same time, equal numbers of potassium ions are secreted into the filtrate. Similarly, the hormone acts on the colonic mucosa to reduce sodium loss in faeces and on the sweat glands to lower the sodium content of sweat. The role of aldosterone in the control of body fluid volumes and composition is discussed elsewhere (p. 745).

Sex hormones. Androgens are produced in considerable quantities by the adrenals of both sexes. The adrenal androgens are all C_{19} compounds. They constitute about two-thirds of the total androgen secretion in the adult male and almost all the secretion in the female. The compounds secreted by the adrenal, dehydroepiandrosterone (DHA) and 4-androstenedione, are much weaker androgens than testosterone, which is secreted by the testis.

Dehydroepiandrosterone (DHA)

4-androstenedione

The physiological significance of the adrenal androgens in the male is unknown. In the female they may stimulate growth of axillary and pubic hair. Small quantities of oestrogens and progestogens are also secreted by the adrenals of both sexes.

Synthesis and metabolism
Only small amounts of the hormones are stored in the adrenal glands and increases in secretion rate depend upon increased synthesis of the hormones. The main synthetic pathways are outlined in Fig. 17.23.

The parent steroid precursor for all steroid hormones is cholesterol. which is converted in all steroid-producing tissues, to the C_{21} steroid pregnenolone, by a complex series of reactions. This is then transformed into progesterone, and it is from these two compounds that the corticosteroids are formed in the zona reticularis and zona fasciculata of the adrenal cortex.

Aldosterone is synthesized specifically in the zona glomerulosa, although its immediate precursor, 18-hydroxycorticosterone, is formed in both fasciculata and glomerulosa. Recent work has shown that, in many species, pregnenolone gives rise mainly (but not exclusively) to 17-hydroxylated corticosteroids like cortisol while

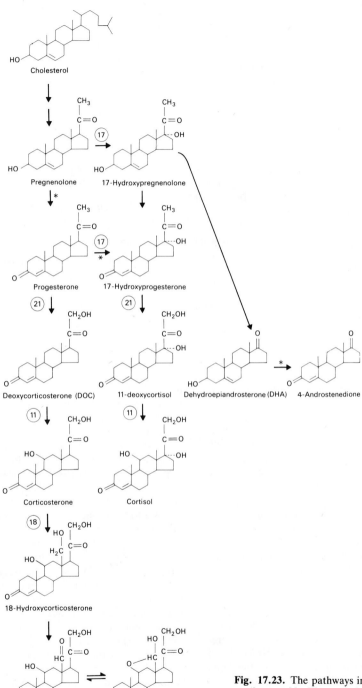

Fig. 17.23. The pathways in the biosynthesis of the corticosteroids. The encircled numbers refer to the position at which hydroxylation takes place.
* indicates minor pathway in human adrenal.

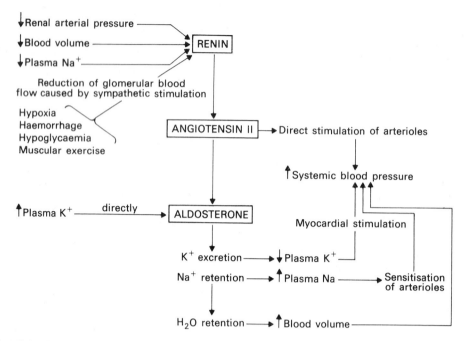

Fig. 17.24. Summary of the control and function of aldosterone.

progesterone gives rise mainly (though again not exclusively) to 17-deoxycorticosteroids such as DOC and corticosterone. Fig. 17.23 summarizes the sequence of hydroxylations of pregnenolone and progesterone at different positions to result in the active corticosteroids.

Neither glucocorticoids nor aldosterone are metabolized by the tissues on which they exert their biological effects. They are mostly degraded in the liver to compounds lacking hormonal activity. These are present in urine, conjugated as glucuronides, and the amounts excreted in 24 hours give a useful index of the mean level of adrenal secretion.

Control of secretion
Removal of the pituitary gland causes marked atrophy of the adrenal cortex and almost complete abolition of cortisol and androgen secretion. Aldosterone secretion is less affected and histological examination shows that the zona glomerulosa has atrophied less than the zonae fasciculata and reticularis. This suggests that aldosterone is largely independent of pituitary ACTH.

Cortisol secretion. A '24-hour clock' within the hypothalamus controls CRF release and causes a marked diurnal variation in the plasma cortisol level; the concentrations being highest early in the morning and lowest in the late evening. Although large variations in the circulating levels of glucocorticoids, such as are caused by removal of the glands or by administration of large quantities of cortisol, may influence CRF or ACTH release, it is unlikely under normal circumstances that cortisol secretion is controlled by a negative feedback effect of the circulating hormone concentration.

Marked increase in cortisol secretion occurs as part of the body's response to a wide variety of stresses. These include severe muscular exercise, general anaesthesia and surgery, haemorrhage, hypoglycaemia and emotional responses such as fear and anxiety. Ability to withstand stress is considerably impaired if a person is unable to raise his plasma cortisol level; a satisfactory explanation of this is still to be found.

Aldosterone secretion. As hypophysectomy causes only a small reduction in aldosterone secretion, the control mechanisms must be located outside the pituitary. This was considered previously (p. 745). Some of the influences on aldosterone secretion and its integrative actions are summarized in Fig. 17.24.

Diseases

In disease states there may be under- or over-secretion of glucocorticoids, mineralocorticoids or the sex hormones. It is important to know whether under or overactivity of the adrenal gland is due primarily to a pathological change in the adrenal or whether the change is secondary to a change of ACTH secretion.

Cushing's Syndrome. In this condition there is increased secretion of both cortisol, which gives rise to the main physiological changes, and the sex hormones. The primary cause can be in the pituitary, leading to excess ACTH or can reside in the adrenal cortex. All cases of hypersecretion of cortisol are covered by this eponym.

The increased cortisol secretion has marked effects on organic metabolism and, as large quantities of cortisol exert mineralocorticoid effects, also on electrolyte metabolism. The pathological changes in this condition can be deduced from the foregoing consideration of this hormone. They include increased protein catabolism leading to muscular wasting and osteoporosis and increased deposition of fat.

Sodium retention leads to water retention and so increases the volume of extracellular fluid. This may be manifested clinically as oedema, and may contribute, with fat deposition, to the 'moon face' appearance commonly seen in patients with Cushing's syndrome. An increase in the volume of ECF may be partly responsible for the arterial hypertension frequently found in the disease. The haemoglobin concentration and the total white cell count are raised but both the eosinophil and lymphocyte counts are lowered.

The excessive secretion of androgens which frequently occurs in Cushing's syndrome may induce some degree of masculinization of female patients.

The commonest cause of a Cushingoid condition at the present time is the therapeutic administeration of cortisol, cortisone or their synthetic analogues. The main reason for giving steroids in larger than physiological amounts is for the treatment of immune disorders such as rheumatoid arthritis, intractable bronchospasm (asthma) and collagen diseases. They are also used to suppress tissue rejection following transplant operations. The side effects of such treatment are similar to those seen in the clinical picture of Cushing's syndrome but one or two additional effects deserve special mention:

1 Because of decreased protein anabolism the healing and repair of tissues is impaired.

2 Impaired immune reactions make the patient more susceptible to infections.

3 With depression of the pituitary–adrenal axis the body no longer responds to stress by increasing adrenocortical secretion. Collapse and possibly death may occur if the patient becomes ill, is injured, or is subjected to surgery.

Hyperaldosteronism. Cases of primary hyperaldosteronism are rare but increased secretion of aldosterone is common in many disorders of body fluid metabolism. Secondary hyperaldosteronism results from increased secretion of renin due to sodium depletion, to reduced plasma volume, or to impaired renal perfusion as in heart failure (Fig. 17.24).

Adrenocortical insufficiency (Addison's disease). The biochemical and physiological changes in Addison's disease have already been described (p. 778). A common feature of adrenocortical insufficiency is brown pigmentation of the skin over certain parts of the body. This results from increased deposition of melanin caused by excessive secretion of MSH and ACTH, resulting from a lack of circulating cortisol.

Enzymic disorders—the adrenogenital syndrome

One cause of reduced cortisol production is a partial or complete deficiency of one of the enzymes required for its synthesis. The commonest deficiency is of 21-hydroxylase (Fig. 17.23). This leads to an accumulation of the precursors of cortisol from which, under these conditions, androgens are synthesized in large amounts. The low levels of cortisol in the plasma cause greåter quantities of ACTH to be secreted leading to a hyperplasia of the gland. The hyperplasia leads to a further increase in the secretion of androgens. In the newborn female child there is a masculinization of the genitalia, giving confusion as to its sex. The male child shows advanced sexual development and may appear to have a precocious (but pseudo) puberty. In both sexes the androgens cause increased muscular development and premature fusion of the epiphyses so that the adult stature is short. The sexually developed and highly muscular boy is often referred to as an 'infant Hercules'.

THE ADRENAL MEDULLA

The secretion of the adrenal medulla is mainly adrenaline (probably 80% adrenaline, 20% noradrenaline). The medulla secretes only in response to stimulation of the splanchnic nerve; after sectioning these nerves secretion falls to a low level. The hormones secreted from the adrenal medulla, in contrast to the neurotransmitters, reach all tissues of the body through the circulation. Adrenaline and noradrenaline are synthesized from tyrosine and are known as catecholamines (p. 288). The methylation of noradrenaline to form adrenaline depends upon the presence of glucocorticoids in relatively high concentrations. These may be achieved locally in the medulla by virtue of the drainage of blood from the adrenal cortex into sinusoids which then pass through the medulla to a central vein. The medullary cells appear to be arranged in columns along these sinusoids. The catecholamines are inactivated partly by uptake into sympathetic nerve endings and partly by metabolism in the liver; the two enzymes involved are o-methyl transferase (COMT) present in effector cells and liver, and monoamine oxidase (MAO) which is also found in sympathetic nerve endings. The derivatives so formed are excreted in urine along with small quantities of the unchanged hormones.

Functions

The classical experiments of Oliver and Shafer in 1895 demonstrated the powerful effects of an extract of the adrenal medulla on the circulation. Later experiments have demonstrated that the extract exerts marked effects on metabolism as well, raising both the plasma glucose and free fatty acid levels, and inhibiting the motility and lowering the tone of intestinal and uterine smooth muscle. The demonstration of increased secretion of adrenaline during stress led W. B. Cannon to put forward his theory that the adrenal medulla, by virtue of the type of actions mentioned above, prepared the body for either 'fight or flight'.

The modern view of the physiological role of the adrenal medulla is that it is of minimal importance. The actions which were quite rightly ascribed to the gland are in practice mainly carried out by the sympathetic nervous system. The fact that the medulla secretes adrenaline whose physiological actions differ slightly from those of the neurotransmitter noradrenaline (p. 716) suggests that medullary secretion may on occasion be the more appropriate response to a stressful situation. Thus psychological and emotional stresses may cause elevation of adrenaline secretion from the adrenal medulla, whereas more physical stresses

such as muscular exercise or arterial hypotension cause activation of the sympathetic-nervous system and the release of noradrenaline.

GENITAL ORGANS

Anatomy

At an early stage in development the genital organs of both the female and male embryo are the same, but during the second month of fetal life the subsequent development of these structures is different and depends on the genetic sex of the individual. This determines whether the germ cells become an ovary or a testis. In the female germ cells then produce feminizing hormones and in the male they produce masculinizing hormones. It is also at this early stage that the close connection between the urinary and genital systems can be seen.

FEMALE GENITAL ORGANS
(Figs. 17.25 & 17.26)

Ovary

The ovary receives its blood supply from the ovarian artery which arises from the abdominal aorta near the origin of the renal artery. On the right the ovarian vein goes to the inferior vena cava and on the left to the left renal vein.

The ovary has an outer layer of cuboidal cells often called the germinal epithelium, although the germ cells are not derived from this outer layer. The ovary consists of an outer cortex in which the germ cells, derived from the yolk sac, are found. The more central part of the ovary is called the medulla and is very vascular. There are numerous spindle-shaped cells in the cortex and medulla and these are involved in the formation of a follicle in which a germ cell becomes

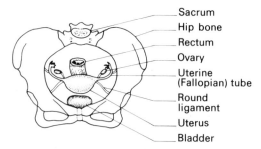

Sacrum
Hip bone
Rectum
Ovary
Uterine (Fallopian) tube
Round ligament
Uterus
Bladder

Fig. 17.25. The arrangement of the female genital organs as seen from above.

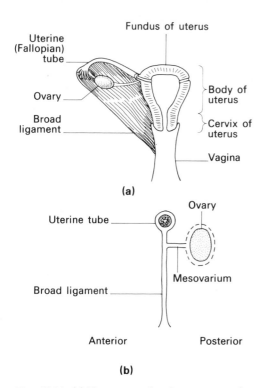

(a)

(b)

Fig. 17.26. (a) The uterus and vagina are more or less sectioned in the coronal plane and the posterior surface of the broad ligament is shown. (b) The broad ligament is sectioned in a parasagittal plane to show the relation of the peritoneum to the uterine tube and ovary.

enclosed and also the production of hormones. At any one time, examination of a section of an ovary shows follicles at various stages of development (Fig. 17.27).

As a follicle develops, the germ cell, about 40 μm in diameter and called an oocyte, becomes larger and reaches its maximum size of 100 μm. Initially the oocyte is surrounded by a number of layers of cells derived from the spindle cells. These are called granulosa cells. At the same time a clear membrane called the zona pellucida develops round the oocyte. Spaces containing fluid (liquor folliculi) begin to appear in the granulosa cells and subsequently coalesce. A mature Graafian follicle consists of a wall of granulosa cells surrounded by two layers of stroma cells, the liquor folliculi and the oocyte attached to one side of the wall. Some of the granulosa cells remain around the oocyte forming the corona radiata. A mature follicle may be 0.5–1 cm in diameter. When mature the follicle lies just under the surface of the ovary.

The oocyte with its corona radiata escapes from the ruptured follicle. This process is called ovulation and occurs about 14 days before the onset of the next menstrual cycle. During the maturation of the follicle the oocyte completes the first meiotic division, a process which apparently begins before puberty, perhaps even in the fetus. The beginning of the second meiotic division takes place about the time of ovulation but is only completed if fertilization takes place. The oocyte is now called an ovum, although this term is frequently used to describe a germ cell throughout its whole process of maturation. In the case of an oocyte, meiotic division results in two cells of very unequal size. The smaller cell is called a polar body and is retained within the zona pellucida.

Following ovulation the oocyte enters the uterine tube through its open lateral end. The collapsed follicle is rapidly filled with large luteal cells, most of which are derived from the granulosa cells of the wall, although some come from the layer immediately surrounding the membrana granulosa. If pregnancy occurs, the corpus luteum continues to grow and persists until about the twentieth week of pregnancy. It then slowly involutes. If pregnancy does not occur, the corpus luteum begins to degenerate a few days before the onset of menstruation. In both cases the corpus luteum is replaced by fibrous tissue which appears white and is therefore called a corpus albicans (white body).

It has been estimated that there are about 400 000 oocytes in each ovary and in her fertile lifetime a woman will produce approximately 400 mature oocytes. Large numbers of the remaining oocytes degenerate after the partial maturation of a follicle. While one follicle is going through the whole process of maturation others begin to mature but eventually undergo degeneration.

The uterine tube

The tube consists of a lining mucosa and muscular coats. The epithelial lining, which is very folded, has two types of cells, ciliated columnar and secretory. The ciliated epithelial cells assist in the movement of the ovum towards the uterus and the secretory cells have a nutritive function.

Peristaltic waves from the lateral towards the medial end of the tube assist the movement of the ovum towards the uterus.

Since the ovum is normally fertilized at the lateral end of the tube, the spermatozoa have to move through the uterine cavity and along the lumen of the tube. This is achieved chiefly by the

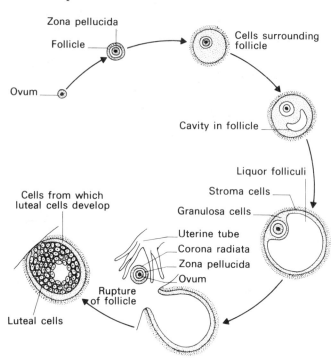

Fig. 17.27. The formation of an ovarian (Graafian) follicle, its rupture and the development of a corpus luteum.

inherent mobility of the spermatoza themselves. After fertilization the zygote takes about 3–4 days to reach the uterine cavity. During this period it divides several times. The secretory cells at the medial end of the tube play an important part in its nutrition.

Uterus

This is a pear-shaped organ lying in the middle of the pelvic cavity in front of the rectum and behind the bladder (Figs. 17.25 & 17.26).

The wall of the uterus consists mainly of smooth muscle, which is about 1.5 cm thick, so that the cavity is relatively small. The uterus has a peritoneal covering and is lined by a mucous membrane called the endometrium. (The muscle layer is called the myometrium.)

The built-up endometrium is shed every 26–35 days from the menarche (the onset of menstruation) until the menopause (the cessation of menstruation). The endometrium consists of an outer layer of columnar cells and several layers of stromal cells containing glands and blood vessels. At the end of menstruation the endometrium is about 0.5 mm thick. Before menstruation it is about ten times thicker due to an increase in the layers of stromal cells. This is accompanied by a great increase in the size and tortuosity of the glands, and an accumulation of

fluid between the stromal cells and of glycogen and lipid in the cells themselves. Just before menstruation there is a slight decrease in the thickness of the endometrium and this is followed by a constriction of the arterioles in the endometrium. Some degeneration of the surface layers of cells takes place and the sudden dilation of the arterioles produces haemorrhages in the superficial part of the endometrium. During menstruation almost the whole of the endometrium is lost. The surviving basal layers next to the myometrium, containing parts of the glands which have been lost, are responsible for the replacement of the lining of the uterus. About 50–100 cm³ of blood is lost during menstruation although this is very variable between individuals and different menstruations in the same person.

Vagina

The vagina (Fig. 17.26) is a tubular structure, extending downwards and forwards from the cervix of the uterus to its opening to the exterior at the vestibule.

Vulva

The term vulva (Latin word meaning a wrapper) refers to the region containing a number of structures collectively known as the external female genitalia (Fig. 17.28).

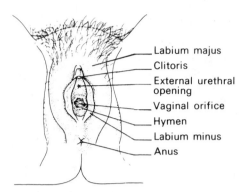

Fig. 17.28. The external female genitalia.

Mammary gland (breast)

This glandular structure is said to develop from modified sweat glands. Before puberty the gland is rudimentary in both the male and female. At puberty, under the influence mainly of oestrogens, the female breast develops. The enlargement is due to the development of some duct tissue and the deposition of fat.

An adult female breast which has never lactated consists mainly of fat (Fig. 17.29). It is divided into about 20 lobes by connective tissue septa. The potential glandular tissue of each lobe is represented by tubules joining to form a lactiferous duct which opens separately on to the nipple. In the early part of pregnancy under the influence of oestrogens the duct tissue proliferates and later in pregnancy, due to progestogens, the secretory tissue develops. The actual production of milk, which occurs about 4 days after the

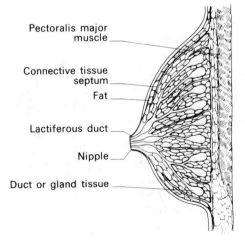

Fig. 17.29. A parasagittal section through a non-lactating, adult, female breast.

birth of the child, is stimulated by prolactin and human growth hormone from the pituitary gland.

MALE GENITAL ORGANS (Fig. 17.30)

Testis

The arterial blood supply and venous and lymphatic drainage of the testis indicate the situation where the testis developed—the posterior abdominal wall. The testis descends into the scrotum late in fetal life.

Both mechanical and hormonal factors are responsible for the descent of the testis, particularly the gonadotrophic hormones of the pituitary gland. The testicular artery comes from the abdominal aorta. The testicular vein on the right side goes to the inferior vena cava and on the left to the renal vein, and the lymphatic vessels go up to the nodes at the side of the abdominal aorta.

Each lobe of a testis contains two or three coiled seminiferous tubules and there are about 250 lobules in a testis. The seminiferous tubules converge towards the connective tissue on the posterior part of the testis. In this connective tissue there is a network of spaces which eventually lead to the upper end of the epididymis through channels called the efferent ductules. A section of a lobe of a testis (Fig. 17.31) shows that the convoluted tubule is embedded in loose connective tissue in which are found the interstitial cells of Leydig. These are large spindle-shaped or polyhedral cells next to the capillary walls. These cells are not fully functional until puberty when under the influence of the hormones of the anterior pituitary they produce testosterone, which is responsible for the development of the secondary sexual characteristics in the male.

The seminiferous tubule itself has a basement membrane on which are the cells from which the spermatozoa develop, and also the cells of Sertoli which, due to their columnar shape and extensive processes, provide mechanical and nutritive support for the germ cells. The peripheral germ cells are called spermatogonia which pass through several stages and finally become spermatozoa (Fig. 17.31). Essentially the changes are the reduction in the number of chromosomes by meiotic division, and the production of a motile cell which consists of a head containing the nuclear material, covered by an acrosomal cap containing the Golgi complex, a connecting piece containing a centriole and a

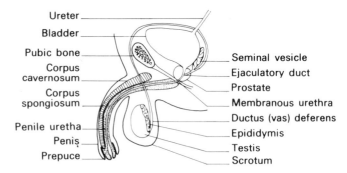

Fig. 17.30. The arrangement of the male genital

complex tail, the first part of which has an outer mitochondrial sheath (Fig. 17.32). The total length of a spermatozoon is about 60 μm, of which the head is about 5 μm. The spermatozoa are finally set free in the lumen of the tubule and make their way towards the head of the epididymis, assisted by some smooth muscle round the efferent ductules.

The epididymis (Fig. 17.31) consists largely of a coiled tubule, about 600 cm long which is continuous with the efferent ductules at the head end and the vas deferens at the tail end. The ductules have tall ciliated cells for helping the movement of the spermatozoa and shorter cells which are secretory and are important in the nutrition of the spermatozoa. The duct of the epididymis has smooth muscle in its wall and tall columnar epithelial cells round the lumen. These are secretory. It is estimated that it takes 12 days for spermatozoa to pass from their connection with the cells of Sertoli to their eventual ejaculation. While in the epididymis the spermatozoa undergo a process of maturation affecting their fertility and motility.

Ductus (Vas) deferens, seminal vesicle and ejaculatory duct

The ductus (vas) deferens passes upwards through the inguinal canal into the abdominal cavity. The seminal vesicles lie on the posterior wall of the bladder and project upwards and laterally on the lateral side of the ductus deferentes (Figs. 17.30 & 17.33). Inferiorly the duct of the seminal vesicle joins the ductus deferens and forms the ejaculatory duct. There is some doubt as to whether spermatozoa are stored in the seminal vesicle. Its secretion is added to the seminal fluid and may be important as a vehicle for the spermatozoa stored in the ductus.

The ejaculatory duct opens posteriorly on either side of the midline into the upper part of the prostatic urethra.

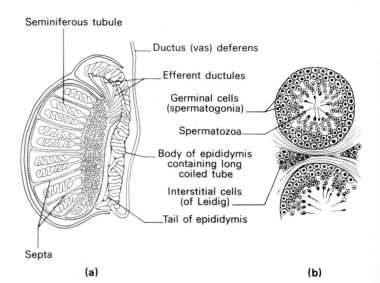

Fig. 17.31. (a) A vertical section through the testis and epididymis. (b) A section through a seminiferous tubule.

(a)   **(b)**

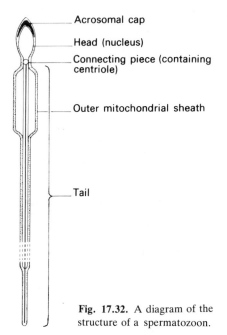

- Acrosomal cap
- Head (nucleus)
- Connecting piece (containing centriole)
- Outer mitochondrial sheath
- Tail

Fig. 17.32. A diagram of the structure of a spermatozoon.

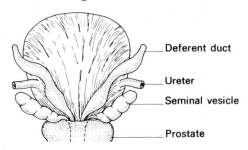

- Deferent duct
- Ureter
- Seminal vesicle
- Prostate

Fig. 17.33. The posterior surface of the bladder seen from behind showing the relations of the uterus, ducti deferentes, seminal vesicles and prostate.

Prostate

The prostate is a fibromuscular, glandular organ lying inferior to the base of the bladder (Figs. 17.30 & 17.33). The urethra passes downwards and slightly forwards from the bladder through the prostate. The ejaculatory ducts enter the prostate superiorly on either side of the midline, posterior to the urethra. They run forwards and medially and open on to the posterior wall of the urethra on either side of a vertical crest. At the side of the crest there is a depression into which the ducts of the prostatic glandular tissue open.

Penis

The parts of the penis are illustrated in Figs. 17.30 & 17.34.

The sex hormones

The female sex hormones, oestrogens and progestogens, are produced by the ovary in the female. The male sex hormones, the androgens, are produced by the testis of the male. Considerable amounts of weaker androgens are also produced by the adrenal cortex of both sexes. During pregnancy the placenta produces a gonadotrophin, oestrogen, progesterone (a progestogen) and a lactogen.

ANDROGENS

The main hormone secreted by the testis is testosterone, which is produced by the interstitial or Leydig cells (Fig. 17.31). It is converted to a more active form, dihydrotestosterone, in many tissues. In the plasma the androgens are bound to sex-hormone-binding globulin (SHBG). These steroids, like the other androgens, are C_{19} compounds derived initially from cholesterol through the intermediaries pregnenolone and progesterone, which are C_{21} steroids (Fig. 17.23).

The androgens are reduced in the liver and are

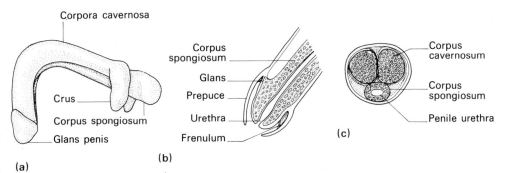

- Corpora cavernosa
- Crus
- Corpus spongiosum
- Glans penis

(a)

- Corpus spongiosum
- Glans
- Prepuce
- Urethra
- Frenulum

(b)

- Corpus cavernosum
- Corpus spongiosum
- Penile urethra

(c)

Fig. 17.34. (a) The structure of the penis. (b) The prepuce in sagittal section. (c) A cross section of the body of the penis.

excreted in the urine as conjugated glucu-
coronides and sulphates.

Functions
Androgens stimulate the growth of the accessory
sex organs (i.e. penis, scrotum, seminal vesicles
and prostate) at puberty and are necessary for
the structural and functional maintenance of
these throughout the reproductive life. They are
essential both for spermatogenesis and for the
secretion of the seminal plasma. They also cause
the development of secondary sexual characteristics at and after puberty. These include the
growth of facial and axillary hair and the characteristic male distribution of the pubic hair, the
breaking of voice and the development of a mas-
culine personality. Associated with this sexual
development is a spurt of growth starting at the
onset of puberty and ending with ossification of
the epiphyseal cartilages at the end of puberty.
Although such a spurt is absent in the prepubes-
cent castrate, growth is slower and continues
longer in such people because the epiphyses of
their long bones do not fuse at the normal time.

The androgens exert a marked anabolic effect
on protein metabolism, which results in greater
muscle mass and heavier bone development in
the male. This leads to the more angular build of
males compared with the more rounded
development of females who have larger quantities of subcutaneous fat.

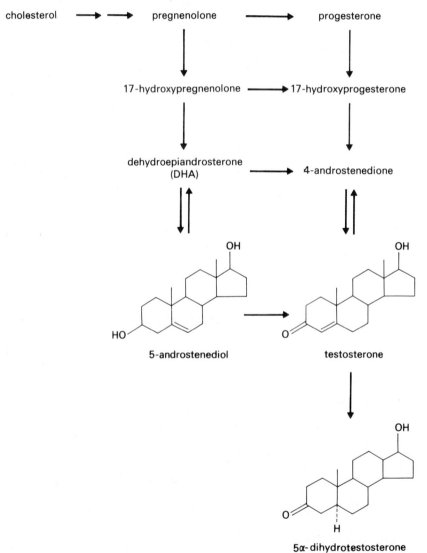

Control of testicular function

The endocrine and exocrine functions of the testis are both stimulated by the gonadotrophins, namely follicle-stimulating hormone (FSH) and luteinizing hormone (LH), which are secreted by the anterior pituitary. LH stimulates testosterone production by the interstitial cells. Spermatogenesis depends on both FSH and testosterone.

OESTROGENS AND PROGESTOGENS

Progesterone is a C_{21} steroid and is produced from cholesterol. It is a precursor of testosterone (Fig. 17.23).

Like the testis in the male, the ovary in the female produces both hormones and the gamete. Small quantities of oestrogens are produced in childhood, and increasing levels are reponsible for the development taking place at puberty. The adult female ovulates at approximately monthly intervals. The development and discharge of the ovum are associated with cyclical changes in secretion of oestrogens and progestogens by the ovary, which lead to cyclical changes in the structure of the uterus and other parts of the genital tract. These structural and hormonal changes are known as the menstrual cycle. In the older woman, following the cessation of menstruation, the ovary produces only miminal quantities of oestrogens.

The oestrogens are secreted in small amounts by the stroma of the ovary and in much larger amounts from the granulosa cells and from the corpus luteum. They are also produced by the adrenals in both sexes, by the testis and the placenta during pregnancy. In plasma the oestrogens are bound to sex-hormone-binding globulin.

Progesterone is produced in large quantities by the corpus luteum and therefore high circulating levels are present only during the secretory phase of the menstrual cycle and during pregnancy. Smaller amounts are secreted by the adrenals and by the testis.

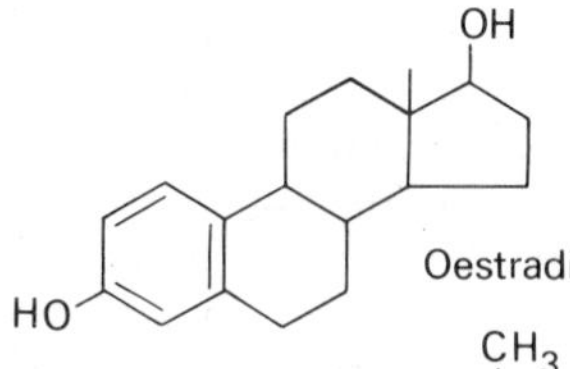

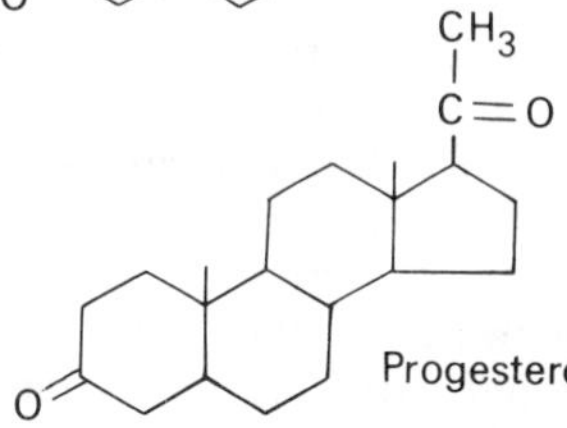

Functions

Oestrogens are necessary for sexual development at puberty and for the maintenance of the sex organs during the reproductive phase of life. Oestrogens and progesterone induce the changes in the reproductive tract and elsewhere which occur during the menstrual cycle. Furthermore they are necessary for the continuance of pregnancy and for the preparation of the breast for lactation. The actions of the two hormones are summarized in Table 17.2.

Table 17.2. The actions of oestrogens and progesterone.

	Oestrogens	Progesterone
Menstrual cycle	Proliferative changes	Secretory changes
Puberty	Development of secondary sex characters and accessory sex organs	–
Implantation	Inhibits	Potentiates
Myometrium	Increases motility and sensitivity to oxytocin	Reduces motility and sensitivity to oxytocin
Breast development	Ducts	Alveoli

THE MENSTRUAL CYCLE

Menstruation occurs at approximately monthly intervals. The actual length of cycles varies from woman to woman and often from one cycle to another in the same woman. We will consider the changes occuring during a cycle of 28 days (Fig. 17.35). The first day of vaginal bleeding is conventionally taken as day 1 of the cycle. Destruction of the endometrium lasts for 3–5 days and vaginal bleeding continues for 1 or 2 days longer. The endometrium then regenerates under the influence of oestrogens from the maturing follicle (proliferative phase). Ovulation occurs on about the 14th day of the cycle, and further development of the endometrium takes place under the influence of hormones secreted from the corpus luteum (secretory phase). From the 25th day onwards the production of these hormones falls rapidly, leading to menstruation.

Oestrogens are secreted by the maturing follicle. Following ovulation the follicular cells undergo rapid structural and biochemical changes, collectively known as luteinization, to form the corpus luteum. This secretes oestrogens and, because of enzymatic changes,

progesterone also. The oestrogens produced by the maturing follicle stimulate growth of the endometrium. The combination of oestrogens and progesterone released by the corpus luteum prepares the endometrium to receive a fertilized ovum and ensure its early development. Failure to fertilize an ovum is followed at a later stage in the cycle by a fall in hormone production by the corpus luteum leading to breakdown of the endometrium. This breakdown and the discharge of the debris and blood via the vagina is known as menstruation. The blood which is shed at menstruation does not usually clot because it contains high levels of fibrinolysins. If the ovum is fertilized, hormone production continues and menstruation does not supervene.

Under the influence of the hypothalamus the anterior pituitary secretes the gonadotrophins, FSH and LH. Levels of FSH are higher in the early part of the menstrual cycle than during the post-ovulatory period (Fig. 17.35), with a sharp peak associated with ovulation. LH levels are relatively constant throughout the cycle except for a pronounced surge immediately prior to ovulation. FSH causes the ovarian follicle to grow and secrete increasing amounts of oes-

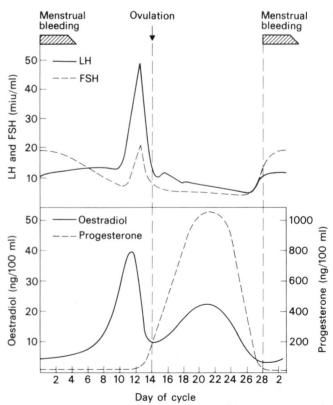

Fig. 17.35. The levels of LH, FSH, oestradiol and progesterone during the menstrual cycle.

trogens. LH, acting together with FSH, induces ovulation and after ovulation it initiates the formation of the corpus luteum and the subsequent production of both oestrogens and progesterone. In consequence of this intermittent release of the gonadotrophins the level of oestrogen rises to a peak just prior to ovulation and there is a further later rise produced by secretion from the corpus luteum. The level of progesterone is low during the proliferative phase and rises rapidly following ovulation.

It is difficult to explain the hormonal changes occurring during the menstrual cycle only in terms of feedback. They are more easily explained by the presence of a monthly clock which may be modulated by the feedback of ovarian hormones.

PUBERTY

Puberty is the period of time extending over several years during which the body is transformed from that of a child into that of an adult. During childhood the levels of sex hormones in the blood are low. Increased secretion of gonadotrophins induced by a process of maturation in the central nervous system causes an increase of the sex hormones and this is responsible for the development of the sexual organs and secondary sex characteristics at puberty.

THE MENOPAUSE

From the age of 40 onwards a woman becomes less fertile; the menstrual cycles first become irregular and longer and then menstruation ceases. The time at which this occurs is called the menopause and marks the end of the woman's reproductive life. The physiological changes during and after the menopause may be directly attributed to the lowered levels of oestrogen in the blood. The reproductive organs and the breasts atrophy: in particular the vaginal epithelium becomes thin and fragile. Failure of the ovary to produce oestrogens results in increased secretion of gonadotrophins which may be responsible for some of the symptoms experienced at the menopause.

There is no male equivalent of the menopause.

PREGNANCY

Hormones
About 6 days after fertilization the embryo implants into the endometrium. The blastocyst,

as it is called at this stage, consists of the formative mass from which the fetus will develop and the trophoblast, which is responsible for implantation and develops into the chorion. The rapidly growing trophoblast first becomes attached to the endometrium and then invades this epithelium until it is almost completely embedded within it (Vol. 1, Book 2).

To ensure continuing development of the newly implanted blastocyst it is clearly essential to prevent the next menstruation which would normally begin some 8 days after implantation. The breakdown of the endometrium is prevented by the persistence of the corpus luteum which continues to secrete progesterone and oestrogen. This persistence is caused by the secretion of the hormone, human chorionic gonadotrophin (hCG) from the developing chorion and placenta. This is the mechanism by which the uterus 'informs' the ovary of a conception. Pregnancy tests depend upon the presence of hCG in the urine of the pregnant woman.

At a later stage in pregnancy the placenta begins to produce progesterone and oestrogens and gradually makes a greater contribution to maintaining the pregnancy than does the corpus luteum. From the sixth week of gestation the placenta also secretes human placental lactogen (hPL) which stimulates breast development and may also act as a gonadotrophin.

Pregnancy normally lasts for 38 weeks from the time of conception, but since the exact date of conception is unknown, the duration of pregnancy is normally counted from the first day of the last menstrual period.

Maternal changes during pregnancy
There are marked changes in the activities of many of the mother's body systems during pregnancy. These are responses to the metabolic demands of the fetus and may be partly induced by ovarian and placental hormones. Body weight gradually increases through pregnancy; the total weight gain by term may be of the order of 11 kg, which may partly be accounted for by the weight of the fetus (3 kg), the placenta and amniotic fluid (2 kg), the uterus (1 kg) and breasts (1.5 kg). The balance is due to a generalized increase in body weight and includes both tissue and fluid.

The high blood flow to the placenta leads to an increase in cardiac output which reaches a maximum 40% greater than prior to pregnancy. Blood volume increases by up to 30% largely as a result of increasing the volume of plasma. This decreases the haemoglobin concentration. The rapidly growing fetus requires a supply of protein, vitamins and minerals which may, on occasion, lead to maternal deficiency. This is more pronounced if the mother was previously deficient or bordering on deficiency. The most likely deficiencies are of calcium, iron and folic acid.

The hormonal control of labour

Until the 36th week of gestation the uterus (not the fetus) is quiescent but during the last weeks the mother may notice weak contractions which suggest increasing excitability of the myometrium.

The onset of labour is now believed to be determined by the fetus rather than by the mother. A normally functioning fetal pituitary adrenal axis appears to be necessary to initiate labour. In the sheep, fetal hypophysectomy or adrenalectomy markedly prolongs pregnancy, and in the human the onset of labour is usually delayed when the fetus is anencephalic and thus has no functioning pituitary. During the last weeks of pregnancy the levels of circulating oestrogens in the mother are increased and the level of progesterone is lowered. This change in the hormonal environment of the uterus leads to increased excitability of the myometrium and increased sensitivity to oxytocin. The increased production of oestrogen by the placenta is dependent upon the production of precursors in the fetal adrenal.

It has been known for many years that the release of oxytocin from the posterior pituitary is essential for labour but attempts to demonstrate elevation of oxytocin levels in the blood were, until recently, unsuccessful. It has now been shown that release of oxytocin increases during the later stages of labour and that this causes uterine contraction through the local release of prostaglandins. Prostaglandin production in the uterus is increased by oestrogens; this probably explains the increased sensitivity of the organ to oxytocin which may be induced by oestrogens.

Lactation

The breasts develop at puberty under the influence of oestrogens. During pregnancy they are prepared for lactation under the influence of oestrogens, progesterone and hPL secreted by the placenta, and prolactin from the anterior pituitary. Small quantities of milky fluid may be expressed from the nipple early in pregnancy.

Following delivery of the placenta the circulat-ing levels of oestrogens or progesterone fall and this appears to allow prolactin to stimulate milk production. Lactation may be suppressed by administration of large doses of synthetic oestrogens. Removal of milk by the suckling infant stimulates production of milk, whereas accumulation of milk inhibits production. The sucking of the nipple by the infant causes a reflex release of oxytocin from the posterior pituitary which contracts the myoepithelial cells of the milk ducts and thus aids the expression of the milk. This is an interesting reflex in that the afferent pathway is nervous but the efferent pathway is humoral.

The first milk produced by the breast is called the 'colostrum' and differs from later secretions in that it contains maternal antibodies. These proteins are absorbed without digestion from the gut of the newborn and confer passive immunity during the early weeks of life.

ORAL CONTRACEPTION—THE 'PILL'

This is at the present time the most convenient and most widely used method of contraception in the UK. Most commercial preparations consist of a mixture of synthetic oestrogens and progestogens, although some contain progestogens only. They probably suppress gonadotrophin secretion from the pituitary thus preventing maturation of the follicle and ovulation. Additional protection may be given by alterations in endometrial development and in the properties of cervical mucus.

HORMONAL CONTROL OF CARBOHYDRATE METABOLISM
(see also p. 179)

The continual utilization of glucose by all body tissues requires that they be replenished from the glucose in the circulating blood. The concentration of glucose in the blood of normal man, 8–12 hours after a meal, is usually 70–90 mg/100 cm³ (4–5 mmol/dm³).

The dependence of various tissues on circulating blood glucose varies widely. The central nervous system is perhaps most critically dependent since glucose is the major energy source that crosses the blood–brain barrier at a rate sufficient to sustain normal function. If the blood glucose falls abruptly, the very low glycogen content of brain is insufficient to sustain its metabolic needs and a hypoglycaemic coma results. However, many tissues can derive a considerable portion of their chemical energy from

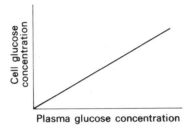

Fig. 17.36. Relationship between external and internal glucose concentration in cells with glucose permeable membranes.

other nutrients; e.g. cardiac muscle can utilize fatty acids and lactic acid from the blood.

The intestinal absorption of the products of carbohydrate digestion provides a very large, but variable, contribution of glucose to the blood. Of course, this is a discontinuous process. In a normal individual, a short period of starvation does not cause a catastrophic fall in blood glucose since glucose can be derived from the breakdown of glucose-6-phosphate by those tissues containing glucose-6-phosphatase (liver, kidney, intestine). This source of blood glucose is derived mainly from glycogen but can be derived from non-carbohydrate sources, e.g. amino acids.

There are three routes by which glucose may be lost from the blood:

1 Glucose may pass into those cells whose membranes are freely permeable to it (liver, kidney, islets of Langerhans, neurons and erythrocytes). The intracellular concentration of free glucose in these cells is in equilibrium with the glucose concentration in the extracellular fluid (Fig. 17.36).

2 Glucose may pass into cells whose membranes are partially impermeable (muscle and adipose tissue). No glucose enters the cells until a certain plasma concentration is reached, and the rate-limiting step in the glucose metabolism appears to be the rate at which glucose is transported across the cell membrane (fig. 17.37).

Glucose, once inside the cells, is phosphorylated into glucose-6-phosphate, which may then be transformed into other products such as glycogen or fat.

3 Glucose may escape into the urine. Under normal circumstances, no more than a trace of glucose is lost in the urine, but if the blood glucose level becomes abnormally high as in diabetes mellitus, the urinary loss of glucose can be a serious problem.

The sources and fates of blood glucose are shown in Fig. 17.38.

For the normal functioning of tissues and organs it is essential for the blood glucose concentration to be maintained. The first line of defence is the control of appetite, which seems to be partially related to the blood glucose level. Several experiments suggest that glucose and insulin are involved in appetite control: (a) intravenous infusion of glucose diminishes eating in animals; (b) insulin injections stimulate appetite and polyphagia (over-eating); (c) blood glucose levels alter the discharge rate of hypothalamic neurons which are thought to be responsible for the regulation of food intake.

Provided the diet is adequate, the blood glucose level depends primarily on the following reaction:

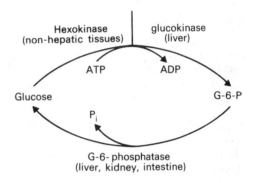

At a glucose concentration of about 100 mg/100 cm^3 the rate of formation of G-6-P equals the rate of breakdown of G-6-P. An increase in glucose concentration speeds the reaction to the right, and a fall in glucose moves the reaction to the left. The blood glucose level is in a position of equilibrium above the glucose threshold of those cells with partially impermeable membranes and therefore glucose can enter these.

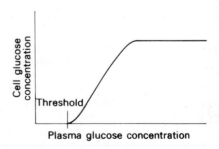

Fig. 17.37. Relationship between external and internal glucose concentration in cells with partially glucose-permeable membranes.

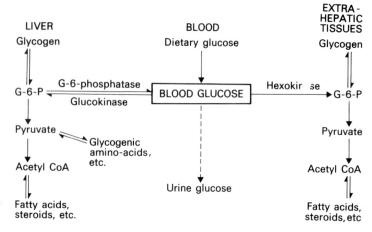

Fig. 17.38. Sources and fate of blood glucose.

HORMONAL CONTROL

As the glucose $\rightleftharpoons$ G-6-P reaction is relatively slow, the blood glucose concentration would tend to fluctuate dramatically between meals. Unfortunately, certain tissues such as the brain cannot tolerate such fluctuations, and hormone control is essential in order to maintain a stable blood glucose level. Insulin, growth hormone and possibly glucagon are continually involved whereas other hormones may have to be recruited during conditions of stress or exercise.

Insulin

Insulin is a large peptide formed in the β-cells of the pancreatic islets of Langerhans (Fig. 13.26). The blood glucose level is the most important single factor in the control of insulin secretion. Since the islet cells are freely permeable to glucose, the intracellular glucose concentration mirrors plasma glucose changes. A rise in blood glucose results in an increased insulin output. It is thought that a metabolite of glucose is responsible, since agents which competitively block glucose metabolism and thereby lower the level of glucose metabolites result in less insulin being released when the plasma glucose concentration increases.

Other factors are known to control insulin output, but their significance is not fully understood:
1   Ingestion of food and the presence of food in the stomach favours insulin release, probably by stimulation of the vagus nerve.
2   The presence of food in the stomach and duodenum releases the hormones gastrin, secretin and pancreozymin. Any one of these, when injected into dogs, causes a very rapid release of insulin.

(1) and (2) are probably anticipatory stimulants in that they make insulin ready and waiting for the forthcoming increase in the plasma glucose level.
3   Certain amino acids (arginine, lysine, leucine and phenylalanine) favour insulin release.
4   The presence of glucagon in the blood stimulates insulin release, but the reason for this is obscure.
5   Adrenaline and noradrenaline inhibit the release of insulin. This is important during exercise when circulating blood glucose is needed by active tissues.

The general effects of insulin secretion (summarized in Figs. 17.39 & 17.40) are as follows:
1   The level of intracellular cyclic-3′,5′-AMP is lowered, particularly in the liver. This subsequently prevents the activation of glycogen phosphorylase and inhibits glycogen breakdown (glycogenolysis).

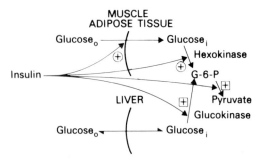

o   Outside cell membrane
i   Inside cell membrane
⊕   Activation
⊞   Enzyme induction

Fig. 17.39. Mode of action of insulin on carbohydrate metabolism.

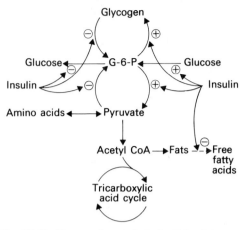

Fig. 17.40. Hormonal control of raised blood glucose levels.

2 The activity of glycogen synthetase in muscle is increased. This favours glycogen synthesis (glycogenesis).

3 Acting on tissue hexokinase it appears that insulin favours the transfer of free hexokinase into mitochondrial-bound hexokinase (more active) resulting in more blood glucose being converted into G-6-P.

4 There is an increase in the rate at which glucose is transferred across muscle and adipose tissue cell membranes. Insulin is not required to assist the transport of glucose into cells with freely permeable membranes—brain, kidney and liver.

5 Insulin induces the activity of liver glucokinase so that more G-6-P is produced.

6 It also induces the activity of glycolytic enzymes responsible for the breakdown of G-6-P.

7 There is a suppression of key gluconeogenic enzymes converting pyruvate into glucose.

8 The breakdown of triglycerides is inhibited such that the free fatty acid content of the blood is lowered. High free fatty acid levels in the blood inhibit glycolytic enzymes. Insulin action lifts this inhibition and thereby favours the breakdown of G-6-P into pyruvate.

In general, an elevated blood glucose concentration is lowered by an increased insulin output. An excessive dose of insulin may cause such a fall in blood glucose levels that the diminished supply of glucose to freely permeable cells, particularly the nervous system, results in a loss of consciousness and even permanent cerebral damage.

Glucagon

Glucagon is a small peptide secreted by the α-cells of the Islets of Langerhans in the pancreas. It is not thought to be essential to life. Glucagon output is inversely proportional to the blood sugar concentration (i.e. it is stimulated by hypoglycaemia) but the control operates slowly in comparison with the control of insulin.

The actions of glucagon are as follows (Fig. 17.41):

1 By increasing the levels of cyclic-3′,5′-AMP via adenyl cyclase activation, glucagon inactivates glycogen synthetase and activates glycogen phophorylase in liver cells (p. 189). In this way glycogen breakdown is stimulated.

2 There is an increase in adipose tissue lipase activity (due to increase in cyclic-3′,5′-AMP levels) and a subsequent rise in plasma free fatty acids. These fatty acids inhibit the enzymes responsible for the breakdown of G-6-P in glycolysis.

3 Gluconeogenesis from lactate and amino acids is increased.

In general, glucagon raises the blood glucose level by inhibiting glycolysis and promoting G-6-P formation which subsequently becomes dephosphorylated. It has been suggested that glucagon, instead of being regarded as opposing insulin should be considered as cooperating with insulin in supplying glucose to peripheral tissues; glucagon raising the blood glucose, or preventing its fall, whilst insulin facilitates glucose entry into tissues. This could explain why glucagon stimulates insulin release.

Growth hormone

The output of growth hormone, like that of glucagon, is inversely related to the blood glucose level. Growth hormone stimulates lipolysis and the subsequent rise in free fatty acids inhibits the breakdown of G-6-P, thereby slowing down glucose utilization (Fig. 17.41). It thus exerts a hyperglycaemic effect.

ACTH and glucocorticosteroids

Under conditions of stress there is an increased release of glucocorticoids. These have been found to retard the oxidation of glucose in peripheral tissues by elevating the levels of free fatty acids in the blood (lipolysis) which inhibit glycolytic enzymes. Carbohydrate precursors are directed into glucose formation by induction of gluconeogenic enzymes.

The steroids also stimulate protein catabolism into amino acids which the induced gluconeo-

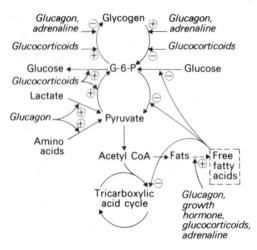

⊕ Stimulation or induction of enzymes

⊖ Inhibition of enzymes

Fig. 17.41. Hormonal control of lowered blood glucose levels.

genic enzymes in the liver and kidney convert into glucose (Fig. 17.41).

The net effect of glucocorticoid release is to elevate the blood glucose concentration and it has been put forward that the steroids are normally involved in maintaining a constant blood sugar level.

Adrenaline
Adrenaline has been found to stimulate the formation of cyclic-3′,5′-AMP in muscle and liver, by adenyl cyclase activation, resulting in an elevated phosphorylase activity and a decreased glycogen synthetase activity. Glucose output therefore increases. Adrenaline has an action on

lipase activity similar to that of glucagon (Fig. 17.41).

The net effect of adrenaline is to increase the glucose supply to tissues, particularly those in the nervous system, which are freely permeable to glucose.

A summary of the hormonal control of glucose metabolism is depicted in Table 17.3.

HORMONAL INTEGRATION

Hormonal integration can be appreciated by following the events after a meal.
1 Levels of blood glucose, fatty acids and amino acids rise.
2 Insulin is released and stimulates glucose entry into cells, glycogenesis, lipogenesis and protein synthesis.
3 Blood glucose gradually falls causing the output of insulin to fall and of growth hormone to rise.
4 Growth hormone causes lipolysis and allows peripheral tissues such as muscle to metabolize the free fatty acids. Protein synthesis also continues.
5 Sustained cellular metabolism of glucose results in liver glycogenolysis to maintain a constant blood glucose.
6 Adrenaline comes into play in emergency situations only.
7 The role of glucagon is obscure.

The capacity of man to dispose of administered glucose is referred to as glucose tolerance, and a typical glucose tolerance curve is shown in Fig. 17.42.

The plasma glucose concentration after the oral administration of glucose (usually about 50 g taken in solution by a subject who has fasted overnight) reaches a peak after about 1

Table 17.3. Summary of the hormonal control of glucose metabolism.

Hormone	Glycogenesis	Glycogenolysis	Gluconeogenesis	Glycolysis	Blood glucose
Insulin	↑	↓	↓	↑	↓
Glucagon	↓	↑	↑	↓	↑
Growth hormone	–	–	–	↓	↑
Glucocorticoids	↑	↓	↑	↓	↑
Adrenaline	↓	↑	↑	↓	↑

hour, and then steadily falls to normal over the next two hours. The fall is due to (a) increased passage of glucose into cells, which is independent of hormonal changes and (b) pancreatic discharge of insulin and its effects.

Diabetes mellitus. In an individual with diabetes mellitus, a condition in which there is a lack of insulin, the fasting blood glucose is elevated and after oral administration of glucose the blood level rises higher than normal. Often the renal threshold is exceeded and glucosuria occurs. Since the insulin response is deficient or lacking, the blood glucose level is extremely slow to return to normal; the patient is said to have a decreased glucose tolerance. Clinical manifestations of diabetes mellitus are: excess urine production (polyuria) because urinary glucose is acting as an osmotic diuretic (p. 741); excess water intake (polydipsia) because dehydration has stimulated the thirst centre in an attempt to replace lost water; and excessive eating (polyphagia) to replace lost glucose. In the absence of insulin the uptake of glucose by the tissues, particularly adipose and muscle, and its storage by the liver is inhibited. Growth hormone mobilizes fatty acids and their oxidation is increased at the expense of carbohydrate oxidation, which is very impaired. Ketone bodies are produced too rapidly for the body to metabolize and, if the diabetes remains untreated, a diabetic coma ensues due to the accumulation of ketone bodies and the acidaemia which may be present.

In contrast, hyperinsulinism causes a lower than normal fasting blood glucose level and after oral administration of glucose the blood glucose concentration may hardly rise at all before falling as low as 40 mg/100 cm³; i.e. there is a high glucose tolerance. The main symptoms are

due to the response of neurons in the central nervous system to the hypoglycaemia. The patient may be confused, anxious, irritable, weak, and may even lose consciousness. There may be marked hunger. In an attempt to remedy the hypoglycaemia, there is activation of the sympathetic system. Other signs include pallor, sweating and tachycardia.

Unfortunately, diabetics who inject themselves each morning with insulin experience a delayed fall in blood glucose, usually between meals, and this must be balanced by diet or by taking glucose tablets. Failure to remedy the situation can lead to a hypoglycaemic crisis in which the symptoms of hyperinsulinism are seen. It is therefore quite possible for a diabetic patient to lose consciousness because of hypo- or hyperglycaemia. Hyperglycaemic coma has a slower onset.

1 Hypoglycaemia may be precipitated by over-injection of insulin or failure to control the delayed fall in sugar level. This condition is the most dangerous of the two.

2 Hyperglycaemia may be due to failure to inject insulin or to take oral hypoglycaemic drugs.

In all instances, it is best to administer a glucose drink (on the assumption that the coma is hypoglycaemic). If the patient recovers within about 20 minutes the hypoglycaemic coma will have been corrected, but if there is no improvement, the hyperglycaemic coma must be corrected by an insulin injection. If insulin was to be injected as soon as an undiagnosed coma precipitated, a hypoglycaemic condition could be made so much worse that irreparable brain damage might result. On the other hand the administered glucose drink will not significantly worsen the hyperglycaemic condition.

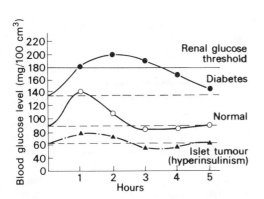

Fig. 17.42. Glucose tolerance curves.

PROSTAGLANDINS

Prostaglandins were originally extracted from seminal fluid but have since been found in many tissues. There are several naturally occurring prostaglandins and many synthetic derivatives, and they elicit a wide range of responses from animal tissues *in vitro* and *in vivo*. Only a brief review of these compounds will be attempted in order to mention some of their possible functions in physiological and pathological processes.

The prostaglandins are analogues of a 20-carbon monocarboxylic acid, prostanoic acid, which consists of a 5-carbon cyclopentane ring with two hydrocarbon chains.

Prostanoic acid

Considerable curiosity is aroused by the nomenclature of the prostaglandins, e.g. PGF$_2\alpha$. Prostaglandins are called by the letters A, B, C, D, E and F according to variation in the constituents of the cyclopentane ring. The number of double bonds in the sidechains is indicated by numerals 1, 2, or 3. The letters α and β refer to the orientation of the hydroxyl group on the cyclopentane ring, the naturally occurring compounds having the α-configuration (Fig. 3.108).

The most abundant mammalian prostaglandins are PGE$_2$ and PGF$_2\alpha$. *In vivo* most cells seem capable of synthesizing prostaglandins from essential fatty acid precursors. This involves a complex of microsomal enzymes called 'prostaglandin synthetase'. Prostaglandins are rapidly metabolized by tissue enzymes; for example, at least 80–90% of circulating prostaglandins are destroyed during a single passage through the liver or lungs.

Prostaglandins differ in their effects on tissues both quantitatively and qualitatively. Some of these differences will be described. The cardiovascular effects are complex but in general PGE$_2$ causes vasodilatation in most vascular beds. Strips of non-pregnant human uterus are induced to contract *in vitro* by PGF$_2\alpha$ and are relaxed by PGE$_2$, but *in vivo* PGF$_2\alpha$ and PGE$_2$ given intravenously cause the contraction of both human pregnant and non-pregnant uterus. PGF$_2\alpha$ causes contraction and PGE$_2$ causes relaxation of human bronchial muscle.

Asthmatics are particularly sensitive to PGF$_2\alpha$. Diarrhoea and abdominal cramps have been caused by some prostaglandins. There is evidence that prostaglandins can depress or facilitate transmission in the autonomic system.

Some selective antagonists of prostaglandins do exist, indicating that there are specific prostaglandin receptors of more than one kind.

Thus PGE and PGF have opposite effects in many instances, and the antagonists are effective against some prostaglandins and not others.

Since prostaglandins occur in so many tissues, practically every pharmacological effect has been scrutinized for a possible function of these substances in physiological or pathological processes. Their possible involvement in reproductive physiology has received considerable attention. They may assist the passage of spermatozoa in the female genital tract. The increase in prostaglandins at term indicates that they may be involved in inducing labour. Indeed labour can be induced by intravenous infusion of prostaglandins. These substances are also used to cause abortions in early pregnancy.

Prostaglandins have also been considered to regulate the tone of other smooth muscles. The high bronchial tone in asthma has been related to a possible predominance of PGF$_2\alpha$ (bronchoconstrictor) over PGE$_2$ (bronchodilator).

Prostaglandins can be released by various means including chemical, mechanical and thermal, and also by nerve stimulation. They are believed to play a part in inflammation by intensifying the effects of chemical mediators of inflammation such as histamine, bradykinin and 5-hydroxytryptamine, thus increasing capillary permeability, swelling and pain. It is now known that anti-inflammatory drugs such as aspirin prevent the synthesis of prostaglandins. This effect has been invoked as an explanation for the beneficial effects of aspirin as an anti-inflammatory agent. It is also suggested that several undesirable effects of aspirin, e.g. gastric ulceration and haemorrhage, are related to the inhibition of prostaglandin synthesis. Some prostaglandins can inhibit gastric secretion, so by reducing the synthesis of prostaglandins, aspirin could cause an increased secretion of gastric juice; this, together with a reduced secretion of protective mucus (also possibly caused by aspirin), could lead to erosion of the mucosa.

HORMONAL INFLUENCES ON ORAL TISSUES

The manifestations of endocrine disturbances (endocrinopathies) are often seen first by an alert dentist. Sometimes a routine bite-wing radiograph reveals unusual alveolar bone changes, but clues are also provided by the appearance of the gingiva, the spacing of the teeth, the condition of the periodontium and so on.

No matter how gross the manifestations of malnutrition and disease are in the body, enamel and dentine are very rarely affected. Teeth are privileged structures. Apart from caries, their integrity can only be significantly affected during their development.

SEX HORMONES

Sex hormones may have a pronounced effect on the gingiva but usually the pathology is not initiated by the hormonal changes; they merely predispose towards the condition. For example, in the presence of local irritation, gingival hyperplasia (swelling) is common about the age of puberty but regresses when the irritation is removed. The hyperplasia is usually attributed to the generalized anabolic effects of the raised levels of circulating androgens and oestrogens.

The hormonal changes during the menstrual cycle are associated with oral changes. The metabolism of the oral flora shows variations which probably correspond with changes in the composition of saliva or gingival crevicular fluid.

Both the incidence and severity of gingivitis increase during pregnancy. This is not considered to be due to an increased amount of dental plaque, but is due to the systemic action of chorionic gonadotrophins, oestrogen and particularly progesterone, which probably act by altering the reaction of peridontal tissues to bacterial products and trauma. The structure of capillaries and venules is altered so that their permeability is increased and this together with a decrease of aggregation of macromolecules in the tissue causes the water content of the gingiva to be increased.

The use of synthetic sex hormones to prevent conception can cause gingivitis. The regular use of the contraceptive pill, which consists of mixtures of synthetic progestogens and oestrogen-like compounds, can lead to inflamed papillae even in subjects with previously perfect gingivae.

After the menopause, keratinization is reduced and an atrophic gingivitis may develop.

DIABETES MELLITUS

The symptoms of diabetes mellitus are the result of a biochemical lesion which affects almost all the tissues of the body. There has been some controversy as to whether there is a causal relationship between untreated diabetes and gingivitis. An enhanced susceptibility to infection is characteristic of the altered protein metabolism in diabetics. A higher incidence of dental plaque has also been reported. These two factors might contribute towards the high incidence of gingivitis in untreated or uncontrolled diabetics.

There is less disagreement about the association between periodontitis and diabetes. The observed rarefaction of bone, the decreased capacity to synthesize collagen and the widening of the periodontal membrane have all been attributed to the effects of impaired microcirculation and vascular stasis. Electron microscope studies have shown that the capillary basement membrane becomes thickened and subendothelial deposits are layed down in the walls of small vessels. These changes are not, of course, confined to the mouth.

The position regarding diabetes and dental caries is confusing. So many diabetic patients control their condition by restricting their diet to what amounts to a non-cariogenic regime that it is now difficult to obtain evidence about this relationship.

GROWTH HORMONE

In pituitary dwarfs, the eruption rate and shedding time are delayed. The dental arch is too small to accomodate all the teeth so that malocclusion develops. The crowns of the teeth appear to be small, but this is only because eruption is incomplete. Excess growth hormone in infancy produces pituitary giants in whom there are larger than normal jaws but average size teeth, so that the teeth are abnormally separated from one another and may overerupt.

The mandible retains into early middle age a potential growth centre beneath its fibrous articular covering. This can respond to an increased level of growth hormone at a time when the long bones are unable to do so. Thus in acromegaly, the length of both the horizontal and ascending ramus of the mandible is increased leading to pronounced prognathism. Often the mandibular angle is markedly obtuse, and this deformity results in a considerable increase in the volume of the mouth. The teeth become widely separated from each other and the increased size of the tongue (macroglossia) probably contributes in causing protrusion of the anterior teeth in both jaws.

PARATHYROID HORMONE

Loss of the lamina dura around the teeth and the margins of the inferior dental canal is often the earliest change to be detected radiographically in cases of hyperparathyroidism. These signs are not specific for this disturbance. In severe hyperparathyroidism multiple cystic spaces affecting the mandible are common.

ADRENOCORTICOTROPHIC HORMONE
(ACTH) AND CORTISONE

Overproduction of ACTH as in Cushing's syndrome and prolonged cortisone therapy cause osteoporosis throughout the skeleton, including the alveolar bone and the lamina dura.

With underactivity of the adrenal cortex (Addison's disease) the characteristic pigmentation of the skin is often seen first in the oral mucosa.

THYROID HORMONE

In the deficiency condition of cretinism the eruption of the teeth is delayed. There is a pronounced retardation in the development of the jaws and the tongue appears abnormally large. The shedding of primary teeth is delayed.

FURTHER READING

MAKIN H.L.J. (Ed.) (1975) *Biochemistry of steroid hormones*. Blackwell Scientific Publications, Oxford.

MONTGOMERY P. & WELLBOURN J.J. (1974) *Medical and Surgical Endocrinology*. Edward Arnold & Co., London.

TEPPERMAN J. (1968) *Metabolic and Endocrine Physiology* (2nd Edition). Year Book Publications, Chicago.

VAUGHAN JANET M. (1970) *The Physiology of Bone*. Oxford University Press, Oxford.

CHAPTER 18

Nutrition

GENERAL PRINCIPLES

The purpose of this chapter is to provide an outline of the principles of nutrition based on the concept of the balanced diet, the main nutrients and their uses. Physiological concepts such as metabolic rate and nitrogen balance are also considered. Nutrition in relation to oral tissues, and fluoride are discussed in more depth.

The balanced diet

In addition to protein, carbohydrates and fats, which are the main energy providers, the diet must supply essential mineral salts including those required in minute quantities (trace elements) and vitamins. Bulk or roughage must be derived from foods in order to promote muscular activity to move unabsorbed materials along the alimentary canal; vegetables and fruit, with their indigestible cellulose, do this particularly well.

The proportion of carbohydrate, protein and fat in the diet is dictated by many factors other than nutritional, the main ones being availability, cost, custom and social pressures such as advertizing.

While these factors will not be considered here, it should be recognized that any attempt to change dietary behaviour (e.g., to reduce sucrose consumption) is unlikely to be successful without an analysis of existing eating habits in a population.

For a typical British diet, an approximate distribution is shown in Table 18.1. Fat intake exceeds the physiological requirements. Some of the fat in our meals is an integral part of foods such as eggs, milk and meat, but much of it is included during cooking merely to improve the palatability.

Recommended daily intakes of all nutrients have been calculated so that national food policies and, at a lower level, catering for large groups of people, can be planned scientifically. It must be emphasized that failure of an individual to fulfill these requirements over a short period (say, a week) does not lead to malnutrition. After a long time, subclinical deficiencies, about which we know little, may be present before the overt signs of malnutrition are observed. (Fig. 18.3).

Tables quoting the nutrient content of foods can be misleading for several reasons. The method of cooking can reduce the nutrient value of a food. Although a diet may appear to contain plenty of a particular nutrient this may be available for absorption in limited quantities either because it is bound, as is some of the niacin in cereals or, as in the case of the fat-soluble vitamins, A, D, E and K, when fat digestion and absorption are impaired for some reason. Table 18.2 provides a comparison between rich

Table 18.1. Proportions of carbohydrate, protein and fat in U.K. diet.

	% total energy	Intake/day (grams)	Principal sources
Protein	10–15	70	Meat, eggs, cheese, fish and milk
Carbohydrate	45–50	400	Potatoes, bread, sugar, rice
Fat	40	80	Butter and margarine, cooking oils and fats; cheese

Table 18.2. Sources and recommended allowances of a few important nutrients.

Nutrient	Rich sources wt. per 100g	Common sources wt. per 100g	Recommended daily allowance for adults
Vitamin D₃ (cholecalciferol) (μg)	Cod liver oil 500	Margarine 7	2.5*
Vitamin C (ascorbic acid) (mg)	Blackcurrants 200	Oranges:Tomatoes:French-fried potatoes 40 25 20	30
Folic acid (μg)	Ox liver : Oysters 300 250	Lettuce : Spinach : Orange juice 20 30 50	100
Calcium (mg)	–	Cheese : Milk : Nuts 750 120 100	500
Iron (mg)	Black sausage : Raw liver : Red meat : Wholemeal flour : Eggs 20 10 5.0 5.0 2.5		10(12†)

*No dietary sources may be necessary for adults who are sufficiently exposed to sunlight.
†In women.

sources and common sources of a few nutrients. When discussing sources in our diet it is necessary to remember that the richest source is rarely the main dietary source. Recommended allowances are usually on the generous side.

Some of the special requirements during infancy, pregnancy, lactation and old age will be discussed later.

ENERGY SUPPLIED BY FOOD AND ENERGY EXPENDITURE

Carbohydrate, protein or fat can be completely oxidized by burning them in a bomb-calorimeter and about 3.9, 5.2, and 9.3 kcal/g are produced respectively. The precise nature of the substance used introduces small variations. The unit of heat is the kilocalorie (kcal), which is defined as the amount of heat necessary to raise the temperature of 1 kg (1000 cm³) of water by 1°C (from 15 to 16°C). During metabolism in the body however, protein is incompletely utilized and energy equivalent to 1.25 kcal/g protein is wasted by excreting large amounts of urea. If it is assumed that about 99, 92 and 95% of the ingested carbohydrate, protein and fat respectively are absorbed from typical mixed diets then it is possible to calculate the calorie or energy equivalent of a particular food. For instance, the protein content of wheat flour is 13%, so the energy supplied by this protein in say 100 g flour, expressed as kcal, is:

$$13 \times \frac{92}{100} \times (5.2 - 1.25) = 47.2 \text{ kcal}$$

It is customary to consider the calorie equivalents of available carbohydrate, protein and fat in the diet as being 4, 4 and 9 kcal/g respectively and this approximation is good enough for most purposes.

Each gram of substrate needs x dm³ of oxygen to produce n calories (where n is characteristic of the substance) and in so doing, y dm³ of carbon dioxide are produced. The ratio y/x is called the respiratory quotient (RQ).   OXYGEN / CO₂ PROD

For glucose, the calculation is as follows:

$$C_6H_{12}O_6 + 6O_2 \rightarrow 6CO_2 + 6H_2O + \text{heat}$$

180 g glucose +
6 × 22.4 dm³ O₂   → 6 × 22.4 dm³ CO₂ + 108 g water + 6730/kcal

∴ 1 g + 0.75 dm³ O₂   → 0.75 dm³ CO₂ + 0.6 g water + 3.74 kcal

or 1 dm³ O₂ ≡ 4.95 kcal and the RQ = 1

For a typical fat, the calculation is:

$$C_{57}H_{104}O_6 + 80 O_2 \rightarrow 57 CO_2 + 52 H_2O + \text{heat}$$

884 g fat +
80 × 22.4 dm³ O₂   → 57 × 22.4 dm³ CO₂ + 936g H₂O + 8309 kcal

1g + 2.03 dm³ O₂   → 1.44 dm³ CO₂ + 1.05 g water + 9.4 kcal

or 1 dm³ O₂ = 4.63 kcal and the RQ is 0.71

The sources of calories in a British diet tend to

vary according to income, as proteins and to some extent fats, are expensive (Table 18.1).

METABOLIC RATE

Shortly after a meal there is a demonstrable rise in the rate of energy expenditure (metabolic rate) which can continue for about two hours. This effect is most pronounced after ingesting protein and can represent an increase of up to 30% over the previous rate. The cause of this specific dynamic action (SDA) of foods is still uncertain. The rise is too quick to be attributed to utilization of the absorbed food but might be due to stimulation of protein metabolism in the liver.

The total calories required from food depend on an individual's energy expenditure (Table 18.3); if intake is less than expenditure there is a loss of body weight. The converse is all too true. Individuals differ in the efficiency with which they utilize food energy. Recent evidence indicates that some individuals are able to convert excess energy to heat by means of brown adipose tissue stores. Others, less fortunate perhaps, convert surplus food energy to fat, and if positive energy balance persists this can lead to obesity.

An enormous amount of data is available on the energy expenditure of different activities and occupations so that it is possible to calculate the food requirements of different groups of people (Tables 18.3 & 18.4). Muscular activity is the main influence on metabolic rate. Even involuntary shivering and muscle tension have an effect. Fever increases metabolism by some 10% for every degree centigrade rise.

The rate at which energy is used at rest is termed the basal metabolic rate (BMR) and is determined under specific conditions: the patient is relaxed, lying down but not asleep (although sleep does not alter the BMR significantly), and lightly clothed at an equitable temperature some 14 hours after eating. The BMR is expressed as kcal (or kJ)/m² of body surface per hour. An individual's energy expenditure bears

Table 18.3. Mean daily energy expenditure (or energy requirement from food) by male individuals with various occupations.

	kcal
University students	2920
Building worker	3000
Army cadet	3476
Coal miner	3666

Table 18.4. Energy expenditure of some physical activities for a 65 kg male.

	kJ/10 min.*
Rest	48
Walking 2 mph	120
4 mph	220
Ballroom dancing	250
Country dancing	350
Fast swimming	400

*1 kcal = 4.2 kJ

less relation to his or her weight than it does to surface area. This is because fat cells, skin and bone contribute little to oxidative metabolism yet form a considerable proportion of the total body weight, and also because heat loss is proportional to surface area. Because of the clothes worn by man, the question of heat loss is less relevant. In fact the BMR is more closely related to the 'lean body mass' than to surface area, but the latter is so easily derived from height and weight measurements that it is customary to use these.

The BMR declines rapidly from a high figure in infants until near puberty then falls gradually. As normally measured, the BMR is lower in women than in men, but this is due to the greater amount of fat in females. An overriding control over the BMR is exerted by the thyroid hormone, probably via respiratory enzymes in the mitochondria. Indeed, measurement of basal metabolic rate was formerly used to assess thyroid function.

Measurement

Methods used to determine energy expenditure depend on several underlying principles.

Total energy expenditure = heat produced plus mechanical work = energy equivalent of food ingested minus energy equivalent of urine and faeces.

The heat output and any work done can be directly measured in a respiration calorimeter, but this method is rarely used because of the expensive apparatus required.

The total energy expenditure is proportional to oxygen consumption and varies according to the substance being oxidized but, because the energy equivalent of 1 dm³ of oxygen is very similar for carbohydrate, fat and protein (5.0, 4.7 and 4.6 kcal), and since a mixture of these normally supplies our energy, a mean value of 4.85 kcal/dm³ O_2 can be used. This corresponds to an RQ of 0.82. Assuming this value, the

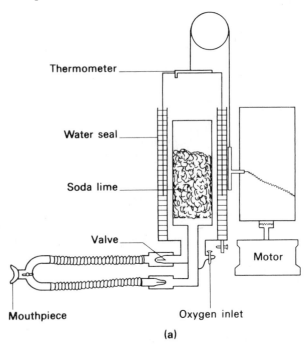

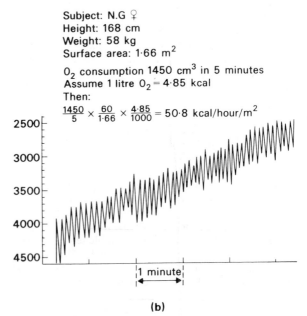

Fig. 18.1. (a) Diagram of the
Benedict-Roth spirometer for
determining oxygen
consumption and metabolic rate;
(b) part of a typical record.

energy expenditure can be assessed from measurements of oxygen consumption alone.

Measurement of oxygen consumption. A Benedict–Roth spirometer (Fig. 18.1) provides a closed circuit in which the subject inspires pure oxygen through a one-way valve from a light-weight cylinder which floats on water (like a gasometer) inside another tank. The expired carbon dioxide is absorbed completely as the air passes back through another one-way valve to the cylinder. As oxygen is used, the cylinder falls and the rate of fall is recorded by an ink-writer on an electrically operated rotating drum. The

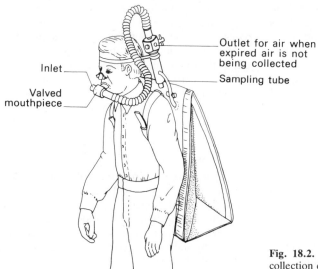

Inlet

Valved
mouthpiece

Outlet for air when
expired air is not
being collected

Sampling tube

Fig. 18.2. The Douglas bag for
collection of expired air.

metabolic rate is calculated as shown (Fig. 18.1).
This method is employed for resting subjects in
hospital laboratories.

Oxygen consumption is measured in subjects
who are undertaking exercise by using a portable
system. In one method expired air is collected
over a timed interval of up to 10 minutes in a
Douglas bag which can be carried on a harness
on the subject's back (Fig. 18.2). Air is breathed
in from the atmosphere and out to the bag via a
valved mouthpiece. The volume of air in the bag
is subsequently measured and a sample is withdrawn to measure its content of O_2 and CO_2;
CO_2 is usually determined by infrared absorption and O_2 by paramagnetic analyser.

PROTEIN REQUIREMENTS AND NITROGEN
BALANCE

Proteins of the body are in a dynamic state; that
is to say they are continually being synthesized
from, and broken down to, amino acids. These
processes occur at very different rates depending
upon the tissue involved.

A person is said to be in positive nitrogen
balance when the protein absorbed, expressed in
terms of nitrogen content, is greater than the
nitrogen excreted in the urine. If absorption is
less than excretion then there is a negative balance and this indicates a loss of tissue protein. To
be meaningful, such balance studies must be
conducted over several days during which time
the diet must be kept constant. On many diets
the faecal nitrogen is small, but some is always
present, as it originates from intestinal cells and

digestive secretions. This 'endogenous faecal
nitrogen' is present even on a protein-free diet.
The urine too contains endogenous nitrogen.
The calculation to determine nitrogen balance
(omitting any sweat contribution) is therefore:

Retained
  nitrogen = Food N − (faecal N + urinary N)

The diet must provide protein well in excess of
the endogenous loss. The actual protein
requirement is determined by many factors, one
of which is the quality of the dietary protein; that
is, its composition with respect to the essential
amino acids (p. 227). These amino acids are
usually defined as those which, in a young animal, cannot be synthesized by the body at rates
commensurate with growth and consequently
have to be supplied in sufficient quantities in the
diet. However, it is now known that except for
lysine and threonine all these amino acids can be
synthesized by transamination reactions from
the corresponding keto acids if these are specially supplied in the diet (p. 216).

Most diets, apart from those eaten by underprivileged communities, contain a mixture of
proteins so that one usually complements a deficiency in another. The daily recommended
amount is about 45 g of good quality protein.
Such protein, which is rich in essential amino
acids, is usually of animal origin and hence it was
formerly termed first-class or animal protein.
These labels have been discarded because several vegetables such as soya bean, peas and nuts
are good sources of high quality proteins.

The subject of protein supply is, of course, one of the most important problems facing scientists and governments throughout the world. Children, because of their relatively greater protein requirements, are most susceptible to protein deficiency (kwashiorkor). Tissues with the fastest turn-over of protein suffer most. Intestinal mucosal cells consequently succumb and soon fail to digest and absorb, with the result that there is a worsening of the nutritional deficiency. The liver fails to synthesize proteins, plasma albumin in particular; this upsets the maintenance of the plasma colloid osmotic pressure and oedema results. Muscle wasting, infections and anaemia also become evident.

FATS

Fats provide a concentrated source of energy and act as a vehicle for fat-soluble vitamins. The adipose tissue acts like a blanket and prevents heat loss as well as acting as a fat store. It is still a little uncertain if there are any fatty acids which are essential in human metabolism. In most other species the polyunsaturated acids, cis-linoleic acid and cis-arachidonic acid, are essential. However, if only one of them is supplied in the diet, the other can then be synthesized. Most diets contain adequate amounts of essential fatty acids (EFA) as they occur widely in vegetable oils. Deficiency of EFA in experimental animals leads to restriction of growth and skin disorders; human infants experimentally deprived of EFA develop an eczematous dermatitis which responds specifically to the ingestion of linoleic acid. One of the metabolic roles of EFA is their incorporation into phospholipids which are vital components of cell membranes (p. 149). Prostaglandins are also synthesized from arachidonic acid (p. 799). According to the USA Food and Nutrition Board, the minimum human requirement of EFA is near 2% of the total energy intake of the diet (see also p. 234).

There have been several reports that diets rich in polyunsaturated fats tend to lower plasma cholesterol, plasma triglycerides and platelet stickiness, all of which suggest a decreased tendency to thrombosis (a condition in which small aggregations of platelets and fibrin trap red blood cells and subsequently block small vessels) and atherosclerosis (a thickening of arteries due to deposition of lipids within the vessel wall).

CARBOHYDRATES

Carbohydrates are the main energy yielding foods for most societies. The chief source is starch from potatoes and cereals, but an increasing amount of sugar in the form of sucrose is now consumed. Lactose is the carbohydrate in milk. Within broad limits the ratio of carbohydrate to fat in the diet is unimportant. If there is a deficiency of carbohydrate or if glucose cannot be metabolized properly, then fat is used to supply the bulk of the energy with the result that ketosis develops (p. 209).

MINERALS

The elements considered essential in the diet can be conveniently grouped according to their availability and properties.

Sodium, potassium and chloride are present as salts in most natural foods but are also added for flavouring and for preserving. They are very soluble and are readily absorbed. Salt is usually consumed in excess of physiological needs and is normally promptly excreted in urine. Small amounts are lost in faeces. Considerable amounts may be secreted in sweat. Despite this excess intake, the kidney has a well-developed mechanism for conserving sodium chloride when body sodium is depleted (p. 745). Calcium, magnesium and phosphorus form much of the skeleton and have important roles in cellular processes. Milk and cheese supply most of the calcium in British diets. Cows' milk contains about 0.12 g/100 cm^3 or 0.70 g/pint. About 0.2 g calcium can be ingested daily from drinking-water in 'hard-water' areas. Figures for the calcium content of food can be misleading in terms of the amount actually absorbed since the efficiency of calcium absorption is usually low (p. 761).

A phosphorus deficiency is unlikely because it is a major constituent of all plant and animal tissues in organic as well as inorganic forms.

Magnesium, like phosphorus, is amply supplied by most diets. Deficiency, like that of potassium, results from severe diarrhoea because of the relatively high concentration of these elements in digestive secretions.

Iron is an essential part of haemoglobin, myoglobin and some enzyme systems. The amount required in the diet is relatively small because only small amounts are lost from the body and because there is an efficient recycling and storage system (p. 673). The availability of iron in some vegetable sources and in eggs is low and, as with calcium, local factors in the intestine sometimes are more important than the content of the food in determining the amount absorbed per day. Red meat, like liver and beef, is a good source of iron. Absorption is higher in iron-deficient subjects.

Of the trace elements, iodine, cobalt, zinc and copper are of particular significance. These and others are discussed more fully later (p. 822). Iodine is contained in the thyroxine molecule and is essential for all vertebrates. The richest sources of iodide are seafoods but most table salt is usually fortified with iodide. Cobalt is a constituent of vitamin B₁₂, a deficiency of which has widespread effects on haemopoietic tissue and the nervous system. Vitamin B₁₂ is needed for the synthesis of DNA.

Fluoride will be considered separately (p. 823) because of its important and unique relationship with dental caries. The argument as to whether or not it is an essential element is likely to continue until ways are found of preparing a fluoride-free diet for experimental animals.

Vitamins will be discussed later (p. 810).

NUTRITIONAL REQUIREMENTS IN
PREGNANCY, LACTATION, CHILDHOOD AND
OLD-AGE

Pregnancy and lactation
More energy must be supplied during pregnancy for the growth of the fetus and placenta, and later for the deposition of fat stores, some of which the mother can subsequently draw upon during lactation. An extra 300 kcal/day are required, but this can be reduced by conserving physical activity. Inadequate food intake results in decreased birth weights and statistically higher infant mortality.

The allowance of calcium must be raised to 1–1.2 g calcium/day. There is some evidence that the percentage absorption is increased during pregnancy.

Throughout the reproductive life of women their iron intake must exceed that of men in order to make good the inevitable losses incurred during menstrual periods. In pregnancy the demands are great because the fetus is supplied with a store of iron so as to withstand dietary deprivation during suckling, which is a time of intense haemopoietic activity. An increase in most vitamins is recommended, particularly vitamins D, B₁₂ and folic acid. Usually these needs are met by eating just a little more of the correct foods, but an additional daily pint of milk goes far in providing the additional calories, protein, calcium, vitamin A and some of the B group as well as fluid which is particularly important in lactation.

Infancy
Arguments in favour of breast-feeding have been waged for years. Lactoferrin is present in human milk but not in cows milk and this has the ability to inhibit growth of pathogenic intestinal microorganisms. Artificial feeds often contain too much salt and phosphate and their fatty acids are more difficult to absorb than those in human milk. The psychological benefits for mother and child of breast-feeding are frequently discussed, but need not concern us here. These arguments apart, milk from the breast or bottle is an excellent food for the infant and provides all its requirements apart from vitamin C and possibly iron. The composition of milk is shown in Table 18.5.

Iron deficiency anaemia is quite common in infants who are suckled or maintained solely on a milk diet for too long, a practice in some societies where it is erroneously thought that lactation safeguards against a further pregnancy. The iron needs of the 1-year old infant who is growing rapidly cannot be satisfied from milk or from the iron store in the liver, therefore mixed feeding should not be delayed beyond 6 months of age.

The protein requirements of an infant per kilogram of body weight are five times that of an adult. A positive nitrogen balance has to be maintained throughout childhood as much body protein is being formed.

The highest demands for calcium are during the spurt of bone growth at puberty when 0.7–1.0 g/day of calcium is recommended in the diet.

Old age
The energy requirements of the elderly are usually less because of reduced physical activity. As

Table 18.5. Composition of milk expressed as weight/100 cm³.

	Human	Cow
kcal.	68	66
Carbohydrate (g)	6.8	5.0
Protein (g)	1.5	3.5
Fat (g)	4.0	3.5
Calcium (mg)	25	120
Phosphorus (mg)	16	95
Iron (mg)	0.1	0.1
Vitamin A (μg)	50	45
Vitamin D (μg)	0.03	0.04
Thiamin (μg)	17	40
Riboflavin (μg)	30	150
Nicotinic acid (μg)	170	80
Ascorbic acid (mg)	3.5	2

Table 18.6. Variation in the composition of flour of different extraction-rates.

Percentage extraction	kcal	Content per 100g of wheat flour (before enrichment)					
		Protein (g)	Fibre (g)	Calcium (mg)	Thiamin (mg)	Nicotinic acid (mg)	Riboflavin (mg)
100 (wholemeal)	328	13.6	2.2	28	0.4	5.0	0.16
85	339	13.6	0.3	19	0.36	1.9	0.08
70 (white)	341	12.8	0.1	13	0.08	1.1	0.05

Most breads are about 1/3 water, and therefore supply about 250kcal/100g and about 8.5g protein/100g.

the total food intake becomes less so the possibility of a lack of certain nutrients becomes greater. Folic acid and ascorbic acid are the most common deficiencies and together are often responsible for anaemia in the elderly. Housebound or infirm people may not get enough sunlight and therefore vitamin D. Additional calcium as well as vitamin D is recommended in an attempt to check the progressive bone resorption in old age (p. 397).

COMPOSITION AND IMPORTANCE OF SOME STAPLE FOODS

Bread and flour supply some 14% of the calories in the national diet in Britain. In sections of the shift-working community where sandwiches, cake and biscuits are eaten several times a day the figure is higher. Most of the flour used for bread comes from wheat and in its milling different proportions of the whole wheat grain are used. The nutritive properties of bread are related to the degree of milling or extraction rate. Much of the outer, largely indigestible, pericarp, the rich protein aleurone layer and the germ, which are rich in protein, fat, minerals and several of the B group of vitamins, are removed from the carbohydrate rich endosperm in 75% (high) extraction white flour. These points are made clear in the analyses shown in Table 18.6. To prevent deficiencies it is customary for white flour to be enriched with thiamin, iron and calcium.

Phytic acid in wholemeal flour can interfere with the absorption of calcium and iron (Table 18.7) but this effect is somewhat reduced by the action of phytase, an enzyme present in the cereal, which is activated during the leavening stage of bread-making (p. 761). To minimize any influence of phytic acid on calcium absorption millers add chalk to wholemeal flour.

Potatoes are an excellent food and certainly are a good cheap alternative to cereals. Because they contain over two-thirds of their weight as water they contribute about one third of the starch and calories which would be provided by the same weight of cereal and about two-thirds of that in bread. The potato supplies carbohydrate, protein, variable quantities of vitamin C, carotene, vitamin B and minerals. It is because of the relatively large amounts eaten rather than the concentration of nutrients in potatoes that they are so useful in the diet.

The composition of milk (Table 18.5) shows it to be almost a complete food for the young. The more rapid growth rate of calves necessitates more protein, calcium and phosphate in cows' milk than human milk. The two major proteins, casein and lactalbumin, are rich in essential amino acids. Milk fat contains in addition to the triglycerides some cholesterol and phospholipids. Lactose is the main carbohydrate. The high calcium and phosphorus content is obviously valuable in the formation of hard tissues. Aided by vitamin D and possibly lactose too, maximum calcium absorption is ensured.

VITAMINS

Vitamins are defined as those naturally-occurring organic substances which are found to be essential in very small amounts for the normal

Table 18.7. Influence of phytic acid in flours of different extraction-rates upon calcium absorption.

Type of bread	Calcium intake mg/day	Absorption of calcium	
		mg/day	% of intake
White (70% extraction)	488	250	51
Dephytinized brown	590	231	39
Brown	550	89	16

functioning of living organisms (this is because they act as co-enzymes in essential biochemical reactions). Traditionally, vitamins have been classified on the basis of their solubility in either water or fats and fat solvents. These solubility differences determine the distribution of vitamins in food and the patterns of absorption, transport, storage and excretion within the body, but the members of each group have little else in common. A more logical alternative classification is based on their nutritional importance. Absence of certain vitamins from the diet results in well recognised deficiency symptoms in human populations, whereas deficiency of other vitamins is so rare that it has only been fully documented in experimental animals given diets which have deliberately been rendered lacking in the vitamins concerned.

In the early days of nutrition research, vitamins were quantified in terms of International Units. With the advent of more sophisticated biochemical methods for separation and measurement, vitamins can now be obtained in pure forms and recommended intakes are more usually expressed in terms of milligrams or micrograms (Table 18.2).

Although it is important to maintain a satisfactory daily intake of vitamins, it should be recognised that it is also possible to suffer from an overdose of vitamins, particularly fat-soluble vitamins. No harm results from higher doses of water-soluble vitamins because any excess is readily excreted.

Water soluble vitamins are readily leached out of vegetables during prolonged boiling in water. For example, cabbage, over-cooked in water, may contain only 10% of its initial vitamin C. Cooking can also improve the nutritive value;

for example, niacin becomes more available for assimilation when cereals are heated.

It is customary to consider thirteen vitamins but, in addition to these, there are a few vitamin-like substances which the body needs but is normally able to synthesize in sufficient quantities. These include para-aminobenzoic acid, myo-inositol and choline.

Vitamin deficiency

Structure, biochemical role and deficiency. Knowing the key role of vitamins in biochemical processes, it might be predicted that deficiency states would lead inevitably to serious ill health and even death. It is true that thousands of deaths have been attributed to scurvy, due to lack of vitamin C; pellagra, associated with an insufficiency of nicotinic acid; beriberi, due to vitamin B_1 (thiamin) deficiency; and pernicious anaemia caused by decreased absorption of vitamin B_{12} or more rarely, lack of folic acid. It is puzzling why serious clinical disturbances do not result from a deficiency of some of the other vitamins, particularly those of the B complex which participate in important metabolic pathways. Perhaps these are required in such small amounts that it is difficult to produce overt deficiency symptoms. It must be realised that such symptoms only appear after a long time. First there is depletion of vitamin stores, the rate of which is variable for different vitamins; cellular metabolic changes follow, and only when these seriously interfere with the cellular machinery do the outward clinical signs present (Fig. 18.3).

Populations at risk. Nutritional education has significantly reduced widespread deficiency in

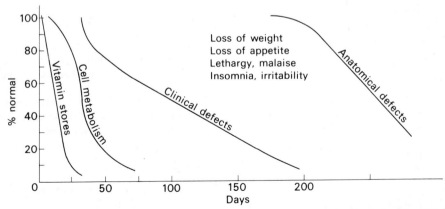

Fig. 18.3. Time course of changes observed in volunteers with vitamin B_1 depletion. Modified from

Marks J. (1968) *The vitamins in health and disease—a modern reappraisal.* Churchill, London.

the industrialized, more affluent countries, though some small sections of the population are still vulnerable. The elderly and housebound, through ignorance, apathy or poverty, often eat the wrong foods. Persons with food fads or particular social customs and those suffering from absorption disorders are also prone to vitamin deficiencies. Many alcoholics become malnourished and show signs of vitamin deficiency particularly of thiamin, nicotinic acid and folic acid.

In underprivileged countries, multiple vitamin deficiencies are common and generally accompany protein and/or calorie deficiencies, which are even more difficult problems to solve.

Deficiency states and their detection. Several techniques are available for diagnosing the vitamin nutritional status of an individual prior to or in conjunction with the rather subjective clinical assessment of the classical symptoms and signs. Several specific biochemical tests have been developed based on the role of the vitamins in metabolic processes.

Clinical manifestations. It is difficult to see the link between the biochemical role of some vitamins and the clinical manifestation of their deficiency. One of the most exciting areas of current research is centred around understanding how specific deficiencies cause the pathological changes associated with them. The areas of the body which most often supply the clue to deficiency are the eyes, skin and mouth. It follows that the dentist can be an important diagnostician of vitamin insufficiency. The relationship between nutrition and oral health will be considered in a separate section (p. 827).

Chemical structure and function
The actual relationship between structure and biochemical role has been clearly established for only some vitamins.

VITAMIN A

Occurrence. The vitamin is present in food as both retinol and β-carotene (provitamin A), its precursor. Retinol occurs in fish liver oils, milk and butter, and β-carotene is present in green vegetables and carrots.

Recommended daily intake. An adult requires 750 μg of retinol per day: 1 μg of retinol is equivalent to 6 μg of β-carotene, which is only poorly absorbed. An enzyme in the mucosa of the small intestine splits some of the dietary β-carotene to yield two molecules of retinol.

The absorption of vitamin A depends upon the presence of an adequate level of fat in the diet. Normally about 150 mg of vitamin A is stored in the liver, sufficient to provide 2 years supply.

Metabolism. Two functions have been elucidated for vitamin A. The one that is best understood concerns its role in vision (p. 964). However, this probably only involves less than 1% of the retinol in the healthy adult; the other role involves growth and maintenance of epithelial tissues. Recent work provides evidence that vitamin A is necessary for the biosynthesis of glycoproteins and glycolipids containing mannose and fucose which are important components of intracellular membranes. It is suggested that monosaccharides such as mannose are transferred from hydrophilic to hydrophobic environments by means of a carrier molecule of retinyl phosphate.

Deficiency. This is frequently seen in young children suffering from protein-calorie malnutrition but is very rare in prosperous societies. The most characteristic signs of hypo-vitaminosis A are in the eye. The ability to see in poor light is impaired (night blindness) because synthesis of the visual pigment rhodopsin, which takes place in the dark, depends upon a supply of retinol (p 964).

All epithelial surfaces including the conjunctiva and cornea show squamous metaplasia (a change in the form of a cell to one which is not characteristic of the tissue), the cells becoming flattened, dried-out and heaped one upon another. This condition in the eye is termed xerophthalmia and is the earliest sign of deficiency. If the deficiency is prolonged, softening of the cornea results, followed progressively by necrosis, ulceration and blindness. According to the WHO some 20 000 young children go permanently blind every year because of a failure to absorb necessary minute amounts of retinol from their diets. With prolonged deficiency, hair follicles develop collars of thickened keratinized cells (follicular keratosis) and sweat glands become blocked with keratin.

THE B VITAMINS

The individual members of the vitamin B complex are usually found together in nature and have the common property of acting as coenzymes (p. 88).

Vitamin B₁—thiamin (formerly aneurine)

Occurrence. Thiamin is found in cereals, yeast, eggs, pulses and nuts. It is thermolabile, and during the baking of bread up to 30% can be lost.

Deficiency has been observed when a diet high in polished rice and milled wheat is consumed because the rejected outer layers of the grain contain most of the vitamin.

An enzyme, thiaminase, found in freshwater fish, destroys thiamin: the Japanese custom of eating raw fish can therefore lead to thiamin deficiency. The enzyme is denatured when fish is cooked. Thiaminase is an example of a vitamin antagonist (or antivitamin).

Recommended daily intake. The daily requirement is related to the amount of carbohydrate in the diet, but 1 mg is usually adequate. The active form of this vitamin is thiamin pyrophosphate (TPP), formed by the phosphorylation of thiamin by ATP.

Metabolism. TPP acts as a coenzyme in several reactions involved in the metabolism of carbohydrates:
1   Oxidative decarboxylation of α-keto-acids to carboxylic acids requires the cofactors TPP, Mg^{2+} or Mn^{2+}, lipoic acid and coenzyme A, e.g.

Pyruvic acid -----------→ Acetyl CoA
α-Ketoglutaric acid -----------→ Succinyl CoA

In the absence of TPP there is a build-up of pyruvic acid which may be responsible for neurological damage in thiamin deficiency.
2   The transketolase reaction of the pentose phosphate shunt also requires TPP (p. 213):

xylulose 5-P		sedoheptulose 7-P
+	→	+
ribose 5-P		glyceraldehyde 3-P

Red cell transketolase activity is measured with and without added TPP in determining the vitamin B₁ nutritional status of a person suspected of suffering from a deficiency.

Deficiency. Although the disease beriberi is generally considered to be the earliest documented deficiency disorder, being recognised in China in 2600 BC, its cause remained unknown until early this century. Beriberi is now much less common in rice-eating communities of South-east Asia because a less polished rice with more of the outer bran is milled and also because a more balanced diet is consumed.

The early signs and symptoms have been reported in several experimental thiamin depletion studies in human volunteers. Many of the clinical features can be attributed to the impaired metabolism of carbohydrate, leading to the accumulation of toxic levels of pyruvic (and lactic) acid. In the peripheral nervous system there is muscular weakness and incoordination, numbness and tingling.

Riboflavin (vitamin B₂)

Occurrence. Riboflavin occurs in milk, meat, cereal products and eggs. It is destroyed by exposure to light and 50% of the riboflavin in a bottle of milk can be destroyed by leaving it for 2 hours on a sunny doorstep. This loss could be reduced by the use of dark brown bottles. It has also been shown that fluorescent lighting in supermarkets destroys riboflavin in milk sold in cartons. Some riboflavin is synthesized by gut bacteria.

Recommended daily intake. In 1979 the following daily allowances for riboflavin in the UK were proposed: adult females, 1.3 mg; pregnant females and adult males, 1.6 mg; lactating females, 1.7 mg. Data from the National Food Survey indicate that actual intakes in the UK population are approximately 30% higher on average than these recommended levels, milk providing the single largest contribution.

Metabolism. Riboflavin forms a part of the two coenzymes: (a) flavin adenine dinucleotide (FAD), and (b) flavin mononucleotide (FMN). These function as hydrogen acceptors in a number of oxidation/reduction reactions

FAD is, for example, vital in the mitochondrial conversion of succinate to fumarate in the Krebs cycle (p. 198).

Deficiency. The early clinical effects of ariboflavinosis have been described in human volunteers on riboflavin deficient diets though certain symptoms seen in people suffering from more general vitamin B deficiency respond to the administration of riboflavin. These include lesions of the lips and tongue, eczema round the sides of the nose and nasolabial folds, and ocular effects such as lachrymation, itching eyes and eyelids and vascularization of the cornea.

Nicotinic Acid (Niacin)

Occurrence. The principal sources of this vitamin are meat, cereal products and dairy produce. It can be formed in the body from the amino acid tryptophan at the rate of 1 mg from 60 mg of dietary L-tryptophan. For this reason the niacin content of foods is conventionally measured as niacin equivalents, being the sum of the nicotinic acid (niacin) plus one-sixtieth of the tryptophan. Deficiency occurs particularly in areas of the world where maize is the staple food. This is because niacin in maize is not available, and maize protein is low in tryptophan.

Recommended daily intake. Eighteen milligrams of niacin equivalents are recommended for an adult man and 15 mg for a woman. In producing white flour from whole wheat there is a considerable loss of nicotinic acid (Table 18.6) so that white flour is often fortified by the addition of thiamin and nicotinic acid. Both free nicotinic acid and nicotinamide are equally active biologically.

Metabolism. Nicotinamide forms a part of the two coenzymes; (a) nicotinamide adenine dinucleotide (NAD^+), and (b) nicotinamide adenine dinucleotide phosphate ($NADP^+$). These function as hydrogen acceptors in oxidation/reduction reactions and are vital in the formation of ATP (p. 196).

In the oxidation of glucose via glycolysis and the citric acid cycle, ten molecules of NAD^+ and two molecules of FAD are reduced: the NADH $+ H^+$ and $FADH_2$ thus formed are subsequently re-oxidised by the electron transport chain which is coupled to phosphorylation of ADP. Examples of reactions involving NAD^+ and $NADP^+$ are:

1   Malate $+ NAD^+$

$$\longrightarrow$$
Malate dehydrogenase
NADH $+ H^+$ + oxalacetate (p.199)

2   Glucose–6–P $+ NADP^+$

$$\longrightarrow$$
G-6-P dehydrogenase
NADPH + 6–P–gluconolactone $+H^+$

3   NADPH behaves as a reducing agent in fatty acid synthesis, e.g.

$$CH_3COCH_2COSCoA + H^+ \longrightarrow$$
$$+ \text{ NADPH}$$

$$NADP^+ + CH_3-\overset{H}{\underset{OH}{C}}-CH_2-CO-SCoA$$

4   When fatty acids are being oxidized, one of the coenzymes for this is NAD^+:

$$CH_3\overset{H}{\underset{OH}{C}}-CH_2CCOSCoA$$

$$\underset{\longrightarrow}{NAD^+ \qquad NADH + H^+}$$

$$CH_3COCH_2COSCoA$$

Deficiency. The symptoms of this now uncommon condition, termed pellagra, vary considerably. The digestive system, skin and nervous system are affected.

There may be inflammation and atrophy of the lining of any part of the digestive tract. Parts of the skin exposed to sunlight become pigmented, roughened and ulcerated. There are mental changes, weakness, tremor and some loss of touch and position sense. Some of these disturbances, particularly depression, may be due to inadequate formation of 5-HT from tryptophan in parts of the brain (p. 289).

Vitamin B_6

Occurrence
This vitamin is found in three forms, which are all equally active. Pyridoxine occurs in plants, while pyridoxal and pyridoxamine are found in animals.

Recommended daily intake. This is thought to be about 2 mg per day, though deficiencies in human diets are rare.

Metabolism. Pyridoxal phosphate which is the active form of this vitamin is a coenzyme for several reactions:

1   *Transamination* (p. 216)

$$R_1CHNH_2COOH \qquad\qquad R_1COCOOH$$
$$+ \qquad \underset{\text{aminotransferase}}{\overset{\text{Vitamin } B_6}{\longrightarrow}} \qquad +$$
$$R_2COCOOH \qquad\qquad R_2CHNH_2COOH$$

2   *Decarboxylation*

$$RCHNH_2COOH \underset{\text{decarboxylase}}{\overset{\text{Vitamin } B_6}{\longrightarrow}} RCH_2NH_2 + CO_2$$

This reaction is important in the production of the neurotransmitter γ-amino-butyric acid (GABA) from glutamic acid.

3 Other reactions in which pyridoxal phosphate is essential include one of the steps in the biosynthesis of haem:

Succinyl CoA

$$\begin{array}{c} + \\ \text{Glycine} \end{array} \xrightarrow[\text{Vitamin B}_6]{\overset{\text{CoASH}}{\underset{\text{CO}_2}{\rightleftarrows}}} \begin{array}{c} \delta\text{-Aminolevulinic} \\ \text{acid} \end{array}$$

Deficiency. Although a genuine dietary deficiency in man is rare, some clinical features, similar to the deficiency signs in experimental animals, have been recognised in patients suffering from tuberculosis who are receiving the drug isoniazid, a pyridoxine antagonist. These people develop a peripheral neuropathy which responds to pyridoxine administration. Other conditions which respond to pyridoxine are some iron-resistant microcytic anaemias, and depression in some women taking 'the pill'.

Pantothenic acid

Occurrence. Pantothenic acid is present in all living cells; the richest sources are liver, kidney and fresh vegetables.

Recommended daily intakes. Dietary shortages practically never arise. It has been calculated that 5 mg/day is sufficient for adults and children and most diets contain two to four times this amount.

Metabolism. Pantothenic acid is a constituent of coenzyme A (see below).

One key reaction of CoASH has been considered in the section dealing with thiamin, i.e. the formation of acetyl CoA from pyruvic acid.

Deficiency. Human deficiency of this vitamin has not been conclusively demonstrated except in experiments in which volunteers were fed a deficient synthetic diet and an antagonist, ω-methyl pantothenic acid. The symptoms included headache, fatigue, impaired motor coordination, muscle cramps and gastrointestinal disturbances.

Biotin

Occurrence. Good sources are liver, kidney and yeast, and it is also present in certain vegetables, pulses and nuts. Deficiency through dietary shortage is unknown.

Recommended daily intake. Biotin conforms to the definition of a vitamin, but since it is readily produced by human intestinal bacteria, there is normally no deficiency disease, as such, in man. The intestinal microbial synthesis of biotin can be disturbed by antibiotic therapy. A daily intake of 150–300 μg of biotin is considered adequate.

Metabolism. Biotin is a coenzyme for a number of carboxylase enzymes, for example, acetyl CoA carboxylase, which is important in fatty acid biosynthesis (p. 231).

$$CH_3 COSCoA + CO_2 + ATP \xrightarrow{\text{Biotin Mg}^{2+}}$$

$$\begin{array}{c} \text{COOH} \\ | \\ CH_2COSCoA + ADP + P \end{array}$$

Malonyl CoA

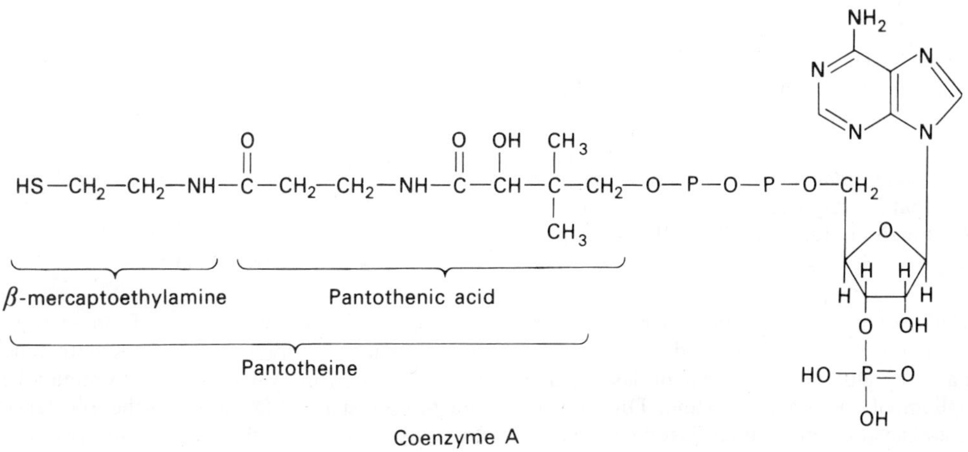

Coenzyme A

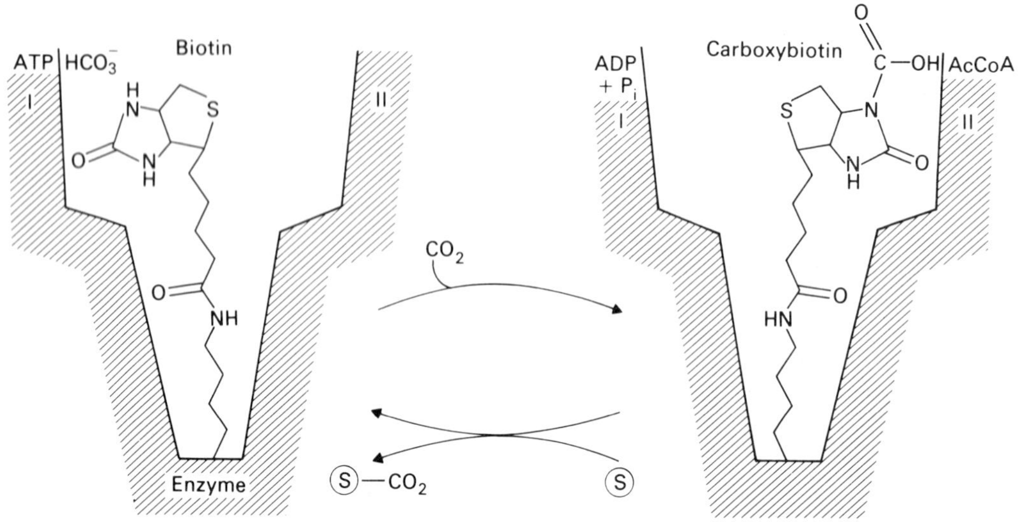

Fig. 18.4. Hypothetical scheme illustrating the translocation of a 1'–N carboxybiotinyl prosthetic group from the carboxylation site (I) to the transcarboxylation site (II) of acetyl CoA carboxylase.

Biotin is covalently bonded to a lysine residue in carboxylase enzymes. It is able to accept and then donate CO_2 as illustrated here; ATP is usually required for carboxybiotin formation.

Biotin, which is covalently attached to the carboxylase enzyme, is able to accept and then pass on CO_2 to substrate molecules (Fig. 18.4).

Deficiency. In an experimentally induced deficiency the subjects became fatigued, depressed and sleepy. They complained of nausea, loss of appetite and muscular pains. There was anaemia and desquamation of the tongue and skin.

Raw egg white contains the protein avidin, which combines with biotin rendering it unavailable. When eggs are cooked, avidin is denatured and biotin liberated.

Folic acid (pteroylglutamic acid)

Occurrence. The vitamin is widely distributed in foods; particularly rich sources are yeast, liver, spinach and lettuce.

Recommended daily intake. Studies on man suggest that the requirement is about 50–100 μg daily, though in pregnancy it may be 400 μg or more.

Metabolism. Most of the folic acid in foods is in a polyglutamyl form but this is hydrolysed to free folic acid by glutamyl carboxypeptidase in the epithelium of the small intestine. During the process of absorption, folic acid is reduced in two

steps to become tetrahydrofolic acid (THF), the active form of the vitamin.

Microorganisms, unlike man, are capable of synthesizing folic acid from p-aminobenzoic acid. Sulphonamides are effective in treating some bacterial infections. They interfere with folic acid synthesis because their structures are similar to p-aminobenzoic acid, a constituent part of the folic acid molecule.

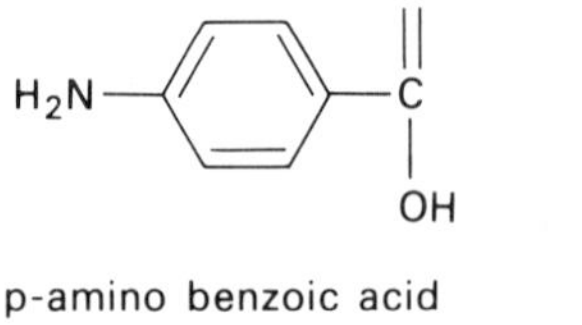

Sulphanilamide

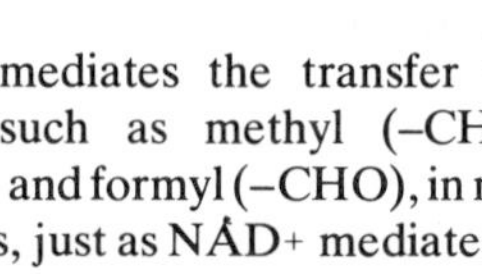

p-amino benzoic acid

THF mediates the transfer of one-carbon groups such as methyl (–CH₃), methylene (–CH₂–) and formyl (–CHO), in many metabolic reactions, just as NAD+ mediates the transfer of two hydrogen atoms. Vital biosynthetic reactions, in which methylated derivatives of THF donate single carbon units include the formation of: methionine, the purine bases adenine and guanine and the pyrimidine base thymine. Formation of the purine and pyrimidine bases is essential for DNA and RNA synthesis. Hence folate deficiency will reduce the ability of bone marrow erythrocyte precursor cells to divide and multiply normally resulting in the typical megaloblastic (pernicious) anaemia characteristic of this condition. THF also serves as an acceptor of single carbon units in certain degradative reactions including those involved in the catabolism of the amino acids serine and histidine.

Two examples of metabolic reactions involving THF are given below:

1 THF + H₂NCH.COOH
          CH₂OH
          Serine

Serine
hydroxymethylase
———————————————→
(pyridoxal phosphate)

Methylene THF + glycine

Methylene THF can be reduced to methyl THF.

2 In the breakdown of histidine to glutamate an intermediate compound, formiminoglutamate ('figlu'), reacts with THF and is converted to glutamate.

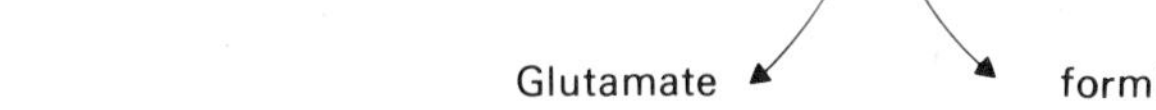

HOOC —CH₂—CH₂— CH —COO⁻   + THF
                        |
                        NH
                        |
                    HC═NH
     formimino-glutamic acid

Glutamate ◄   ► formimino-THF

Patients lacking either folic acid or vitamin B_{12} excrete elevated levels of 'figlu' in urine following a loading dose of histidine; this is a useful diagnostic test for the deficiency.

Deficiency. The most common cause of the deficiency in prosperous countries is malabsorption, as for example in old age or following surgical removal of part of the small intestine. Pregnancy makes large demands on the maternal stores of folic acid (in the liver) and, if the diet is poor, often results in a deficiency in the later stages. Oral contraceptives, anticonvulsants and some other drugs impair folate metabolism.

The typical response to folic acid deficiency is a megaloblastic anaemia because nuclei in red cell precursors do not mature properly and cell division is impaired.

Vitamin B_{12} (cobalamin)

Occurrence. Vitamin B_{12} occurs only in association with animal proteins, one of the richest sources being liver.

Recommended daily intake. Because of its wide distribution in meat and other animal products, information concerning the dietary requirement is not easily obtained. Estimates range from 1–5 μg/day.

Structure. This is a complex molecule built around a porphyrin ring resembling haem, but containing cobalt not iron.

Metabolism. Patients with a deficiency of vitamin B_{12} have elevated plasma levels of $N^5/$ methyl tetrahydrofolic acid and it has been suggested that this is because vitamin B_{12} is necessary for the conversion of methyl THF to THF as shown overleaf (top):

Methionine serves as the principal methyl donor in the body. A major consequence of B_{12} deficiency is that folic acid (THF) is not available to participate in the biosynthesis of DNA nucleotide bases (p. 236).

B_{12} is a coenzyme for the enzyme methyl malonyl CoA isomerase. Methyl malonyl CoA is formed from propionyl CoA, the end product of β-oxidation of fatty acids of odd chain length (some 1–2% of the total fatty acids in body lipids). (See overleaf.)

Deficiency. A few cases of dietary deficiency have been reported among strict vegetarians but shortage of vitamin B_{12} usually results from fail-

Homocysteine → Methionine (via N5-methyl THF, THF, Vitamin B₁₂ transmethylase)

$$\text{Homocysteine} \xrightarrow[\text{transmethylase}]{\text{Vitamin B}_{12}} \text{Methionine}$$

Fatty acyl CoA (containing 2n + 3 carbon atoms) → β oxidation → Propionyl CoA $CH_3.CH_3.CO\text{-}SCoA$ (nCoASH, nAcetyl CoA)

Propionyl CoA carboxylase (a biotin enzyme): CO_2, ATP, ADP + P_i → Methyl malonyl CoA

Methyl malonyl coenzyme A isomerase B_{12} → Succinyl CoA → TCA cycle

ure in absorption. This can be due to inadequate secretion of intrinsic factor in gastric juice.

B₁₂ deficiency is manifested in those parts of the body in which cells are rapidly dividing, e.g. blood-cell forming tissue, the oral mucosa and gastrointestinal tract. The most characteristic feature of the deficiency is anaemia in which the bone marrow contains many megaloblasts and a dearth of normoblasts. Nerve fibres often degenerate both in dorsal and lateral tracts of the spinal cord and in the peripheral system (subacute combined degeneration). Symptoms include tingling and numbness, motor weakness, ataxia and some loss of reflex activity.

Vitamin C (*ascorbic acid*)

Occurrence. Vitamin C occurs in citrus fruits, blackcurrants, and vegetables, particularly tomatoes and new potatoes.

Recommended daily intake

Thirty milligrams is the quantity recommended in the UK. Some sections of the community, particularly old people living alone, do not receive adequate amounts of the vitamin during the winter months. Infantile scurvy is now rare because mothers supplement the milk diet with orange or blackcurrant juice or vitamin preparations.

Metabolism

Ascorbic acid is a vitamin necessary only in the diet of man and other primates and the guinea pig; most mammals possess the enzyme L-gulonolactone oxidase (L-gulonoxidase) which converts L-gulonolactone to ketogulonolactone, which then undergoes spontaneous molecular rearrangement, forming ascorbic acid (p. 124).

Ascorbic acid functions as a reducing agent, being itself easily oxidized to dehydroascorbic acid:

Ascorbic acid ⇌ (H_2) Dehydroascorbic acid

1 Ascorbic acid has one important metabolic role as a coenzyme in the hydroxylation of certain proline and lysine residues in the biosynthesis of collagen (p. 248). For example:

Proline in
protocollagen

| |
| Proline hydroxylase |
| Fe^{2+}, O_2, α-ketoglutaric acid |
| Ascorbic acid |

Hydroxyproline
in procollagen

In the absence of ascorbic acid, collagen synthesis is impaired, and this leads to failure to form connective tissues.
2 Ascorbic acid increases the absorption of iron.
3 Other oxidation-reduction reactions requiring vitamin C include:

Tryptophan → 5-hydroxytryptophan

Dopamine → Noradrenaline

p(OH) Phenyl pyruvate → Homogentisic acid

Vitamin C is also involved in steroid metabolism (p. 780).

Deficiency. The association between scurvy and the prolonged lack of fresh fruit and vegetables goes back several hundred years and the success or failure of many sea ventures and explorations was often determined by the incidence of scurvy. There have been several successful attempts to induce scurvy in volunteers.

The principal disturbance is in the connective tissues: the activity of fibroblasts, odontoblasts and osteoblasts is impaired (Fig. 18.8). The heal-ing of wounds in soft tissues and bones (fractures) is poor and scar tissue can break down so that old wounds open and become infected. As the synthesis of the basement membrane around capillaries and the adhesion of capillary endothelial cells are dependent on the vitamin, spontaneous bleeding is common in scurvy.

In many cases of scurvy, anaemia is present. The defect is attributed to an accelerated rate of cell destruction rather than defective formation and is one cause of a condition designated as haemolytic anaemia.

Vitamin D

Occurrence. Vitamin D can be synthesized in the body when the skin is exposed to ultraviolet light. In areas of the world where there is not much sunlight the diet has to supply the vitamin, particularly during the winter months.

Fish, eggs, butter and milk provide vitamin D and it is added to some foods such as margarine and canned milk.

Recommended daily intake. A daily intake of 10 μg is recommended for young children and adolescents in the winter months, but when the contribution from sunlight is likely to be great, no specific recommendations are now made.

Structure. There are several forms of vitamin D:
1 *Vitamin D_2* (ergocalciferol), which is the form of the vitamin normally used to fortify foods, is produced by exposing ergosterol, found in yeast, to ultraviolet radiation.
2 *Vitamin D_3* (cholecalciferol) is the form normally produced in the skin by the action of sunlight on the provitamin, 7-dehydrocholesterol, which in turn is formed from acetate by several complex reactions leading to the formation of cholesterol (p. 155). Vitamin D_3 is present in foods, particularly fish oils.

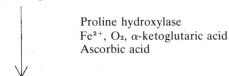

7-Dehydrocholesterol   Cholecalciferol (Vitamin D_3)

Metabolism. Ergocalciferol and cholecalciferol are provitamins and are converted first to 25-hydroxycholeciferol in the liver where it is then stored. Some of the 25-hydroxy-derivative is carried to the kidney where it is further oxygenated at the 1 carbon atom to give 1, 25-dihydroxy D₃. This is released and taken in the blood to the mucosal cells of the small intestine where it promotes the formation of polyribosomes. The mRNA of these is coded for the synthesis of the specific 'calcium binding protein' whose function is to increase intestinal calcium absorption (p. 766). Vitamin D₃ metabolites accumulate in the hypertrophic zone of cartilage cells in epiphyseal growth plates, in osteoblasts, osteocytes and in calcifiable cartilage and osteoid, but their precise role remains uncertain. It is probable that they affect the synthesis and structure of collagen and proteoglycans. They are required for the resorption of old bone and the deposition of new bone.

irritability. The most easily identifiable signs are the characteristic skeletal lesions. These vary according to the time of onset of the deficiency. In babies there is often craniotabes (a softening of the membranous bones of the skull). Frequently, closure of the anterior fontanelle is delayed. In cartilaginous bones, the epiphyses are enlarged and widened because the cartilage is only slowly replaced by bone-forming cells and osteoid tissue. When this affects costochondral junctions it produces the so-called 'rickety rosary'. If rickets continues into the second year of life the lower ends of the femur, tibia and fibula are unable to take the strains imposed by standing and the leg bones become bowed.

Several hypotheses have been proposed to explain osteomalacia in some Asian immigrants in the UK. It could be that specialized cooking procedures are responsible. For example, it is possible that some of the vitamin originally present in butter is destroyed during ghee making. In addition, most Asians make chapattis with flour

25-(OH) D₃
(25-Hydroxycholecalciferol)

1,25-(OH)₂ D₃
(1,25-Dihydroxycholecalciferol)

Deficiency. The deficiency diseases are rickets in the young child and osteomalacia in adults. At the beginning of this century rickets was known as the disease of 'poverty and darkness'; poverty because the main dietary sources were too expensive for many to buy and darkness because of inadequate exposure to sunlight due to several factors such as poor housing and smoky atmospheres. It is probable that even today there is a deficiency amongst many old incapacitated people in northern latitudes particularly during the winter months. Unfortunately the normal glass in windows filters out the ultraviolet light necessary for vitamin D synthesis in the skin.

The first symptoms of rickets to attract attention are a lack of muscle tone affecting postural and abdominal muscles, gastrointestinal disturbances, diarrhoea, delayed development and

containing phytate which might reduce the absorption of calcium in the gut (p. 762). Social customs, such as the observance of purdah amongst orthodox Muslim women, and the nature of the clothes worn by Sikh women, restrict exposure to sunlight. This is less likely to be serious in the more sunny Indian subcontinent than in northern countries.

Vitamin D supplements have been available since 1945 and have contributed to the dramatic decrease in the incidence of rickets in British children. However, the reluctance of some of the more traditional Asian women to attend welfare and baby clinics in the UK to obtain the vitamin preparations might be partly responsible for cases of rickets among this ethnic group.

Hypervitaminosis D. This condition is not just of academic interest since several cases of hypervitaminosis D have been reported in patients who have attempted to treat themselves with large doses of the vitamin, and in children whose mothers were tempted by the availability of unlimited supplies at welfare centres and pharmacies. The principal consequence is metastatic calcification (soft tissues, such as tendons and blood vessels) and gastrointestinal disturbances. Some fatalities have been reported.

Vitamin E (α-tocopherol)

Occurrence. The richest sources are certain vegetable oils. The common sources are vegetables, cereals, dairy produce and animal products.

Recommended daily intake. Although the US National Research Council recommends 30 mg/day of DL-α-tocopherol acetate or its equivalent, according to some authorities there are no good grounds to support any recommended intake of vitamin E. This is because the

cauliflower, green tomatoes, peas and cereals. A second form, vitamin K_2, is synthesized by bacteria including *E. coli* of the human colon. Cows' milk contains significant quantities of vitamin K_2. The biological activity of K_2 is less than that of K_1.

Recommended daily intake. Estimates suggest that about half the daily requirement is derived from plant sources, the remainder coming from gut flora. In clinical situations associated with malabsorption of fat, a daily oral supplement of 50–100μg is recommended. No definite dietary requirements have been set for vitamin K under normal circumstances.

Metabolism. Vitamin K participates in the synthesis of several proteins involved in blood clotting, namely, factors II (prothrombin), VII, IX and X. During prothrombin formation, glutamic acid residues in the N-terminal region are carboxylated to form γ-carboxyglutamic acid, as follows:

$$
\begin{array}{ccc}
\text{COOH} & & \text{COOH COOH} \\
| & & \diagdown \diagup \\
\text{CH}_2 & \xrightarrow[\text{reduced vitamin K}_1]{\text{Carboxylase HCO}_3^-} & \text{CH} \\
| & & | \\
\text{CH}_2 & & \text{CH}_2 \\
| & & | \\
\text{--- NH —CH—CO---} & & \text{---NH — CH — CO - - -} \\
\text{Glutamic acid} & & \gamma\text{-Carboxyglutamic acid}
\end{array}
$$

tocopherol requirement increases with increasing intake of polyunsaturated fatty acids.

Metabolism. Vitamin E functions as an antioxidant. It is oxidized in preference to polyunsaturated fatty acids and its action is similar to that of substances used in the food industry to prevent fats from going rancid.

Deficiency. The most probable cause of the deficiency in the human is impaired fat absorption and not a dietary insufficiency. In such patients a form of haemolytic anaemia develops possibly because of decreased stability of the erythrocyte membrane to hydrogen peroxide. There are also degenerative conditions in muscles leading to creatinuria.

Vitamin K

Occurrence. Vitamin K_1 is widely distributed in dark green vegetables such as spinach, kale and the outer leaves of cabbage. It is also present in

The other vitamin K-dependent proteins are believed to be activated by a similar mechanism.

Deficiency. A primary dietary deficiency of this vitamin has never been clearly demonstrated in adults, probably because most diets contain an amount, which, together with that synthesized by the bacterial flora in the large intestine, satisfies their requirements. Intestinal production of vitamin K_2 can be abolished by antibiotic therapy, and in this situation patients are more dependent upon dietary vitamin K_1. Normally 1–1.5 mg of vitamin K are stored in the liver so that the body possesses a reserve supply for periods of shortage. Newborn babies have a sterile gut and receive little vitamin K from human milk so that during the first few weeks of life it is not uncommon for babies to have a low plasma prothrombin level. Bleeding occurs into the skin, brain, peritoneal cavity or alimentary tract and is aggravated by trauma at birth. Deficiency in adults is caused by conditions associated with reduced fat absorption. In such people it is difficult to stop bleeding after injury and surgery.

To prevent thrombosis anticoagulant drugs may be administered and many of these act by antagonizing or competing with vitamin K. Within this group are dicoumarol, phenylindanedione and warfarin.

TRACE ELEMENTS

The term trace elements describes a group of minerals which is known to exist in plant or animal tissues in small or trace amounts; the word trace was originally used because the particular element was in such small quantities that it could not be accurately measured. It is still used today even though there are now many analytical methods which can accurately determine the concentration of these microconstituents. In any sample of human or animal tissue, 20–30 trace elements can be detected, ranging in concentration from a few milligrams to less than 1 $\mu g/100$ g tissue. Some of these are known to have an essential role in metabolism, i.e. they are required as a dietary factor for the normal growth, development, and maintenance of the health of the individual. Some of the essential trace elements act as cofactors or regulators in enzyme reactions. Withdrawal of any of these elements is known to produce deficiency states which are corrected only by supplementing the diet with the missing element. Eight trace elements are known to be essential in animal nutrition; iron, iodine, copper, zinc, manganese, cobalt, molybdenum and selenium. Others, such as fluorine, bromine, barium and strontium can be classified as probably essential but are not yet proved to be so. A third group; cadmium, chromium, nickel, vanadium and rubidium are always found in significant amounts in tissues and are at present being studied particularly to see if any trace element–enzyme relationships are formed. A fourth group, comprising the remainder of the known trace elements consists of aluminium, silver, lead, gold, bismuth, tin, titanium, and gallium. These are found in tissues, but since they are not known to play a role in metabolic processes, are considered to have been acquired from contaminants in the diet.

Analytical methods
Since 1950 there has been a considerable advance in the study of the distribution and role of the trace elements mainly because of the availability of improved experimental techniques.
These consist of:
1   Refinements in the methods of producing purified diets containing very low levels of the element concerned but adequate in all other dietary requirements. In this way it was possible to show that molybdenum and selenium were essential trace elements in animal nutrition.
2   Improvements in the analytical methods available for estimating sub-microgram quantities of trace elements present in organs, tissues and diets. Spectrographic analysis, involving the study of the spectra produced when a dry-ashed sample of tissue is burned in a carbon arc, has been largely superseded by more sensitive atomic absorption and radioactive methods.

Ingestion and absorption
Most of man's daily intake of trace elements is supplied by food though in some cases significant amounts of certain elements are ingested from water. Only a portion of the trace elements in food is usually absorbed and utilized. Precise figures are not available but studies on very young infants show that the daily requirement for copper is approximately a fifth of that in the diet. Many factors in the digestive tract may influence the absorption of trace elements. Thus, the biological availability of any element depends upon:
1   The relative concentration of other trace elements present in the diet. For example, the copper concentration in the liver of the sheep is markedly affected by the levels and proportions of copper, zinc, molybdenum and inorganic sulphate in the diet.
2   The properties of the compounds in which the trace element is present in the food. For example the element must be in solution before it can be absorbed.
3   Adsorption, chelation, or complex formation with substances such as amino acids.
4   The presence of oxidizing or reducing agents in the diet. For example iron is absorbed from the duodenum only in the ferrous state. Reducing agents such as vitamin C and cysteine are required to convert any ferric iron into the ferrous form.

Biological action
The majority of the biologically active trace elements serve as key components of enzyme systems or of proteins with vital body functions.

In 1959 it was shown that chromium, nickel and manganese were present in various preparations of nucleic acid and that their concentration was related to the concentration of phosphate. It is thought that these metals help to stabilize the secondary helical structure of the nucleic acid and if so must play a vital role in protein biosynthesis and therefore the transmission of genetic information.

Many interrelationships exist between two or more trace elements. Classical experiments with Australian sheep showed that storage of copper in the liver of these animals was significantly reduced by an increased dietary intake of molybdenum. In fact, copper deficiency states can be induced in many species by deliberately increasing the soluble molybdenum salts in the diet.

In the biosynthesis of haemoglobin both iron and copper are required. The iron is incorporated into the porphyrin ring to form the haem molecule and copper, in the form of the copper-containing dehydrase enzyme, is required to facilitate the condensation of two molecules of γ-aminolaevulinic acid to form a precursor of protoporphyrin, porphobilinogen.

Those trace elements which have been implicated in affecting dental caries prevalence are discussed later (p. 829).

Fluoride

Fluoride is the ionic form of the element fluorine and is of particular interest because of its unique relationship with dental caries. The widespread advocation of the use of water fluoridation as a public health measure makes it essential for the health scientist to be conversant with the systemic effects of fluoride.

Availability

Although fluoride is found in rocks, mineral deposits, soils, fertilizers and sea water (1 mg/dm^3), remarkably little is present in human diets. Drinking water usually contains fluoride, ranging in concentration from trace amounts of about 0.1 mg/dm^3 in many areas to high levels of 1–3 mg/dm^3 and even over 8 mg/dm^3 in a few places. Fluoride concentrations are more usually expressed as parts/10^6 (1 mg F per dm^3 is 1 part/10^6 and so forth). The optimum level of fluoride from a dental health point of view is 0.7–1.0 part/10^6, and in order to achieve this, some communities have added fluoride to their water supplies. Concentrations above 2 parts/10^6 can cause mottling of enamel in the permanent teeth. At higher levels of fluoride, mottling becomes unsightly and for this reason it has become customary to reduce naturally occurring high levels to more acceptable values.

Fluoride salts dissolve in water and freely dissociate to yield fluoride ions; e.g.

$$NaF \rightleftharpoons Na^+ + F^-$$

Even with the relatively insoluble calcium fluoride (CaF_2), which is often the source of naturally occurring fluoride ions in water, the enormous dilutions involved ensure that the salt is completely dissociated to free calcium and fluoride ions.

The tea plant is unusual in its ability to accumulate high concentrations of fluoride in its leaves (40–200 parts F/10^6, dry weight). The beverage, as normally prepared (with low F tap water) contains about 1.5–2.0 parts F/10^6, which is equivalent to about 0.3 mg fluoride per cup of tea. Indeed a large proportion of the daily fluoride intake in this country comes from tea (Table 18.8). Fish might be expected to be another major dietary source, but in fact only dried fish, fish skin, and fish with soft edible bones like canned salmon and sardines provide significant amounts.

No other common items of food contain appreciable quantities of fluoride. Human milk and cows' milk contain extremely small amounts (0.05 mg/dm^3 or less) and raising the dietary fluoride intake of the mother (human and cow) has a negligible effect on the milk fluoride level. Artificial milk feeds prepared from milk powder and fluoridated drinking water (containing 1 part F/10^6) supply about 30 times the fluoride of normal milk and can raise the daily F intake to 0.8 mg. Surprisingly, this has little effect on caries incidence.

It is difficult to assign representative figures for the mean daily fluoride intake of any age group because of variations in water and tea-drinking habits, in fluoride concentrations in different water supplies and to a lesser extent in the foods eaten. In hot climates, the consumption of water is obviously higher and this affects the amount of fluoride ingested. Little information is available about the water intake of children. The most conservative estimates for total water intake range from 0.32 dm^3/day in 1-year-olds to 0.6 dm^3 in 9-year-olds. If it is assumed that all this water is fluoridated at the 1 part/10^6 level, then 0.32 and 0.6 mg/day of fluoride would be contributed from water alone.

As a dental health measure, tablets containing about 2.2 mg sodium fluoride (=1 mg F) are

mg F/L → 1/10^6

Table 18.8. Mean daily fluoride intakes in 12–15 year old children in UK in a fluoridated area (1 part F/10⁶).

	mg fluoride
Drinking water (including that used in making tea, coffee and fruit drinks)	0.85
Tea	0.45
Fluoride derived from toothpaste	0.20†
Food* and Water used in cooking*	0.50
Total	2.00

* Estimates rather than actual determinations
† Estimated as amount absorbed rather than ingested.

often given to children who do not have the benefit of water fluoridation. In some countries fluoride has been added to table-salt with beneficial effects in reducing caries.

Recent reports have drawn attention to a hitherto unsuspected source of fluoride intake, namely fluoride-containing toothpaste. It seems that it is the practice among many children to swallow some paste after brushing their teeth (Table 18.8). Some young teenagers ingest as much as 5 mg F/day in this way but this is not all absorbed. Small amounts of toothpaste are inevitably swallowed even after spitting-out and

this also contributes marginally to the overall fluoride intake (Table 18.8.).

Smoke from some factory chimneys and the dust from brick-works can contain appreciable amounts of fluoride in particulate form. In the neighbourhood of such areas, grazing cattle can apparently ingest sufficient fluoride to affect their milk yields and induce symptoms of skeletal fluorosis.

Fluoride requirement. Because of the difficulties of preparing experimental diets which are specifically and exclusively fluoride-free, there has been disagreement on whether fluoride should be labelled an essential trace element. However, recent experimental studies on rats show that fluoride appears to be an essential dietary factor (at very low levels) in relation to their normal growth and reproduction.

Distribution of fluoride in the body
Providing fluoride is in solution its absorption in the intestine is relatively rapid and complete. By following, over a period of several hours, the change in the plasma fluoride concentration, it has been found that after absorption, fluoride is rapidly diluted by fluid in the extracellular compartment; a slower uptake by the skeleton follows and then, later, excretion by the kidney (Fig. 18.5). Small quantities of fluoride are lost in sweat and milk and some is taken up by the fetus. The plasma fluoride is kept relatively constant and at a low level by an efficient process of renal excretion and skeletal deposition. After some 1–3 years of living in an area with a constant level of fluoride in the water supply, the body attains an approximate equilibrium condition in which the urine has about the same fluoride concentration as the drinking water,

Fig. 18.5. Plasma fluoride concentrations (log. scale) following a single dose of sodium fluoride by mouth (●) and intravenously (▲). 10 ng/cm³ = 0.01 parts/10⁶). The fluoride levels during a control period in the same subjects are also shown (■). The curves indicate that the bioavailability of sodium fluoride tablets taken by mouth is 100% in a fasted subject. By using mathematical models to describe absorption, distribution and excretion of fluoride it has been concluded from the shape of these curves and areas enclosed by them that plasma fluoride (a) becomes distributed rapidly to the various fluid compartments (b) is taken up by the skeleton (c) is excreted by the kidney and, if the administered dose is high (d) is later affected by a back diffusion of F from bone crystallites. (After Ekstrand J. (1977) *Studies on the pharmacokinetics of fluoride in Man.* Almquivst Wiksell, Stockholm.)

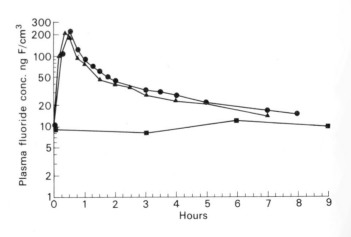

and the daily urinary fluoride output almost equals the fluoride intake. However, the actual percentage of a single fluoride test dose which is excreted by the kidneys varies according to the past history of fluoride exposure and age, both of which affect the skeletal component of the homeostatic mechanism. In young children, with little previous exposure to fluoride, only about 20–30% of a small dose of ingested fluoride is excreted; the proportion of ingested fluoride incorporated in hard tissues is high and reflects the greater degree of bone growth and turnover. In young adults this rises to 50–60% and can be raised further by increasing the total fluid intake. The tubular reabsorption of fluoride in the kidney is less efficient than that of chloride and is reduced by a high urinary flow.

When individuals leave a high fluoride area for a low one, or when patients cease therapeutic measures involving prolonged ingestion of large quantities of fluoride, only a small amount of the fluoride stored in the skeleton gradually comes out and is excreted.

 Saliva contains very low concentrations of fluoride which parallel, and are similar to, the plasma fluoride levels (0.01 parts $F/10^6$). Soft tissues in general do not accumulate fluoride. Dental plaque is unusual in concentrating fluoride.

As analytical methods have become more refined, so the reported values for fluoride in plasma have become less. Some recent figures are presented in Table 18.9. It is now thought that all the fluoride is ionized in human plasma. Shortly after drinking a cup of fluoridated water there is a small peak in the serum fluoride level (Fig. 18.6), the height of which is related to the concentration of fluoride ingested.

Table 18.9. Serum fluoride level in relation to fluoride concentration in water supply.

Fluoride in water supply	Fluoride in serum	
(parts/10^6)	parts/10^6	μmol
0.1	0.008	0.41
1.0	0.017	0.88
5.6	0.08	4.3

From Taves D.R. (1975) *British Nutrition Foundation Bulletin*, **15**, 193.

Incorporation into hard tissues. Although this topic has already been considered (p. 400), it is important to emphasize that there is a high affinity between fluoride and hydroxyapatite and that fluoride incorporation into bones continues throughout life.

The distribution of fluoride in bone is related to the pattern of growth and remodelling so that levels vary in different bones and even within different parts of any one bone. Fluoride is probably translocated from bone undergoing

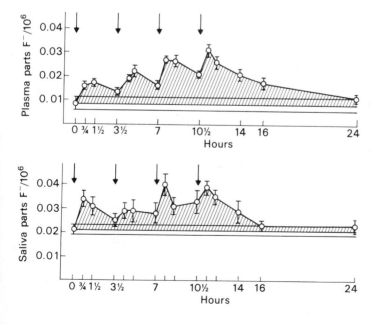

Fig. 18.6. Mean plasma and salivary fluoride concentrations following the ingestion of fluoride in drinking water. At intervals, shown by the arrows, 250 cm³ water containing 2 parts $F/10^6$ ($= 0.5$ mg F) was drunk by the six subjects. (After Henschler D., Buttner W and Patz J. (1975) Absorption, distribution in body fluids and bioavailability of fluoride. In *Calcium metabolism, bone and metabolic bone diseases*. Editors, Kuhlencordt and Kruse. Springer-Verlag, Heidelberg.)

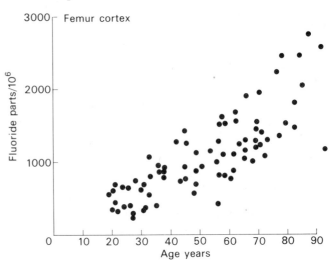

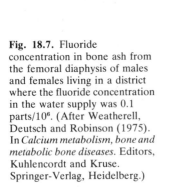

Fig. 18.7. Fluoride concentration in bone ash from the femoral diaphysis of males and females living in a district where the fluoride concentration in the water supply was 0.1 parts/10^6. (After Weatherell, Deutsch and Robinson (1975). In *Calcium metabolism, bone and metabolic bone diseases.* Editors, Kuhlencordt and Kruse. Springer-Verlag, Heidelberg.)

resorption to new bone which is being laid down. Analyses have been carried out on comparable bone specimens from humans of different ages living in districts supplied with drinking water containing different concentrations of fluoride. For any one age group the content of bone fluoride reflects the level of water fluoride, but there is some disagreement concerning the rate of skeletal fluoride deposition in the elderly. Some reports suggest that a plateau is reached whereas others, with a greater number of observations, show no evidence for this (Fig. 18.7). It has been shown recently that plasma fluoride levels are positively related to age and to the amount of fluoride in the skeleton. Patients with chronic renal insufficiency accumulate larger fluoride levels in their bones.

The bulk of fluoride entering enamel does so during formation, apart, of course, from any which is applied topically to the tooth surface by the dentist or by use of a fluoride-containing dentifrice. In the dentine of permanent teeth, fluoride continues to be deposited at the pulpal dentine surface and in secondary dentine.

Placental transfer. Results in experimental animals suggest that fluoride does not pass freely across the placenta. Passage is probably easier in the human since the fluoride concentration in blood from the umbilical cord is almost the same as that in maternal blood. However, variations in fluoride intake by mothers during pregnancy cause only small differences in the fluoride levels in the teeth of their children; probably too small to alter significantly their resistance to dental caries (Table 18.10).

Table 18.10. Fluoride content of ashed fetal femur and teeth in the full term fetus from low and high fluoride areas.

Fluoride (parts/10^6) in drinking water	Mean F (parts/10^6)	
	Femur	Teeth
0.1	43.8	40.8
0.55	92.5	69.7
1.00	85.2	53.8

From Gedalia (1970) *Fluorides and human health*, p. 128, WHO, Geneva.

Effects of fluoride on enzymes and metabolism. It must always be remembered that the effects of fluoride on isolated enzyme systems and tissues may not be the same as effects *in vivo.* Above all, it is the actual fluoride ion concentrations in the experimental media which must be compared with those in body fluids. In human studies, it is not only the fluoride concentration in the water supplies but the total daily intake and the duration of exposure to fluoride which must be carefully noted.

The ingestion of naturally occurring fluoride in water by large numbers of people throughout the world at concentrations ranging from 1 to 8 parts/10^6 has afforded an unparalleled opportunity for studying any longterm effects of this element on human health. Examination of disease and death-rate statistics provides a consensus of evidence that fluoride at these levels constitutes no major health hazard.

Fluoride is known to be a potent inhibitor of the activity of several enzymes and this forms the basis for some of the objections to fluoridating water supplies as a dental health measure. However, the levels of fluoride needed to bring about such enzyme inhibition *in vitro* are usually 10–100 times higher than those in plasma of people in high fluoride areas.

Comparatively little is known of the in-vivo effects, if any, of fluoride at the low levels found in blood and soft tissues. There is no substantial evidence that fluoride at 1–2 parts/10^6 in water supplies has any marked disadvantageous overall effect on the adult. That relatively low levels of fluoride in drinking water can influence cellular metabolism is an inescapable conclusion from the observation that mottling of enamel is seen in the permanent teeth of children who drink water containing over 2 parts F/10^6 during tooth development. Mottling is due to an effect on the ameloblasts which leads first to a disturbance in matrix-formation and then mineralization. Remarkably high concentrations of fluoride can be accommodated in the skeleton without incurring any histological changes or measurable effects upon bone cells (p. 401).

Nutrition and oral tissues

INTRODUCTION

It is important to distinguish truly nutritional or systemic effects of diet on the teeth, supporting tissues and oral epithelium from local environmental effects as food passes through the mouth. The type of food in the mouth may influence the metabolism of the bacteria-containing dental plaque which is the primary agent in the initiation of both caries and periodontal disease, but nutritional factors, acting systemically, can make the teeth and periodontium either more or less resistant to this agent. However, a systemic influence can only affect the structure of teeth during their development while the other tissues in the mouth, because they are continuously being renewed, are always susceptible. An exception to these generalizations is a systemically induced alteration in the composition of saliva, which, by altering the local environment, alters the oral disease processes. Some idea of the many components of oral tissues which can be targets for nutritional disturbances are shown below:

1 *Developing tooth.* Ameloblasts and odontoblasts, hydroxyapatite crystals and 'foreign' ions like F^+, Mg^{2+}, CO_3^{2-}; proteins, lipids and citrate in the organic matrix of enamel and dentine.

2 *Periodontal ligament.* Collagen fibres.

3 *Oral epithelium.* Cell growth and differentiation, keratin and mucin synthesis.

4 *Alveolar bone.* Mineral, collagen and ground substance.

5 *Connective tissue.* Collagen, elastin and ground substance.

Nutritional deficiencies can be due to direct dietary insufficiencies or they can be indirect, as for example, when there is impaired intestinal absorption or defective metabolism. A poor dentition or a painful mouth can lead to the rejection of certain nutritious items such as fruit or meat, and childish food fads, to rejection of milk or vegetables.

The relationship between nutrition and oral health is said to be primarily non-specific. This means either that one change, for example atrophy of ameloblasts and enamel hypoplasia, can result from several different deficiency states, or that one deficiency might produce several different disturbances.

The danger in drawing conclusions about human nutrition from the results of studies in animals must be emphasized. Not only are experimental diets in animals grossly abnormal when compared with the natural diets, they are also very different from human diets. In addition, the oral flora, the feeding patterns, the times of tooth eruption relative to birth and weaning and so on are unlike those in man.

RELATIVE IMPORTANCE OF PRE- AND POST-ERUPTIVE FACTORS ON CARIES SUSCEPTIBILITY

The ravaging effects of westernized 'commercial' diets upon the teeth of persons who previously had a more natural unrefined diet have been seen throughout the world and bear witness to the view that the 'arch criminal' in dental caries is refined carbohydrate, particularly sucrose. The relative freedom from caries previously enjoyed by some communities was not necessarily due to superior nutrition as we understand the term, nutritional deficiencies were often present (in fact), but rather to a less cariogenic oral environment. Tooth surfaces may remain unaffected by caries because of the absence of a cariogenic challenge rather than because of a built-in resistance. It seems that modern man's high susceptibility to caries does not result from faulty tooth structure caused by abnormalities in diet during tooth development;

in other words, dental caries is not due primarily to inadequate nutrition but to faulty eating habits.

It is outside the scope of this section to consider in detail the local dietary factors which are so important in causing dental caries; these will merely be summarized. The prime concern will be the systemic effects of nutrients on the structure of oral tissues. Because of the overwhelming evidence showing the protective effects of fluoride against caries, this trace element is discussed separately (Vol. 1, Book 2 p. 208).

Local environmental factors

Physical consistency. Theoretically it would be anticipated that hard foods and those requiring much chewing would be beneficial to the oral tissues, due to the mechanical cleansing action on the teeth and adjacent soft tissues and the stimulating effects on gingival circulation, alveolar bone turnover, keratinization of epithelium and salivary flow. Support for this view comes from animal studies and there is limited circumstantial evidence in man. Certainly, the converse situation, a nutritionally adequate but soft diet, frequently promotes more bacterial plaque, gingivitis and periodontal disease in experimental animals; the same has been observed in some relatively caries-free communities in various parts of the world.

There seems little doubt that the harmful effect of certain forms of confectionery on tooth surfaces is due to both their physical properties and their sugar content. Proof of this was obtained in the now famous Vipeholm study in Sweden in which the dental condition of institutionalized subjects given various amounts and types of sugar supplements over many months was examined.

Frequency of eating. The Vipeholm study also showed that the frequency of eating sugar-containing foods was related to caries prevalence. Carefully controlled experiments in rats have substantiated these results. The habit of eating between-meal snacks and sweets must account for much of the high prevalence of caries in Britain.

Carbohydrates. Many studies on rodents show that sucrose is the most cariogenic of the simple carbohydrates, probably on account of its key role in the synthesis of extracellular polyglycans by some microorganisms in bacterial plaque.

Starchy foods produce little or no caries as they are not readily broken down to simple fermentable sugars in the mouth.

Protective factors. Although laboratory experiments demonstrate that unrefined cereals and crude sugars contain factors capable of reducing the rate at which powdered enamel is dissolved by acid it has proved more difficult to show their effectiveness in the mouth. Phytate and other organic phosphates have been implicated as being responsible. Surveys in different communities, as well as experimental studies in animals, indirectly support the concept of these protective factors, but so many other variables are present that it is difficult to assess their significance. For example, some experiments in rats and hamsters have given rather surprising results. It was found that certain foodstuffs when unrefined were more cariogenic than when refined. The probable explanation is that the unrefined food has a higher vitamin and nutrient value and is better able to support cariogenic bacteria than the less nutritive refined food.

Considerable interest was aroused by the finding that addition of inorganic ortho- and pyrophosphates to cariogenic diets in rats significantly lowered the incidence of dental caries, but this post-eruptive effect has not been consistently observed in clinical trials.

Fats. It is almost impossible to achieve a reduction in the fat content of an experimental diet without at the same time changing the physical consistency so that much more food is lodged in fissures and gingival crevices. It is not unexpected therefore that the addition of a small amount of groundnut oil to a fat-free, high sucrose diet, significantly reduced caries in rats.

Systemic effects of nutrients

Proteins, carbohydrates and fats. Although protein deprivation is common in many parts of the world it is usually accompanied by other nutritional deficiencies, inadequate hygiene and infections by bacteria, viruses and protozoa. The pre-eruptive effect of protein deficiency on caries susceptibility is generally difficult to determine because of the relatively low cariogenicity of the foods eaten after tooth eruption. However, in a study in Guatemala it was found that the deciduous teeth of undernourished children were more susceptible to caries than those of the better-fed. The deciduous incisors of the deprived children were hypo-

Table 18.11. Pre-eruptive influence of a purified, high sucrose diet on caries susceptibility of rat molars.

Duration of feeding purified high sucrose diet prior to conception	Mean caries incidence in teeth of offspring		
	Molars	Cavities	Score
2 months	3.3	5.6	7.0
4 months	5.1	8.6	13.7

From Sognnaes R.F. (1948) *Journal of the American Dental Association* **37**, 676.

plastic and this was probably responsible for some of the increased caries.

Trace elements other than fluoride. In the late 1940s Sognnaes showed, in a small number of rats, that a purified, high sucrose diet given during pregnancy and lactation increased caries susceptibility in the offspring. Even more important was the finding that the longer the females were fed this diet, the higher was the caries incidence in their young (Table 18.11). This suggested that the purified diet, although nutritionally adequate for general health, lacked some factor, which in the stock diet was producing caries protection in the developing teeth. The mothers fed on the purified diet were gradually becoming depleted of this factor. Since a further study showed that the ash of the stock diet contained the missing factor it seemed that a single or multiple element deficiency was involved. Although this reasoning was possibly incorrect, the concept that trace elements are involved in caries has been amply confirmed.

Many clinical surveys have shown that certain elements in soil, vegetation, milk and drinking water are associated with caries prevalence. In

Table 18.12. Comparison of percentage caries-free first permanent molars of children from high and low molybdenum areas in Somerset, England.

	High molybdenum	Low molybdenum
Boys	28.2	8.3
Girls	17.9	6.6

From Anderson (1965). In *Advances in Fluorine Research and Dental Caries Prevention* **3**, 165.

Britain, attention has been mainly restricted to molybdenum, whose presence in relatively high concentrations in soil of some rural areas of Somerset is associated with a lower caries incidence (Table 18.12). A study in New Zealand revealed marked differences in the composition of soils and vegetation and in caries incidence in two nearby towns; high caries was associated with low levels of barium, strontium and magnesium and low caries with high levels of molybdenum, aluminium and titanium. The fluoride concentrations in the drinking waters were similar. Several reports from different parts of the world point to high levels of manganese and copper in the water supplies of areas with high caries prevalence. Vanadium has been shown to reduce caries in animal experiments and has been associated with lower caries rates in epidemiological surveys. A systematic search for a common factor to explain very low caries figures seen in the records of some naval recruits in the USA led to the finding that high strontium levels in water supplies were responsible. Caries incidence is higher in areas of Wyoming and Oregon, known by agriculturists to be high selenium areas. Children living there have raised levels of selenium in their urine. It is not known how these trace elements act, but it is almost certainly systemic rather than local.

Calcium, phosphorus and magnesium. After tooth formation has been completed there is no apparent withdrawal of minerals in response to a mineral deficient diet, whereas there is pronounced mobilization of alveolar bone. Such diets affect the composition of the developing teeth of rats to a much smaller extent than the supporting bone. It seems that teeth are formed 'at the expense of bones'. Some histological changes were noted in these rat teeth but they were confined to the dentine. The abnormally low levels of calcium and phosphorus in these diets are unlikely to have a parallel in human nutrition. Despite admonitions about the need for extra dietary calcium for the development of 'strong' teeth there is remarkably little proof that increased consumption of calcium-rich dairy products has any benefit in preventing caries.

Closely linked with calcium in the diet is the question of the hardness of water and caries prevalence. It is difficult to isolate hardness from other variables in different water supplies and the position is still rather uncertain.

Vitamin A. One of the essential features of this vitamin is its control over differentiation of ectodermal cells and in providing the signal for production of mucin.

In rats fed a vitamin A deficient diet, decreased amounts of sialic acid and hexosamines are incorporated into salivary glycoproteins from the sublingual glands.

Deficiency, which is rare in humans, causes keratinization of salivary ducts and impaired secretion of mucin, hyperplasia (increased production of cells) of the gingival epithelium and hyperkeratosis. In developing teeth the ectodermal enamel organ becomes keratinized and this causes enamel hypoplasia (Fig. 18.9).

Vitamin B group. Although no cell is exempt from nutrient deprivation, overt reactions to nutritional deficiencies are often tissue-orientated. Those tissues which are repeatedly exposed to mechanical, thermal, chemical and microbial insults and therefore have a rapid cell-turnover are particularly vulnerable. Such tissues are to be found lining the oral cavity and these are sensitive to vitamin B deficiency. A key stage is in the mitotic and maturation processes in cells.

The basic fault lies in the failure of cell division and maturation to keep pace with the needs of the tissues for protection. As a consequence, the tissues become damaged and inflammation follows. They frequently become infected. The stimulus given to increased regeneration of the cells cannot properly be met and so the situation progressively deteriorates. Common complaints include soreness and a burning sensation of the lips, mouth and tongue accompanied by discomfort in eating and swallowing. These conditions fortunately respond rapidly to treatment with vitamin supplements. It is worth noting, however, that iron-deficiency anaemia and infection cause oral changes which are not dissimilar to those described here.

Vitamin C. The importance of this vitamin in the formation of collagen and some constituents of connective tissues such as chrondroitin sulphate manifests itself in the oral disturbances seen in scurvy. In an extensive study in monkeys, the effects of a scorbutic diet (one which produces scurvy) included a breakdown of the collagen fibres in the periodontal ligament, atrophy of alveolar bone (Fig. 18.8), and bleeding of the gums. Such symptoms have been observed in humans. Loosening of the teeth aggravates the resorption of alveolar bone. In elderly edentulous patients, in whom the vitamin deficiency is most common, the residual alveolar mucosa is unaffected. In developing teeth of the guinea pig there is marked atrophy of the odontoblasts and consequently defective dentine formation.

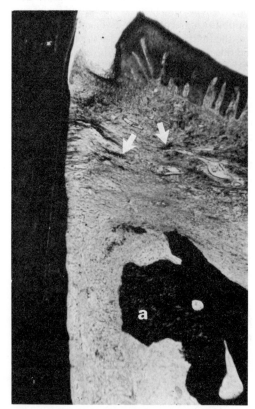

Fig. 18.8. Degeneration of periodontal fibres in an experimental monkey after several months on a vitamin C deficient diet. Only the principal fibres adjacent to the epithelial cuff remain intact. There are signs of bleeding within the connective tissue (arrows) and loss of the alveolar bone (a) adjacent to root.

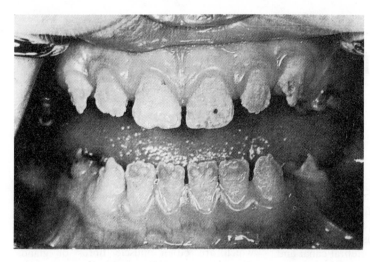

Fig. 18.9. Very severe enamel hypoplasia in a 13½ year old male who has had rickets (vitamin D deficiency). (After Pindborg (1970). In *Pathology of Dental Hard Tissues*, p. 156. Munksgaard, Copenhagen.)

The spectrum of disturbances seen in vitamin C deficiency is attributable to the essential role of the vitamin in the metabolism of mesodermal tissues, the nature of which is still uncertain. Epidemiological studies suggest that there is no relationship between the prevalence of caries or periodontal disease and vitamin C dietary status.

Vitamin D. Although deficiency in young rats and dogs produces an excess of osteoid in alveolar bone, there is a remarkable lack of data on the state of the periodontium in conditions of rickets and osteomalacia in man. Reports that the enamel and dentine besides being poorly calcified are also thinner, suggest that the vitamin is concerned in matrix formation as well as in its calcification. The classical work by Mellanby showing enamel hypoplasia in rachitic puppies supports this view. How the vitamin affects ameloblast function is not known. Enamel hypoplasia (Fig. 18.9) has recently been seen in the deciduous teeth of some children who had experienced neonatal tetany because of lack of vitamin D during late fetal development.

Unfortunately, studies on dogs do not provide information to link vitamin D deficiency and caries as dogs are caries-immune. There seems no doubt that hypoplasia potentiates carious attack because of the retention and stagnation areas created on the roughened, pitted surfaces of teeth, but it is uncertain if the association between vitamin D deficiency and caries can be taken much further. The value of vitamin D supplements for all children and expectant mothers as far as dental health is concerned is very questionable.

FURTHER READING

BENDER A.E. (1973) *Nutrition and Dietetic Foods.* Leonard Hill Books, Intertext, Aylesbury.

COOK-MOZAFFARI P., DOLL R. *et al.* (1981) *Journal of Epidemiology and Community Health*, Vol. 35, p. 227. Fluoridation of water supplies and cancer mortality.

DAVIDSON, Sir S. *et al. (1979) Human Nutrition and Dietetics* (7th Edition). Churchill Livingstone, Edinburgh.

D.H.S.S. (1979) *Recommended Daily Amounts of Food Energy and Nutrients for Groups of People in the United Kingdom.* H.M.S.O., London.

NIZEL A.E. (1981) *Nutrition in Preventive Dentistry, Science and Practice* (2nd Edition). W. B. Saunders Co., Philadelphia.

Royal College of Physicians of London (1976) *Fluoride, Teeth and Health.* Pitman Medical, London.

CHAPTER 19

The Nervous System

ANATOMY

The nervous system for descriptive convenience is divided into peripheral and central parts. The central nervous system comprises the spinal cord and brain, which lie in the vertebral canal and cranial cavity respectively. The peripheral nervous system consists of sensory (afferent) and motor (efferent) fibres; these are distributed to all regions of the body in bundles termed nerves. It also includes sensory and autonomic ganglia which are collections of neuronal bodies associated with the nerves.

The sensory fibres of the peripheral nerves convey information, in the form of nervous impulses, from receptors to the central nervous system. Receptors are elements capable of detecting changes in the external and internal environment, and are found throughout the body (for details of their structure and function, see p. 308). Thus, through the agency of sensory nerve fibres a wealth of information is continu-

ously brought to the central nervous system from a vast array of different kinds of receptors.

Motor fibres of the peripheral nerves transmit instructions in the form of nervous impulses from the central nervous system to effectors which are either muscle fibres or glands. Through the medium of effectors various responses are evoked such as movements of the limbs, alterations in the activities of the various internal organs and changes in the secretory activities of glands.

The central nervous system is a compact mass of tissue composed of nerve cells and their fibres, supporting cells or neuroglia, and vascular elements. The nerve cells or neurons number many thousand millions—(the number of neuroglial cells far exceeding them). Through their fibres or processes, neurons communicate with other neurons by means of synapses (see pp. 281 & 295). Some fibres are short and connect to neighbouring cells, others form long tracts or pathways which connect to more remotely situ-

Table 19.1. The development of the three primary vesicles of the brain.

Primary vesicles		
Rhombencephalon (hindbrain) { Myelencephalon Metencephalon		Medulla oblongata Pons and cerebellum
Mesencephalon (midbrain)	–	Midbrain
Prosencephalon (forebrain) {	Diencephalon (interbrain) {	Thalamus Hypothalamus Epithalamus Subthalamus Retina and optic nerve
	Telencephalon (endbrain) {	Cerebral cortex Corpus striatum Internal capsule Lamina terminalis and associated commissures Olfactory lobe

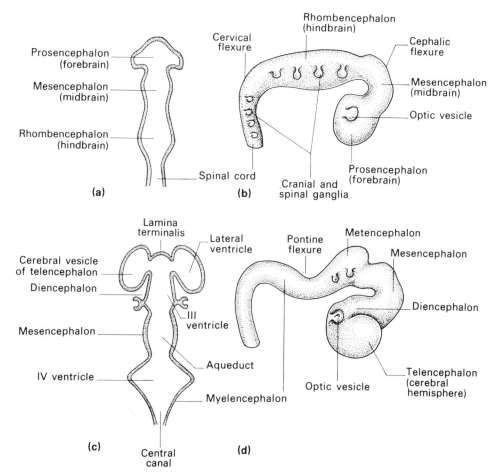

Fig. 19.1. Diagrams of the developing, human brain vesicles and ventricular system. (a and b) Three primary brain vesicles of a four week old embryo. Note the cervical flexure demarcating the spinal cord from the hindbrain, and the cephalic flexure forming the boundary between hindbrain and midbrain. (c and d) Six week old embryo showing five brain vesicles.

ated nerve cells. In essence, the central nervous system receives through receptors, via sensory fibres, information which is then relayed through various pathways to specific regions in the spinal cord or brain for 'decoding' and analysis. New impulses are then directed through different pathways and conveyed ultimately by motor fibres of the peripheral nerves to effectors. Thus, on the basis of information received the nervous system is able to initiate the most appropriate response.

Neurons, neuroglia and nerve fibres are described on p. 276.

Major divisions of the central nervous system

The central nervous system, consisting of brain and spinal cord, originates from the neural tube (Book 2) which is a derivative of the ectodermal layer of the embryonic disc, appearing at the end of the third week of gestation. The rostral end of the tube grows rapidly and differentiates into three hollow expansions, the primary vesicles, which will form the major divisions of the brain. The rest of the tube retains its simple tubular form and develops into the spinal cord.

The three primary vesicles in ascending order from the spinal cord are the hindbrain, the midbrain and the forebrain, which are all clearly recognizable by the end of the fourth week (Fig. 19.1a & b). Their further development is shown in Figs. 19.1, 19.2 and Table 19.1.

By the end of the fifth week the hindbrain becomes divided by the pontine flexure into the myelencephalon (medulla oblongata), and the

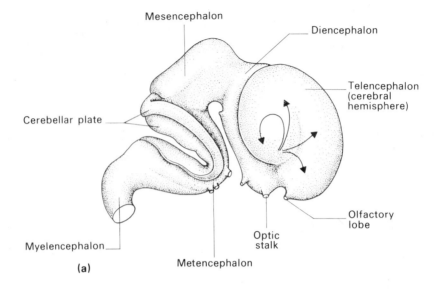

Mesencephalon

Diencephalon

Telencephalon
(cerebral
hemisphere)

Cerebellar plate

Olfactory
lobe

Myelencephalon

Optic
stalk

Metencephalon

(a)

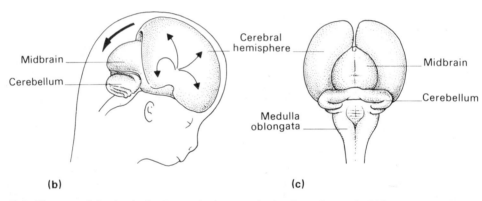

Midbrain

Cerebellum

Cerebral
hemisphere

Midbrain

Cerebellum

Medulla
oblongata

(b)   **(c)**

Fig. 19.2. Diagrams of the developing human brain. (a) Lateral view of the brain vesicles of an eight week old embryo. (b) Lateral view and (c) posterior view of a brain of a twelve week old fetus. Arrows show the direction of growth and enlargement of the cerebral hemisphere.

metencephalon, which gives rise to the pons and cerebellum (Fig. 19.1d). At the same time the forebrain vesicle undergoes considerable modification. On each side it develops a lateral evagination called the cerebral vesicle, the future cerebral hemisphere. The rostral wall (lamina terminalis) of the forebrain together with the cerebral vesicles constitute the telencephalon, whilst the central part forms the diencephalon. Subsequently the cerebral vesicles expand in a complex manner, overgrowing the roof of the diencephalon and fusing with its lateral walls (Figs. 19.2 & 19.3). They eventually bury the dorsal and lateral aspects of the midbrain and encroach onto the superior surface of the developing cerebellum.

Despite the embryololgical upheaval, the cavities of the neural tube remain connected, although much altered in size and shape. Collectively they constitute the ventricular system, the general plan of which is shown in Fig. 19.1c. The cavity of the hindbrain forms the fourth ventricle; that of the midbrain develops into a narrow canal, the cerebral aqueduct; and the diencephalic cavity becomes compressed into a narrow cleft termed the third ventricle. The lateral ventricles and the anterior part of the third ventricle are derived from the telencephalic cavity; each lateral ventricle communicating with the third ventricle through the interventricular foramen.

The major derivatives of the diencephalon are the paired thalami, the hypothalamus and the

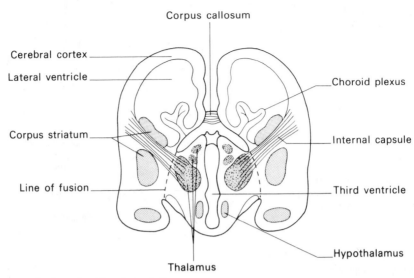

Fig. 19.3. Diagram of a frontal section through the fetal brain, showing the site of the line of fusion between the diencephalon and telencephalon.

pineal body. Each thalamus arises in the lateral wall of the third ventricle, developing into a large mass of grey matter (Fig. 19.3). The hypothalamus develops in the floor of the third ventricle and extends into the lower part of each lateral wall (Fig. 19.3). Hypothalamic derivatives include the mamillary bodies, infundibulum and posterior lobe of the pituitary gland (neurohypophysis). The pineal body arises as a caudal evagination of the diencephalic roof and comes to lie above the midbrain. In addition, the retina and optic nerve of each eye develop from outgrowths on either side of the diencephalon (see optic vesicles, Fig. 19.1d).

The cerebral cortex arises in the walls of the cerebral vesicles and develops into a highly convoluted layer of grey matter covering the outer aspect of the cerebral hemispheres. The corpus striatum also develops in the cerebral vesicle but is restricted to the floor of the lateral ventricle near the site of the secondary fusion of diencephalon with telencephalon. It differentiates into a large mass of grey matter which subsequently becomes divided into lentiform and caudate nuclei by an important group of projection fibres termed the internal capsule (Fig. 19.3). Two commissures of note develop in the lamina terminalis. These are bundles of fibres which cross the midline to link cortical regions of one side with those of the opposite side. The larger commissure is a massive bundle, the corpus callosum, which in sagittal section of the mature

brain arches from the lamina terminalis over the roof of the diencephalon (Fig. 19.37). Its size parallels the enormous growth of the cerebral cortex. The anterior commissure, much smaller, lies in the lower part of the lamina terminalis (Fig. 19.37).

The major regions of the adult brain are shown in Fig. 19.4, and the major derivatives of the brain vesicles are summarized in Table 19.1. Note that the midbrain and hindbrain exclusive of the cerebellum are referred to as the brainstem, and that the two cerebral hemispheres constitute the cerebrum.

Spinal cord

The spinal cord lies within the vertebral canal surrounded by protective membranes, the meninges. In the adult it extends from about the level of the first or second lumbar vertebra to the lower border of the foramen magnum at the base of the skull where it becomes continuous with the medulla oblongata. In length the cord is about 45cm; in width about 1.0–1.5 cm. During the early stages of fetal development the spinal cord occupies the entire length of the vertebral canal but due to the different growth rates of the neuraxis and the vertebral column, the caudal tip comes to lie at the level of the third lumbar vertebra at birth, and later assumes the adult level.

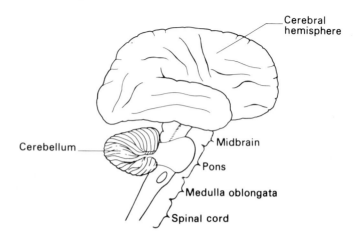

Fig. 19.4. Semi-diagrammatic scheme of the major divisions of the brain, viewed from the lateral side.

EXTERNAL FEATURES

The cord is cylindrical but not uniform in diameter, being somewhat flattened antero-posteriorly in the cervical region. It also has two fusiform swellings, the cervical and lumbar enlargements or intumescences (Fig. 19.5), which represent those parts of the cord whose nerve roots innervate the upper and lower limbs respectively. The end of the cord rapidly tapers, and forms the conus medullaris out of which projects a thin fibrous filament called the filum terminale. This structure continues down the vertebral canal to the level of the second sacral vertebra where it pierces the dura mater. Here it becomes invested in dural tissue and continues caudally to be attached to the coccyx.

The spinal cord is grooved longitudinally by sulci or fissures (Fig. 19.6). On the posterior surface the posteromedian sulcus marks the site of a pial invagination, the posteromedian septum, which extends deeply into the substance of the cord. On the anterior surface is a deep cleft, the anteromedian fissure, which contains blood vessels. Lying laterally on each side of cord are the posterolateral and anterolateral sulci, which mark the sites at which the dorsal root fibres enter and the ventral root fibres leave the cord respectively.

Attached at intervals along each side of the spinal cord are pairs of dorsal and ventral spinal roots which join in their appropriate interver-tebral foramina forming spinal nerves. Because the spinal cord only occupies the upper two thirds of the vertebral canal and the interverte-bral foramina are regularly spaced along the entire length of the canal, the roots become progressively longer and more obliquely

inclined as the cord is descended (Fig. 19.5). The longest roots therefore emerge from the conus medullaris. Bundles of ventral and dorsal roots which descend beyond the caudal tip of the spinal cord are collectively known as the cauda equina (Fig. 19.5), so named because of its fancied resemblance to a horse's tail. Each dorsal root is characterized by a fusiform swelling, the spinal or dorsal root ganglion, which is situated just proximal to the spinal nerve.

The spinal cord is divided into segments which, although not morphologically obvious, are indicated by the emergence of groups of rootlets forming nerve roots. Each segment is defined as that portion of the cord which contributes dorsal and ventral root fibres to a single pair of spinal nerves. In total there are 31 segments corresponding to 31 pairs of spinal nerves which comprise 8 cervical, 12 thoracic, 5 lumbar and 5 sacral pairs and usually one coccygeal pair.

GENERAL ARRANGEMENT OF GREY
AND WHITE MATTER

Internally the cord consists of a central core of grey matter surrounded by an outer mantle of white matter. The latter is composed of bundles of myelinated and non-myelinated nerve fibres, mostly longitudinally directed, together with supporting neuroglial cells. Grey matter consists of cell bodies of neurons, dendrites, axons and terminal arborizations of neuronal processes, as well as neuroglial cells. In the fresh, unfixed state it appears slightly pink, indicating a rich blood supply. The core of grey matter is organized in long columns and appears H shaped in transverse section. The crossbar of the H corresponds

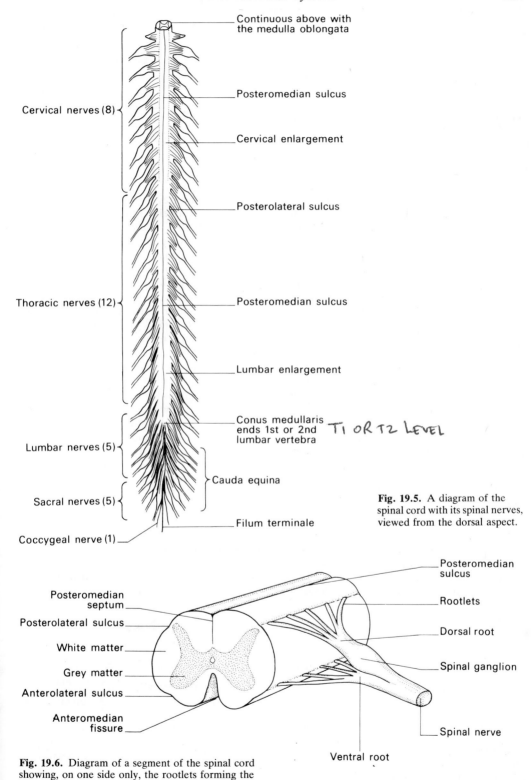

Continuous above with
the medulla oblongata

Posteromedian sulcus

Cervical nerves (8)

Cervical enlargement

Posterolateral sulcus

Thoracic nerves (12)

Posteromedian sulcus

Lumbar enlargement

Conus medullaris
ends 1st or 2nd   T1 OR T2 LEVEL
lumbar vertebra

Lumbar nerves (5)

Cauda equina

Sacral nerves (5)

Filum terminale

Coccygeal nerve (1)

Fig. 19.5. A diagram of the
spinal cord with its spinal nerves,
viewed from the dorsal aspect.

Posteromedian
sulcus

Posteromedian
septum

Rootlets

Posterolateral sulcus

Dorsal root

White matter

Grey matter

Spinal ganglion

Anterolateral sulcus

Anteromedian
fissure

Spinal nerve

Ventral root

Fig. 19.6. Diagram of a segment of the spinal cord
showing, on one side only, the rootlets forming the
ventral and dorsal roots.

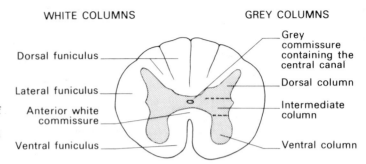

WHITE COLUMNS   GREY COLUMNS

Dorsal funiculus

Lateral funiculus

Anterior white commissure

Ventral funiculus

Grey commissure containing the central canal

Dorsal column

Intermediate column

Ventral column

Fig. 19.7. Transverse section of the spinal cord, showing the major subdivisions of white and grey matter.

to the grey commissure; the vertical limbs represent the dorsal and ventral columns with the intervening intermediate column (Fig. 19.7). In the thoracic region and the upper lumbar region the intermediate column is expanded laterally to form the lateral column. White matter is also organized into long columns or funiculi (Fig. 19.7), namely: dorsal, lateral and ventral. The ventral funiculi join in the midline forming the anterior commissure which consists of crossing fibres arising from various neurons of the grey matter.

The central canal runs through the entire length of the cord and extends into the lower part of the medulla oblongata where it communicates with the fourth ventricle. Caudally the canal ends in an expansion which sometimes opens into the subarachnoid space. The canal is lined with ciliated epithelium, the ependyma, and is filled with cerebrospinal fluid.

ORGANIZATION OF GREY MATTER
(Figs. 18.8 & 19.9)

The grey matter of the cord contains numerous multipolar neurons which show considerable variation in the size and shape of their cell body processes. These neurons fall into two broad categories; small neurons whose processes are confined to the grey matter, and larger neurons whose long axons either form fibre tracts or project peripherally as efferent fibres of the ventral spinal roots. Many of the smaller neurons are intrasegmental; that is they connect contralateral and ipsilateral cells of the same segment; these are mostly Golgi type II cells. Other cells give rise to axons of varying length which ascend or descend to form ipsilateral and contralateral connections at various segmental levels.

Examination of transverse sections of the cord reveals that nerve cells are neither randomly nor uniformly distributed, but are organized into groups or nuclei (Fig. 19.8), some of which extend throughout the length of the cord whilst others are confined to specific regions only. However, recent quantitative histological and electrophysiological studies in animals show a laminar arrangement of neurons throughout the length of the cord; the laminae lying roughly parallel with the dorsal and ventral surfaces of the grey matter (Fig. 19.9).

Dorsal grey columns
The dorsal grey columns consist of the following cell groups: the substantia gelatinosa, the dorsal funicular nucleus and the thoracic nucleus. All these groups save the last mentioned are found at all levels of the cord. The substantia gelatinosa

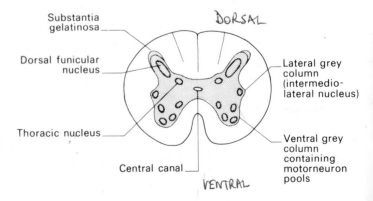

Substantia gelatinosa

Dorsal funicular nucleus

Thoracic nucleus

DORSAL

Lateral grey column (intermediolateral nucleus)

Ventral grey column containing motorneuron pools

Central canal

VENTRAL

Fig. 19.8. Transverse section of the spinal cord, showing the arrangement of nuclei in the grey matter.

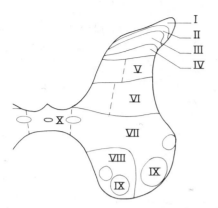

Fig. 19.9. Lamination in the grey matter of the spinal cord. Laminae I to VI represent the dorsal column, II and most of III forming the substantia gelatinosa, whilst the rest of III together with IV are equivalent to the dorsal funicular nucleus. Lamina VII represents the intermediate column including the thoracic nucleus. Lamina IX comprises the α and γ motoneuron pools of the ventral column.

consists of numerous small interneurons and some larger cells. The small cells receive connections from both large and small diameter fibres or the dorsal spinal roots and in turn are connected directly or indirectly with neurons which give rise to the spinothalamic pathways. It is suggested that the substantia gelatinosa is functionally concerned with pain mechanisms (p. 317).

The dorsal funicular nucleus is a poorly defined cell column containing small and medium sized interneurons as well as larger neurons which give rise to the long crossed spinothalamic tracts. A group of strikingly large neurons, the thoracic nucleus of Clarke, is present in the thoracic and upper lumbar segments only. Axons of these large neurons form the dorsal spinocerebellar tract.

Lateral grey columns
These columns extend from the first thoracic segment as far as the second lumbar segment. Most of the nerve cells situated here are preganglionic sympathetic neurons whose axons leave the cord in the ventral spinal roots and pass via white rami communicantes into the ganglionated sympathetic trunk.

In the second, third and fourth sacral segments there are preganglionic parasympathetic neurons whose axons emerge as 'pelvic' splanchnic nerves and synapse with postganglionic cells located in parasympathetic ganglia of the pelvic viscera.

Ventral grey columns
The ventral grey columns contain multipolar neurons of varying size: large alpha (α) motor neurons and small gamma (γ) motor neurons, as well as numerous small interneurons. The motor neurons have long axons which pass out of the spinal cord through the ventral spinal roots as motor fibres, to be distributed via spinal nerves to striated skeletal muscles.

The α-motor neurons innervate extrafusal muscle fibres. They have cell bodies which are 25–100 μm in diameter and contain large 'chunky' Nissl granules. These cells are arranged in elongated columns or nuclei within the ventral grey columns. Small motor neurons (cell body diameter 10–25 μm) give rise to gamma (γ) efferent fibres which supply intrafusal fibres of muscle spindles located in skeletal muscle (p. 330). These nerve cells lie in and around the nuclear groups of α-motoneurons.

The columnar groups of motoneurons are not haphazardly arranged, but are somatotopically organized although the precise arrangement, especially in man, is controversial. Generally speaking, it appears that medial cell groups which are present through the length of the cord supply muscles of the trunk and neck; the lateral cell groups, located in the cervical and lumbar enlargements, innervate muscles of the limbs.

FIBRE TRACTS OF THE SPINAL CORD

The ascending and descending fibres of the spinal cord are organized into bundles which are more or less confined to specific regions in the white columns or funiculi (Fig. 19.10). Fibre bundles having the same source, course and termination are known as tracts or fasciculi, and are usually named according to their origin and destination. For example the spinocerebellar tracts denote bundles of fibres which arise from neurons in the spinal cord and terminate in the cerebellum; the vestibulospinal tracts arise from cells of one of the vestibular nuclei and end by synapsing with neurons of the spinal cord.

Ascending tracts
Dorsal white columns (Fasciculus cuneatus and Fasciculus gracilis) (Fig. 19.10). These columns are composed of heavily myelinated axons which originate from unipolar cells (primary afferent neurons) situated in dorsal root ganglia. The axons enter the spinal cord through the medial part of each and every dorsal root. Each dorsal column in the upper region of the cord is divided by a pial septum into a medial fasciculus gracilis

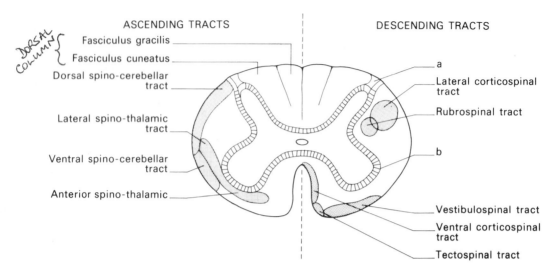

Fig. 19.10. Diagram of a transverse section of the spinal cord, showing the major tracts. Ascending tracts are shown on the left: descending on the right. (a) is the posterolateral tract and (b), the hatched region, indicates the intersegmental tracts lying around the periphery of the grey matter.

which carries sensory information from the lower limb and lower part of the trunk, and a lateral faciculus cuneatus which conveys sensory information from the upper trunk and upper limb. Each fasciculus continues into the medulla where its fibres end by forming synapses on nerve cells (secondary afferent neurons) of the nucleus gracilis and nucleus cuneatus respectively. Axons of these secondary neurons constitute the internal arcuate fibres which after crossing the midline ascend through the brainstem as a discrete bundle known as the medial lemniscus (Fig. 19.11). The latter then terminates in neurons of the ventroposterolateral nucleus of the thalamus. These neurons constitute the tertiary afferent neurons in this sensory pathway and in turn are the source of axons which relay to the postcentral gyrus (sensory cortex).

Functionally, the fasciculi gracilis and cuneatus convey impulses from receptors in muscles, tendons, ligaments and joints which give rise to sensations of movement and position (conscious proprioception). They also conduct impulses concerned with tactile localization and discrimination as well as pressure and vibration sensibilities.

Lateral and ventral spinothalamic tracts (Fig. 19.12). The neurons whose axons form the spinothalmic tracts are found in the dorsal funicular nucleus. They are usually regarded as secondary afferent neurons which receive input directly from axons of dorsal root ganglionic cells (primary afferent neurons) via dorsal roots (but see substantia gelatinosa: p. 839). Axons from these secondary neurons ascend one or two cord segments then cross obliquely in the anterior white commissure to form the spinothalamic tract on the opposite side of the cord.

The lateral spinothalamic tract runs the length of the cord, gradually accumulating more and more fibres as it ascends. In the brainstem the tract becomes known as the spinal lemniscus which in the region of the midbrain lies superficially in the tegmentum closely related to the medial lemniscus. The fibres terminate in the thalamus, by synapsing with neurons (tertiary neurons) of the ventroposterolateral nucleus which then relay to the postcentral gyrus (sensory cortex). This pathway conveys impulses from the limbs and trunk concerned with pain and thermal sense (p. 314).

The ventral spinothalamic tract ascends through the brainstem and at pontine levels joins the medial lemniscus and continues rostrally to end in the thalamus. Here, neurons of the ventroposterolateral nucleus relay to the sensory cortex. Functionally, this tract is chiefly concerned with crude tactile and possibly pressure sensations.

Ventral and dorsal spinocerebellar tracts (Fig. 19.13). The spinocerebellar tracts are situated

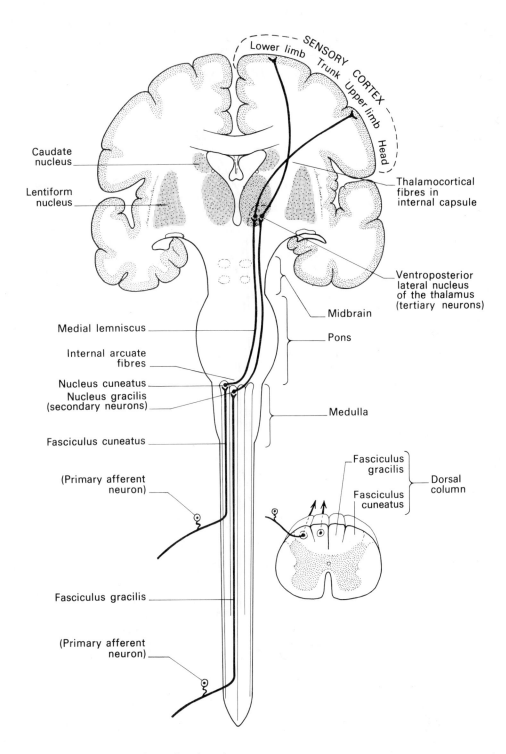

Fig. 19.11. Schematic diagram of a section through the brain and spinal cord, showing the dorsal column – medial lemniscal pathway.

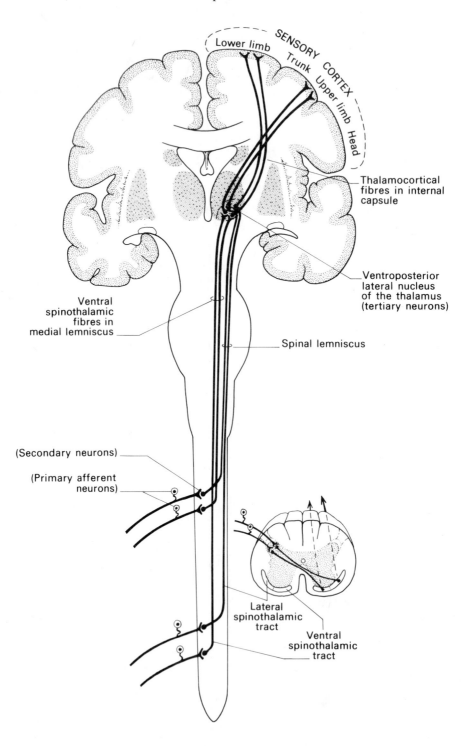

Fig. 19.12. Schematic diagram of the spinothalamic
pathways. See Fig. 19.11 for the names of the
main regions of the brain.

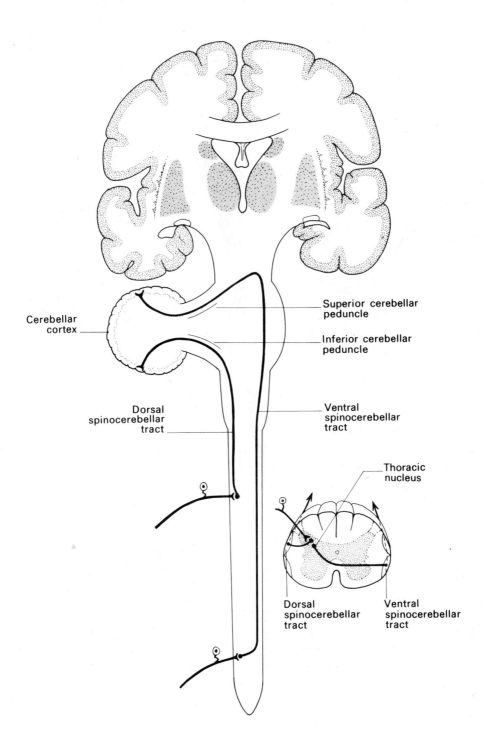

Fig. 19.13. Schematic diagram of the spinocerebellar pathways. See Fig. 19.11 for the names of the main regions of the brain.

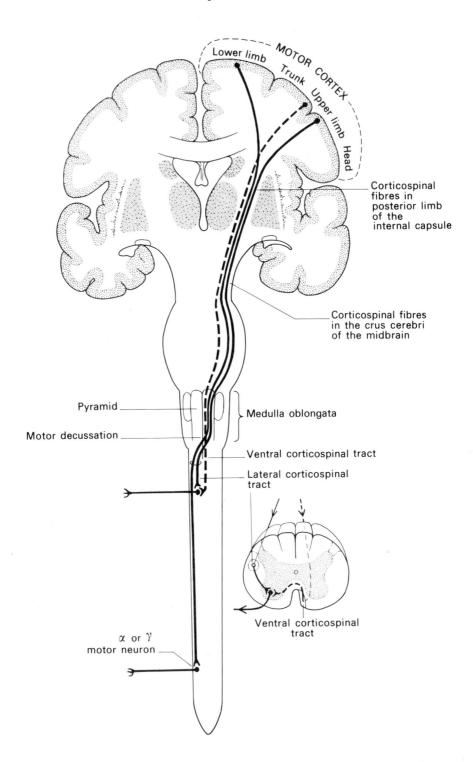

Fig. 19.14. Schematic diagram of the corticospinal tracts.

close to each other in the peripheral zone of the lateral funiculus. The dorsal spinocerebellar tract lies in front of the incoming fibres of the dorsal roots: the ventral spinocerebellar lies behind the outgoing fibres of the ventral roots.

The dorsal tract consists predominantly of uncrossed fibres arising from secondary neurons in the dorsal grey columns. These neurons form a distinct nucleus, the thoracic or dorsal nucleus, which is confined mainly to the thoracic region of the cord. The tract ascends as far as the medulla oblongata, then passes via the inferior cerebellar peduncle to end in the cerebellar cortex.

The ventral spinocerebellar tract is principally composed of crossed fibres arising from secondary neurons situated in the dorsal grey columns of the lumbosacral region of the cord. The tract takes a more circuitous route than its partner, for it ascends to the level of the upper pons before passing to the cerebellar cortex via the superior cerebellar peduncle.

Neurons contributing fibres to the spinocerebellar tracts receive proprioceptive and exteroceptive information from the lower limbs and trunk via afferent fibres of primary neurons which are situated in the dorsal root ganglia. However information of a similar nature from the upper limbs and neck is partly relayed in the dorsal white columns to nuclei in the medulla and thence to the cerebellum via the inferior cerebellar peduncles.

Descending tracts
Corticospinal tracts (Fig. 19.14). The corticospinal tracts are important motor pathways extending from the cerebral cortex to the spinal cord. Fibres forming these tracts descend from the cortex through the internal capsule of the cerebrum (p. 872), traverse the cerebral crus of the midbrain, then pass through the pons and enter the pyramid of the medulla oblongata. At the caudal level of the medulla the majority (70–90%) of corticospinal fibres cross in the motor or pyramidal decussation and descend in the cord as the lateral corticospinal tract; the remainder of the fibres pass through the pyramid without crossing and enter the spinal cord as the ventral corticospinal tract. Fibres of this tract then descend and cross the midline in the anterior white commisure to terminate on the opposite side of the cord.

The ventral corticospinal tract is confined to the cervical region of the cord, whereas the lateral corticospinal tract extends through the length of the cord. Fibres of both tracts termi-nate by synapsing on motor and interneurons. The corticospinal pathways convey impulses to the spinal cord which result in voluntary movements (p. 472).

Rubrospinal, vestibulospinal and tectospinal tracts (Fig. 19.15). All these tracts arise from specific groups of neurons situated in the brainstem. They convey impulses to the spinal cord and influence, either directly or indirectly through interneurons, the activity of α and γ motor neurons (p. 470, Fig. 10.48).

The rubrospinal tract consists of crossed fibres arising from cells of the red nucleus which are situated in the midbrain. The fibres descend in the lateral funiculus as a compact bundle lying ventral to the lateral corticospinal tract.

The vestibulospinal tract is derived from axons of cells in the lateral vestibular nucleus, located in the region of the pontomedullary junction. This nucleus receives impulses from the vestibular apparatus and cerebellum and plays a role in balance and postural activities. The tract is composed of uncrossed fibres which descend in the peripheral zone of the ventral funiculus.

The tectospinal tract lies sandwiched between the ventral corticospinal and vestibulospinal tracts. Fibres of the tract arise from neurons of the contralateral superior colliculus. The superior colliculus is situated in the tectum of the midbrain and is an important centre for visual as well as auditory reflexes. Tectospinal fibres mediate reflex postural and head turning movements in response to visual and auditory stimuli.

Intersegmental tracts and the posterolateral tract
Ipsilateral and contralateral connections between cord segments are maintained by short ascending and descending fibres which arise from dorsal column neurons. These fibres form intersegmental tracts which lie around the margins of the grey matter. The posterolateral tract (of Lissauer) is a small bundle lying between the tip of the posterior column and the surface of the cord. It is composed mainly of intersegmental fibres, but also contains fine myelinated fibres of the lateral division of the dorsal root which bifurcate into short ascending and descending branches before terminating on cells in the substantia gelatinosa. These tracts are shown in Fig. 19.10.

The brainstem

The spinal cord is connected to the forebrain by

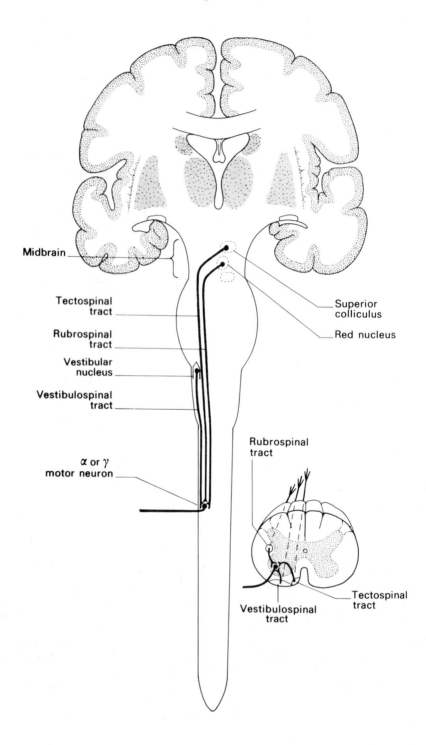

Fig. 19.15. Schematic diagram of the tectospinal,
rubrospinal and vestibulospinal tracts.

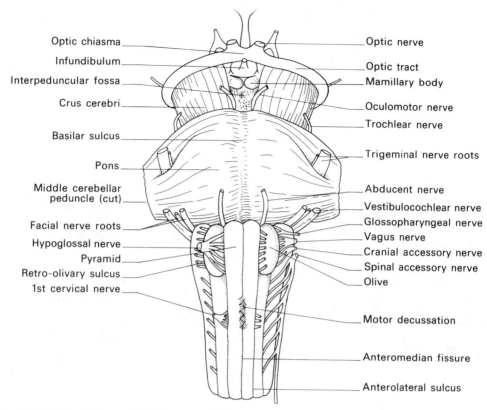

Optic chiasma — Optic nerve
Infundibulum — Optic tract
Interpeduncular fossa — Mamillary body
Crus cerebri — Oculomotor nerve
— Trochlear nerve
Basilar sulcus — Trigeminal nerve roots
Pons — Abducent nerve
Middle cerebellar peduncle (cut) — Vestibulocochlear nerve
— Glossopharyngeal nerve
Facial nerve roots — Vagus nerve
Hypoglossal nerve — Cranial accessory nerve
Pyramid — Spinal accessory nerve
Retro-olivary sulcus — Olive
1st cervical nerve — Motor decussation
— Anteromedian fissure
— Anterolateral sulcus

Fig. 19.16. Ventral aspect of the brainstem and the interpeduncular fossa.

the brainstem, composed of the medulla oblongata, pons and midbrain. The greater part of the dorsal and to some extent the lateral surfaces of the brainstem are hidden from view in the intact brain. But, when the forebrain and the cerebellum are removed all the surfaces are exposed. The ventral and dorsal surfaces are illustrated in Figs. 19.16 and 19.17 which show the main external features. Most of the brainstem, together with the cerebellum, lies in the posterior cranial fossa, save for the midbrain which projects into the middle cranial fossa. All the cranial nerves with the exception of the olfactory and optic are attached to the brainstem.

MEDULLA OBLONGATA

The medulla oblongata is the cranial continuation of the cervical part of the spinal cord, and extends from the lower border of the foramen magnum to the lower border of the pons. In shape it is somewhat conical: in length, about 30mm.

External features
The medulla oblongata, seen from the ventral aspect (Fig. 19.16), possesses sulci which are in continuity with those of the spinal cord. Thus, the anteromedian fissure extends rostrally to the lower border of the pons. Flanking each side of the fissure is the pyramid, a bundle composed of corticospinal fibres. Most of these fibres cross obliquely in the lower part of the medulla forming the motor or pyramidal decussation which partly obliterates the anteromedian fissure. The anterolateral sulcus separates the pyramid from the olive, formed by the underlying inferior olivary nucleus. Through this sulcus emerge rootlets forming the hypoglossal nerve (in the region of the olive) and the root of the abducent nerve (at the pontomedullary junction). Emerging from the retro-olivary sulcus are the rootlets of the cranial accessory, vagus and glossopharyngeal nerves in caudorostral sequence.

The dorsal aspect of the medulla oblongata (Fig. 19.17) presents the posteromedian sulcus, flanked on each side by the dorsal column of

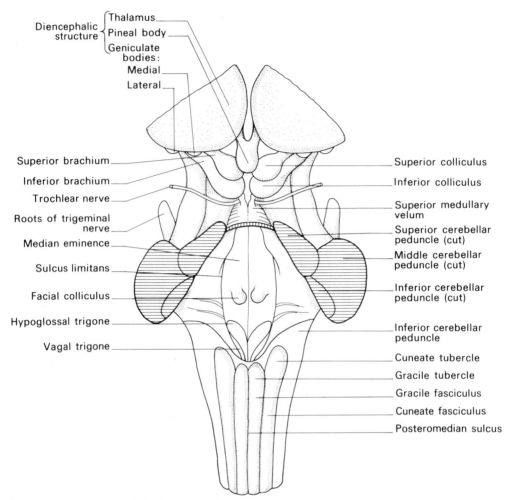

Diencephalic structure
- Thalamus
- Pineal body
- Geniculate bodies:
  - Medial
  - Lateral

Superior brachium
Inferior brachium
Trochlear nerve
Roots of trigeminal nerve
Median eminence
Sulcus limitans
Facial colliculus
Hypoglossal trigone
Vagal trigone

Superior colliculus
Inferior colliculus
Superior medullary velum
Superior cerebellar peduncle (cut)
Middle cerebellar peduncle (cut)
Inferior cerebellar peduncle (cut)
Inferior cerebellar peduncle
Cuneate tubercle
Gracile tubercle
Gracile fasciculus
Cuneate fasciculus
Posteromedian sulcus

Fig. 19.17. Dorsal aspect of the brainstem. The cerebellum has been removed to show the floor of the fourth ventricle.

white matter consisting of the gracile and cuneate fasciculi. Each fasciculus ends in a similarly named tubercle, composed of grey matter (see gracile and cuneate nuclei, p. 840). The upper part of the medulla is bounded posterolaterally on each side by the inferior cerebellar peduncle, a bundle of nerve fibres which enters the cerebellum. The dorsal medullary surface lying between these peduncles and bounded below by the cuneate and gracile tubercles forms the caudal part of the floor of the fourth ventricle (p. 858).

Internal structure of the medulla oblongata
The internal structure of the medulla oblongata whilst showing many features of spinal cord

organization at caudal levels, undergoes considerable modifications as cranial levels are approached. The major changes involved are the following:
1   The disruption of the central grey matter by the decussation of the corticospinal fibres;
2   The termination of the fasciculi cuneatus and gracilis in their respective nuclei which in turn give rise to crossed fibres forming the medial lemnisci;
3   The development of cranial nerve nuclei, and also relay nuclei;
4   The development of the fourth ventricle.

(It must be remembered that a nucleus in the central nervous system refers to a collection of cell bodies and usually implies a relay station

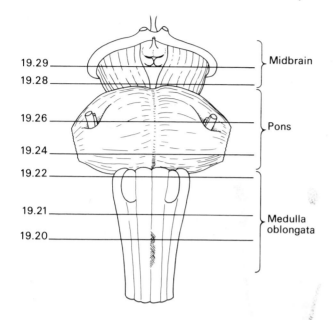

19.29 — Midbrain
19.28 —

19.26 — Pons
19.24 —

19.22 —

19.21 — Medulla
19.20 — oblongata

Fig. 19.18. Ventral aspect of the brainstem, showing the approximate levels of transverse sections represented in later figs.

between different neurons by means of a synapse.)

The above and other features will be examined in more detail by reference to transverse sections at appropriate levels through the medulla oblongata. The levels of these sections and the disposition of the cranial nerve nuclei in profile in the brain stem are shown in Figs. 19.18 & 19.19.

A transverse section through the lowest part of the medulla oblongata shows several noteworthy features (Fig. 19.20). Most conspicuous is the pyramidal decussation. Fibres leave each pyramid, cross in the median plane anterior to the central grey matter, and reach the lateral funiculus of the opposite side where they descend as the lateral corticospinal tract. Some fibres leave the pyramid without crossing and descend into the anterior funiculus of the spinal cord to form the ventral corticospinal tract.

The dorsal columns of white matter also undergo changes. The dorsal funiculus is gradually replaced by two dorsal expansions of grey matter, the gracile and cuneate nuclei. The substantia gelatinosa enlarges and is now termed the nucleus of the spinal tract of the trigeminal nerve. It receives primary afferent fibres from the trigeminal sensory root. These fibres descend from the pons as a bundle, the spinal tract.

Just above the pyramidal decussation (Fig. 19.21) the gracile and cuneate nuclei are very prominent and receive the terminating fibres of the gracile and cuneate fasciculi. Cells of these nuclei are the source of internal arcuate fibres which sweep across the midline to form a narrow bundle or fillet of ascending fibres, the medial lemniscus, destined to end in the thalamus.

The spinal nucleus and the spinal tract of the trigeminal nerve extend through this section. Within the central grey matter new coextensive cell columns associated with cranial nerves appear and continue cranially to the upper level of the medulla. They are the nucleus of the tractus solitarius, the dorsal nucleus of the vagus, the nucleus ambiguus and the hypoglossal nucleus, the latter two being continuous with the cell columns of the spinal accessory nerve and the first cervical nerve respectively.

A transverse section through the upper medulla (Fig. 19.22) shows an expansion in width due to an increase in grey matter associated with nuclei of olive and cranial nerves. The central canal has moved dorsally to open into the fourth ventricle, the grey matter surrounding it now forming the floor of the ventricle and containing certain cranial nerve nuclei.

The hypoglossal nucleus lies subjacent to the hypoglossal trigone, and close to the median plane. Axons from cells of the hypoglossal nucleus pass ventrally to emerge as a series of rootlets on the surface in the anterolateral sulcus between the pyramid and olive. The rootlets form the hypoglossal nerve which supplies stri-

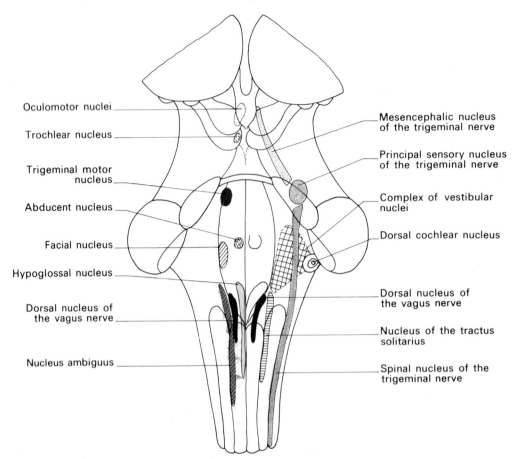

Oculomotor nuclei

Trochlear nucleus

Trigeminal motor nucleus

Abducent nucleus

Facial nucleus

Hypoglossal nucleus

Dorsal nucleus of the vagus nerve

Nucleus ambiguus

Mesencephalic nucleus of the trigeminal nerve

Principal sensory nucleus of the trigeminal nerve

Complex of vestibular nuclei

Dorsal cochlear nucleus

Dorsal nucleus of the vagus nerve

Nucleus of the tractus solitarius

Spinal nucleus of the trigeminal nerve

Fig. 19.19. Surface projection of the nuclei of the cranial nerves on the dorsal aspect of the brainstem. Motor nuclei are shown on the left side; sensory nuclei on the right.

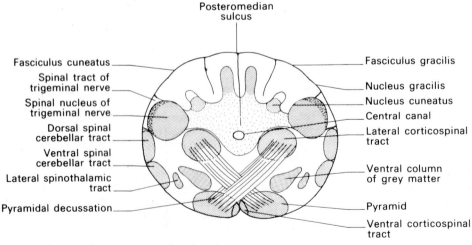

Posteromedian sulcus

Fasciculus cuneatus

Spinal tract of trigeminal nerve

Spinal nucleus of trigeminal nerve

Dorsal spinal cerebellar tract

Ventral spinal cerebellar tract

Lateral spinothalamic tract

Pyramidal decussation

Fasciculus gracilis

Nucleus gracilis

Nucleus cuneatus

Central canal

Lateral corticospinal tract

Ventral column of grey matter

Pyramid

Ventral corticospinal tract

Fig. 19.20. Diagram of a transverse section through the motor or pyramidal decussation, see Fig. 19.18 for the level.

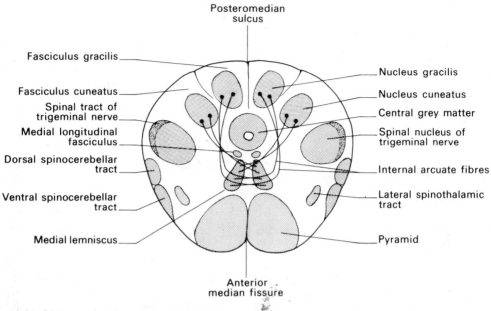

Fig. 19.21. Diagram of a transverse section of the medulla oblongata through the sensory decussation formed by crossing internal arcuate fibres. See Fig. 19.18 for the level.

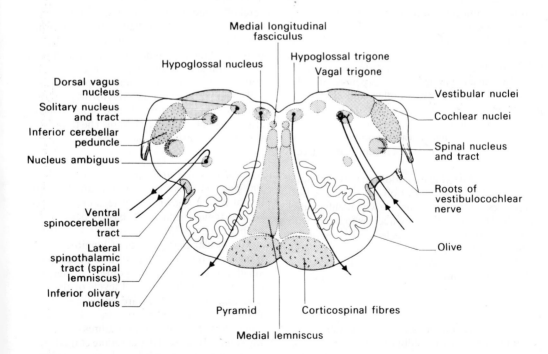

Fig. 19.22. Diagram of a transverse section of the medulla oblongata through the upper part of the olive. See Fig. 19.18 for the level.

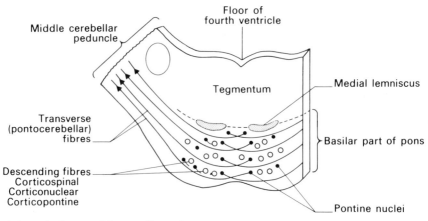

Floor of
fourth ventricle

Middle cerebellar
peduncle

Tegmentum

Medial lemniscus

Transverse
(pontocerebellar)
fibres

Basilar part of pons

Descending fibres
Corticospinal
Corticonuclear
Corticopontine

Pontine nuclei

Fig. 19.23. Schematic diagram of the pons illustrating the main regions and the components of the basilar part.

ated muscles of the tongue. The dorsal nucleus of the vagus lies lateral to the hypoglossal nucleus and subjacent to the vagal trigone. It is the source of the preganglionic vagal fibres which are distributed to terminal parasympathetic ganglia innervating thoracic and abdominal viscera.

A distinctive bundle of descending fibres, the tractus solitarius is intimately associated with a group of neurons, the nucleus of the tractus solitarius. The tract is formed by primary afferent fibres of the facial, glossopharyngeal and vagus nerves. It is concerned with taste sensation.

The nucleus ambiguus lies deep in the medulla between the olivary complex and the spinal nucleus of the trigeminal nerve. It contains motor neurons whose axons are distributed by the glossopharyngeal, vagus and cranial accessory nerves to striated muscles derived from certain branchial arches.

The most striking new addition to the medulla at this level is the inferior olivary nucleus which appears as a sac-like structure with highly folded walls. The inferior olivary nucleus together with the accessory olivary nuclei form important medullary cerebellar relay centres, receiving afferent fibres from the spinal cord, subcortical and cortical sources.

PONS

The pons is continuous with the medulla oblongata below, and the midbrain above. It lies ventral to the cerebellum and the fourth ventricle.

External features
Seen from the ventral aspect the pons is convex

from above downwards and from side to side (Fig. 19.16); and it is clearly demarcated from the medulla oblongata by a transverse groove out of which the abducent, facial and vestibulocochlear nerves escape. Closer inspection of this surface shows transversely orientated bundles of fibres which sweep across the midline to form on each side a large bundle, the middle cerebellar peduncle. The midline of this pontine surface is marked by a shallow furrow in which runs the basilar artery. The two roots, motor and sensory, of the trigeminal nerve emerge through the ventral surface of the pons, the motor root being smaller and more medially placed.

The dorsal aspect of the pons forms part of the floor of the fourth ventricle and is only exposed after removal of the cerebellum. The floor of the ventricle is considered on p. 858).

Internal structure of the pons
The pons in transverse section is divided into a dorsal region known as the tegmentum, and a ventral region termed the basilar part or pons proper (Fig. 19.23).

The basilar part consists of longitudinal and transverse fibres interspersed with numerous small islets of cells, the pontine nuclei. This arrangement is found at all levels of the pons. The longitudinal fibres are corticospinal, corticonuclear and corticopontine. From their names it is clear that all these fibres originate in the cerebral cortex. They enter the cranial end of the pons as a compact bundle but in the midpontine region this is broken up into numerous smaller bundles by the transversely orientated pontine fibres. The corticospinal fibres reform at the

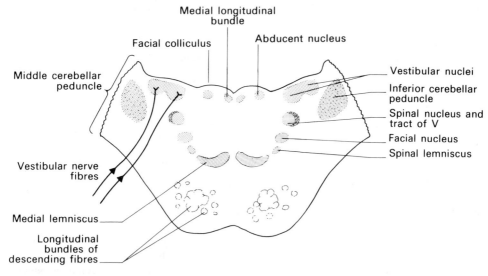

Medial longitudinal bundle

Facial colliculus

Abducent nucleus

Middle cerebellar peduncle

Vestibular nuclei

Inferior cerebellar peduncle

Spinal nucleus and tract of V

Facial nucleus

Spinal lemniscus

Vestibular nerve fibres

Medial lemniscus

Longitudinal bundles of descending fibres

Fig. 19.24. Diagram of a transverse section of the pons through the facial colliculus. See Fig. 19.18 for the level.

caudal end of the pons into a large, discrete bundle which enters the medulla oblongata as the pyramid. Corticonuclear fibres end by synapsing, either directly or indirectly (via interneurons), on motor neurons of cranial nerve nuclei. The majority of these fibres cross to the opposite side before terminating. Corticonuclear fibres like corticospinal fibres are part of the motor system; whereas corticopontine fibres are concerned with cerebellar activities. They establish synapses with homolateral pontine nuclei. The transverse fibres of the pons (pontocerebellar fibres) leave these nuclei and cross the median plane to form the middle cerebellar peduncle.

The tegmentum of the pons, unlike the basilar part, shows variation throughout its length which will be illustrated by two transverse sections through the pons.

At the level of the facial colliculus (Fig. 19.24) are the motor nuclei of the abducent and facial nerves, and also nuclei associated with the vestibulocochlear nerve. The abducent nucleus lies close to the median plane beneath the facial colliculus (Fig. 19.25). Its fibres leave at the lower border of the pons to supply the lateral rectus muscle.

The motor nucleus of the facial nerve is situated laterally in the tegmentum. Its fibres supply striated muscles derived from the second branchial arch which include the 'muscles of facial expression.' These outgoing fibres take a curious

'looped' course before leaving the brainstem at the lower pontine border (Fig. 19.25). Near the rostral pole of the abducent nucleus the facial nerve bundle turns sharply; this loop together with the abducent nucleus form a bulge, the facial colliculus, in the floor of the fourth ventricle.

The nucleus of the spinal tract of the trigeminal nerve is still present at this level and continues to the upper part of the pons where it is replaced by the principal sensory nucleus of the trigeminal nerve. The associated spinal tract is formed of descending sensory root fibres derived from unipolar cells of the trigeminal ganglion (Fig. 19.71). These fibres terminate on cells of the spinal nucleus whose axons cross to the opposite side of the pons forming an ascending bundle, the trigeminal lemniscus, which is destined for the thalamus. The connections and function of the trigeminal motor and sensory nuclei are considered on p. 904.

The cranial part of the pons (Fig. 19.26) shows several noteworthy features which include the appearance of the motor and principal sensory nuclei of the trigeminal nerve, and also the convergence of the medial, spinal and trigeminal lemniscal pathways.

The lemnisci unite into one transversely orientated bundle. This lies in the ventral part of the tegmentum, and is gradually moving laterally as it ascends to terminate in the thalamus. All these lemnisci consist of crossed axons of secondary

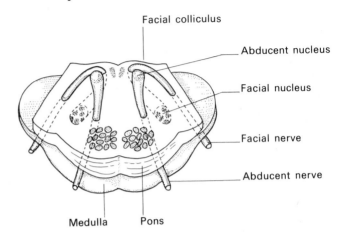

Facial colliculus

Abducent nucleus

Facial nucleus

Facial nerve

Abducent nerve

Medulla   Pons

Fig. 19.25. Diagram of the internal course of the facial nerve and its relationship to the abducent nucleus, viewed from the superior aspect of a transverse section of the pons.

neurons on the sensory pathways and therefore bring information from the opposite side of the body. The medial lemniscus together with axons from the principal sensory nucleus of the trigeminal nerve convey impulses subserving pressure and tactile modalities as well as proprioceptive information; the spinal lemniscus (lateral spinothalamic tract) and the trigeminal lemniscus mediate impulses concerned with pain and thermal sensation. Thus, the lemnisci are functionally organized; furthermore, they are also somatotopically arranged in the following manner. Fibres conveying impulses from the head and neck lie in the medial part of the lemniscal bundle, those from the upper limb and trunk are centrally placed, whilst those from the lower limb are laterally situated.

Another bundle, the lateral lemniscus, accompanies the united lemniscal bundles. It forms part of the cochlear pathways which are considered elsewhere (p. 883).

MIDBRAIN

The midbrain is the smallest part of the brainstem, being only about 2 cm in length. It connects the pons and cerebellum to the forebrain. Running through the midbrain is a canal, the cerebral aqueduct (Fig. 19.27), which opens into the fourth ventricle below and the third ventricle above. For descriptive purposes the midbrain is divided into a dorsal part or tectum, and a ventral part which is composed of two symmetrical halves, the cerebral peduncles. The plane of

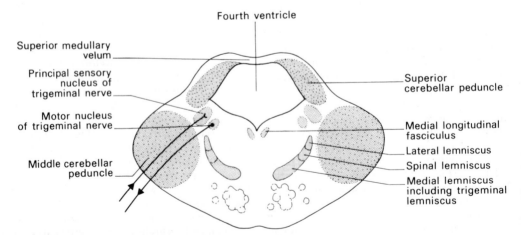

Fourth ventricle

Superior medullary velum

Principal sensory nucleus of trigeminal nerve

Motor nucleus of trigeminal nerve

Middle cerebellar peduncle

Superior cerebellar peduncle

Medial longitudinal fasciculus

Lateral lemniscus

Spinal lemniscus

Medial lemniscus including trigeminal lemniscus

Fig. 19.26. Diagram of a transverse section of the pons through the motor nucleus of the trigeminal nerve. See Fig. 19.18 for the level.

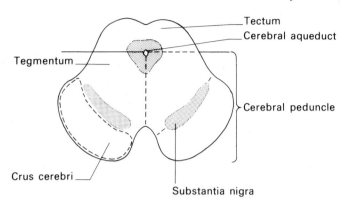

Tectum
Cerebral aqueduct

Tegmentum

Cerebral peduncle

Crus cerebri

Substantia nigra

Fig. 19.27. Diagram showing the major regions of the midbrain in transverse section.

division is taken through the cerebral aqueduct. The ventral part is further subdivided into the tegmentum, continuous below with the pontine tegmentum, and the crura cerebri consisting of a massive pair of fibre bundles.

External features

Seen from the ventral aspect (Fig. 19.16) the crura cerebri appear as pillar-like structures which converge on to the upper border of the pons. They form the lateral borders of the *interpeduncular fossa*, which is limited rostrally by the optic tracts and chiasma. The surface of the upper part of the fossa, though not derived from the midbrain, is included here for convenience. It shows a pair of rounded elevations, the mamillary bodies, and also a median eminence out of which arises the stalk of the pituitary gland (hypophysis cerebri).

The dorsal aspect of the midbrain (Fig. 19.17) consists of the tectum which comprises four rounded elevations, the colliculi. Caudally the tectum becomes continuous with the superior cerebellar peduncles and the intervening superior medullary velum which form the roof of the superior part of the fourth ventricle. Cranially the tectum merges with the diencephalic part of the forebrain, and is partly overlapped by the pineal body in the midline and also the pulvinar of the thalamus on each side.

The colliculi forming the tectum are arranged in pairs, the inferior and superior colliculi, which are centres concerned with auditory and visual reflexes respectively. Each colliculus is connected with the thalamus by a superficially placed bundle of fibres, the brachium, which arises from the lateral margin of the colliculus. The brachium of the inferior colliculus runs to the medial geniculate body; whilst the brachium of the superior colliculus is formed partly of

optic tract fibres and also of fibres from the visual cortical area. Both geniculate bodies form elevations on the caudal part of the undersurface of the thalamus and are closely apposed to the dorsolateral surface of the midbrain. The trochlear nerves are also seen on the dorsal surface of the midbrain, emerging caudal to the inferior colliculus.

Internal structure of the midbrain

The major features of the internal structure of the midbrain are illustrated by two transverse sections, one through the inferior colliculus, the other through the superior colliuculus (Figs. 19.28 & 19.29).

Certain elements, namely the crus cerebri consisting of corticospinal, corticonuclear and corticopontine fibres (see p. 845), and in addition the mesencephalic nucleus and the substantia nigra extend throughout the midbrain.

The mesencephalic nucleus of the trigeminal nerve consists of unipolar cells which are found in isolated groups around the lateral margin of the periaqueductal grey (for connections and function, see p. 904).

The substantia nigra is a layer of neurons containing melanin pigment and forms part of the extrapyramidal motor system (p. 473).

It has connections with the cerebral cortex, basal ganglia, brainstem and spinal cord. One of the major efferent pathways (nigrostriatal) terminates principally in the caudate nucleus (p. 866).

At the level of the inferior colliculus (Fig. 19.28) the superior cerebellar decussation and the trochlear are seen, the latter supplying efferent fibres to the superior oblique muscle. The decussation of the superior cerebellar peduncles occupies the central region of the tegmentum. The fibres, after crossing, terminate in the red

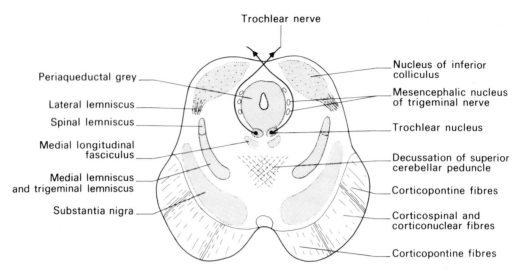

Trochlear nerve

Periaqueductal grey

Lateral lemniscus

Spinal lemniscus

Medial longitudinal fasciculus

Medial lemniscus and trigeminal lemniscus

Substantia nigra

Nucleus of inferior colliculus

Mesencephalic nucleus of trigeminal nerve

Trochlear nucleus

Decussation of superior cerebellar peduncle

Corticopontine fibres

Corticospinal and corticonuclear fibres

Corticopontine fibres

Fig. 19.28. Diagram of a transverse section of the midbrain through the inferior colliculus. See Fig. 19.18 for the level.

nucleus and also in the ventrolateral nucleus of the thalamus, thus establishing dentato-rubro-thalamic connections. The lemniscal pathways form a curved bundle in transverse section on the lateral side of the tegmentum just dorsal to the substantia nigra. The lateral lemniscus is most superficially placed, some of its fibres terminating at this level in the inferior collicular nucleus, the remainder passing via the inferior

brachium to the medial geniculate body. The spinal, trigeminal and medial lemnisci continue through the midbrain and terminate in the ventroposterior nucleus of the thalamus.

At the level of the superior colliculus the red nucleus is a conspicuous structure (Fig. 19.29), readily seen in section with the unaided eye. It receives afferent fibres from the cerebral cortex and the dentate nucleus of the cerebellum. It

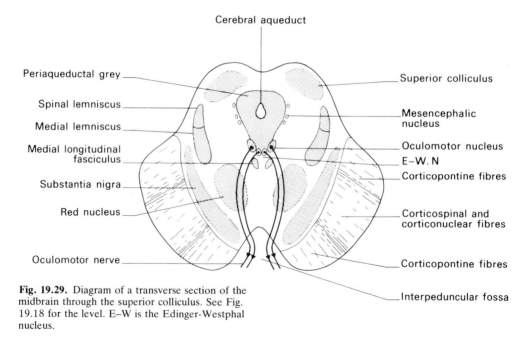

Cerebral aqueduct

Periaqueductal grey

Spinal lemniscus

Medial lemniscus

Medial longitudinal fasciculus

Substantia nigra

Red nucleus

Oculomotor nerve

Superior colliculus

Mesencephalic nucleus

Oculomotor nucleus

E–W. N

Corticopontine fibres

Corticospinal and corticonuclear fibres

Corticopontine fibres

Interpeduncular fossa

Fig. 19.29. Diagram of a transverse section of the midbrain through the superior colliculus. See Fig. 19.18 for the level. E–W is the Edinger-Westphal nucleus.

projects fibres to the ventrolateral nucleus of the thalamus, and sends axons which cross the median plane to descend as the rubrospinal tract. Also found at this level are the oculomotor and Edinger–Westphal nuclei. The former supplies certain extraocular muscles and also the levator palpebri superioris; the latter gives rise to preganglionic parasympathetic fibres destined for the ciliary ganglion (p. 882).

The medial longitudinal fasciculus extends throughout the length of the brainstem, some of its fibres descending into the spinal cord. It consists of ascending and descending fibres from several sources, but the majority are efferent fibres from the vestibular nuclear complex, which terminate on motor nuclei supplying ocular muscles, and on motor neurons innervating cervical muscles. Functionally, this system coordinates movements of the eyes and head in response to stimuli from the vestibular apparatus.

Tectum of the midbrain

The inferior colliculus (Fig. 19.17) consists internally of a compact mass of neurons termed the inferior collicular nucleus which receives impulses from the cochlear via the lateral lem-niscus and relays them to the medial geniculate body and subsequently to the auditory cortex (p. 884). The nucleus also receives information from the medial geniculate body and the auditory cortex, as well as establishing connections with all the other colliculi, superior and also inferior. Functionally, the inferior colliculi are cochlear reflex centres concerned with localizing the direction of sound and also with head turning movements in response to auditory stimuli. The cochlear system is considered on p. 969.

The superior colliculus receives impulses from a wide variety of afferents which include fibres from the retina (visual input), from the spinal cord (tactile, thermal and pain stimuli), from the inferior colliculi (auditory input) and from the occipital cortex. It projects mostly crossed fibres to the brainstem, particularly to nuclei innervating ocular muscles, to the cerebellum and to the spinal cord. The latter structure receives efferents from the superior colliculus via the tectospinal tract. Electrophysiological evidence from animal experiments suggests that the superior colliculi are integrating centres responsible for movements of eyes, ears, head, trunk and limbs in response to visual and also auditory stimuli.

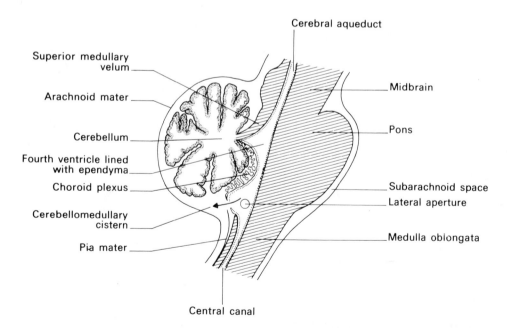

Fig. 19.30. Diagram of a sagittal section through the hindbrain, showing the fourth ventricle. Note that the ventricle is continuous with the cerebral aqueduct above and the central canal below; and that the ventricle opens into the subarachnoid space through apertures, a median one (see arrow) and two lateral ones.

Fourth ventricle

The position of the fourth ventricle of the hindbrain is shown in Figs. 19.17 and 19.30. It is a shallow cavity lined with ependyma.

The roof is formed from two sloping laminae or vela which meet at an acute angle to make a tent-like dorsal recess. The more rostrally situated lamina consists of a thin layer of white matter, the superior medullary velum, bounded on each side by the superior cerebellar peduncles, which also contribute to the formation of the roof (Fig. 19.26). The other lamina, termed the inferior medullary velum, consists mainly of a thin sheet of non-nervous tissue composed of pia mater and ependyma. The pia mater is arranged as a double fold, the tela choroidea, which contains vascular fringes forming the choroid plexus of the fourth ventricle. The inner aspect of the tela choroidea is covered by ependyma lining the ventricular cavity. The ventricle opens into the subarachnoid space through deficiencies in the caudal part of the roof.

The floor or rhomboid fossa is diamond-shaped, and is formed by the dorsal surface of the pons and upper part of the medulla oblongata. It is bounded on each side by the superior cerebellar peduncles above, and the cuneate and gracile tubercles below.

The hypoglossal trigone (Fig. 19.17) marks the site of the subjacent upper part of the hypoglossal nucleus and the vagal trigone lies over nuclei associated with the vagus nerve. The facial colliculus is formed by underlying root fibres of the facial nerve and also the abducent nucleus.

Cerebellum

The cerebellum, a part of the hindbrain, is situated in the posterior cranial fossa. In essence, it consists of two lateral cerebellar hemispheres joined by a narrow median portion, the vermis (Fig. 19.31). The entire surface of the cerebellum is marked by transversely running fissures with intervening folds known as folia. Some fissures are deeper than others and divide the cerebellum into lobes and numerous lobules. For our purpose the cerebellum may be regarded as consisting of three lobes, each receiving one of the three major cerebeller input channels. These do not correspond exactly to the morphological lobes and are best understood by tracing the evolution of the cerebellum (Fig. 19.32).

The primitive cerebellum or archicerebellum was probably formed by the elaboration of one of the vestibular nuclei which expanded into the roof of the primitive hindbrain. It receives mainly vestibular impulses and is primarily concerned with balance mechanisms. At a later stage in evolution more effective equilibratory mechanisms became necessary possibly as a consequence, amongst other factors, of more advanced methods of locomotion. This led to the development of an additional lobe, the paleocerebellum, which mainly receives spinocerebellar pathways. A further lobe, the neocerebellum, was later introduced. This developed hand-in-hand with the cerebral neocortex and basilar part of the pons and became a prominent feature of the mammalian cerebellum. It has connections with the cerebral cortex through the corticopontocerebellar

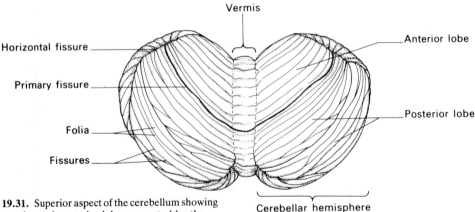

Fig. 19.31. Superior aspect of the cerebellum showing the anterior and posterior lobes separated by the primary fissure. The third morphological lobe, the flocculonodular complex, is situated on the inferior aspect of the cerebellum.

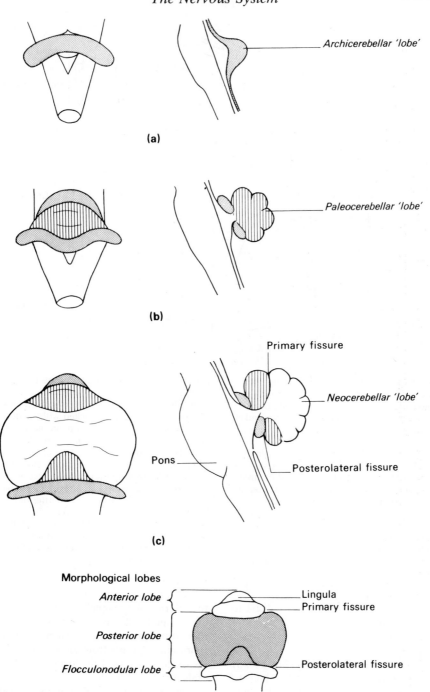

(a)

Archicerebellar 'lobe'

(b)

Paleocerebellar 'lobe'

(c)

Primary fissure

Neocerebellar 'lobe'

Pons

Posterolateral fissure

(d)

Morphological lobes

Anterior lobe

Posterior lobe

Flocculonodular lobe

Lingula
Primary fissure

Posterolateral fissure

Fig. 19.32. Diagrams showing the hypothetical stages in the evolution of the cerebellum. (a) Archicerebellum which receives vestibular input; (b) addition of paleocerebellum receiving spinocerebellar input; (c) addition of neocerebellum receiving input from the cerebral cortex via the corticopontocerebellar pathways. The cerebellum is represented in dorsal aspect on left and in sagittal aspect on the right. (d) Diagram illustrating the three morphological lobes of the cerebellum and their relationship to the 'evolutionary lobes', compare with (c).

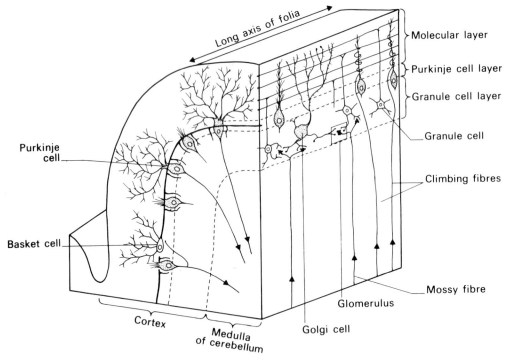

Long axis of folia

Molecular layer

Purkinje cell layer

Granule cell layer

Granule cell

Climbing fibres

Purkinje cell

Basket cell

Mossy fibre

Glomerulus

Cortex

Medulla of cerebellum

Golgi cell

Fig. 19.33. Diagram of the general organization of the cerebellar cortex represented by a slice through a folium. The cortex consists of the following three layers. (1) The molecular layer is mainly composed of processes derived from cell bodies of the deep layers, ascending afferent fibres and basket cells. The processes of basket cells are orientated in a plane perpendicular to the long axis of the folia; their dendrites are profuse; and their axons end in many collaterals which form basket-like networks around the bodies of Purkinje cells. One basket cell forms synapses with about 100 Purkinje cells. (2) Purkinje cells have flask-shaped bodies which form a single stratum between the molecular and granule cell layers. Their dendrites branch profusely into the molecular layer and are orientated, like basket cell dendrites, perpendicular to the long axis of the folia. Axons of Purkinje cells form the output pathway of the cerebellum, ending mainly on cells of roof nuclei. (3) The granule cell layer is packed with small cells, interspersed with large Golgi neurons. The small or granule cells possess short dendrites which form synaptic glomeruli with the endings of other cerebellar components. Axons of granule cells enter the molecular layer and bifurcate into long processes which run parallel with the long axis of the folia. These parallel fibres synapse on the dendrites of basket and Purkinje cells, each Purkinje cell receiving as many as 300 000 parallel fibres. Golgi cells have large dendritic fields and profuse axonal arborizations. They either form links between parallel fibres and glomeruli or inter-connect numbers of glomeruli.

pathways (p. 862). It is no longer realistic to ascribe discrete functions to particular lobes of the cerebellum (p. 473).

Internal structure of the cerebellum (Fig. 19.33) The cerebellum is composed of a surface layer of grey matter, the cortex, and a deep core of white matter, the medulla. The cortex is uniform throughout, consisting of three layers of different cell types. A very complex neuronal circuitry has been described, but its functional significance is still uncertain.

Input to the cerebellar cortex is through climbing and mossy fibres. Climbing fibres arise from the inferior olivary nucleus and end by branching around the dendrites of Purkinje cells where numerous synapses are formed. Mossy fibres represent afferents from all sources other than the olivary nucleus. They form numerous collaterals which end in glomeruli.

Output from the cerebellar cortex is through Purkinje cell axons, most of which terminate on cells of the roof nuclei situated in the medullary white matter. There are four such nuclei on each side, namely, the dentate nucleus, which is the largest and most lateral, the fastigial nucleus which is the most medial, and the emboliform and globose nuclei which form intervening col-

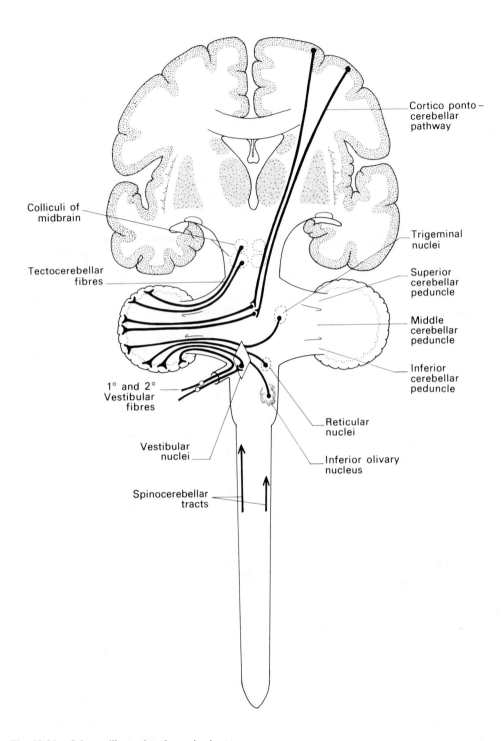

Cortico ponto-
cerebellar
pathway

Colliculi of
midbrain

Trigeminal
nuclei

Tectocerebellar
fibres

Superior
cerebellar
peduncle

Middle
cerebellar
peduncle

Inferior
cerebellar
peduncle

1° and 2°
Vestibular
fibres

Reticular
nuclei

Vestibular
nuclei

Inferior olivary
nucleus

Spinocerebellar
tracts

Fig. 19.34a. Schema illustrating the major input
(afferent pathways) of the cerebellum.
Spinocerebellar pathways are shown in more detail in
Fig. 19.13.

lections of neurons. Efferent fibres from the roof nuclei are considered below.

Connections of the cerebellum

The cerebellum is joined to the brainstem by three pairs of peduncles (Fig. 19.17) composed of afferent and efferent cerebellar fibres. The inferior cerebellar peduncles connect the upper and dorsal part of the medulla oblongata to the cerebellum, and contain fibres, mostly afferent, which arise from spinal and medullary sources. The middle cerebellar peduncles are massive bundles and emerge in continuity with the dorso-lateral parts of the pons. Curving dorsally they overlap the more medially placed superior and inferior peduncles to enter the cerebellum. They are exclusively composed of afferent fibres from the pons. The superior cerebellar peduncles are directed cranially out of the cerebellum and enter the midbrain just caudal to the inferior colliculi. They help to form the roof of the fourth ventricle and are mostly composed of fibres leaving the roof nuclei.

Afferent connections (Fig. 19.34a)

1 The *vestibulocerebellar tract* consists of primary afferent fibres of the vestibular part of the eighth cranial nerve and also secondary afferent fibres from cells of the vestibular nuclei. These are mainly distributed to the flocculonodular lobe and lingula (archicerebellum).

2 The *spinocerebellar tracts* carry proprioceptive information from the trunk and lower limbs (Fig. 19.13) and terminate in the paleocerebellum.

3 The *olivocerebellar tract* originates from the inferior olivary nucleus and the accessory olivary nuclei which are important medullary relay centres receiving afferent fibres from cerebral cortical, subcortical and spinal cord regions.

4 *Pontocerebellar fibres* form part of the corticopontocerebellar pathway through which the cerebral cortex influences the cerebellum.

5 *Trigeminocerebellar fibres* arise from all three of the sensory trigeminal nuclei (p. 904). Those from the mesencephalic nucleus are primary afferent fibres conveying proprioceptive information from the head, the others from the spinal and principal sensory nuclei are secondary afferent fibres relaying exteroceptive information from the head through the inferior cerebellar peduncle.

6 *Tectocerebellar fibres* convey both auditory and visual impulses from the midbrain to the cerebellum.

7 *Reticulocerebellar fibres* from the medullary reticular nuclei enter through the inferior peduncle.

Efferent connections (Fig. 19.34b)

The roof nuclei (dentate, emboliform, globose and fastigial) receive impulses from the cerebellar cortex through axons of Purkinje cells and give rise to efferent cerebellar fibres. The vast majority of these fibres leave in the superior cerebellar peduncle, most of them crossing in the midbrain tegmentum before passing to their various destinations. However, some fibres from the fastigial nucleus leave in the inferior cerebellar peduncle.

1 *Dentatothalamic fibres* form part of a pathway linking the neocerebellum with 'motor' areas of the cerebral cortex. They stem from cells of the dentate nucleus and cross in the decussation of the superior cerebellar peduncles in the midbrain to end in the ventrolateral nucleus of the thalamus.

2 *Cerebellorubral fibres* originate from cells of the globose and emboliform nuclei, cross in the midbrain to synapse on neurons of the red nucleus. In turn the red nucleus gives rise to the rubrospinal tract which influences the pattern of activity of α and γ motor neurons.

3 *Cerebellovestibular fibres* leave the cerebellum through the inferior peduncle and terminate in neurons of the vestibular nuclei. Many of the fibres originate in the flocculonodular lobe and parts of the vermis, others stem from the fastigial nucleus.

4 *Cerebelloreticular fibres* arise from the fastigial nucleus and are distributed through the inferior and superior cerebellar peduncles to reticular nuclei of the brainstem and thalamus. Some of these reticular nuclei give rise to reticulospinal tracts which influence the activities of α and γ motor neurons.

Functional and clinical considerations

The cerebellum receives information from a variety of sources (proprioceptive from muscles, joints, tendons and the vestibular apparatus; exteroceptive from skin, eye and cochlea; and input from the cerebral cortex and reticular system) which is then integrated and subsequently modifies the cerebellar efferent discharge pattern to the motor control centres. Through these centres the cerebellum exerts a controlling influence on (a) posture and balance, (b) the regulation of muscle tone and (c) the coordination of

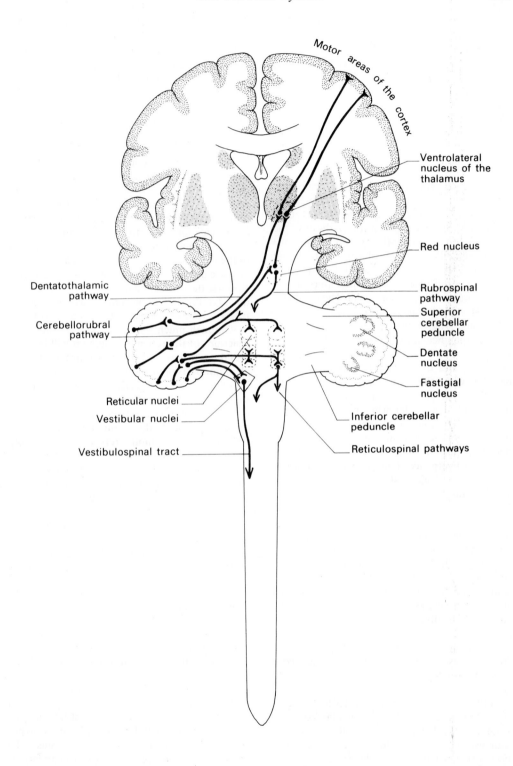

Motor areas of the cortex

Ventrolateral
nucleus of the
thalamus

Red nucleus

Dentatothalamic
pathway

Rubrospinal
pathway

Superior
cerebellar
peduncle

Cerebellorubral
pathway

Dentate
nucleus

Fastigial
nucleus

Reticular nuclei

Vestibular nuclei

Inferior cerebellar
peduncle

Vestibulospinal tract

Reticulospinal pathways

Fig. 19.34b. Scheme illustrating the major output
(efferent pathways) of the cerebellum

individual muscles necessary for smooth voluntary movements.

Clinically, the most marked effects of cerebellar lesions seen in man may include (a) disequilibrium, (b) dystonia (disturbances in muscle tone), and (c) ataxia or asynergia (muscular incoordination), which in the case of unilateral cerebellar involvement are all confined to the same side as the lesion.

Reticular system

The reticular system is phylogenetically the oldest part of the chordate central nervous system, having evolved long before the advent of the major sensory and motor pathways, the thalamus and the cerebral cortex. It consists of a core of reticular neurons, disposed throughout the brainstem and diencephalon, which is arranged as a diffuse network, interspersed with loosely organized reticular nuclei. The geometry of most reticular neurons is such that their numerous, long dendrites are orientated in a plane perpendicular to the long axis of the brainstem, whereas their axons bifurcate into long ascending and descending branches, arranged parallel with the long axis. These axonic branches give rise to many collaterals. Each neuron through its dendrites receives synaptic contacts from some 4 000 neurons, and through its axonic branches connects to about 25 000 neurons; thus a remarkable convergence of input and divergence of output is achieved which enables the reticular system to function as a central integrator of nervous activity.

The reticular core may be regarded as two functionally interconnected regions, namely: a lateral zone, confined to the medulla and pons; and a medial zone, extending throughout the brainstem. The lateral zone is mainly a 'sensory' or associative region receiving input from many sources and, in turn, projecting on to the medial zone which acts as a 'motor' or effector zone connected to diverse regions of the brain and spinal cord.

The input to the reticular system is derived from the ascending fibres of the spinal cord which include the spinoreticular tracts and collateral branches from other long tracts, particularly the spinothalamic pathways (p. 840). Other significant afferents to the reticular core are from trigeminal, cochlear, vestibular and retinal sources. Descending influences from the cerebral cortex reach the reticular system through corticoreticular fibres, and collaterals derived from the corticospinal and corticonuclear tracts.

The reticular system also receives fibres from the limbic system, various thalamic and hypothalamic nuclei, and also from the corpus striatum and cerebellum.

The output of the reticular system is extensive, providing efferent fibres to diverse regions of the central nervous system. The reticular system influences the activities of the α and γ motor neurons of the spinal cord and brainstem (p. 471), either directly through pathways (reticulospinal and reticulonuclear) arising from pontine and medullary nuclei, or indirectly through reticular projections to the cerebellum, red nucleus, corpus striatum and cerebral cortex. Visceral activities are influenced through reticular connections with the hypothalamus and by direct reticular fibres to lower autonomic centres of the brainstem and cord. Other reticular efferents are directed to various thalamic nuclei, particularly the intralaminar and medial nuclei, and nuclei of the midline which, in turn, project diffusely to most regions of the cerebral cortex.

Although much remains unknown about the functions of the reticular system, it will be seen that the reticular core receives information from all major parts of the nervous system, and in turn influences either directly or indirectly these same regions. The reticular system participates in the control of visceral and motor activities as previously noted; thus, stimulation of certain reticular areas inhibits reflex and cortically induced movements whereas facilitation of movements is produced by stimulation of other reticular areas. In addition, stimulation of the reticular system may induce either a state of alertness in a sleeping animal by excitation of the cerebral cortex, or sleep in a wakeful animal by inhibition of the cortex (p. 936); moreover, bilateral lesions of the reticular core may result in an irreversible coma.

The forebrain

DIENCEPHALON

The diencephalon (Figs. 19.1 & 19.2) is part of the forebrain. Caudally it is continuous with the midbrain, and is encased on each side by the cerebral hemispheres. It consists of structures lying around the third ventricle, some of which help to form the walls and floor of this midline cavity. These include the thalamus, hypothalamus, subthalamus and epithalamus. The roof of the diencephalon is formed mainly of ependyma overlayed with a layer of vascular pia mater, but caudally it consists of the epithalamus

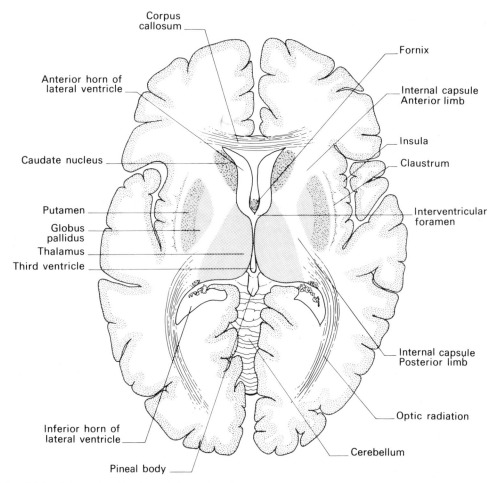

Corpus
callosum

Fornix

Anterior horn of
lateral ventricle

Internal capsule
Anterior limb

Insula

Caudate nucleus

Claustrum

Putamen

Interventricular
foramen

Globus
pallidus

Thalamus

Third ventricle

Internal capsule
Posterior limb

Optic radiation

Inferior horn of
lateral ventricle

Cerebellum

Pineal body

Fig. 19.35. Horizontal section through the brain at the
level of the frontal and occipital poles of the cerebral
hemispheres.

which comprises the habenular complex, the
posterior commissure and the pineal body.
Diagrams of the horizontal, coronal and sagittal
sections of the brain (Figs. 19.35, 19.36 &
19.37) should be consulted in order to understand the topographical relationship of these
various diencephalic structures.

The thalamus

The thalami are two masses of grey matter lying
one on either side of the third ventricle so forming the upper part of the lateral walls of this
cavity. Each thalamus is ovoid in shape (Fig.
19.38a) and possesses a pointed anterior end
which forms the posterior border of the interventricular foramen (p. 875), and a blunt posterior end, the pulvinar, which overhangs the ros-

tral part of the midbrain tectum. Usually the two
thalami are joined across the midline of the third
ventricle by the thalamic adhesion (massa
intermedia). Above, from lateral to medial, the
thalamus is related to the caudate nucleus, the
body of the lateral ventricle, and the fornix;
below, it lies on the hypothalamus and subthalamus. On the lateral side of the thalamus run
bundles of fibres forming part of the internal
capsule.

The thalamus consists of several nuclear complexes which are further subdivided into nuclei.
The major nuclear groups and their principal
connections are shown diagrammatically in Fig.
19.38a and b. The internal medullary lamina,
comprising intrinsic and extrinsic thalamic
fibres, separates the nuclei into three major

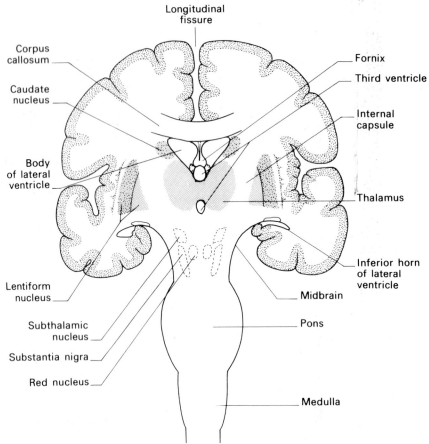

Fig. 19.36. Diagram of an oblique coronal section
through the brain.

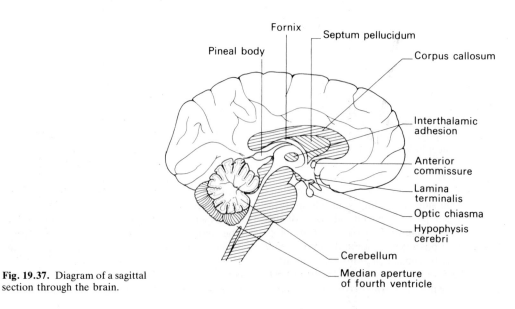

Fig. 19.37. Diagram of a sagittal
section through the brain.

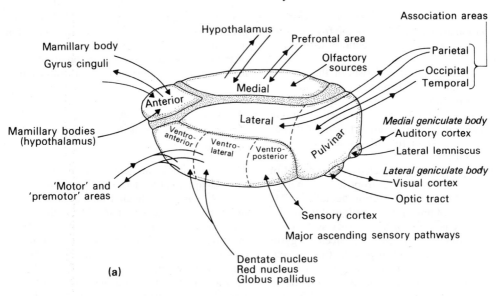

(a)

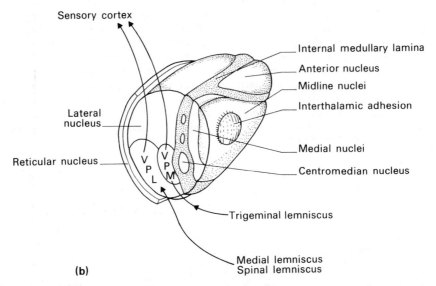

(b)

Fig. 19.38. The main thalamic nuclei with their major connections. (a) The thalamus seen from the superolateral aspect; (b) the anterior half of the thalamus, also seen in transverse section. The heavily stippled region represents the internal medullary lamina.

groups, namely: anterior, medial and ventro-lateral (Fig. 19.38).

The anterior nuclei receive fibres from the mamillary body via the mamillothalamic tract and make reciprocal connections with the cingu-late gyrus. These structures also form part of the limbic system (p. 878).

The medial nuclei appear to be responsible for the integration of somatic, visceral and olfactory information which influences the activities of various forebrain structures. Damage to these nuclei by disease or by the surgical destruction of their frontal connections (prefrontal leucotomy) results in gross disturbances in personality, motivation and intellect.

The ventrolateral nuclear complex consists of two tiers: the lateral and ventral divisions. The lateral division which includes the pulvinar has reciprocal connections with most cortical association areas, save those of the frontal lobe. It also has many interconnections with other thalamic nuclei.

The ventral division consists of the ventro-anterior, ventrolateral and ventroposterior nuclei. The first two nuclei influence the motor control systems, and surgical destruction of the ventrolateral nucleus is undertaken to reduce rigidity and tremor in patients suffering from Parkinsonism.

The ventroposterior nucleus is composed of several subnuclei, the ventroposterior lateralis (VPL) and the ventroposterior medialis (VPM) being the most noteworthy. Cells of this nucleus are tertiary neurons of the sensory system and project to the sensory cortex postcentral gyrus (Fig. 19.38b). Lesions involving this nucleus result in contralateral loss of tactile and proprioceptive sensation, sometimes associated with disturbances of pain and temperature sensibilities.

In addition, the thalamus has other nuclear groups (sometimes termed 'non-specific' nuclei) which include the reticular, midline and intralaminar groups. The reticular nucleus is part of the reticular system, sending axons to many thalamic nuclei and receiving fibres from most areas of the cerebral cortex. The intralaminar nuclei lie within the internal medullary lamina. One such nucleus is the centromedian which receives terminals or collateral fibres of

the spinothalamic tracts, the medial and trigeminal lemnisci. It is associated with pain mechanisms, and bilateral surgical destruction of the centromedian nucleus is sometimes performed in man for the relief of intractable pain.

The hypothalamus

The hypothalamus forms the floor and lower part of the lateral walls of the third ventricle (p. 869), as its name implies it lies under (below) the thalami.

The hypothalamus contains many nuclei, some clearly demarcated, others less so, but, in general, it may be divided into an anterior or supraoptic region situated above the optic chiasma, a middle or tuberal region lying above the tuber cinereum, and a posterior or mamillary region associated with the mamillary bodies (Fig. 19.39). Certain nuclei are noteworthy for they are directly involved in hormone production. Thus, the neurons of the supraoptic and paraventricular nuclei produce respectively vasopressin and oxytocin which are transported by their axons to the neurohypophysis (p. 769). In addition, certain tuberal nuclei produce hormone release or inhibiting factors (p. 774).

The hypothalamus may be considered as the highest centre of the brain concerned with the integration of autonomic activities (p. 925). It receives inputs from ascending visceral (autonomic) fibres carrying interoceptive information, and from collaterals of the lemniscal pathways

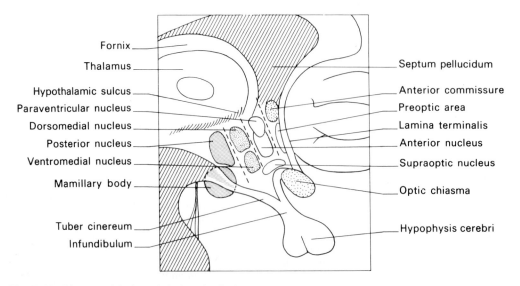

Fig. 19.39. Diagram of the hypothalmic region in the left wall and floor of the third ventricle, showing some of the hypothalamic nuclei.

concerned with exteroceptive information. The hypothalamus is extensively interconnected with the limbic system, one of the major pathways being the fornix from the hippocampus to the mamillary bodies (p. 878); with the reticular system (p. 864), and parts of the thalamus (see above) which indirectly link the cortex with the hypothalamus.

Outgoing hypothalamic connections influence the activities of the peripheral autonomic system, e.g. through connections with the dorsal nucleus of the vagus nerve and with the preganglionic cells of the intermediolateral column of the thoracic cord which is part of the sympathetic outflow. In addition, the hypothalamus influences the hormonal secretions of the hypophysis cerebri (pituitary gland) through nervous and vascular connections (p. 769).

Functionally the hypothalamus, through its multiplicity of connections and its influence on the secretory activities of the hypophysis cerebri, plays many roles, some of which are briefly discussed below.

General autonomic effects. The hypothalamus influences the motility and secretory activities of the gut, the heart rate and cardiac output, as well as vasomotor tone, peripheral resistance and blood pressure. In general, parasympathetic effects are carried out by cell groups situated in the anterior portion of the hypothalamus and sympathetic effects by cells located more posteriorly, but this distinction is by no means absolute.

Endocrine regulation. The hypothalamus synthesizes the hormones, vasopressin and oxytocin. Additionally, it produces hormones or releasing factors as they are termed which are specific in controlling the release of one or other of the hormones from the anterior lobe of the hypophysis (p. 774). It plays an important part in reproduction by regulating the secretion of the gonadal (sex) hormones.

Regulation of water balance and food intake. The hypothalamus is concerned with conservation of body water and water intake (p. 744). A group of cells lying in the lateral zone of the hypothalamus is termed the thirst or drinking 'centre'. Prolonged stimulation of these cells in experimental animals causes copious drinking (hyperdipsia) leading to overhydration.

Similarly there is a feeding or hunger 'centre' located in the lateral zone and a satiety 'centre' in the medial zone of the hypothalamus (p. 799).

The hypothalamus also plays an important role in the control of temperature regulation (p. 724).

Subthalamus and epithalamus

The subthalamus forms the ventrocaudal part of the diencephalon, lying below the thalamus and merging with the tegmentum of the midbrain (Fig. 19.36). It contains, on each side, the subthalamic nucleus and the cranial extensions of the red nucleus, and the substantia nigra (p. 855). Passing through the subthalamic region are bundles of fibres, destined for the thalamus.

The epithalamus which forms the caudal part of the roof of the third ventricle consists of the pineal body, the habenular complex and the posterior commissure. The pineal body (Fig. 19.17) is a pear-shaped structure, almost 1.0 cm long, which projects backwards from the roof of the third ventricle. Functionally, the pineal body is an endocrine gland and is probably concerned with the development of the gonads, influencing (through the hypothalamus) the output of follicular stimulating and luteinizing hormones. The habenular complex is part of the limbic system (p. 878), whilst the posterior commissure is a complex of crossing fibres connecting various diencephalic nuclei.

The third ventricle

The third ventricle is a midline cavity interposed between the two thalami. In horizontal and transverse sections it appears as a narrow slit. Anteriorly it communicates with each lateral ventricle through the interventricular foramen (Fig. 19.35), whilst posteriorly it opens into the cerebral aqueduct of the midbrain. The floor of the ventricle is formed mainly by the hypothalamus and is prolonged downwards as a recess into the infundibulum to which is attached the hypophysis. The roof consists of a layer of ependyma covered by a fold of pia mater, the tela choroidea, which contains a pair of vascular fringes called the choroid plexuses of the third ventricle. Each lateral wall is composed of a smaller, lower part formed by the medial surface of the hypothalamus and a larger, upper part consisting of the medial surface of most of the thalamus which are separated from each other by the hypothalamic sulcus (Fig. 19.39).

TELENCEPHALON

The telencephalon consists principally of the cerebral hemispheres with their associated commissures, but also includes the anterior parts

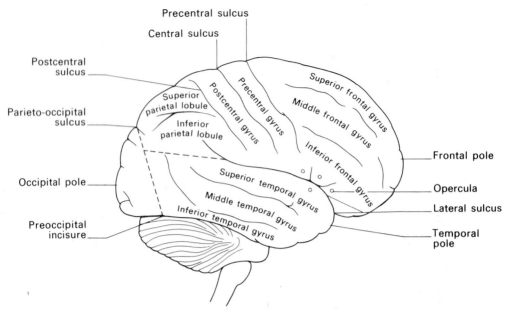

Fig. 19.40. View of the right side of the brain showing the major sulci and gyri of the superolateral surface of the cerebral hemisphere. The interrupted lines indicate the artificial boundaries between the occipital, parietal and temporal lobes.

of the third ventricle and the adjacent preoptic areas. Seen from above the two cerebral hemispheres are incompletely separated by a median cleft named the longitudinal cerebral fissure which contains a sickle-shaped fold of dura mater, the falx cerebri (p. 888). The central region of the cleft is limited below by the corpus callosum, a massive fibre bundle connecting the hemispheres across the midline. Taken together the cerebral hemispheres constitute the cerebrum.

Each cerebral hemisphere consists of an outer layer of grey matter named the cortex, a central mass of white matter, and a deep core of grey matter forming the basal ganglia or nuclei. Within the substance of the cerebral hemisphere and partly surrounding the basal nuclei is a cavity, termed the lateral ventricle, which communicates with the third ventricle.

Surfaces and lobes of the cerebrum (Fig. 19.40)
The surfaces of the cerebrum are characterized by numerous, irregular elevations called convolutions or gyri which are separated by deep furrows named fissures or sulci. This elaborate infolding of the outer layer of the cerebrum considerably augments both the volume and the surface area of the cortex of which only a third of the area is visible on the surface.

Superolateral surface of the cerebral hemisphere
The lateral and central sulci help to divide the hemisphere into regions which are the frontal, parietal, occipital and temporal lobes—their names corresponding to the vault bones of the skull which more or less overlie them.

The frontal lobe contains the precentral gyrus positioned between the central sulcus and the precentral sulcus. This strip of cortex is the 'motor' area which gives rise to some of the fibres forming the corticonuclear and corticospinal tracts.

The parietal lobe is separated from the frontal lobe by the central sulcus, its other boundaries are artificial. The postcentral gyrus, interposed between the central and postcentral sulci, is the sensory area which receives fibres from some of the thalamic nuclei.

The occipital lobe terminates posteriorly in the occipital pole, the extreme tip of which contains a small part of the visual or striate cortex representing the macular area of the retina.

The temporal lobe is separated from the frontal and parietal lobes by the lateral sulcus and a line drawn in continuity with this sulcus (Fig. 19.40). The central part of the upper surface of the superior temporal gyrus is the auditory area and receives fibres from the medial geniculate body.

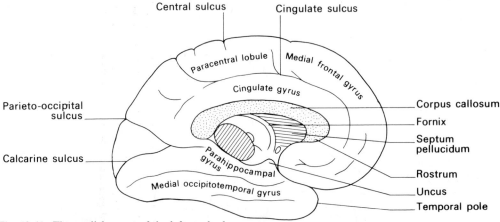

Fig. 19.41. The medial aspect of the left cerebral hemisphere showing some of the sulci and gyri, the brainstem has been removed.

The insula is a buried portion of the cortex, situated deep to the anterior part of the lateral sulcus and overlapped by three 'lids' or opercula contributed by the lower regions of the frontal and parietal lobes and the upper part of the temporal lobe. Lying deep to, and almost co-extensive with, the insula, are the claustrum and the lentiform nucleus (Fig. 19.35). The functional role of the insula is uncertain, but stimulation in man produces visceral effects, e.g. increase in salivation and gastric motility, and abdominal discomfort such as nausea and belching.

Medial and inferior surfaces of the cerebral hemispheres

When both hemispheres are *in situ* in the skull, the medial surface (Fig. 19.41) is separated from that of the opposite hemisphere by the longitudinal cerebral fissure and falx cerebri. It displays a large, curved bundle of commissural fibres named the corpus callosum. Lying below, and attached to the corpus callosum is the septum pellucidum which joins an arched band of fibres named the fornix. The septum pellucidum forms part of the septal area.

The central sulcus, already seen on the lateral surface of the hemisphere, ends in the paracentral lobule into which extend the motor and sensory areas. The cingulate gyrus is part of the limbic system and makes reciprocal connections with the anterior nuclear group of the thalamus. The lips on each side of the posterior part of the calcarine sulcus in the occipital lobe represent the striate cortex or primary visual area and receive fibres from the lateral geniculate body.

The inferior surface of the cerebral hemisphere (Fig. 19.42) is divided by the lateral sulcus into anterior and posterior parts situated at different levels. The anterior part or orbital surface of the frontal lobe rests on the floor of the anterior cranial fossa and is indented by several sulci. The olfactory sulcus is a longitudinally running groove which lodges the olfactory tract and bulb; other sulci divide the orbital surface into orbital gyri. The posterior part consisting of the undersurfaces of the temporal and occipital lobes rests on the floor of the middle cranial fossa anteriorly and the tentorium cerebelli posteriorly. Its surface is divided into a number of longitudinally running gyri. The most medial of these is the parahippocampal gyrus which ends anteriorly in a hook-shaped projection named the uncus, a part of the olfactory system.

The cerebral cortex

The cerebral cortex is a layer of grey matter forming the surface of the hemispheres. It varies in thickness from 4.5 mm in the precentral gyrus to about 1.5 mm in the occipital lobe. The number of neurons in the human cortex is reckoned in astronomical terms, variously estimated at 2.6 to 14.0 thousand millions.

Cortical neurons show considerable variation in size, shape and position (Fig. 19.43). Most numerous are pyramidal and stellate cells which are present at most levels and in most regions of the cortex. Pyramidal cells vary in size from small through to giant neurons (of Betz). Each

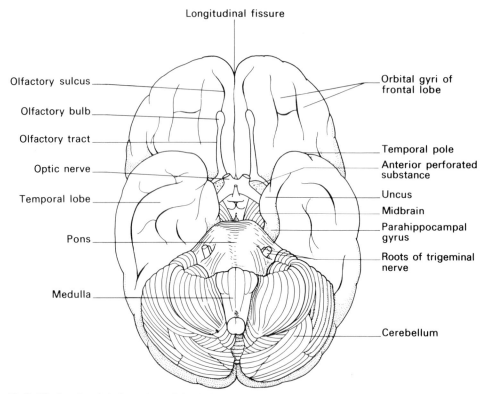

Fig. 19.42. The basal or inferior aspect of the brain.

possesses an apical dendrite extending towards the surface of the cortex, and several laterally spreading basal dendrites. Many of the axons of pyramidal cells are projection fibres which leave the cortex and end by synapsing in subcortical structures, e.g. basal nuclei, thalamus, brainstem nuclei and grey matter of the spinal cord. Other pyramidal axons either form bundles of long and short association fibres which end in various cortical regions of the ipsilateral hemisphere, or cross as commissural fibres which terminate in the cortex of the contralateral hemisphere. Stellate (granule) cells have small, star-shaped cell bodies, numerous short branching dendrites and a single axon. They form synapses with other cortical cells and are associative in function.

On the basis of the arrangement and density of the various cell types a conspicuous banded or laminated pattern is seen in the cortex. Six layers arranged parallel to the cortical surface are recognized but these are not found over the cortex as a whole (Fig. 19.43).

Afferent fibres to the cortex include ascending projection fibres from the thalamus, association fibres from other cortical regions of the same hemisphere, and commissural fibres from the cortex of the opposite hemisphere.

NERVE FIBRES OF THE CEREBRUM

White matter forms a large part of the hemisphere, packing all the available space between the cortex and those more deeply placed structures, the lateral ventricle and basal ganglia. It is composed of three types of fibres: association, commissural and projection fibres. Some of the association fibre bundles are named and illustrated in Fig. 19.44.

Commissural fibres cross the median sagittal plane and interconnect the cortex of one hemisphere to that of the other. The topography of one such bundle of commissural fibres, the corpus callosum, has already been described.

Projection fibres connect the cerebral cortex with subcortical structures, such as the thalamus, basal ganglia, and grey matter of the brainstem and spinal cord. They consist of ascending fibres to, and descending fibres from the cortex. The majority of these fibres converge above the basal ganglia where they form a fan-like array of

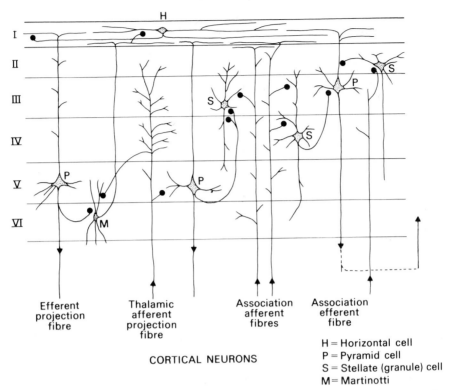

I

II

III

IV

V

VI

Efferent
projection
fibre

Thalamic
afferent
projection
fibre

Association
afferent
fibres

Association
efferent
fibre

CORTICAL NEURONS

H = Horizontal cell
P = Pyramid cell
S = Stellate (granule) cell
M = Martinotti

Fig. 19.43. Diagrammatic representation of the layers of the cerebral cortex, showing some of the cortical neurons and their interconnections. Layers I–III contain many stellate cells and are concerned with association and higher functions such as the interpretation of sensory input, memory and discrimination. Layer IV is largely receptive, receiving fibres from the thalamus. Layers V and VI contain large pyramidal cells which give rise to corticofugal projection fibres.

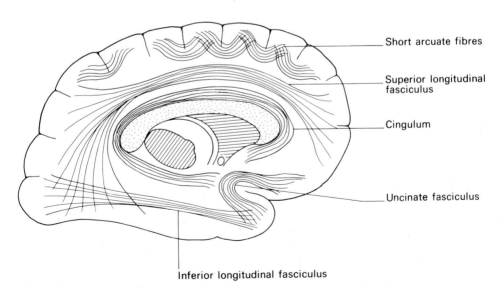

Short arcuate fibres

Superior longitudinal fasciculus

Cingulum

Uncinate fasciculus

Inferior longitudinal fasciculus

Fig. 19.44. Diagram of some of the association fibre bundles, projected onto the medial aspect of the left cerebral hemisphere. Short arcuate fibres interconnect adjacent gyri: long association bundles (e.g. the cingulum) form connections between more remote regions.

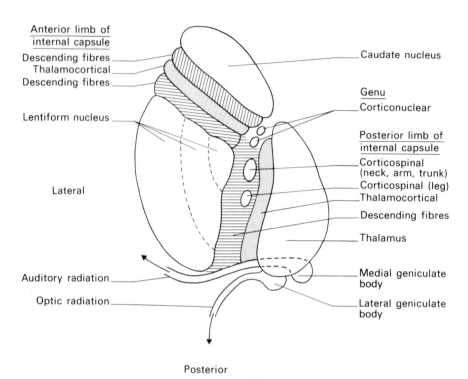

Anterior

Anterior limb of
internal capsule
Descending fibres
Thalamocortical
Descending fibres

Lentiform nucleus

Lateral

Auditory radiation
Optic radiation

Caudate nucleus

Genu
Corticonuclear

Posterior limb of
internal capsule
Corticospinal
(neck, arm, trunk)
Corticospinal (leg)
Thalamocortical
Descending fibres
Thalamus

Medial geniculate
body
Lateral geniculate
body

Posterior

Fig. 19.45. Diagram showing the relations and main components of the internal capsule in horizontal section. Note that descending fibres in the cross-   hatched regions include corticopontine, corticothalamic and others.

bundles known as the corona radiata; many of the fibres then pass through the basal ganglia as a compact, large bundle called the internal capsule and then continue into the brainstem as the crus cerebri of the midbrain.

THE INTERNAL CAPSULE

The internal capsule is a compact bundle of projection fibres lying medial to the lentiform nucleus. In horizontal section it consists of an anterior limb situated between the head of the caudate nucleus and the lentiform nucleus, and a posterior limb interposed between the thalamus and the lentiform nucleus (Figs. 19.35 & 19.45). The two limbs converge and meet to form a junctional region called the genu.

The various sets of projection fibres are located in the internal capsule as shown in Fig. 19.45.

Due to the compact nature of the internal capsule, a small lesion of this fibre bundle produces widespread neurological disturbances.

Thus, haemorrhage or thrombosis involving the posterior limb results in contralateral paralysis (hemiplegia) of the upper and lower limbs, and trunk owing to injury of the corticospinal fibres. In addition, lesions at this site damage the thalamocortical fibres causing contralateral sensory loss. Involvement of the posterior part of the posterior limb of the capsule affects vision and hearing because of injury to the optic and auditory radiations.

THE BASAL NUCLEI

The basal nuclei or ganglia are a heterogenous group of nuclei lying in the deep part of the cerebral hemisphere. They include the caudate and lentiform nuclei which are functionally linked and collectively known as the corpus striatum. This during early development is a single mass of grey matter but later becomes separated by the fibres of the internal capsule into the caudate and lentiform nuclei. The caudate nucleus comprises: a head which forms the floor of the anterior horn of the lateral ventricle; a body overlying the superolateral part of the thalamus; and a tail which forms the roof of the inferior horn of the lateral ventricle. The tip of the tail is fused to a small mass of grey matter, the amygdala (p. 881), which is usually included as a component part of the basal ganglia.

In section the lentiform nucleus consists of the putamen, and the globus pallidus or pallidum (Figs. 19.35 & 19.36). Structurally, the putamen and caudate nucleus are similar, together they form the striatum.

The connections of the corpus striatum are various and complex but in outline the striatum receives the main input and projects to the pallidum which in turn gives rise to the major output pathways.

The main afferent fibres to the striatum come from the cerebral cortex, the intralaminar and midline groups of thalamic nuclei, and the substantia nigra. Efferent fibres from the pallidum synapse in ventral thalamic nuclei, which then project to the premotor area situated in front of the motor area in the frontal lobe. Other pallidofugal fibres end in the subthalamic nucleus, the red nucleus, the substantia nigra and nuclei of the reticular system.

Functionally the corpus striatum together with various nuclei forms part of an elaborate motor control system often called the extrapyramidal system. Pathological lesions of these structures result in two basic types of disturbance which are (a) various kinds of abnormal, unwanted movements, termed dyskinaesia, and (b) changes in muscle tone, called dystonia. The dyskinaesia, which usually disappear during sleep, are: (a) tremor at rest; (b) slow, writhing movements usually involving the limbs (athetosis); (c) brisk, graceful movements of considerable complexity involving the distal parts of the limbs or muscles of the face and tongue (chorea); or (d) violent, forceful movements of the limbs (ballism). The most common condition affecting the extrapyramidal system is paralysis agitans or Parkinsonism caused by degeneration of the substantia nigra.

THE LATERAL VENTRICLES

The two lateral ventricles are ependymal-lined cavities lying in the cerebral hemispheres. They are filled with cerebrospinal fluid and communicate with the third ventricle through the interventricular foramina. Seen in lateral profile each ventricle consists of a central part or body with three prolongations or horns (Fig. 19.46). The roof of the anterior and central part is formed by the corpus callosum, its floor by the caudate nucleus and the lateral part of the thalamus. The caudate nucleus helps to form the roof of the inferior or temporal horn. The floor consists mainly of the hippocampus.

Olfactory system

The olfactory system consists of the olfactory epithelium, the olfactory nerves, bulbs and tracts, and the olfactory cortex. In most mammals and lower vertebrates the olfactory system is well developed, but in man it is considerably reduced—only a small area of cortex being primarily concerned with the sense of smell.

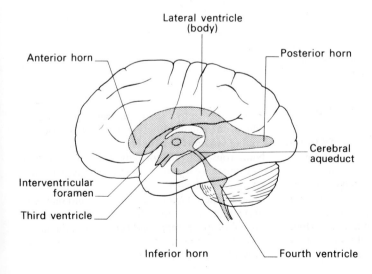

Lateral ventricle (body)

Anterior horn

Posterior horn

Interventricular foramen

Third ventricle

Cerebral aqueduct

Inferior horn

Fourth ventricle

Fig. 19.46. Diagram illustrating the ventricular system, projected onto the left surface of the brain.

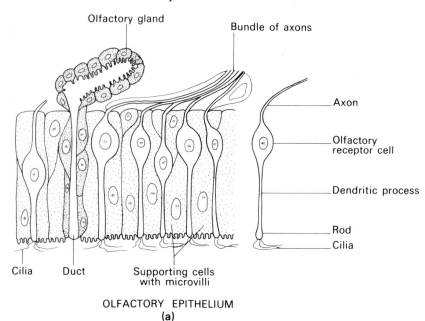

Fig. 19.47. (a) Section through olfactory epithelium. (b) Diagram of the olfactory bulb, tract and striae, showing some of the connections of the olfactory system.

OLFACTORY EPITHELIUM, OLFACTORY NERVES, BULBS AND TRACTS

The olfactory epithelium lines an area of 2.0–3.0 cm² in the roof of the nasal cavity, extending a short way on to the nasal septum and the lateral wall of the cavity. It consists of olfactory receptor cells, which are bipolar neurons, and columnar supporting cells whose external surfaces possess many elongated microvilla (Fig. 19.47). The cell bodies of the olfactory receptors lie near the basal aspect of the epithelium and each gives rise to a single, unbranched dendrite which on reaching the external surface of the epithelium ends in a bulbous projection or rod. Numerous long olfactory cilia emerge from each rod, and these together with the microvilli form a complex meshwork which is bathed in fluid secreted by the olfactory glands. The fluid plays an important role in olfaction, by allowing odoriferous substances to diffuse from the nasal airstream to the olfactory receptors; it also possesses bactericidal properties.

Stemming from each receptor cell body is a fine (0.2 μm) non-myelinated axon which courses with other olfactory axons to form slender bundles, each bundle being encased with Schwann cells. The bundles then aggregate into 20 or so branches which pass through foramina in the cribriform plate of the ethmoid bone and end in the olfactory bulb. These branches collectively form the olfactory nerve, and during their passage through the foramina are supported by meningeal investments.

The olfactory bulb is a small, ovoid mass of grey matter lying on the floor of the anterior cranial fossa, above and just lateral to the cribriform plate. It is continuous with the olfactory tract, a flat, white band, which runs backwards in the olfactory sulcus on the orbital surface of the frontal lobe to reach the anterior perforated substance where the tract divides into the lateral and medial olfactory striae. Structurally, the bulb contains a variety of neurons including large mitral cells and small granule cells (Fig. 19.47b). Entering fibres of the olfactory nerve converge on to dendrites of the mitral cells and together with processes of other cells in the bulb form synaptic complexes called glomeruli. Collateral fibres of the mitral cells synapse with granule cells whose axons also end in the glomeruli and so form reverberating circuits. Axons of the mitral cells pass in the olfactory tract and are then distributed to:

1 The primary olfactory cortex via the lateral olfactory stria.
2 The septal area via the medial olfactory stria and
3 The opposite olfactory bulb through the medial stria and anterior commissure.

A few mitral axons leave the olfactory tract and end directly in the anterior perforated substance.

PHYSIOLOGY OF OLFACTION

The olfactory receptors are responsible for detecting odours conveyed to the olfactory area by respiratory currents, including odours from food in the buccal cavity. Their action on the receptor endings causes electrical depolarizations which are conducted to the base of the receptor cells to initiate action potentials in their axons. These nerve fibres converge on the second order mitral cells of the olfactory bulb in a ratio of about 25 000:1, so that very small electrical changes in the olfactory epithelium can be collected and concentrated by the central nervous system; this is probably the chief reason

for the great sensitivity of the sense of smell.

The olfactory system can also discriminate a wide range of odorants (unlike the taste system which can only discern four classes). Odour qualities such as 'floral', 'minty', 'musky', 'camphoraceous' and 'pungent', can be correlated with certain molecular properties of odorants (molecular shape, presence of certain chemical groups, etc.), suggesting that there is 'key and lock' relationship between odorous molecules and the receptor proteins present in the olfactory cell membranes. It is thought that different groups of receptor cells are 'tuned' to different classes of odorants, so that mixtures of odours give rise to complex patterns of neural activity which are then analysed by the central nervous system. It should also be noted that noxious odours such as that of ammonia, may be detected by an entirely different system, namely the trigeminal sensory endings of the nasal cavity, even in the absence of a functional olfactory system, for example after fracture of surrounding bones has severed the olfactory nerves (see below).

OLFACTORY CORTICAL AREAS AND THE SEPTAL AREA

The anterior perforated substance (Figs. 19.42 & 19.47b) is a small, thin layer of grey matter which forms part of the olfactory cortex. It lies between the diverging lateral and medial olfactory striae, and is bounded caudally by the uncus and the optic tract. Numerous small vessels, the central arteries, pierce the substance to supply the underlying corpus striatum.

The primary olfactory cortical area includes:
1 Most of the anterior perforated substance,
2 The uncus which is a hook-shaped projection on the medial border of the temporal lobe, and
3 The corticomedial part of the amygdala.
This area receives fibres from the olfactory bulb through the lateral olfactory stria as previously noted, and has profuse connections with the secondary olfactory cortical area (entorhinal area) which is located in the anterior part of the parahippocampal gyrus (Fig. 19.48). In addition, it makes connections with other limbic structures and with the hypothalamus and thalamus. Both primary and secondary olfactory areas are held to be responsible for the conscious appreciation of odours.

The septal area lies on the medial aspect of the frontal lobe, below the genu and rostrum of the corpus callosum and in front of the lamina terminalis. It includes the paraterminal gyrus,

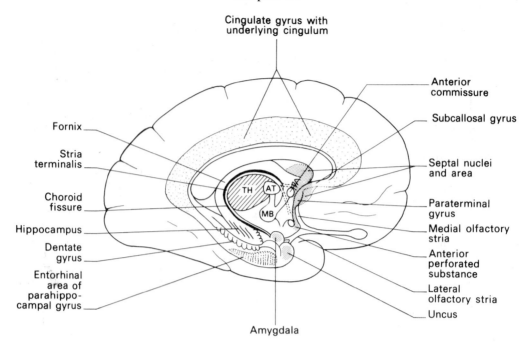

Cingulate gyrus with
underlying cingulum

Anterior
commissure

Subcallosal gyrus

Fornix

Stria
terminalis

Septal nuclei
and area

Choroid
fissure

TH   AT

MB

Paraterminal
gyrus

Hippocampus

Medial olfactory
stria

Dentate
gyrus

Anterior
perforated
substance

Entorhinal
area of
parahippo-
campal gyrus

Lateral
olfactory stria

Uncus

Amygdala

AT = Anterior thalamic nuclei
TH = Cut part of thalamus
MB = Mamillary body

Fig. 19.48. (a) Schematic diagram illustrating many of
the structures included in the limbic system.

and a deeper lying collection of cells, called the
septal nuclei, which extend into the septum
pellucidum. The septal area receives afferent
fibres from the primary olfactory area and also a
small number of fibres from the olfactory bulb
via the medial olfactory stria. It also makes
reciprocal connections with the hippocampus
through the fornix and with hypothalamic nuclei
and the midbrain tegmentum through the medial
forebrain bundle.

It is doubtful whether the septal area appreci-
ates olfactory stimuli at a conscious level but
functions rather as a zone of communication
between olfactory, hypothalamic and limbic
structures. Through descending fibres of the
medial forebrain bundle and through complex
pathways via the habenular complex, the septal
nuclei connect with the brainstem tegmentum,
and influence autonomic nuclei, e.g. the salivatory nuclei and the dorsal vagal nucleus. It is
through some of these pathways that the olfactory system triggers salivation and gastric secretion in response to aromas associated with food.

Applied anatomy. Permanent loss of the sense

of smell (anosmia) is commonly caused by the
interruption of the delicate fibres of the olfactory nerves due to fracture of the cribriform
plate of the ethmoid bone. But, anosmia may
also be caused by tumours involving the olfactory bulb or tract. Damage to the uncus may
result in 'uncinate fits', characterized by olfactory hallucinations of a disagreeable nature.

Limbic system

The limbic lobe is a term used to denote a group
of cortical structures bordering the junctional
region between the diencephalon and the telencephalon. Many of these structures are
phylogenetically old and assume an arched form
in the medial wall of the cerebral hemisphere
(Fig. 19.48). They include the subcallosal, cingulate and parahippocampal gyri, as well as the
hippocampal formation underlying the parahippocampal gyrus. The limbic lobe forms part of a
more extensive neural organization, termed the
limbic system, which in addition includes certain
nuclei of the hypothalamus and thalamus, the
amygdala and components of the olfactory sys-

tem, and also interconnecting fibre bundles such as the fornix, mamillothalamic tract and stria terminalis.

The limbic system receives information from visceral, somatic and olfactory sources, and is functionally concerned with the emotional aspects of behaviour related to the survival of the individual and the species, together with the visceral and somatic responses, evoked by these emotions. It also plays an important role in mechanisms involved with memory.

HIPPOCAMPAL FORMATION

This consists of the hippocampus, dentate gyrus and an adjoining strip of the parahippocampal gyrus known as the subiculum; all lie close to the outer convex border of the choroid fissure on the medial aspect of the temporal lobe (Fig. 19.48a). Their relationships are best shown in transverse section (Fig. 19.48b).

The hippocampus forms a curved elevation in the floor of the inferior horn of the lateral ventricle, its anterior part ending in a paw-like swelling, the pes hippocampi. The ventricular aspect of the hippocampus is covered by a subependymal layer of white matter, the alveus, composed of fibres mostly originating from the hippocampal cortex. These converge medially to form a bundle, the fimbria of the hippocampus, which then continues as the fornix.

The dentate gyrus is a narrow strip of cortex, characterized by tooth-like projections on its medial border. It is interposed between the fimbria and the parahippocampal gyrus, being continuous with the hippocampus but separated from the parahippocampal gyrus by hippocampal sulcus.

Histologically, the cortical zones from the parahippocampal gyrus, through the subicular region of the latter gyrus, and then to the hippocampus and dentate gyrus show a gradual transition from a six to a three layered organization of cells. The trilaminar arrangement represents phylogenetically the oldest part of the cortex. The three layers of the hippocampus are: polymorphic, pyramidal and molecular. The pyramidal layer is composed of large and small pyramidal neurons whose elaborate dendrites, apical and basal, extend into the adjacent layers (see below), whilst their axons enter the alveus and continue in the fornix as the main efferent pathway from the hippocampus. The polymorphic layer, situated deep to the alveus, consists of basal dendrites of the pyramidal neurons, and also basket cells whose axons

ramify on the cell bodies of the pyramidal neurons. The molecular layer comprises apical dendrites together with recurrent collaterals of the pyramidal neurons which synapse on these dendrites; it also harbours interneurons. Both polymorphic and molecular layers receive afferent fibres which terminate mainly on the dendrites of the pyramidal cells but also on the processes of certain interneurons located in these layers.

The dentate gyrus, like the hippocampus, is structurally organized in three layers, similarly named except that the pyramidal one is replaced by a layer of granule cells. These cells give rise to distinctive axons (mossy fibres) which enter the hippocampus and synapse with the apical dendrites of the pyramidal cells. The other two layers of the dentate gyrus contain various interneurons and receive afferent fibres from external sources. Some cells give rise to efferent fibres which leave the hippocampal formation in the fornix.

Connections of the hippocampal formation. The principal source of afferent fibres to the hippocampus and the dentate gyrus is from the parahippocampal gyrus (subiculum and entorhinal cortex). The latter gyrus is connected with widespread areas of the cerebral cortex through association fibres. One of the more noteworthy bundles of association fibres is the cingulum which runs in the deep part of the cingulate gyrus connecting, in particular, the septal region, cingulate and parahippocampal gyri.

Efferent fibres from the hippocampus and dentate gyrus are exclusively distributed by a highly arched bundle, the fornix (Fig. 19.48a). The fibres after entering the alveus collect medially to form a flattened bundle, the fimbria, which makes up the inferior margin of the choroid fissure. Gradually curving backwards, upwards and medially, the fimbria reaches the undersurface of the corpus callosum and then continues as the crus of the fornix. Here, the two crura meet in the midline and form the body of the fornix which arches forwards and downwards, being attached at first to the corpus callosum and then to the laminae of the septum pellucidum. Finally, the body of the fornix diverges into right and left bundles which pass behind the anterior commissure, each bundle penetrating the lateral wall of the third ventricle to end in the mamillary body. Topographically, the lateral border of the body forms the superior margin of the choroid fissure and is separated from the upper surface of the thalamus by the

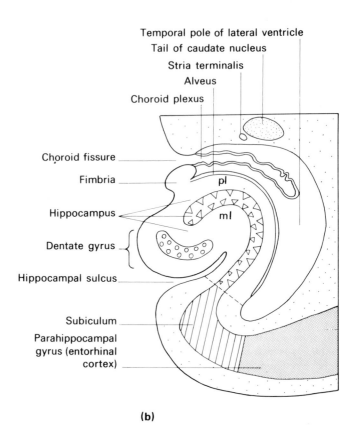

Temporal pole of lateral ventricle
Tail of caudate nucleus
Stria terminalis
Alveus
Choroid plexus

Choroid fissure

Fimbria

pl

Hippocampus

ml

Dentate gyrus

Hippocampal sulcus

Subiculum
Parahippocampal
gyrus (entorhinal
cortex)

(b)

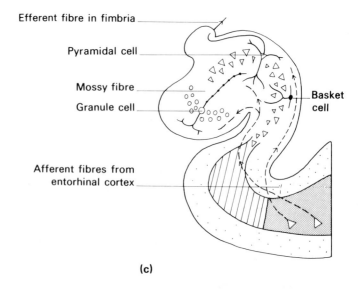

Efferent fibre in fimbria

Pyramidal cell

Mossy fibre

Granule cell

Basket
cell

Afferent fibres from
entorhinal cortex

Fig. 19.48. (b and c) Diagrams of the major formation features and connections of the hippocampus. (b) A coronal section of the inferior horn of the lateral ventricle showing the hippocampus and its related structures. Note the molecular layer (m.l.) and polymorphic layer (p.l.) with the intervening layer of pyramidal cells. (c) Schemic diagram showing some of the connections of the hippocampal formation. Triangular and circular profiles represent cell bodies of the pyramidal and granule neurons respectively.

(c)

laterally projected choroid plexus of the third ventricle. The bundles of the fornix form the anterior boundaries of the interventricular foramina.

Efferent fibres from the hippocampus mostly end in the hypothalamus, especially the mamillary body, but some are distributed to the septal area. In addition, the two hippocampi are interconnected by fibres crossing in the commissure of the fornix, situated between the two crura. The mamillary body is connected through the mamillothalamic bundle with the anterior thalamic nuclei which in turn are reciprocally connected with the cingulate gyrus. Through the cingulum (see above) connections are established between the cingulate gyrus and the hippocampus. This circuitous pathway from hippocampus to mamillary body to thalamus to cingulate gyrus and back again to the hippocampus is known as the 'Papez circuit'.

AMYGDALA

The amygdala is a small mass of grey matter, almond-shaped as its name indicates, which is situated in the pole of the temporal lobe at the tip of the inferior horn of the lateral ventricle (Fig. 19.48). It lies deep to the uncus, closely related to the ventral part of the hippocampus, and is fused to the tip of the tail of the caudate nucleus.

The amygdala consists of two functionally interconnected parts: the corticomedial part of the amygdala blends with the cortex of the uncus, and forms part of the primary olfactory cortex, receiving fibres from the olfactory bulb; the basolateral part receives no direct olfactory fibres but is in communication with the secondary olfactory area (entorhinal cortex), situated in the anterior part of the parahippocampal gyrus. The amygdala also receives afferents from other sources, namely the hypothalamus, thalamus and reticular system.

Efferent fibres from the amygdala leave in a discrete bundle, termed the stria terminalis, which ends principally in the septal area and anterior part of the hypothalamus. Topographically, this outflow pathway follows the arched-form of the caudate nucleus. At first it runs backwards in the roof of the inferior horn of the lateral ventricle, then continues in the floor of the body of the lateral ventricle, occupying the groove between the thalamus and the caudate nucleus. Finally, in the region of the interventricular foramen it distributes fibres to their destinations.

SOME FUNCTIONAL CONSIDERATIONS

Stimulation or ablation of parts of the limbic system in man and experimental animals leads to a variety of complex changes in behaviour which are only briefly considered here. Bilateral removal of the temporal lobes including the hippocampal formation and amygdala results in docility, hypersexuality, and lack of emotional responses such as fear or anger in situations which would normally warrant these reactions. Dietary habits are altered and food is often consumed in excess. In monkeys and cats, stimulation of the amygdala results in an aggressive, vicious animal which will attack any approaching object; in man, such stimulation produces feelings of anger or fear. A wide variety of visceral responses have been produced in animals by stimulation of the hippocampus, amygdala or cingulate gyrus. These include changes in gastro-intestinal movements, changes in respiratory patterns, pilo-erection and pupillary dilatation.

The role of the limbic system in memory is considered elsewhere (p. 943).

Visual system

The retina and its nerves are described on p. 949.

OPTIC NERVE, CHIASMA AND OPTIC TRACT

Each optic nerve is formed by axons of ganglionic cells of the retina. The axons, numbering about one million, collect at the optic disc and pierce the choroidal and scleral coats of the eyeball, the sclera in this region forming a thin, fenestrated membrane, the lamina cribrosa. Here, the fibres acquire myelin sheaths and become organized into numerous bundles which collectively make up the optic nerve.

In its intraorbital course the optic nerve passes backwards and medially inside the cone of muscles formed by the four recti and enters the cranial cavity through the optic canal. The nerve is pierced in the posterior part of the orbital cavity by the central artery of the retina (a branch of the ophthalmic artery). From the eyeball to the posterior opening of the optic canal the nerve is encased by all three meningeal investments.

The intracranial course of the optic nerve is short. After emerging from the optic canal it continues backwards and medially to the optic chiasma. The internal carotid artery lies lateral

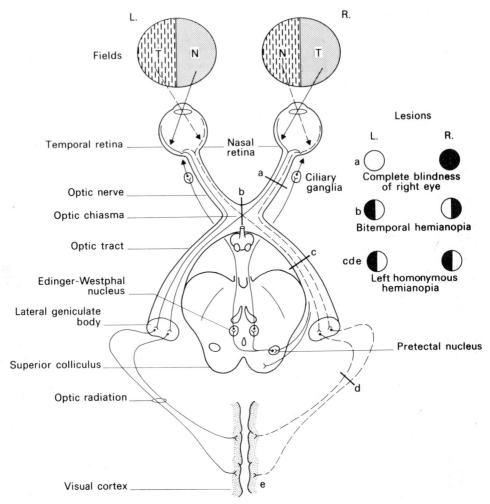

Fig. 19.49. Diagram of the visual pathways. T and N stand for the temporal and nasal fields respectively.

to the nerve and the anterior cerebral artery crosses above the optic nerve.

The optic chiasma appears to be formed by the union of the two optic nerves and to give rise on each side to the optic tracts. However, within the chiasma a partial decussation occurs, the fibres from the nasal (medial) halves of the retina crossing to the opposite side and those from the temporal (lateral) halves of the retina remaining uncrossed (Fig. 19.49). Thus, each emerging optic tract consists of 'temporal fibres' from the retina of the same side and 'nasal fibres' from the opposite retina. About 55% of optic nerve fibres cross in the chiasma. Topographically, the chiasma forms the lowest part of the anterior wall of the third ventricle (Fig. 19.39). Above, it

is continuous with the lamina terminalis: behind, with the tuber cinereum (of the hypothalamus) and below lies the hypophysis, separated by a membrane, the diaphragma sellae.

The optic tracts pass backwards and laterally along the sides of the tuber cinereum where they form the anterolateral boundaries of the interpeduncular fossa (Fig. 19.16). Each tract then sweeps around the upper part of the cerebral peduncle of the midbrain and enters the lateral geniculate body.

The lateral geniculate body is a small, ill-defined eminence situated on the undersurface of the posterior part of the thalamus and close to the medial geniculate body (Fig. 19.17). Internally it is composed of neurons, arranged in laminae, which give rise to fibres of the optic radiation which pass to the visual cortex.

The visual (striate) cortex occupies the walls, upper and lower lips of the posterior calcarine fissure, situated on the medial aspect of the occipital lobe, and extends for variable distance on to the occipital pole. In section the grey matter of this region is unusually thin and is divided by a white line, the visual stria, readily seen with the unaided eye.

CLINICAL CONSIDERATIONS

A lesion destroying all the fibres of an optic nerve obviously results in total blindness in the eye of the affected side. Damage to the crossing fibres of the chiasma will involve the nasal halves of both retinae (Fig. 19.49), causing a bilateral temporal field defect termed bitemporal hemianopia. The commonest cause of this defect is pressure on the chiasma from a pituitary tumour. Unilateral lesions of the optic pathway beyond the chiasma (tract, radiation or visual cortex) impair transmission of impulses from the temporal part of the retina on the same side and the nasal part of the retina of the opposite side, resulting in a visual defect confined to the contralateral half of the binocular field. This disturbance is termed homonymous hemianopia.

Vestibulocochlear pathways

The vestibulocochlear or eighth cranial nerve transmits impulses from special sense organs of the internal ear to the hindbrain. It consists of two functionally distinct parts:
1   The cochlear part which carries auditory impulses from the cochlea; and
2   The vestibular part which conveys impulses from the vestibular apparatus (utricle, saccule and semicircular canals: p. 970) concerned with equilibrium, postural mechanisms and muscle tone. Both parts leave the internal ear through the internal acoustic meatus and then separate to enter the dorsolateral aspect of the hindbrain at the caudal border of the pons. During most of its course the eighth nerve is accompanied by the facial nerve and the labyrinthine artery.

COCHLEAR PATHWAYS

The primary neurons of the cochlear pathway are bipolar cells whose cell bodies form the cochlear (spiral) ganglion located in the modiolus of the bony cochlea. Their peripheral processes end in relation to hair cells which are the audi-

tory receptors of the organ of Corti situated on the basilar membrane of the cochlear duct (Fig. 20.31); their central processes form the cochlear part of the eighth nerve and end by synapsing in the dorsal and ventral cochlear nuclei which are respectively situated on the dorsal and ventral aspects of the inferior cerebellar peduncle (Fig. 19.50). Axons from the cochlear nuclei terminate in the nuclei of the trapezoid body on the same and opposite sides. Tertiary neurons give rise to efferent fibres which form on each side of the pontine tegmentum a longitudinal bundle termed the lateral lemniscus. Each lemnicus then ascends to the midbrain where most of the fibres terminate in the nucleus of the inferior colliculus, the rest of the lemniscal fibres together with axons from the collicular nucleus run to the medial geniculate body which is a small eminence on the undersurface of the posterior part of the thalamus (Fig. 19.17). The medial geniculate body is the final relay nucleus on the cochlear pathway, its emerging axons form the auditory radiation (geniculotemporal tract) which passes in the posterior limb of the internal capsule before terminating in the auditory area of the temporal cortex.

Damage to either the cochlear nerve or both cochlear nuclei results in deafness on the corresponding side whereas unilateral destruction of the cochlear pathway beyond the cochlear nuclei produces partial loss of hearing which is worse in the contralateral ear.

VESTIBULAR APPARATUS AND VESTIBULAR PATHWAYS

The vestibular apparatus lies in the vestibule of the osseous labyrinth of the internal ear. It consists of:
1   The semicircular canals,
2   The utricle and
3   The saccule.
These together with the cochlear duct (part of the auditory system) form an enclosed, fluid-filled compartment termed the membranous labyrinth (Fig. 20.30).

Impulses are conveyed from the vestibular apparatus by bipolar neurons whose cell bodies form the vestibular ganglion situated in the depths of the internal accoustic meatus. The peripheral processes of these neurons innervate the hair cells in the canals, utricle and saccule; whilst the central processes form the vestibular part of the eighth nerve which enters the hindbrain slightly rostral and medial to the cochlear

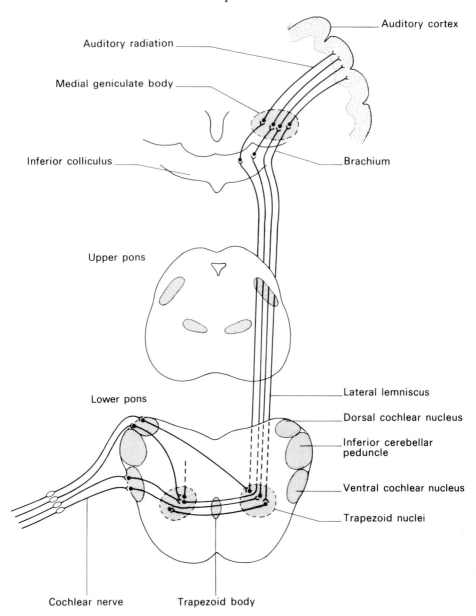

Fig. 19.50. Diagram of the cochlear pathways.

nerve. The majority of entering vestibular fibres terminate differentially in all four of the vestibular nuclei, the remainder being distributed to the archicerebellum and fastigial nuclei.

The vestibular nuclear complex consisting of inferior, superior, medial and lateral nuclei occupies the vestibular area in the floor of the fourth ventricle (Fig. 19.19). In addition to receiving fibres of the vestibular nerve all nuclei

of the vestibular complex receive fibres from the archicerebellum and fastigial nuclei. The main pathways arising from the vestibular complex are shown in Fig. 19.51. These are:
1 Vestibulocerebellar fibres.
2 Vestibulospinal fibres (p. 845).
3 Fibres from all four vestibular nuclei which enter the medial longitudinal fasciculus to be distributed to nuclei of the extraocular muscles

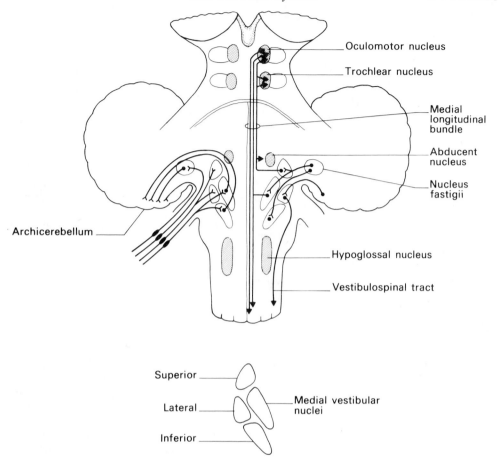

Fig. 19.51. Schematic diagram showing some of the connections of the vestibular nerve and its nuclei, together with some of the components of the medial longitudinal bundle.

(i.e., abducens, trochlear and oculomotor), cervical motor neurons and to the brainstem reticular system. The vestibulo-ocular components are necessary for conjugate eye movements in response to stimulation of the vestibular apparatus.

Damage to the vestibular apparatus or pathways results primarily in disturbances of equilibrium and posture. Since the vestibular system is intimately connected with the cerebellum, some of the signs produced by vestibular damage are similar to those of cerebellar malfunction. Unilateral lesions produce forced movements of the body and also deviations of the eyes, head and body to the affected side. There is a tendency to stagger or fall to the affected side, and the eyes may show conjugate and patterned rhythmic oscillations (nystagmus), features common to cerebellar disturbance. Irritative lesions of the vestibular apparatus result in vertigo (a subjective sensation of rotation) and visceral disturbances (nausea, vomiting, sweating and vasomotor changes). The nausea and vomiting associated with motion sickness are the result of stimulation of the maculae of the vestibular apparatus.

The meninges

Within the skull and vertebral column, the brain and spinal cord are further protected and supported by three membranes, collectively termed the meninges. The dura mater (pachymeninx) forming the outermost membrane is thick and inelastic, being composed mainly of collagen fibres. Deep to it lies the arachnoid mater, a delicate membrane consisting of loose connective tissue. The innermost membrane or pia mater is highly vascular and closely invests the subjacent nervous tissue. The latter two mem-

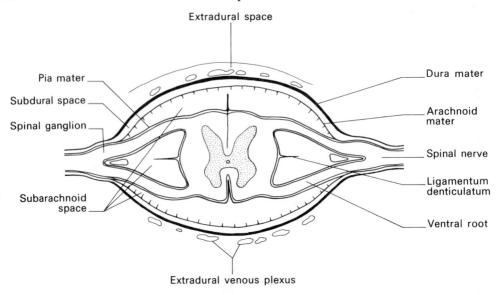

Fig. 19.52. A transverse section through the spinal
cord and its membranes.

branes are sometimes regarded as a single entity,
the pia-arachnoid or leptomeninx. The general
arrangement of the meninges is shown in Fig.
19.52.

DURA MATER

The spinal dura mater (Fig. 19.53) extends as a
tubular sheath from the margins of the foramen
magnum to the second sacral vertebra below. At
this lower level the dura then invests the filum
terminale of the spinal cord, forming a thin fibrous strand which is anchored to the coccyx
below. As the nerve roots pass to the intervertebral foramina, each collects a dural coat which
becomes continuous with the epineurium of the
spinal nerve. The outer surface of the spinal dura
is separated from the walls of the vertebral canal
by the extra-dural space containing a plexus of
veins and some fatty tissue. Between the inner
surface of dura and the underlying arachnoid
mater is the subdural space. This contains only a
thin film of serous fluid which just separates the
two membranes.

The cranial dura mater covers the brain and is
usually regarded as two layers:
1 An inner or meningeal layer, continuous
with and corresponding to the spinal dura; and
2 An outer or endosteal layer which is really
the periosteum lining the inner aspect of the
bones of the cranial cavity.

The two layers are tightly adherent at the base of
the skull and along the sutures, but are easily
separated in the vault region. At certain sites,
intracranial venous sinuses and meningeal blood
vessels run between the two layers.

The meningeal layer of the dura provides
sheaths around the cranial nerves as they issue
from the skull. Outside the cranial cavity the
sheaths blend with the epineurium of the nerves
or, in the case of the optic nerve, with the sclera
of the eyeball. In addition, the meningeal layer
forms inwardly projecting septa, the falx cerebri
and the tentorium cerebelli, which mechanically
support the brain.

The falx cerebri (Fig. 19.54), named on
account of its sickle-like shape, is a median
partition which projects downwards into the
longitudinal fissure between the cerebral hemispheres. It is attached in front to the crista galli of
the ethmoid bone, and behind to the upper
surface of the tentorium cerebelli. The upper
margin of the falx is fixed to the inner surface of
the skull along the margins of the groove for the
superior sagittal sinus; its lower margin, free and
concave, contains the inferior sagittal sinus.

The tentorium cerebelli (Figs. 19.54 & 19.55)
is a crescentic partition projecting between the
cerebellum below and the occipital lobes of the
cerebral hemispheres above. Its outer convex
border is attached on each side to (a) the margins
of the groove for the transverse sinus on the

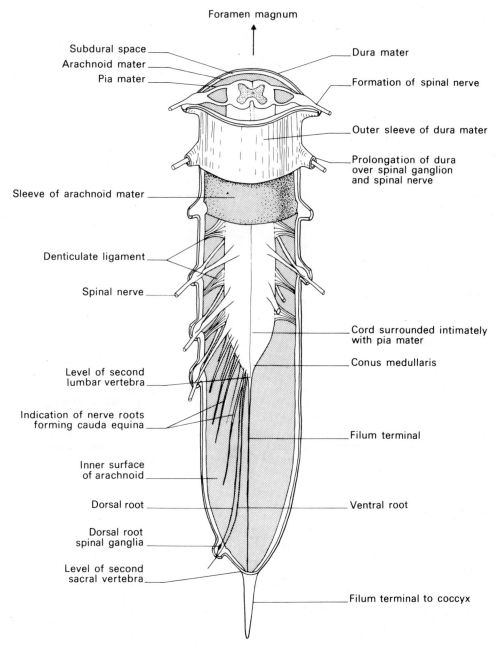

Foramen magnum

Subdural space
Arachnoid mater
Pia mater

Dura mater

Formation of spinal nerve

Outer sleeve of dura mater

Prolongation of dura
over spinal ganglion
and spinal nerve

Sleeve of arachnoid mater

Denticulate ligament

Spinal nerve

Cord surrounded intimately
with pia mater

Conus medullaris

Level of second
lumbar vertebra

Indication of nerve roots
forming cauda equina

Filum terminal

Inner surface
of arachnoid

Dorsal root

Ventral root

Dorsal root
spinal ganglia

Level of second
sacral vertebra

Filum terminal to coccyx

Fig. 19.53. Diagram to show the general arrangement of the spinal meninges.

occipital and parietal bones, (b) the superior border of the petrous temporal bone and (c) the posterior clinoid process of the sphenoid bone. Its concave inner border is free, extending from one anterior clinoid process to the other; this border together with the dorsum sellae of the sphenoid bone forms the boundary of a large

oval opening, the tentorial notch, which contains the midbrain and part of the cerebellar vermis. As previously noted the falx cerebri is attached in the midline to the upper surface of the tentorium cerebelli and within this line of attachment runs the straight sinus.

The meningeal layer of the dura mater also

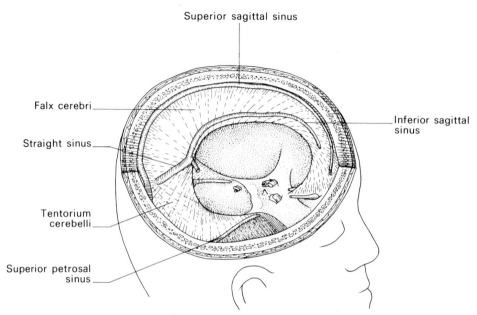

Fig. 19.54. The reflections of the cerebral dura mater, shown by removal of part of the right side of the skull and the entire brain.

provides a roof to the sella turcica which encloses the hypophysis cerebri (pituitary gland). This roof, called the diaphragma sellae, is pierced centrally by the infundibulum or pituitary stalk.

The nerve supply of the cranial dura mater is derived from all three divisions of the trigeminal nerve, the upper three cervical nerves and postganglionic sympathetic (vasomotor) fibres from the superior cervical ganglion. Although there is much overlap in the areas of distribution of the meningeal branches of the trigeminal nerve, in general those of the ophthalmic division supply the tentorium cerebelli, the dura of the vault and

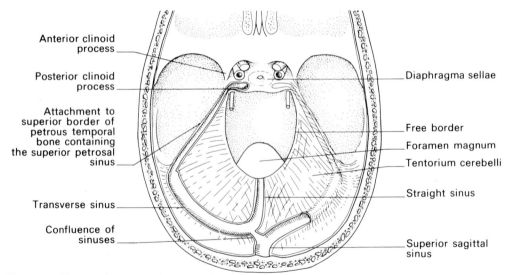

Fig. 19.55. The superior aspect of the tentorium cerebelli, exposed by the removal of the vault bones and brain.

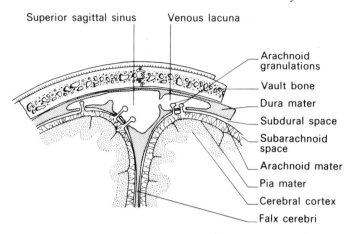

Superior sagittal sinus   Venous lacuna

Arachnoid granulations

Vault bone

Dura mater

Subdural space

Subarachnoid space

Arachnoid mater

Pia mater

Cerebral cortex

Falx cerebri

Fig. 19.56. A coronal section through the vertex of the skull showing the cerebral meninges and the arachnoid granulations.

anterior cranial fossa, whilst the meningeal branches of the maxillary and mandibular divisions innervate the dura of the middle cranial fossa. Ascending meningeal branches of the cervical nerves supply the dura of the posterior cranial fossa. They enter the skull through the foramen magnum as direct branches or through the jugular foramen and hypoglossal canal as indirect branches (see meningeal branches of the vagus and hypoglossal nerves, pp. 917, 901).

The arterial supply of the cranial dura mater is derived from branches of the internal carotid, vertebral, occipital and maxillary arteries. The latter gives rise to a large and clinically important branch, the middle meningeal artery, which enters the middle cranial fossa through the foramen spinosum of the sphenoid bone and supplies the bones and dura of the temporal and parietal regions. Fractures of the temporal region may tear branches of this artery causing extradural haemorrhage which leads to rapid compression of the brain, impairment of cerebral blood flow and consequent coma.

ARACHNOID MATER

The arachnoid mater (Figs. 19.52, 19.53 & 19.56) is a delicate, avascular membrane, lying between the dura mater and the pia mater. It consists of flattened mesothelial cells and also interlacing fibres composed of collagen, elastin and reticulin. The arachnoid appears to be in direct contact with the inner surface of the dura mater but as previously noted is separated from this surface by the narrow subdural space. The inner surface of the arachnoid is separated from the underlying pia mater by another, but considerably more capacious, space termed the sub-

arachnoid space. This contains cerebrospinal fluid, and in certain regions is bridged by strands (trabeculae) of connective tissue which connect the arachnoid to the pia mater.

PIA MATER

The pia mater is the innermost layer of the meninges. It entirely covers the outer surface of the brain and spinal cord, and also forms sheaths around the cranial nerves and the roots of the spinal nerves as they traverse the subarachnoid space. Structurally the pia mater consists of cells and fibres similar to those of the arachnoid, but in addition abounds with blood vessels which supply the underlying nervous tissue. Its deepest stratum is firmly attached to a well defined basement membrane which is apposed to a subjacent layer formed by expanded endings of astrocytic processes (see external limiting membrane, p. 871).

The pia mater not only covers the brain but is also invaginated into the ventricles to form the tela choroidea and choroid plexuses. The plexuses are highly vascular structures and are responsible for the production of cerebrospinal fluid. The spinal pia mater also shows modifications in the form of certain fibrous extensions which help to maintain the position of the spinal cord within the subarachnoid space. These extensions are the filum terminale and the ligamentum denticulatum (Fig. 19.53). Each ligament is a long, narrow sheet of pia extending from the lateral side of the cord, midway between the rows of ventral and dorsal roots. Its medial border is continuous with the pia of the side of the cord, whilst its lateral border ends in a

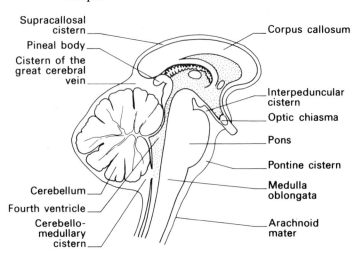

Fig. 19.57. A diagram showing the principal subarachnoid cisterns.

Labels: Supracallosal cistern, Pineal body, Cistern of the great cerebral vein, Cerebellum, Fourth ventricle, Cerebello-medullary cistern, Corpus callosum, Interpeduncular cistern, Optic chiasma, Pons, Pontine cistern, Medulla oblongata, Arachnoid mater

series of tooth-like projections which are attached to the dura mater.

SUBARACHNOID SPACE

The subarachnoid space surrounds the brain and spinal cord, and lies between pia and arachnoid mater. It contains cerebrospinal fluid as well as blood vessels and nerve bundles which cross the space to enter or leave the central nervous system. Due to the incongruities between the surfaces of the brain and the surrounding cranial cavity the width of the cranial part of subarachnoid space is very variable. The space is almost obliterated on the summits of gyri, especially those underlying the vault of the skull, but is deep in the fissures and sulci. Certain regions of the subarachnoid space are more capacious and form subarachnoid cisterns some of which are depicted in Fig. 19.57.

The cerebello-medullary cistern (cisterna magna) is clinically important, for samples of cerebrospinal fluid are obtained from it by inserting a needle through the posterior atlanto-occipital membrane in the nape of the neck (cisternal puncture).

The spinal part of the subarachnoid space lies within the vertebral canal, extending from the level of the foramen magnum to the second sacral vertebra where the dural sac ends. It surrounds the spinal cord which terminates at the level of the second lumbar vertebra. Below this level the space contains the cauda equina and the filum terminale and is used clinically to obtain samples of cerebrospinal fluid by means of lumbar puncture. This is carried out by inserting a needle in the midline, usually between the spinous processes of the fourth and fifth lumbar vertebrae.

ARACHNOID VILLI AND ARACHNOID GRANULATIONS

The subarachnoid space receives a continuous supply of cerebrospinal fluid from the ventricular system through three openings, the median aperture and the lateral apertures of the fourth ventricle. The circulating fluid is absorbed from the subarachnoid space through numerous arachnoid villi which are closely associated with the larger intradural venous sinuses, particularly with the superior sagittal sinus and its lacunae (Fig. 19.56). Each villus (Fig. 19.58) is a small pouch of arachnoid tissue which protrudes through a dural opening into a venous sinus; its cavity, containing cerebrospinal fluid and a network of fibres, is connected with the main subarachnoid space by a small stalk. It is lined internally by mesothelial cells and externally by vascular endothelium, through which cerebrospinal fluid is drawn into the surrounding blood stream by osmosis.

Arachnoid villi show marked changes with age. At birth the villi are few and microscopically small. About the age of three years, more villi are present, many of which can now be seen macroscopically, appearing as small white bodies situated in clusters in the walls of the venous sinuses. These bodies are termed arachnoid granulations or Pacchionian bodies, and with advancing age become more numerous and hypertrophied. They commonly calcify, and frequently cause erosion of bone which results in a series of small pits on the inner aspect of the

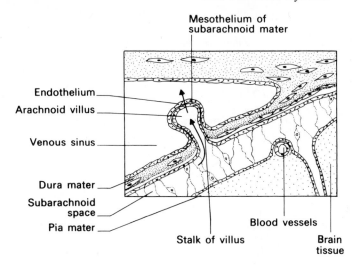

Mesothelium of subarachnoid mater

Endothelium

Arachnoid villus

Venous sinus

Dura mater

Subarachnoid space

Pia mater

Stalk of villus

Blood vessels

Brain tissue

Fig. 19.58. A diagram showing the structure of an arachnoid villus and its relationship to the venous sinus and subarachnoid space.

skull, close to the groove for the superior sagittal sinus.

Arachnoid granulations are not the only routes through which cerebrospinal fluid escapes from the subarachnoid space. Some fluid is probably absorbed into epineurial lymphatics which drain the extensions of the subarachnoid space surrounding the cranial and spinal nerves as they leave the skull and vertebral column.

The composition and physiology of cerebrospinal fluid is considered on p. 932.

The ventricular system and the circulation of cerebrospinal fluid

The overall plan of the ventricular system is shown in Fig. 19.59. Cerebrospinal fluid is produced by the choroid plexuses of all the ventricles, those of the lateral ventricles being the most extensive.

A choroid plexus is formed of vascular pia mater (the tela choroidea) which is invaginated into the ventricular cavity and there picks up a layer of ependyma (Fig. 19.60). To the naked

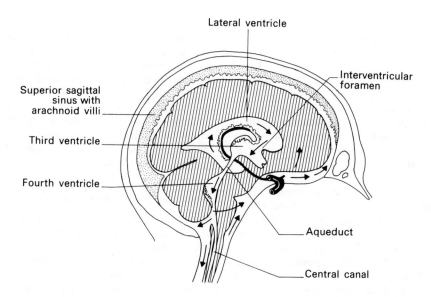

Lateral ventricle

Superior sagittal sinus with arachnoid villi

Third ventricle

Fourth ventricle

Interventricular foramen

Aqueduct

Central canal

Fig. 19.59. A diagram illustrating the flow of cerebrospinal fluid in the ventricles and subarachnoid space. The arrows indicate the flow pattern of the fluid.

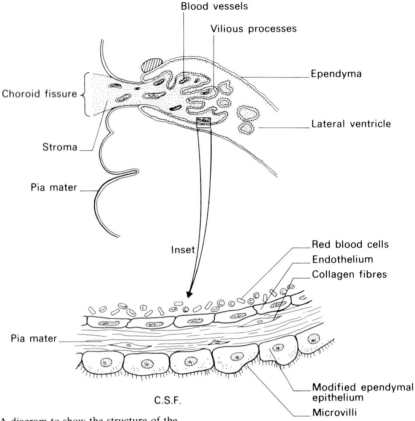

Fig. 19.60. A diagram to show the structure of the choroid plexus in the inferior horn of the lateral ventricle.

eye the surface of the plexus consists of highly irregular fringes which microscopically are studded with numerous villous processes. Each process contains an inner core of connective tissue or stroma, a capillary bed with afferent and efferent vessels, and an outer layer of ependyma. The ependymal cells, which are often ciliated, possess microvilli and thus an enormous surface area is availabe for the formation of cerebrospinal fluid.

Cerebrospinal fluid flows from the lateral ventricles to the third ventricle through the interventricular foramina, and thence to the fourth ventricle through the aqueduct of the midbrain. The fluid leaves the ventricular system to enter the subarachnoid space by way of three openings, a median and two lateral apertures situated in the fourth ventricle. From these sites there is a slow movement of fluid along the subarachnoid cisterns on the base of the brain, and then upwards over the medial and superolateral sur-

faces of the brain; some fluid is also directed downwards into the spinal subarachnoid space. The flow of cerebrospinal fluid is influenced by movements of the head and vertebral column, and possibly by the pulsations of the superficial cerebral arteries.

Cerebrospinal fluid is absorbed by arachnoid villi. The production, absorption and other physiological aspects of cerebrospinal fluid is considered elsewhere (p. 932).

Blood supply of the brain (see also p. 718)

Blood is delivered to the brain by conducting or superficial arteries, represented by the large arteries and their branches which lie in the pia mater covering the brain. These give rise in turn to numerous smaller vessels termed penetrating or nutrient arteries which pass into the substance of the brain to form extensive capillary networks. The conducting vessels form anastomoses which may be sufficient to support an adequate supply of blood in the event of the occlusion of a small vessel. Anastomoses also occur between the penetrating vessels, but these are generally ineffective, and occlusion of such arteries results in necrosis of tissue in the affected region.

ARTERIAL BLOOD SUPPLY

The brain receives blood through two pairs of large arteries, the vertebral and internal carotid, situated on the base of the brain.

Vertebral arteries
The vertebral artery enters the cranial cavity through the foramen magnum, passing at first lateral and then ventral to the medulla oblongata. At the lower border of the pons it unites in the midline with the opposite vertebral artery to form the basilar artery.

In the neck the vertebral arteries give rise to a variable number of spinal radicular arteries which pass through the intervertebral foramina to supply the spinal cord and dura mater. These spinal vessels freely anastomose with the anterior and posterior spinal arteries.

Inside the skull the vertebral arteries supply branches to the spinal cord, medulla and cerebellum.

Basilar artery
The basilar artery gives off two cerebellar vessels, the anterior inferior and superior cerebellar arteries which supply the lower and upper surfaces of the cerebellar hemispheres. The labyrinthine artery may arise from the basilar artery or, more frequently, from the anterior inferior cerebellar artery; it enters the internal acoustic meatus in company with the facial and vestibulocochlear nerves, being distributed to the inner ear. Pontine arteries are numerous, stemming from the basilar trunk or from its branches. At the upper pontine border the basilar artery divides into two posterior cerebral arteries.

Branches of the posterior cerebral artery (and incidently other major cerebral arteries) are divided into central and cortical sets. Central arteries are small perforating vessels, arising in groups along the commencement of the major artery, whereas cortical arteries are conducting vessels which ramify over the surface of the cerebrum. More specifically, central branches of the posterior cerebral artery provide the major blood supply to the thalamus, and also distribute to the midbrain, pineal body and the choroid plexuses of the third and lateral ventricles. Cortical branches supply the occipital lobe and much of the temporal lobe (i.e. gyri on the medial and inferior aspects of the latter, but excluding the temporal pole: Fig. 19.61). Note that the visual cortical area lies within the region supplied by the posterior cerebral artery.

Internal carotid artery
The internal carotid artery begins at the bifurcation of the common carotid artery in the neck, and ascends to the base of the skull where it passes through the carotid canal in the petrous part of the temporal bone. Within the cranial cavity it traverses the cavernous sinus and then divides into two major vessels, the anterior and middle cerebral arteries, which supply the greater part of the cerebral hemisphere. For descriptive purposes the artery is divided into cervical (p. 645), petrous, cavernous and cerebral parts.

The petrous part of the internal carotid artery passes through the carotid canal where it initially lies in front of the cochlea and tympanic cavity. It is surrounded by the carotid plexus of nerves, derived from the internal carotid nerve of the superior cervical ganglion.

The cavernous part of the internal carotid artery runs through the cavernous sinus (Fig. 19.62), passing at first upwards towards the posterior clinoid process, then forwards on the medial side of the body of the sphenoid bone; finally it curves upwards on the medial side of the anterior clinoid process and pierces the dural roof of the sinus. Situated lateral to the artery are the oculomotor, trochlear, abducent nerves and also the ophthalmic and maxillary divisions of the trigeminal nerve, while medially and above the artery lies the pituitary gland, ensconced in the fossa of the sphenoid bone. Postganglionic sympathetic fibres of the carotid plexus accompany the artery and are distributed to its cerebral branches and also along the ophthalmic artery to orbital structures. The cavernous part of the internal carotid artery supplies branches to the pituitary gland and also to the surrounding meninges. On leaving the sinus it gives off the ophthalmic artery, the distribution of which is considered on p. 645.

The cerebral part of the internal carotid artery turns sharply backwards below the optic nerve to reach the anterior perforated substance, where it lies lateral to the optic chiasma and medial to the anterior part of the lateral fissure. It then divides into the anterior and middle cerebral arteries.

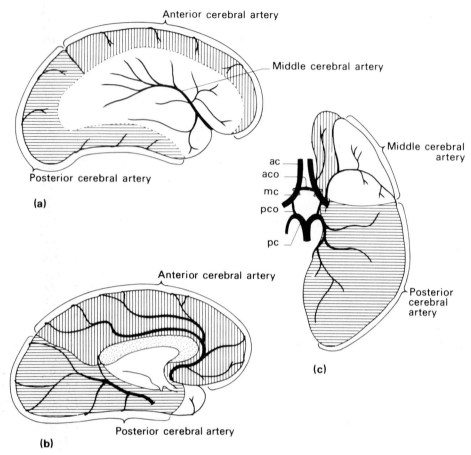

Fig. 19.61. Diagrams of the blood supply of the cerebral cortex. (a) Lateral aspect; (b) medial aspect and (c) inferior aspect. ac — anterior cerebral artery; aco — anterior communicating artery; mc — middle cerebral artery; pco — posterior communicating artery; and pc — posterior cerebral artery.

The anterior cerebral artery passes medially and forwards above the optic nerve to reach the longitudinal fissure between the two cerebral hemispheres. Here it curves around the genu of the corpus callosum and then runs backwards on the surface of this commissure. At the beginning of the longitudinal fissure the anterior cerebral artery is joined to its fellow artery of the opposite side by a short trunk, the anterior communicating artery. (Fig. 19.61).

Occlusion of the anterior cerebral artery results in paralysis of the contralateral lower limb (monoplegia), for the 'leg area' of the motor cortex, situated in the medial aspect of the frontal lobe, is supplied by this artery.

The middle cerebral artery runs laterally into the lateral fissure between the frontal and temporal lobes where it divides into branches which are distributed over the lateral surface of the cerebral hemisphere (Fig. 19.61). Its central branches (anterolateral group), also known as striate arteries, enter the anterior perforated substance to supply most of the corpus striatum (caudate and lentiform nuclei) and also the internal capsule. The largest of the striate arteries is particularly prone to rupture, and is termed the 'artery of cerebral haemorrhage'. Bleeding or occlusion of the central arteries damages fibres of the internal capsule, resulting in paralysis of the contralateral side of the body (hemiplegia). It is important to note that the middle cerebral artery supplies the auditory area and the greater part of the motor and sensory cortical areas.

Circulus arteriosus (of Willis)
The circle is in fact a heptagonal arrangement of major cerebral arteries and communicating ves-

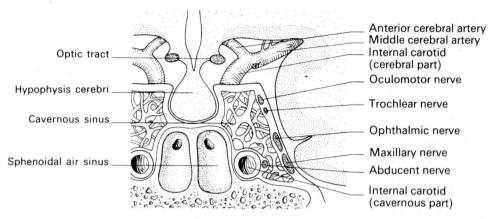

Optic tract

Hypophysis cerebri

Cavernous sinus

Sphenoidal air sinus

Anterior cerebral artery
Middle cerebral artery
Internal carotid
(cerebral part)
Oculomotor nerve

Trochlear nerve

Ophthalmic nerve

Maxillary nerve
Abducent nerve

Internal carotid
(cavernous part)

Fig. 19.62. A coronal section through the middle cranial fossa showing the cavernous and cerebral parts of the internal carotid artery, together with the cavernous sinus and its contents.

sels (Fig. 19.61). It lies on the base of the brain in the interpeduncular cistern, surrounding the optic chiasma, pituitary stalk and mamillary bodies. The circle is formed in front by the two anterior cerebral arteries and the short anterior communicating artery, and behind by the two posterior cerebral arteries, derived from the basilar artery. On each side the circle is completed by the posterior communicating artery which connects the internal carotid artery with the posterior cerebral artery.

VENOUS DRAINAGE OF THE BRAIN AND
VENOUS SINUSES OF THE DURA MATER

Veins of the brain have thin walls, little or no muscle, and no valves. For descriptive purposes they may be divided into two main groups:
1 External and internal cerebral veins which drain the superficial and deep parts of the cerebral hemispheres respectively; and
2 Veins draining the brainstem and cerebellum.
Both groups principally drain into the internal jugular veins through a system of interconnecting venous sinuses running in the dura mater.

Venous sinuses of the dura mater
These sinuses, like the veins of the brain, contain little muscle and no valves. They lie between the two layers of the dura mater and drain blood from the brain, the meninges and bones of the skull. Some are also associated with arachnoid villi (Fig. 19.56) and therefore absorb cerebrospinal fluid.

The superior sagittal sinus (Fig. 19.54) lies in the attached margin of the falx cerebri. It starts in front of the crista galli, runs backwards and ends near the internal occipital protuberance where it usually turns to the right to enter the right transverse sinus. The sinus in its course grooves the inner aspect of the frontal bone, the adjacent margins of the parietal bones and squamous part of the occipital bone.

It receives blood from the superior cerebral veins and is connected on each side with three blood filled spaces or venous lacunae into which drain diploic and meningeal veins. Both the sinus and lacunae possess numerous arachnoid granulations.

The inferior sagittal sinus (Fig. 19.54) is also associated with the falx cerebri and runs backwards in its free border to the junction of the falx with the tentorium cerebelli. Here, it is joined by the great cerebral vein to become the straight sinus which then continues backwards and downwards within the line of attachment of the falx with the tentorium. On reaching the internal occipital protuberance the straight sinus usually passes to the left and enters the left transverse sinus. In this region a small vein connects the left transverse sinus with the terminal part of the superior sagittal sinus (confluence of the sinuses) as it enters the right transverse sinus.

Each transverse sinus, being the continuation of either the superior sagittal sinus or the straight sinus, lies in the attached margin of the tentorium cerebelli and passes laterally and then forwards to the base of the petrous part of the temporal bone where it leaves the tentorium to become the sigmoid sinus. In its course it grooves the inner surface of the squama of the occipital bone and a small part of the parietal bone. It receives the inferior cerebral veins and also the superior petrosal sinus.

The sigmoid sinus is a direct continuation of the transverse sinus and curves downwards and medially in a groove on the mastoid part of the temporal bone. It then turns forwards to reach the jugular foramen where it leaves the skull to become the internal jugular vein. In the upper part of its course it is related anteriorly to the mastoid antrum and mastoid air cells, being separated from them by only a thin shell of bone.

The cavernous sinuses (Fig. 19.62) are situated on each side of the body of the sphenoid bone. Each extends from the superior orbital fissure in front to the apex of the petrosal part of the temporal bone, and lies between the inner and outer layers of the dura mater. The sinus is about 2 cm long and 1 cm wide. Its lumen is spongy in appearance, being divided into irregular spaces by bridging strands of connective tissue (trabeculae); its walls are lined internally by endothelium which also invests the trabeculae. Passing forwards through the cavernous sinus is the internal carotid artery accompanied by the abducent nerve and the carotid plexus of sympathetic nerves, all of which are separated from the cavity of the sinus by endothelium. Lying in the lateral wall between the endothelium and the dura are the oculomotor and trochlear nerves and also the ophthalmic and maxillary divisions of the trigeminal nerve. The hypophysis cerebri (pituitary gland) and the body of the sphenoid bone are medial relations of the sinus whilst the trigeminal ganglion lies lateral to the posterior part of the sinus.

The cavernous sinus receives blood from the orbit through the superior and inferior ophthalmic veins, and from the brain via the inferior cerebral veins and one of the middle cerebral veins. The sinus drains into the transverse sinus through the superior petrosal sinus (Figs. 19.54 & 19.55) which runs backwards in a groove on the superior border of the petrosal part of the temporal bone; it also drains into the internal jugular vein via the inferior petrosal sinus which travels backwards along the groove between the temporal and occipital bones. Both the cavernous sinuses are linked across the midline by veins (intercavernous sinuses) in the diaphragma sellae.

Diploic, meningeal and emissary veins
The diploic veins form a network of channels in the diploë of the skull. They connect with meningeal veins, the venous sinuses of the dura

and also with veins lying outside the skull. Regular routes exist between the diploë of the frontal bone and the cavernous sinus, whilst more posteriorly the diploic veins of the parietal and occipital bones terminate in the transverse sinus.

The meningeal veins are arranged as plexuses of small vessels in the dura mater which drain through larger veins into the venous sinuses. An important drainage channel is provided by the middle meningeal veins which accompany the middle meningeal arteries in grooves on the inner surface of the parietal and temporal bones. These veins connect with the lacunae of the superior sagittal sinus, and may drain into the cavernous sinus and its tributaries, or leave the skull through the foramen ovale to join the pterygoid venous plexus.

The emissary veins pass through small foramina of the skull, forming connections between the intracranial venous sinuses and the extracranial veins. They are numerous and occur at various, often inconstant, sites. Some of the more constant ones include: a mastoid emissary vein, connecting the sigmoid sinus with the posterior auricular vein; a posterior condylar emissary vein which passes through the condylar foramen, linking the sigmoid sinus with veins of the suboccipital region; and a network of veins which unites the cavernous sinus with the pterygoid plexus through the foramen ovale.

Applied anatomy. Connections between the extracranial venous system and venous sinuses provide routes for the spread of suppurative infection from the face, scalp, orbit, paranasal air sinuses, middle ear or mastoid air cells which may result in septic thrombosis of the venous sinuses and/or brain abscess. The cavernous sinus is particularly prone to thrombosis from facial sepsis, for its tributaries (the ophthalmic veins) communicate with the veins of the face.

The cranial nerves

There are twelve pairs of cranial nerves and they are numbered in rostrocaudal sequence as follows:
(1) Olfactory, (2) Optic, (3) Oculomotor, (4) Trochlear, (5) Trigeminal, (6) Abducent, (7) Facial, (8) Vestibulocochlear, (9) Glossopharyngeal, (10) Vagus, (11) Accessory, (12) Hypoglossal.

The first two pairs (olfactory and optic) are connected to the ventral aspect of the forebrain whereas the remaining ten pairs, excepting part of the accessory nerve, are attached to the brainstem. Some cranial nerves are similar to spinal nerves in that they are mixed, that is, they contain considerable numbers of both motor (efferent) and sensory (afferent) fibres; others are composed predominantly of either motor or sensory fibres. Motor fibres of the cranial nerves arise within the brain from groups of neurons termed nuclei of origin. Sensory fibres, on the other hand, project into the brain and end by synapsing on cell groups called nuclei of termination. Some of these sensory fibres arise from cell bodies of unipolar neurons which form ganglia (cranial sensory ganglia), situated on the nerve trunk close to the base of the skull; others arise from cell bodies found more peripherally in special sense organs such as the eye, nose and ear. Both, motor as well as sensory fibres, are further subdivided into functional components; their corresponding nuclei of origin and termination are arranged within the brainstem as a series of discontinuous longitudinal columns. This arrangement is more easily understood by a brief examination of the embryological development of cord and brainstem (p. 833).

The nervous system is derived from ectoderm. In the midline of the dorsal surface of the embryonic plate the neural groove appears and sinks below the surface of the plate forming the neural tube (Fig. 19.63a). During this process some neuroectodermal cells become separated forming the neural crest. These cells migrate and differentiate into the following neural elements: unipolar neurons of dorsal root ganglia of spinal nerves, unipolar neurons of cranial sensory nerve ganglia, bipolar neurons of ganglia of the vestibulocochlear nerve, and multipolar neurons of autonomic ganglia (Book 2).

The cranial end of the neural tube undergoes considerable modification, so forming the cerebral hemispheres, brainstem and cerebellum; whilst the remaining part of the neural tube forms the spinal cord. The basic tubular structure, although obscured in the cerebral hemispheres, persists in the spinal cord and brainstem; here, proliferating cells become arranged in longitudinal columns. The lateral walls of the primitive spinal cord thicken, each developing two distinct masses, the dorsal (alar) lamina and the ventral (basal) lamina. These project into the lumen of the central canal and are separated by a longitudinal groove, the sulcus limitans (Fig. 19.63b).

Cells of the dorsal lamina develop into sensory (afferent) neurons. Some become interneurons with short axons responsible for segmental reflexes, others give rise to long axons which form ascending tracts of the cord. They are arranged into two longitudinal columns, a somatosensory column and a viscerosensory column (Fig. 19.63c). Cells of the somatosensory column receive incoming dorsal root fibres which convey impulses from the skin, striated muscles, joints and ligaments of the body walls and limbs; those of the viscerosensory column receive impulses via the dorsal root fibres from blood vessels, glands of the skin, and visceral structures (e.g., smooth muscle and glands of the gut).

Cells of the ventral lamina differentiate into motor (efferent) neurons whose axons grow out of the cord to supply peripheral structures. Two longitudinal columns of cells are formed, a somatomotor one which innervates striated muscle derived from myotomes and somatopleure, and a visceromotor column whose fibres are destined to terminate by synapsing with autonomic ganglionic cells.

The dorsal and ventral laminae and the sulcus limitans continue throughout the brainstem. The laminae differentiate into four functional columns, continuous and homologous with those of the primitive cord; but owing to the development of the branchial arches and special senses in the cranial region additional columns of cells are formed. These include a branchiomotor column which supplies striated muscle derived from branchial arch mesoderm, and a gustatory (branchiosensory) column which receives fibres concerned with taste sensation. This columnar arrangement is shown diagrammatically in Fig. 19.63d. As development proceeds the brainstem columns become broken up into nuclei associated with specific cranial nerves.

Cranial nerves may be broadly divided into three groups, namely: somatomotor nerves, branchial arch nerves and nerves of the special senses.

1 Somatomotor nerves comprise the oculomotor, trochlear, abducent and hypoglossal. They supply muscles derived from the cranial myotomes and their axons arise from cells of the somatomotor column which lie close to the midline of the brainstem. They are homologous with the ventral roots of the spinal nerves and all except the trochlear nerve arise in line with them on the ventral aspect of the brainstem.

2 Nerves of the branchial arches comprise the trigeminal, facial, glossopharyngeal, vagus and accessory. They are characterized by containing branchiomotor fibres which supply striated muscle derived from the branchial arches; in addition, these nerves (save the accessory which

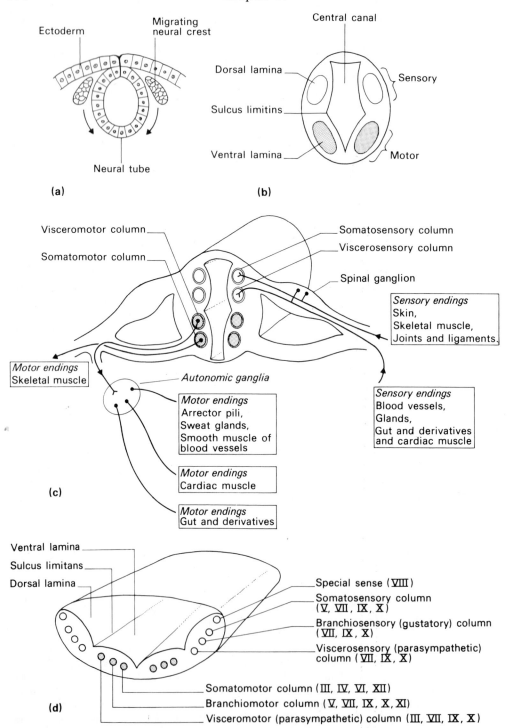

Fig. 19.63. Diagrams illustrating the development of the functional columns of neurons forming the various components of spinal and cranial nerves. (a) Transverse section of the primitive neural tube with neural crest. (b) Development of the sensory and motor columns of the spinal cord. (c) Functional components of the spinal nerves. (d) Functional columns of neurons of the brainstem showing their associations with the cranial nerves.

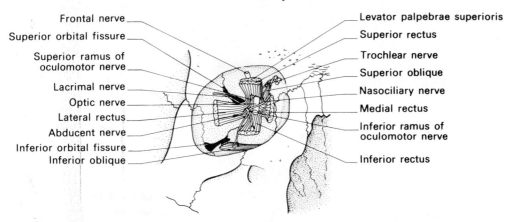

Frontal nerve
Superior orbital fissure
Superior ramus of oculomotor nerve
Lacrimal nerve
Optic nerve
Lateral rectus
Abducent nerve
Inferior orbital fissure
Inferior oblique

Levator palpebrae superioris
Superior rectus
Trochlear nerve
Superior oblique
Nasociliary nerve
Medial rectus
Inferior ramus of oculomotor nerve
Inferior rectus

Fig. 19.64. Dissection of the right orbit, seen from the front, showing the relationship of the nerves to the orbital muscles.

is believed to be solely branchiomotor) possess other functional components such as somatosensory, viscerosensory, gustatory and visceromotor fibres.

3 Nerves of the special senses include the olfactory, optic and vestibulocochlear nerves. Apart from being sensory in function these nerves have little in common. The olfactory nerve is unusual in being solely derived from ectodermal cells lying outside the neural tube and crest. The optic nerve arises from retinal ganglion cells and resembles a fibre tract of the brain rather than a peripheral nerve; this is substantiated by its failure to regenerate following injury. The developmental origin of the vestibulocochlear nerve is controversial, some

evidence suggests that it is derived from the neural crest and can be regarded as homologous with a somewhat modified dorsal root.

These nerves are described in their respective systems; olfactory system (p. 875), visual system (p. 881) and vestibulocochlear pathways (p. 883).

SOMATOMOTOR CRANIAL NERVES

The abducent, trochlear and oculomotor nerves (Figs. 19.64, 19.65 & 19.66)

The abducent nerve supplies the lateral rectus muscle of the eyeball. Fibres of the nerve arise from the abducent nucleus (Fig. 19.25) in the pontine part of the floor of the fourth ventricle.

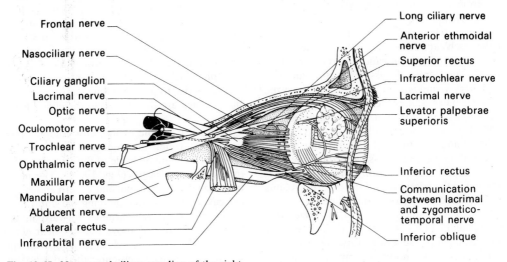

Frontal nerve
Nasociliary nerve
Ciliary ganglion
Lacrimal nerve
Optic nerve
Oculomotor nerve
Trochlear nerve
Ophthalmic nerve
Maxillary nerve
Mandibular nerve
Abducent nerve
Lateral rectus
Infraorbital nerve

Long ciliary nerve
Anterior ethmoidal nerve
Superior rectus
Infratrochlear nerve
Lacrimal nerve
Levator palpebrae superioris
Inferior rectus
Communication between lacrimal and zygomatico-temporal nerve
Inferior oblique

Fig. 19.65. Nerves and ciliary ganglion of the right orbit, seen from the right side.

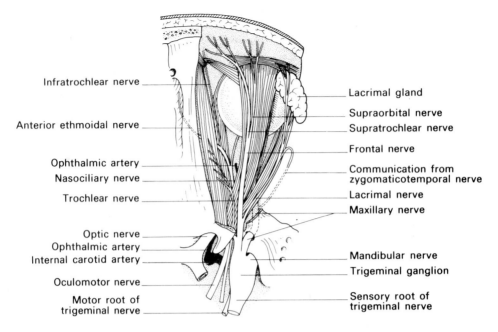

Fig. 19.66. Nerves of the right orbit, seen from the superior aspect.

The fibres emerge as a nerve bundle from the sulcus separating the pons from the medulla oblongata on the ventral aspect of the brainstem (Fig. 19.16). The nerve pierces the dura mater close to the apex of the petrous temporal bone and dorsum sellae of the sphenoid bone. Next, it traverses the cavernous sinus (Fig. 19.62), then passes into the orbital cavity through the superior orbital fissure and common tendinous ring from which the recti muscles arise.

The trochlear nerve innervates the superior oblique muscle of the eyeball. Its fibres originate in the trochlear nucleus (Fig. 19.28) which lies in the tegmentum of the caudal part of the midbrain. The fibres decussate in the anterior medullary velum with trochlear fibres from the opposite nucleus; they then emerge as the trochlear nerve on the dorsal surface of the brainstem behind the inferior colliculus (Fig. 19.17). The nerve continues forward around the lateral aspect of the midbrain passing through the dura mater behind the posterior clinoid process. It now lies in the lateral wall of the cavernous sinus accompanied by the oculomotor nerve, above, and the ophthalmic division of the trigeminal nerve, below (Fig. 19.62). It then enters the orbit through the superior orbital fissure.

The oculomotor nerve is composed primarily of somatomotor fibres which innervate all extra-ocular muscles except the superior oblique and lateral rectus; in addition, it supplies the striated muscle of the levator palpebrae superioris. The nerve also contains visceromotor fibres which indirectly supply the smooth muscle of the ciliary body and sphincter pupillae through connections with the ciliary ganglion. All these fibres arise from the oculomotor complex, an elongated nucleus, situated just ventral to the periaqueductal grey of the cranial part of the midbrain (Fig. 19.29). The nucleus contains a number of cell groups, each of which is specifically responsible for the innervation of a particular eye muscle. One such group, the Edinger-Westphal nucleus, lies dorsal to the main nucleus and gives rise to preganglionic parasympathetic fibres which are distributed to the ciliary ganglion.

Fibres leaving the oculomotor complex pass ventrally through the midbrain tegmentum to emerge on the medial side of the crus cerebri as the oculomotor nerve (Fig. 19.16). The nerve traverses the interpeduncular cistern and enters the cavernous sinus by piercing the dural roof. Inside the sinus it continues forward in the lateral wall, situated above the trochlear nerve (Fig. 19.62). It then divides into a superior and an inferior ramus which enter the orbit accompanied by the nasociliary and abducent nerves.

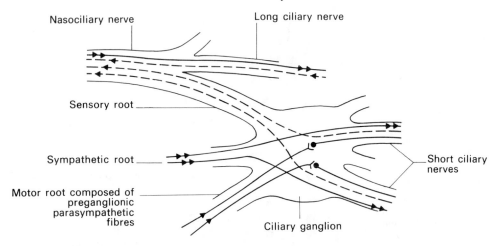

Fig. 19.67. Diagram of the ciliary ganglion showing its roots and distributing branches. Continuous lines with single arrows represent preganglionic parasympathetic fibres which synapse in the ganglion; the ganglionic cells giving rise to postganglionic parasympathetic fibres. Continuous lines with double arrows are postganglionic sympathetic fibres. Interrupted lines indicate sensory fibres.

The superior ramus supplies the levator palpebrae superioris and the superior rectus: individual branches of the inferior ramus supply the medial rectus, inferior rectus and inferior oblique muscles. The branch to the inferior oblique also carries preganglionic fibres supplying the ciliary ganglion.

The ciliary ganglion (Figs. 19.65 & 19.67) is a collection of parasympathetic, multipolar cells situated near the apex of the orbit between the lateral rectus muscle and the optic nerve. Preganglionic parasympathetic fibres from the Edinger–Westphal nucleus synapse with the ganglion cells, from which postganglionic parasympathetic fibres travel in the short ciliary nerves to supply the sphincter pupillae and ciliary body. Passing through the ganglion without interruption are postganglionic sympathetic fibres, derived from the superior cervical ganglion, which are conveyed to the orbit through a branch of the internal carotid plexus termed the sympathetic root of the ganglion. These fibres are distributed by the short ciliary nerves to blood vessels of the eyeball. Also passing through the ciliary ganglion without synapsing are sensory fibres from the eyeball including the cornea. These travel in the short ciliary nerves through the ciliary ganglion and form the sensory root of the ganglion which communicates with the nasociliary nerve. The short ciliary nerves are some eight to ten in number, but these further divide and are then distributed to the eyeball.

Clinical anatomy (p. 947). Damage to the abducent, trochlear or oculomotor nerves results in double vision (diplopia) which shows as a squint (strabismus) due to the paralysis of one or more extra-ocular muscles. Complete lesions of the oculomotor nerve result in the following signs: drooping of the upper eyelid (ptosis) owing to paralysis of levator palpebrae superioris; pupillary dilatation (mydriasis) and loss of the light reflex (p. 961) due to paralysis of the sphincter pupillae; and loss of the accommodation reflex (p. 961) on account of paralysis of the sphincter pupillae and ciliaris muscle.

The hypoglossal nerve

The hypoglossal nerve is the motor nerve to muscles of the tongue. Fibres forming the nerve arise from the hypoglossal nucleus (Fig. 19.22) which extends the length of the medulla. They emerge from the anterolateral sulcus of the medulla as a series of rootlets issuing between the pyramid and the olive (Fig. 19.16). The rootlets pass laterally behind the vertebral artery, then fuse to form a common trunk in the anterior condylar (hypoglossal) canal before leaving the skull. At this point in its course the hypoglossal nerve lies deep to the internal jugular vein, the ninth, tenth and eleventh cranial nerves. It then enters the carotid sheath, hooks around the inferior ganglion of the vagus nerve and descends vertically in front of the vagus nerve (Fig. 19.68). Leaving the sheath the nerve appears below the posterior belly of the digastric

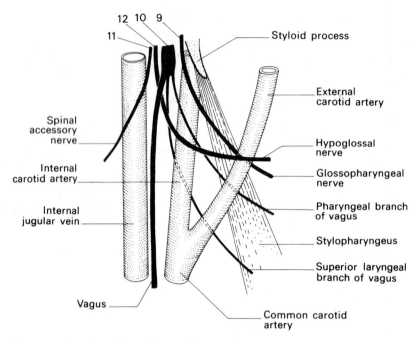

12 10 9

11

Styloid process

Spinal
accessory
nerve

External
carotid artery

Internal
carotid artery

Hypoglossal
nerve

Glossopharyngeal
nerve

Internal
jugular vein

Pharyngeal branch
of vagus

Stylopharyngeus

Superior laryngeal
branch of vagus

Vagus

Common carotid
artery

Fig. 19.68. Diagram to show the relations of some of
the cranial nerves and their branches to the internal
and external carotid arteries.

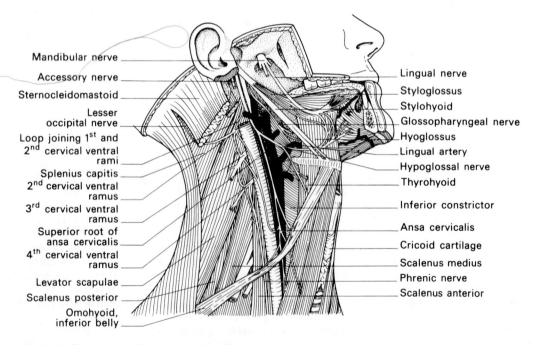

Mandibular nerve

Accessory nerve

Sternocleidomastoid

Lesser
occipital nerve

Loop joining 1st and
2nd cervical ventral
rami

Splenius capitis

2nd cervical ventral
ramus

3rd cervical ventral
ramus

Superior root of
ansa cervicalis

4th cervical ventral
ramus

Levator scapulae

Scalenus posterior

Omohyoid,
inferior belly

Lingual nerve

Styloglossus

Stylohyoid

Glossopharyngeal nerve

Hyoglossus

Lingual artery

Hypoglossal nerve

Thyrohyoid

Inferior constrictor

Ansa cervicalis

Cricoid cartilage

Scalenus medius

Phrenic nerve

Scalenus anterior

Fig. 19.69. Drawing of a dissection to show the
disposition of the right hypoglossal and lingual nerves,
and part of the cervical plexus.

muscle, winds around a branch of the occipital artery, and then passes forward crossing superficial to the internal and external carotid arteries and the loop of the lingual artery (Fig. 19.69). The nerve now lies just above the greater cornu of the hyoid bone and runs forward on the hyoglossus where it lies deep to the stylohyoid and tendon of the digastric muscle. Here the hypoglossal nerve is related to the mylohyoid below and to the deep part of the submandibular gland and its duct above.

The hypoglossal nerve communicates with branches of the lingual, the vagus, with the sympathetic trunk, and also with the first and second cervical nerves. The cervical elements join the hypoglossal trunk opposite the atlas vertebra. The hypoglossal nerve gives many branches which are detailed below, see also Fig. 19.70.

1 Meningeal branches supply the dura mater of the posterior cranial fossa. They pass through the anterior condylar canal and consist of sympathetic fibres and cervical sensory fibres.

2 The descending branch contains fibres from the first cervical nerve only, and constitutes the upper root of the ansa cervicalis. This branch unites with the lower root of the ansa cervicalis, derived from the second and third cervical nerves to form a loop, the ansa cervicalis (ansa hypoglossi), which is situated on the lateral side of the carotid sheath. Branches from the ansa cervicalis supply the sternohyoid, omohyoid and sternothyroid strap-muscles.

3 Muscular branches innervate styloglossus, hyoglossus, genioglossus, as well as all the intrinsic muscles of the tongue. Two other muscular branches also arise from the hypoglossal

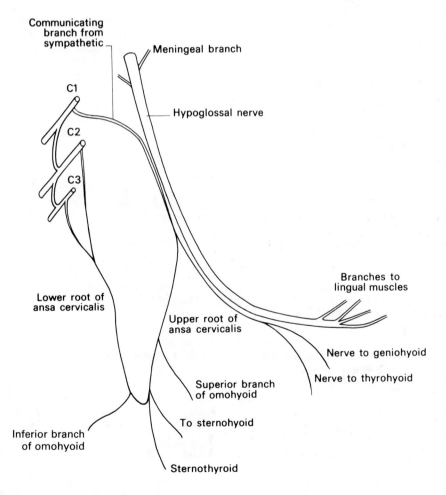

Fig. 19.70. Diagram of the right hypoglossal nerve and the ansa cervicalis.

nerve trunk but contain fibres originating from the first cervical nerve only. These supply the genioglossus and thyrohyoid.

Clinical anatomy. Damage to the hypoglossal nerve results in unilateral paralysis and hemiatrophy of the tongue musculature; on protrusion, the tongue deviates to the paralysed side due to the unopposed action of the muscles on the sound side. The larynx also may deviate on swallowing, but to the unaffected side, owing to unilateral paralysis of some of the infrahyoid strap-muscles which are depressors of the hyoid bone and are supplied by the descending branch (C1) of the hypoglossal nerve. Bilateral nerve lesions produce dramatic disabilities. The tongue muscles are completely paralysed and atrophy; speech is disturbed and mastication affected; swallowing is so impaired that the patient has to push (manually) the bolus of food into the pharynx before swallowing can be achieved.

BRANCHIAL ARCH NERVES

The trigeminal nerve

The trigeminal (fifth) nerve is the largest cranial nerve. It is a mixed nerve consisting predominantly of sensory fibres. These supply most of the face and scalp, part of the external ear and tympanic membrane, the nasal and oral cavities including the oral part of the tongue, the teeth and their supporting tissues. The motor fibres innervate striated muscle derived from the first branchial arch which includes amongst others the muscles of mastication. Proprioceptive fibres from these muscles, and from the temporomandibular joint and periodontal ligaments of the teeth are also contained in the trigeminal nerve.

The nerve is connected to the ventral surface of the pons by a large sensory root and a much smaller motor root, the former lying lateral and slightly posterior to the latter (Fig. 19.16). Both roots pass forwards to enter the trigeminal cave, a recess in the dura mater which is situated near the tip of the petrous part of temporal bone. Within the cave the sensory root expands forming the trigeminal ganglion, a crescentic shaped structure consisting of unipolar neurons (Fig. 19.71). The peripheral processes of these cells form the ophthalmic and maxillary nerves, and the sensory part of the mandibular nerve, all of which issue from the ganglion; the central processes constitute most of the fibres of the sensory root. This arrangement, whereby a collection of unipolar cells on the nerve trunk distributes sensory fibres to the periphery, is typical of most of the nerves belonging to the branchial group, e.g. the seventh, ninth and tenth cranial nerves. But, in addition, the trigeminal nerve contains sensory fibres derived from unipolar cells located within the central nervous system; these fibres which arise from the mesencephalic nucleus (p. 855) are concerned with proprioception and are distributed through the sensory root and trigeminal ganglion to the periphery; i.e. they are not functionally connected to the ganglion.

All fibres of the sensory root enter the pons where they mostly bifurcate into ascending and descending branches. All the descending elements form the spinal tract of the trigeminal nerve which passes through the pons and medulla oblongata to the upper level of the second cervical segment of the cord. During its descent, fibres of the tract terminate at various levels by synapsing on cells of the spinal nucleus of the trigeminal nerve. It has been shown experimentally, in animals and man, that both the fibres of the tract and the cells of the spinal nucleus are somatotopically organized. Fibres of the ophthalmic nerve lie in the ventral part of the tract and terminate in the lower or cervical part of the nucleus; those of the maxillary nerve are situated centrally in the tract and end in the intermediate part of the nucleus; mandibular fibres are placed in the dorsal part of the tract and synapse on cells in the upper part of the nucleus. Fibres of the spinal tract primarily subserve pain and temperature sensation; thus, the knowledge of the organization of the tract has considerable surgical importance in the relief of intractable pain arising from the 'trigeminal area'. Owing to the superficial disposition of the tract in the medulla and upper spinal cord it may easily be interrupted surgically.

Most of the ascending fibres of the sensory root synapse on cells of the principal sensory nucleus (Fig. 19.71), situated in the upper part of the pons. They are mainly concerned with tactile and pressure sensation. Other ascending fibres of the root are peripheral processes of unipolar cells of the mesencephalic nucleus, which carry impulses concerned with proprioception from the masticatory muscles, the temporomandibular joint, and the periodontal ligaments of the teeth, and probably from the facial and extraocular muscles as well. The central processes or collaterals of cells of the mesencephalic nucleus connect with neurons of the trigeminal motor nucleus forming monosynaptic reflex arcs for proprioceptive control of

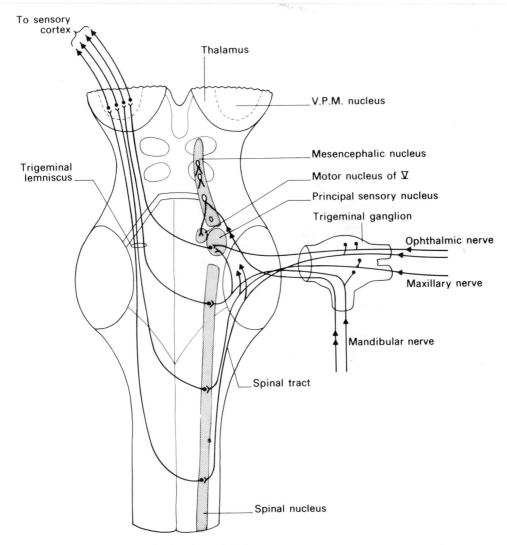

To sensory cortex

Thalamus

V.P.M. nucleus

Mesencephalic nucleus

Motor nucleus of V

Principal sensory nucleus

Trigeminal ganglion

Ophthalmic nerve

Maxillary nerve

Trigeminal lemniscus

Mandibular nerve

Spinal tract

Spinal nucleus

Fig. 19.71. Schematic diagram showing the nuclei of the trigeminal nerve and their main connections. V.P.M. is the ventroposterior nucleus of the thalamus.

the masticatory muscles (p. 574); others terminate in the cerebellum, and some in the principal sensory nucleus.

Connections of the sensory nuclei (Fig. 19.71). Neurons of the spinal and principal sensory nuclei give rise to axons which ascend and terminate in the ventroposterior nucleus of the thalamus. The majority of the fibres cross the midline; those from the spinal nucleus form the trigeminal lemniscus; those from the principal nucleus travel in the medial lemniscus. Thus, the trigeminal sensory pathway from the periphery

to the cerebral cortex consists of three orders of neurons viz; the primary neurons are unipolar cells of the trigeminal ganglion, the secondary neurons are found in the spinal or principal nuclei, and the tertiary neurons—whose fibres relay impulses to the sensory cortex—are situated in the thalamus.

The motor nucleus of the trigeminal nerve lies in the upper part of the pons on the medial side of the principal sensory nucleus. It consists of large multipolar cells interspersed with smaller interneurons. Axons of the large cells collectively form the motor root and are distributed

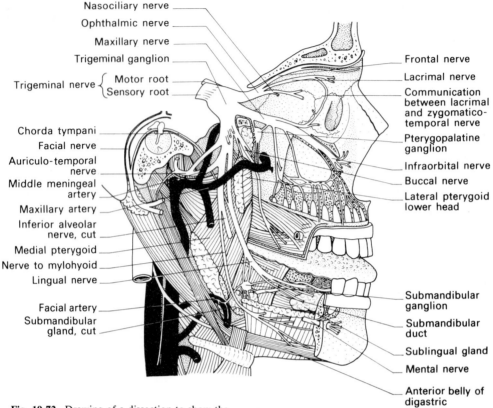

Nasociliary nerve
Ophthalmic nerve
Maxillary nerve
Trigeminal ganglion
Trigeminal nerve { Motor root
                  { Sensory root
Chorda tympani
Facial nerve
Auriculo-temporal nerve
Middle meningeal artery
Maxillary artery
Inferior alveolar nerve, cut
Medial pterygoid
Nerve to mylohyoid
Lingual nerve
Facial artery
Submandibular gland, cut

Frontal nerve
Lacrimal nerve
Communication between lacrimal and zygomatico-temporal nerve
Pterygopalatine ganglion
Infraorbital nerve
Buccal nerve
Lateral pterygoid lower head
Submandibular ganglion
Submandibular duct
Sublingual gland
Mental nerve
Anterior belly of digastric

Fig. 19.72. Drawing of a dissection to show the disposition of the right ophthalmic, maxillary and mandibular nerves.

principally to masticatory muscles, through the mandibular nerve. The motor nucleus receives ipsilateral and contralateral fibres from the corticonuclear tracts which influence the activity of the large neurons either directly or indirectly through local interneurons.

The ophthalmic nerve (Figs. 19.64, 19.65, 19.66 & 19.72)
This nerve is composed entirely of sensory fibres. It supplies the eyeball, the lacrimal gland, the mucous membrane of part of the nasal cavity, and the conjunctiva. Additionally it innervates the skin of the nose, eyelids, forehead and most of the scalp (Fig. 19.73). The nerve arises from the trigeminal ganglion and passes forwards through the cavernous sinus where it lies in the lateral wall between the trochlear nerve above and the maxillary nerve below. On leaving the sinus it divides into three branches, namely, lacrimal, frontal and nasociliary. These nerves enter the orbit through the superior orbi-

tal fissure in company with the cranial nerves supplying the muscles of the eye.

The lacrimal nerve runs forwards along the lateral wall of the orbit, above the upper border of the rectus lateralis. It often receives through the zygomaticotemporal branch of the maxillary nerve, parasympathetic secretomotor fibres destined for the lacrimal gland. It enters the lacrimal gland to supply it, and then gives terminal branches to the conjunctiva and skin of the upper eyelid.

The frontal nerve divides into the supra-trochlear and supraorbital nerves.

The supratrochlear nerve gives filaments to the conjunctiva and skin of the upper eyelid, and then continues upwards towards the midline of the forehead to supply the skin of the surrounding region. The supraorbital nerve gives twigs to the conjunctiva and skin of the upper eyelid and then supplies the forehead and scalp as far back as the lambdoid suture.

The nasociliary nerve enters the orbit through

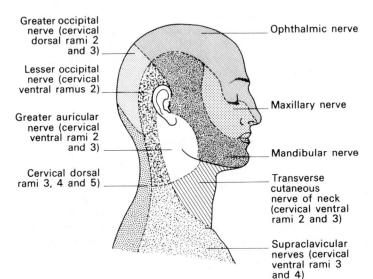

Greater occipital nerve (cervical dorsal rami 2 and 3)

Lesser occipital nerve (cervical ventral ramus 2)

Greater auricular nerve (cervical ventral rami 2 and 3)

Cervical dorsal rami 3, 4 and 5)

Ophthalmic nerve

Maxillary nerve

Mandibular nerve

Transverse cutaneous nerve of neck (cervical ventral rami 2 and 3)

Supraclavicular nerves (cervical ventral rami 3 and 4)

Fig. 19.73. Diagram to show the cutaneous supply of the face, scalp and neck. Compare with Fig. 19.78.

the medial part of the superior orbital fissure with the abducent nerve and the two divisions of the oculomotor nerve. All these nerves now lie within the 'cone' formed by the recti muscles of the eye. Crossing above the optic nerve the nasociliary nerve leaves the muscle cone and runs along the medial wall of the orbit. It gives a terminal branch, the infratrochlear nerve, which runs below the trochlea of the superior oblique to supply the skin of the medial angle of the eye and adjoining side of the nose, the conjunctiva, lacrimal sac and upper part of the nasolacrimal duct. Within the orbit the nasociliary nerve gives rise to the long ciliary, the posterior and anterior ethmoidal nerves.

The long ciliary nerves arise from the nasociliary nerve as it crosses above the optic nerve. There are two, sometimes three, branches which enter the eyeball to supply the sclera and cornea with sensory fibres. These nerves also contain postganglionic sympathetic fibres from the internal carotid plexus, destined to innervate the dilator pupillae of the iris. The posterior ethmoidal nerve when present passes through the posterior ethmoidal foramen in the medial wall of the orbit and supplies the ethmoidal and sphenoidal sinuses. The anterior ethmoidal nerve leaves the orbit through the anterior ethmoidal foramen and canal and runs medially over the upper surface of the cribriform plate of the ethmoid bone. It then enters the nasal cavity through a slit in the plate adjacent to the crista galli and gives rise to lateral and medial internal nasal branches which supply the mucous mem-

brane of the anterosuperior quadrant of the lateral wall of the nose and the front part of the nasal septum respectively. It terminates as the external nasal nerve which runs forwards on the under surface of the nasal bone to supply the skin of the tip and adjoining side of the nose including the vestibule.

The maxillary nerve (Figs. 19.65, 19.66, 19.72 & 19.73)

This nerve is entirely sensory. It runs forwards from the trigeminal ganglion, and traverses the cavernous sinus where it lies in the lower part of the lateral wall of the sinus. It then passes through the foramen rotundum and enters the upper part of pterygopalatine fossa. It leaves the fossa through the inferior orbital fissure, as the infraorbital nerve, and continues forwards in the floor of the orbit. Finally, it emerges on the face through the infraorbital foramen and divides into terminal branches, the palpebral, nasal and superior labial which supply the lower eyelid, the skin of the side of the nose, and the skin and mucous membrane of the anterior part of the cheek and upper lip respectively.

The branches of the maxillary nerve are: meningeal, ganglionic, zygomatic, superior alveolar, and the infraorbital which has been considered above.

The meningeal branch is composed of sensory fibres from the maxillary nerve and sympathetic fibres derived from the internal carotid plexus. It arises in the cranial cavity and supplies the dura mater of the middle cranial fossa.

The ganglionic branches, usually two in number, form connections with the pterygopalatine (sphenopalatine) ganglion which lies in the pterygopalatine fossa. They contain sensory fibres from the mucous membrane of the nose, palate and pharynx which are distributed in branches of the ganglion (see below); in addition they carry secretomotor fibres destined for the lacrimal gland which often travel in the zygomaticotemporal nerve (see below).

The zygomatic nerve arises in the pterygopalatine fossa, passes through the inferior orbital fissure and then runs on the inner aspect of the lateral wall of the orbit where it divides into two branches, zygomaticofacial and zygomaticotemporal. The zygomaticofacial nerve passes forwards to enter a small canal in the zygomatic bone, and emerges on the face. It supplies an area of skin overlying the zygomatic bone. The zygomaticotemporal nerve passes into the temporal fossa through a canal in the zygomatic bone, pierces the temporalis fascia to supply the overlying skin of the temple. Within the orbit it communicates with the lacrimal nerve conveying postganglionic parasympathetic (secretomotor) fibres from the pterygopalatine ganglion to the lacrimal gland. These postganglionic fibres may run an isolated course.

The posterior superior alveolar (dental) nerves arise in the pterygopalatine fossa and descend in the periosteum covering the posterior surface of the maxilla. Here, they break up into further branches which enter the posterior dental foramina and pass forwards in bony canals to form a plexus with fibres from the middle and anterior superior alveolar nerves. The posterior superior alveolar nerves and their ramifications supply the permanent molar teeth, the adjoining gingiva and mucous membrane of the cheek; in addition they supply the mucous membrane of the maxillary sinus.

The middle superior alveolar (dental) nerves are inconstant in number, sometimes absent or as many as three. When present they arise from the infraorbital nerve as it lies in the infraorbital groove, and incline downwards and forwards in the lateral wall of the maxillary sinus. They contribute to the formation of the superior dental plexus, supplying the upper premolar teeth and the mesiobuccal root of the first molar and also the mucous membrane of the maxillary wall.

The anterior superior alveolar (dental) nerve arises from the infraorbital nerve at a point situated about halfway along the infraorbital canal. It runs in a tortuous bony tunnel, the canalis sinuosus, lying in the anterior wall of the maxillary sinus. At first the nerve passes laterally but soon turns medially beneath the infraorbital canal; then it follows the curve of the margin of the anterior nasal aperture; finally, it ends besides the nasal septum. The nerve contributes fibres to the superior dental plexus and supplies the upper incisor and canine teeth. It also gives rise to nasal branches which supply the mucous membrane of the lateral wall (anteroinferior quadrant) and floor of the nasal cavity including the adjacent part of the nasal septum.

The pterygopalatine (sphenopalatine) ganglion (Figs. 19.72 & 19.74) consists of parasympathetic neurons, functionally connected with the facial nerve, and many fibres of passage, mostly associated with the maxillary nerve. It is situated in the upper part of the pterygopalatine fossa.

The ganglion receives autonomic fibres through the nerve of the pterygoid canal (p. 448). The preganglionic parasympathetic fibres arise from the superior salivatory nucleus in the pons and travel in the greater petrosal nerve before joining the nerve of the pterygoid canal. These fibres relay in the ganglion, and postganglionic fibres are distributed to the mucous glands of the nasal cavity, palate and pharynx, through branches of the ganglion (see below); other postganglionic parasympathetic fibres are delivered to the lacrimal gland via ganglionic branches of the maxillary nerve and thence through the zygomaticotemporal (see above) and may continue in the lacrimal nerves. Postganglionic sympathetic (vasomotor) fibres pass through the pterygopalatine ganglion without interruption and are distributed by branches of the ganglion. These fibres are derived from the superior cervical ganglion and travel in the internal carotid plexus, and thence in the deep petrosal nerve which joins the nerve of the pterygoid canal.

In summary, it follows that branches of the pterygopalatine ganglion contain three types of fibres from their different sources, namely: sensory fibres derived from the maxillary nerve, postganglionic sympathetic (vasomotor) fibres, and postganglionic parasympathetic (secretomotor) fibres derived from cell bodies contained in the ganglion.

The course and distribution of the major branches are considered below (Figs. 19.74 & 19.75).

The greater (anterior) palatine nerve passes down through the greater palatine canal and runs in a shallow groove on the inferior surface of the hard palate towards the incisive foramen.

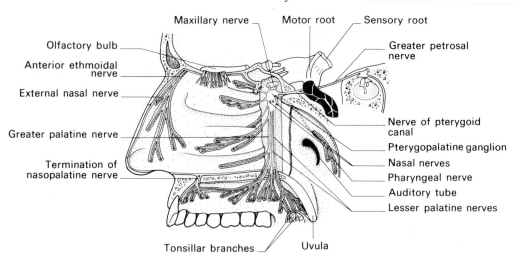

Fig. 19.74. The right pterygopalatine ganglion and its branches.

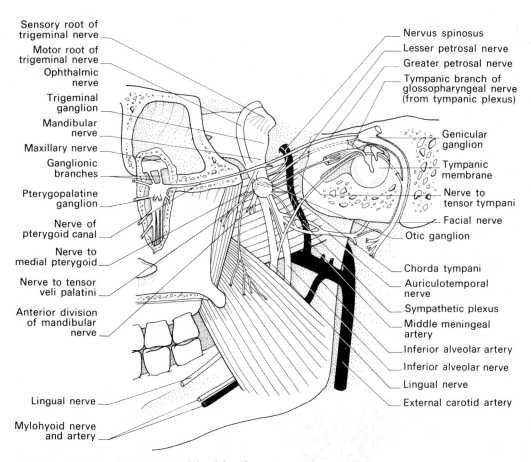

Fig. 19.75. Drawing of a dissection of the right otic ganglion, the lingual and inferior alveolar nerves, seen from the medial aspect.

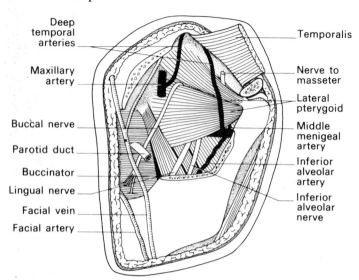

Deep temporal arteries

Maxillary artery

Buccal nerve

Parotid duct

Buccinator

Lingual nerve

Facial vein

Facial artery

Temporalis

Nerve to masseter

Lateral pterygoid

Middle menigeal artery

Inferior alveolar artery

Inferior alveolar nerve

Fig. 19.76. Drawing of a dissection of the left pterygoid region, seen from the lateral aspect, which shows some of the branches of the mandibular nerve.

It supplies the mucous membrane of the hard palate and the gingival tissue on the lingual side of the upper teeth. Within the greater palatine canal the nerve gives rise to posterior inferior nasal branches which pass through foramina in the lateral wall of the nose and supply the mucous membrane of its posteroinferior quadrant.

The lesser (middle and posterior) palatine nerves, two in number, descend behind the greater palatine nerves and emerge through the lesser palatine foramina. They supply the soft palate including the uvula, and the tonsil. Nerves from the soft palate contain fibres subserving taste which pass via the pterygopalatine ganglion, the nerve of the pterygoid canal and the greater petrosal nerve. These fibres are the peripheral processes of unipolar cells, located in the (genicular) ganglion of the facial nerve, whose central processes end in the nucleus of the tractus solitarius.

The lateral posterior superior nasal nerves pass through the sphenopalatine foramen to supply the mucous membrane of the posterosuperior quadrant of the lateral wall of the nose and also the mucosa of the posterior ethmoidal air cells.

The medial posterior superior nasal nerves consist of two short nerves and one long nerve, all of which pass through the sphenopalatine foramen and cross the roof of the nasal cavity to reach the nasal septum. The short nerves supply the posterior part of the roof and septum. The long nerve is the nasopalatine (long spheno-

palatine) nerve which inclines along the nasal septum to enter the roof of the mouth through the incisive foramen. It supplies the nasal septum and the mucous membrane of the anterior part of the hard palate including the supporting tissue of the central and usually the lateral incisor teeth.

The pharyngeal nerve passes backwards through the palatinovaginal canal and innervates the mucous membrane of the nasopharynx.

The mandibular nerve (Figs. 19.72, 19.73, 19.75 & 19.76)

The mandibular nerve is a mixed nerve. It supplies many of the structures concerned with mastication; these include the teeth and gingivae of the mandible, the mucous membrane of the oral (presulcal) part of the tongue and the floor of the mouth, the temporomandibular joint and the masticatory muscles. It also supplies the skin of part of the temple and pinna of the ear, and the skin of the lower part of the face including the lower lip.

The nerve is formed from a large sensory root, arising from the trigeminal ganglion, and the whole of the motor root of the trigeminal nerve. Both leave the trigeminal cave by descending through the foramen ovale, the motor root lying medial to the sensory. Immediately below the foramen the roots unite to form the main trunk of the mandibular nerve which lies between the upper head of the lateral pterygoid laterally and the tensor veli palatini medially. After a short descending course the main trunk divides into a small anterior and a large posterior trunk.

Branches of the main trunk (Fig. 19.75). The meningeal branch or nervus spinosus is a recurrent branch which enters the middle cranial fossa through the foramen spinosum or sometimes through the foramen ovale. It mainly supplies the dura mater of the middle cranial fossa but also sends filaments to the mucous membrane lining the mastoid antrum and air cells.

The nerve to the medial pterygoid runs forwards to supply the muscle; it also sends fibres which traverse the otic ganglion without synapsing to supply the tensor tympani and tensor veli palatini.

Branches of the anterior trunk. These are all motor branches apart from the buccal nerve; all are initially related to the lateral pterygoid muscle.

The deep temporal nerves run over the upper border of the lateral pterygoid to supply the temporalis. There are usually two, anterior and posterior, but sometimes a third or middle nerve is present passing between the two heads of the lateral pterygoid.

The masseteric nerve passes above the lateral pterygoid and through the mandibular notch, lying between the tendon of the temporalis and the posteriorly situated temporomandibular joint to which it sends some sensory filaments. The nerve then innervates the masseter.

The nerve of the lateral pterygoid runs with the buccal nerve before entering the deep surface of the muscle.

The buccal nerve is the longest of the nerves arising from the anterior trunk and is entirely sensory. It passes forwards between the heads of the lateral pterygoid and gradually inclines forwards and downwards in a fascial tunnel on the deep surface of the temporalis muscle. It reaches the superficial surface of the buccinator where it is crossed superficially by the parotid duct. The nerve supplies the skin of the cheek and its lining of mucous membrane including the buccal gingivae adjoining the lower molar and premolar teeth.

Branches of the posterior trunk. This trunk is wholly sensory, except for fibres distributed by the nerve to the mylohyoid. It gives rise to three major branches all of which are intimately related to the mandible.

The auriculotemporal nerve is usually formed from two roots which embrace the middle meningeal artery. The nerve passes backwards between the neck of the mandible and the sphenomandibular ligament, then winds laterally behind the temporomandibular joint where it lies on the deep surface of the parotid gland; finally it ascends over the posterior root of the zygoma before dividing into superficial temporal branches. It gives auricular branches which supply the tragus, and branches which supply the skin of the external acoustic meatus and part of the tympanic membrane. As the nerve winds around the temporomandibular joint it supplies the joint and also sends branches to the parotid gland. The parotid branches contain vasomotor fibres from the sympathetic root of the otic ganglion and also secretomotor (postganglionic parasympathetic) fibres derived from the cell bodies forming the otic ganglion. The superficial temporal branches supply the skin of the temporal region, accompanied by the superficial temporal artery and its branches.

The lingual nerve descends on the deep surface of the lateral pterygoid in company with the inferior alveolar nerve which lies more posteriorly. Emerging below the lateral pterygoid the lingual nerve inclines forwards between the ramus of the mandible and the medial pterygoid. It then comes into direct contact with the medial side of the mandible where it lies below and behind the third molar tooth, and between the attachments of the mylohyoid below and the superior constrictor above. Here, the medial side of the nerve is only covered by mucous membrane and is readily felt with the finger. Leaving the mandible the nerve passes forwards and slightly medially on to the side of the tongue. It crosses in turn the lateral surfaces of the styloglossus and hyoglossus before dividing into terminal branches which enter the substance of the genioglossus. On the surface of the hyoglossus the lingual nerve lies above the deep part of the submandibular gland and its duct, further forward it becomes intimately related to the duct. Here, the nerve, gradually inclines downwards and forwards on the lateral side of the duct, crosses below it, and finally runs upwards and forwards on the medial side.

The lingual nerve distributes sensory fibres to the mucous membrane or the oral (presulcal) part of the tongue and the floor of the mouth including the lingual gingivae. In addition, it carries fibres from taste buds of the presulcal part of the tongue excluding those of the vallate papillae, and also takes preganglionic parasympathetic (secretomotor) fibres to the submandibular ganglion. Both taste and secretomotor fibres are carried in the chorda tympani (p. 913), a branch of the facial nerve, which joins the lingual nerve as it descends across the lateral pterygoid.

The inferior alveolar (dental) nerve through its branches supplies all the teeth of the lower jaw, part of the buccal gum, the skin and mucous membrane of the lower lip, and the skin over the chin; moreover, it gives motor fibres to two muscles—the mylohyoid and the anterior belly of the digastric. It descends to the mandibular foramen, at first on the deep surface of the lateral pterygoid and then between the ramus of the mandible and the sphenomandibular ligament. Before entering the mandibular canal through the foramen it gives off the nerve to mylohyoid; within the canal it travels below and close to the roots of the molar and premolar teeth which it supplies. Its intraosseous course and distribution are detailed on p. 457.

The incisive nerve runs in a small intraosseous tunnel in the mandible and usually supplies the first premolar, canine and incisor teeth; although these teeth may be innervated solely or additionally by fibres of the incisor plexus which re-enter the labial surface of the mandible. The mental nerve leaves the mental foramen and distributes branches to the skin of the chin, and to the skin and mucous membrane of the lower lip. Some of the fibres emerging from the foramen form the incisor plexus which supplies the labial periodontium and gingiva of the incisor and canine teeth.

The nerve to the mylohyoid arises from the inferior alveolar nerve just before it enters the mandibular foramen. It pierces the sphenomandibular ligament, runs downwards and forwards (in a groove) on the medial side of the mandible, and reaches the inferior surface of the mylohyoid, supplying it and the anterior belly of the digastric.

Clinical anatomy. Damage to the whole of the sensory root of the trigeminal nerve produces an ipsilateral anaesthesia of most of the scalp, the face (save for an area of skin over the angle of the mandible), the mucous membrane of the nasal and oral cavities (excluding the postsulcal part of the tongue, and the fauces); in addition, corneal sensation is lost with the associated absence of the corneal reflex. Involvement of the motor root causes paralysis accompanied by wasting of the masticatory muscles on the corresponding side of the lesion. Fractures through the foramen ovale may result in paralysis of the muscles of mastication together with sensory

loss confined only to areas supplied by the mandibular nerve. The inferior alveolar nerve may also be involved in fractures of the mandible, resulting in denervation of the teeth distal to the lesion with sensory loss of areas supplied by the mental nerve.

Pain due to the involvement of various branches of the trigeminal nerve is common and is frequently of the type termed 'referred pain'. The most common causative factors are infections of the nasal cavity and paranasal sinuses, as well as affections of the teeth and their supporting tissues. For example: maxillary sinusitis may irritate the infra-orbital nerve or its branches, particularly the superior alveolar nerves, producing pain referred to the upper teeth; dental caries or an impacted third molar tooth in the lower jaw may cause pain in the lower part of the face, ear, temporomandibular joint or temple.

The facial nerve

The facial (seventh) nerve is composed of a large motor and a smaller sensory root which emerge from the lower border of the pons between the olive and the inferior cerebellar peduncle (Fig. 19.16). The motor root supplies muscles derived from the second branchial arch. These comprise muscles of the face, scalp and auricle, the platysma, stapedius, the stylohyoid, and the posterior belly of the digastric. The sensory root (intermediate nerve) contains fibres subserving taste from the mucosae of the presulcal part of the tongue and the soft palate. It also carries preganglionic parasympathetic (secretomotor) fibres from the superior part of the salivatory nucleus in the pons to the submandibular and pterygomandibular ganglia. Postganglionic parasympathetic fibres go from the submandibular ganglion to supply the submandibular and sublingual salivary glands and from the pterygomandibular ganglion to supply the lacrimal gland and glands of the mucosae of the nasal cavity, palate and nasopharynx.

The motor nucleus of the facial nerve lies in the caudal part of the pons; efferent fibres leaving it take a circuitous route (Fig. 19.25) before passing out of the brainstem as the motor root. Incoming fibres concerned with taste descend in the tractus solitarius and end in the nucleus of the tractus solitarius in the medulla oblongata.

The two roots of the facial nerve accompanied by the vestibulocochlear nerve leave the brainstem and enter the internal acoustic meatus of the petrotemporal bone (Fig. 19.77). The facial components occupy the anterosuperior region of the meatus, the sensory root between the motor

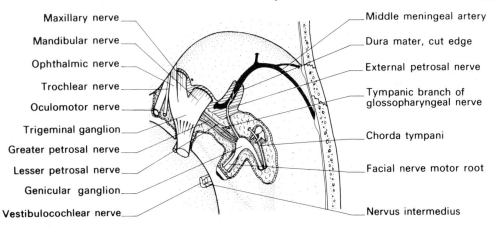

Maxillary nerve
Mandibular nerve
Ophthalmic nerve
Trochlear nerve
Oculomotor nerve
Trigeminal ganglion
Greater petrosal nerve
Lesser petrosal nerve
Genicular ganglion
Vestibulocochlear nerve

Middle meningeal artery
Dura mater, cut edge
External petrosal nerve
Tympanic branch of glossopharyngeal nerve
Chorda tympani
Facial nerve motor root
Nervus intermedius

Fig. 19.77. Drawing of a dissection of the right middle cranial fossa showing the course of the facial nerve and some of its connections within the petrous temporal bone.

root and the eighth nerve—hence its synonym intermediate nerve. At the end of the meatus it enters the facial canal lying above the vestibule. Within the canal the sensory root possesses a small swelling, situated where the nerve turns sharply backwards. This is the genicular ganglion which is composed of unipolar neurons whose processes convey impulses concerned with taste. The nerve leaves the skull through the stylomastoid foramen.

The extracranial course of the facial nerve in the neck is short for on leaving the stylomastoid foramen the nerve passes forwards into the substance of the parotid gland. Here it lies superficial to the retromandibular vein which separates it from the more deeply placed external carotid artery. Within the gland the nerve divides into branches which reunite on the anteromedial surface of the gland to form the parotid plexus. From this network of nerve fibres further branches are distributed to muscles of the face.

Branches of the facial nerve may be arranged into three groups:
1 Those formed within the petrotemporal bone: the greater petrosal nerve, nerve to stapedius and chorda tympani.
2 Those arising in the neck before the nerve enters the parotid gland: the posterior auricular nerve, the nerve to the posterior belly of digastric, and to stylohyoid.
3 Branches distributed to muscles of the face: temporal, zygomatic, buccal, marginal mandibular and cervical.

The greater petrosal nerve (Fig. 19.79) con-

sisting of taste and secretomotor fibres arises from the genicular ganglion and runs forwards to emerge in a groove on the anterior surface of the petrotemporal bone directed towards the foramen lacerum. In the foramen it is joined by the deep petrosal nerve formed by postganglionic sympathetic fibres, derived from the internal carotid plexus. The conjoined nerves now enter the pterygoid canal forming the nerve of the pterygoid canal which proceeds to the pterygopalatine ganglion.

The fibres concerned with taste pass through the pterygopalatine ganglion without interruption to be distributed through the lesser palatine nerves to the soft palate.

The nerve to stapedius (Fig. 19.79) arises from the facial nerve as it descends vertically through the petrotemporal bone. It passes forwards through a small canal to supply the muscle.

The chorda tympani (Figs. 19.72, 19.77 & 19.79) arises from the facial nerve a short distance above the opening of the stylomastoid foramen. It curves upwards in a small canal in the posterior wall of the tympanic cavity, crosses the deep aspect of the tympanic membrane where it lies between the fibrous and mucous layers. Here, it is related to the upper part of the handle of the malleus. Leaving the substance of the membrane it enters another bony canal which opens into the medial part of the petrotympanic fissure. Next, the nerve descends on the medial side of the spine of the sphenoid—which it sometimes grooves—and

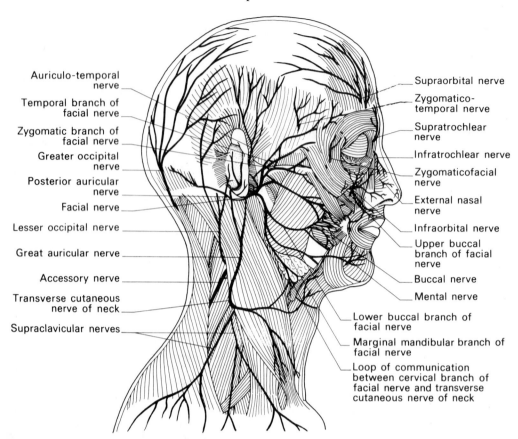

Auriculo-temporal nerve

Temporal branch of facial nerve

Zygomatic branch of facial nerve

Greater occipital nerve

Posterior auricular nerve

Facial nerve

Lesser occipital nerve

Great auricular nerve

Accessory nerve

Transverse cutaneous nerve of neck

Supraclavicular nerves

Supraorbital nerve

Zygomatico-temporal nerve

Supratrochlear nerve

Infratrochlear nerve

Zygomaticofacial nerve

External nasal nerve

Infraorbital nerve

Upper buccal branch of facial nerve

Buccal nerve

Mental nerve

Lower buccal branch of facial nerve

Marginal mandibular branch of facial nerve

Loop of communication between cervical branch of facial nerve and transverse cutaneous nerve of neck

Fig. 19.78. Drawing of a dissection of the nerves of the right side of the face, scalp and neck. Compare with Fig. 19.73.

runs down the medial surface of the lateral pterygoid muscle to join the lingual nerve. The chorda tympani consists of fibres subserving taste—the peripheral processes of unipolar cells of the genicular ganglion—which are distributed through the lingual nerve to tastebuds on the presulcal part of the tongue, excluding the vallate papillae. In addition, it contains preganglionic parasympathetic fibres derived from the salivatory nucleus. These travel in the lingual nerve to synapse on cells of the submandibular ganglion from which postganglionic parasympathetic fibres are distributed to the submandibular and sublingual salivary glands.

The digastric and stylohyoid branches leave the facial nerve trunk just below the stylomastoid foramen and supply the posterior belly of digastric and stylohyoid respectively (Fig. 19.78). The posterior auricular nerve arises close to the opening of the stylomastoid fora-

men. It ascends behind the external acoustic meatus where it branches to supply the posterior auricular muscle and the occipital belly of occipitofrontalis.

The temporal branches (Fig. 19.78) ascend across the zygomatic arch. They supply the orbicularis oculi, the frontal belly of occipitofrontalis and the corrugator, as well as the anterior and superior auricular muscles.

The buccal branches pass forwards into the cheek to supply the buccinator, the orbicularis oris, the muscles of the upper lip, both zygomatic muscles and the muscles of the nose.

The marginal mandibular branch runs forwards below the angle of the mandible and enters the neck deep to the platysma. Here it follows the lower border of the mandible which it crosses to supply the risorius and muscles of the lower lip and chin.

The cervical branch also passes into the neck.

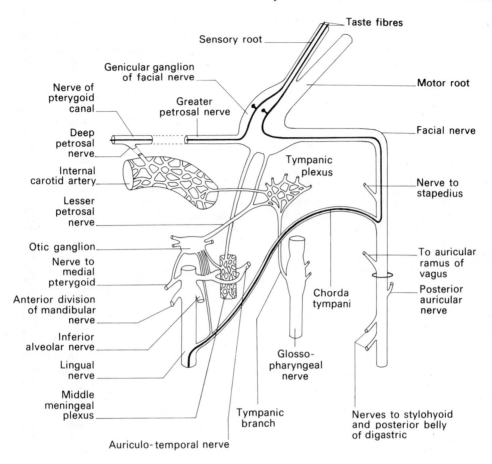

Fig. 19.79. Schematic diagram of the connections and branches of the facial nerve within the petrous temporal bone.

It curves downwards and forwards deep to the platysma which it supplies.

The submandibular ganglion (Fig. 19.72) is a peripheral ganglion of the parasympathetic system (functionally) associated with the facial nerve. It lies on the hyoglossus immediately below the lingual nerve to which it is attached by nerve fibres. The ganglion is fusiform in shape and contains multipolar neurons. It receives preganglionic parasympathetic fibres derived from the salivatory nucleus which travel via the chorda tympani and lingual nerve. These fibres end in synapses on the ganglionic cells which in turn give rise to postganglionic parasympathetic (secretomotor) fibres. The latter are distributed to the submandibular and sublingual salivary glands and also to glands of the tongue and the floor of the mouth. Postganglionic sympathetic (vasomotor) fibres derived from the superior cervical ganglion pass through the submandibular ganglion without synaptic interruption. They are distributed to blood vessels of the submandibular and sublingual glands.

Clinical anatomy. Damage to the motor root of the facial nerve results in loss of the normal symmetry of the face, owing to paralysis of the ipsilateral facial muscles.

Paralysis of the orbicularis oculi leads to widening of the palpebral fissure, inability to close the eye and to loss of the blink reflex.

Paralysis of the orbicularis oris allows saliva to dribble out of the corner of the mouth due to lack of lip seal, and drooping of the corner of the mouth.

Paralysis of the buccinator muscle leads to

accumulation of food in the vestibule of the mouth during mastication.

Damage to the sensory root results in loss of taste sensibility of the ipsilateral side of the pre-sulcal part of the tongue excluding the vallate papillae. Facial paralysis accompanied by taste loss indicates a lesion situated distal to the emerging roots but proximal to the point of departure of the chorda tympani from the facial nerve, that is in the facial canal or internal acoustic meatus.

The facial nerve may be interrupted by fractures through the petrous temporal bone but, more commonly, is involved by an inflammatory process of unknown aetiology, termed Bell's palsy.

The glossopharyngeal nerve

The glossopharyngeal (ninth) nerve is a mixed nerve. It receives fibres concerned with general sensation from the posterior part of the tongue, the tonsil and the pharynx; it also carries fibres subserving taste from the mucosa of the posterior part of the tongue including the vallate papillae. The glossopharyngeal nerve supplies the stylopharyngeus, and in addition sends preganglionic parasympathetic fibres to the otic ganglion which in turn supplies the parotid gland with secretomotor fibres.

The intracranial course of the glossopharyngeal nerve is short. It is formed from several rootlets which emerge from the upper part of the medulla oblongata in a groove placed between the olive and the inferior cerebellar peduncle (Fig. 19.16). The rootlets amalgamate leaving the skull through the jugular foramen where they are related to but separated from the vagus and accessory nerves by the inferior petrosal sinus. Within the foramen the glossopharyngeal nerve possesses two swellings; a small superior ganglion and a much larger inferior ganglion. Both contain typical unipolar cells whose peripheral processes are distributed by branches of the glossopharyngeal nerve, and whose central processes connect with sensory nuclei in the medulla. Those processes concerned with visceral sensation including taste end in the nucleus of the tractus solitarius: those subserving general sensation are believed to terminate in the nucleus of the spinal tract (Fig. 19.22).

Motor fibres supplying the stylopharyngeus arise from cells of the upper part of the nucleus ambiguus, whilst preganglionic parasympathetic fibres originate in the inferior salivatory nucleus.

After leaving the skull the glossopharyngeal nerve descends in the upper part of the carotid sheath, lying between the internal carotid artery and the internal jugular vein (Fig. 19.68); it inclines forward crossing superficial to the former vessel but deep to the styloid process with its attached muscles. It now leaves the carotid sheath and follows the deep surface of the stylopharyngeus to enter the pharynx between the adjacent borders of the superior and middle constrictor muscles where it divides into branches for distribution to pharynx, tongue and tonsil.

The major branches of the glossopharyngeal nerve are: tympanic, carotid, pharyngeal, muscular, tonsillar and lingual. They are described below.

The tympanic branches (Fig. 19.79) arise from the inferior ganglion and enter the tympanic cavity through a tiny canal, the opening of which is found in the petrous temporal bone between the carotid canal and the jugular foramen. In the tympanic cavity they ramify on the surface of the promontory to form the tympanic plexus (with fibres from the facial nerve) which also receives sympathetic fibres from the carotid plexus. The tympanic plexus supplies fibres to the mucous membrane of the tympanic cavity including the auditory tube and the mastoid air cells; in addition it gives rise to the lesser petrosal nerve. This nerve, largely composed of autonomic fibres, leaves the tympanic cavity through a groove in the anterior surface of the petrous temporal bone, and then passes through the foramen ovale to join the otic ganglion (see below).

The carotid branches (sinus nerves) originate from the main nerve trunk immediately below the jugular foramen and descend on the internal carotid artery to supply baroceptors contained in the carotid sinus, a dilatation found at the beginning of the inernal carotid artery. They play an important role in the regulation of blood pressure (p. 711).

The pharyngeal branches are given off as the glossopharyngeal nerve crosses the middle constrictor muscle of the pharynx. They unite with pharyngeal branches of the vagus and laryngopharyngeal branches from the sympathetic trunk to form the pharyngeal plexus. The glossopharyngeal component of the plexus is entirely sensory, supplying the mucous membrane of the pharynx.

The muscular branch supplies the stylopharyngeus only.

The tonsillar branches ascend deep to the hyoglossus to supply the tonsil. With the lesser

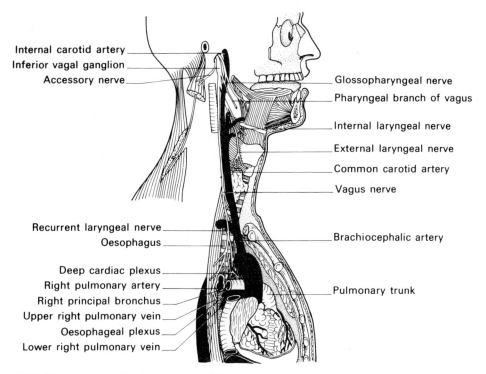

Internal carotid artery
Inferior vagal ganglion
Accessory nerve

Glossopharyngeal nerve
Pharyngeal branch of vagus
Internal laryngeal nerve
External laryngeal nerve
Common carotid artery
Vagus nerve

Recurrent laryngeal nerve
Oesophagus

Brachiocephalic artery

Deep cardiac plexus
Right pulmonary artery
Right principal bronchus
Upper right pulmonary vein
Oesophageal plexus
Lower right pulmonary vein

Pulmonary trunk

Fig. 19.80. The course and distribution of the right vagus nerve in the neck and thorax. The glossopharyngeal and spinal accessory nerves are also shown.

(middle and posterior) palatine nerves they form a plexus whose branches supply the soft palate and the pillars of the fauces.

The lingual branches also pass deep to the hyoglossus and innervate the mucous membrane of the postsulcal part of the tongue and the vallate papillae. These branches convey impulses concerned with general sensation as well as taste from these regions.

The otic ganglion (Fig. 19.75) is a collection of autonomic cells, functionally connected with the glossopharyngeal nerve. It is situated below the foramen ovale, lying medial to the motor root of the mandibular nerve and lateral to the tensor veli palatini. Preganglionic parasympathetic fibres from the lesser petrosal nerve end in synapses on the ganglionic cells which send postganglionic parasympathetic (secretomotor fibres) to the parotid gland. Passing through the ganglion without interruption are postganglionic sympathetic (vasomotor) fibres derived from the superior cervical ganglion which are also destined for the parotid gland. Both sets of postganglionic fibres reach the gland through the

auriculotemporal nerve. Other fibres of passage in the ganglion arise from the motor root of the mandibular nerve. These supply the tensor veli palatini and tensor tympani, as well as the medial pterygoid.

Clinical anatomy. The chief signs of interruption of the glossopharyngeal nerve are sensory loss in the postsulcal part of the tongue, the tonsil, the palatal arches and the soft palate on the affected side. Taste sensation is absent in the postsulcal part of the tongue including the vallate papillae. The gag reflex (p. 581) is also lost on the affected side.

The vagus nerve (Fig. 19.80)

The vagus (tenth) nerve has an extensive course, being distributed not only to structures in the head and neck but to viscera in the thorax and abdomen. It is a mixed nerve containing a variety of fibre components. These comprise branchiomotor and visceromotor fibres, as well as viscerosensory, somatosensory and gustatory (taste) fibres; the visceromotor and viscerosensory moieties form a major contribution of the cranial parasympathetic system.

The nerve is formed by about ten rootlets which issue from the medulla oblongata in a groove lying between the olive and the inferior cerebellar peduncle (Fig. 19.16). It leaves the skull through the jugular foramen in company with the accessory and glossopharyngeal nerves. Two swellings are found on the vagus nerve as it passes into the neck. These are senory ganglia and consist of unipolar neurons whose peripheral processes are distributed in branches of the vagus nerve whilst their central processes connect to sensory nuclei in the medulla oblongata. The superior ganglion which lies in the jugular foramen is small and spherical. The peripheral processes of cells contained in this ganglion form the auricular nerve, the central processes are believed to terminate in the spinal nucleus of the trigeminal nerve. These processes are concerned with somatic sensation. The inferior ganglion is fusiform (some 2–3 cm long) and is situated below the jugular foramen. The cells forming this ganglion are concerned with visceral sensation including taste, their central processes end in the nucleus of the tractus solitarius.

Branchiomotor fibres arise from the caudal part of the nucleus ambiguus (Fig. 19.22). They enter the vagus nerve by two routes. The majority of fibres descend in the cranial part of the accessory nerve which joins the vagal trunk just beyond the inferior ganglion; the others pass directly to the vagus nerve. Branchiomotor fibres supply striated muscle of the palate pharyngeal constrictors and the intrinsic muscles of the larynx. Visceromotor fibres originate from the dorsal nucleus of the vagus (Fig. 19.22). They are preganglionic parasympathetic fibres which are distributed through vagal branches to peripheral parasympathetic ganglia. Postganglionic fibres from the ganglia supply smooth muscle and glands of the oesophagus, stomach, small intestine and part of the colon, and in addition supply the heart and lungs.

Entering the neck the vagus nerve descends vertically in the carotid sheath, lying at first between the internal carotid artery and the internal jugular vein and then, at the level of the thyroid cartilage, between the common carotid artery and the same vein (Fig. 19.68). At the root of the neck the course of the right and left vagal nerves differ. On the right side (Fig. 19.80) the nerve crosses anterior to the first part of the subclavian artery and enters the thorax, lying at first posterior to the right brachiocephalic vein

and then between the superior vena cava and the right side of the trachea. Next, it continues down behind the root of the lung and reaches the side of the oesophagus where it breaks up into branches which contribute to the formation of the pulmonary and oesophageal plexuses.

On the left side the vagus nerve enters the thorax by descending between the left common carotid and left subclavian arteries, and behind the left brachiocephalic vein. It crosses the left side of the arch of the aorta and runs behind the root of the lung. At the upper level of the aortic arch it is crossed superficially by the phrenic nerve. Behind the root of the lung the vagus nerve breaks up into branches which help to form the pulmonary and oesophageal plexuses.

The oesophageal plexuses are situated around the lower part of the thoracic oesophagus. They give rise to the anterior and posterior vagal trunks which enter the abdomen through the oesophageal opening of the diaphragm. The anterior vagal trunk, mostly composed of fibres from the left vagus, supplies the lesser curvature and anterior aspect of the stomach, the proximal part of the duodenum, the head of the pancreas and the liver. The posterior vagal trunk, mostly consisting of fibres from the right vagus, innervates the greater curvature and posterior surface of the stomach. It also gives a large coeliac branch which ends in the coeliac plexus but additionally supplies fibres to the splenic, hepatic, renal and superior mesenteric plexuses.

The vagus nerve gives rise to the following branches in the neck and thorax (Fig. 19.80).

The meningeal branches arise in the jugular foramen and consist of sympathetic and sensory cervical fibres which run in the vagus nerve for a short distance before entering the posterior cranial fossa. They supply the dura and meningeal vessels of this region.

The auricular branch is also given off in the jugular foramen. Arising from the superior ganglion, it passes backwards behind the jugular vein to enter the petrous temporal bone through the lateral wall of the jugular fossa, and then emerges through the tympanomastoid fissure. It supplies the skin of part of the cranial side of the auricle and the posterior wall of the external acoustic meatus, and also the outer surface of the tympanic membrane.

The pharyngeal branch leaves the inferior ganglion and curves forwards between the internal and external carotid arteries to reach the upper border of the middle constrictor muscle. Here, it breaks up into branches which unite with branches from the glossopharyngeal nerve and the sympathetic trunk to form the pharyngeal plexus. The vagal contribution to the plexus is mainly derived from the cranial part of the accessory nerve and supplies the pharyngeal constrictors and all the muscles of the soft palate save tensor veli palatini.

The superior laryngeal nerve arises from the inferior ganglion and inclines forwards on the side of the pharynx, deep to the internal carotid artery. It divides into a large sensory branch, the internal laryngeal nerve, and a smaller motor branch, the external laryngeal nerve. The former pierces the thyrohyoid membrane and supplies the mucous membrane of the pharynx, the valleculla and the vestibule of the larynx, as well as innervating the stretch receptors of intrinsic muscles of the larynx. The external laryngeal nerve accompanied by the superior thyroid artery descends deep to the sternothyroid, and then pierces the constrictor muscle supplying its lower fibres (cricopharyngeus). It finally winds around the inferior thyroid tubercle and innervates the cricothyroid.

The recurrent laryngeal nerve has a different origin and course on the two sides of the body. On the left the nerve arises from the vagus nerve on the left side of the arch of the aorta, and hooks below the arch and behind the ligamentum arteriosum. On the right it comes off the vagus nerve in front of the first part of the subclavian artery, and then turns below and behind the artery. Each nerve now ascends in the groove between the trachea and the oesophagus, pursuing a similar course to reach the larynx. Before entering the larynx the nerve passes on the medial side of the thyroid gland where it is intimately related to the inferior thyroid artery or its branches. It then runs upwards deep to the inferior constrictor muscle to enter the larynx behind the cricothyroid joint. The recurrent laryngeal nerves innervate all the intrinsic muscles of the larynx except cricothyroid; they also supply sensory fibres to the mucous membrane of the larynx below the vocal folds and to the mucosa of the trachea.

The cardiac branches consist of two groups of nerves, the superior and inferior cardiac, which arise from the vagus nerve in the upper and lower regions of the neck; additional cardiac branches emerge from the vagus nerve or its branches in the thorax. All cardiac branches contribute to the deep part of the cardiac plexus, except the left inferior branches which are distributed to the superficial part of the plexus.

The pulmonary branches unite with sympathetic fibres to form pulmonary plexuses which send branches to the root of the lung and bronchi, the vagal fibres supplying bronchial constrictor muscle.

The oesophageal branches supply the smooth muscle and mucosa of the oesophagus but many are large branches forming the oesophageal plexuses from which emerge the anterior and posterior vagal trunks.

The accessory nerve

The accesssory (eleventh) nerve is a motor nerve formed from two roots, each having a separate origin and distribution. The cranial root consists of efferent fibres arising from cells of the lower part of the nucleus ambiguus (Fig. 19.22). The fibres leave the side of the medulla oblongata between the olive and the inferior cerebellar peduncle in line with the rootlets of the vagus and glossopharyngeal nerves (Fig. 19.16). The spinal root has a more extensive origin, and consists of axons whose cell bodies are situated in the lateral part of the anterior grey column of the upper five cervical cord segments. The axons emerge on the lateral surface of the cord as a row of rootlets placed behind the denticulate ligament, midway between the dorsal and ventral spinal roots. The rootlets ascend in the subarachnoid space forming a trunk which enters the skull through the foramen magnum, behind the vertebral artery. Both cranial and spinal roots then pass into the jugular foramen accompanied by the vagus nerve. Within the foramen the roots join for a short distance only to separate. The cranial part unites with the vagus nerve, its fibres being distributed via vagal branches to the muscles of the soft palate (excluding tensor veli palatini) and the larynx. The spinal part (Fig. 19.68) on leaving the jugular foramen crosses the transverse process of the atlas, and is usually situated deep to the internal jugular vein. It then enters the upper part of the sternomastoid being joined by fibres of the second cervical nerve, traverses that muscle, and emerges in the posterior triangle of the neck where it picks up fibres from the second and third cervical nerves (Fig. 19.80). Finally, it passes under the anterior border of trapezius forming a plexus on the deep aspect of the muscle with fibres of the third and fourth cervical nerves. The spinal part of the accessory nerve supplies motor fibres to the sternomastoid and trapezius, cervical fibres supplying these muscles are generally regarded as being concerned with proprioception.

Spinal nerves

There are 31 pairs of spinal nerves arranged on the following regional basis: 8 cervical, 12 thoracic, 5 lumbar, 5 sacral and 1 coccygeal. Each nerve emerges from an inervertebral foramen (Fig. 19.81) where it is formed by the union of a ventral and dorsal root, the latter being associated with a spinal (or dorsal root) ganglion.

 Efferent

The ventral roots are composed of motor (afferent) fibres, derived from neurons of the anterior and lateral grey columns of the spinal cord. These fibres leave the cord through the anterolateral sulcus as a series of rootlets which then unite to form the ventral root. The dorsal roots consist of sensory (afferent) fibres which are the central processes of cells situated in the spinal ganglion. On leaving the ganglion the fibres form two main bundles which then divide into a series of rootlets to enter the spinal cord through the posterolateral sulcus.

The spinal ganglia are fusiform swellings containing the cell bodies of unipolar neurons whose central processes form the dorsal root as previously noted, while their peripheral processes are directed into the spinal nerves. Each ganglion lies on the dorsal root just proximal to the junction of the ventral and dorsal roots, and is usually situated in the intervertebral foramen.

The roots of the spinal nerves are not of uniform length or inclination, for the spinal cord only extends in the vertebral canal as far as the second lumbar vertebra. The upper cervical roots are short and run almost horizontally, but as the spinal cord is descended the roots become progressively longer and more steeply inclined downwards. Roots issuing from the spinal cord below the second lumbar segment are long and almost vertically disposed, collectively forming the cauda equina (Fig. 19.5).

FUNCTIONAL FIBRE COMPONENTS OF THE SPINAL NERVES

A typical spinal nerve (Fig. 19.82) consists of the following functional components.

1   Somatosensory fibres convey exteroceptive and proprioceptive information from a variety of receptors in the skin, fasciae, skeletal muscle, joints, etc.
2   Viscerosensory fibres (autonomic afferents) bring interoceptive information from receptors situated in blood vessels, glands and viscera. Both kinds of fibres (1 and 2) are the peripherally directed processes of unipolar cells contained in the spinal ganglia.
3   Somatomotor fibres are the axons of α and γ motor neurons of the anterior grey columns of the spinal cord; they innervate skeletal muscle.
4   Visceromotor fibres are sympathetic and parasympathetic efferent fibres. (a) The preganglionic sympathetic fibres arise from cells of the lateral grey column of the thoracic and upper two lumbar segments of the spinal cord. They leave the spinal nerve through a white ramus communicans (Fig. 19.82) to synapse with ganglionic neurons of the sympathetic trunk. These cells then send postganglionic sympathetic fibres through a grey ramus communicans for distribution to sweat glands and arrector pili muscles of

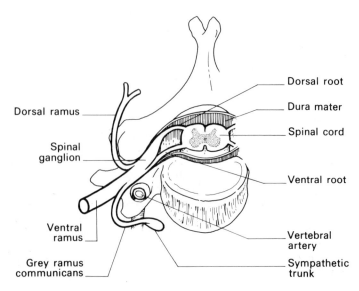

Fig. 19.81. Diagram showing the relations of a cervical nerve and its spinal ganglion to a cervical vertebra.

Dorsal ramus

Spinal ganglion

Ventral ramus

Grey ramus communicans

Dorsal root

Dura mater

Spinal cord

Ventral root

Vertebral artery

Sympathetic trunk

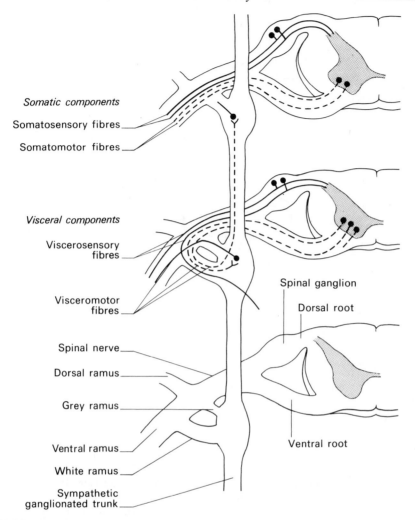

Somatic components
Somatosensory fibres
Somatomotor fibres

Visceral components
Viscerosensory fibres
Viceromotor fibres
Spinal nerve
Dorsal ramus
Grey ramus
Ventral ramus
White ramus
Sympathetic ganglionated trunk

Spinal ganglion
Dorsal root
Ventral root

Fig. 19.82. Plan showing the functional components of a typical spinal nerve. The upper part of the diagram shows the somatic components. The middle part depicts the visceral components; here, preganglionic sympathetic fibres (interrupted lines) enter the trunk through the white ramus to synapse on ganglion cells which give rise to postganglionic fibres (see text). The lower part of the diagram shows the rami associated with the spinal nerves.

the skin, and smooth muscles of blood vessels. (b) The preganglionic parasympathetic fibres are axons of cells situated in the lateral columns of the second, third and fourth sacral segments of the spinal cord. They run in the ventral roots and spinal nerves associated with these segments, and then relay in pelvic ganglia where emerging postganglionic fibres supply smooth muscle and glands of the pelvic viscera and descending colon.

DORSAL AND VENTRAL RAMI

On leaving the intervertebral foramen each spinal nerve gives rise to small recurrent meningeal branches and then divides into a dorsal and a ventral ramus. The meningeal branches re-enter the intervertebral foramen to supply sensory and sympathetic fibres to vertebral joints, blood vessels and the dura mater, those of the upper three cervical nerves also supply the dura mater of the posterior cranial fossa.

The dorsal rami run posteriorly and then divide into lateral and medial branches which innervate muscles and skin of the dorsum of the neck and trunk. The ventral rami, for the most part, unite to form plexuses for the supply of limbs: but in the thoracic region they run an

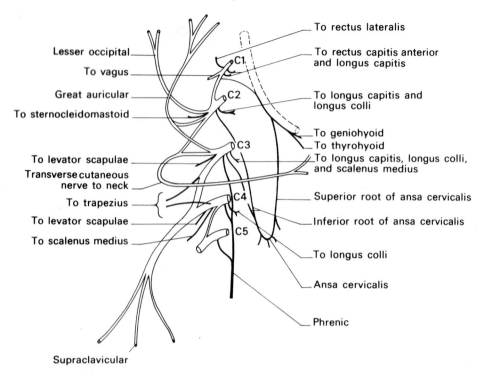

Fig. 19.83. Scheme of the cervical plexus. Muscular branches are shown as solid lines: the hypoglossal nerve in interrupted lines.

independent course, innervating the muscles and skin of the lateral and ventral walls of the trunk.

CERVICAL PLEXUS

The cervical plexus (Fig. 19.83) is formed from the ventral rami of the upper four cervical nerves, and innervates some of the muscles of the neck as well as supplying cutaneous branches to the head, neck and chest. It lies opposite the four upper cervical vertebrae, deep to the sternomastoid and in front of the scalenus medius.

These rami, save the first (see p. 902), divide into ascending and descending branches which then reform into a series of communicating loops, each loop being composed of fibres from two adjacent trunks. Branches of the cervical plexus arise from the loops and also directly from the rami. They are organized into a superficial set (largely cutaneous) and a deep set (mainly supplying muscles).

Superficial branches (Fig. 19.78)

These consist of (a) a group of ascending nerves: the lesser occipital (C2), greater auricular (C2,3) and transverse cutaneous (C2,3); and (b) a group of descending nerves, the supraclavicular (C3,4). All these superficial branches pass through the posterior triangle of the neck and penetrate the deep cervical fascia before supplying the skin.

The lesser occipital nerve stems from the second cervical nerve and loops below the spinal accessory nerve before ascending along the posterior border of the sternomastoid to the side of the head behind the auricle. The skin of this region and the upper part of the medial surface of the auricle is supplied by this nerve.

The greater auricular nerve arises from the second and third cervical nerves. It curls round the posterior border of the sternomastoid and ascends on that muscle to reach the parotid gland. It supplies the skin over the gland and the angle of the mandible, and also the skin covering the mastoid process. Other branches supply the medial surface of the auricle, except its upper part, and some of the lateral surface of the auricle, including the concha and lobule.

The transverse (anterior) cutaneous nerve of the neck originates from the second and third cervical nerves. After curving round the posterior border of the sternomastoid it crosses the middle of that muscle, deep to the external jugular vein and platysma, and then divides into ascending and descending branches which supply the skin of the front and side of the neck.

The supraclavicular nerves emerge beneath the posterior border of the sternomastoid muscle as a common trunk derived from the third and fourth cervical nerves. The trunk then divides into lateral, intermediate and medial branches which descend and diverge beneath the platysma, and finally pierce the fascia just above the level of the clavicle. The lateral supraclavicular branches pass downwards and laterally across the surface of the trapezius and acromion, supplying the skin of the upper and posterior parts of the shoulder. The intermediate supraclavicular branches descend over the clavicle, and supply the skin over the pectoralis major as far as the level of the second rib. The medial supraclavicular branches cross the sternal attachments of the sternomastoid and supply the skin of this region down to the level of the second rib. Some fibres also innervate the sternoclavicular joint.

Deep branches

These consist of communicating and muscular branches.

The communicating branches pass from the first and second cervical nerves to the vagus and hypoglossal nerves, those passing to the vagus forming a meningeal branch. The contribution to the hypoglossal nerve gives rise to a meningeal branch, the superior root of the ansa cervicalis and nerves to the geniohyoid and thyrohyoid.

The muscular branches are numerous (Fig. 19.83) and form lateral and medial groups. The lateral group of nerves supplies motor fibres to the levator scapulae (C3,4) and the scalenus medius (C3,4), and proprioceptive fibres to the sternomastoid (C2,3,4) and trapezius (C2). The medial group supplies rectus capitis lateralis, rectus capitis anterior, longus capitis and longus colli; in addition, it includes the inferior root of the ansa cervicalis and the phrenic nerve.

The inferior root of the ansa cervicalis (Fig. 19.70) is composed of fibres from the second and third cervical nerves. It descends on the lateral side of the internal jugular vein for a variable distance to form a loop, the ansa cervicalis (Fig. 19.69), with the superior root of the ansa cervicalis (see p. 903). From the ansa muscular branches are distributed to the sternohyoid, sternothyroid and both bellies of the omohyoid.

The phrenic nerve (Figs. 19.69 & 19.83) arises mainly from the fourth cervical nerve but also receives fibres from the third and fifth cervical nerves. It supplies motor fibres to the diaphragm and distributes sensory fibres to the certain parts of the pleura and pericardium. The nerve appears on the upper part of the lateral border of the scalenus anterior and descends along the front of that muscle, deep to the prevertebral fascia. In the lower part of the neck it is crossed superficially by the inferior belly of the omohyoid, the internal jugular vein and the transverse cervical and suprascapular arteries and, on the left side, by the thoracic duct—all these structures lying beneath the sternomastoid. At the root of the neck the phrenic nerve passes behind the subclavian vein and in front of the subclavian and internal thoracic arteries, to enter the thorax just medial to the inner border of the first rib. Within the thorax the course of the right and left phrenic nerves are similar, each descends in front of the root of the lung between the fibrous pericardium and the mediastinal pleura to reach the diaphragm; however their relations are different.

The right phrenic nerve leaves the medial border of the scalenus anterior and descends successively on the lateral side of the right brachiocephalic vein, the superior vena cava and the fibrous pericardium bordering the right atrium and inferior vena cava. It then pierces central tendon of the diaphragm close to the inferior vena caval opening and supplies inferior surface of the diaphragm.

The left phrenic nerve passes downwards from the medial border of the scalenus anterior on to the front of the first part of the subclavian artery. It then continues between the left common carotid and the subclavian arteries where it passes forwards and medially, superficial to the vagus nerve. Next, it crosses the left side of the arch of the aorta and passes in front of the root of the lung to descend between the mediastinal pleura and the fibrous pericardium covering the left ventricle. Finally it pierces the muscular portion of the diaphragm and supplies the lower surface.

Apart from being the only source of motor fibres to the diaphragm, the nerves carry pro-

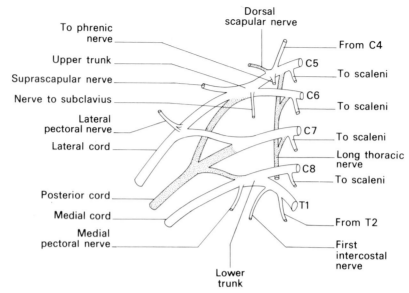

Fig. 19.84. Schema of the brachial plexus. The stippled bundles represent the posterior divisions of the nerve trunks, and also the long thoracic nerve.

prioceptive fibres from this muscle, and in addition supply sensory fibres to the fibrous and parietal serous pericardium and also the mediastinal and diaphragmatic pleura.

THE BRACHIAL PLEXUS (Fig. 19.84)

The brachial plexus is formed in the neck by the union of the ventral rami of the fifth, sixth, seventh and eighth cervical nerves and the greater part of the ramus of the first thoracic nerve. These constitute the roots of the plexus. In addition, the plexus receives variable contributions from the ventral rami of the fourth cervical and second thoracic nerves.

The roots emerge between the scalenus anterior and scalenus medius muscles and unite into trunks. The ventral rami of the fifth and sixth cervical nerves join at the lateral border of the scalenus medius to form the upper trunk of the plexus; the ventral rami of the eighth cervical and the first thoracic nerves unite behind the scalenus anterior to form the lower trunk; whilst the seventh cervical ventral ramus continues as the middle trunk. All three trunks run downwards and laterally in the posterior triangle of the neck, the upper two trunks lying above the third part of the subclavian artery, the lower trunk passing posterior to the artery. Behind the clavicle each trunk divides into an anterior and a posterior division. The anterior divisions of the upper and middle trunks unite to form the lateral cord, a bundle which passes into the arm on the lateral side of the axillary artery. The anterior division of the lower trunk continues as the medial cord, placed at first behind and then on the medial side of the axillary artery. The posterior divisions of all three trunks join to form the posterior cord which lies at first above and then behind the axillary artery.

The roots of the brachial plexus have connections with the sympathetic trunk.

Branches of the brachial plexus may be grouped into (a) supraclavicular branches which arise in the neck from the roots or upper trunk, and (b) infraclavicular branches which arise in the arm from the cords of the plexus. The latter group supplies muscles, joints and skin of the upper limb, and includes such nerves as the radial, ulnar and median. The supraclavicular branches supply the scaleni, longus cervicis and certain muscles of the pectoral girdle and shoulder.

THORACIC VENTRAL RAMI

There are twelve thoracic ventral rami on each side. The upper eleven run between the ribs forming the intercostal nerves, the twelfth or subcostal nerve lies below the last rib. Near to its point of origin each ramus is connected with a corresponding ganglion of the sympathetic trunk by white and grey rami communicantes.

The first thoracic ventral ramus sends most of its fibres to the brachial plexus (see above), but also gives off a small intercostal nerve to the first intercostal space.

The second to the sixth intercostal nerves are more typical. Each nerve runs forwards in its respective space, lying undercover of the lower margin of the rib and between the internal and innermost layers of intercostal muscles. Near the sternum the nerve leaves the space and ends as the anterior cutaneous nerve. During its course the intercostal nerve and its collateral branch supply the muscles of the space. The trunk of the nerve also gives rise to the lateral cutaneous nerve.

The seventh to the eleventh intercostal nerves run forwards in their respective spaces and then continue into the abdominal wall. They also give rise to collateral, lateral and anterior cutaneous branches.

The intercostal nerves supply the intercostal muscles, and muscles of the anterior and lateral regions of the abdominal wall. They also distribute cutaneous fibres to the thorax and abdomen, as well as sensory fibres to the parietal pleura and peritoneum.

LUMBAR AND SACRAL VENTRAL RAMI

The ventral rami of the upper three lumbar nerves and the greater part of the fourth form the lumbar plexus, while the rest of the fourth lumbar ramus and the ventral rami of the fifth lumbar and upper three sacral nerves constitute the sacral plexus. The two plexuses are collectively termed the lumbosacral plexus. The ventral rami of the fourth and fifth sacral nerves together with that of the coccygeal nerve form the coccygeal plexus.

The lumbar and sacral plexuses give rise to major nerves (such as the femoral, obturator and sciatic) which are distributed to the lower limb. The lumbar plexus also supplies branches to the lower trunk, while the sacral and coccygeal plexuses give off branches to pelvic and pudendal structures.

The autonomic nervous system

The autonomic (visceral or vegetative) nervous system is concerned with the innervation of cardiac muscle and smooth muscle of the vascular, respiratory, alimentary and urogenital systems, the eye and orbit, as well as smooth muscles (arrectores pilorum) of the skin. The glands supplied by autonomic fibres are those of the respiratory, urogenital, alimentary systems (including the salivary glands), and also the lacrimal glands, sweat glands, and others.

The autonomic system consists not only of efferent (visceromotor) components but also afferent (viscerosensory) ones. Primary afferent autonomic neurons, like those of the afferent somatic pathway, are unipolar cells whose cell bodies are found in the sensory ganglia of spinal and cranial nerves. Their peripheral processes are distributed to the viscera through spinal nerves and some of the cranial sensory nerves; their central processes pass into the central nervous system through the dorsal roots of spinal nerves or through the sensory roots of cranial nerves.

The efferent autonomic pathway differs from that of the somatic one, for it employs two neurons for the transmission of impulses from the neuraxis to the peripherally placed effectors. The primary or preganglionic neurons lie in the visceromotor nuclei of the cranial nerves and in the intermediate grey columns of the spinal cord. They are small multipolar neurons. Their axons, termed preganglionic fibres, leave the central nervous system in cranial and spinal nerves to pass to outlying autonomic ganglia. Here, they end by synapsing on secondary or ganglionic neurons whose axons termed postganglionic fibres are then distributed to the viscera. Preganglionic fibres are thinly myelinated, whereas postganglionic fibres are usually nonmyelinated. One preganglionic fibre synapses with some 15–20 ganglionic cells each of which gives rise to one postganglionic fibre. This arrangement accounts for the diffusion of autonomic responses, especially in the sympathetic division.

On the basis of the distribution of the outflowing preganglionic fibres the autonomic system is divided into functionally distinct parts, the sympathetic and parasympathetic divisions. Preganglionic fibres of the sympathetic division leave the spinal cord in thoracic and lumbar spinal nerves and constitute the thoracolumbar outflow (Fig. 19.85). They mostly end in ganglia of the sympathetic trunks which lie close to the spinal cord though some fibres are carried through the sympathetic trunks and terminate in subsidiary sympathetic ganglia situated in the prevertebral autonomic plexuses of the abdomen. In contrast, parasympathetic preganglionic fibres pass out of the neuraxis in certain cranial and sacral spinal nerves. They constitute the

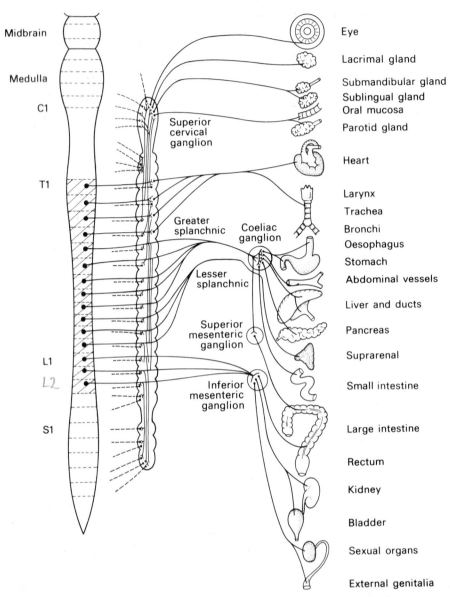

Fig. 19.85. Plan of the efferent part of the sympathetic division (thoraco-lumbar outflow) of the autonomic nervous system. Interrupted lines indicate postganglionic fibres which pass in grey rami to the spinal nerves: other postganglionic and also preganglionic fibres are represented by continuous lines.

craniosacral outflow (Fig. 19.86) and terminate in ganglia which are situated some distance from the neuraxis, close to or within the walls of the visceral organs. Thus postganglionic fibres arising from parasympathetic ganglia tend to run a shorter course than those arising from ganglia of the sympathetic system.

Most viscera have a dual innervation, receiv-ing postganglionic fibres from sympathetic as well as parasympathetic sources. But, smooth muscle of some blood vessels, the arrectores pilorum and sweat glands of the skin appear to be innervated only by the sympathetic division.

The efferent parts of the autonomic system are influenced through various descending pathways, both direct and indirect, which origi-

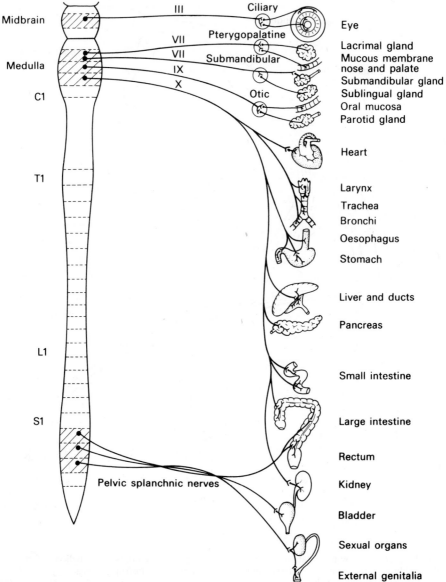

Fig. 19.86. Plan of the efferent part of the parasympathetic division (craniosacral outflow) of the autonomic nervous system.

nate from the hypothalamus, the limbic system and also the reticular system. Stimulation of the prefrontal cortex also results in autonomic responses. Furthermore, autonomic acitivities are modified by sensory input from visceral as well as somatic sources.

The functional roles of the two divisions of the autonomic system are complementary. For example, parasympathetic activity results in cardiac slowing, bronchoconstriction, and increase in peristalsis and glandular secretions of the intestinal tract. Sympathetic activity, on the other hand, results in cardiac acceleration, bronchodilatation and a reduction in intestinal tract activities.

PARASYMPATHETIC DIVISION

Only the general arrangement of the efferent parasympathetic division is described below.

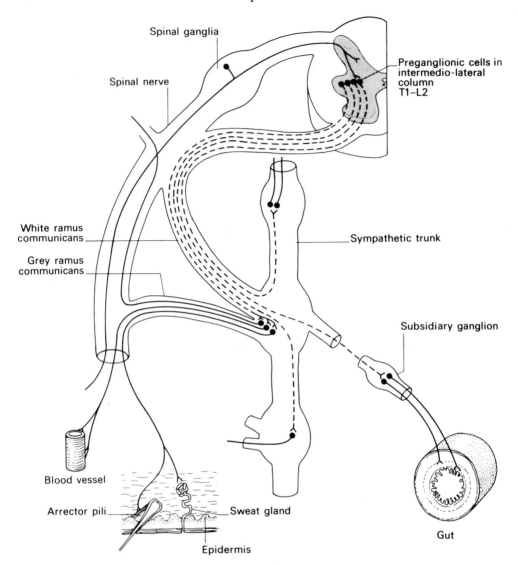

Spinal ganglia

Spinal nerve

Preganglionic cells in
intermedio-lateral
column
T1–L2

White ramus
communicans

Grey ramus
communicans

Sympathetic trunk

Subsidiary ganglion

Blood vessel

Arrector pili

Sweat gland

Epidermis

Gut

Fig. 19.87. Diagram to show the relationship of preganglionic fibres to the sympathetic trunk and ganglia, and the subsequent distribution of postganglionic fibres. Preganglionic fibres are indicated by interrupted lines.

Details of individual cranial autonomic ganglia and their connections are considered in the section on cranial nerves. These parasympathetic ganglia consist of the ciliary, submandibular, pterygopalatine and otic which share the following features (Fig. 19.86). All contain the cell bodies of postganglionic neurons which form synapses with incoming preganglionic parasympathetic fibres. They also contain fibres of passage which run through the ganglia without synapsing. These consist of postganglionic sympathetic fibres, sensory fibres from somatic and

visceral sources, and sometimes fibres subserving taste. The cranial nerves which constitute the parasympathetic division (Fig. 19.86) are the oculomotor, facial, glossopharyngeal and vagus nerves. The pelvic splanchnic nerves are formed from the second, third and sometimes the fourth sacral nerves. These sacral fibres arise from preganglionic parasympathetic cells of the intermediate column of the corresponding sacral segments of the cord. They relay in ganglia found in either the pelvic autonomic plexuses or the walls of the viscera. Postganglionic fibres then innervate the smooth muscle and glands of the distal part of the large intestine including the rectum. In addition they supply the bladder, being excitatory to the smooth muscle of the wall and inhibitory to the sphincter, and are thus concerned with the control of filling and emptying this viscus. Other postganglionic fibres are distributed to the gonads, smooth muscle and glands of the genital tracts, and erectile tissue of the external genitalia.

THE SYMPATHETIC DIVISION

Preganglionic sympathetic fibres arise from cell bodies lying in the intermediate grey columns of all thoracic and the upper two lumbar segments of the spinal cord (Fig. 19.85). They leave the cord in the ventral roots of the corresponding segments and travel a short distance in the spinal nerves before emerging in the white rami communicantes which then join the sympathetic trunks. On entering the trunk the preganglionic fibres end in the following ways (Fig. 19.87): (a) some synapse in ganglia situated at the level of the entering fibres; (b) others ascend or descend to synapse in ganglia situated in the upper or lower parts of the chain, whilst (c) others, after ascending or descending, leave the trunk without synapsing as splanchnic nerves destined for ganglia situated in some of the autonomic plexuses.

The sympathetic trunks are two ganglionated chains (Fig. 19.88). Each extends from the base of the skull to the coccyx and lies more or less anterolateral to the vertebral column. More specifically, in the neck the trunk lies in front of the transverse processes of the cervical vertebrae and behind the carotid sheath, whilst in the thorax it runs anterior to the heads of the ribs and is covered by parietal pleura. The ganglia vary in number and position. Usually there are 3 cervical, some 10 to 12 thoracic and 8 or 9 lumbosacral ones.

Postganglionic fibres derived from the cell bodies of ganglia of the sympathetic trunk are distributed to their effectors in various ways (Fig. 19.87). Some fibres emerge as bundles termed grey rami communicantes. They enter the initial parts of all spinal nerves to be distributed through branches of the ventral and dorsal primary rami to sweat glands, arrector muscles and smooth muscles of blood vessels. Thus every spinal nerve contains postganglionic fibres from corresponding ganglia or parts of the sympathetic trunk. Other postganglionic fibres pass out as branches which join certain autonomic plexuses

to supply such organs as the heart and lungs. Others pass on to neighbouring blood vessels and travel with them to supply outlying structures. They also innervate these vessels.

Cervical and cranial parts of the sympathetic division (Fig. 19.88)

The cervical part of each sympathetic trunk consists of the superior, middle and cervicothoracic ganglia together with their intervening fibre connections. Preganglionic fibres supplying these ganglia ascend in the sympathetic trunk and arise mainly from the upper three or four thoracic segments.

The superior cervical ganglion is the largest of the three ganglia and lies behind the carotid sheath opposite the second and third cervical vertebrae. Its cell bodies give rise to numerous postganglionic branches which include:
1   Grey rami communicantes to the upper four cervical nerves,
2   A laryngopharyngeal branch destined for the pharyngeal plexus,
3   Cardiac branches and
4   The internal carotid nerve.

The internal carotid nerves and their ramifications constitute the cranial part of the sympathetic division. Each nerve extends from the superior cervical ganglion and accompanies the internal carotid artery into the skull. Here, the nerve ramifies around the artery forming the internal carotid plexus. Branches of the plexus composed mostly of vasomotor fibres are then distributed either in certain cranial nerves or by branches of the cerebral blood vessels. They include the deep petrosal nerve, branches to the tympanic plexus and ocular branches which contain fibres to the dilator pupillae as well as vasomotor fibres (see ciliary ganglion and short ciliary nerves, p. 882).

The middle cervical ganglion is the smallest of the cervical ganglia and is variable in position. Usually it lies at the level of the sixth cervical vertebra, close to the inferior thyroid artery. It is connected above to the superior cervical ganglion by a solitary cord and below to the cervicothoracic ganglion by several cords, one of which loops around the first part of the subclavian artery and is called the ansa subclavia.

The thoracic and lower parts of the sympathetic division

The thoracic part of the sympathetic division consists of a row of ganglia linked by intervening portions of the trunk. The number of thoracic ganglia is usually less than that of the thoracic

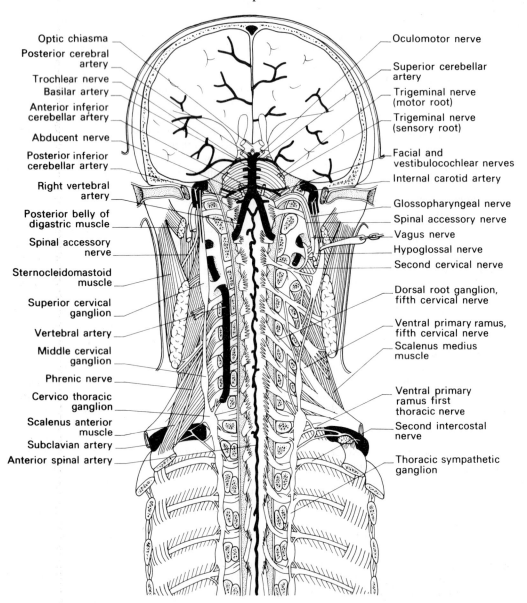

Optic chiasma

Posterior cerebral
artery

Trochlear nerve

Basilar artery

Anterior inferior
cerebellar artery

Abducent nerve

Posterior inferior
cerebellar artery

Right vertebral
artery

Posterior belly of
digastric muscle

Spinal accessory
nerve

Sternocleidomastoid
muscle

Superior cervical
ganglion

Vertebral artery

Middle cervical
ganglion

Phrenic nerve

Cervico thoracic
ganglion

Scalenus anterior
muscle

Subclavian artery

Anterior spinal artery

Oculomotor nerve

Superior cerebellar
artery

Trigeminal nerve
(motor root)

Trigeminal nerve
(sensory root)

Facial and
vestibulocochlear nerves

Internal carotid artery

Glossopharyngeal nerve

Spinal accessory nerve

Vagus nerve

Hypoglossal nerve

Second cervical nerve

Dorsal root ganglion,
fifth cervical nerve

Ventral primary ramus,
fifth cervical nerve

Scalenus medius
muscle

Ventral primary
ramus first
thoracic nerve

Second intercostal
nerve

Thoracic sympathetic
ganglion

Fig. 19.88. Drawing to show the general relationship of the upper part of the sympathetic trunk. The bodies of the vertebrae have been removed to expose the spinal cord and the roots of the spinal nerves.

spinal nerves, for the first and sometimes the second thoracic ganglia are incorporated in the cervicothoracic ganglion (Fig. 19.88).

The second to the fifth ganglia inclusive contribute postganglionic fibres to the pulmonary and cardiac plexuses, and also supply fibres to the aorta, trachea and oesophagus. Branches composed mainly of preganglionic fibres emerge through the fifth to the ninth, tenth and

eleventh, and twelfth thoracic ganglia forming respectively the greater, lesser and least splanchnic nerves. These nerves descend and are distributed to sympathetic ganglia located in the abdominal autonomic plexuses.

The lower part of each sympathetic trunk consists of a number of lumbar and sacral ganglia and intervening parts of the trunk. From the lumbar ganglia emerge lumbar splanchnic nerves, mostly composed of preganglionic fibres, which then relay in ganglia of the abdominal autonomic plexuses. Small sacral splanchnic nerves consisting of postganglionic fibres run from some of the sacral ganglia to pelvic viscera via pelvic autonomic plexuses.

AUTONOMIC PLEXUSES

Autonomic plexuses consist of two elements, fibres and ganglionic cells, which are derived from both divisions of the autonomic system. The fibres include preganglionic and postganglionic axons as well as autonomic afferent fibres. The ganglionic cells are organized as discrete, dissectable ganglia or are diffusely arranged within the plexuses.

The major prevertebral plexuses include pulmonary, cardiac, coeliac and mesenteric. They lie near the midline, in front of the vertebral column and are closely associated with the major arteries. Subsidiary plexuses extend from them along the smaller arteries and distribute fibres, not only to the blood vessels, but also to muscle and glands of the viscera.

The pulmonary plexuses lie around the pulmonary vessels and bronchi in the roots of the lungs and receive preganglionic parasympathetic fibres from the dorsal vagal nucleus via branches of the vagus nerve. Stimulation of parasympathetic efferents results in bronchoconstriction, vasodilatation and secretion of mucus from bronchial glands. Postganglionic sympathetic fibres pass to the pulmonary plexuses from the second to the fifth thoracic ganglia of the sympathetic trunk. Stimulation of these fibres produces bronchodilatation and vasoconstriction.

The superficial and deep cardiac plexuses innervate the heart and its associated blood vessels. The plexuses are composed of fibres from the cardiac branches of the cervical and upper four thoracic ganglia of both sympathetic trunks, and cardiac branches from both vagi and both recurrent laryngeal nerves. Sympathetic fibres of the plexus are mostly postganglionic, whereas parasympathetic fibres (from vagal sources) are preganglionic and terminate on ganglionic cells which contribute postganglionic parasympathetic fibres to the plexuses. Fibres travel from the cardiac plexuses to the heart along major blood vessels. The sinoatrial node and atrial muscle are supplied by parasympathetic and sympathetic fibres, whilst ventricular muscle is supplied by sympathetic fibres only. Stimulation of sympathetic cardiac nerves increases the heart rate, the speed of conduction and tension of cardiac muscle, and also causes vasodilatation of the coronary vessels. On the other hand, parasympathetic stimulation decreases the heart rate and also the excitability of the junctional tissue, especially that surrounding the atrioventricular node.

Autonomic afferent fibres also course through the cardiac plexuses. Sympathetic afferents pass in all cardiac branches of the sympathetic trunk ganglia except those of the superior cervical ganglia. They monitor sympathetic responses, but are also concerned with signalling cardiac pain—felt as a constricting pain encircling the chest (angina pectoris) which also radiates down the arm and sometimes up into the neck and jaw. Vagal afferent fibres are largely responsible for important cardiovascular reflexes.

The coeliac, superior and inferior mesenteric plexuses are interlinked networks of autonomic fibres situated on the anterior and lateral aspects of the abdominal aorta. Through subsidiary plexuses they deliver fibres to some of the abdominal viscera. All three plexuses contain ganglia composed of cell bodies of sympathetic neurons. They also consist of:
1   Preganglionic and postganglionic fibres from the sympathetic trunks,
2   Preganglionic fibres from vagal sources and
3   Many autonomic afferent fibres.

More specifically, the coeliac and mesenteric plexuses receive sympathetic fibres (mostly preganglionic) through splanchnic nerves (greater, lesser and least) which emerge from thoracic ganglia of the sympathetic trunks. The inferior mesenteric plexus also receives additional sympathetic fibres (mostly preganglionic) from splanchnic nerves coming from the first two lumbar ganglia of the trunks. Many of the preganglionic fibres relay in the ganglia of these plexuses which in turn give rise to postganglionic sympathetic fibres. However, some preganglionic sympathetic fibres pass through the plexuses and synapse directly on cells of the suprarenal medulla which functionally and developmentally may be regarded as modified postganglionic sympathetic neurons. Also traversing these plexuses without interruption are preganglionic parasympathetic fibres from the posterior vagal trunk. These, together with postganglionic sympathetic nerves are distributed to certain abdominal viscera through the following periarterial plexuses:
1   Plexuses surrounding the branches of the coeliac artery distribute fibres to the stomach, duodenum, liver, gall bladder and spleen.

2   Those associated with branches of the superior mesenteric artery distribute fibres to the duodenum, jejunum, ileum and the proximal part of the colon up to the splenic flexure.

3   Those of the renal and gonadal arteries distribute to the kidneys and gonads (testes and ovaries) respectively.

4   Plexuses associated with branches of the inferior mesenteric artery, reinforced with fibres from pelvic splanchnic nerve (sacral outflow of the parasympathetic), distribute fibres to the descending colon, sigmoid colon and upper part of the rectum.

Fibres (preganglionic parasympathetic, postganglionic sympathetic and autonomic afferent) of the periarterial plexuses then enter the walls of the alimentary tract and form intrinsic plexuses which lie between the circular and longitudinal muscle (myenteric plexuses) and also in the submucosa (submucous plexuses). Here, the parasympathetic fibres synapse on ganglionic cells which furnish postganglionic fibres.

The hypogastric plexus is a downward extension of the prevertebral abdominal plexuses. Its lower part descends and diverges around the sides of the pelvic viscera to form right and left pelvic plexuses. Each consists mainly of

1   Preganglionic parasympathetic fibres from the pelvic splanchnic nerves (sacral outflow),

2   Postganglionic sympathetic fibres from lumbar and sacral ganglia of the sympathetic trunk and

3   Autonomic afferent fibres.

These fibres are distributed to pelvic viscera through subsidiary plexuses, the preganglionic elements first relaying on postganglionic parasympathetic neurons contained in or about the walls of the viscera. Pelvic viscera supplied include the lower part of the rectum and also the anal canal, the bladder, the internal genital organs (prostate, seminal vesicles and ducti deferentia in the male; uterus, uterine tubes and vagina in the female) and also the external genitalia. In addition, the distal part of the large intestine and the upper part of the rectum are supplied with parasympathetic fibres from the sacral outflow which ascend through the hypogastric plexus to the inferior mesenteric plexus.

Blood brain barrier

The concept of a blood-brain barrier began to be formulated towards the end of the last century when workers noticed that certain dyes introduced into the circulation of experimental animals failed to stain the central nervous system, but when introduced into the cerebrospinal fluid (CSF) caused staining and damage of the cerebral tissue. Our modern concept must explain not only the phenomenon of an absolute barrier as in the case of some dyes, but also the remarkable degree of selectivity that is necessary to account for the composition of the CSF and the fact that this remains extraordinarily constant in the face of severe fluctuations in the composition of the other body fluids. A purely passive barrier could not account for these findings. Constancy of composition is essential for the proper functioning of the central nervous system and it is not therefore surprising that a complex mechanism has been evolved for its protection.

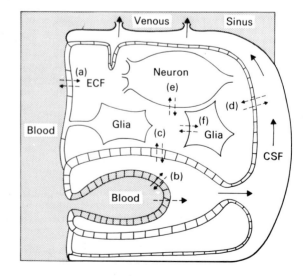

Fig. 19.89. Scheme illustrating exchanges within the central nervous system between (a) blood and cerebral ECF across the blood-brain barrier, (b) blood and CSF across the choroid plexus, (c) and (d) CSF and brain ECF in the ventricles (c) and subarachnoid space (d), (e) and (f) brain ECF and brain cells. Solid arrows indicate flow of CSF from choroid plexus to arachnoid villi where drainage takes place into venous sinuses. After Davson H. and Bradbury M. W. B. (1964) The fluid exchange of the central nervous system *Symp. Soc. Exp. Biol.* **19**, 349–364.

Table 19.2. Concentrations of various solutes in plasma and lumbar CSF of human subjects given in mmols unless otherwise indicated. Data from various authors (after Davson 1967).

	CSF	Plasma	CSF/Plasma
Na	147	150	0.98
K	2.86	4.63	0.62
Mg	1.12	0.81	1.40
Ca	1.14	2.35	0.49
Cl	113	99	1.10
HCO3	22.30	26.80	0.87
Inorg.P (mg/100cm^3)	3.40	4.70	0.73
Protein (mg/100cm^3)	28	6800	0.004
Glucose (mg/100cm^3)	65	110	0.60
Osmolality (m osmol)	289	289	1.00
pH	7.307	7.397	0.99
P$_{CO_2}$	50.50	41.10	1.23

Fig. 19.89 shows the relationship between blood, brain and cerebrospinal fluid. The barriers between blood and brain ECF, and between blood and CSF, serve to isolate the CNS and its fluid environment from the blood. Both barriers exhibit a high degree of selectivity and low permeability towards many of the plasma constituents and so facilitate the establishment of the observed concentration differences between blood and CSF (Table 19.2).

In adult man the CSF has a volume of about 140 cm^3, of which some 25 cm^3 is in the ventricles. This is continuously secreted by the choroid plexuses (Fig. 19.60). The composition of the secreted fluid is constant and is modified little as it circulates through the ventricular and subarachnoid spaces to be finally eliminated through the villi of the arachnoid granulations (Fig. 19.58) by a bulk flow mechanism. In addition to serving as a stable environment for neuronal metabolism, the CSF of the cerebral and spinal subarachnoid spaces protects the CNS against mechanical injury. The brain and the spinal cord are suspended in the CSF and as a result of buoyancy, the brain, which weighs on average 1400 grams in adult man, has an apparent weight of only 50–100 grams. This hydraulic medium also serves to protect the CNS from the effects of rapid acceleration. In the absence of CSF there would be a much greater incidence of rupture to the suspending meninges and meningeal blood vessels. The falx cerebri (Fig. 19.54) and tentorium cerebelli also stabilize the brain against twisting. Since blood vessels ramify throughout the nervous tissue the blood-brain barrier must be anatomically diffuse if it is to isolate the neural elements from the blood.

The astroglia, whose end-feet processes are seen to form a sheath around the cerebral capillaries, have been postulated as the barrier but it is more likely to be the capillary endothelium itself since microperoxidase (mw 1900) introduced into the CSF is able to gain access to the space between the glial sheath and the capillary, but is unable to penetrate into the blood across the capillary endothelium. In addition electron microscopy has revealed that not only are the cerebral capillaries of the continuous type, but they also have 'tight' junctions by which the adjacent cells are fused by zonulae occludens. The resistance to passage of material between blood and the brain is therefore greatest at the level of the endothelium. Another barrier with tight junctions is seen at the choroidal ependyma. At the blood-CSF barrier the capillaries are permeable to markers introduced into the blood. Some brain tissue seems to be outside the blood-brain barrier in as much as it is more permeable. This includes the pineal, posterior pituitary, and part of the hypothalamus. It is probable that some of these areas contain chemoreceptors which monitor changes in the composition of plasma.

The concentrations of various solutes in plasma and lumbar CSF of normal human subjects is given in Table 19.2.

Only magnesium and chloride are in higher concentrations in CSF than in normal plasma; sodium is almost identical in both fluids and the rest are in significantly lower concentrations in CSF than in normal plasma. These concentrations in CSF are maintained even during substantial changes in plasma levels. The brain barrier systems behave as a cell membrane —the solutes, being unable to pass between adjacent cells, have to pass the transcellular route.

It is therefore possible to predict that lipophobic substances and species which are charged at physiological pH will not easily penetrate the barrier whereas lipophilic species will do so with relative ease. Charged species will show selectivity on the basis of their physicochemical properties as they enter through water filled channels in the cell membrane. Carbon dioxide in the blood can freely diffuse through the barrier into the CSF where it becomes hydrated, then dissociates to form bicarbonate and hydrogen ions. Bicarbonate and hydrogen ions diffuse much less readily than CO_2. The H^+ concentration in CSF plays a vital role in the regulation of respiration through its action on the central chemoreceptors.

In addition to these purely passive restrictive phenomena the brain barrier systems also have facilitatory functions. Specific transport mechanisms are located at the barriers to facilitate the entry or removal of a variety of substances. D-Glucose, which is extremely lipophobic, is transferred across the barrier by a facilitated transport mechanism specific to it and other similar hexoses. The barrier also has outwardly directed 'pumps' which serve to restore normal concentrations in the event of a disturbance. Like other carrier mediated processes those in the barrier are saturable and stereospecific. In addition the CSF serves as a 'sink' into which the byproducts of brain metabolism can diffuse before being finally eliminated from the CNS through the bulk-flow mechanism for the drainage of CSF.

The presence of a barrier between the blood and CSF necessarily limits the entry of therapeutic agents as these substances are subjected to the same selectivity. Consequently, massive doses may have to be administered parenterally in order to achieve the desired concentrations in the CNS if they cannot be given intrathecally (into the CSF). In this connection it is interesting to note that anaesthetics are lipid soluble. The physical characteristics of many centrally acting drugs are such as to facilitate their entry across the barrier.

CONDITIONED REFLEXES

In his classical studies of conditioned reflexes, Pavlov discovered that if a bell were rung just prior to meat being placed in a dog's mouth, the dog soon associated bell-ringing with presentation of meat. Repetition of this procedure caused the dog to salivate in response to the bell-ringing alone, the conditioned stimulus (CS), without presentation of the meat which was the unconditioned stimulus (US). A conditioned reflex, then, is a reflex response to a stimulus that does not normally produce a response which is meaningful in terms of the quality of the stimulus. It is acquired by repeatedly applying the conditioned stimulus just prior to a stimulus which is normally associated with the response.

Using this sort of protocol, conditioning can develop in response to many unusual conditioning stimuli. Excess repetition of the conditioned stimulus without periodic reinforcement by the unconditioned stimulus can lead progressively to loss of the conditioned response. This process is termed extinction or, as Pavlov himself called it, 'internal inhibition'. A conditioned response can be prevented by interposing an external strong stimulus unrelated to the response, such as a loud noise, a situation which is known as 'external inhibition'. The conditioned response can readily be re-established by pairing the CS with the appropriate US once again.

There is usually a critical interval between CS and US beyond which the conditioned response will fail to be established. Periods exceeding about two minutes lead to failure of the conditioned response.

Animals can be taught to discriminate between conditioning stimuli if only one of these leads to a reward (presentation of food usually). The degree of discrimination can be quite remarkable. The ability of animals to discriminate potentially rewarding stimuli has been widely used in the procedure known as operant conditioning. An extension of this is where an animal is taught to carry out a task for a reward; in this case, the discriminative task is the conditioned stimulus, the reward may be the animal's favourite food. For example, blindfolded monkeys have been conditioned to discriminate between degrees of roughness. This technique has been used to determine the somesthetic or stereognostic abilities of animals with CNS lesions. Such investigations have been invaluable in determining sensory loss after lesions of particular parts of the nervous system. Operant conditioning is invaluable in such investigations since animals are, of course, incapable of communicating their deficiencies to human observers in any abstract way.

Similarly animals can be taught conditioned

avoidance reflexes, the most common example being the avoidance of minor electric shocks which are received when a particular response is made by the animal. In studies on taste perception (p. 545), an animal can be given a shock each time it drinks one of three solutions which differs slightly in taste, but in no other way, from the other two. After a few attempts, the animal becomes conditioned and its ability to discriminate between solutions can be used in neurophysiological studies.

Clearly, conditioning involves a simple form of learning, and most psychologists would agree that conditioning and learning share common mechanisms. Past experience is a prerequisite for both. Many conditioned reflexes are established in everyday life, and often it is academic whether we label these as learned behaviour or conditioned responses. As an example, we can consider the circus animal which is trained to carry out a complex series of tasks in order to obtain a relatively minor reward. The reward need not always involve something as basic as food. Many animals, and children too, can be trained to carry out tasks by being rewarded with affection. Correspondingly, learning in human beings often involves reward in terms of long-term goals, such as the acquisition of status, power or a high standard of living. The dividing line between conditioning and learning is, therefore, usually in terms of the simplicity of the learning situation. Usually, in conditioning, the rewards are immediate, whereas in learning the rewards are less easily apparent.

EEG AND DIFFERENT CONSCIOUS STATES

If two disc electrodes are placed on the surface of the skull, oscillations in potential difference between the electrodes can be recorded of the order of 50–200 μV at variable frequencies and amplitudes depending upon the conscious state of the subject and the positions of the electrodes on the scalp. These waves are known as the electroencephalogram (EEG). As the form of the EEG changes with different mental states of the subject as well as disease, electroencephalography is a powerful diagnostic tool. Absence of the EEG is indicative of brain death.

The origin of these waves is somewhat complex. In part, they arise from summated excitatory and inhibitory potentials generated in the dendrites of cortical cells, as well as from discharges of these cells. However, it is now known that major components are also produced by referred potentials from eye muscles and slow changes in potential from superficial glial cells.

The most easily detectable EEG rhythm is known as the α-rhythm and it can be readily obtained from the parietooccipital region of a quiescent relaxed subject with his eyes closed. This rhythm varies somewhat in amplitude and frequency between different individuals. The frequency range is from 8–14/sec. However, in any particular individual it is extraordinarily constant in frequency, the amplitude waxing and waning periodically. The EEG is said to be synchronized during the α-rhythm (Fig. 19.90). If the subject is given a mental task to perform the α-rhythm is replaced by higher frequency, low amplitude, irregular acitivity with frequency components of 14–25/sec, commonly known as the β-rhythm. The cortex is said to be desynchronized in this alert mental state (Fig. 19.90). Any significant sensory stimulus leading to the alert state causes cortical desynchronization, or, as it is often termed, α-blocking. Desynchronization is, therefore, associated with arousal leading to the alert state.

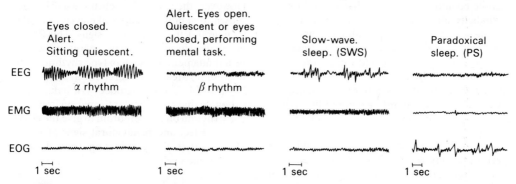

Fig. 19.90. Electroencephalogram (EEG), electromyogram (EMG) and electrooculogram (EOG) signals in different states of consciousness.

When a subject adopts the behavioural symptoms of going to sleep, such as lying down, relaxing and closing the eyes, synchronization of the EEG occurs leading to a condition of slow-wave sleep (SWS). This is characterized by high amplitude, low frequency delta waves, at 4/sec, interspersed with α-like oscillations at 10–14/sec. Potentials from the orbit, the electrooculogram (EOG), reflecting the activity of the eye muscles, are absent. A second stage of sleep which is now considered to be associated strongly with dreaming is known as paradoxical sleep (PS). PS is associated with rapid eye movements (REM) and is sometimes referred to as REM sleep. During paradoxical sleep, the EEG shows a desynchronized rhythm similar to the alert state although responses to sensory stimuli are absent, and indeed the depth of sleep is very intense. During PS, the EMG is generally entirely absent for long periods with the exception of the ocular muscles and occasional movements of the digits which occur during dreaming. Subjects abruptly awoken during this state often recall dreams.

Sleep

Sleep is associated with a large decrease in skeletal muscle tone, a loss of motor reactions to environmental changes, a large increase in threshold to sensory stimuli, and finally an ability to be aroused to the waking state. The last factor distinguishes sleep from anaesthesia, narcosis or coma. Sleep is also associated with large decreases in respiratory and cardiac rate, as well as a considerable fall in blood pressure.

Sleep is a natural phenomenon, even in animals low in the phylogenetic scale. For example, earthworms exhibit a 24-hour sleep–wake cycle and will even continue to do so when transected into their separate halves. A 24-hour periodicity of consciousness is exhibited in people who are deprived of all clues as to the time of day, such as lighting changes from day to night, meal times etc., and cannot therefore be related solely to external environmental changes. A circadian sleep rhythm therefore exists which is apparently governed by cyclical changes in the internal environment of animals and man.

It is known that when one is fatigued after performing physical exercise, sleep comes more readily but there is not the slightest evidence that metabolic by-products of 'muscular tiredness', such as an increase in lactic acid, can cause sleep. The feeling of being tired prior to sleep is psychological, not physical, although this does not rule out the theory that a specific sleep 'toxin' is produced in the CNS. Recently, some well controlled experiments have implied that a short chain peptide is released into the cerebrospinal fluid in sleep deprived animals and this initiates the events which lead to sleep. The peptide is claimed to cross the blood brain barrier in a small group of cells known as the area postrema in the IVth ventricle. Activity here then influences nuclei of the ascending reticular formation, whose role in sleep is discussed later in this section. It would seem possible that a peptide builds up in concentration during the day and eventually 'triggers' the sleep-inducing system.

The change from wake to sleep and vice versa is known as the sleep–waking cycle, and the factors responsible for this fundamental rhythm are still not well understood despite the discovery of numerous areas in the brain which can regulate the cycle.

Experiments on chronic decerebrate cats have indicated that neural mechanisms are present in the reticular formation (p. 864) of the brainstem, which can produce the alternate states of consciousness after isolation from the cerebrum. Two antagonistic systems are present in the reticular formation; a more rostral activating reticular system stretches into the rostral pons area, whilst a lower brainstem deactivating system induces sleep and cortical sychronization. These systems interact both with one another and with structures in the cerebrum which they innervate. It is the balance between the activities of these reticular systems that appears to determine whether sleep or the awake state predominates. The brainstem is not of course the only area of brain which shows a sleep–wake cycle; it may impose its rhythm on cerebral structures. However, the isolated cerebrum itself has been shown to exhibit a sleep–wake cycle, as judged by neural activity and EEG signs. This 24-hour alternation in consciousness, therefore, seems to be a fundamental circadian type rhythm existing in all brain areas; the search for a 'sleep centre' has possibly been misguided. On balance, it is probable that the reticular formation imposes its basic rhythm on the cerebrum to give the characteristic EEG and behavioural signs of the two states and is the dominating control on the sleep–wake cycle.

MECHANISMS OF SLEEP

In recent years, it has been found that the brain-

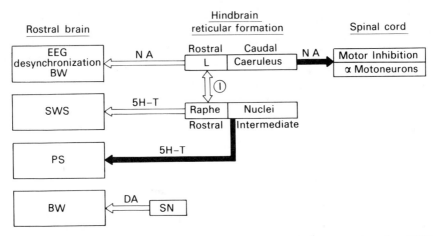

Fig. 19.91. Interactions between areas of CNS involved in changing states of consciousness. BW, behavioural waking; SWS, slow-wave sleep; PS, paradoxical sleep; NA, noradrenaline; 5H-T, 5-hydroxytryptamine; DA, dopamine; SN, substantia nigra. (See text for further explanation).

stem reticular formation liberates well identified neurotransmitter substances among which are 5-hydroxytryptamine (5–HT) and nor-adrenaline (NA). Basically, the more rostral activating reticular system is capable of liberating NA at non-specific thalamic and cortical sites to induce the arousal response with appropriate desynchronization of the EEG, whereas the lower brainstem system produces EEG synchronization and behavioural sleep by the liberation of 5–HT (Fig. 19.91).

THE RAPHE SYSTEM

A distinct group of cells in the rostral portion of the Raphe nuclei in the floor of the IVth ventricle liberates 5–HT from their axon terminals in the cerebrum causing EEG synchronization and behavioural sleep of the slow-wave variety (SWS).

In the intermediate Raphe on the other hand are found another group of neurones which liberate 5–HT at the terminals in the cerebrum to generate PS with concomitant cortical desynchronization and rapid eye movements. It seems that in the normal animal the intermediate and rostral Raphe co-operate in some way since paradoxical sleep cannot be produced unless a preceding phase of slow-wave sleep occurs.

THE LOCUS CAERULEUS AND WAKING

The Locus Caeruleus has been delineated into two distinct functional zones, rostral and caudal. Enhanced activity in the rostral zone is associated with the waking state through the dorsal noradrenergic pathway. Activation of rostral Locus Caeruleus is thought to inhibit in some way 5–HT release initiated by the rostral Raphe system, but it is not known whether the reverse occurs. A descending noradrenergic path arises from the caudal Locus Caeruleus and produces powerful inhibition of spinal cord motoneurons. This inhibition of motor activity is a particular manifestation of paradoxical sleep. The quiescent EMG in PS may therefore be a function of caudal Locus Caeruleus activity 'shutting off' motor behaviour resulting from dreams.

An additional pathway contributes to behavioural waking. This arises from the substantia nigra and is anatomically associated with the ascending noradrenergic path from the rostral Locus Caeruleus. The transmitter liberated rostrally in the brain by this pathway is dopamine (Fig. 19.91).

ABNORMAL SLEEP STATES

Individuals who exhibit abnormal periods of sleep during the day are said to be suffering from narcolepsy. Amphetamines are usually used in high doses for the treatment of this condition. Although they have structures which are very similar to adrenaline, their effect is considerably larger because they are not readily inactivated in the brain. They are presumed to potentiate the action of the ascending activating reticular formation which in turn suppresses the Raphe nuclei sufficiently to dampen down sleep mechanisms.

The condition of sleeplessness is very common, particularly amongst the elderly. Barbiturates are the drugs most preferred to induce sleep in this condition. Their action is to cause a general depression of the nervous system, reducing polysynaptic activation especially in ascending sensory pathways that contribute to wakefulness. Chlorpromazine, the best known tranquillizer, has now become a most commonly used drug and is known to depress the ascending reticular activating system cells whose output is noradrenergic. It antagonizes noradrenaline, leaving the effect of 5–HT unabated, thus promoting a condition of forebrain inactivation.

BRAIN MECHANISMS AND BEHAVIOUR

Most of the brain mechanisms to be discussed in this section can be classed as cognitive; that is, they are concerned with those mechanisms which we use to process information about the world we live in. They have been chosen because it is in the fields of perception, memory, reasoning and language that man surpasses other mammals. Wherever possible, evidence is cited from studies of humans rather than animals in the belief that the most helpful insights into man's behaviour nearly always come from studies of man. There are some obvious excep-

tions to this principle, such as the work on the response characteristics of single cells in the visual system, which will be described later. Another potentially important contribution from animal work is the provision of a basis for comparison with studies on man. From these comparisons it may be possible to identify the brain structures responsible for what can be considered as characteristically human behaviour.

Brain and behaviour: some basic considerations of structures

The importance of understanding relationships between the structure and function of the brain has been recognized for a long time. Human ability however is not related to crude structural differences such as the 'bumps' on the skull (phrenology) or cranial capacity. These somewhat crude measurements completely fail to take into account such factors as the organization within the brain, cell density and the total numbers of nerve cells. Comparisons of various brain regions do indeed reveal those that are associated with phylogentic development. Quantitative analyses of various cortical structures have shown that, apart from the olfactory centres, all structures have enlarged during phylogeny and that the most marked development has been in the neocortex. Since the

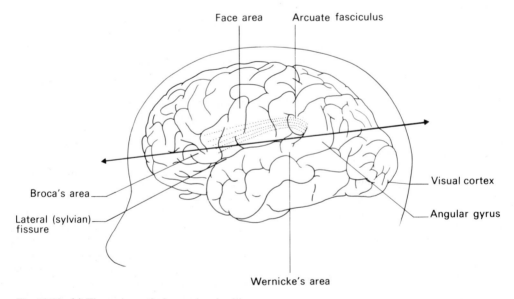

Fig. 19.92. (a) The main cortical areas involved in language production (Broca's area) and language reception (Wernicke's area).

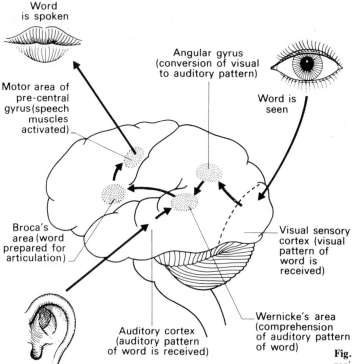

Word
is spoken

Angular gyrus
(conversion of visual
to auditory pattern)

Motor area of
pre-central
gyrus (speech
muscles
activated)

Word is
seen

Broca's
area (word
prepared for
articulation)

Visual sensory
cortex (visual
pattern of
word is
received)

Auditory cortex
(auditory pattern
of word is received)

Wernicke's area
(comprehension
of auditory pattern
of word)

Word is heard

Fig. 19.92. (b) A summary of the main regions involved in the various aspects of language processing in the left cerebral hemisphere.

neocortex appears to be the area involved in those behaviours which distinguish the higher mammals, the greater part of this review will consider the cortical functions of the cerebral hemispheres.

One very important distinction demonstrated in recent years between the brain of man and of lower mammals is a difference between the functions of the left and right cerebral hemispheres in man. On the whole it would appear that the two hemispheres share mirror-imaged functions in all mammals except man.

In the early 1960s it was concluded that there was little evidence of differences between the hemispheres in such gross measures as weight, specific gravity, surface area and length. More recently detailed anatomical comparisons have demonstrated differences which probably account for the well-demonstrated localization of speech controls to the left cerebral hemisphere. This work has been based on comparisons of those regions around the lateral fissure (Fig. 19.92) which are known to be involved with speech in the left hemisphere. Notably it has been shown that there is a significant enlargement of the planum temporale (the posterior

region of the superior surface of the temporal lobe: Fig. 19.92a) on the left side in neonate brains and in 65% of a sample of 100 adult brains. This is part of the classically described posterior speech area. The finding that auditory stimuli evoke greater electrical potentials in the left than the right hemisphere of the neonate, strongly suggests that in the majority of individuals the superior surface of the left temporal lobe is an area with pre-programmed language functions.

Left hemisphere damage in the adult, particularly to the inferior frontal and posterior temporoparietal regions (Fig. 19.92), produces various linguistic defects, whereas damage to the corresponding areas in the right hemisphere rarely does so. Moreover, direct stimulation of these areas in the left hemisphere has been shown to interfere directly with speech (Fig. 19.93). However it must be added that language is not permanently impaired if this region is damaged early in childhood. This is an important point: although regions having a specific function can be demonstrated in young and old, these regions are not necessarily fixed in the young; some plasticity exists.

Hemisphere differences in cognitive functions

The above findings gave rise to the notion that the hemisphere containing the speech functions dominated the other hemisphere, but more recent work has shown that each hemisphere contributes different but complementary functions.

In so-called 'split brain' patients the corpus callosum has been cut in the treatment of intractable epilepsy. The commissures are cut to prevent the spread of epilepsy across the hemispheres, but this eliminates direct cross-communication between the functionally intact hemispheres. Thus it is possible to test the functions of each hemisphere separately if care is taken to present test information unilaterally (i.e. to one hand, ear or visual field only). Following surgery, an object which has been identified by touch with one hand is not recognized as having already been identified when it is presented to the other; and the same is true for smells identified through one nostril. Moreover the patient cannot provide a verbal description for information which has been presented selectively to the left side and therefore to the right hemisphere (speech control is in the left hemisphere). Whereas there appears to be no transfer of factual information, emotionally loaded stimuli (e.g. risqué photographs) are transferred, possibly via subcortical connections.

In all right-handed patients it has consistently been confirmed that the left hemisphere dominates speech, writing and calculation. The right hemisphere can be seen to dominate various non-linguistic functions involving the perception and processing of spatial patterns, relations and transformation.

Recent work in which information is fed in to right or left channel in normal subjects has demonstrated the superiority of the right-visual field (i.e. left hemisphere) in perceiving words, letters and familiar objects, and superiority of the left visual-field in perceiving the location and quantity of dot patterns, in detecting the slopes of lines, in depth perception and in recognizing faces. These are not all-or-none differences since both hemispheres are able to process each type of stimulus but one is better than the other. The picture emerging from work with normal subjects is that there is hemisphere specialization but that this is by no means absolute and may best be conceived in terms of biases.

Studies of patients with unilateral lesions also suggest differences in the psychological functions of each hemisphere. Damage to the temporal lobes has often been found to result in impaired memory, but it can now be demonstrated that the side of the damage determines the type of memory defect. Taken as a whole, several different approaches to the investigation of interhemispheric differences yield a consistent picture (Fig. 19.93). In a normally functioning man the hemispheres obviously work together and in a sense the above section has avoided the most interesting question, namely the role of interactions between the hemispheres and the functions of the corpus callosum in these interactions.

THE LOCALIZATION OF CORTICAL FUNCTIONS

Until fairly recently there has been a widely accepted subdivision of the cerebral neocortex into three functionally distinct areas, namely the sensory, motor, and association areas. Sensory areas were deemed to be solely involved with the reception of sensory information, motor areas with the organization and execution of responses and the association areas with functions lying between these, particularly those concerned with higher cognitive processes such as memory, language and problem solving. Although this subdivision is still widely accepted and will be used here, it should be noted that recent findings make it increasingly difficult to accept this three-way classification of cortical areas.

Sensory and motor areas
Visual cortex. Following recent revisions, the sensory areas remain perhaps the most aptly named, particularly the visual cortex. There is widespread agreement concerning the location of the visual cortex both in terms of function and anatomy. The main optic pathways project via the lateral geniculate body of the thalamus to areas 17 and 18 (the visual cortex). Removal of, or damage to, these areas produce visual impairments of varying degrees of severity. In non-primates, such as cats and rabbits, removal of the visual cortex leads to a reduction in visual acuity but the animals still seem to be capable of some normal visual behaviour. In primates the same experiment produces much more serious visual faults. It was originally claimed that removal of the visual cortex led to a complete inability to discriminate between vertical and horizontal lines but more recent work casts doubt on this. Monkeys without a visual cortex have been shown to be capable of accurately

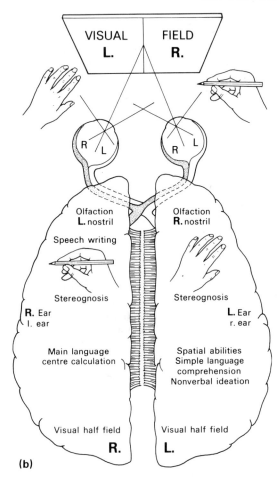

VISUAL FIELD
L. R.

R / L   R / L

Olfaction
L. nostril

Olfaction
R. nostril

Speech writing

Stereognosis

Stereognosis

R. Ear
l. ear

L. Ear
r. ear

Main language
centre calculation

Spatial abilities
Simple language
comprehension
Nonverbal ideation

Visual half field
R.

Visual half field
L.

(b)

Fig. 19.93. A simple summary of the functions associated with the left and right cerebral hemispheres.

locating objects in space after appropriate training. Similar results have recently been demonstrated in man: though unable to discriminate between different patterns these patients were able to judge the position and the orientation of objects in space. Incredibly, they reported that they were totally unaware of these objects at a conscious level; that is, they certainly could not see them. Hence the description of this ability as 'blindsight'. These results raise the possibility that there might be two distinct visual systems each involved in a functionally separate aspect of vision, one cortical and the other subcortical. A number of investigators have argued that the main visual pathway (retina $\longrightarrow$ lateral geniculate body $\longrightarrow$ visual cortex) relays information from the fovea of the eye and hence is predominately concerned with resolving pattern discrimination etc. A second system, based on the superior colliculus, brings material to our atten-

tion and is therefore involved in eye movements and peripheral vision. Thus the two systems might be characterized as being involved in 'seeing what' and 'seeing where' respectively. A further suggestion is that the subcortical system, which is phylogenetically more primitive, is fully operational at birth and that the young infant uses this system until the main cortical system has fully developed.

The processes underlying pattern discrimination within the visual cortex are gradually beginning to be understood as the result of studies which monitor the activity of single cells in the visual cortex, particularly in area 17. This work has shown that single cells in the visual cortex only fire in response to a very specific stimulus. Thus cells can be found which only respond when the eye 'sees' lines of specific orientations or of particular lengths or objects in particular parts of the visual field and at particular depths, and movements in certain directions. These 'feature analysing' cells have been found to be organized in columns, all the cells in a column having the same firing pattern (Fig. 20.21). These cells are involved in the first stages of decoding the incoming visual stimuli by analysing the various features present in any one retinal image. This initial 'feature analysis' stage is assumed to be followed by processing in the visual association areas, particularly in area 19 and in the inferotemporal regions. Thus damage to these areas in man can result in bizarre visual disorders known as the visual agnosias. Patients with visual agnosias show no sensory loss; all the information available in the retinal image can be detected, but they may be totally unable to understand what any particular object is or to recognize faces or to see more than one object at a time.

The various feature analysing cells are present from birth, at least in the cat and monkey, and probably in man but their specificities are not particularly well defined and can be modified during the earlier periods of development.

Auditory cortex. The auditory cortex is neither as well defined nor as well investigated as the visual cortex. Electrophysiological recordings from single cells have revealed a variety of 'feature analysers' which are organized in columns similar to the visual system. However the functional significance of these 'feature analysers' is undecided.

It has been argued that the auditory cortex is involved with processing various features of sound rather than merely responding to specific physical characteristics, such as tonal changes. Ablation of the auditory cortex in mammals does not affect the capacity to discriminate between sound and silence, nor does it reduce the capacity to discriminate the intensity or frequency of tones. The main impairments are related to the localization of sounds and to the discrimination between more complex sounds, such as tonal patterns and voice sounds. On this basis it is assumed that the auditory cortex is particularly concerned with processing biological rather than physical attributes of sound stimuli.

Somatosensory and motor cortex. Many researchers feel that it is now untenable to distinguish between a somatosensory and a motor cortex in any clearly defined way. Somatosensory stimulation has been shown to evoke electrical potentials in the motor as well as in the somatosensory cortex. Moreover movements can be produced by direct stimulation of the somatosensory cortex as well as the motor cortex. In both areas it has been well demonstrated that there is a mapping of the body surface and that body areas which are more richly innervated have a larger cortical projection area. These two 'homunculi' or 'cortical representations' of the body surface were once assumed to be quite separate (Fig. 19.94), one representing the dermatomes and the other controlling the myotomes. Recent evidence of linkage and overlaps between the motor and somatosensory areas tends greatly to weaken this view.

Cells in the somatosensory cortex have feature analysing properties in that they can be shown to respond to specific somatosensory stimuli. They are also organized in columns but as with the auditory cortex, the functional significance of these cells is not really understood.

A complete understanding of motor functions can only be derived from a consideration of all the areas known to be involved in the control of movement, namely the motor cortex, cerebellum and basal ganglia (p. 472). Motor commands are generated in the cortex as the result of information processed in sensory, association or motivation areas. The intricate timing of rapid movements is now thought to be preprogrammed in the cerebellum whereas the basal ganglia serve as a ramp generator for slow voluntary movements. For movements needing a complicated analysis of tactile objects, the output patterns of the cerebellum and basal ganglia are further processed in the motor cortex.

Association areas

The main association areas of the neocortex are the frontal regions and the parietal–temporal–occipital regions. These areas are largest in man and as their name implies they are involved with correlating and elaborating intracortical events, particularly such aspects of behaviour as memory, learning, language, and the timing and organization of responses.

Repeated errors are characteristic of the behaviour of human patients with frontal lobe lesions. These patients do not necessarily perform badly on general intelligence tests, but they tend to be bad at maze tests and card sorting tests which involve such skills as planning ahead, grouping of objects and the ability to change from one approach to another.

Lesions in the dorsolateral region of the frontal association cortex have also been found to

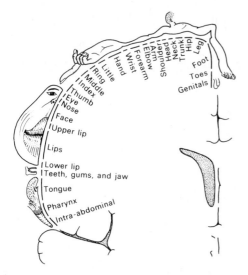

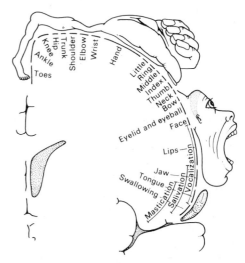

Fig. 19.94. A graphic representation showing how much of the cortex is allocated to sensation and control of different parts of the body. (After Penfield W. and Rasmussen T. (1950) *The Cerebral Cortex of Man.* New York: MacMillan.)

affect motivation and emotions as well as certain perceptual skills. In addition, mechanisms involved in the control of voluntary eye movements have been shown to be localized in the frontal areas. Whereas normal subjects can be shown to scan pictures in a systematic and orderly fashion, patients with frontal lesions are much more erratic. This inevitably results in a poorer selection of information which may in turn diminish the accuracy of subsequent analysis.

Both the frontal and the more posterior association areas are involved with speech (Fig. 19.92b).

From the evidence available it is clearly very difficult to describe a simple unitary concept of frontal lobe functions. In addition to the impairments described above, frontal lesions have also been shown to interfere with such functions as judging sequences of events, word fluency and spatial memory (e.g. learning a route). There is some differentiation between the functional attributes of the left and right frontal areas. Perhaps the most parsimonious view of the frontal lobes ascribes to them an executive role, and a role in coordinating and arranging in sequence various cortical processes. This view is consistent both with the behavioural evidence and with neuroanatomical studies of cell connections which have shown that the frontal cortex receives indirect and partially overlapping afferents from all the major sensory

areas as well as having reciprocal connections with the other association areas.

In primates there is good evidence that the inferotemporal regions are involved in visual perception. Damage to these areas does not appear to interfere with basic visual processes, such as the ability to detect the presence or absence of an object or to discriminate between different patterns or shades of grey, but leads to defects in more complex aspects of vision. Removal of this area interferes with visual learning but does not affect learning in other modalities.

LIMBIC SYSTEM

The Limbic system (p. 878) consists of a group of structures forming a ring on the inner surface of each hemisphere; the septal area, the cingulate gyrus, the hippocampus and the amygdala (Fig. 19.95). Phylogenetically these are the most primitive of the cerebral regions and are associated with olfactory functions in lower order animals, but in man this area is involved in a range of behavioural functions from memory to emotions.

Hippocampus

In man the hippocampus has been traditionally associated with short-term memory but recent theories stress its role in focussing attention. Rats whose hippocampi have been removed are

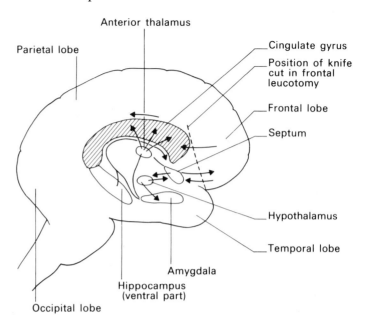

Anterior thalamus

Parietal lobe

Cingulate gyrus

Position of knife
cut in frontal
leucotomy

Frontal lobe

Septum

Hypothalamus

Temporal lobe

Fig. 19.95. A diagram showing
the approximate position of the
hypothalamus and the main
structures of the limbic system.

Occipital lobe

Hippocampus
(ventral part)

Amygdala

easily distracted and less able to ignore irrelevant or redundant stimuli in test situations. The hippocampus is probably involved in focussing attention by a mechanism which filters 'relevant' stimuli.

Amygdala

Removal or electrical stimulation of the amygdala typically changes emotional and motivational states. After a brief period in which an animal's activity is reduced, amygdalectomy often results in increased activity which may be reflected in general behaviour or in such specific activities as eating or sexual behaviour. Lesions in the amygdala can also produce a range of emotional changes. Animals can either become quite tame and docile or can show increased aggressiveness. Moreover fear and rage can be produced by stimulation as well as by lesions of the amygdala.

The other parts of the Limbic system have also been implicated in emotional behaviour particularly the cingulate gyrus which it has been suggested might underlie the experience of emotion. A more recent interpretation of the Limbic system has suggested a functional division between the lower part (amygdala and hippocampus) concerned with those emotional states associated with biological survival (fighting and eating) and the upper part (cingulate gyrus) concerned with emotions related to sexual and social behaviour.

It is clearly unwise to think that the control of emotional behaviour is exclusively located in the Limbic system. The Limbic system has major connections with other cortical areas and with the reticular formation (Fig. 19.96). Emotional behaviour involves many areas of the brain since human emotional responses depend on the degree of arousal and the interpretation of the situation giving rise to the emotional change. Even so it is interesting to note that in recent years there has been an increased interest in surgery of the Limbic area for the treatment of chronic emotional disturbances such as severe aggressive behaviour.

THE HYPOTHALAMUS

One key to understanding the functions of the hypothalamus is its position. It lies between the higher regions and the brainstem, below the thalamus and close to the pituitary gland and the Limbic system (Fig. 19.39, 19.95 and 19.96). It has connections with these and many other brain regions and with sensory pathways, and has a very rich blood supply. The hypothalamus plays a vital role in regulating and integrating a range of behaviours. It is involved in the control of water balance and in regulating body temperature, in activity of the autonomic nervous system, and in various endocrine processes.

Behavioural changes follow electrical stimulation or induced lesions in the hypothalamus. If

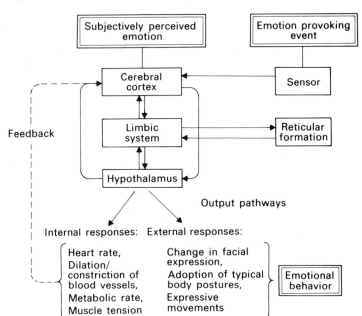

Internal responses:

- Heart rate,
- Dilation/constriction of blood vessels,
- Metabolic rate,
- Muscle tension

External responses:

- Change in facial expression,
- Adoption of typical body postures,
- Expressive movements

Emotional behavior

Fig. 19.96. A schematic diagram of the brain regions involved in control of emotion.

the posterior hypothalamus is stimulated sympathetic activity is evoked together with such behavioural changes as increased arousal and rage. In contrast, stimulation of more anterior areas tends to evoke parasympathetic activity resulting in such changes as decreased arousal and lowered heart-rate. This suggests that the posterior hypothalamic regions are associated with 'fight and flight' type reactions to threat situations, and the anterior regions with more vegetative functions. More recent research has confirmed and refined these findings and supports the idea of two discrete hypothalamic controls over emotional aspects of behaviour. This dualism, an opposition between excitatory and inhibitory functions, can be seen in other behavioural investigations involving this area. Lesions placed in the ventromedial part of the hypothalamus consistently lead to overeating (hyperphagia) and therefore to obesity, whereas lesions in the lateral part of the hypothalamus produce the opposite effect: animals stop eating (aphagia) and would starve if not force-fed. These complementary effects gave rise to a theory of feeding involving a 'feeding centre' and a 'satiety centre' which exert a reciprocal control on each other. Direct electrical recording from the ventromedial region has shown it to be affected by such factors as blood glucose levels and stomach distension. Direct electrical stimulation has resulted in marked reductions in

food intake. The aphagia which follows lateral lesions is probably due to a greatly decreased motivation to eat rather than to any motor impairment. Electrical stimulation in this region results in marked hyperphagia. A striking finding has been the demonstration that separate neurochemical pathways are involved in eating and drinking. Direct injections into rats' hypothalamic regions have shown that feeding is activated by noradrenaline and drinking by acetylcholine.

General conclusions

1 Man is characterized by a uniquely expanded neocortex.
2 In man the two cerebral hemispheres have differences in structure and function. The left side is more competent at processing linguistic and temporal information, the right side at processing visual and spatial information.
3 Within each hemisphere there are clearly defined areas set aside for sensory, motor and higher cognitive (association) functions, although this strict sub-division may well be outliving its usefulness.
4 Subcortical regions appear to be largely concerned with more basic functions, particularly emotion, motivation, eating, sexuality and general arousal, but these areas operate in conjunction with higher cortical regions.

This last point is critical since a brief overview of this sort tends to isolate and delineate functions whereas in life human behaviour depends on the unity of the whole brain and the complex interplay of all the structures involved. Clearly a complete understanding of the functions of the brain is still a long way off, but it is hoped that the present review will at least convey a general picture of the current state of some of our knowledge.

FURTHER READING

BROADBENT D. (1974) Division of functions and integration of behaviour. In F. O. Schmidt and F. G. Worden (eds.) *The Neurosciences*: Third Study Program. Massachusetts Institute of Technology, Boston.

DAVSON H. (1967) *Physiology of the Cerebrospinal Fluid*. London; Churchill.

KIMURA D. (1973) The Asymmetry of the Human Brain, *Scientific American* **228**, 70.

KORNHUBER H.H. (1974) Cerebral cortex, cerebellum and basal ganglia; an introduction to their motor functions. In F. O. Schmidt and F. G. Worden (eds.) *The Neurosciences*: Third Study Program. Massachusetts Institute of Technology, Boston.

MASTERTON R.B. & BERKLEY M.A. (1974) Brain Functions: changing ideas on the role of sensory, motor and association cortex on behaviour. In M. R. Rosenzweig and L. W. Porter (eds.) *Annual Review of Psychology* **25**, 277.

CHAPTER 20

Vision and Hearing

VISION

ANATOMY

Bony orbit

The walls of the orbit have already been described.

The orbit is a socket for the eyeball. The eyeball is connected with the brain by the optic nerve, and supported in the orbit by a packing of fatty connective tissue. In starvation and advanced disease, the fat is metabolized with the result that the eyeball sinks into the socket producing a haggard appearance. The eyeball is moved within the orbit by muscles passing from the bone to the outer fibrous coat of the eyeball and its function is to transduce light stimuli into action potentials which pass along the optic nerve. It is protected by upper and lower eyelids which contain a sphincter muscle for their closure (orbicularis oculi): the upper is attached to a muscle which elevates it and opens the eye.

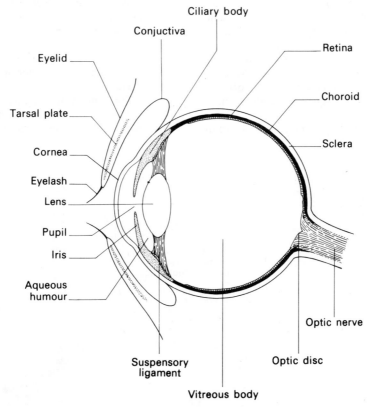

Fig. 20.1. Vertical sagittal section through the eyeball and eyelids.

Eyeball

The eyeball is a spherical structure with a wall which has three coats. The inside of the eyeball contains fluid which is under pressure. The fluid is divided into two by a vertical circular partition so that there is a large posterior and small anterior compartment (Fig. 20.1).

THE FIBROUS COAT

The outer coat, the white of the eye, is called the sclera which becomes the transparent cornea at the front. The sclera and cornea are continuous with each other at the corneoscleral junction (or limbus) of the eyeball. The scleral spur projects behind this junction (Fig. 20.2). The sclera consists of white fibrous tissue which varies in thickness and is almost surrounded by a fascial sheath. Anteriorly, the conjunctiva, a thin transparent modified skin, is reflected from the eyelids on to the sclera to which the extrinsic muscles of the eye are attached. The sheath of the optic nerve, a continuation of the dura mater of the brain, fuses with the sclera.

The cornea projects relative to the sclera and is about 11 mm in diameter. It is the major refractive medium of the eyeball and largely consists of transparent connective tissue fibres which are continuous with those of the sclera. The outer aspect of the cornea is covered by epithelial cells similar to those of non-keratinized stratified squamous epithelium.

The cornea is avascular and is richly innervated by the ophthalmic nerve. Abrasions of the cornea are particularly painful and its sensitivity is the basis of the corneal reflex.

VASCULAR COAT

The middle coat of the eyeball, the vascular coat, or uveal tract, consists of the choroid which lines the sclera as far forwards as the region of the corneoscleral junction where it is called the ciliary body. The ciliary body becomes the iris which is the coloured part of the eyeball and forms a circular structure behind the cornea separate from it. In the middle of the iris is the pupil.

The ciliary body contains smooth muscle which is attached to the scleral spur. The lens of the eye is suspended by fibres which attach it to the posterior surface of the ciliary body. These fibres, the suspensory ligament of the lens, are normally tensed. When the ciliary muscle contracts it pulls the ciliary body inwards so that the suspensory ligament is relaxed, the lens becomes more convex, and the eye can focus on near objects.

The posterior surface of the ciliary body is covered by epithelium which is an anterior continuation of the retina, but is not light-sensitive. Between the ciliary epithelium and the muscle there is a considerable quantity of loose vascular connective tissue whose function is related to fluid circulation in the anterior part of the eyeball. This tissue also contains a large number of nerve fibres, many of which are sensory to the cornea. The smooth muscle is innervated by postganglionic parasympathetic fibres from the

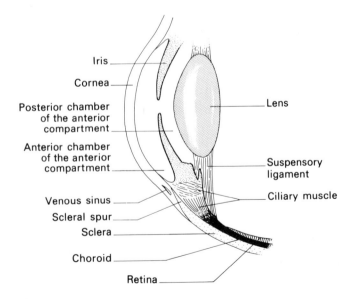

Fig. 20.2. Enlarged view of the corneoscleral junction.

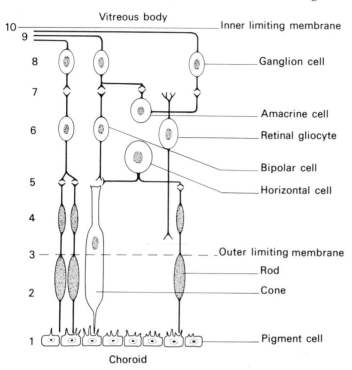

Fig. 20.3. The cellular elements of the retina and its ten layers. (1) Pigment cell layer; (2) layer of rods and cones; (3) outer limiting membrane; (4) outer nuclear layer; (5) outer plexiform layer; (6) inner nuclear layer; (7) inner plexiform layer; (8) layer of ganglion cells; (9) layer of nerve fibres; (10) inner limiting membrane.

ciliary ganglion. The preganglionic fibres are branches of the oculomotor (third cranial) nerve.

The iris divides the anterior part of the eye into an anterior chamber and a posterior chamber (Fig. 20.1). It contains smooth muscle arranged as an inner sphincter (sphincter pupillae) round the edge of the pupil and an outer dilator pupillae whose fibres are radially arranged and peripherally merge into the ciliary body. Most of the iris consists of a stroma containing vessels and nerves.

Arteries and nerves enter the iris from the ciliary body. The nerves are postganglionic parasympathetic and sympathetic. The parasympathetic fibres have their cell bodies in the ciliary ganglion and end in the sphincter pupillae. The sympathetic fibres have their cell bodies in the superior cervical ganglion. They end in the dilator pupillae and in the blood vessels. Their preganglionic fibres have their cell bodies in the first thoracic segment of the spinal cord.

The colour of the iris is due to the connective tissue cells and pigment cells.

INTERNAL (NERVOUS) COAT

The third or inner coat of the eyeball is the light-sensitive retina. Its nerve elements do not extend on to the ciliary body and iris. The retina is about 0.5 mm at its thickest and 0.1 mm in its anterior part. The optic disc is slightly medial to the posterior pole of the eyeball and is the region where the fibres forming the optic nerve come together and pass backwards through the choroid and sclera. The disc is paler than the rest of the retina; it has no light sensitive elements and is called the blind spot. In the centre of the disc are the central artery and vein of the retina. About 3 mm lateral to the optic disc is a small yellowish area, the macula lutea (yellow spot) with a central depressed part called the fovea centralis where vision is most acute.

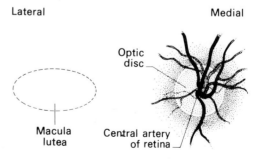

Fig. 20.4. The posterior part of the right retina as seen with an ophthalmoscope.

Ten different layers can be distinguished in histological sections of the retina (Fig. 20.3).

The retina is supplied by arterial blood from two sources. The central artery of the retina, a branch of the ophthalmic artery, has already divided at the optic disc into four branches each supplying a quadrant (Fig. 20.4). The central artery is an end artery and if blocked there is a total loss of retinal function (blindness of that eye). The outer layers of the retina are supplied by choroidal vessels. Veins more or less correspond to the retinal and choroidal arteries.

CONTENTS OF THE EYEBALL

The contents of the eyeball are the aqueous humour in front of the lens, the lens with its suspensory ligament and the vitreous body (Fig. 20.1). The aqueous humour in the anterior compartment is itself divided into anterior and posterior parts by the iris. The fluid, clear and watery, is produced by the ciliary processes of the ciliary body. This fluid passes through the pupil into the anterior chamber whence it is absorbed at the iridocorneal angle into the connective tissue spaces. From there it goes to the venous sinus of the sclera and back to the circulation. The aqueous humour is important in the nutrition of the avascular cornea and lens. It is under pressure and is constantly being produced. If its circulation and/or absorption is interfered with the intra-ocular pressure rises. This results in a condition called glaucoma, in which there is a loss of the peripheral parts of the fields of vision due to the pressure effects on the retina.

The lens consists largely of a series of concentric laminae made up of lens fibres surrounded by a capsule. The capsule is elastic and like the rest of the lens, is also transparent. The lens has no blood vessels. The capsule is attached peripherally to the suspensory ligament of the lens which is in turn attached to the ciliary body beyond the ciliary processes. Behind the lens is the vitreous body. Up to the age of about 40 years the curvature of the lens can be readily increased and this allows near objects to be focussed on the retina. After about 40–45 years the ability to accommodate is gradually lost due to physicochemical changes in the lens. Another not uncommon change is the progressive loss of transparency of the lens, a condition called cataract.

The vitreous body occupies about four-fifths of the interior of the eyeball and lies behind the lens and its suspensory ligament. It is colourless, transparent and jelly-like, consisting of water (99%) with a small amount of mucoprotein. The vitreous body cannot be regenerated. If some of it is lost due to a penetrating wound, the eyeball shrinks and vision is lost.

Muscles and Ligaments

MUSCLES

The ciliary muscle and sphincter and dilator pupillae are the intrinsic muscles of the eyeball. The muscles in the orbit which move the eyeball are called the extrinsic muscles. These include the levator palpebrae superioris, the elevator of the upper eyelid (Fig. 20.5). It is attached to the roof of the orbit posteriorly, above the fibrous ring which includes the opening of the optic canal and the medial end of the superior orbital fissure. The muscle passes forwards towards the front of the orbit and spreads out forming an

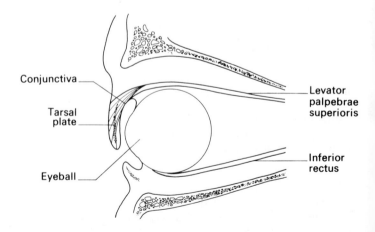

Conjunctiva

Tarsal plate

Eyeball

Levator palpebrae superioris

Inferior rectus

Fig. 20.5. The levator palpebrae superioris.

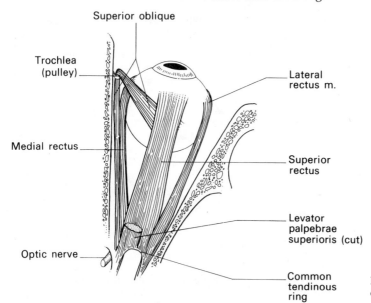

Fig. 20.6. The extrinsic muscles of the right orbit, from above.

aponeurosis which is attached to the upper edge of the tarsal plate and, after passing through the orbicularis oculi, to the skin of the upper eyelid. There are some smooth muscle fibres in the lower part of the levator palpebrae superioris and these are supplied by sympathetic nerve fibres. As its name suggests the muscle elevates the upper eyelid and has the opposite effect to the orbicularis oculi which closes the eyelids. Its nerve supply is the oculomotor nerve and sympathetic fibres to the smooth muscle.

The muscles which move the eyeball fall into two groups, the four recti and the two obliques (Figs. 20.6–2.09). The four recti are attached to a fibrous ring at the back of the orbit. Each rectus (superior, inferior, lateral and medial) is attached to the equivalent part of the ring. Each

runs forwards and ends in a tendinous expansion which is attached to the sclera, about 0.5 cm, behind the edge of the cornea. The two oblique muscles are the superior and the inferior. The superior oblique muscle lies in the superomedial part of the orbit above the medial rectus. It is attached to the bone above and medial to the optic canal and passes forwards towards the front of the orbit where just within the orbital margin superomedially it hooks round the trochlea, a fibrocartilaginous pulley on the frontal bone. The muscle then passes laterally and backwards inferior to the superior rectus muscle and is attached to the sclera above and behind the equator of the eyeball, lateral to a vertical axis through the middle of the eyeball.

The inferior oblique muscle, unlike all the

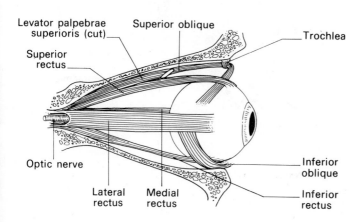

Fig. 20.7. The extrinsic muscles of the right orbit from the lateral side.

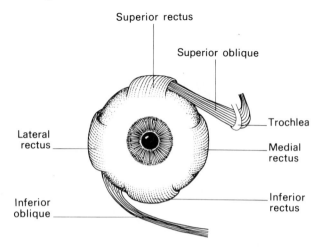

Fig. 20.8. The extrinsic muscles
of the right orbit from the front.

others lies entirely in the front of the orbit and is
attached medially to the orbital surface of the
maxilla, lateral to the nasolacrimal canal. The
muscle passes laterally and backwards inferior to
the inferior rectus muscle and is attached to the
sclera below and behind the equator, lateral to
the vertical axis of the eyeball.

The oculomotor nerve supplies the superior,
medial and inferior recti and inferior oblique
muscles. The abducent nerve supplies the lateral
rectus and the trochlear nerve supplies the
superior oblique.

The actions of the extrinsic muscles are usually described in the following way (Figs. 20.10
and 20.11). The lateral rectus pulls the eyeball
outwards and the medial rectus inwards. The
superior rectus pulls it upwards and inwards and
the inferior rectus downwards and inwards. The
superior oblique pulls it downwards and outwards and the inferior oblique upwards and
outwards. Upward movement is produced by the
combined actions of the superior rectus and
inferior oblique and downward movement by
the inferior rectus and superior oblique. This

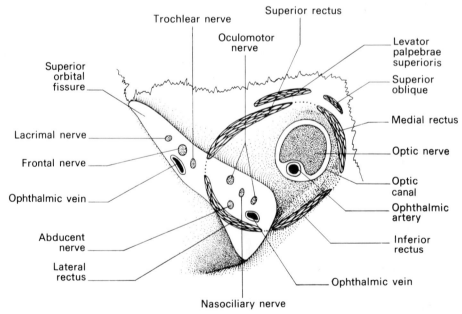

Fig. 20.9. The structures related to the superior
orbital fissure and the optic foramen, right side.

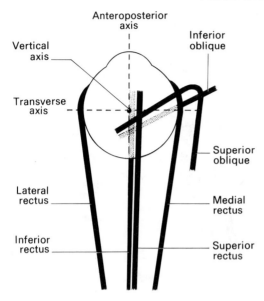

Fig. 20.10. The actions of the extrinsic muscles of the left eyeball, seen from above.

description of the movements assumes that movements only occur about a transverse axis (upward and downward movement) and a vertical axis (outward and inward movement). Rotatory movements, that is, movements about an anteroposterior axis also occur; for example the inferior oblique of the left eyeball produces a clockwise rotation and the superior oblique of the same eyeball produces a counter-clockwise rotation (Fig. 20.11). In addition it should be emphasized that almost any movement of the eyeball involves at least three and even more muscles.

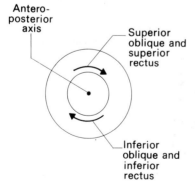

Fig. 20.11. Rotatory actions about an anteroposterior axis of the extrinsic muscles of the left eyeball seen from in front.

LIGAMENTS

The eyeball is enveloped in a fascial covering which extends from the cornea to the optic nerve and fuses with the sclera adjacent to both these structures (Fig. 20.12). If followed backwards from the sclera, the muscles pass through this fascial covering and take with them a sheath which fuses with the connective tissue covering of the muscle. These sheaths have attachments to other structures. That of the lateral rectus is attached laterally to the zygomatic bone and the sheath of the medial rectus is attached medially to the lacrimal bone. These constitute the check ligaments. The suspensory ligament of the eyeball is a thickening of the fascia of the inferior rectus which is attached on each side to a check ligament. The sheath of the superior rectus is attached to the levator palpebrae superioris and through this to the tarsal plate of the upper eyelid and that of the inferior rectus to the sheath of the inferior oblique and the tarsal plate of the lower eyelid.

The orbit contains a variable amount of fat which more or less surrounds the eyeball, muscles, vessels and nerves. Strands of smooth muscle are found in the fat.

Nerves and vessels

Apart from branches of the maxillary division of the trigeminal nerve which cross the orbit (infraorbital and zygomatic branches, the latter including the parasympathetic secretomotor fibres to the lacrimal gland), five cranial nerves enter or leave the orbit to supply its contents. These are the optic (II), the oculomotor (III), the trochlear (IV), the ophthalmic division of the trigeminal (Va), and the abducent (VI).

The vessels and nerves entering and leaving the orbit posteriorly are usually grouped according to whether they pass inside or outside the fibrous ring (Fig. 20.9). The optic nerve and ophthalmic artery enter through the optic canal inside the ring. Usually one ophthalmic vein leaves the orbit outside and one inside the ring on their way to the cavernous sinus. The distribution of the artery and vein has been described (p. 646 and 653).

The ophthalmic branch of the trigeminal nerve is the nerve of general sensation to the orbit and its contents (p. 906).

Eyelids

Each eyelid (Latin, palpebra) is a movable fold containing a tarsal plate of dense connective tis-

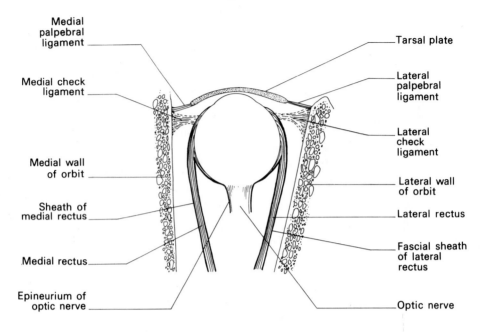

Medial palpebral ligament

Medial check ligament

Medial wall of orbit

Sheath of medial rectus

Medial rectus

Epineurium of optic nerve

Tarsal plate

Lateral palpebral ligament

Lateral check ligament

Lateral wall of orbit

Lateral rectus

Fascial sheath of lateral rectus

Optic nerve

Fig. 20.12. Horizontal section of the right orbit and eyeball to show the orbital fascia from above.

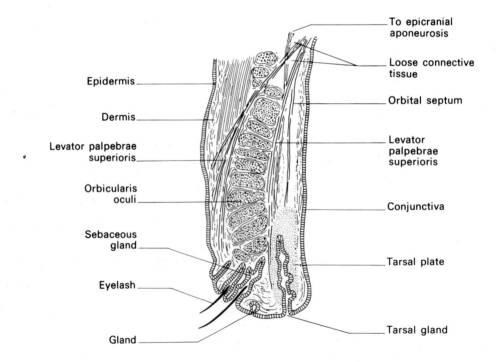

To epicranial aponeurosis

Loose connective tissue

Orbital septum

Levator palpebrae superioris

Conjunctiva

Tarsal plate

Tarsal gland

Epidermis

Dermis

Levator palpebrae superioris

Orbicularis oculi

Sebaceous gland

Eyelash

Gland

Fig. 20.13. The structure of the eyelid.

sue. A thin orbital septum connects the periphery of these plates to the orbital margin. Superficially these plates are covered by the orbicularis oculi (Fig. 20.13) muscle which is in turn covered by loose connective tissue supporting a very thin, freely movable skin. On the deep surface of the eyelid the skin is modified and known as the conjuctiva. The edge of each eyelid contains eyelashes and the openings of ducts of glands lying within the lids.

Several varieties of gland are contained within the eyelids and pass their secretion through ducts on to the free edges of the eyelids (Fig. 20.13). Many of these secrete sebum or modified sebum which, due to its surface tension, is said to prevent the tears overflowing on to the cheeks.

Both eyelids are supplied by the ophthalmic artery while the lower is additionally supplied by the maxillary and facial arteries. The sensory supply to the upper eyelid is from the ophthalmic nerve and to the lower eyelid from the infra-orbital branch of the maxillary nerve. The orbicularis oculi muscle is supplied by the facial nerve.

The conjunctiva lining the inside of the eyelids consists of a non-keratinized stratified squamous epithelium overlying a thin transparent layer of connective tissue containing a large number of small blood vessels. From all around the eyelids, the conjunctiva is reflected on to the sclera. Over the cornea the epithelium consists of about five layers of cells. In the condition of conjunctivitis the blood vessels in the conjunctiva become engorged giving the eye a pink appearance.

SURFACE ANATOMY

Examination of the eyelids and conjunctiva can be easily carried out with a mirror (Fig. 20.14).

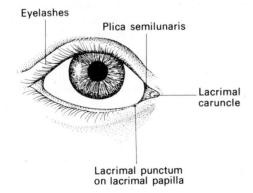

Fig. 20.14. Surface anatomy of the right palpebral fissure (space between the eyelids).

The thinness of the skin is fairly obvious. At the edge of the lids are the eyelashes. The openings of modified sweat glands near the attachment of the eyelashes can be seen. When infected a stye results. About 4–5 mm from the medial angle (or canthus) of the eye on each eyelid there is a small elevation, the lacrimal papilla, on which opens the lacrimal canaliculus at the lacrimal punctum. The carunculus lacrimalis is a small reddish body at the medial angle between the edges of the eyelids. It consists of modified skin and has a few fine hairs projecting from it. Lateral to the caruncle is a semilunar fold of modified conjunctiva, the plica semilunaris, most easily seen if the eyeball is turned laterally. This may be homologous with the nictitating membrane of some reptiles and mammals. If the lower eyelid is pulled downwards and the eyeball turned upwards the reflection of the conjunctiva from the eyelid to the sclera can be readily seen. The line of the reflection is called the inferior fornix. The superior fornix cannot be seen because the upper eyelid cannot be everted to the same extent as the lower. The tarsal glands and their openings, shining through the conjunctiva, can be seen on the inner surface of the eyelid. If the eye is turned downwards it is fairly easy to evert the upper eyelid round the upper edge of its tarsal plate. This is a useful and important manoeuvre for inspecting the inner surface of the upper eyelid if the presence of a foreign body is suspected.

Lacrimal apparatus

The lacrimal apparatus includes the lacrimal gland, lacrimal canaliculi, lacrimal sac and nasolacrimal duct (Fig. 20.15). The lacrimal gland is a tubulo-alveolar gland. It consists of a larger orbital part (2.5 cm × 1 cm) which lies in the lacrimal fossa of the frontal bone just inside the superolateral edge of the orbit, and a smaller palpebral part in the lateral region of the upper eyelid. The gland produces the tears which are almost entirely water and contain inorganic salts and a bactericidal enzyme. The secretomotor nerve supply of the gland comes from the facial nerve and the postganglionic fibres have their cell bodies in the sphenopalatine ganglion. These fibres enter the orbit through the inferior orbital fissure or with the zygomatic branch of the maxillary nerve. In the orbit the fibres either pass directly to the lacrimal gland or join the lacrimal nerve and then go to the gland.

The lacrimal canaliculi begin at the lacrimal papillae of the eyelids. Superior and inferior

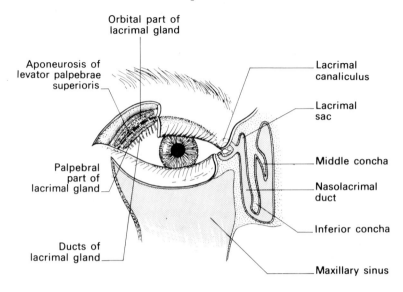

Orbital part of
lacrimal gland

Aponeurosis of
levator palpebrae
superioris

Lacrimal
canaliculus

Lacrimal
sac

Palpebral
part of
lacrimal gland

Middle concha

Nasolacrimal
duct

Inferior concha

Ducts of
lacrimal gland

Maxillary sinus

Fig. 20.15. The right lacrimal apparatus.

canaliculi enter the lacrimal sac. The lacrimal sac is the upper part of the canal which leads from the orbit to the inferior meatus of the nasal cavity. In front of the sac just below its upper end is the medial palpebral ligament and behind the sac at the same level are some fibres of the orbicularis oculi. The sac lies in the fossa formed by the lacrimal and maxillary bones in the anterior part of the medial wall of the orbit. It is continuous with the nasolacrimal duct which lies in a canal in the lateral wall of the nose. The canal is formed laterally by the maxilla and medially by the lacrimal bone and inferior concha. The duct opens into the anterior part of the inferior meatus of the nose.

Normally the tears produced by the lacrimal gland pass across the conjunctival sac from the lateral to the medial side due to capillary attraction and the blinking movements of the eyelids. By the time the tears have reached the canaliculus most of them have evaporated. The remainder enters the canaliculi due to capillary attraction and possibly a sucking action of the lacrimal part of the orbicularis oculi on the upper end of the lacrimal sac. The production of tears is a carefully balanced process and requires the repeated closure of the eyelids to prevent excess evaporation. If the lids are held open for twenty to thirty minutes the cornea can become dry with serious consequences to the viability of its superficial cells.

THE PHYSIOLOGY OF VISION

Adequate illumination is a prerequisite for the functioning of the cones in central, clear colour vision. The periphery of the retina, on the other hand, which contains most of the rods, is better adapted for vision in poor light. The rods and cones also differ in their wavelength sensitivities.

The photosensitive pigment of the rods, rhodopsin, when illuminated, breaks down into retinine and opsin, a photochemical reaction which initiates depolarization of the rod. In the presence of bright light most of the rhodopsin is broken down so that the rods become less sensitive. In the absence of light, the stores of rhodopsin are maximal, and the rods are most sensitive. Under normal conditions the breakdown products of this light-sensitive reaction are resynthesized into more visual pigment via a cyclic chain of events (Fig. 20.22).

If a person is placed in a totally dark room, having been previously adapted to bright light, a strong stimulus is needed to give the sensation of light, in other words there is a 'high visual threshold'. Repeated testing shows that there is a ten-fold increase in sensitivity during the first six minutes, after which there is a sudden further increase, which continues for some 25–30 minutes (Fig. 20.16). During this latter phase, vision becomes monochromatic and colour vision is lost. By the end of this period a light

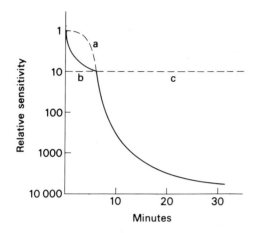

source which is some 6000–8000 times less powerful can be detected; a remarkable adaptation.

Wavelength and receptors

RODS

Recordings from microelectrodes inserted into retinal ganglion cells (Fig. 20.17) show that while there are responses to a range of wavelengths, they are greatest at 500 nm if the stimulus is low intensity light (to exclude stimulation of the cones). The curve obtained by plotting responses to different wavelengths of low intensity light corresponds to the absorption spectrum of rhodopsin.

Fig. 20.16. The dark adaptation curve. (a) Curve obtained in 'rod only' retina, (b) is the level below which vision is monochromatic, (c) is the curve obtained in 'cone only' retina.

CONES

Similar recordings, but with high intensity light, show that different groups of cones respond to

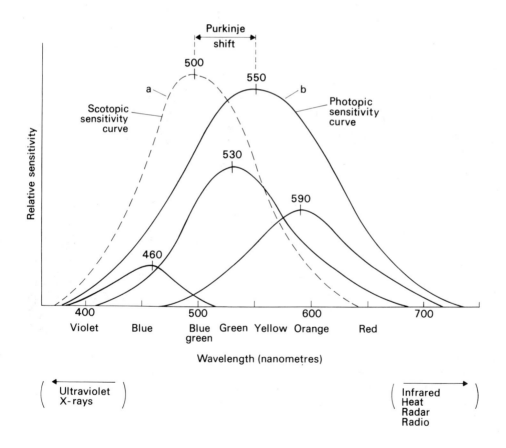

Fig. 20.17. Relative sensitivities at different light wavelengths. (a) Is the dark adapted (scotopic) sensitivity curve, which coincides with absorption curve of rhodopsin though on a different scale. (b) Is the summed curve of 3 cone groups (photopic sensitivity curve).

wavelengths which peak at about 460, 530 and 590 nm. These correspond to violet-blue, bluish green-yellow and orange-red and could broadly be described as 'blue,' 'green' and 'red' groups. Stimulation of one, two or more combinations of these groups gives rise to colour sensations ('hue'). The peak response is at 550 nm (Fig. 20.17), the wavelength to which the human eye is most sensitive in good light and which gives the sensation of 'white' if the different components are combined in the correct proportion.

As light progressively fades in the evening, the cones adapt ten-fold (as shown in Fig. 20.16) but then become ineffective, since there is insufficient light to stimulate them. As the rods take over, the cone sensitivity (550 nm) gives way to the rod sensitivity (500 nm). This change in wavelength sensitivity related to light intensity is called the Purkinje shift or phenomenon.

Colour vision

Normal people have the correct proportions of the three types of colour-sensitive cones, and are called 'trichromatic'. If an individual has a deficiency of say the 'red' type, he (it is nearly always a male) has difficulty separating the different red hues. If he has a complete absence of the red type, when presented with a multi-coloured selection of wool and given a red strand to match, he may choose a red or grey piece of wool of a similar shade intensity—he does not distinguish them as separate colours ('red blind'). A person with a defect of 'green' cones has like problems. 'Blue blindness' is very rare. The most common type of colour blindness occurs in those individuals whose 'red' and 'green' cone groups are not functionally differentiated. They see these colours as similar and are 'red-green' colour blind.

It is important to realise that colour blindness is only a noticeable defect when colours have to be compared. Thus people may be unable to detect cyanosis or jaundice, may mistake the colour of pills, gas cylinders, electric wiring, the colours in urine testing, titrations, etc.

Colour blindness is a recessive X-linked inherited condition. Of the population, some 8% show some type of colour blindness and only 0.4% are female.

Visual acuity

Clear vision, optical considerations aside, can only occur using the cones at the macula, and the image of any object we look at (the fixation point) always falls on this area. The grain of the cones here is very fine and with their 'straight-through' connections to the ganglion cells and to the optic nerve, would appear very suitable for fine discrimination of separate points of light.

The foveal cones are 2–3 μm in diameter, and so subtend an angle of about 40 seconds of arc from the optical centre of the eye. A gap of 40 seconds of arc could be appreciated as one unstimulated cone separating two stimulated ones. It has been known since ancient times that stars 1 minute of arc apart could just be seen as separate.

In practice, visual acuity is measured by reference to 'normal' or 'average'. If a person reads from 6 metres (20 feet) a row of letters normally read at 6 metres, then he has '6/6 (20/20) visual acuity'. At this distance the rays of light are virtually parallel, and the test is constructed so that the size of the letters subtends an angle of 5 minutes, and the thickness of the lines 1 minute. If a person only reads at 6 metres the row that would normally be read at 18 metres, then they only have '6/18 acuity'. To have '6/5 acuity' is therefore better than average.

It goes without saying that at the exit of the optic nerve, where there are no rods or cones, there is no visual sensation: the 'blind spot'.

When rays of light pass from one medium to a more optically dense medium they are deviated (refracted), being bent towards the 'normal'—a plane perpendicular to the surface. The actual amount of bending depends on the 'refractive indices' of the media (Fig. 20.18).

The 'refractive index' (n) of a medium is obtained by the formula:

$$n = \frac{\sin i \ (\text{vacuum})}{\sin r \ (\text{medium})}$$

Fortunately the refractive index of air is virtually the same as a vacuum.

Examples are: $n_{(air)} = 1.00$; $n_{(crown \ glass)} = 1.52$; $n_{(flint \ glass)} = 1.66$; $n_{(aqueous)}$ and $n_{(vitreous)} = 1.33$; $n_{(lens \ of \ eye)} = 1.41$.

When light rays pass back from the high refractive index medium to the low, the same ratios apply, but are reversed.

A lens bringing parallel rays of light to a focus at

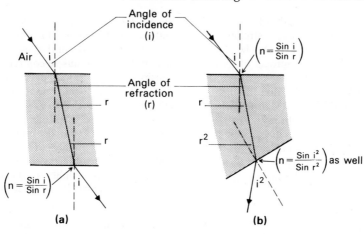

Fig. 20.18. Refraction and refractive index in (a) plate glass and (b) a prism.

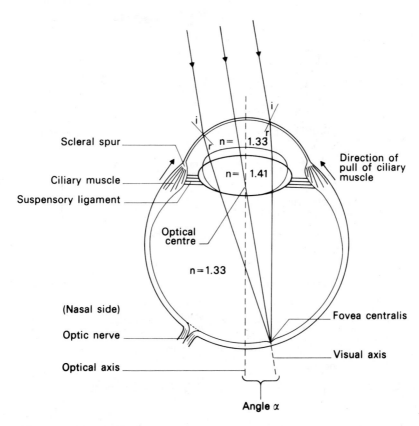

Fig. 20.19. Diagrammatic horizontal section of eye (iris omitted for simplicity) showing refraction and accommodation.

half a metre has a strength of 2 dioptres ('2D')—at quarter of a metre, a strength of 4 dioptres (4D), at 1/10 metre-10D. The dioptric strength of a lens is the reciprocal of its focal length, in metres.

Fig. 20.19 makes the point that the main refracting surface of the eye is the cornea, which is curved, and so converges light rays. The lens of the eye can adjust the focus because it has a different refractive index—but only by about 10D out of a total refractive power of 60+D, and this only in a young person.

ACCOMMODATION

The adjustment that gives the additional focal strength needed for seeing a near object clearly is called accommodation. This is effected in a surprising way. The lens is normally stretched out flatter than it would otherwise be by the tension of the fibres of the suspensory ligament. When the ciliary muscle contracts it relaxes the tension of these fibres, partly by a sphincteric action, but also by moving the peripheral insertion forwards (Fig. 20.19) so that the lens can become rounder. With increasing age the lens becomes harder and so does not change shape so readily, until eventually it is no longer possible to focus on near objects—'presbyopia'. Lenses then have to be supplied in spectacles for near vision, as when reading a book or newspaper.

HYPERMETROPIA, MYOPIA AND ASTIGMATISM (Fig. 20.20)

In the normal eye distant objects fall naturally

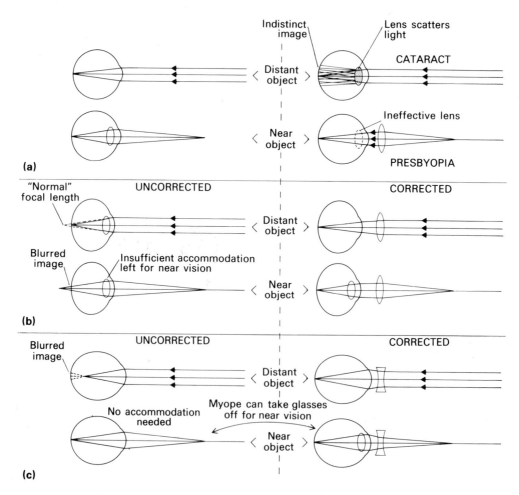

Fig. 20.20. A simplified representation of light paths in visual perception in (a) normal vision, (b) hypermetropia and (c) myopia. Where a lens is drawn in the eye, it indicates accommodation.

into focus on the macula without any effort of accommodation. If the eye is smaller than normal, or the curve of the cornea less than normal, then a constant effort of accommodation has to be made to keep even a distant object in focus. This means that some of the range of accommodation is already used, and there may then be insufficient range left to focus on near objects. Such people see distant objects more easily, and are called 'hypermetropic' or long-sighted. A biconvex ('+', plus, magnifying) lens of appropriate strength in spectacles would do this extra focussing for them.

Conversely should the eye be larger than normal (larger diameter), then the image of distant objects falls in front of the retina, and since there is no mechanism for reducing the focusing in the eye, distant objects therefore appear blurred. Only the image of near objects can fall into focus on the retina—such a person is 'myopic' or 'near-sighted'. Wearing a biconcave ('−', minus, diminishing) lens would enable distant objects to be clearly focussed.

Astigmatism is either of these conditions, but in one plane only, so that, as the name implies, light does not come to a focus at a point. A cylindrical correcting lens would be needed. A contact lens works on a different principle. It provides an artificial anterior refracting surface for the eye, and by adjusting the curvature of the contact lens the effective focussing strength of this surface can be suitably altered.

NORMAL DEVELOPMENT AND THE ONSET OF MYOPIA

Children, being small people, have small eyes, and so are naturally longsighted. On first going to school they have to look at close things, and often complain of aching eyes. As they grow, mostly at puberty, their eyes become larger, and their longsightedness disappears.

Some children, with adult-sized eyes, therefore have unusually good eyesight for their age, and their large eyes are thought very pretty. When they grow up, though, their eyes become abnormally large, and so they become short-sighted. Their relative lack of ciliary tone (less accommodation needed) extends to the constrictor of the pupils which are widely dilated. These large eyes, with dilated pupils, coupled with a rather vague, misty look, because they cannot see clearly, are very attractive, particularly in young ladies! (See right—Pupil dilator reflexes). It is sad that the diminishing lenses needed in their spectacles abolish these benefits!

Pupillary reflexes

The light reflex

If a light is shone into one eye, the pupil of that eye constricts (miosis). This is the 'direct' light reflex. At the same time the contralateral pupil responds equally (the 'indirect' or 'consensual' light reflex). This reflex gives an immediate reduction of light entering the eye, but as the retina slowly adapts, these pupillary reactions are no longer necessary, and the pupil returns to its previous state.

The neural elements involved in these reflexes are: (a) retinal neurons; (b) optic fibres which travel via the optic nerve and tract to the superior colliculus and pretectal nucleus to connect with axons which end in the Edinger–Westphal nucleus; (c) preganglionic fibres from the latter nucleus which pass via the oculomotor nerve to the ciliary ganglion and (d) postganglionic ciliary fibres which innervate the pupillary sphincters.

Pupil dilator reflexes

Dilation of the pupils is caused by stimulation of the sympathetic nerves, and is normally overridden by the constrictor (parasympathetic) reflexes. However, it is brought about on arousal, as with pain, fright or fear. Dilation of the pupil (mydriasis) is recognized as an unspoken sign of approving interest! Atropine drops in the eyes (by blocking tonic parasympathetic activity) produced the same effect in olden days—hence the name 'bella-donna' for this drug.

In the unphysiological state of anaesthesia however, remember that a dilating pupil may be a sign of hypoxia.

Accommodation–convergence reflex

A shift in gaze from distant to close objects results in the following ocular changes. These constitute the near response. (a) Contraction of the ciliaris muscle shortens the focal length of the lens (accommodation); (b) contraction of the sphincter pupillae lessens chromatic and spherical aberration and increases the depth of field necessary for close vision and (c) contraction of the medial recti muscles causes convergence of the optical axes. The triad of changes is called the accommodation–convergence reflex. Unlike the light reflexes; it involves parts of the cerebral cortex. The sensory side of the reflex arc includes the visual pathway from retina to visual cortex, as well as association fibres connecting the visual cortex to the motor cortex; the motor side consists of descending corticonuclear fibres which end on the oculomotor nuclear complex and relay impulses through oculomotor nerve fibres to the medial recti muscles and also to the ciliary ganglion whose postganglionic fibres then innervate the ciliaris and sphincter pupillae muscles.

Fusion, binocular vision and stereoscopic vision

The bony orbits face forwards and outwards, diverging by 45°. Without any effort of the extraocular muscles, the eyes also tend to assume this position—as in blindness or death. The position of the eyes is however normally maintained by a fine balance of these muscles, and the two sides are normally co-ordinated.

A person with normal vision tends to 'fuse' the images from both eyes. Once 'fusion' is established, it provides a powerful stimulus to keep the eyes properly aligned and a person then has 'binocular vision'. Though the view from each eye is not exactly the same, the slightly different images can still be fused, and it is the additional information so obtained that gives the sense of solidity or depth—'stereoscopic vision'. Stereopsis cannot occur without binocular vision, and binocular vision cannot occur in someone with only one functional eye.

VISUAL FIELD

Though peripheral vision may not be clear, it is excellent for sensing movement, so attracting the attention. The monocular visual field is normally limited by the soft tissue margins of the orbit—eyebrow, nose and cheek—except laterally. Hence it is possible to see even more than 90° from the sagittal plane while looking ahead. You can easily check this.

The two eyes together, with their central fields fused, therefore give a considerable forward view, the central, greater part of the binocular field of vision being common to both eyes—the lateral parts belonging to the separate eyes.

Neurological snippets

The motor and sensory nerve supplies to the eyes and associated structures are extensive.

If dust gets into your eyes you blink. This is a reflex involving the ophthalmic branch of the trigeminal and the facial nerve to the orbicularis oculi via their central connections. Since you also blink at a loud noise, sensed via the auditory nerve or at a sudden movement at the periphery of your visual field sensed via the optic nerve this

is a good example of one nerve—the facial in this case, being the 'final common pathway' in more than one reflex. It also demonstrates the extensive interconnections of the cranial nerve nuclei.

It is interesting that the very primitive reflexes involving sudden movements, and the light reflexes, are mediated by nerve fibres that leave the optic tract early, passing straight to the pretectal area and superior colliculi, whence they complete the reflex circuits with the appropriate cranial nerves. This means that they are rapid—you blink before you 'see' a spark shooting towards your eye (blind vision; p. 941).

The rest of the fibres of the optic tract pass, as with all sensory input, to a part of the thalamus—in this case the lateral geniculate bodies, where they relay to the occipital cortex, spreading out on the way as the 'optic radiation'.

Central processing of retinal image

Retinal ganglion cells project to the lateral geniculate nuclei (LGN) and thence to the occipital cortex which contains a highly ordered stereoscopic topographical representation of the retina. Whereas there are approximately equal numbers of LGN and retinal ganglion cells there are about 100 cortical cells for each projecting LGN cell.

Both LGN cells and ganglion cells respond to roughly circular fields of light projected on the retina but cortical cells, according to Hubel and Wiesel, respond best to bars, or slits of light (Fig. 20.21). Each cortical cell is best activated by a bar of light projecting on to a particular area of the retina at a particular orientation. Most cells react to horizontal but some to vertical bars of light, although all orientations are catered for. Furthermore the cortical cells are arranged in narrow vertical columns. An individual column only responds to an image which falls on a particular part of the retina in a particular orientation. Thus each retinal area is represented in several columns of cortical cells. Within each column different classes of cells exist such that some (simple cells) respond best to stationary and moving bars of light and others (complex) to a moving edge in a preferential direction. In the latter it is difficult to locate the receptive field. A third class (hypercomplex) responds best to a moving bar of specific length only.

The interactions of this complex arrangement allow the cortex to reconstruct the visual image piecemeal within the specific columns of cells activated (p 941).

Foveal cones

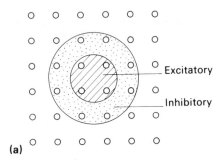

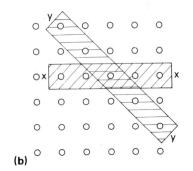

(a)

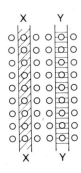

(b)

Fig. 20.21. Central processing of retinal image, (a) a small circle of light in the 'centre receptive field' excites a single ganglion cell and lateral geniculate cell. Light falling on an area surrounding the 'centre receptive field' excites other cells but inhibits those fired by the centre receptive field. (b) A bar of light (x–x) falling on a particular part of the retina excites a column of cells in the visual cortex (X–X). If the bar is at an angle (y–y) cells in a different column (Y–Y) are excited.

BIOCHEMISTRY OF THE EYE TISSUES

The cornea contains protein fibres embedded in a glycosaminoglycan matrix, the protein fibres being arranged regularly and in parallel to allow the passage of light. As there is no blood supply to the tissue itself, oxygen is supplied and metabolites are transported via the aqueous humour.

The lens is also transparent and is composed of macroscopic cells called lens fibres which contain a protein gel. The nuclei and mitochondria of the cells are concentrated at the equator of the lens. There is a steady turnover of the lens proteins (crystallins) during life, the energy required being supplied by glucose. The metabolism of lens tissue is mainly anaerobic glycolysis, with some 8 mg of glucose per day being metabolized. Material diffuses in to and out of the non-vascular lens via the aqueous and vitreous humours.

A high concentration of the tripeptide glutathione is present in the lens, and the cysteine residues with their free –SH groups, act as a reducing agent. The lens also contains a high concentration of ascorbic acid, another strong reducing agent. The role of the glutathione seems to be to maintain the lens protein in a reduced state by means of the free –SH groups. Any fall in the content of the reduced glutathione is associated with a fall in the protein –SH and consequent development of a cloudiness of the lens which is referred to as cataract. This cataract is considered to be due to polymerization of the lens proteins resulting from the oxidative formation of –S–S– bridges arising from the lowered content of reductive –SH groups. The physical structure and transparency of the tissue is therefore altered.

Photochemical processes in vision

The photochemical reaction may be divided into three stages;
1 Photochemical reaction of the visual pigment.
2 Subsequent initiation of the nerve impulse.
3 Regeneration of the visual pigments.

The first stage in the reaction is the break-

Chapter 20

down of rhodopsin to give opsin (protein) and retinal (vitamin A₁ aldehyde), the latter then being reduced to the vitamin A₁ alcohol, retinol. Retinol is then reoxidized to retinal and this recombines with opsin to form rhodopsin (Fig. 20.22).

The critical point of this cyclic reaction is the cis-trans isomerization of the vitamin A₁ side chain. This is in the cis form in rhodopsin, and when rhodopsin is broken down by light the all-trans form results.

This rearrangement causes a marked change in the size and shape of the molecule, thereby altering the permeability of the cell membrane which allows calcium to move out. This efflux alters the membrane potential and triggers a nerve impulse.

Alcohols affect visual pigment metabolism

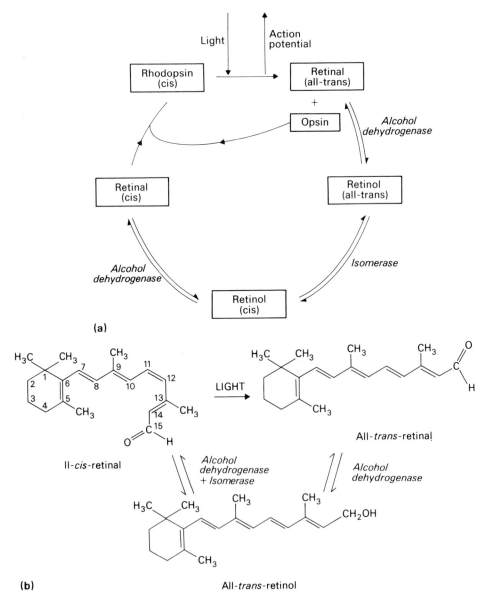

Fig. 20.22. (a) Flow diagram of the breakdown and reformation of rhodopsin. (b) Isomerization, oxidation and reduction of vitamin A₁.

and may seriously impair vision. The alcohol dehydrogenase involved in the oxidation–reduction reactions to reconstitute rhodopsin (Fig. 20.22) is non-specific and competition for the enzyme occurs in the presence of other alcohols. The formation of rhodopsin is therefore inhibited, one reason—amongst others—for not drinking and driving!

Methyl alcohol in very small doses (1–2 cm³) can cause blindness. This is considered to be due to the formation of formaldehyde which inhibits tissue respiration and denatures proteins.

$$CH_3OH \quad \underset{\substack{\text{Alcohol} \\ \text{dehydrogenase}}}{\overset{NAD^+}{\rightleftharpoons}} \quad \begin{array}{l} HCHO + NADH \\ \quad\quad + H^+ \end{array}$$

Ethyl alcohol may be used as an antidote to methyl alcohol poisoning because ethyl alcohol competes with methyl alcohol for the active site of the alcohol dehydrogenase, forming acetaldehyde, which does not affect respiration.

HEARING

ANATOMY

The organ of hearing is located in the temporal bone and can be divided into three parts, the external ear, the middle ear (tympanic cavity) and the internal ear (Fig. 20.23 a & b). The internal ear, however, also contains the vestibular apparatus which is associated with responses to the position of the head in space and its movements, linear, rotatory and angular. The external ear funnels sounds to the tympanic membrane 'ear-drum' which separates the external from the middle ear. A chain of ossicles in the middle ear transmits the movements of this membrane to the internal ear. The movements of the ossicles are transmitted in the internal ear via fluid to a structure in which there are nerve endings, the organ of Corti. These endings are stimulated and the resulting impulses are conveyed to the brain (see p. 977).

External ear

This consists of two parts, the auricle or pinna (Fig. 20.24) and the external acoustic (auditory) meatus (pinna in Latin means a wing). There are fine hairs on the surface of the skin and thicker hairs round the orifice of the meatus which help to protect the internal structures. Several ridges, grooves and hollows can be seen on the lateral surface. The lobule of the ear is its most dependent part and is structurally different from the rest of the auricle in that it has no cartilage and consists of skin covering fibrofatty tissue.

The cartilage of the auricle extends inwards as a partial cylinder, deficient above and behind, and forms the outer part of the external acoustic meatus. It is attached to the bony medial part of the meatus. The auricle is attached to the skull by means of ligaments. There is skeletal muscle related to the auricle in the form of extrinsic and intrinsic muscles. The extrinsic may move the auricle and the intrinsic may change its shape. These muscles are supplied by the facial nerve.

The external acoustic meatus is partly cartilaginous (outer one-third) and partly osseous (inner two-thirds). The osseous part consists of an incomplete cylinder of bone formed by the tympanic part of the temporal bone. The deficiency above and behind is filled by the squamous temporal bone. From concha to tympanic membrane the canal is about 2.5 cm long in the adult, and as it passes medially it curves upwards and backwards. At its medial end the tympanic membrane is lodged in a groove. The membrane is oblique (the lower anterior part is more medial than the upper posterior part). The canal is lined by skin firmly adherent to the underlying cartilage and bone—any infection is very painful because of this. There are hairs and special wax (ceruminous) glands, looking like modified sweat glands, in the skin of the cartilaginous part. Together with the hairs the wax may trap foreign bodies. Its main function may be to cover the surface of the skin with a greasy layer impervious to water.

The main features of the tympanic membrane are shown in Fig. 20.25 a & b.

Middle ear (tympanic cavity)

This cavity in the temporal bone is about 1.5 cm high, 1.5 cm anteroposteriorly and only 0.5 cm from its lateral to its medial wall. Opposite the middle of the tympanic membrane this last measurement is reduced to about 0.2 cm because of the curving inwards of the membrane. The cavity is lined by ciliated, mucous, columnar epithelium continuous with that of the auditory (Eustachian) tube and the nasopharynx. The middle ear is said to have six sides—a roof, floor and anterior, posterior, lateral and medial walls. (See Figs. 20.25 & 20.26.)

The anterior wall has two openings in its

superior part, an upper which transmits the tendon of the tensor tympani and a lower which is the lateral end of the auditory tube (Fig. 20.26). The roof is formed by a thin plate of bone, the tegmen tympani and the floor is related to the bulb of the internal jugular vein.

There are two openings on the medial wall. The upper is oval in shape is called the fenestra vestibuli. The footpiece of the stapes lies in it. The lower which is round is called the fenestra cochleae. It is closed by a membrane. The promontory is a projection on the medial wall lying in front of the two openings. It lies over the first turn of the cochlea, and on it there is a plexus of nerves. The lateral wall (Fig. 20.27) contains the tympanic membrane.

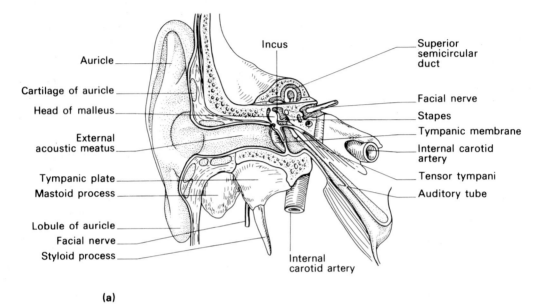

(a)

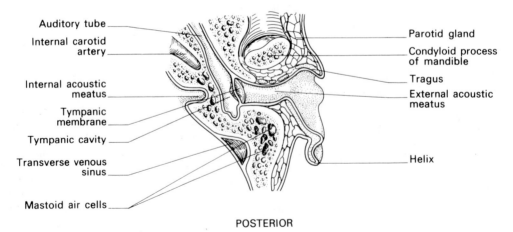

(b)

Fig. 20.23. (a) A coronal section through the right external, middle and internal ears. (b) A horizontal section through the right petrous temporal bone looked at from above showing the relation of the condyloid process of the mandible to the ear.

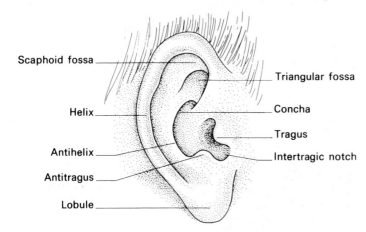

Scaphoid fossa

Helix

Antihelix

Antitragus

Lobule

Triangular fossa

Concha

Tragus

Intertragic notch

Fig. 20.24. The lateral surface of the right auricle.

The tympanic membrane forms an angle of about 50° with the floor of the meatus (Fig. 20.25). The membrane is approximately round and is about 1 cm in diameter. The appearance of the membrane as seen with a speculum is shown in Fig. 20.25a. The handle of the malleus is attached to its inner surface as far as its centre which is called the umbo. Apart from the

flaccid part which is superior, the membrane is taut and bulges into the tympanic cavity.

The tympanic membrane consists of three layers. The inner, which is part of the lining of the tympanic cavity, is said to be covered by ciliated, mucous, columnar cells although the presence of cilia has been questioned. The outer layer, continuous with the lining of the meatus,

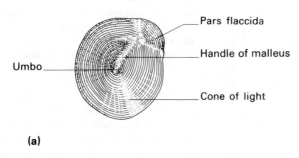

Umbo

Pars flaccida

Handle of malleus

Cone of light

(a)

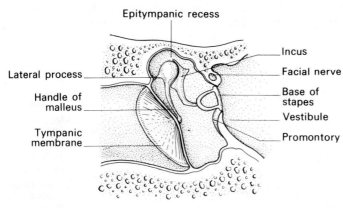

Epitympanic recess

Lateral process

Handle of malleus

Tympanic membrane

Incus

Facial nerve

Base of stapes

Vestibule

Promontory

(b)

Fig. 20.25. (a) The right tympanic membrane as seen with an auroscope. (b) The medial surface of the right tympanic membrane.

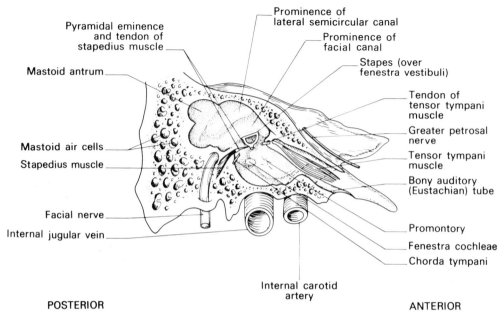

Pyramidal eminence
and tendon of
stapedius muscle

Mastoid antrum

Mastoid air cells

Stapedius muscle

Facial nerve

Internal jugular vein

Prominence of
lateral semicircular canal

Prominence of
facial canal

Stapes (over
fenestra vestibuli)

Tendon of
tensor tympani
muscle

Greater petrosal
nerve

Tensor tympani
muscle

Bony auditory
(Eustachian) tube

Promontory

Fenestra cochleae

Chorda tympani

Internal carotid
artery

POSTERIOR

ANTERIOR

Fig. 20.26. The medial wall of the right tympanic cavity (the middle ear). The main features of the anterior and posterior walls can also be seen.

resembles the epidermis of skin but is modified and consists of layers of superficial flattened cells and deeper layers resembling prickle cells. There are no hairs nor glands. The middle layer of the membrane is fibrous with its fibres arranged radially and circularly. The fibres are of a special composition and are unlike normal collagen or elastin.

The membrane is innervated externally by the auriculotemporal and vagus nerves and internally by the glossopharyngeal nerve.

The mastoid antrum (Figs. 20.26 & 20.27) is a cavity in the temporal bone lying posterior to the middle ear and communicating with it by an opening called the aditus to the antrum. The antrum is covered by the tegmen tympani which separates it from the temporal lobe of the brain. The mastoid air cells lie in the mastoid process of the petrous temporal bone and are usually closely related to the mastoid antrum laterally and posteriorly. They are extensions of the antrum but, unlike the antrum which is present at birth, they develop mainly after the second year when the mastoid process develops.

The importance of the antrum and air cells lies in the possibility of the spread of infection into them from the middle ear which is frequently infected especially in children, because of its

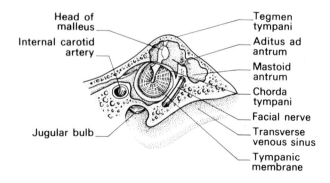

Head of
malleus

Internal carotid
artery

Jugular bulb

Tegmen
tympani

Aditus ad
antrum

Mastoid
antrum

Chorda
tympani

Facial nerve

Transverse
venous sinus

Tympanic
membrane

Fig. 20.27. The lateral wall of the right middle ear as seen from its medial side.

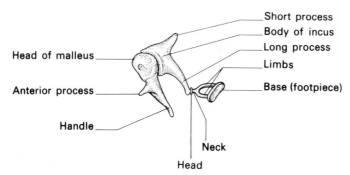

Short process
Body of incus
Long process
Limbs
Base (footpiece)

Head of malleus

Anterior process

Handle

Neck

Head

Fig. 20.28. The right auditory ossicles looked at from in front.

communication via the auditory (Eustachian) tube with the nasopharynx. Infection of bone is difficult to eradicate.

The auditory ossicles (Figs. 20.25 & 20.28) are the three small bones which extend across the cavity of the middle ear from the lateral to the medial wall. The lateral bone, about 1 cm long, is the malleus and consists mainly of a head and a handle. The head lies in the epitympanic recess, that is above the level of the tympanic membrane, and has a posterior articular area which forms a synovial joint with the body of the middle ossicle, the incus. This facet has a large upper part which is almost at a right angle to the lower part. The handle extends to about the middle of the membrane (the umbo). The tensor tympani supplied by the mandibular nerve is attached to the handle near the body. The chorda tympani branch of the facial nerve passes forwards on the tympanic membrane medial to the handle.

The middle ossicle, the incus, is somewhat shorter than the malleus and consists of a body and two widely diverging processes. The body lies in the epitympanic recess and has on its anterior surface a convex articular facet which articulates with the back of the body of the malleus.

The medial ossicle is called the stapes. It is about half the length of the malleus and it has a head, two limbs and a base. The head points laterally and forms a synovial joint with the long process of the incus. The limbs, anterior and posterior, separate from the head and pass medially. They are joined by the oval base which lies in the fenestra vestibuli to the edges of which it is attached by an annular ligament. The stapedius muscle is attached to the stapes at the junction of the head and limbs and is innervated by the facial nerve.

Movements of the ossicles are due to the movements of the tympanic membrane caused by sound waves passing along the external acoustic meatus. These movements are transferred to the fluid on the inner side of the fenestra vestibuli. The malleus moves inwards and outwards and these movements are transferred to the incus. Because the long process of the incus is bent at a right angle there is a rocking movement of the stapes in the fenestra vestibuli, and not an inward and outward movement. The waves are amplified about fifty times since the tympanic membrane is about twenty times the area of the fenestra vestibuli and the lever action of the ossicles increases the movements by a factor of two or three.

Internal ear

The internal ear consists of an osseous labyrinth (Figs. 20.29 a & b) which is a series of cavities in the petrous temporal bone, and a membranous labyrinth inside the bony cavities (Fig. 20.30). The fluid outside the membranous labyrinth is called perilymph and the fluid inside, the endolymph. The osseous labyrinth has three parts. The middle is called the vestibule, the anterior, the cochlea and the posterior, the semicircular canals. The vestibule is medial to the middle ear, is ovoid and has a diameter of about 4–5 mm. Its medial wall has perforations for the vestibular part of the vestibulocochlear (eighth cranial) nerve and is at the lateral end of the internal acoustic meatus. On the lateral wall of the vestibule are the openings of the fenestra vestibuli (superior) and fenestra cochleae (inferior). The five openings of the semicircular canals are seen on the posterior wall. The cochlear canal opens on to the anterior wall.

The cochlea, resembling a snail's shell, is about 5 mm from base to apex and 10 mm broad at its base (Figs. 20.30 & 20.31). The cochlea lies on its side with the basal turn inferior and the apex directed laterally. The basal turn produces

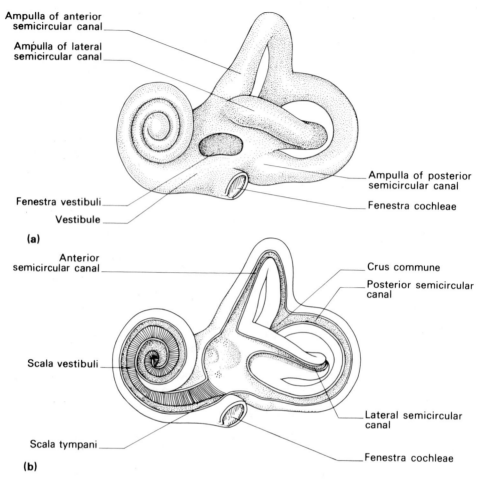

Ampulla of anterior semicircular canal

Ampulla of lateral semicircular canal

Ampulla of posterior semicircular canal

Fenestra cochleae

Fenestra vestibuli

Vestibule

(a)

Anterior semicircular canal

Crus commune

Posterior semicircular canal

Scala vestibuli

Lateral semicircular canal

Scala tympani

Fenestra cochleae

(b)

Fig. 20.29. (a) The left osseous labyrinth from its lateral aspect. (Note that the cochlea is anterior to the semicircular canals.) (b) The interior of the left osseous labyrinth.

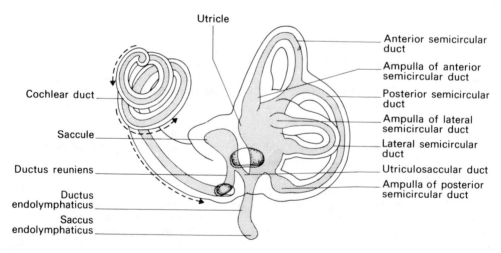

Utricle

Anterior semicircular duct

Ampulla of anterior semicircular duct

Posterior semicircular duct

Cochlear duct

Ampulla of lateral semicircular duct

Lateral semicircular duct

Saccule

Ductus reuniens

Utriculosaccular duct

Ampulla of posterior semicircular duct

Ductus endolymphaticus

Saccus endolymphaticus

Fig. 20.30. Superimposition of the membranous labyrinth on the bony labyrinth on the left side.

the projection of the promontory on the medial wall of the middle ear. There are about two and three-quarter turns and if unravelled the cochlea would be about 30 mm long. Internally the cochlea has a central pillar of bone, the modiolus, which has a perforated base next to the lateral end of the internal acoustic meatus. The cochlear part of the vestibulocochlear nerve passes through the perforations. Projecting from the modiolus is a bony shelf which winds spirally round the modiolus from the base to the apex, like the thread of a screw. This is called the osseous spiral lamina. Attached to the edge of the lamina is the vestibular membrane. Together with the basilar membrane which extends from the edge of the lamina to the outer wall of the cochlear canal, it divides the canal into upper and lower channels, the scala vestibuli and scala tympani. In the lowest coil of the cochlea the scala tympani is continuous with the fenestra cochleae and the scala vestibuli with the fenestra vestibuli. At the apex of the modiolus the scala vestibuli is continuous with the scala tympani at the helicotrema. The cochlear nerve and ganglion lie in the modiolus and the peripheral processes of the cochlear nerve pass outwards in the osseous spiral lamina (Fig. 20.31).

There are three semicircular canals, anterior, posterior and lateral (Figs. 20.29 a & b). The anterior and posterior are vertical and at right angles to each other. They are however at an angle of 45° to the sagittal plane with the

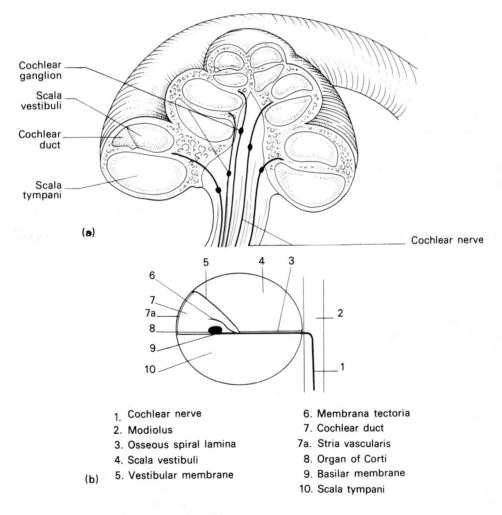

Cochlear ganglion
Scala vestibuli
Cochlear duct
Scala tympani

(a)

Cochlear nerve

5 4 3
6
7
7a   2
8
9   1
10

1. Cochlear nerve
2. Modiolus
3. Osseous spiral lamina
4. Scala vestibuli
5. Vestibular membrane

6. Membrana tectoria
7. Cochlear duct
7a. Stria vascularis
8. Organ of Corti
9. Basilar membrane
10. Scala tympani

(b)

Fig. 20.31. (a) Section through the cochlea. (b) Structures within the bony cochlea.

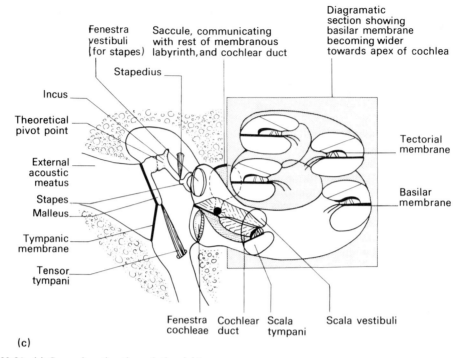

Fig. 20.31. (c) Coronal section through the right middle ear, showing in detail the structure of the cochlea.

anterior directed forwards and outwards and the posterior backwards and outwards (Fig. 20.29). The lateral semicircular canal is horizontal. The anterior and posterior canals have a common opening into the medial part of the vestibule. The opposite ends of these two canals which open into the upper and lower parts of the vestibule are dilated to form ampullae. The ampulla of the horizontal canal is at the end which opens into the vestibule above the fenestra vestibuli. The other end opens below the common opening of the anterior and posterior canals. The canals are about 1 mm and the ampullae about 2 mm in diameter. Each canal is about 15–20 mm long.

Contained within the bony labyrinth is the membranous labyrinth which consists of three semicircular ducts in the canals, the cochlear duct in the bony cochlea and the utricle and saccule in the vestibule (Figs. 20.30 & 20.32). It is important to realise that these structures do not lie in the middle of the spaces within the bony labyrinth but are attached to the wall. The semicircular ducts are arranged in the same way as the canals with a dilated ampulla at one end. Where the duct is attached to the bony wall in the ampulla there is a thickening of the duct wall on the middle of which there is a longitudinal

ampullary crest. Fibres of the vestibular nerve end in relation to this crest (Fig. 20.33). The three ducts open into the utricle. On the lateral part of the utricle the wall is thickened to form the macula which is innervated by the vestibular nerve. The utricle leads into the saccule through a fine duct.

The saccule is in the anterior part of the vestibule near the lower end of the scala vestibuli. The saccule communicates anteriorly with the duct of the cochlea by means of a short duct, the ductus reuniens. There is a diverticulum from this duct called the ductus endolymphaticus, which passes through the petrous temporal bone towards the internal acoustic meatus. The ductus lies just behind this meatus.

The semicircular ducts, utricle and saccule, consist of an outer layer of fibrous tissue, a middle layer of vascular connective tissue and an inner layer of squamous or cuboidal epithelium. Electron microscopic studies have shown that there are two types of epithelial cell, one of which is the type associated with control of the ionic composition of fluids. The cristae of the ampullae are thickened areas of the wall and have two types of cell, hair and supporting. The hair cells are the sensory cells. They have nerve

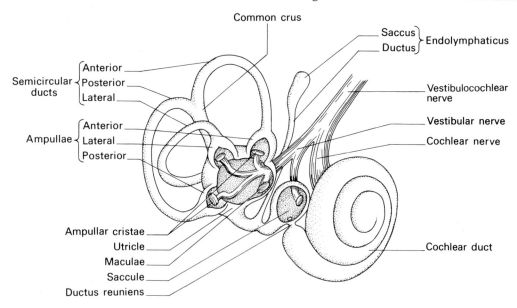

Fig. 20.32. The different parts of the membranous labyrinth.

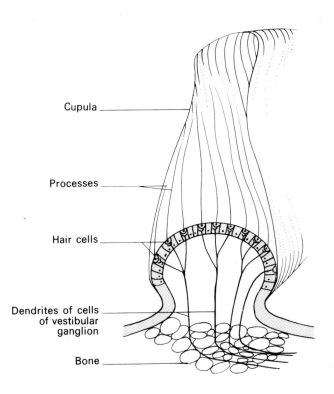

Fig. 20.33. Diagram of the structure of the crest of the ampulla of a semicircular duct. (Section across crista.)

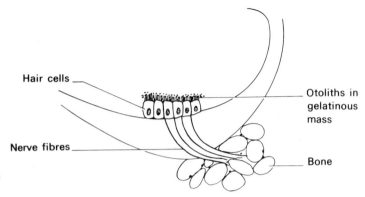

Fig. 20.34. Diagram of a macula
of the saccule and utricle.

endings related to their base and fifty or more
projecting hairs on their free surface (Fig.
20.33). The processes of the hair cells and also
those of the supporting cells project into a gelatinous mass, the cupula. Movement of the fluid
within the ducts moves the cupula. This results in
stimulation of the hair cells which in turn stimulate the nerve fibres. The maculae of the utricle
and saccule also consist of hair cells and supporting cells with their processes projecting into a
gelatinous mass (Fig. 20.34). In addition, small
but heavy crystals of calcium carbonate called
otoliths are embedded in this mass.

The cochlear duct is a spiral tube in the body
cochlea. This duct, which lies between the scala

vestibuli and the scala tympani, is triangular in
cross section (Fig. 20.31). Its floor is formed by
the basilar membrane and its roof by the vestibular membrane of Reissner which is attached
medially to the osseous spiral lamina and laterally to the bony wall of the cochlear canal (Fig.
20.31b). The upper end of the cochlear duct is
closed and its lower end opens into the narrow
duct which joins it to the saccule. The outer wall
of the cochlear duct is formed by the thickened
endosteum of the bony canal covered by a layer
of thin vascular tissue called the stria vascularis.
The vestibular membrane consists of outer and
inner layers of epithelial cells separated by a
basal lamina, but the basilar membrane is more

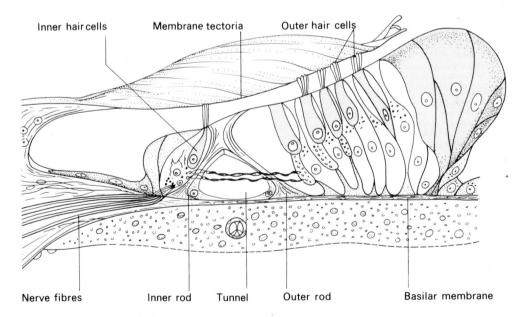

Fig. 20.35. Diagram of the organ of Corti.

complex because it has the spiral organ of Corti on it.

The spiral organ consists of inner and outer rods which meet at an angle so that they enclose a tunnel (Fig. 20.35). Medial to the inner rods is a single row of inner hair cells and lateral to the outer rods are three or four rows of outer hair cells. Lateral to the outer hair cells there are supporting cells. Covering the spiral organ is the membrana tectoria which consists of very fine fibres in a gelatinous matrix (tectoria in Latin means a roof). The fibres of the cochlear nerve pass from the osseous spiral lamina to the basilar membrane where the majority of them make synaptic contact with the bases of the inner hair cells. A minority of the fibres make contact with the outer hair cells.

The perilymph which fills the spaces in the osseous labyrinth outside the membranous labyrinth is similar to cerebrospinal fluid and the space in which it lies is believed to communicate with the subarachnoid space through the cochlear canaliculus. This canaliculus is at the medial end of the anterior wall of the jugular foramen formed by the petrous temporal bone. The source of the perilymph may be the cerebrospinal fluid. The perilymph of the vestibule is continuous with that in the semicircular canals. Movements of the stapes produce pressure waves in the perilymph. These waves pass through the fluid in the scala vestibuli through the helicotrema to the fluid in the scala tympani and result in movements of the basilar membrane.

Movements of the basilar membrane as small as 10^{-11}cm may act as a stimulus to the hair cells.

The endolymph, the fluid within the membranous labyrinth, is very different in composition from that of the perilymph. It is thought that some of the cells of the lining of the semicircular ducts as well as the stria vascularis are responsible for the production of the endolymph and that it is absorbed in the cells of the dilated end of the ductus endolymphaticus. There is probably a continuous production and removal of this fluid.

PHYSIOLOGY

The outer and middle ear

The outer ear in humans is not important in focussing sounds into the external acoustic meatus. The tympanic membrane vibrates readily when sound waves impinge upon it because there is air on both sides of it. The geometry and angulation of the ossicles are responsible for a large increase in the force of the vibration transmitted to the fenestra vestibuli (oval window) and the fluid of the inner ear.

The tensor tympani tends to pull the handle of the malleus inwards if reflexly sent into contraction by a loud noise, and similarly the stapedius tends to pull the stapes out of the fenestra vestibuli. These protective reflexes, by damping vibrations, are responsible for the temporary relative deafness after, say, a loud explosion.

Anything that prevents conduction of sound to the tympanic membrane, for example waxy secretion or water in the external acoustic meatus, produces a degree of deafness. Inappropriate middle ear pressure, as occurs in ascending aircraft, also causes deafness but this is because vibration of the membrane is reduced.

Vibrations, especially low frequencies, are to some extent transmitted through the bones of the skull—this is termed 'bone conduction'. A vibrating tuning fork with the handle held against the mastoid process can be heard. As the vibration fades it is no longer heard, but if then immediately held next to the outer ear it is heard again because 'air conduction' is normally better than bone conduction. Many hearing aids used to compensate for conductive deafness work by simply transferring the amplified vibration to the bone, thereby by-passing the middle ear. The vibrations produced on drilling a tooth are transmitted directly to the skull, and so to the cochlea by bone conduction, and it is this that makes the noise so unpleasantly loud to the patient.

The inner ear

It is the rocking of the stapes in the oval window that transfers the vibrations of the sound to the fluid of the inner ear. The resultant pressure waves are not necessarily transmitted throughout the length of the cochlea, but may take a short cut by deforming the structures in it. Since fluid is virtually incompressible, an equal transmission of energy along or across the fluid compartments of the cochlea is ensured, and any movement has to be dissipated back to the middle ear by the fenestra cochleae. Endolymph is rather like intracellular fluid in composition and perilymph is more like extracellular fluid. There is a difference of potential between the cochlear duct and surrounding structures but, surprisingly, within the duct there is a positive charge. This potential difference is maintained by

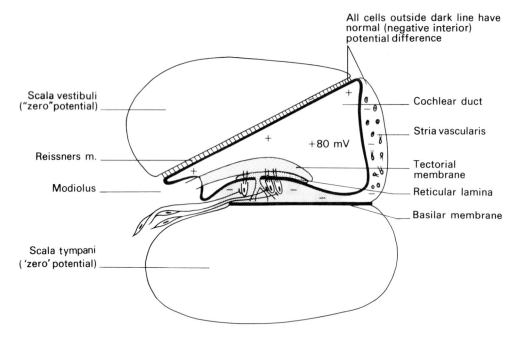

All cells outside dark line have normal (negative interior) potential difference

Scala vestibuli ("zero" potential)

Reissners m.

Modiolus

Scala tympani ('zero' potential)

Cochlear duct

Stria vascularis

Tectorial membrane

Reticular lamina

Basilar membrane

+80 mV

Fig. 20.36. The cochlear duct and surrounding area.

metabolic activity of the stria vascularis (Fig. 20.31), and by the structural separation of the endolymph from the perilymph. If any of these limiting membranes are destroyed then the 'endolymphatic potential' is abolished.

The limits of this region are shown in Fig. 20.36 (cf. Fig. 20.31). Outside this area the cells are bathed, as usual, in extracellular fluid, and, of course, have the normal arrangement of transmembrane potential with the inside relatively negative to the outside.

The endolymphatic potential is about +80 mV relative to the perilymph, but it varies. If the basilar membrane moves towards the scala vestibuli ('up' on our diagram) then the potential difference falls, and if it moves 'down' (on the diagram), it rises. The effect is that of transducing the mechanical movement of the basilar membrane into changes in electrical potential. These changes in potential can be picked up by a nearby electrode and if the signal is amplified and fed into a speaker the original sound is reproduced. This system has been termed 'cochlear microphonics'. However, it must be pointed out that this cannot be the mechanism of converting sound into nervous impulses, for many of the sound frequencies are far too high to be carried by nerve fibres. The most that can be said

is that this effect may augment the normal method of converting the movements of the basilar membrane into nerve impulses.

The basilar membrane and the organ of Corti

Both the basilar and tectorial membranes are attached at the modiolus to solid structures, and are held evenly apart by the structures between them. Movements of the basilar membrane are detected by the hair cells in the organ of Corti (Fig. 20.35). The processes of the hair cells are embedded in the tectorial membrane so that when the basilar membrane oscillates the processes are sheared. This shear causes a change in the electrical potential of the hair cells, which, if sufficient, leads to depolarization. The depolarization is transmitted to the peripheral dendrite of the cells of the spiral ganglion thereby initiating nerve impulses which indicate local displacement of the basilar membrane.

PHYSICS OF SOUND

Sound has two components—loudness and pitch. Excessive noise is now recognized as a cause of hearing injury, most usually in industry and is limited by law.

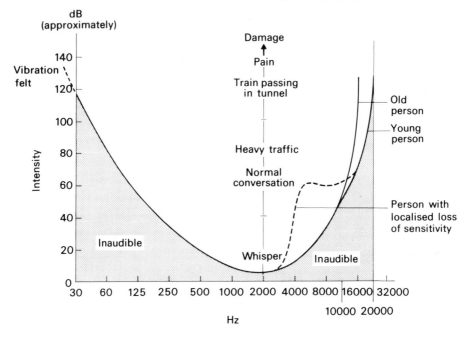

Fig. 20.37. Threshold intensity/frequency.

Sound intensity, loudness, pitch and noise

Sound intensity can be measured, and expressed as the energy needed to cause a diaphragm to oscillate (the units are pressure/area). The least sound that can be heard is in the region of 0.000204 dynes/cm² (10^{-16} watts/cm²) which is accepted as the reference level (= 0 bel, the unit of sound intensity). An intensity of ten times this reference level, i.e. × 10 to the power of 1, = 1 bel or 10^{-15} watts/cm². One hundred times the reference level, i.e. × 10 to the power of 2 = 2 bels. (A sound one million (10^6) times the reference level would be one of 6 bels intensity). Curiously the unit normally used is the decibel (dB), of which there are 10 to the bel, so 6 bels = 60 dB. We hear sounds with an intensity range of 0–140 (±) dB. (140 dB = 14 bels = 10^{14} × 0.0002 dynes/cm².)

'Loudness' however, is not quite the same thing; it is the subjective appreciation of sound intensity, which may vary from person to person according to their pitch sensitivity.

The pitch of a note is defined as the number of cycles per second or hertz (Hz) producing that note. A high pitch has a high frequency.

It is possible to generate sounds of known frequency, free from harmonics, and using these pure tones or notes, the sensitivity to various frequencies can be measured (audiometry).

Noise refers to sound which does not have an orderly repeating wave form; it is random and carries no useful information.

Fig. 20.37 shows that man is most sensitive to frequencies around 1000–3000 Hz, and that outside this range we hear less easily. Beyond our frequency range we are deaf, no matter how much energy a vibration contains.

To produce notes of equal loudness outside the most sensitive range requires increased energy. As age increases there is a loss of the upper frequencies. Knowing the 'normal' curve it is possible to plot individual graphs and to demonstrate any loss of sensitivity to particular frequencies. An amplifying hearing aid should really only amplify the range that is deficient.

THEORIES AND MECHANISM OF HEARING

As the basilar membrane, carrying the organ of Corti, spirals to the apex of the cochlea, it becomes much wider (Fig. 20.31). It is known that prolonged exposure to loud sound with a narrow frequency range (experimentally this can be a known frequency) produces localized damage to the organ of Corti. High frequencies damage areas on the basal turns and lower frequencies damage more apical areas. Confirmation that high frequencies are sensed by the

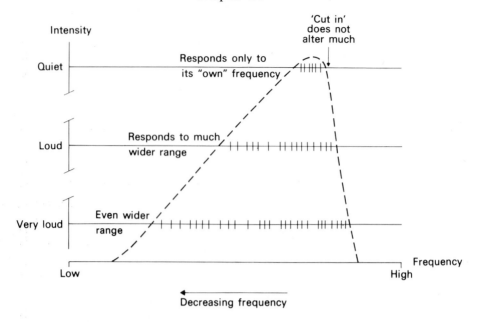

Intensity

Quiet — Responds only to
its "own" frequency

'Cut in'
does not
alter much

Loud — Responds to much
wider range

Very loud — Even wider
range

Low   High   Frequency

← Decreasing frequency

Fig. 20.38. Diagrammatic representation of three recordings from one fibre of the spiral ganglion.

basal turns, and low frequencies by the apex of the cochlea comes from recordings of nerve impulses from various parts of the spiral ganglion.

These observations have led to the 'resonance' hypothesis which suggested that the basilar membrane is 'tuned' and that the 'strings' of the membrane vibrate in sympathy with the frequency of the sound vibration. Thus a complex waveform could be 'sorted' into the frequency components which would be sensed at the respective points along the length of the organ of Corti, the 'place' hypothesis. This physical theory, together with the finding that, under deep anaesthesia, it is possible to demonstrate a point-to-point projection from the organ of Corti on to the primary auditory cortex in the superior temporal gyrus, was accepted as a reasonable explanation for the mechanism of hearing.

Then it was found that the basilar membrane is not under tension. If incised the hole does not gape, and if indented the membrane does not take up the shape of a structure under tension. Even more interesting is the observation that recordings from individual fibres of the spiral ganglion (from discrete areas of the organ of Corti) show that the fibres are not as specific as might be expected (Fig. 20.38). With a quiet

stimulus there is indeed a response to a very limited frequency range. However, louder sounds cause the same fibre to respond to a greater range of frequencies below that initially demonstrated, with only a slight increase in response to higher frequencies. Frequencies outside this range are cut off.

Standing waves
A steady note has a simple repetitive waveform. If the handle of a vibrating tuning fork is dipped into a tank of water, the surface is distorted into a pattern of stationary waves, which is related amongst other factors to the frequency of the vibration. In the same way the basilar membrane is distorted into a 'standing wave' whose shape depends on the frequency of the sound. A complex waveform makes a more complex standing wave with a series of points of maximum deflection. The complexity is compounded by the fact that the basilar membrane is not of uniform width. The result is that high frequency components produce deflection of the basilar membrane in the basal turns of the cochlea and the lower frequency components produce their standing waves in the apical turns. Thus the place hypothesis is correct in that progressively lower frequencies are sensed towards the apex of the cochlea but the resonance hypothesis is

incorrect in that the membrane is not caused to vibrate like a series of differently tuned strings.

Increasing loudness causes a greater length of membrane to be deflected for each frequency, though the points of maximum deflection remain the same. Cochlear microphonic effects are initiated at these points so that the threshold of the hair cells is lowered and they are readily stimulated. The troughs on either side of the wave tend to cut out adjacent frequencies. The cerebral cortex has to make a 'best estimate', from all the information presented to it, both of pitch and loudness.

A lesion of any part of the neurological pathway causes 'perceptive deafness', sometimes called nerve deafness. Consider, for example, a localized lesion of the organ of Corti. A quiet sound that causes a small displacement of the basilar membrane in this region is not sensed. However, if the sound is amplified, then a greater length of membrane is displaced, and in this case some information can be obtained—perhaps sufficient to allow some details of the sound to be estimated. Unfortunately nearby frequencies are also amplified, so that there may be considerable distortion of the sound.

Stereophonic sensation

A sound source to one side is heard by both ears, but with unequal loudness, and not at exactly the same time. The pinnae act as rear sound-baffles, and by turning the head it is usually easy to decide if a sound comes from in front or behind. It is the time lag between the two sides that enables the cerebral cortex to produce a sense of 'position' for the source—a stereophonic sensation.

CENTRAL CONNECTIONS

The cells of the spiral ganglion correspond to the cells of the dorsal root ganglia of peripheral nerves. The central axons of these pass as the cochlear part of the auditory nerve (VIII) to the cochlearnuclei in the medulla, where they synapse. Further neurons (both crossed and uncrossed) pass up the brainstem to the inferior colliculi and also to the primary auditory areas in the superior temporal gyri by way of relay stations in the medial geniculate bodies. In the brainstem, branches are given off to the reticular formation, or arousal system. A sudden sound is one of the few stimuli that can send one almost immediately from deep sleep to wakefulness.

THE MEMBRANOUS LABYRINTH AND BALANCE

Apart from the cochlea, the rest of the membranous labyrinth is concerned with sensing position and movement of the head. Static orientation and linear acceleration are sensed by the maculae of the utricle and saccule, respectively, whereas rotation is sensed by the cristae of the ampullae of the semicircular canals.

UTRICLE AND SACCULE (Figs. 20.32 & 20.34)

The otoliths within the maculae are moved by forces of acceleration (including gravity) and so deform the hair cells thereby initiating depolarization. These sensors tend not to adapt. If the head is tilted on to one shoulder this displacement is sensed by the maculae, which continue to produce nervous impulses for as long as the position is maintained.

THE SEMICIRCULAR CANALS (Figs. 20.32 & 20.33)

Rotating the head tends to leave the endolymph behind, that is, it produces an inertial movement of endolymph in at least one semicircular canal on each side (Fig. 20.39). The planes of the 3 canals are arranged so that rotation in one direction in any one plane can readily be distinguished from the opposite rotation, for although both cristae are deflected in each case, the deflections are oppositely directed (Figs. 20.39 a & b).

'Rotation' does not refer to being whirled around by mechanical devices, but to small movements in the ordinary motion of the body during normal activity like looking to one side, turning a corner, and so on.

Should the rotation continue at a uniform rate (as on a roundabout) the endolymph soon catches up with the head, the natural resilience of the cristae returns them to their neutral positions, and the impulses die away. On stopping there is again an inertial flow of endolymph. This deflects the cristae and gives rise to certain postural reflexes, but in this unphysiological circumstance they produce 'dizziness'—including 'vertigo', which is the false sense of rotation.

'Balance'

'Balance' is the result of co-ordination of sensory input from diverse sources such as labyrinth, eyes, proprioceptors of muscles and joints, pressure receptors of the skin (soles of feet, weight of clothes); in fact any sensor that can provide clues to position in space. The input is connected with a motor outflow to muscles which constantly adjusts posture to maintain a stable position (p. 470). A changing pattern of sensory information accompanies every movement and must be correctly interpreted so that the motor efforts do not occur on a background of bodily instability.

Vestibular reflexes

The reflexes originating from the inner ear are extremely widespread, reaching perhaps every voluntary muscle. Some reflexes involve the muscles of the eyes. If the head is turned to the left, the eyes move to the right, and vice versa. But for these 'eye-fixing' reflexes our field of vision would bounce up and down as we walked. If the head is rotated too far, as when a person is rotated in a chair, the eyes snap back to the 'ahead' position, to a new fixation point. In such continuing rotation, the slow reflex movement and quick, correcting movement constitute 'nystagmus'.

In true rotation, the field of vision moves past

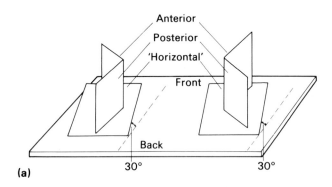

(a)

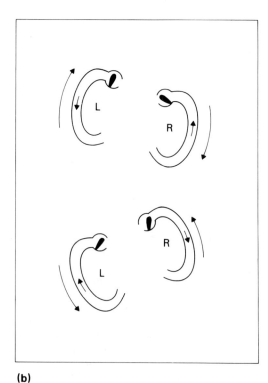

(b)

Fig. 20.39. (a) The planes of the semicircular canals. (b) The effects on the cristae of rotation in opposite directions.

the eyes, and confirms the direction of the rotation. After continuous rotation has stoppped the visual and proprioceptor information confirms that movement has stopped but apparent movement is sensed by the semicircular canals due to distortion of hair cells in the maculae. This situation, or any other like it in which there is conflicting information, gives the sense of instability or dizziness. This can induce very disturbing sensations, nausea or vomiting, and the inability to remain upright.

CENTRAL CONNECTIONS

The hair cells induce nervous impulses in the peripheral dendrites of the cells of the vestibular ganglion on the vestibular part of the auditory (VIII) nerve. The central axons pass to the vestibular nuclei. The connections of these are:

1   Ascending, to the medial longitudinal bundle, (to influence eye movements), the cerebral cortex, and the cerebellum, and

2   Descending, via the vestibulo-spinal tracts for postural balance.

APPENDIX 1

Essentials of Physical Biochemistry

THE CHEMICAL ELEMENTS OF LIFE

Living organisms only use some of the elements surrounding them. Table A.1 reflects this natural selection at an atomic level.

The universe appears to be 99% hydrogen and helium. Eight elements provide more than 98% of the atoms in the earth's crust. Of these eight elements, six account for more than 99.9% of the atoms in the human body. Of the 90 naturally occurring elements on earth, 24 play an essential role in living organisms. These 24 elements can be conveniently considered functionally in terms of three groups (Table A.2).

Biochemistry is the study of the organization and inter-relationship of these elements as components of living organisms. An elementary understanding of chemical bonding is therefore fundamental to any such study.*

CHEMICAL BONDING

All chemical bonds owe their existence to some specific distribution of electrons in the vicinity of the participating atoms. The strength with which these electrons hold atoms together is measured in terms of the amount of energy consumed or liberated when a bond is broken or formed. This is called the bond dissociation energy or more properly, the bond dissociation enthalpy. The

---

* Measurement of atoms, molecules and bond lengths: Two units are used: The nanometre ($1nm = 10^{-9}$ m) (preferred) and the Ångström ($1\text{Å} = 10^{-10}$m = 10^{-1}nm).

Table A.1. The selective use of elements.

Composition of universe		Composition of earth's crust		Composition of seawater		Composition of human body	
Per cent of total number of atoms							
H	90	O	47	H	66	H	63
He	9.1	Si	28	O	33	O	25.5
O	.057	Al	7.9	Cl	.33	C	9.5
N	.042	Fe	4.5	Na	.28	N	1.4
C	.021	Ca	3.5	Mg	.033	Ca	.31
Si	.003	Na	2.5	S	.017	P	.22
Ne	.003	K	2.5	Ca	.006	Cl	.03
Mg	.002	Mg	2.2	K	.006	K	.06
Fe	.002	Ti	.46	C	.0014	S	.05
S	.001	H	.22	Br	.0005	Na	.03
		C	.19			Mg	.01
All others	.01	All others	.1	All others	.1	All others	.01

Table A.2. The 24 essential elements.

The basic 6		The principle cations and anions		The trace elements	
These account for 99.9% of total protoplasmic mass		Components of the ionic milieu		Act as key components of enzyme systems and other proteins with vital functions	
Hydrogen	H	Phosphorus	HPO_4^{2-}	Iron	Fe
Oxygen	O	(3 ionic forms)		Copper	Cu
Nitrogen	N		$H_2PO_4^-$	Manganese	Mn
Carbon	C			Zinc	Zn
Phosphorous	P		OPO_3^{2-}	Cobalt	Co
Sulphur	S			Chromium	Cr
		Sulphur	SO_4^{2-}	Selenium	Se
		(2 ionic forms)		Molybdenum	Mo
			OSO_3^-	Silicon	Si
		Sodium	Na^+	Tin	Sn
		Potassium	K^+	Vanadium	V
		Calcium	Ca^{2+}	Fluorine	F
		Magnesium	Mg^{2+}	Iodine	I
		Chlorine	Cl^-		

word enthalpy means heat content and for a constant pressure process, the enthalpy change (ΔH) is the heat evolved or absorbed. Sometimes so-called bond energies are quoted. These are average values for types of bonds and do not refer to bonds in specific molecules. The units for all three parameters are kilojoules per mole (kJ/mol) or kilocalories per mole (kcal/mol).

Of the attractive forces that hold atoms together, the strongest are covalent bonds, which are shared pairs of electrons. Their energies vary from approximately 200–400 kJ/mol. Since the kinetic energy of heat motion is about 2–5 kJ/mol, these bonds rarely break spontaneously at physiological temperatures. The number of covalent bonds that a single atom can form is dictated by the valency of the atom (the number of electrons available to form pairs with electrons from the other atom). Thus hydrogen can form one; oxygen, two; nitrogen, three and carbon, four covalent bonds.

Noncovalent bonds are based on electrostatic interactions between atoms. They are weak, with energies from 4–30 kJ/mol, and can therefore break and reform easily at physiological temperatures. The number of noncovalent bonds that any atom can form is usually restricted only by the availability of space around that atom.

Table A.3 summarizes the differences between covalent and non-covalent bonds.

Table A.3. The differences between covalent and non-covalent bonds.

Covalent	Non-covalent
Atoms joined by covalent bonds necessarily belong to the same molecule	Participating atoms need not belong to the same molecule
Strong	Weak
Bond energy = 210–420 kJ/mol (50–100 kcal/mol)	Bond energy = 4–30 kJ/mol (1–7 kcal/mol)
Bond length < 1.8Å	Bond length > 2.5Å
Little variation possible in strength or direction	Capable of precise and infinite variation.
Inflexible	Flexible
Formation very often catalyzed by enzymes	Formation never catalyzed by enzymes

Non-covalent bonds

The three types of non-covalent bonds in biological systems differ according to the source of the electrostatic force. The low energy of these bonds means that they participate in all reversible molecular interactions in living organisms.

ELECTROSTATIC BONDS

These are the electrostatic forces that act between oppositely charged groups.

In aqueous solution they have an average bond energy of about 20 kJ/mol. The charged side chains or end groups of proteins, nucleic acids and lipids are often involved in bonding of this type. Electrostatic bonds are also known as ionic bonds, salt linkages, salt bridges or ion pairs.

A typical interaction is that between an anionic carboxylate ion and a cationic amino group, shown in Fig. A.1.

H——————————H

O·25nm

Fig. A.1. Interaction between an anionic carboxylate ion and a cationic amino group.

HYDROGEN BONDS

These occur when hydrogen is shared by two other atoms.

Molecular groups containing an electronegative atom attached to hydrogen are polarized; in other words they have an unequal distribution of electrons. Examples include $>N^{\delta-}-H^{\delta+}$ and $-O^{\delta-}-H^{\delta+}$.

Here the delta signs (δ) imply that the atom to which they refer has either a slight excess of charge ($\delta-$) or a slight deficit of charge ($\delta+$).

Groups like these, with a slight charge separation are called dipoles. Hydrogen bonds are the electrostatic interactions of these dipoles with other dipoles of which the most common is $>C^{\delta+} = O^{\delta-}$. Bond energies range upwards from 20 kJ/mol (3–7 kcal/mol).

An important feature of hydrogen bonds is that they are directional. The strongest hydrogen bond is one in which the three participating atoms lie on a straight line.

The solubility of sugar in water results from the ability of the many hydroxyl groups in the sugar to form hydrogen bonds with water molecules.

One fundamental biochemical role of hydrogen bonds came to the fore in 1957 when Watson and Crick showed that these bonds not only maintain the structural integrity of the genetic material (DNA), but also enable the genetic information stored within the nucleus as DNA to be transferred to the sites of protein synthesis in the cytoplasm in the form of RNA (p. 240).

VAN DER WAALS BONDS

These are nonspecific attractive forces which arise when two atoms come close (but not too close!) together.

Three distinct types of force contribute to what is now collectively known as the Van der Waals force between two atoms or molecules: the orientation (or dipole-dipole) force, the induction (or Debye) force and the dispersion (London or charge fluctuation) forces. The net result of these forces may be attractive or repulsive depending on the distance between the atoms concerned. Attraction is optimum at the

Table A.4. Van der Waal's radii of atoms.

Atom	Radius Å
H	1.2
O	1.4
N	1.5
C	2.0
P	1.9
S	1.85

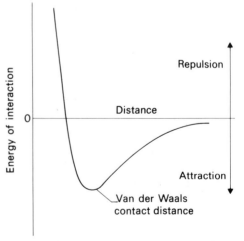

Fig. A.2 Energy of a Van der Waal's interaction as a function of the distance between the two atoms.

Van der Waals contact distance or Van der Waals radius (Table A.4, Fig. A.2).

At distances closer than the Van der Waals radius the orbital electrons of the respective atoms repel each other strongly. (The contact distance for two atoms is obtained by adding the values for the participating atoms.) Thus these bonds occur between atoms separated by about 0.3–0.4 nm.

As with the other types of noncovalent bonds, Van der Waals bonding is electrostatic in origin. The charge separation necessarily arises from a redistribution of electrons, which can occur for a variety of reasons.

Dispersion forces

Of the contributing forces mentioned, the dispersion forces are always present even in apolar molecules such as methane and carbon dioxide. This is because although on average the dipole moment is zero, at any instant in time there will be a dipole moment whose direction and magnitude depends on the particular positions of the electrons in their orbits. This dipole then polarizes another atom nearby.

Orientation forces. These arise between molecules such as water which have permanent electric dipoles. This interaction is analogous to the attraction of two small magnets.

Induction forces. These arise between polar and nonpolar molecules. A polar molecule can induce a dipole in a nearby nonpolar molecule. This is analogous to the attraction between a magnet and an iron bar.

THE HYDROPHOBIC EFFECT

The hydrophobic effect is due to the tendency of nonpolar chemical groups and molecules to associate together.

It has been suggested that this is perhaps the most important single factor in the organization of the constituent molecules of living matter into complex structural entities such as cell membranes and organelles.

Water molecules have an asymmetric distribution of electrons. The electronegative oxygen attracts electrons, leaving the hydrogen with a slight electron deficit. Such molecules, which carry separated positive and negative charges, are said to have electric dipole moments and are known as polar molecules. Non-polar molecules have essentially no dipole moment, although

because of dispersion forces, they may carry transient dipoles.

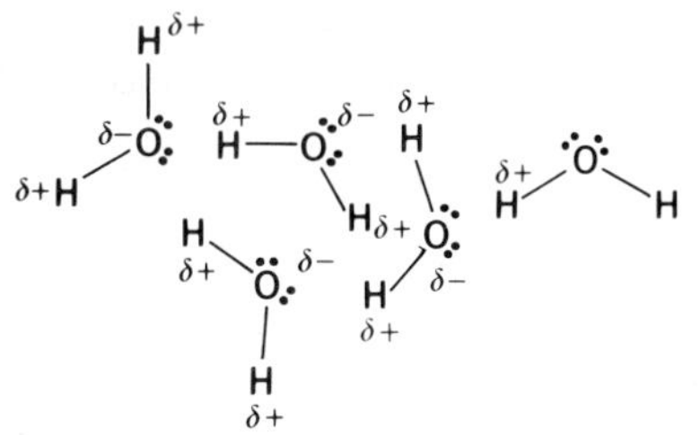

Fig. A.3. A representation of a cluster of water molecules.

The representation of a cluster of water molecules in Fig. A.3 shows that they have a high affinity for each other. They are subject to both strong Van der Waals orientation forces (because they are polar) and hydrogen bonding. This strong affinity that water molecules have for each other is in contrast to apolar molecules such as methane which do not have any special mutual affinity (apart from weak Van der Waals attractive forces). Nevertheless, in the presence of water, apolar molecules do associate (bonding energy = 4–8 kJ/mol) for the following reason. Water molecules surrounding apolar molecules are constrained in that they are unable to form all the bonds they would otherwise make in the absence of the apolar molecule. The existence of this constraint implies that the water molecules are more ordered (have less entropy) in the presence of the apolar solute. This constraint is minimized and the entropy of the water molecules maximized by the clustering of the apolar molecules: this is the driving force behind the hydrophobic interaction.

Covalent chemical bonding

Electrons around atoms occupy three-dimensional atomic orbitals or energy levels which can be said to represent the size and shape of the space around the nucleus in which there is the greatest probability of finding a particular electron. In 1925 Wolfgang Pauli published theoretical reasons for stating his exclusion principle whereby only two electrons can occupy any given orbital and these must have opposite spins. Bond formation between two atoms involves the overlapping of the atomic orbitals of the two atoms. Once the two atomic orbitals overlap sufficiently they become two molecular orbitals. One of these is the bonding orbital which has reduced energy compared to the atomic orbital. The other is an antibonding orbital and is of no further concern in this discussion.

Orbitals have characteristic shapes and are numbered according to their distance from the nucleus. The 1s orbital is spherically symmetrical and nearest to the nucleus. The 2s orbital is the same shape but further away. In addition to the spherical 2s orbital there are also three 2p orbitals, all of the same energy and shape, arranged at x, y and z axes and therefore termed $2p_x$, $2p_y$ and $2p_z$ orbitals. (Representations of these orbitals can be found in standard chemistry texts).

An atom which takes up the maximum electron space available on the first and second major energy levels will possess 10 electrons. Their disposition is described as $1s^2\, 2s^2\, 2p_x{}^2\, 2p_y{}^2\, 2p_z{}^2$. Larger atoms can accommodate electrons in orbitals available at increasing distances from the nucleus. Major energy levels are labelled from 1 to 7 and each level has one or more prescribed orbitals termed s, p, d and f. The detailed electronic configuration of the elements is described in standard chemistry texts.

ISOMERISM AND CONFIGURATION

The chemistry of carbon allows the formation of an almost unlimited number of different compounds from a limited number of kinds of atoms. Many of these compounds are isomers, in that although they differ in some respect, they have the same molecular formulae.

Two important terms relating to molecular structure are configuration and conformation.

A molecular configuration is a specific arrangement of atoms in a molecule such that it cannot be converted to any other arrangement unless a covalent bond or bonds are broken. Configurations can exist in various forms known as conformations. These are interconvertible without breaking covalent bonds.

The simplest form of isomerism is based on different ways of ordering the same collection of atoms. The two alcohols below are isomers of this kind.

$$CH_3{\diagdown}{}$$
$$CHOH \qquad\qquad CH_3CH_2CH_2OH$$
$$CH_3{\diagup}{}$$

Isopropyl alcohol   n-Propyl alcohol
(Propan-2-ol)   (Propan-1-ol)

Of much more interest are compounds which differ only in the arrangement of their constituent atoms in space. These compounds are called stereoisomers and they are of two kinds.

1 Enantiomers (formerly known as optical isomers) are stereoisomers which differ in only one physical characteristic: their ability to rotate plane-polarized light clockwise or anticlockwise.

2 Diastereoisomers. Under this heading come stereoisomers which differ in some other physical or chemical characteristic independent of any ability to rotate plane-polarized light.

Enantiomerism

Molecules which exhibit the characteristic of enantiomerism have the property of handedness, i.e they are chiral (Greek: cheir, hand) and are not superimposable on their mirror images.

Fig. A.4 is a representation of the amino acid alanine ($CH_3\, CH\, NH_2\, COOH$) together with its reflection in a mirror.

It is evident that those two forms of alanine cannot be superimposed one upon the other anymore than your right hand can be superimposed upon your left hand. The configuration of the two molecules is different.

In this example the property of chirality is endowed by the presence of four different substituents attached to the central carbon atom which under such circumstances is termed an asymmetric carbon atom. These two stereoisomers of alanine are called an enantiomeric pair.

As noted, enantiomers can be distinguished physically only by their effect on a beam of monochromatic plane-polarized light. Normal white light is an electromagnetic vibration which consists of wave motions in many directions and of all wavelengths in the visible region. Monochromatic light has waves of only a single wavelength, and plane-polarized light has all wave motions in parallel planes. A solution of an enantiomer of known concentration has the ability to rotate the plane of the wave motion of polarized light clockwise or counterclockwise by a specific angle. Fig. A.5a illustrates this effect in a schematic way.

This angle (Θ), which can be measured in a polarimeter, depends upon the nature of the molecule, the amount of solution in the beam, the solvent, the temperature, the concentration of the solution and the wavelength of the light beam. A characteristic value can identify a given substance if a fixed amount of material is used under specified conditions. The specific rotation $[\alpha]_D^t$, is

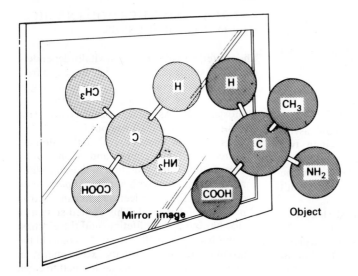

Fig. A.4. A representation of the amino acid alanine together with its mirror image.

defined as the rotation caused by 1 gram of substance per cubic centimetre in a sample tube of 10 cm (1 dcm).

$$[\alpha]_D^{t°C} = \frac{\Theta}{l.d}$$

Θ = observed rotation (in dcm)
l = length of light path through solution
d = density of solution in g/cm³
t = temperature in °C
D symbolizes the sodium line of the spectrum which has a wavelength of 589nm.

Substances which cause clockwise rotation are called dextrorotatory (symbolized by the (+) sign or d): substances which rotate light counterclockwise are called laevorotatory (symbolized by the (−) sign or l) (Fig. A.5b).

A mixture of equal amounts of (+) and (−) isomers is optically inactive since the rotation caused by the (+) enantiomer is exactly cancelled by the rotation caused by the (−) enantiomer. This effect is termed external compensation and such a solution is termed a racemic mixture.

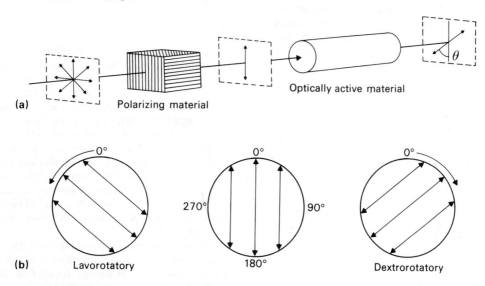

Fig. A.5. (a) Diagrammatic representation of a polarimeter. (b) The directions of rotation of plane-polarized light by enantiomers.

Diastereoisomerism

Diastereoisomers, in general, may either be enantiomers that are not mirror images of each other or they may be geometric isomers.

ENANTIOMERIC DIASTEREOISOMERS

Molecules which contain two or more asymmetric centres can exist in more than two stereoisomeric forms. The maximum number of different configurations is 2^n where n is the number of asymmetric carbon atoms (Van't Hoff's rule).

For example: if a compound has five asymmetric carbon atoms a total of $2^5 = 32$ isomers can exist. Such diastereoisomers will not have identical physical properties and will probably undergo chemical changes at slightly different rates.

GEOMETRIC ISOMERS

A carbon atom linked to another carbon by a single (sigma) covalent bond can rotate with respect to the other carbon atom. A double bond (pi) cannot act as a rotation axis because rotation of 90° would move the p orbitals on the two adjacent carbons to a position where they would no longer overlap. In other words the energy required to rotate an atom about a double bond would have to be sufficient to break the pi bond.

This restriction on rotation means that a given compound can exist in two different configurations depending on the position of substitution. An example is fumaric acid, which is an important intermediate in the tricarboxylic acid (TCA) cycle (p. 198).

$$COO^- \diagdown \diagup COO^-$$
$$C = C$$
$$H \diagup \diagdown H$$

Cis-fumaric acid

$$H \diagdown \diagup COO^-$$
$$C = C$$
$$COO^- \diagup \diagdown H$$

Trans-fumaric acid

These so-called cis and trans forms are not interconvertible and are geometric isomers.

In the body only trans-fumarate is formed.

ENERGY AND THERMODYNAMICS IN LIVING PROCESSES

The existence of life on earth is vitally dependent on certain subtle reactions which occur in a fraction of a microsecond, namely the capturing of light energy by plant life in the process of photosynthesis. As Albert Szent-Gyorgi (the discoverer of vitamin C) has put it:

'It is common knowledge that the ultimate source of all our energy and biomolecular organization is the radiation of the sun. When a photon interacts with a material particle on our globe it lifts one electron from an electron pair to a higher level. This excited state as a rule has but a short lifetime and the electron drops back within 10^{-7} to 10^{-8} seconds to the ground state, giving off its excess energy in one way or another. Life has learned to catch the electron in its excited state, uncouple it from its partner and let it drop back to the ground state through its biological machinery, utilizing its excess energy for life processes.'

Thermodynamics (literally 'heat movement') is the science of energy transformation. It is of fundamental importance in biochemistry which is much concerned with the mechanisms whereby energy is captured, stored, transformed and utilized for a range of activities — chemical, locomotive, contractile, electrical. Two thermodynamic concepts, entropy and free energy are essential in understanding the way in which biological machinery utilizes energy.

Entropy

A given amount of heat energy, although it may be quantitatively equivalent to some other form of energy is nevertheless qualitatively inferior. Heat is a degraded form of energy. It is degraded in the sense that although work can be completely turned to heat, one cannot take heat energy and convert it *solely* into work as the only net product of the process. If this were possible, it would be tantamount to taking heat out of a cold body and putting it into a hot body without any extra energy expenditure. Thus spontaneous heat energy transfer between the cubes of metal represented in Fig. A.6 is always in the direction indicated.

While it cannot be proved that this will always occur it is our experience of the physical universe that spontaneous heat energy transfer in the reverse direction is never observed.

This recognition that heat energy has a decreased capacity for work when compared

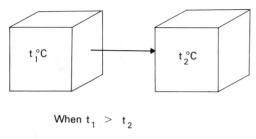

When $t_1 > t_2$

Fig. A.6. Spontaneous heat energy transfer.

with equivalent amounts of other forms of energy is so important that it is accepted as a law — the second law of thermodynamics. This law can be expressed in several ways one of which is:

A cyclical process whose only net result is to take heat from a reservoir and convert it to work is impossible.

A clue to the underlying molecular events responsible for this observation lies in the absolute temperature scale.

Experimentally it is found that for each degree Celsius that a gas is cooled, its volume shrinks by 1/273.16th of the volume it occupies at 0°C. This finding implies that reducing the temperature to −273.16°C would cause the gas to have no volume.

Actually, at −273.16°C the gas volume would reflect the space taken up by perfectly motionless gas molecules, a small but nevertheless finite volume. Thus −273.16°C is the *absolute zero* of a temperature scale known as the Kelvin scale after Lord Kelvin (1824–1907) the Scottish physicist who established its theoretical importance in thermodynamics.

$$t°K \rightleftharpoons t°C + 273.16$$

Heat is related to the kinetic or 'moving' energy of atoms. But atoms move at random and since work is the expenditure of energy in a specified direction it is clear that the thermal energy of atoms cannot be transformed into work on a one to one basis. This is why heat energy has a decreased capacity for work.

This decreased capacity for work is measured in terms of entropy (S). Changes of entropy are written as ΔS (delta S).

ΔS, (the heat energy per degree that is unavailable for useful work at constant temperature) is equal to the heat absorbed or evolved reversibly, divided by the absolute temperature at which the process occurs.

$$\Delta S = Q_{reversible}/T$$

The heat changes must be reversible because

entropy is a state function. A state function is any measurable aspect of a system which depends only on its properties and not on its previous history.

Since thermal energy is zero at 0°K, atoms at this temperature cannot dissipate energy as heat. Thus their entropy is also zero. At any temperature above 0°K, a spontaneous physical or chemical transformation will involve some kind of random motion on the part of the component atoms or molecules. Thus such a transformation must be accompanied by a positive change of entropy.

From this discussion it follows that all spontaneous changes involve an increase in the total entropy of the system. The laws of thermodynamics, put in a succinct, summary form, now become:

First law: The total energy of an isolated system is constant.

Second law: The entropy of an isolated system can never decrease.

ENTROPY AND DISORDER

Since work can be regarded as a manifestation of ordered energy and heat as disordered energy, entropy can also be used as a measure of disorder within a system. At 0°K entropy is zero and order is maximal.

In our universe, disorder rules. Chaos is more probable than order. There may indeed be local areas of organization (as in living matter) but only at the expense of disorder elsewhere.

A refrigerator certainly lowers the entropy of the water in the ice compartment (ice has an ordered structure) but only at the cost of the heat (and therefore increased entropy) generated by the pump that compresses the refrigerant.

These theoretical concepts, perhaps somewhat difficult to grasp in the abstract, may be clearer in the context of the following practical example.

Imagine putting a spoonful of sugar in a cup of tea. After a short time, the distribution of sugar molecules in the tea will be rather as in the diagram below (Fig. A.7), where the circles represent sugar molecules.

The molecules spread from the crowded region at the bottom of the cup where the sugar was added, towards the less crowded region. But why should this happen? There is no driving force that tends to make molecules move in this way. Every molecule is driven quite independently, by Brownian motion. These molecular movements are not governed by the presence or

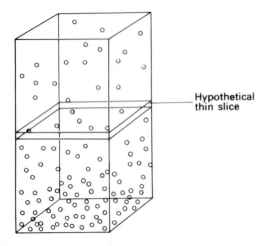

Hypothetical
thin slice

Fig. A.7. Diagrammatic representation of the distribution of sugar molecules in a cup of tea showing a hypothetical thin slice whereby the number of molecules passing up or down could be counted.

absence of neighbouring molecules and yet this random molecular movement eventually produces a uniform distribution of sugar within the tea. If attention is focussed on a thin section it is true that by virtue of their random movement molecules will be carried with equal probability to the top and to the bottom. But for this very reason the section will be crossed by more molecules coming from the bottom than from the top merely because there are more randomly moving molecules on the bottom. Eventually there will be equal numbers of randomly moving molecules on either side of any hypothetical slice through the tea-cup. At this point, when there is no possibility of further disorder of sugar molecules, disorder is maximal. The system has spontaneously changed in such a way as to decrease its capacity for further change. Its entropy is maximal. This is the second law in action.

Since heat causes molecules to move in a random fashion it is not surprising to learn that there is a close connection between entropy and probability. Entropy is related to the probability of an event as disorder is more probable than order. To reverse the process — in other words to reconcentrate the sugar at the bottom of the cup, so increasing the order (decreasing the entropy) of the system — could involve any of a variety of procedures, all of which would utilize energy of some form, to reverse the spontaneous tendency for the sugar molecules to randomly distribute themselves throughout the cup. This tendency of the universe to randomization is

appreciated not least by owners of betting shops and casinos, who obviously have a good grasp of the second law. It is evident that most people lack this knowledge for as Bernard Shaw observed 'a passion for games of chance is common, but whoever heard of someone addicted to buying-up casinos!'

Table A.5 illustrates how entropy values reflect molecular disorder. Graphite is less ordered than diamond; ice more ordered than steam.

Table A.5. Entropy values for some different forms of carbon and water.

Substance	Entropy (S, in J/°K/mol)
Carbon (diamond)	2.3
Carbon (graphite)	5.7
Water (ice)	41
Water (liquid)	70
Water (vapour, 1 atm)	189

Free energy

Compare the First and Second laws of thermodynamics. The First law states that all forms of energy are interconvertible but in the process energy can neither be created nor destroyed. This provides an overall balance sheet of what is going on but says nothing about the direction of energy interconversion. This latter topic is the domain of the Second law which tells us that certain processes can or cannot occur spontaneously. Under certain circumstances ΔS can be used to predict whether or not a reaction may proceed spontaneously. Despite this potential usefulness, it is rather inconvenient to use in practice. (Its use involves making measurements of reversible changes in a system and in the surroundings). To get over these difficulties Gibbs introduced the concept of the change in free energy, ΔG of a reaction. (We now use 'G' to commemorate Gibbs, though the term ΔF, which is synonymous with it, is also widely used).

Free energy (G) is energy that has the ability to do work, i.e. $\Delta G = \Delta H - T \Delta S$

ΔH is known as the change in enthalpy and is equivalent, providing there are no net pressure or volume changes, to the total heat change during the reaction. T is the absolute temperature.

Thus the useful energy made available by a reaction is equal to the change in heat content (ΔH) of the system minus the change in entropy (ΔS) of the system multiplied by the absolute temperature (T) at which the reaction occurs.

TΔS is the energy which is degraded and un-available for work.

UNITS

ΔH is measured in joules, T in degrees Kelvin and ΔS in joules per degree Kelvin. The units of G or ΔG are therefore joules.

$$1J = \text{one Kg m}^2/s^2$$
$$= \text{one Nm (newton metre)}$$
$$= \text{one Ws (watt second)}$$

Conveniently, ΔG values are expressed as kilojoules per mole (kJ/mol) of the substance of interest. (1 mole is the molecular weight in grams of the substance.)

The older terminology of kilocalories per mole (kcal/mol) is still extensively used. It is advisable to become familiar with both forms.

$$1 \text{ kcal/mol} = 4.184 \text{kJ/mol}$$

INTERPRETATION OF FREE ENERGY CHANGES

Changes in free energy are the driving force behind all biochemical reactions. As a result, the value of ΔG can be used to predict the occurr-ence and direction of a reaction. But observe that nothing is stated here about the possible rate of the reaction. That is the province of kine-tics (p. 993). The predictive rules for ΔG are as follows:

For a given reaction: $X \rightleftharpoons Y$, ΔG may be positive, negative or zero

1 If ΔG is negative ($\Delta G < O$) the reaction will proceed spontaneously to the right and will yield energy. In other words, the reaction is exergonic and is capable of doing work.

2 If ΔG is zero the reaction is at equilibrium and there is no net reaction in either direction. Thus the reaction neither yields nor requires energy.

3 If ΔG is positive ($\Delta G > O$) the reaction will not proceed spontaneously to the right (the reverse reaction is spontaneous) and will require energy. Such a reaction is termed endergonic.

In general then, reactions characterized by a large negative ΔG proceed nearly to comple-tion—those characterized by large positive ΔG occur to only a very limited extent (or, in the presence of products, go backwards) unless there is an external driving force.

For example, if the reactants are present at molar concentrations at 25°C then a ΔG value of about -20kJ/mol will drive the reaction to vir-tual completion. But again, it is emphasized that the magnitude of ΔG predicts only the extent to which it proceeds and the amount of energy available from it.

A spontaneous reaction certainly occurs immediately but may proceed at a rate imper-ceptible to the human observer.

Since the magnitude of ΔG depends on experimental conditions, biochemists use $\Delta G^{o\prime}$ (delta G nought prime) which is the difference between the free energies of products and re-actants in their standard states (pressure of 1 atmosphere and concentration of 1 mol per litre) at pH 7.0. The temperature at which the $\Delta G^{o\prime}$ value was obtained must be specified.

A $\Delta G^{o\prime}$ value for a particular reaction is a measure of the driving force with which the con-centrations of the reactants and products change from the standard concentrations of 1 molar to the concentrations they each have when the reaction has reached equilibrium (defined as the point at which there is no further change in the concentrations of the reactants with time). Once equilibrium has been achieved $\Delta G = O$ (note *not* $\Delta G^{o\prime} = O$).

This means that there will be no change in the ratio of the products to the reactants. This cons-tant ratio is termed the equilibrium constant. The close relationship between ΔG and the equilibrium constant for a reaction is discussed in detail on p. 993.

Many biochemical reactions are sequential. That is, two (and often many more) reactions are coupled together in such a way that an appar-ently unfavourable reaction is driven to favour the formation of a desired end product. Thus an exergonic second reaction in a sequence may drive an endergonic first reaction.

One example occurs in the breakdown of sugar and involves the formation of pyruvate from phosphoglycerate. In this context the chemical nature and significance of these subs-tances do not matter (they are discussed in detail on p. 185). Attention here is given only to the free energy changes that drive the reactions.

The reaction sequences concerned are as follows:

1. 3–phospho-glycerate $\rightleftharpoons$ 2–phospho-glycerate
    $$\Delta G^{o\prime} = +4.45 \text{ kJ/mol}$$

2. 2–phospho-glycerate $\rightleftharpoons$ 2–phosphoenol-pyruvate
    $$\Delta G^{o\prime} = -2.69 \text{ kJ/mol}$$

3. 2–phosphoenol-pyruvate + ADP + H$^+$ $\rightleftharpoons$ Pyruvate + ATP
    $$\Delta G^{o\prime} = -21.00 \text{ kJ/mol}$$

Reaction 1 is not favoured energetically because it has a positive $\Delta G^{o\prime}$. However reactions 2 and 3 occur spontaneously since they have negative $\Delta G^{o\prime}$ values.

The sum of reactions 1, 2 and 3 is:

$$\text{3–phospho-} \quad \rightleftharpoons \quad \text{Pyruvate + ATP}$$
$$\text{glycerate + ADP} \qquad\qquad + H_2O$$
$$\Delta G^{o\prime} = -19.24 \text{ kJ/mol}$$

Thus the reaction sequence is driven to completion.

It is not a valid objection to say that reactions 2 and 3 will not proceed because $\Delta G^{o\prime}$ for reaction 1 is positive. The equilibrium will indeed lie to the left but there will still be some 2–phosphoglycerate present. Reaction 2 will remove this rapidly thus inducing reaction 1 to shift to the right. Thus 3–phosphoglycerate will be continuously removed from the system as pyruvate is formed.

This example of a sequential reaction illustrates the danger of deciding the direction of a reaction merely on the basis of its $\Delta G^{o\prime}$ value. One may be certain that standard conditions do not exist in a cell and the most likely source of variation is the concentration of the reactants. Metabolism is the totality of chemical processes that occur in a cell and all of these processes are sequentially linked in some way. This does not mean that biochemical energetics is necessarily always complex, merely that some caution should be used in applying the simple rules of thermodynamics to such processes.

INTRODUCTION TO EQUILIBRIA AND KINETICS

A living organism is a discrete interacting system of some 24 chemical elements which participate in a very large number of simultaneously and sequentially operating chemical reactions. Whether chemical processes take place in a cell or in a test-tube they are subject to the same overall constraints; the same basic chemical principles apply whatever the reaction.

The basic principles governing a chemical reaction are the reaction equilibria and kinetics. With respect to any specific reaction, the concepts of equilibria are concerned with the question 'how much?' and kinetics with the problem 'how fast?'

Chemical equilibrium

It is virtually certain that all chemical reactions take place in both directions.

$$\text{Reactants} \rightleftharpoons \text{Products}$$

In many cases the reverse reaction occurs to such a small extent that it is negligible. Reactions of this kind are said to proceed to completion.

In cases where both forward and reverse reactions occur to a noticeable extent, the process is regarded as a reversible reaction. Very often, such a situation can be set up merely by altering the conditions of the reaction. Providing reaction conditions are held constant, all reversible reactions exist in a state of chemical equilibrium. This is a state in which there is no change in the composition of the reaction mixture with time. In other words, the ratio of the amount of products formed to the amount of reactants present, is a constant. This ratio can be constant for only two reasons. Either all chemical reactions have ceased or the formation of products is taking place at exactly the same rate as the formation of reactants.

It has been found that it is this latter state of dynamic equilibrium that accounts for the constancy of the ratio. The direction of a reaction depends upon the concentration of the various components. More precisely, the rate of a chemical reaction is proportional to the molar concentration of the reacting substance. This is termed the law of mass action and is a fundamental concept in consideration of chemical processes.

EQUILIBRIUM CONSTANTS

The most valuable item of information one can have about any equilibrium reaction is its equilibrium constant. This is a ratio (i.e. a pure number) which reveals the extent to which a given reaction has proceeded under specified conditions. The expression for this constant is derived using the law of mass action.

Consider the process by which substances A and B react to form products C and D:

$$A + B \rightleftharpoons C + D$$

By the law of mass action the rate at which A and B react will be proportional to the product of the molar concentrations of A and B ([A] and [B]) (it is the product because in this case the rate is proportional to the 'pairs' of A and B available for reaction).

Rate of forward reaction $\propto$ [A] [B]

or

Rate of forward reaction $= K_f$ [A] [B]

where K_f is a proportionality constant for the forward reaction.

Similarly

Rate of reverse reaction $\propto$ [C] [D]

or

Rate of reverse reaction = K_r [C] [D]

where K_r is a proportionality factor for the reverse reaction.

At the equilibrium position, the rate of the forward reaction equals the rate of the reverse reaction therefore:

$$K_f[A] [B] = K_f[C] [D]$$

or

$$\frac{K_f}{K_r} = \frac{[C] [D]}{[A] [B]}$$

The ratio of the two constants K_f and K_r is termed K, the equilibrium constant of the reaction.

$$K = \frac{[C] [D]}{[A] [B]}$$

If K is very large (much greater than 1) then the reaction concerned has virtually proceeded to completion. Conversely, if K is much less than 1 then the reaction has taken place to only a small extent.

Relationship between K and ΔG

The thermodynamic criterion for equilibrium states that ΔG for the reaction in question must be zero. Put another way, at equilibrium there is no driving force to effect net changes in the concentrations of reactants or products. One might therefore guess that there should be a connection between a 'measure of the extent to which a reaction occurs' (which is K) and the 'change in free energy of a reaction' (which is ΔG).

The equation relating K and ΔG is:

$$\Delta G_\circ = \Delta G^{\circ\prime} + RT \ln K$$
when $$\Delta G^{\circ\prime} = -RT \ln Keq$$
$$= -2.303 \; RT \; \log_{10} K$$

In this equation, $\Delta G^{o\prime}$ is the standard free energy change of a reaction (p. 991) and K is the equilibrium constant under the same conditions. R is the gas constant and is equal to 8.3144 J/deg/mol. T is the absolute temperature. (0°C = 273.16°K). The numerical relationship is shown in Table A.6.

When K is less than 1.0, $\Delta G^{o\prime}$ is a positive value and the reaction is endergonic. When K is greater than 1.0 the reaction is exergonic.

Influence of other variables on K

Clearly, K is only a constant if the reaction conditions remain the same: usually this means pressure, volume and temperature. A general rule concerning the way in which conditions

Table A.6. The relationship between the $G^{\circ\prime}$, the standard free energy change at 25°C, pH 7.0, and K measured under the same conditions.

K	$\Delta G^{o\prime}$
0.001	+ 17.12
0.01	+ 11.42
0.1	+ 5.71
1.0	0
10.0	− 5.71
100.0	− 11.42
1000.0	− 17.12

affect a reaction was enunciated by Henri le Chatelier (1850–1936) who in 1888 stated:

'Every change of one of the factors of an equilibrium brings about a rearrangement of the system in such a direction as to minimize the original change'.

In other words, if a system under equilibrium is put under increased pressure then it rearranges itself in such a way as to take up as little room as possible. Because of this the pressure does not increase as much as might be expected. Similarly if the temperature is raised, the system tends to absorb heat so that the temperature does not go up by as much as would be indicated.

So far, these general comments about chemical reactions have centred on equilibrium processes. The law of mass action, however, also applies to a different aspect of the reaction, namely reaction rates or kinetics. Almost all biochemical reactions are influenced by specialized proteins termed enzymes. Enzymes can influence the rate at which a chemical reaction proceeds. The topic of enzyme kinetics is dealt with in Chapter 4 but the following observations provide some background for that discussion.

Kinetics and rate equations

The term rate implies a change in some quantity with time. Take the reaction

$$A \underset{}{\overset{K}{\rightleftharpoons}} B$$

where K is the rate constant for the formation of B.

It has already been shown that the rate of formation of B is equal to K[A]. It is also equal to the amount of A that disappears (to form B) per unit time. As so:

Rate of formation of B $$= \frac{\Delta[B]}{\Delta t} = K \, [A] = - \frac{\Delta[A]}{\Delta t}$$

Where Δ denotes 'the change in' and the minus sign expresses the fact that [A] is decreasing with time.

The equation above is called the rate law for the conversion of A into B and implies that the number of molecules of A disappearing per second depends only upon the number of molecules of A present. Such a process is called a first order reaction. In other words the rate law depends on the concentration of one constituent — a fact stressed in the equation below by explicitly writing the exponent of A which in this case is 1.

$$\frac{\Delta[B]}{\Delta t} = K \, [A]^1$$

This leads to a definition of reaction order:

The order of a reaction is a number equal to the sum of the exponents of the concentration terms in the rate equation.
A reaction can be zero, first, second, third or nth order.

Rate equations for reactions governed by zero order kinetics do not have a concentration term. The velocity of such reactions will therefore be essentially independent of the substrate concentration and for all practical purposes constant.

Usually only zero and first order kinetics are encountered in biochemistry.

BIOCHEMICAL EQUILIBRIA

Thermodynamics is the key to an understanding of why chemical or physical processes are driven in one direction or another. The preceding discussion has centred on chemical changes. Energy is also needed for the physical transport of water and other molecules within and across cell membranes. Osmosis and Donnan equilibria are two general phenomena which underlie inter and intracellular transport of molecules and ions.

Osmosis

For biological systems osmosis is the passage of water and small ions across membranes in response to a solute concentration gradient (i.e. the solute will have an appreciably larger molecular weight than the small ions or water). Flow is in the direction of highest solute concentration.

Fig. A.8 shows a container divided into sections, a and b. Section a contains pure water whilst b contains in addition a solute which is unable to pass through the membrane. Because of this selectivity on the basis of molecular size

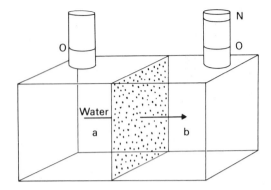

Fig. A.8. The passage of water through a semi-permeable membrane, accumulating on the side containing solute.

the membrane is termed semi-permeable.

Experimentally it is found that water will flow from a to b; this is indicated by the liquid level rise from O to N.

Initially the two identical volumes of liquid in compartments a and b differ only in that b contains water and solute molecules. For this reason there will be fewer water molecules in b than in a since some will be displaced by the solute molecules. Consequently, per unit volume, there is a higher concentration of water in a than in b. Making use of the argument that was applied in the case of diffusion in the absence of a membrane we may conclude that water will pass from a (region of high concentration) to b (region of lower concentration).

If a sufficient counterpressure is applied at N, this flow of water can be prevented. The magnitude of the pressure required to stop any net flow of water between a and b is equal to the osmotic pressure of the solution in b and is usually designated by Π. An empirical equation relates osmotic pressure to the concentration of the solute is as follows:

Π = CRT

where: Π is the osmotic pressure
C is the concentration of the solution in mols of solute per litre of solution
R is the gas constant
T is the absolute temperature
This equation is only valid in dilute solutions. The equation breaks down at higher concentrations because other molecular forces come into play.

Fig. A.9 illustrates this effect. Curves 2 and 3 show marked deviation from the theoretical (straight line) curve 1. The marked difference between the experimental and hypothetical

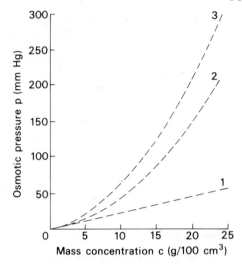

Fig. A.9. The relationship between protein concentration and osmotic pressure. Curve 1 is the hypothetical plot for a macromolecule of molecular weight 68 000 which obeys the Van't Hoff equation; curve 2 is the experimental plot for serum albumin (molecular weight 68 000) at pH 5.4; curve 3 is the experimental plot for serum albumin at pH 7.4.

plots reflect certain macromolecular interactions which act to increase the osmotic pressure of the serum albumin solution at higher protein concentrations.

There are two principal explanations of this behaviour:
1   The excluded volume effect. This is discussed in the context of carbohydrate polymers (p. 144), but also applies to other macromolecules.
2   Donnan equilibria. This is responsible for the difference between curves 2 and 3 in Fig. A.9.

THE DONNAN EQUILIBRIUM

So far in this discussion, it has been assumed that the solute molecules are neutral. However, many biological macromolecules carry functional groups which are ionized at physiological pH values. Such charged macromolecules markedly affect the transport of the small ions and water which surround them.

Increasing the pH from 5 to 7 will in general promote further ionization of the functional groups present in proteins. It is this increase in the net charge on the protein that is responsible for curve 3.

Imagine yet another container divided by a semi-permeable membrane which is permeable to both water and small ions. This corresponds to the membranes of vascular systems where inorganic salts can diffuse through, but proteins, as a rule, cannot.

Let P^- represent a macromolecule such as a protein carrying charged groups. Such a macromolecule is called a polyelectrolyte. Most body polyelectrolytes are polyanions that carry net negative charges at physiological pH. Since electrostatic forces are extremely strong, P^- will always be found in association with some small ions of opposite charge called counterions. In this example the counterion is sodium (Na^+).

P^- together with its counterions is placed in one portion of the container. A second solute $Na^+ Cl^-$ is added to the water on the other side. The initial concentration of salt is Cs. P^{z-} indicates that the polyelectrolyte has z negative charges and will therefore be associated with z Na^+ ions.

The initial state of the system is depicted in Table A.7. Since the membrane is permeable to small ions, chloride ions will migrate from the salt compartment (left) to the polyelectrolyte compartment (right) i.e. from high to zero concentration. If only the chloride ions moved there would soon be a predominance of sodium ions (and a net positive charge) on the left hand side. Because electrostatic forces are so powerful, this situation does not arise. Each chloride ion that migrates across the membrane is accompanied by a sodium ion. Eventually an equilibrium state is reached at which time there is no net movement of ions through the membrane.

If x represents the concentration of chloride ions that pass through the membrane to the polyelectrolyte compartment, then the final state the system attains is as shown in Table A.7.

From a thermodynamic point of view, at equilibrium there is no remaining driving force

Table A.7. The distribution of small ions in the presence of a polyanion.

	Salt Compartment				Polyelectrolyte Compartment			
	Initial		Final		Initial		Final		
Species	Na^+	Cl^-	Na^+	Cl^-	Na^+	P^{z-}	Na^+	P^{z-}	Cl^-
Concentration	Cs	Cs	Cs–x	Cs–x	zCp	Cp	zCp+x	Cp	x

that will allow net transfer of ionic species across the membrane. Thus the free energy of the left hand system (LHS) is equal to that of the **right** hand system (RHS)!

$$\Delta G_{LHS-RHS} = O$$

The equation for this transfer of diffusible ion is:

$$Na^+{}_{LHS} + Cl^-{}_{LHS} \rightleftharpoons Na^+{}_{RHS} + Cl^-{}_{RHS}$$

$$\therefore \quad K \text{ eq.} = \frac{[Na^+{}_{RHS}] \; [Cl^-{}_{RHS}]}{[Na^+{}_{LHS}] \; [Cl^-{}_{LHS}]} = 1$$

So $[Na^+{}_{LHS}] \; [Cl^-{}_{LHS}] = [Na^+{}_{RHS}] \; [Cl^-{}_{RHS}]$

So at equilibrium the product of the concentrations of the sodium and chloride ions on one side of the membrane equal the product of the similar concentrations on the other side. Since the polyelectrolyte P^- is associated with sodium counterions the concentration of sodium ions on the right hand side will not be equal to the concentration of chloride ions.

Using the terms for the concentrations at equilibrium:

$$(Cs - x)(Cs - x) = (zCp + x)(x)$$

which becomes: $x = \dfrac{Cs^2}{zCp + 2Cs}$

x is the amount of chloride ion (or sodium ion) that diffuses across the semipermeable membrane into the polyelectrolyte compartment. The difference between the total salt concentration in the salt compartment and that in the polyelectrolyte compartment is the sum of the sodium and chloride ions on the right hand side minus the sum of the sodium and chloride ions on the left hand side:

Net difference
in diffusible $= [zCp + 2x] + [2(Cs - x)]$
electrolyte

At any specific polyelectrolyte concentration (except at very low values) the salt concentration in the polyelectrolyte increases markedly as the initial salt concentration, Cs, is decreased. Osmotic pressure experiments, in effect, measure the number of molecules restrained by the semipermeable membrane.

Clearly, at low salt concentrations there will be a contribution to the osmotic pressure by the redistributed salt in addition to that by the polyelectrolyte.

Returning to Fig. A.9 it will now be apparent why curve 3 is so steep. The rise of pH from 5.4 to 7.4 results in increased ionization which will therefore bring into play an increased Donnan equilibrium contribution.

Here we have examined the effect of the Donnan equilibrium on osmotic pressure experiments. Many physicochemical determinations are subject to this Donnan phenomenon and so most measurements on biological polyelectrolytes are carried out either in high concentrations of electrolyte (usually salt) or at very low concentrations of the macromolecule.

ACID–BASE EQUILIBRIA

The concept of an acid and a base

An acid can donate protons; a base can accept protons.

This view of acid-base behaviour, proposed in 1923 stresses proton transfer. Previously, acids were regarded as substances that released hydrogen ions (H^+ ions) in solution and bases, hydroxyl ions (OH^- ions).

It is important to realize that once a molecule has donated a proton (behaved as an acid), it is then clearly in a position to accept a proton back again. In other words it can act as a base. Thus any substance which has acidic properties will also possess, under certain circumstances, basic properties as well. This is illustrated symbolically for molecules R and S in the equation below:

$$HR \quad + \quad S \rightleftharpoons R \quad + \quad HS$$
conjugate   conjugate   conjugate   conjugate
acid of R   base of S   base of R   acid of S

The word conjugate reminds us of this dual aspect of acids and bases.

Strong and weak electrolytes

Strong electrolytes ionize immediately and completely on dissolving in water. This means that there is no question of any equilibria being set up between a strong acid/base and a proton under normal aqueous conditions. ('Normal' here means conditions of interest to a biochemist.) Weak electrolytes do not necessarily ionize on dissolving. Their degree of ionization (the percentage of molecules in a given population which will donate or accept protons) is dependent on the number of protons already in the solution. Weak electrolytes can be classified as either mono- or polyprotic acids or bases depending on whether they can donate or accept one or several protons. Acetic acid, for example, is a monoprotic acid while proteins act as polyprotic bases. Almost all molecules of biological interest are weak electrolytes.

Ionization of water

All biochemical reactions take place in the presence of water. The way in which water splits up into charged species is therefore of fundamental interest. Ionization can be shown using the ideas of conjugate acid and base just mentioned:

$$HOH + HOH \rightleftharpoons H_3O^+ + OH^-$$

| About to act as a conjugate base | About to act as a conjugate acid | Acting as an acid | Acting as a base |

It can be seen that one water molecule acts as an acid (donates a proton) while another acts as a base (accepts a proton). To avoid writing H_3O^+ each time, H^+ can be used as an abbreviation. The ionization can then be written as if it were a dissociation:

$$HOH \rightleftharpoons H^+ + OH^-$$

The net result is, of course, the same. These equations reflect an equilibrium reaction (the reaction is going from right to left as well as from left to right). The number of ions present at any single instant will depend on the position of the equilibrium. Experimentally this number can be found by conductivity measurements and is exactly 10^{-7} mols per litre of each ion at 25°C. The ratio of the concentrations of the products of a reaction to the concentrations of the reactants is called the equilibrium constant for that reaction. (See p. 992).

The dissociation equilibrium constant for water is therefore:

$$K_d = \frac{[H^+][OH^-]}{[HOH]}$$

In this case, the concentrations of the products are known. The concentration of the reactant, water, is its concentration in moles per litre of water:

$$= \frac{\text{wt. of 1 litre } H_2O/mw}{1 \text{ litre}}$$

$$= \frac{1000/18}{1}$$

$$= 55.6M$$

$$\therefore K_d = \frac{(10^{-7})(10^{-7})}{55.6}$$

Since the molarity of water compared to the concentrations of most solutes is essentially constant, a new constant K_w can be defined which combines the two constants K_d and the non-varying value of 55.6M for water.

$$K_w = K_d \times M_{H_2O}$$

$$= \frac{10^{-14}}{55.6} \cdot (55.6)$$

and $K_w = 10^{-14}$

K_w is termed the ionic product of water. K_w is more conveniently expressed by taking the negative logarithm of this number ('p' denotes the operation of taking the negative logarithm of a number). The result is termed pK_w. The magnitude of pK_w varies inversely with temperature.

Ionization of weak monoprotic acids

This can be treated in exactly the same way as water ionization.

$$HA + HOH \rightleftharpoons H_3O^+ + A^-$$

| conjugate acid | conj. base | conj. acid | conj. base |

$$HA \rightleftharpoons H^+ + A^-$$

Both equations amount to the same result. The acidic ionization constant K_a is:

$$K_a = \frac{[A^-][H^+]}{[HA]}$$

Ionization of weak monoprotic bases

Amines ($R-NH_2$) are the most frequently encountered bases in biochemistry. Again, they ionize following the pattern seen previously.

$$R-NH_2 + HOH: \rightleftharpoons R-NH_3^+ + OH^-$$

| conj. base | conj. acid | conj. acid | conj. base |

$$R-NH_2 \rightleftharpoons R-NH_3^+ + OH^-$$

Notice that in this latter permutation it is not clear where the OH^- ion comes from. In other words, the ionization must be considered as it actually occurs. However in calculations there is no error in working with the simpler equation and K_b is defined:

$$K_b = \frac{[R-NH_3^+][OH^-]}{[R-NH_2]}$$

The pH scale

This is used as a convenient way of reporting the number of hydrogen ions present in a solution compared to the number of hydroxyl ions. pH is defined as the negative logarithm of the activity of the hydrogen ion. Activity is a term which expresses the effective concentration of a species. It is not always the same as the actual concentration, but for most practical purposes, the activity is equivalent to the concentration. Activity and concentration are not equivalent at extremely high or very low hydrogen ion concentrations. For most biochemical applications pH is defined as the negative logarithm of the hydrogen ion concentration.

$$pH = - \log [H^+]$$

Example. What is the pH of a solution of 0.002M HCl? HCl is a strong acid and therefore ionizes completely. Thus 0.002M HCl contains 0.002 moles of H^+ ions and 0.002 moles of Cl^- ions.

$$pH = - \log (0.002)$$
$$pH = + \log \frac{1}{0.002}$$
$$= \log 5.0 \times 10^2$$
$$= 2.699$$

A useful relationship can be derived by using the 'p' notation. It has already been shown that:
$$[H]^+][OH^-] = K_w$$
Taking logarithms

$$\log [H^+] + \log [OH^-] = \log K_w$$
$$\therefore \quad -\log [H^+] -\log [OH^-] = -\log K_w$$
$$\therefore \quad pH + pOH = pK_w$$
$$\therefore \quad pH + pOH = 14$$

This relationship means that if any one of the values H^+, OH^-, pH or pOH are known, then the other three can be readily calculated.

The concept of pK

It has already been shown in the case of pK_w, pH and pOH that the operation of taking the negative logarithm of a number can be of great use in coping with numbers which vary enormously in magnitude. The same principle is applied to equilibrium constants. Thus:

pK_a is defined as $- \log K_{a-}$
and
pK_b is defined as $- \log K_b$

where K_a and K_b are the acid and base dissociation constants as previously defined. These pK equilibrium (abbreviated to 'pK') values vary from around zero to 14. pK values are a measure of the strength of an acid or base. Strong acids or bases have low pK_a or pK_b values. The 'p' scale is logarithmic, thus for example, formic acid (pK = 3.75) is almost exactly ten times stronger as an acid than acetic acid (pK = 4.76). Hydrocyanic acid (pK = 9.31) is nearly a million times weaker in acidic strength than formic acid.

A more intuitively useful definition of pK is given in the discussion on the Henderson–Hasselbalch equation.

Relationship between pK_a and pK_b

The concept of the conjugate acid/base has constantly been stressed in this discussion (once an acid has acted as an acid it can then act as a base). Labelling a substance as an acid or base is therefore only a means of describing its behaviour under certain specified conditions. Any ionizable group can therefore be described in terms of its pK_a or its pK_b. These two parameters are related as follows:

Writing the ionization of a weak acid:

$$HA + HOH \rightleftharpoons H_3O^+ + A^-$$
$$\therefore \quad K_a = \frac{[H_3O^+] [A^-]}{[HA]}$$

and $[H_3O^+] = \dfrac{K_a \, HA}{[A^-]}$

The conjugate base A^- reacts with water to form the conjugate acid again.

$$A^- + HOH \rightleftharpoons HA + OH^-$$
$$K_b = \frac{[HA] [OH^-]}{[A^-]}$$

and $[OH^-] = \dfrac{K_b \, [A^-]}{[HA]}$

but $[H_3O] [OH^-] = K_w$

and $\dfrac{K_a \, [HA]}{[A^-]} \cdot \dfrac{K_b \, [A^-]}{[HA]} = K_w$

$$\therefore \quad K_a \times K_b = K_w$$

Taking logarithms

$$\log K_a + \log K_b = \log K_w$$

and $- \log K_a - \log K_b = - \log K_w$

or in other words

$$pK_a + pK_b = pK_w = 14.00 \text{ at } 25°C$$

Ionization of polyprotic acids and bases

Many molecules of biological interest are polyprotic. The K_a values for each dissociation are numbered in order of decreasing acid strength. (K_{a1}, K_{a3} etc.) Thus a triprotic acid/base will dissociate as shown below:

$$\overset{K_{b3}}{\underset{K_{a1}}{H_3A \rightleftharpoons H_2A^-}} + H^+ \overset{K_{b2}}{\underset{K_{a2}}{\rightleftharpoons HA^{2-}}} + H^+ \overset{K_{b1}}{\underset{K_{a3}}{\rightleftharpoons A^{3-}}} + H^+$$

K_b values are also numbered in order of strength and so K_{a3} and K_{b1} are the equilibrium constants referring to the same ionization. The same relationship previously derived apply in the same way and thus for a triprotic acid/base:

$$pK_{a1} + pK_{b3} = pK_w$$
$$pK_{a2} + pK_{b2} = pK_w$$
$$pK_{a3} + pK_{b1} = pK_w$$

Relationship between pH and K_a/K_b (The Henderson–Hasselbalch equation)

This is a most important equation fundamental to all considerations of acid–base equilibrium states in biological systems. It relates the pH of the solution of a weak acid/base to its pK_a or pK_b. Only the equation relating pH and pK_a will be derived here. The relationship between pOH and pK_b can however be derived in an analogous way.

By definition
$$K_a = \frac{[H^+][A^-]}{[HA]}$$

$\therefore$
$$[H^+][A^-] = K_a[HA]$$

and
$$[H^+] = K_a\frac{[HA]}{[A^-]}$$

Taking logarithms

$$\log[H^+] = \log K_a + \log\frac{[HA]}{[A^-]}$$

and
$$-\log[H^+] = -\log K_a - \log\frac{[HA]}{[A^-]}$$

and
$$pH = pK_a - \log\frac{[HA]}{[A^-]}$$

or
$$pH = pK_a + \log\frac{[A^-]}{[HA]}$$

Notice that when the ratio of conjugate base to acid is 1, then $pH = pK_a$. Turning this round one can therefore state that:

with respect to a specific ionizing group in a population of molecules, pK is the pH at which 50% of these groups will be ionized and 50% will be unionized.

This definition is one of the most useful to bear in mind when dealing with any problem in acid-base equilibria. The Henderson–Hasselbalch equation makes it possible to

1 Calculate the pH that will be given by a particular weak acid from a knowledge of its pK_a value and a determination of the molar ratio of its unionized proton donor (HA) and proton acceptor conjugate base (A^-) present.

or

2 Determine the pK_a for any particular acid from a measurement of the amounts of salt $[A^-]$ and acid $[HA]$ present at a particular pH.

FURTHER READING

MORRIS J.G. (1974) *A Biologist's Physical Chemistry*, 2nd edn. Edward Arnold, London.

APPENDIX 2

Some Common Abbreviations used in Biochemistry

A	adenine	Hb	haemoglobin
ACP	acyl carrier protein	HbO₂	oxyhaemoglobin
Acetyl CoA	acetyl coenzyme A	His	histidine
(acetyl-S-CoA)		Hyl	hydroxylysine
ACTH	adrenocorticotrophic	Hyp	hydroxyproline
	hormone	IgG (M,D,E,A)	immunoglobulin G
ADP	adenosine diphosphate		(M,D,E,A)
Ala	alanine	Ile	isoleucine
AMP	adenosine monophosphate	ITP	inosine triphosphate
cAMP	cyclic AMP (adenosine 3',	LDH	lactic dehydrogenase
	5'-cyclic	Leu	leucine
	monophosphate)	Lys	lysine
Arg	arginine	Mb	myoglobin
Asn	asparigine	MbO₂	oxymyoglobin
Asp	aspartate	Met	methionine
ATP	adenosine triphosphate	NAD⁺	nicotinamide adenine
ATPase	adenosine triphosphatase		dinucleotide (oxidized
C	cytosine		form)
CoA	coenzyme A	NADH	nicotinamide adenine
CoQ	coenzyme Q		dinucleotide (reduced
Cys	cysteine		form)
CyS	cystine	NADP⁺	nicotinamide adenine
DNA	deoxyribonucleic acid		dinucleotide phosphate
DNP	2,4-dinitrophenyl		(oxidized form)
FAD	flavin adenine dinucleotide	NADPH	nicotinamide adenine
	(oxidized form)		dinucleotide phosphate
FADH₂	flavin adenine dinucleotide		(reduced form)
	(reduced form)	Phe	phenylalanine
FDNB	fluorodinitrobenzene	PEP	phosphoenolpyruvate
fMet	formylmethionine	Pi	inorganic orthophosphate
FMN	flavin mononucleotide	PPi	inorganic pyrophosphate
	(oxidized form)	Pro	proline
FMNH₂	flavin mononucleotide	PTH	phenylthiohydantoin
	(reduced form)	PRPP	phosphoribosylpyrophosphate
FPPC	filter paper partition	RNA	ribonucleic acid
	chromotography	mRNA	messenger RNA
G	guanine	rRNA	ribosomal RNA
Gln	glutamine	tRNA	transfer RNA
Glu	glutamate	RNase	ribonuclease
Gly	glycine	Ser	serine
GDP	guanosine diphosphate	T	thymine
GMP	guanosine monophosphate	Thr	threonine
GSH	glutathione	TLC	thin layer chromatography
GTP	guanosine triphosphate	TPP	thiamine pyrophosphate

Trp	tryptophan	UDP-glucose	uridine diphosphate glucose
Tyr	tyrosine	UMP	uridine monophosphate
U	uracil	UTP	uridine triphosphate
UDP	uridine diphosphate	Val	valine
UDP-galactose	uridine diphosphate galactose		

APPENDIX 3

Units and Definitions

The mole (mol) is the unit of quantity and always contains the same number of particles.

e.g. 1 mole of H^+ has a mass of 1.008 grams
1 mole of H_2 has a mass of 2.016 grams
1 mole of $CO(NH_2)_2$ has a mass of 60.06 grams

The unit of volume is the LITRE (l) and is defined as one decimetre cubed (dm^3).

Concentrations are given in moles per litre (mol/dm^3). One mole of solute in one litre of solvent is a molar (M) solution.

Osmolarity of a molar solution of a non-ionizable substance is an osmole (osmol).

One molar NaCl, if ionized completely in solution, has an osmolarity of two osmoles.

Equivalent (Eq) is that quantity of substance which will combine with or displace one mole of hydrogen ion.

Equivalent × valency = Mole.

micron (μm)	= 10^{-6} m
nanometre (nm)	= 10^{-9} m
Ångstrom (Å)	= 10^{-10} m = 10^{-1} nm
calorie (kcal)	= 4.186 kJ
mm Hg	= 0.133 kPa = 1 Torr
pascal (Pa)	= newton (N) per square metre (Nm^{-2})

Watt (W)	= 1 Joule/sec
horsepower (hp)	= 746 Watts = 746 J sec^{-1}
log_e or ln	= log to base e (log_e x = log_{10} x × 2.3026)
isotope	= nuclide of same element but different atomic mass
iu (sometimes IU)	= international unit (must be defined)
hertz (Hz)	= frequency of repetition of cyclic phenomena
kilopond	= kilogram force ≈ 9.8 N
newton (N)	= 1 joule acting over 1 metre ($J m^{-1}$)
Ci	= Curie = 3.7 × 10^{10} disintegrations per second (MBq, megabequerel)
P	= partial pressure, e.g. P_{CO_2}, also referred to as gas tension

The following prefixes may be used to indicate decimal fractions or multiples of the basic or derived units.

Fraction	Prefix	Symbol	Multiple	Prefix	Symbol
10^{-1}	deci	d	10^3	kilo	k
10^{-2}	centi	c	10^6	mega	M
10^{-3}	milli	m			
10^{-6}	micro	μ			
10^{-9}	nano	n			
10^{-12}	pico	p			

Index